Surgery of the Alimentary Tract

SECOND EDITION

Stomach and Duodenum
Incisions
Sutures

RICHARD T. SHACKELFORD, M.D.

Associate Professor Emeritus of Surgery
and the Department of Surgery
The Johns Hopkins University School of Medicine

GEORGE D. ZUIDEMA, M.D.

Warfield M. Firor Professor of and Director
Section of Surgical Sciences
The Johns Hopkins University School of Medicine
Surgeon-in-Chief, The Johns Hopkins Hospital

W. B. SAUNDERS COMPANY
Philadelphia London Toronto
Mexico City Rio de Janeiro Sydney Tokyo

W. B. Saunders Company: West Washington Square
Philadelphia, PA 19105

1 St. Anne's Road
Eastbourne, East Sussex BN21 3UN, England

1 Goldthorne Avenue
Toronto, Ontario M8Z 5T9, Canada

Apartado 26370—Cedro 512
Mexico 4, D.F., Mexico

Rua Coronel Cabrita, 8
Sao Cristovao Caixa Postal 21176
Rio de Janeiro, Brazil

9 Waltham Street
Artarmon, N.S.W. 2064, Australia

Ichibancho, Central Bldg., 22-1 Ichibancho
Chiyoda-Ku, Tokyo 102, Japan

Library of Congress Cataloging in Publication Data (Revised)

Shackelford, Richard T.

Surgery of the alimentary tract.

Vols. by R. T. Shackelford and G. D. Zuidema.

Previous 1955 ed. by R. T. Shackelford, based on Bickham's Operative surgery, is entered under Bickham, Warren Stone.

Includes bibliographies and index.

Contents: v. 1. Esophagus.—v. 2. Stomach and duodenum, incisions, sutures.—v. 3. Colon, anorectal tract.—[etc.]

1. Alimentary canal—Surgery.   I. Bickham, Warren Stone, 1861-   . Surgery of the alimentary tract.   II. Zuidema, George D.   III. Title. [DNLM: 1. Digestive system—Surgery. W1900 S524s]

RD540.B5 1978   617'.43   75-44606

ISBN 0-7216-8084-4 (v. II)   AACR 1

Surgery of the Alimentary Tract (Volume 2)   ISBN 0-7216-8084-4

© 1981 by W. B. Saunders Company. Copyright 1955 by W. B. Saunders Company. Copyright under the Uniform Copyright Convention. Simultaneously published in Canada. All rights reserved. This book is protected by copyright. No part of it may be reproduced, stored in a retrieval system, or transmitted in any form or by any means, electronic, mechanical, photocopying, recording, or otherwise, without written permission from the publisher. Made in the United States of America. Press of W. B. Saunders Company. Library of Congress catalog card number 75-44606.

Last digit is the print number: 9   8   7   6   5   4   3   2

CONTRIBUTORS

THOMAS R. GADACZ, M.D.
Associate Professor of Surgery, The Johns Hopkins University School of Medicine; Chief, Surgical Service, Veteran's Administration Medical Center, Baltimore, Maryland

ANTHONY L. IMBEMBO, M.D.
Associate Professor of Surgery, The Johns Hopkins University School of Medicine, Baltimore, Maryland

RICHARD S. JOHANNES, M.D.
Assistant Professor of Medicine and Gastroenterology, The Johns Hopkins University School of Medicine, Baltimore, Maryland

FRANCIS D. MILLIGAN, M.D.
Associate Professor of Medicine, The Johns Hopkins University School of Medicine, Baltimore, Maryland

MARK M. RAVITCH, M.D.
Surgeon-in-Chief, Montefiore Hospital, Pittsburgh, Pennsylvania

W. ROBERT ROUT, M.D.
Assistant Professor of Surgery, The Johns Hopkins University School of Medicine, Baltimore, Maryland

RICHARD T. SHACKELFORD, M.D.
Associate Professor of Surgery, Emeritus, The Johns Hopkins University School of Medicine, Baltimore, Maryland

DENNIS W. SHERMETA, M.D.
Professor and Chief, Division of Pediatric Surgery, University of Chicago, Pritzker School of Medicine, Chicago, Illinois

FELICIEN M. STEICHEN, M.D.
Director, Department of Surgery, Lenox Hill Hospital, New York, New York

MICHAEL J. ZINNER, M.D.
Assistant Professor of Surgery, State University of New York, Downstate Medical Center, Brooklyn, New York

GEORGE D. ZUIDEMA, M.D.
Professor and Director, Section of Surgical Sciences, The Johns Hopkins University School of Medicine, Baltimore, Maryland

PREFACE

The first edition of Surgery of the Alimentary Tract was published in 1955, and this three volume set proved to be invaluable to thousands of practicing general surgeons and residents in training over the following years. Through the stimulus of Robert B. Rowan, who at the time was the Medical Editor of the W. B. Saunders Company, Dr. Richard T. Shackelford agreed to work on a second edition. Because of the rapid growth and development of surgical technic and new approaches to the treatment of disease, it soon became obvious that the second edition would have to be expanded substantially. At that time, Dr. Shackelford agreed to complete the work on the first volume, dealing with surgery of the esophagus, and to participate actively in preparation of the text on surgery of the stomach and duodenum as well. At this point, Dr. George D. Zuidema was invited to join the enterprise, and he enlisted the help of several individuals, most of whom either were or had been members of the faculty at Johns Hopkins Medical School. In a few instances, we had to go farther afield to obtain the services of individuals with special expertise in other areas, particularly those dealing with pediatric surgery.

At the time of this writing, we have completed work on Volume II, which deals with the stomach and duodenum, incisions useful in approaching the alimentary tract, and the choice of suture material as well as the use of stapling devices. Volume III deals with the colon and the anorectal tract, and includes material on inflammatory disease, malignancies, and trauma. Although we have incorporated new authors and new ideas, we have tried to maintain the approach that was so successful in the first edition — namely, dealing with the embryology, physiology, and anatomy, as well as with surgical diseases and technical considerations. We would like to express our appreciation to the many individuals who have contributed chapters or sections of these volumes, for their dedication and commitment to what has truly become a departmental effort. It is difficult to adequately express the gratitude which we feel for them and for the quality of their participation.

We would also like to thank Robert B. Rowan for his contributions to the enterprise while he was associated with the Saunders Company; Elizabeth Taylor, who was responsible for the entire make-up of the book; Susan Hunter, who worked with us during the early phases; and Lisette Bralow, who has taken over more recently. We would also like to thank a number of other individuals for their help: Kitty Shackelford, Loraine Loss, and Diane Benson for their help, and Lisa Witlin for her many long hours in working on the manuscript as well. We can simply state that this has been a project which all of us have enjoyed, but it is also a project that would not be possible without the cheerful cooperation and goodwill of everyone involved.

RICHARD T. SHACKELFORD, M.D.
GEORGE D. ZUIDEMA, M.D.

CONTENTS

PART TWO   THE STOMACH AND DUODENUM

Chapter 1
ANATOMY AND PHYSIOLOGY OF THE STOMACH 3
   Embryology 3
      Congenital Malformations of the Stomach 4
   Surgical Anatomy of the Stomach 6
   Physiology of the Stomach 13
      Gastric Secretion 13
         Gastric Mucosa 13
         Gastric Juice 15
         Gastric Mucosal Barrier 18
         Regulation of Gastric Secretion 18
         Measurement of Gastric Acidity 27
   Digestive Function of the Stomach 32

Chapter 2
SURGICAL ANATOMY AND PHYSIOLOGY OF THE DUODENUM 38
   Surgical Anatomy of the Duodenum 38
      Divisions 38
      Fixation 40
      Circulation 42
   Physiology of the Duodenum 45

Chapter 3
INTUBATION 46
   Peroral Gastric Intubation 48
   Nasal Gastric, Gastroduodenal, and Lower Gastrointestinal
      Intubation 49
         Levin Tube 49
         Bilumen Gastrojejunostomy Tube 51
         Bilumen Gastroduodenal Tube 52
         Miller-Abbott Tube 53
         Harris and Cantor Single-Lumen Mercury-Weighted Tubes 54
      Complications Attending Use of Indwelling Gastrointestinal
         Tubes 54
   Postoperative Gastric Decompression 59
   Routine Postoperative Nasogastric Intubation 63
      Omission of Routine Postoperative Gastric Intubation 64

Chapter 4
GASTROSCOPY AND PERITONEOSCOPY 66
Peroral Gastroscopy 66
Esophagogastroduodenoscopy (EGD) 68
Indications and Contraindications 68
Preparation and Procedure 68
Duodenoscopy 70
Endoscopic Retrograde Cholangiopancreatography (ERCP) 72
Other Reported Experiences with Upper GI Endoscopy 75
Fiberoptic Endoscopic Therapeutic Procedures in Upper GI Tract 80
Fiberendoscopic Complications 88
Anterior Gastroscopy and Duodenoscopy Through a Gastrotomy or Gastrostomy Stoma 89
Peritoneoscopy or Laparoscopy 90
Advantages and Limitations 91
Indications and Contraindications for Diagnostic Peritoneoscopy 92
Technic 94
Special Examinations 101
Operative Procedures 102
Regional Examination from the Usual Site of Puncture 102
Wound Closure 107
Examination in Children 107
Precautions 108
Postoperative Care 108
Complications 108
Results 109
Conclusions 110

Chapter 5
OBSTRUCTIVE DISORDERS 111
Acute Dilatation of the Stomach 111
Gastrolysis and Duodenolysis (Freeing of Adhesions) 113
Atresia and Stenosis of the Stomach (Neonatal Gastric Outlet Obstruction) 114
Combined Congenital Gastric and Duodenal Obstruction 120
Congenital Antral Membrane in Older Children and Adults 123
Antral Mucosal Diaphragm Associated with Esophageal Hiatal Hernia 126
Congenital Duodenal Atresia 128
Biliary Tract Abnormalities Associated with Duodenal Atresia 136
Congenital Duodenal Stenosis 141
Congenital Intrinsic Duodenal Stenosis Presenting After Infancy 144
Megaduodenum 147
Congenital Aganglionic Megaduodenum 147
Megaduodenum Due to Congenital Absence of Duodenal Musculature 150
Hereditary Megaduodenum without Anatomic Explanation 150

Congenital Extrinsic Obstruction of Duodenojejunal Junction 152
  Superior Mesenteric Artery (SMA) Syndrome 155
  SMA Syndrome without Associated Peptic Ulcer Disease 162
  SMA Syndrome with Associated Severe Peptic
    Ulcer Disease 163
  Congenital Duodenal Diaphragm Plus SMA Syndrome 165
  Pediatric Patients 167
  Burned Children 168
  Bedridden Combat Casualties 169
  Cast Syndrome 170
  Association with Scoliosis 171
Volvulus of the Stomach 171
  Secondary Volvulus 180
  Idiopathic or Primary Volvulus 181
Gastric Volvulus in Pediatric Patients 183

Chapter 6
OBSTRUCTION-LIKE DISORDERS 184
  Gastropexy 184
  Gastric Plication 185
    Technics 185
  Bilocular Stomach or Hourglass Contraction of Stomach 188
    Etiology 188
    Pathology 189
    Symptoms 189
    Diagnosis 189
    Treatment 190
  Cascade Stomach 195

Chapter 7
INJURIES OF THE STOMACH 197
  Gastric Injuries by Blunt Trauma 197
    Diagnosis 198
    Laceration of the Gastric Mucosa 204
    Transmural Perforation 204
    Intramural Hematomas of the Stomach 205
  Gastric Injuries by Penetrating Trauma 206
    Missile Wounds of the Stomach 206
      Diagnosis 207
      Management of Missile Wounds of Stomach 208
      Operation 210
  Gastric Injuries by Stab Wounds 212
    Operative Treatment 216
  Foreign Bodies of the Stomach 216
    Symptoms 217
    Treatment 217

Corrosive Injuries of the Stomach 217
    Types of Injury 217
    Factors Determining Severity of Injury 217
    Diagnosis 217
    Treatment 218
    Complications... 218

Chapter 8
INJURIES OF THE DUODENUM 219
Types of Injuries 219
    Blunt Trauma 220
    Penetrating Wounds 220
    Associated Injuries... 221
    Corrosive Injuries and Foreign Bodies of the Duodenum............. 222
Diagnosis 222
    Radiologic Studies... 222
    Other Diagnostic Aids... 223
Treatment 224
    Blunt Trauma 224
        Retroperitoneal Rupture... 224
        Injuries of the Duodenum and Pancreas 225
        Rupture of Duodenum with Avulsion of the Ampulla of Vater.. 226
        Transection of Duodenum with Avulsion of the Common Duct... 227
        Traumatic Pyeloduodenal Fistula 228
        Influence of Previous Gastrectomy on Major Blunt Duodenal Injury... 230
        Intramural Hematoma of the Duodenum..................................... 233
        Methods of Treatment... 236
        Operative Technics... 242
        Pediatric Duodenal Hematoma 243

Chapter 9
TUMORS OF THE STOMACH AND DUODENUM............................. 246
Benign Gastric Tumors... 246
    Leiomyoma 246
    Gastric Polyps... 246
    Miscellaneous Benign Tumors of the Stomach 247
Benign Tumors of the Duodenum.. 247
Malignant Tumors of the Stomach 247
    Carcinoma... 247
    Gastric Lymphoma 250
    Leiomyosarcoma 250
Malignant Tumors of the Duodenum.. 250

CONTENTS

Chapter 10
GASTRIC AND DUODENAL ULCERS 251
    Gastric Ulcers 251
        Etiology 251
        Pathology 251
        Clinical Findings 252
        Diagnostic Studies 252
        Treatment 253
    Duodenal Ulcers 254
        Etiology 254
        Pathology 255
        Clinical Findings 255
        Diagnostic Studies 255
        Treatment 256
        Giant Duodenal Ulcer 258
        Diagnosis 258
        Treatment 259
    Complications of Gastric and Duodenal Ulcer 259
        Perforation 259
            Symptoms and Diagnosis 259
            Treatment 260
        Obstruction 260
            Symptoms and Diagnosis 261
            Treatment 261
        Hemorrhage 261
            Symptoms and Diagnosis 262
            Treatment 262
    Zollinger-Ellison Syndrome (Gastrinoma) 263
        Symptoms and Findings 264
        Treatment 264
    Post-Traumatic Stress Ulceration 265
        Treatment 267
        Prevention 268
    Summary of Operative Treatment of Ulcer Disease 269
        Gastric Ulcers 269
        Duodenal Ulcer 269

Chapter 11
GASTRIC AND DUODENAL FISTULAS AND PERFORATIONS 270
    Causes of Gastric and Duodenal Fistulas 270
    Types of Fistula 270
        Gastrojejunocolic Fistula 271
        Duodenal Fistula 272
    Diagnosis 273
    Treatment 273
    Neonatal Gastric Perforations 274

Chapter 12
PYLORIC STENOSIS AND OTHER GASTRIC DISORDERS 277
- Congenital Hypertrophic Pyloric Stenosis 277
  - Incidence and Etiology 277
  - Clinical Signs and Symptoms 278
  - Diagnosis 278
  - Physical Examination 278
  - Surgical Procedure 279
- Congenital Hypertrophic Pyloric Stenosis in Adults 280
  - Causes 280
  - Diagnosis 280
  - Treatment 280
- Gastric Duplication 281
  - Surgical Management 281
- Spontaneous Rupture of the Stomach in Adults 281
  - Etiology 282
  - Clinical Characteristics 284
  - Treatment 285
- Gastritis 285

Chapter 13
GASTRIC RESECTION AND RECONSTRUCTION 287
- Gastrectomy 287
  - History 287
  - Extent of Gastrectomy in Relation to Disease 289
  - Reconstruction 289
  - Technic 289
    - Billroth I Operation 296
    - Von Haberer Modification 297
    - Horsley Modification 300
    - Kocher Modification 301
    - Von Haberer-Finney Modification 301
    - Billroth II Operation 301
    - Polya-Balfour Modification 306
    - Devine Exclusion 306
    - Finsterer Partial Gastrectomy with Antral Exclusion 306
    - Roux-en-Y Modification 308
    - Sleeve Resection 309
- Total Gastrectomy and Reconstruction 309
  - Technic 309
    - Longmire Method 310
    - Lahey Method 315
    - Orr Method 315
    - Graham Method 323
    - Roux-en-Y Total Gastrectomy 325
    - Jejunal Interposition 328
    - Reconstruction with a Reservoir or Pouch 328
- Total Gastrectomy with Esophagoduodenostomy 328
  - Technic 328
    - Transposition of Terminal Ileum and Ascending Colon for Substitute Gastric Reservoir (Lee) 331

CONTENTS

Transposition of Transverse Colon for Substitute
  Gastric Reservoir 331
Gastrostomy 332
  Definition 332
  Indications 332
  Types of Gastrostomy 333
    Stamm Gastrostomy 333
    Witzel Gastrostomy 334
    Permanent Gastrostomies 334
Pediatric Gastrostomy 341
  Comments on Gastrostomy 342
Gastroenterostomy 343
  History 343
  Indications 344
  Technics 344
    Gastroduodenostomy 344
    Gastrojejunostomy 344
    Comments on Gastrojejunostomy 353
Complications after Gastrointestinal Anastomosis 354
  Hematemesis 354
    Methods of Treatment 354
    Technic for Ligation of Bleeding Point 355
  Postoperative Gastric Retention 355
    Diagnosis and Methods of Treatment 356
    Prevention 357
    Jejunoplasty 357
  Leakage from Duodenal Stump 362
  Rupture of Abdominal Incision 362
  Jejunal Ulcer 362
  Marginal Ulcer 363
    Disconnection of Gastrojejunostomy 364
  Repair of Gastroileostomy 367

Chapter 14
VAGOTOMY, PYLOROPLASTY, AND GASTRIC BYPASS 368
  Vagotomy 368
    Types of Vagotomy 370
      Truncal Vagotomy 370
      Selective Vagotomy 371
      Proximal Gastric Vagotomy 371
      Transthoracic (Supradiaphragmatic) Vagotomy 372
    Postoperative Complications of Vagotomy 374
    Comments 374
  Pyloroplasty 375
    Indications 375
    Types of Pyloroplasty 376
      Heineke-Mikulicz Pyloroplasty 376
      Finney Pyloroplasty 377
      Judd Pyloroplasty 381
      Moschel Pyloroplasty 381
    Comments on Pyloroplasty 383

Gastric Procedures for Morbid Obesity 384
    Gastric Bypass 384
    Comparison of Gastric and Jejunoileal Bypass in the
        Treatment of Morbid Obesity 393
    Gastric Partitioning for Morbid Obesity 394

PART THREE INCISIONS

INTRODUCTION 402

Chapter 15
EXPOSURE OF THE CERVICAL ALIMENTARY TRACT 403
    Anatomy 403
        Veins 409
        Arteries 412
        Nerves 413
    Approaches to the Cervical Esophagus 418
        Technic of Anterolateral Approach (Left Side) 420

Chapter 16
EXPOSURE OF THE THORACIC ALIMENTARY TRACT 423
    Anatomy 423
        Thoracic Walls 423
        Blood Vessels and Nerves 427
        Muscles and Mammary Gland 430
        Fasciae of the Thoracic Wall 438
        Thoracic Cavity and Its Contents 439
        Diaphragm 442
    Approaches to the Thoracic Esophagus 442
    Minor Thoracotomy Incisions 443
        Selection of Incisions 443
        Technic 444
        Comments 444
    Major Thoracotomy Incisions 444
        Standard (Posterolateral) Thoracotomy Incision 445
            Technic 449
        Closure of Incisions 449
        Anterolateral Thoracotomy Incision 449
            Technic 449
        Posterior Extrapleural Thoracotomy Incision 451
            Technic 451
        Thoracicoabdominal (Abdominothoracic) Incision 452
            Technic 453

Chapter 17
EXPOSURE OF THE STOMACH AND DUODENUM 455
    Gastrotomy 462
        Indications 462
        Technic 462
        Technic of Closure of Gastrotomy Incision 465
    Gastrorrhaphy 465

Chapter 18
ABDOMINAL INCISIONS 467
    Anatomy.. 467
        Layers of the Abdominal Wall.. 467
            1. Skin 468
            2. Subcutaneous Tissue 468
            3. Deep Fascia... 468
            4. Muscle-Bone Layer... 469
            5. Fifth Layer or Transversalis Fascia 483
            6. Sixth or Extraperitoneal Fat Layer 484
            7. Seventh Layer—Peritoneum.. 485
        Linea Alba 485
        Umbilicus 486
    Types and Choice of Incisions 486
        Upper Midline Incisions 488
            Technic 488
            Methods of Upward Extension 490
            Extension by Lateral Transverse Abdominal Incision 495
        Lower Midline Incision.. 497
            Technic 497
            Comment 498
            Methods of Extension 498
        Paramedian Incision 499
            Technic 500
            Methods of Extension 500
        Midrectus (Transrectus) Incision 502
            Technic 502
            Methods of Extension 502
        Pararectus Incision (Kammerer-Battle)..................................... 503
            Technic 503
            Methods of Extension 504
    Transverse Abdominal Incisions... 504
        Upper Abdominal Transverse Incision 504
        Modified Upper Abdominal Transversus Incision by
            Retracting Instead of Severing the Rectus Muscles (Sanders) 506
            Lateral Upper Abdominal Transverse Incision
                (Singleton) 508
            Transverse Midabdominal Incision 509
            Transverse Low Abdominal Incision 511
        Pfannenstiel Incision 511
            Technic 512
            Methods of Extension 513
        Left Transverse Incision for Abdominoperineal Excision of
            Rectum (Coller).. 515
            Technic 515
        Oblique Incisions 515
            Subcostal Incision (Kocher) 515
            McBurney Gridiron Incision 519
            Rockey-Davis Incision.. 521
            Lateral Oblique Abdominal Incision with Division of
                Muscles in Same Direction as Skin Incision (Kocher)............ 524
    Comments on Abdominal Incisions 524

Chapter 19
DRAINAGE OF ABDOMINAL WOUNDS.. 525

Chapter 20
COMPLICATIONS OF INCISIONS 529
    Contaminated Wounds.. 529
    Delayed Closure 530
    Other Complications 532
        Disruption.. 532
        Wound Infection 532
        Wound Hematoma... 532

PART FOUR   SUTURES

Chapter 21
CLOSURE OF WOUND 535
    The Genesis of Suturing... 535
    Absorbable and Nonabsorbable Sutures 536
        Monofilament and Multifilament Sutures 539
        Infection 539
        Principles of Suture Selection.. 540
    Anatomic Considerations 540
    Types of Wound Closures.. 544

Chapter 22
GASTROINTESTINAL SUTURING... 556
    Materials... 559
        Suture Materials.. 559
        Needles... 561
    Fundamental Forms of Simple Suturing 562
    Standards for Satisfactory Intestinal Suturing.................................... 562
    Types of Sutures 562
        Interrupted Lembert Suture 562
        Continuous Lembert Suture 564
        Halsted Interrupted Quilt (Mattress) Suture 564
        Pursestring Suture... 564
        Cushing Suture 565
        Connell Suture... 566
        Parker-Kerr Stitch.. 566
        Through-and-Through U-Stitch 566
        Marshall U-Stitch 571
        Furrier Suture.. 571
        Simple Overhand Continuous or Interrupted Suture (Albert)........... 571
        Lock-Stitch (Glover Stitch) 573
        Czerny Interrupted Sutures.. 573
        Continuous Through-and-Through Marginal (Albert)
            Suture and Interrupted Gould Inverted Mattress Suture
            for Enterorrhaphy... 573
        Three-Layer Suture Line... 574
        Gambee Single-Layer Open Intestinal Anastomosis 574
        Navy Single-Layer Everting Anastomosis 577

CONTENTS

Chapter 23
MECHANICAL SUTURES 579
    The Healing of Intestinal Wounds 579
    Mechanical Sutures in the Healing of Intestinal Wounds 580
    Experimental and Clinical Comparative Studies of
        Manual and Mechanical Suture Technics 581
    History of Stapling Instruments.. 581
    The Contemporary American Instruments............................. 583
  Surgical Technics with Stapling Instruments 587
    Precautions and Safeguards 594
    Reported Experience with Autosuture Instruments 595
    Comments 600

BIBLIOGRAPHY... 601
INDEX 619

Part 2

THE STOMACH AND DUODENUM

Chapter 1

ANATOMY AND PHYSIOLOGY OF THE STOMACH

EMBRYOLOGY

The embryonic foregut at first is largely pharyngeal, but with growth it elongates to form the primordia of the esophagus and stomach cranial to the anterior intestinal portion (Gray and Skandalakis, 1972). Up to the fifth or sixth week of gestation the gastrointestinal tract is a straight midline tube. "The stomach and duodenum, from which the other supramesocolic viscera will develop, are suspended by ventral and dorsal mesenteries [Fig. 1-1]. The celiac artery, the main artery to this segment of the gut as well as the derived viscera, reaches these organs through the dorsal mesogastrium" (Edwards, Malone, and MacArthur, 1975). Dilatation in the region of the future stomach appears during the fifth week of gestation at segments C-3 to C-5. With further development the stomach descends. Lateral flattening of the gastric lumen occurs; the stomach and duodenum change from a straight tube to their postnatal S-shaped form.

As the foregut grows, the ventral mesogastrium and the anterior edge of the gastroduodenal tube rotate to the right about the long axis; the dorsal mesogastrium and posterior edge rotate to the left. This also involves the terminal esophagus. The left vagus nerve comes to lie anterior to the terminal esophagus and the stomach while the right vagus positions posterior.

The greater and lesser curvatures of the stomach become established during the sixth and seventh weeks of gestation (Fig. 1-2). Most investigators state that the dorsal border grows faster than the ventral border and moves to the left to become the greater curvature, but this matter is controversial (Fig. 1-3) (Gray and Skandalakis, 1972).

Within the ventral mesogastrium the liver grows from the ventrally located hepatic bud. The duodenal end of the bud, which becomes the bile and main pancreatic ducts, shifts farther to the right and then behind the duodenum. The budding head of the pancreas rotates in the same way and fuses with the anlage of the body of the pancreas growing from the dorsal pancreatic bud.

As rotation of the gastroduodenal segment is concluded, these organs and their dorsal mesenteries become fixed by fusion to adjacent portions of the posterior abdominal wall. "In some places there is also fusion to already rotated parts of the gut, as where the greater omentum is in contact with the transverse colon, or where the transverse mesocolon crosses the already rotated duodenum" (Gray and Skandalakis, 1972). According to these investigators, the gastric rugae and circular muscular layer appear by the eighth intrauterine week, the longitudinal layer appears between the eighth and tenth weeks, and the oblique layer, between the twelfth and fourteenth weeks. Parietal cells are recognizable at about 11 weeks. Chief cells appear about the twelfth week but no pepsinogen can be identified in them until their birth. Pepsin is present in the mucosa by the last half of the sixth month, but neither pepsin nor hydrochloric acid appears in the gastric contents until near term. The stomach contents are nearly neutral at birth, but gastric acid increases within a few hours. This occurs in the absence of food and may be due to increased oxygen tension of the blood acting on the parietal cells.

At birth an infant's stomach contains a gray mucous material composed of gastric secretions and desquamated cells mixed with amniotic fluid. Maternal blood swallowed during parturition may be sufficient to give a positive test for occult blood during the first few days of life.

Congenital Malformations of the Stomach

Congenital malformations of the stomach are uncommon. The only frequent serious gastric disorder of infancy is hypertrophic pyloric stenosis, which is not of embryonic origin.

According to Gray and Skandalakis (1972), "The stomach is never completely absent except in nonviable monsters, and rarely is it grossly hypoplastic." However, Gerbeaux and associates (1971) reported that during investigations for failure to thrive in an infant who had been premature, they discovered congenital absence of the stomach by means of a barium meal. Peroral stomach biopsy produced only fragments of esophageal mucosa and no gastric mucosa. Further studies showed rapid passage of the

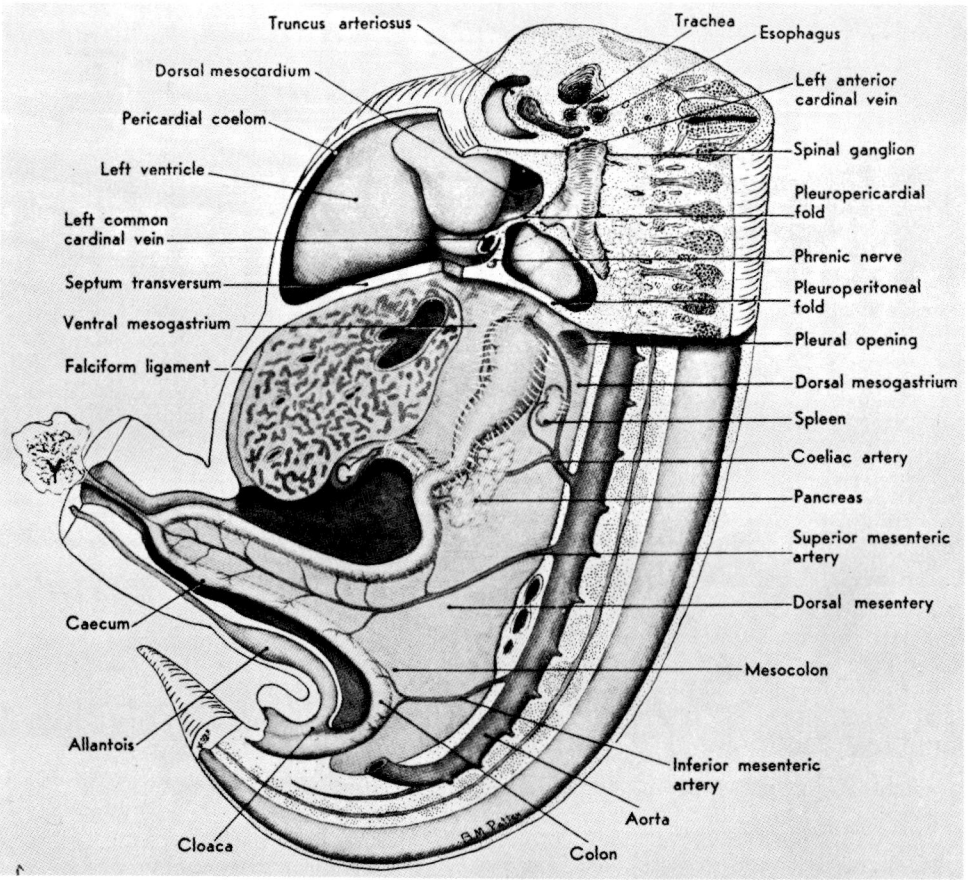

Figure 1–1. The human embryo in the seventh week of gestation, in diagrammatic longitudinal section. (From Patten, B. M.: Human Embryology. 3rd ed. New York, McGraw-Hill Book Company, 1968.)

EMBRYOLOGY

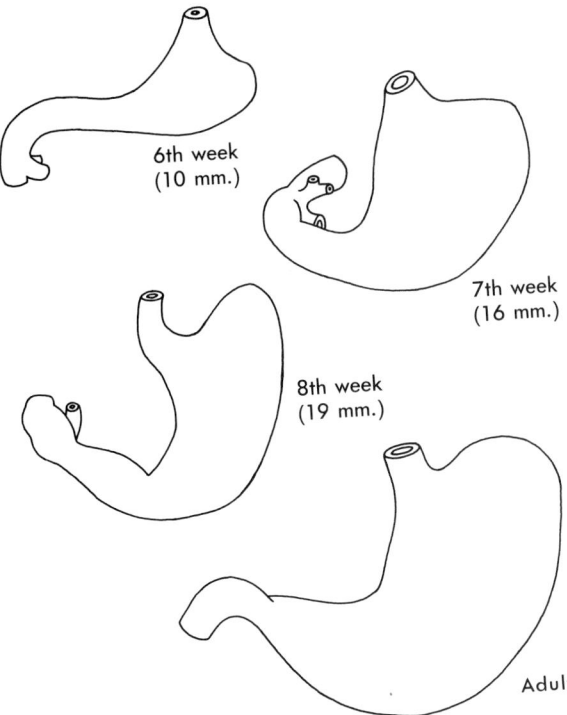

Figure 1–2. The shape of the stomach in prenatal stages and in the adult. (From Gray, S. W., and Skandalakis, J. E.: Embryology for Surgeons. Philadelphia, W. B. Saunders Company, 1972.)

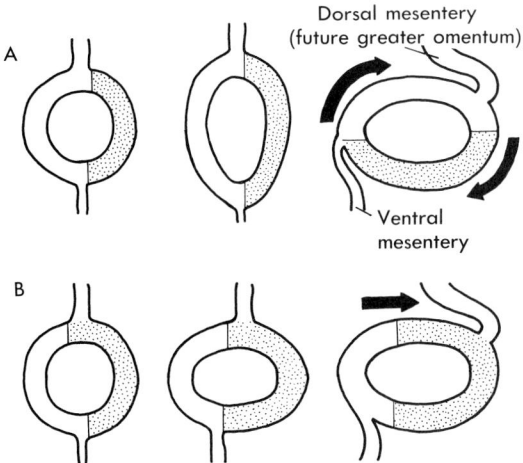

Figure 1–3. Cross sectional diagrams through the embryonic stomach during the seventh week, illustrating two hypotheses for the rotation of the stomach. *A*, Classic view, in which the dorsal border rotates to the left to become the greater curvature; *B*, view of Dankmeijer and Miete, in which the left side becomes the greater curvature as a result only of increased growth — that is, no actual rotation occurs. (From Gray and Skandalakis, cited in previous figure.)

food bolus toward the duodenum. Absence of megaloblastic anemia and normal serum levels of folic acid and vitamin B_{12} were evidence that the endocrine function of the stomach was normal. During surgical construction of an artificial stomach by interposition of a loop of intestine, a rudimentary stomach of antropyloric type with normal histology was found. There was no malrotation.

"Transposition [of the stomach] to the right side of the abdomen, as in a mirror-image, sometimes occurs in conjunction with the reversal of other asymmetrically placed organs. Some or all of the stomach may be located above the diaphragm *(thoracic stomach)*. It is accompanied by a short esophagus and represents an arrested descent. Stenosis results from an overdevelopment of the pyloric sphincter" (Arey, 1974).

MICROGASTRIA. This extremely rare abnormality is defined as "congenital smallness of the stomach" (Dorland's, 1974). "It is a rare abnormality in which the stomach does not differentiate normally and does not undergo normal rotation" (Blank and Chisolm, 1973). Previous cases have been associated with prematurity, oligodactylia, radial and ulnar hypoplasia, and dolichocephaly.

Gray and Skandalakis (1972) state that microgastria was reported in the necropsy of a child in one of the earliest descriptions of congenital pyloric stenosis, by Blair in 1717. Another child, described by Hoyt in 1924, had a stomach with a capacity about one-tenth that of normal. In 1956 Caffey described an anomalous stomach which lay in the midline of a 6-month-old infant. The curvatures were not developed and there was no differentiation into regions. The gastroesophageal junction was incompetent and the esophagus was dilated. The child suffered from secondary anemia and weight loss.

Tubular stomachs have been reported at least twice in association with agenesis of the spleen, congenital cardiac defects, and partial situs inversus. One such infant lived for 6 months (Putschar and Manion, 1956).

In 1973 Blank and Chisolm reported a 27-year-old woman who had congenital microgastria that was apparent on roentgenographic examination when she was 1 year old. Despite inability to eat anything but puréed foods for her first 13 years and despite persistent vomiting during that time, she attained normal adult size and had three healthy children.

I have been unable to find any reports of attempts to treat this anomaly surgically.

Schulz and Niemann (1971) presented a new syndrome in a 4-day-old premature female who underwent exploratory laparotomy for persistent vomiting and radiographic evidence of high intestinal obstruction. At surgery a Type I malrotation was found, and there was much difficulty in identifying the stomach; initially gastric aplasia was suspected. Barium meal revealed an extremely small, normally rotated stomach with normal anatomy, associated with a dilated esophagus and a small sliding hiatal hernia. In addition the infant had unilateral shortened forearm, homolateral thumb aplasia, and dolichocephaly.

OTHER CONGENITAL MALFORMATIONS. A case of congenital cystic dysplasia of the stomach and esophagus was reported in 1970 as an incidental finding at autopsy in a 35-day-old male baby who died of bronchopneumonia. The walls of the stomach and esophagus contained numerous epithelial-lined cysts located in the submucosa with partial atrophy of the surrounding mucosa and muscularis (Traversa, Nibbi, and Bossù, 1970).

Cohen presented five cases of intrathoracic stomach volvulus in children. In each case the repair was done through a right lateral thoracotomy. Two cases were associated with absent hemidiaphragm and another case was associated with paraesophageal hernia (Cohen, 1970).

A review of all cases of acute volvulus of the stomach up to 1971 disclosed 43 patients. Cole and Dickinson, the investigators, emphasize the need for *complete* obstruction of the lumen of the stomach to fulfill the criteria for volvulus. Associated diaphragmatic defects were seen in 28, or 65 per cent, of these patients. Vomiting associated with abdominal distention and inability to pass a nasogastric tube are the usual clinical findings. The recommended treatment is transabdominal reduction of the volvulus and fixation of the stomach by a gastrostomy. Overall mortality has been 68 per cent; however, since 1950 only 2 of 26 patients have died.

SURGICAL ANATOMY OF THE STOMACH

The stomach is the musculomembranous expansion of the alimentary canal between the esophagus and the duodenum. The end that connects with the esophagus is the *cardiac* end, and that nearest the duodenum is the *pyloric* end, or *pylorus*. The upper concave surface or edge is the *lesser curvature;* the lower convex edge is the *greater curvature*. The coats of the stomach are four: an outer peritoneal or *serous* coat; a *muscular* coat, made up of longitudinal, oblique, and circular fibers (the latter forming a pyloric sphincter); a *submucous* coat lined with a muscular layer, the *muscularis mucosae;* and the *mucous* coat or membrane forming the inner lining. Gastric glands in the mucous coat secrete gastric juice containing hydrochloric acid, pepsin, and various other digestive enzymes into the cavity of the stomach. Food mixed with this secretion forms a semifluid substance (chyme) suitable for further digestion by the intestine.

For ease of description the stomach is divided arbitrarily into three portions (Fig. 1–4): (1) the fundus, the part extending above and to the left of the junction of the esophagus with the stomach (cardia); (2) the body, the portion that lies between the fundus above and the pyloric antrum below; and (3) the pyloric antrum, the distal portion of the stomach, beginning at the level of the angular notch and narrowing in caliber as it approaches the pyloric sphincter (pylorus). The pyloric canal is the portion of the alimentary canal that passes through the pyloric sphincter; it is about 2.5 cm. long.

The stomach measures about 25 cm. in length and 10 cm. in diameter and ordinarily has a capacity of from 0.9 to 1.4 liters of fluid. However, these dimensions and capacities may vary greatly in different individuals and also in the same individual at different times and with changed conditions. The volume of an empty gastric lumen may be only 50 ml. or less, but the stomach has great compliance since about 1000 ml. can be ingested before intraluminal pressure begins to rise.

Although the shape of the stomach varies among individuals, some fairly constant external anatomic features can be recognized (Fig. 1–5).

SURGICAL ANATOMY OF THE STOMACH

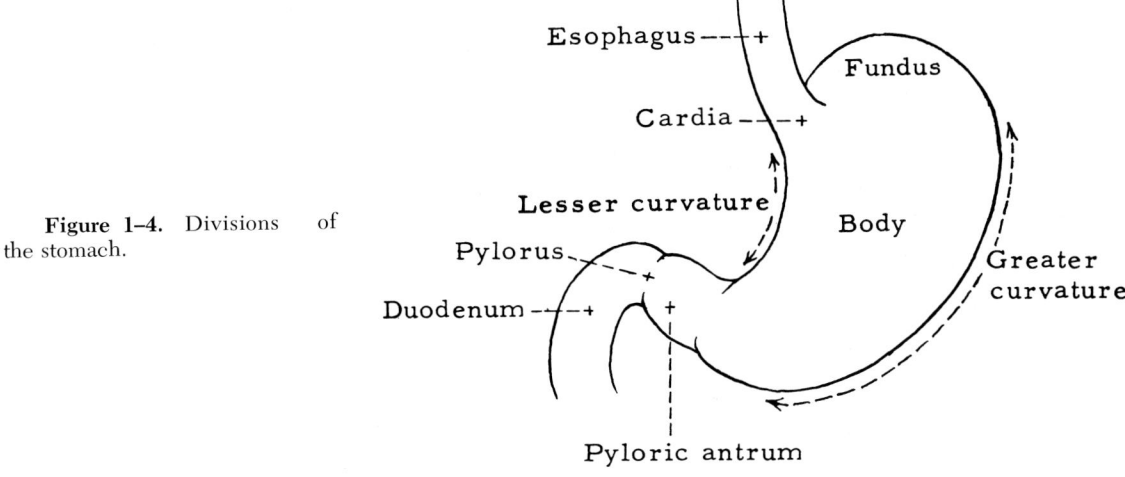

Figure 1–4. Divisions of the stomach.

The *incisura* is the angular notch on the lesser curvature that separates the antrum on the right from the body of the stomach on the left. The *cardia* is the zone adjacent to the esophagus; the *fundus* is the dome-shaped part that extends to the left and above the esophagogastric junction. The *antrum* is that part of the stomach distal to the incisura, and the term usually includes the distally contiguous pyloric canal ending at the pylorus, which is the distal aperture of the stomach through which the gastric contents are emptied into the duodenum. The *pylorus* is surrounded by a strong band of circular muscle, the pyloric sphincter, which can be palpated. Contracted muscle situated proximal to the sphincter and beneath an occasional indentation can be mistaken for the sphincter itself. The *pyloric vein* (Fig. 1–6) is usually visible externally and marks the gastric margin of the pylorus. This vessel crosses the anterior aspect of the pylorus and is a valuable landmark, for it is larger and more constant at the greater curvature. It is helpful in distinguishing a gastric from a duodenal ulcer.

Position

Allowing for differences in age, body build, visceral support, and peristalsis of the individual subject, the stomach may be said to lie in the epigastric and left hypochondriac regions, about five-sixths of it to the left and one-sixth to the right of the median line (Fig. 1–7). The anterior gastric wall lies in the greater peritoneal cavity, and the posterior wall in the lesser cavity.

The *fundus* extends to the left sixth chondrosternal articulation, or the fifth rib in the mammary line, and to the cupula of the diaphragm; this is slightly above and behind the apex of the heart, and is 3 to 5 cm. higher than the cardiac orifice.

The *cardiac orifice* lies opposite the left seventh chondrosternal articulation, about 2.5 cm. from the sternum on a level with the ninth dorsal spine. It is situated from 2 to 3 cm. below the esophageal opening in the diaphragm, about 7.5 cm. medial to the left extremity of the stomach, and 11 cm. from the anterior abdominal wall.

The *pylorus* is located on a level with the seventh costochondral junctions (which are 5 to 7.5 cm. below the sternoxiphoid

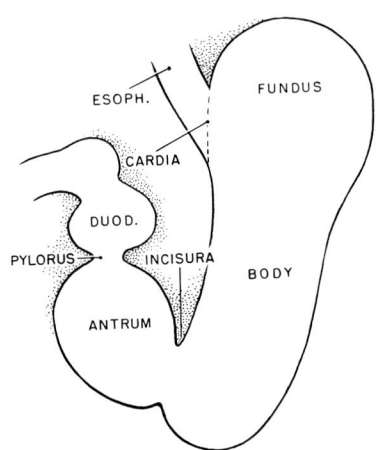

Figure 1–5. External features of the stomach.

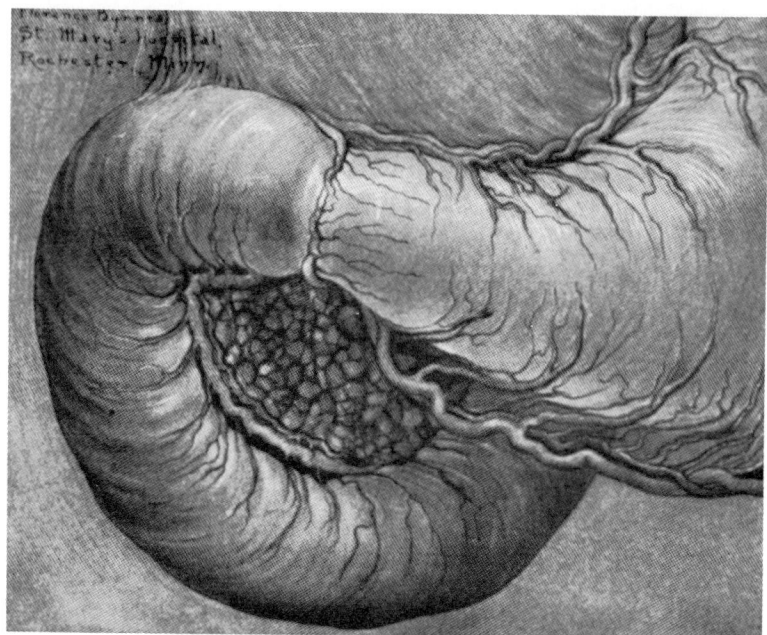

Figure 1–6. Blood vessels about the pyloric end of the stomach and duodenum with special reference to the pyloric vein.

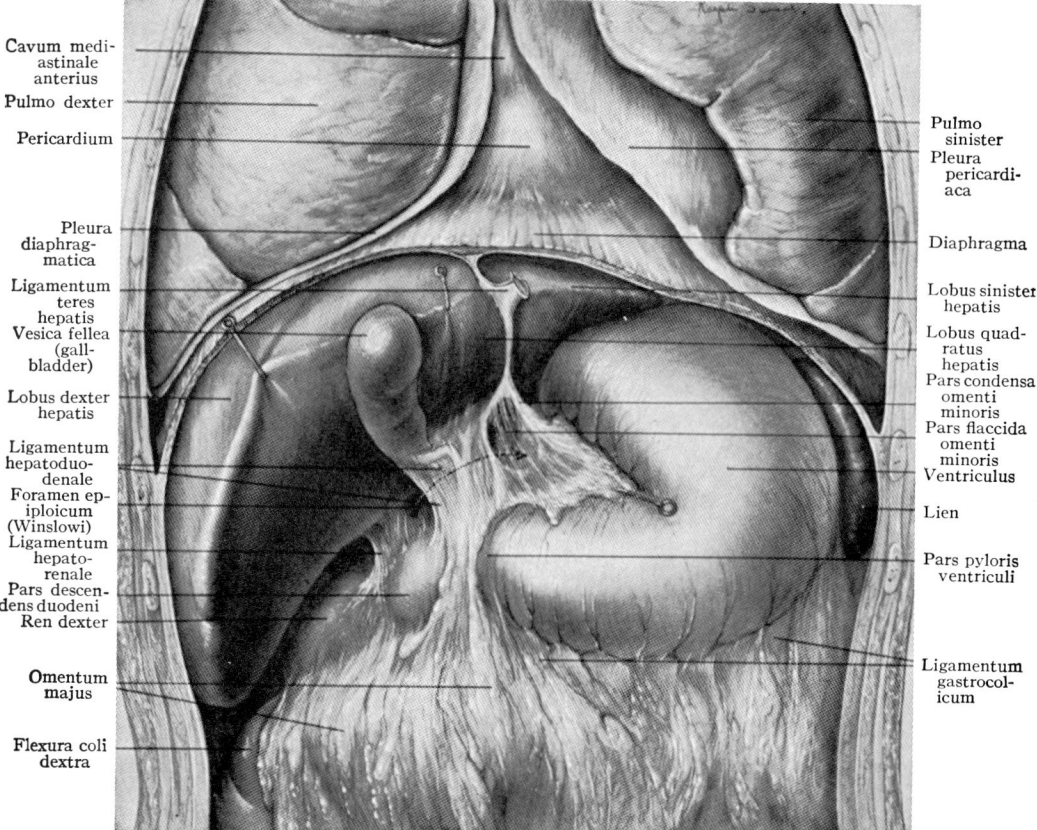

Figure 1–7. Supramesocolic viscera and their relations with the thoracic contents.

SURGICAL ANATOMY OF THE STOMACH

joint). It is at the right of the median line and on a level with the twelfth dorsal spine (upper border of the first lumbar vertebra).

Relations

The stomach lies under the liver and diaphragm, above the jejunum, ileum, and transverse colon, and upon the transverse mesocolon. *Anteriorly and superiorly* it lies against the diaphragm, thoracic wall (anterior portions of the seventh, eighth, and ninth ribs), the left and quadrate lobes of the liver, the anterior abdominal wall, and the lesser omentum. *Posteriorly and inferiorly* (Fig. 1–8) it is related to the diaphragm and its crura, the aorta and inferior vena cava, first lumbar vertebra, celiac axis, lesser peritoneal sac, splenic flexure of the colon, transverse colon, transverse mesocolon, left kidney and suprarenal capsule, the pancreas, splenic vessels, duodenum (fourth or ascending portion), and the solar plexus. The *right end* is adjacent to the transverse colon and the inferior surface of the liver. The *left end* reaches the spleen and the diaphragm.

Fixation Points and Ligaments

The stomach is bound to the diaphragm by the esophagus, and to the vertebral column by the duodenum. The phrenicogastric ligament connects the cardia to the diaphragm. The gastrohepatic (lesser) omentum unites the lesser curvature to the liver.

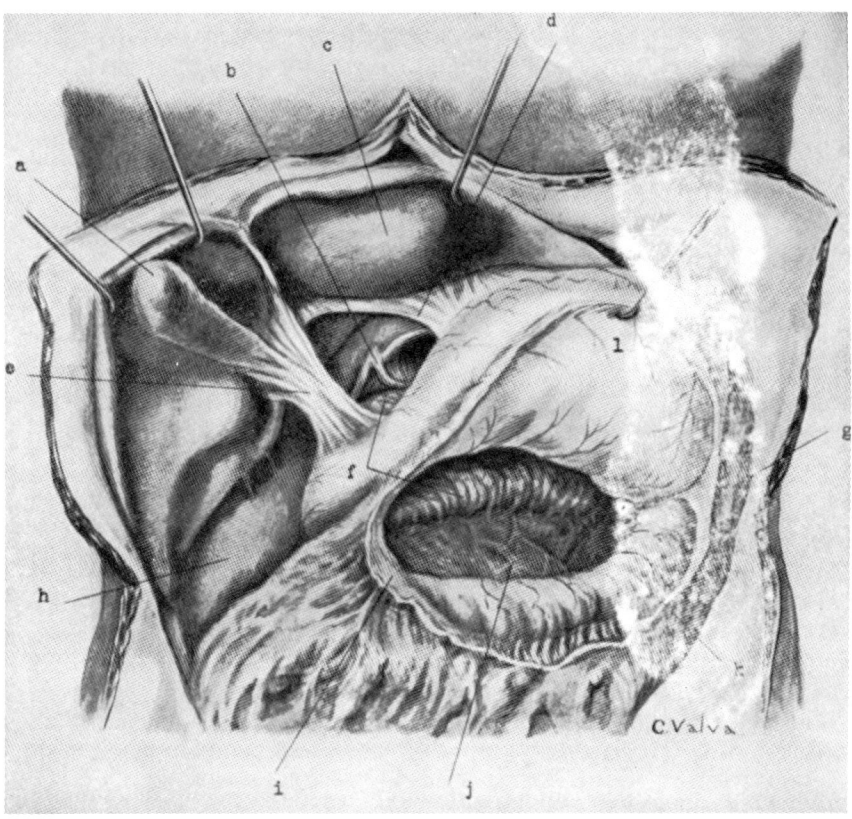

Figure 1–8. The stomach, in relation to some of the deeper, adjacent structures. *a*, Gallbladder; *b*, celiac axis, with the splenic, gastric, and hepatic arteries in view; *c*, left lobe of the liver; *d*, incised margin of the gastrohepatic omentum; *e*, hepatoduodenal ligament; *f*, pancreas, its upper portion being seen through the incised gastrohepatic omentum — and the lower part, through the incised gastrocolic omentum; *g*, spleen; *h*, right kidney, behind the peritoneum; *i*, margin of the incised anterior wall of the gastrocolic omentum; *j*, posterior wall of the lesser omental cavity; *k*, transverse colon; *l*, stomach, displaced to expose the supragastric and infragastric incised openings into the lesser omental cavity.

The hepatoduodenal ligament connects the pylorus and duodenum to the liver. The gastrosplenic omentum binds the greater curvature to the spleen. The gastrocolic ligament (part of the greater omentum) (Fig. 1–7) unites the stomach to the transverse colon. Normally the stomach is freely movable in an anteroposterior direction.

Peritoneal Coverings

The stomach is covered with peritoneum everywhere except exactly at the lesser and greater curvatures and upon the posterior triangular areas at each end (Figs. 1–9 and 1–10).

Circulation and Innervation

The *arteries* of the stomach are the right gastric and right gastroepiploic from the hepatic, the left gastroepiploic and vasa brevia from the splenic, and the left gastric (coronary) from the celiac axis (Fig. 1–11). These arteries communicate grossly and also by communications between small branches within the gastric wall. However, the short gastric arteries supplying the fundus may be incapable alone of supplying distant portions of the stomach.

Womack (1969) warned that variations in the origin of the larger arteries to the stomach are frequent and need to be considered in gastric surgery.

The stomach is the most richly vascularized part of the gut. Its arterial supply is so abundant that it is generally considered safe, when mobilizing the stomach for anastomosing the stomach to the esophagus, to ligate all but one of the four major arteries. However, Nakayama (1954) concluded from his extensive clinical experience and injection studies that it is essential to preserve either the right gastric or the right gastroepiploic arteries and leave the arterial arches along the two curvatures completely intact in order to maintain adequate circulation in the proximal part of the mobilized stomach.

"Beyond the pylorus the profuse arterial anastomoses of the stomach abruptly yield to a paucity of such arterial connections in the remainder of the gut until the

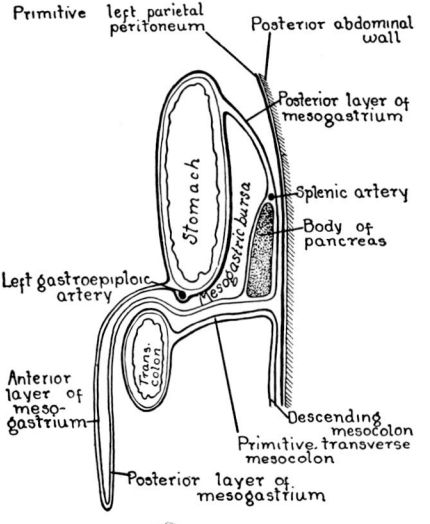

Figure 1–9

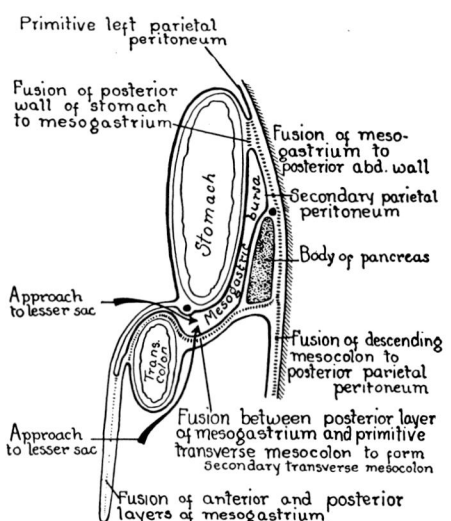

Figure 1–10

Figure 1–9. Left paramedian sagittal section through the upper abdomen before posterior peritoneal fixation occurs of the mesogastric bursa to the left parietal peritoneum and to the transverse colon and mesocolon.

Figure 1–10. Left paramedian sagittal section through the upper abdomen after peritoneal fixation has taken place. The posterior layer of the mesogastrium has fused with the left primitive parietal peritoneum, thus anchoring the splenic artery and the body of the pancreas; the mesogastrium has fused with the superior peritoneal layer of the transverse mesocolon and the serosa on the transverse colon to form the ultimate transverse mesocolon. The apposed serosal layers within the cavity of the greater omentum have fused to a point on a level with the transverse colon. The two arrows indicate the most anatomic surgical approaches to the mesogastric bursa (lesser peritoneal sac).

SURGICAL ANATOMY OF THE STOMACH

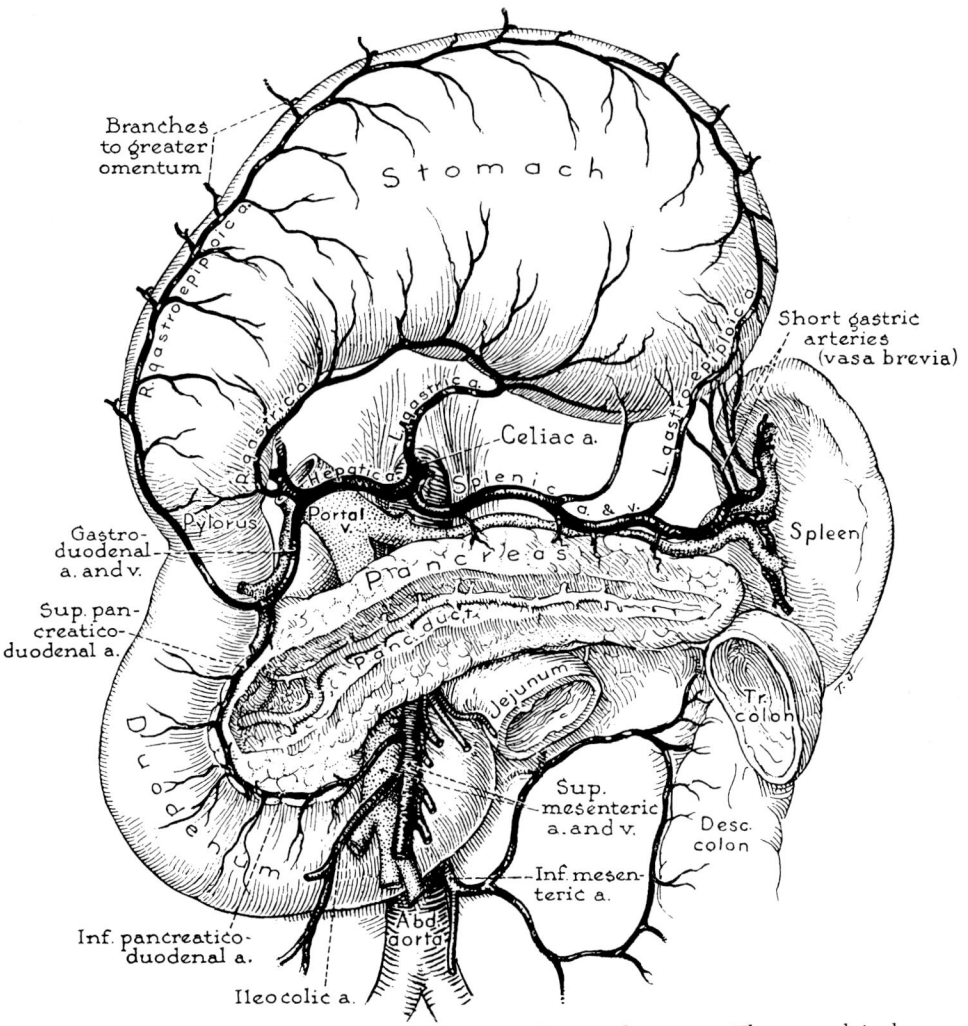

Figure 1-11. Blood supply of the stomach, duodenum, spleen, and pancreas. The stomach is shown reflected upward and the pancreatic duct is exposed.

lower rectum" (Edwards, Malone, and MacArthur, 1975).

The *veins* of the stomach are the left gastric (coronary) and the right gastric (pyloric) (Fig. 1-6), which are tributaries of the portal vein; the right gastroepiploic, which empties into the superior mesenteric; and the left gastroepiploic, which drains into the splenic. The veins accompany their corresponding arteries. At the lower end of the esophagus the left gastric vein (portal system) anastomoses freely in the submucous layer with the lower esophageal veins. These anastomose with the upper esophageal veins, which are tributary through the azygos veins with the vena cava, thus forming an important anastomosis between the portal and systemic venous systems.

The anatomic presence of true non-nutrient arteriovenous communications ("shunts") in the stomach has been controversial. Delaney (1975), using a microsphere method, has shown that such connections comprise less than 2 per cent of the gastric blood flow, if they exist at all. Therefore it seems unlikely that true arteriovenous shunting can be invoked as an explanation for mucosal ischemic states. On the other hand, the intramural gastric circulation may be arranged in parallel circuits like

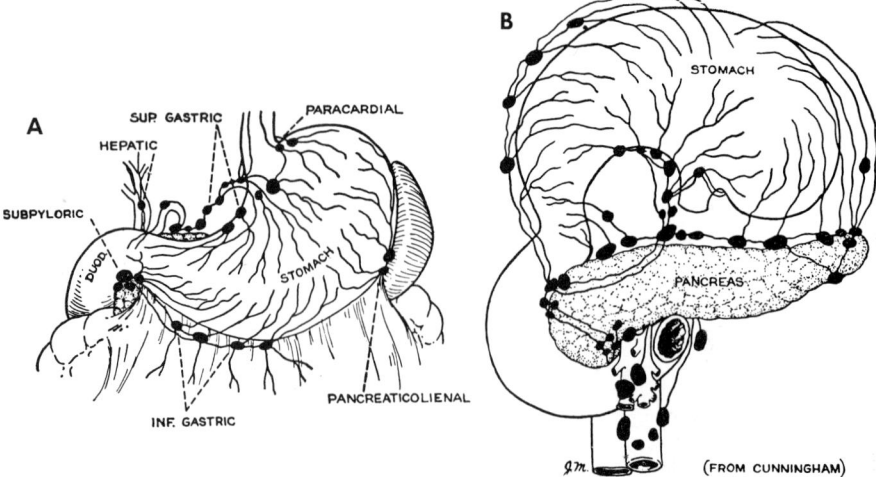

Figure 1-12. Lymph drainage of the stomach in relation to gastrectomy for cancer. *A,* Perigastric groups of nodes are abundant. In cancer the subpyloric glands must be carefully dissected; to remove those along the greater curvature, the entire greater omentum should be excised. Including the spleen in the dissection cuts out the pancreaticolienal glands. *B,* The extensive lymph node field presents posterior to the stomach and with many connecting channels. Portions of the pancreas and transverse colon may require excision. For possible cure, resections of the stomach for carcinoma may include all or part of several surrounding organs and should be nearly total, or total, gastrectomies.

those demonstrated in the small intestine (Kampp, Lundgren, and Sjostrand, 1968). Thus blood entering the stomach wall could be diverted preferentially from one flow compartment to another. Diversion of blood flow from the superficial mucosal layer to the muscularis, for example, could result in the same degree of mucosal ischemia as true shunting. In light of the rather extensive evidence for the existence of ischemic mucosal states, this provides a plausible but as yet undemonstrated mechanism for their development.

The *lymph nodes* lie along the greater and lesser curvatures and at the pyloric and cardiac ends of the stomach (Fig. 1–12).

The *nerves* of the stomach are the right vagus (posterior surface), the left vagus (anterior surface), and the solar plexus of the sympathetic system (Fig. 1–13).

Identification

The stomach is recognized by its relation to the inferior surface of the liver, its continuity with the anterior layer of the gastrohepatic omentum, its thick wall, the direction (Fig. 1–6) of its vessels, its lack of longitudinal taeniae and haustrations, and by its pinkish-white color and absolute opacity. The stomach and the transverse colon have been mistaken for each other.

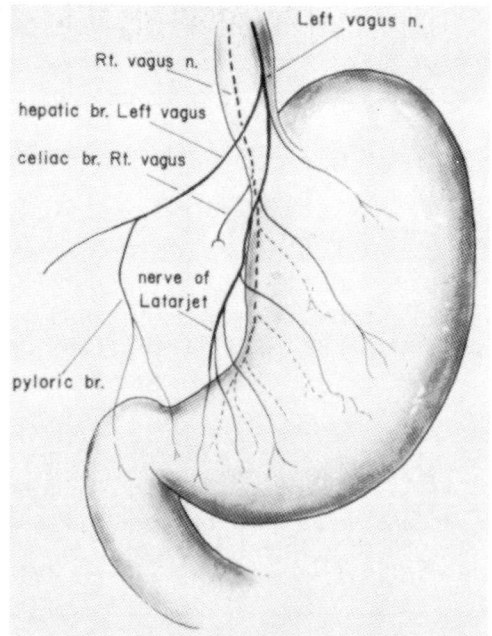

Figure 1-13. Diagram of vagal innervation of the human stomach. (From Menguy, R.: Surgery of Peptic Ulcer. Philadelphia, W. B. Saunders Company, 1976.)

PHYSIOLOGY OF THE STOMACH

Some functions of the stomach are known but of many there is only partial knowledge or no knowledge at all. It is important to the surgeon to know that all or part of the stomach may be removed with only mild and tolerable disturbance of the patient's well-being. Some of the better understood facts concerning the functions may be enumerated as follows:

1. The stomach is a storehouse for macerating, churning, and preparing food in the early part of the process of digestion.
2. The stomach does not assimilate food.
3. Gravity does not play a part in emptying the stomach.
4. The stomach is innervated by the vagus and sympathetic nerves. The vagus nerves increase the tone and force of contractions of the gastric muscles and pyloric sphincter. The sympathetic nerves have an opposite effect on each. Section of the vagus nerves reduces the volume of gastric juice and the tone and activity of gastric muscle.
5. Digestion in the stomach is produced by a combination of *mechanical* churning plus *chemical* solution of food. Symptoms of indigestion may be caused by a disturbance of either process.
6. Agents that reduce gastric secretion are fats, oils, acids, and atropine. Agents that increase gastric secretion are histamine, pentagastrin, alcohol, and condiments.
7. After removal of the whole or part of the stomach, a moderate anemia has developed in 30 to 35 per cent of the patients. It may be macrocytic (more common after total gastrectomy) or of secondary type. Liver and iron therapies according to the type of anemia have proved effective.
8. The stomach is an important secretory organ. Its mucosal lining contains an estimated 35 million secretory glands which are capable of secreting up to 5 liters of fluid in 24 hours. The output of gastric juice in a fasting subject varies between 500 and 1500 ml./24 hr. After each meal about 1000 ml. are secreted by the stomach. Secretory rates depend on the balance of stimulant and inhibitory influences.

Gastric Secretion

GASTRIC MUCOSA

The gastric mucosa is surfaced with columnar epithelial cells which contain and secrete mucus and an alkaline fluid. Over the fundus the mucosa is lush and forms numerous rugal folds that increase its secretory surface. The antral mucosa is relatively thin and almost completely flat.

"The surface of the gastric mucosa is studded with depressions forming gastric pits, into each of which the lumens of the glands empty. The area occupied by the pits is 50 per cent of the total surface. There are about 100 pits per mm." (Davenport, 1971). The functions of the glands and types of cells lining them vary according to the region of the stomach.

The gastric mucosa is divided into three parts: the cardiac gland area, the fundic gland area, and the pyloroantral area.

The *cardiac gland area* (Fig. 1–14, Area 3) is a 0.5- to 4.0-cm. zone beginning at the esophagogastric junction and lined with cardiac glands. These tubular glands are lined mainly with mucous cells and have few or no chief (zygomatic) or parietal (oxyntic) cells. Cardiac glands are characterized by shallow pits and a short length. Their secretion is almost entirely mucus.

The *fundus and body (parietal cell) area* (Fig. 1–14, Area 1) occupies the proximal three-quarters of the gastric mucosa and is primarily responsible for secretion of acid and pepsin. In this area the lumens of three to seven glands empty into each pit and the glands contain three main types of cells: mucous, chief (zygomatic), and parietal (oxyntic), and several other types (Fig. 1–15).

The mucosal surface and the pits are lined with surface mucous cells containing numerous granules of mucin. Mucous cells, termed *mucous neck cells* (neck chief cells), are present in the neck of the gland tubule at the junction of the body of the gland with the gastric pit and at the transition between surface epithelial cells and the glands. These mucous cells and the surface cells of the gastric mucosa between the glands secrete a viscid and alkaline mucus that coats the mucosa with a mucous gel layer over 1 mm. thick. Thus a shell of protection is

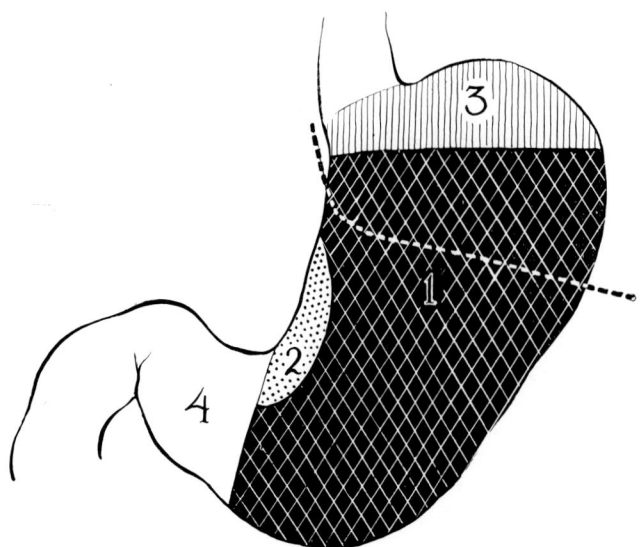

Figure 1–14. Distribution of parietal (acid-secreting) cells in the human stomach. The broken line shows the level for 75 per cent resection. 1, Parietal cells are maximal in this area, and rated 100 per cent. 2, Narrow area on lesser curvature has parietal cells, 75 per cent. 3, Fundus parietal cells, 50 per cent. 4, Prepyloric area, 0 to 1 per cent.

provided for the underlying epithelium against unlimited contact with gastric juice. How effective this protection is remains moot. Mucus also contributes "to lubrication of food transport. Even the slightest irritation of the mucosa directly stimulates the mucus cells to secrete copious quantities of this thick, viscid mucus" (Guyton, 1981).

The chief (zygomatic) cells are cube shaped, with a basally situated nucleus and a basophilic cytoplasm. They are the predominant cells in the deeper portion of the fundic glands. Chief cells secrete pepsinogen, the ferment that is a precursor to pepsin, which is active only in an acid medium and plays a part in protein digestion. Rennin, a milk-curdling enzyme, which is abundant in infants but meager in adults, and lipase, a weak, fat-splitting enzyme, are also assumed to be secreted by the chief cells. Chief cells are stimulated to secrete by cholinergic impulses and by the hormones gastrin and secretin.

The parietal (oxyntic) cells are large, pyramid-shaped cells that have bases on the basement membrane of the gland, a centrally placed nucleus, and a finely granular eosinophilic cytoplasm. They do not form a continuous layer but lie here and there along the gland tubule. They are the predominant cell in the upper portion of the gland and are found exclusively in the fundus and body of the stomach. They produce hydrochloric acid and, in humans, intrinsic factor (a glycoprotein secreted by gastric glands, necessary for absorption of vitamin B_{12}). The HCl combines with pepsinogen secreted by the chief cells to form pepsin.

In addition to these three types of cells just described, "true argentaffin and argyrophilic cells, whose functions are not known, are found" (Menguy, 1974).

The pyloroantral area (Fig. 1–14, Area 4) is covered by surface mucous cells similar to those lining the remainder of the stomach. The pits are deeper than in the fundus, and the deeper portions of the glands are coiled. The cells lining the glands in this area resemble the mucous neck cells in the fundic glands. They secrete mucus. Parietal and chief cells are rare or absent.

Small cells in the antral mucosa have been shown by immunohistochemical methods to be the source of production of the hormone gastrin. Such cells are part of the APUD (amine precursor uptake, decarboxylase) cell system, which includes a number of peptide-hormone secretory cells such as those that elaborate insulin, glucagon, secretin, somatotropin, and others. Gastrin is the prime mediator of the gastric phase of gastric secretion; its primary effect is the stimulation of hydrogen ion and pepsin secretion from parietal and chief cells, respectively. It also profoundly influences gastric motility; for example, delaying gastric emptying while stimulating the churn-

PHYSIOLOGY OF THE STOMACH

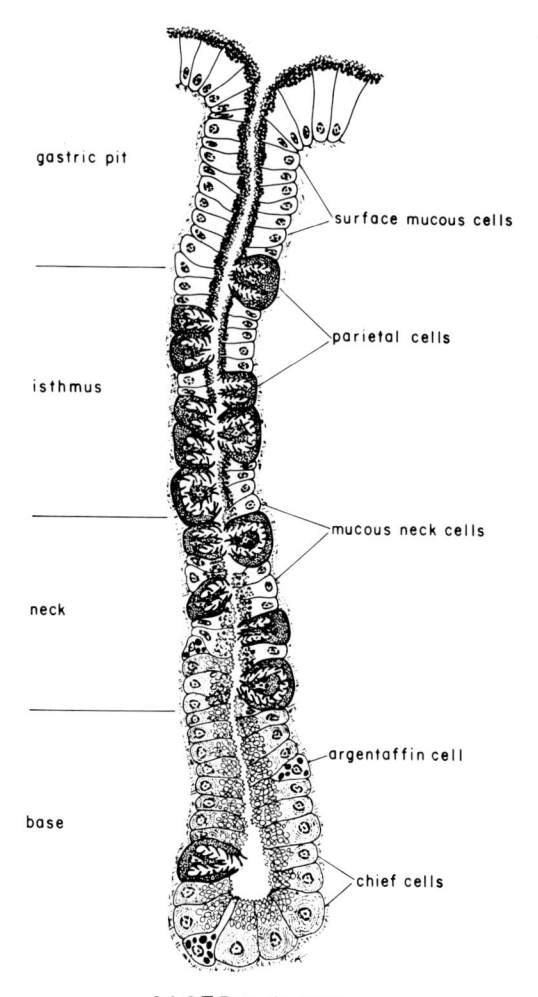

Figure 1-15. A gastric gland. (From Ito, S., and Winchester, R. J.: The fine structure of the gastric mucosa in the bat. J. Cell Biol. 16:541, 1963. Reproduced by courtesy of the authors.)

ing of the acid chyme. Gastrin has been shown to exert a wide variety of other effects in the gastrointestinal tract and elsewhere, but it remains unclear to what extent these effects have physiologic significance.

Dragstedt (1967) pointed out that the antrum, in addition to its internal secretory function, secretes into the lumen of the stomach a faintly alkaline juice exceedingly rich in tenacious mucus.

GASTRIC JUICE

Gastric juice has both organic and nonorganic components.

Organic

1. *Mucus* is secreted predominantly by the prepyloric glands but also by the surface epithelial cells lining the stomach and by mucous cells in the fundic and cardiac gland areas. It is a heterogeneous mixture of glycoproteins with the characteristic properties of adhesiveness, cohesiveness, and high viscosity, which allow it to form a protective thin layer adherent to the mucosa that is resistant to enzymatic proteolysis.

Although once considered to be an important barrier to the diffusion of acid from the gastric lumen to the mucosal surface, gastric mucus has been shown to have no effect whatever on the diffusion of small molecules such as H^+, and little if any effect on the diffusion of larger molecules such as pepsin. Its only effect may well be to provide an "unstirred" layer immediately adjacent to the mucosa, within which a stable pH gradient is set up that affords some protection to the mucosa. It is likely that the primary function of gastric mucus is the same as that of mucus elsewhere in the gastrointestinal tract: that is, to act as a simple lubricant.

On the other hand, Davenport (1971) and others have clearly demonstrated a "gastric mucosal barrier" to ion diffusion that allows the concentration of hydrogen ions in the gastric lumen to exceed that of the mucosal extracellular and intracellular fluid by a factor of 10 million to 1 under normal conditions. Although yet to be defined in clear anatomic terms, this barrier is in some way related to the superficial mucosa, and its selective damage by chemical agents such as alcohol, aspirin, bile salts, and urea allows the back-diffusion of hydrogen ions into the mucosa, resulting in many forms of diffuse superficial hemorrhagic gastritis. More recently, the loss of this barrier function has been shown to be associated with the development of hemorrhagic gastritis under conditions of severe physiologic stess. Whether these changes are the primary cause or only reflect the ischemic mucosal injury that develops in these patients remains unanswered.

2. *Pepsinogens* are inactive zymogens synthesized predominantly in the chief cells of the fundic glandular area and in some cells of the pyloric glandular area. They are stored in granules within the cells.

"Chief cells are stimulated to secrete by cholinergic impulses and by the hormones gastrin and secretin. The most powerful stimulus is vagal stimulation. Ten minutes after the cells are stimulated, most of these granules are discharged. None are present in the cells 3 hours after feeding, although the continuous small basal secretion of pepsinogen continues. The granules begin to reappear after 6 hours and are maximally concentrated after 72 hours.

"Pepsinogen is converted to proteolytically active pepsin when it mixes with acid secreted by the oxyntic cells. Activation occurs more rapidly the lower the pH and is almost instantaneous at pH 2. Pepsin itself activates pepsinogen. Pepsin is maximally active as a proteolytic enzyme between pH 1 and 3. Although pepsinogen is stable in neutral solution, pepsin rapidly and completely loses its catalytic activity when the solution in which it is dissolved is neutralized. Peptic activity of gastric juice is destroyed by neutralization" (Davenport, 1971).

Human gastric juice contains several heterogeneous types of pepsins with different optimal pH levels, but there is no agreement on the physiologic significance of the various types.

Pepsinogen is also found in the blood and is secreted into the urine where it is termed uropepsinogen. This is derived from the stomach, as evidenced by its disappearance from the urine after a total gastrectomy. Although the finding of uropepsinogen in the urine is qualitative evidence that the gastric mucosa is secreting pepsinogen, uropepsinogen levels cannot be used to quantify gastric secretory activity because of a poor correlation between the two. The rate of uropepsinogen secretion is not a measure of gastric secretion.

The simplest method for determining whether the gastric mucosa secretes pepsinogen is to examine the urine for uropepsin activity. Uropepsin activity is usually below normal or absent in patients with chronic atrophic gastritis and absent in cases of complete atrophy (Segal, 1969).

3. *Intrinsic factor* (IF) is a glycoprotein in the mucus secreted into the gastric lumen by the glands in the fundus and body of the stomach. It combines with vitamin B_{12} in the food and thus makes this vitamin available for its absorption in the ileum. "It does this in the following way: First, the intrinsic factor binds tightly with the vitamin B_{12}. In this bound state the B_{12} is protected from digestion by the gastrointestinal enzymes. Second, still in the bound state, the B_{12} and intrinsic factor become adsorbed to the membranes of the mucosal cells in the ileum. Third, the combination is then transported into the cells in pinocytotic vesicles [where dissociation occurs], and about four hours later free vitamin B_{12} is released into the blood" (Guyton, 1981). The fate of the intrinsic factor is unknown.

Lack of intrinsic factor, therefore, causes loss of much of the vitamin because of enzyme action in the gut and also results in failure of absorption.

Vitamin B_{12} absorbed from the gastrointestinal tract is stored in large quantities in the liver and then released slowly as needed to the bone marrow and other tissues in the body. It is an essential nutrient for all cells of the body and for normal erythropoiesis.

The daily requirement of vitamin B_{12} to maintain normal red cell maturation is about 1 μg; a normal liver stores approximately 2 mg. Hence many months of defective B_{12} absorption are required to cause maturation-failure anemia.

Malabsorption of vitamin B_{12} occurs in patients with pernicious anemia whose stomachs do not secrete intrinsic factor, and after total gastrectomy. Vitamin B_{12} deficiency appears only after 3 to 7 years following total gastrectomy since the daily amount needed is small and the liver stores about 1000 times this amount. Total gastrectomy creates a dependence on parenteral administration of vitamin B_{12}.

Subclinical deficiencies in vitamin B_{12} may occur after operations that reduce gastric acid secretion. Abnormal Schilling tests in these patients can be corrected by the administration of intrinsic factor.

Intrinsic factor secretion is enhanced by stimuli that produce H^+ output from parietal cells.

4. *Blood group substances.* About 75 per cent of people secrete into their gastric juice "the major blood group antigens A, B, and H(O) as well as minor blood antigens such as the Lewis substances (Le^a and Le^b). Individuals who have the Le^{a+} substance on their red blood cells (about 25 per cent of the population are Le^{a+}) in addition to their major blood group antigen do not secrete their major blood group antigens into their gastric juice or saliva, but secrete similar amounts of Lewis[a] antigen. For unknown

reasons, these individuals, called 'nonsecretors' are more liable to duodenal ulceration than 'secretors' "(Menguy, 1974).

The trait is genetically determined.

Bacterial Content of Gastric Juice

Wide variations in the proportion of patients with viable bacteria in the stomach have been reported by various investigators. According to Bornside and associates (1978), the gastric juice in a normal human fasting stomach has a total bacterial count of about 2.5×10^3 per ml. of aspirated gastric fluid, equally divided between aerobes and anaerobes. This flora may be augmented by the bacteria in food and saliva and in proximal intestinal contents refluxed through the pylorus. Approximately 1 to 1.5 liters of saliva enter the stomach per day. The upper small bowel contains a sparse bacterial population similar to that of the stomach, so its contribution to the stomach by reflux is insignificant compared with that from the saliva.

Few bacteria survive in the normal fasting stomach because of the pH–hydrochloric acid–dependent gastric bactericidal barrier which promptly kills bacteria at pH values of less than 4.0. Other factors regulating the number of bacteria in the stomach are the number of organisms ingested, the vehicle in which they are ingested (water, milk, and other) and the physical protection of food, the buffering of gastric contents, and the rate of gastric emptying.

Bornside and associates also studied the relation of microbial flora in stomach contents and stomach wall in paired specimens and found they were similar. A survey of the literature showed that most specimens from patients with gastric ulcers or gastric malignancies are positive for bacteria, while only about 60 per cent of specimens from patients with duodenal ulcers are positive.

Macgregor and Ross (1972) performed bacteriologic studies on the gastric aspirates obtained from 280 preoperative and postoperative secretion studies. In the preoperative group viable bacteria were isolated from 41 per cent of patients, whereas in the postoperative group they were isolated from 73 per cent. The nature of the bacterial flora also differed in the two groups.

Preoperative and postoperative bacteriologic studies were done in 46 patients. In 10 there was no growth pre- or postoperatively. In 21 there was no growth preoperatively but growth postoperatively. One patient showed growth preoperatively but no growth postoperatively. In 14 patients there was growth pre- and postoperatively, but of these only 2 retained postoperatively the same bacteria that had been cultured preoperatively. The flora were different in 12 patients; also, the preoperative growth was scanty and the postoperative growth was heavier.

The researchers concluded that infected stomach contents may lead to local sepsis postoperatively, and that the loss or partial loss of the hydrochloric acid barrier of the stomach may facilitate infection by pathogenic gut bacteria.

Greenlee and colleagues (1971) reported on 20 patients with duodenal ulcer requiring elective surgery in whom vagotomy and antrectomy were performed. Gastroduodenostomy reconstruction was used in 16 patients and gastrojejunostomy in 4 patients. Quantitative aerobic and anaerobic bacteriology of the jejunum demonstrated a consistent and marked increase in the number of microorganisms comprising the bacterial flora. Correlation of basal and stimulated gastric secretory output with postoperative bacterial overgrowth failed to demonstrate any definite control by gastric acid over bacterial proliferation in the jejunum. They suggested that the presence of large numbers of microorganisms in the small bowel might relate to several of the postgastrectomy syndromes.

Nonorganic Gastric Juice Components

Hydrochloric acid is an important, and the most characteristic, nonorganic constituent of gastric juice. It is secreted by the parietal cells which are found exclusively in the fundus and body of the stomach. "These cells secrete an electrolytic solution containing 160 millimoles of HCl per liter, which is almost exactly isotonic with body fluids. The pH of this acid solution is approximately 0.8" (Guyton, 1981). The finding of less acidity is believed to be due to neutralization and dilution by other juices.

On the surface of the mucosa this HCl secreted by the parietal cells "is admixed with varying amounts of secretions from other gastric mucosal cells, so that aspirated gastric juice contains Na^+, K^+, and HCO_3, in addition to HCl. Although the levels of the ions are constantly changing, the average concentrations are Na, 65 mEq.; K, 13 mEq.; Cl, 100 mEq.; and H, 90 mEq. The molar concentration of Cl^- exceeds that of H^+, because a small amount of 'neutral' Cl^- is secreted as KCl and NaCl" (Menguy, 1974). As the concentration of H^+ rises during secretion, that of Na^+ and K^+ decreases reciprocally. Chloride concentration remains nearly constant. Some chloride may also be secreted by other than parietal cells. The upper limit of acid concentration in gastric juice is about 150 mEq./L. which is a concentration gradient over 2 million times greater than that in the blood bathing the gastric cells, yet gastric juice maintains its isotonicity at various secretory rates.

GASTRIC MUCOSAL BARRIER

The ability of the stomach to maintain such an enormous concentration gradient of hydrogen ion between the lumen and the plasma is explained by the presence of a gastric mucosal barrier, the integrity of which permits the stomach to hold a high concentration of HCl in its lumen and away from the mucosal tissues. This ability has been shown to be greatly impaired when the gastric mucosa is injured by such agents as acetic acid or aspirin in HCl, thus breaching the integrity of the mucosal barrier and enormously increasing its permeability to hydrogen ion.

"The gastric mucosa barrier is broken by many compounds; among them are HCl in high enough concentration (about 300 mN); and aliphatics such as acetic, propionic and butyric acids, which, because they are un-ionized and fat soluble, diffuse through cell membranes. Other compounds breaking the barrier are detergents, natural (bile salts and lysolecithin) or synthetic (lauryl sulfate), ethanol in a concentration of about 10 per cent by weight, salicylic and acetylsalicylic acids in acid solution but not in neutral solution, some phospholipases and some local anesthetics. Contact of all these compounds, for the appropriate time and in the appropriate concentration, with the gastric mucosa results in a large increase in mucosal permeability" (Davenport, 1971).

Silen (1977) summarized the new concepts of the gastric mucosal barrier and concluded that "whether mucus is anything more than a lubricant remains unsolved. Clearly its protective effect against acid is in doubt since it has weak neutralizing and buffering power and the impedance of diffusion of acid through the mucus is virtually nil. . . . I believe there has begun to accrue a significant body of data which supports the concept that the barrier is no one specific anatomic structure, but rather a dynamic ever-changing capacity of the stomach to withstand injury depending upon circulatory factors, secretory state, and acid-base balance."

Renewal of Gastric Surface Epithelium

"The surface mucous cells lining the lumen of the stomach undergo continuous renewal due to mitotic acitivity confined to mucous neck cells. The daughter cells migrate up the walls of the foveolae, reach the surface of the mucosa, and eventually die and are shed into the lumen of the stomach. Although the neck mucous cells differentiate primarily into surface mucous cells, they also differentiate (much more rarely) into parietal cells and chief cells" (Menguy, 1976). According to Davenport (1971), cells are shed by the normal human gastric mucosa at a rate of a half million cells a minute, and in normal circumstances the time required for renewal of surface epithelial cells is 1 to 3 days.

A normal rate of renewal of the surface epithelium is essential for the maintenance of the integrity of the lining of the stomach. Max and Menguy (1970) have shown that this rate of renewal is significantly reduced by steroids.

The mucosa responds to mild injury by desquamation of its surface layer, followed by regeneration. The actual state of the mucosa, healthy or not, at any one instant or place is the result of a balance between protective and restorative forces and destructive forces.

REGULATION OF GASTRIC SECRETION

In the absence of extraneous stimuli, the stomach secretes acid at a low rate.

Stimuli for gastric secretion die out during the night-time hours. Acid secretion becomes minimal about 2:00 A.M. and the pH of gastric contents rises toward neutrality (Davenport, 1971). Gastric hydrochloric acid output is significantly greater in males than in females, and in patients with duodenal ulcer. It decreases after age 50, except in patients with duodenal ulcer, and may be absent in normal persons as well as in patients with a gastric ulcer, carcinoma, or pernicious anemia.

An increase in blood flow does not stimulate secretion, but blood flow is permissive in the sense that adequate flow is required if the stomach is to secrete. Profound vasoconstriction caused by sympathetic stimulation or by vasoconstrictor drugs is followed by depression of secretion (Davenport, 1971).

Gastric secretion is regulated by both nervous and hormonal mechanisms. Nervous regulation is via the parasympathetic fibers of the vagus nerves as well as through local myenteric plexus reflexes. Hormonal regulation is by gastrin, a hormone formed principally in unidentified cells in the antral mucosa. Small amounts of gastrin are formed in the gastric fundus and the proximal small intestine.

There are factors that increase gastric secretion and other factors that decrease it. Their interaction results in the levels of gastric secretion that are present during fasting and after meals.

VAGAL STIMULATION OF GASTRIC SECRETION. This originates in the dorsal motor nuclei of the vagi and passes via the vagus nerves to the myenteric plexus of the stomach and thence to the gastric glands, causing these glands to secrete large quantities of both pepsin and acid, with a higher proportion of pepsin than in gastric juice produced by other stimuli. In addition, it causes some increase in secretion of mucus by the pyloric and cardiac glands and by the mucous neck cells of the gastric glands. Vagal stimulation also causes the antral mucosa to secrete the hormone gastrin, which then causes the gastric glands to augment the flow of highly acid gastric juice. Thus, vagal stimulation excites stomach secretion both directly, by stimulating the gastric glands, and indirectly, by stimulating gastrin production by the antral mucosa.

"Vagal stimulation of gastric secretion can be induced by the administration of insulin (0.2 µg./kg. body weight). The resulting hypoglycemia stimulates vagal centers with a resulting increase in vagal tone. Characteristically, gastric juice secreted in response to vagal stimulation has a high concentration of pepsin" (Menguy, 1974).

The sight, thought, smell, and taste of food, and also strong emotional stimuli, can cause vagal stimulation of gastric secretion.

Gastrin

According to the collective review of Rayford and Thompson (1977) on this subject, gastrin was discovered in 1905 by Edkins, who reported that extracts of antral mucosa stimulated acid secretion from the gastric fundus. He named the active principle in these extracts "gastrin." Almost 60 years later pure gastrin was first isolated from the antral mucosa of hogs; the chemical structure and physiologic actions of gastrin were determined; and the compound was synthesized.

The hormone gastrin is probably the most potent stimulant of gastric acid secretion known. Its physiologic effects include stimulation of (1) gastric secretion of hydrochloric acid and pepsinogen; (2) gastric, intestinal, and gallbladder mobility; and (3) pancreatic enzyme and bicarbonate ion secretion. It also enhances the tone of the lower esophageal sphincter.

Gastrin is formed mainly in the antral portion of the gastric mucosa. Small amounts are formed also in the gastric fundus and in the proximal small intestine.

Secretion of gastrin and its release into the circulation by the antral mucosa occur in response to (1) vagal stimulation; (2) distention of the antrum; and (3) the presence in the gastric lumen of secretagogues such as food extractives, partially digested proteins, alcohol (in low concentration), caffeine, and so on" (Guyton, 1981).

Food entering the stomach causes release of gastrin in two ways: (1) through physical distention of the stomach by the bulk of the food; and (2) through chemical action of the secretagogues. Both these stimuli elicit gastrin release by stimulating sensory nerve fibers in the gastric epithelium, which synapse with the myenteric plexus, which transmits the stimulus to the gastrin-secreting cells. Hence anything that blocks this myenteric reflex will also block the formation of gastrin: anesthetization of the gastric mucosa, to block the sensory stimuli, and administration of atropine, which blocks the action on the gastrin cells of the acetylcholine released by the myenteric plexus, will each prevent gastrin release.

Gastrin is absorbed into the blood and carried to the gastric glands, where it stimulates mainly the parietal cells and, to a much lesser extent, the chief cells. According to Guyton (1981), "The parietal cells increase their rate of hydrochloric acid secretion as much as eight-fold, and the chief cells increase their rate of enzyme secretion two- to four-fold. The rate of secretion in response to gastrin is somewhat less than to vagal stimulation, 200 ml. per hour in contrast to about 500 ml. per hour... However, the gastrin mechanism usually continues for several hours in contrast to a much shorter period of time for vagal stimulation. Therefore, as a whole, it is likely that the gastrin mechanism is equally as important as, if not more important than, the vagal mechanism for control of gastric secretion. Yet, when both of these work together, the total secretion is much greater than the sum of the individual secretions caused by each of the two mechanisms... [They] *multiply each other rather than simply add to each other.*"

In addition to a synergism between vagal innervation of the antrum and gastrin release during mechanical or chemical stimulation of the antrum, gastrin and vagal stimuli act synergistically on the parietal cell. Denervated parietal cells respond less to exogenous gastrin. Also, a vagally denervated antrum releases less gastrin in response to a given degree of distention than when its vagal innervation was intact. Since the stimuli interact synergistically, separation into a cephalic, or neural, phase of gastric secretion is no longer justified (Davenport, 1971; Menguy, 1974).

These stimuli of gastrin release are strengthened when the antral contents are alkaline. When the acidity of the gastric juice increases to a pH of 2.0, the gastrin mechanism for stimulating gastric secretion becomes totally blocked.

Histamine also stimulates gastric secretion in the same way as gastrin does but it is only about 80 per cent as potent.

Dragstedt and associates (1968) have described the mechanism for gastrin release in greater detail than space permits being included here.

Walsh and Grossman (1975) have published a thorough and well-organized collective review of the world literature pertaining to the subject of gastrin.

Turnipseed and Keith (1976) measured the fasting serum gastrin levels and gastrin response to calcium and secretin infusion in 15 patients with histamine-fast achlorhydria. The patients were sorted into the following subgroups according to the presence or absence of antral gastritis: group I, pernicious anemia without antral gastritis (4 patients); group II, pernicious anemia with antral gastritis (2 patients); group III, atrophic gastritis without antral involvement (1 patient).

They reported that hypergastrinemia occurs in achlorhydric states if the antrum is not diseased and suggested that antral gastritis diminishes gastrin levels in achlorhydric patients. There is a dramatic gastrin response to calcium challenge in patients with pernicious anemia. Only minimal response was observed in patients with atrophic gastritis. Unlike the response observed in the Zollinger-Ellison syndrome, secretin challenge suppresses gastrin in achlorhydric states. The authors pointed out that these findings add a new dimension to the utility of serum gastrin determinations.

Wilson and colleagues (1976) studied 31 patients with hyperparathyroidism and found no support for the hypothesis that peptic ulcer disease seen in some patients with hyperparathyroidism results from calcium-induced hypergastrinemia causing gastric hypersecretion.

Tobe and associates (1976), using highly specific immunofluorescence, studied the distribution of gastrin in the digestive organs of dogs, cats, and human beings. In all three species, gastrin-containing cells were found only in the antrum and in the duodenum. There were no gastrin-containing cells in the parotid, submandibular, or sublingual glands, nor in the esophagus, pancreas, jejunum, ileum, or colon.

Wesdorp and coworkers (1977) pointed out that gastrin-containing G cells have been demonstrated in the human duodenum and that duodenal gastrin makes a considerable contribution to the basal circulating levels of this hormone in human beings. The concentration of gastrin in human duodenal mucosa has been variously reported as being equal to, or less than, the concentration in the antral mucosa. Clinical studies by Stern and Walsh (1973) demonstrated significantly higher basal and postprandial plasma gastrin levels after Billroth I gastrectomy with vagotomy than after Billroth II gastrectomy with vagotomy, suggesting a major contribution of duodenal gastrin to basal and postprandial plasma gastrin levels.

Whether or not the characteristics of release of duodenal gastrin are similar to, or different from the extensively investigated characteristics of release of antral gastrin in people is not known. Wesdorp studied the release of duodenal gastrin in dogs and demonstrated distinct differences in characteristics of canine duodenal gastrin release compared with canine antral gastrin release.

Sauberli (1976) pointed out that gastrin plays a crucial part in human gastric acid secretion, but its role in the pathogenesis of peptic ulceration remains uncertain. The mean plasma gastrin levels, basal as well as stimulated, in patients with duodenal ulcers are only slightly higher than in normal patients. Only in patients with Zollinger-Ellison syndrome has it been shown that there is a direct relation between the high plasma gastrin levels, the extremely elevated rates of gastric acid secretion, and severe gastrointestinal ulcer disease. Sauberli studied 50 consecutive patients with peptic ulcers who were operated upon with proximal selective vagotomy. They were randomly divided into two groups of 25 with, and 25 without, the addition of pyloroplasty.

Three months after the operation radioimmunoassay showed no difference between the two groups in the basal levels as well as the stimulated levels of plasma gastrin. The gastrin levels prior to feeding were significantly higher after operation than before operation. During the meal, gastrin values increased in all three patients and the response to the test meal was significantly higher postoperatively compared with the values before operation. Two hours after the test meal, gastrin levels were still 50 per cent above the preoperative levels in all patients who were operated upon. No difference was found between patients treated with highly selective vagotomy and those treated with highly selective vagotomy plus pyloroplasty. Six and 12 months after the operation, a moderate decrease of gastrin secretion was observed, but basal as well as stimulated levels were still elevated after 12 months compared with the values before operation.

Herbst (1977) summarized what is known about the relationship of gastrin to duodenal ulcer disease in human beings and described the effects of surgery on circulating gastrin:

"There is well-documented evidence indicating inappropriately high basal gastrins in patients with duodenal ulcer disease. After stimulation by protein meals, calcium infusion, and/or insulin-induced hypoglycemia there appears to be an exaggerated release of gastrin in patients with duodenal ulcers compared to control subjects. Vagotomy in general tends to increase serum gastrin by decreasing acid secretion and allowing less inhibition for antral gastrin release. This increase appears less with selective vagotomy and parietal cell vagotomy, compared to truncal vagotomy, suggesting vagal inhibition of gastrin release outside the antrum. Antrectomy may decrease serum gastrins by removing a major source of the hormone. However, extra antral gastrin sources, if stimulated properly, may result in little postoperative change."

Gastric Secretion During Interdigestive Period

During the interdigestive period, when no digestion is occurring anywhere in the gut, the stomach secretes only a few milliliters of gastric juice per hour, and that which is secreted is almost entirely the so-called nonparietal type, comprising mainly mucus, very little pepsin, and either no or very little acid. Occasionally the gastric juice may be slightly alkaline. "However, strong emotional stimuli frequently increase the interdigestive secretion to 50 ml. or more of highly peptic and highly acidic gastric juice per hour, in much the same manner that the cephalic phase of gastric secretion excites secretion at the onset of a meal. This increase of secretion by emotional stimuli is believed to be one of the factors in the development of peptic ulcers" (Guyton 1981).

Gastric Secretory Response to Feeding

This response has been described as occurring in three separate phases: cephalic, gastric, and intestinal (Fig. 1–16). However, the division into three separate phases which are named from the loci where the stimuli act is of value principally for descriptive purposes. Actually the three phases fuse together and "a classification of the stimulatory mechanisms into two phases, vagal-antral and intestinal, is more in agreement with modern physiologic data" (Menguy, 1974).

CEPHALIC PHASE. The sight, smell, taste, or thought of appetizing food may initiate the cephalic phase of gastric secretion even before the food enters the stomach. The stimuli originate in the brain and are transmitted through the vagus nerve to the stomach. The vagal stimuli have the direct effect on the parietal cells of increasing acid output. Impulses via vagal fibers to the antrum release gastrin and thereby indirectly enhance acid secretion. The direct parietal cell stimulation is quantitatively more important (Maher and associates, 1975).

The cephalic phase of secretion produces perhaps 10 per cent of the gastric secretion normally associated with eating a meal (Guyton, 1981). Vagal stimulation of gastric secretions is abolished by successful vagotomy.

GASTRIC PHASE. When the food arrives in the stomach, gastric secretion is enhanced by:

1. Mechanical stimuli by antral distention, which further stimulates the production and release of gastrin initiated previously by vagal stimulation of the antrum.

2. Chemical stimulation by secretagogues which liberate gastrin when in contact with the antral mucosa.

3. Local reflexes in the myenteric plexus of the stomach, and vagovagal reflexes that pass to the brain stem via vagal afferents and return via vagal efferents to the stomach. Both reflexes are caused by the presence of food in the stomach; they cause parasympathetic stimulation of the gastric glands, thus adding to the secretion caused by the gastrin mechanism.

"The gastric phase of secretion accounts for more than two-thirds of the total gastric secretion associated with eating a meal and, therefore, accounts for most of the total daily gastric secretion of about 2000 ml." (Guyton, 1981).

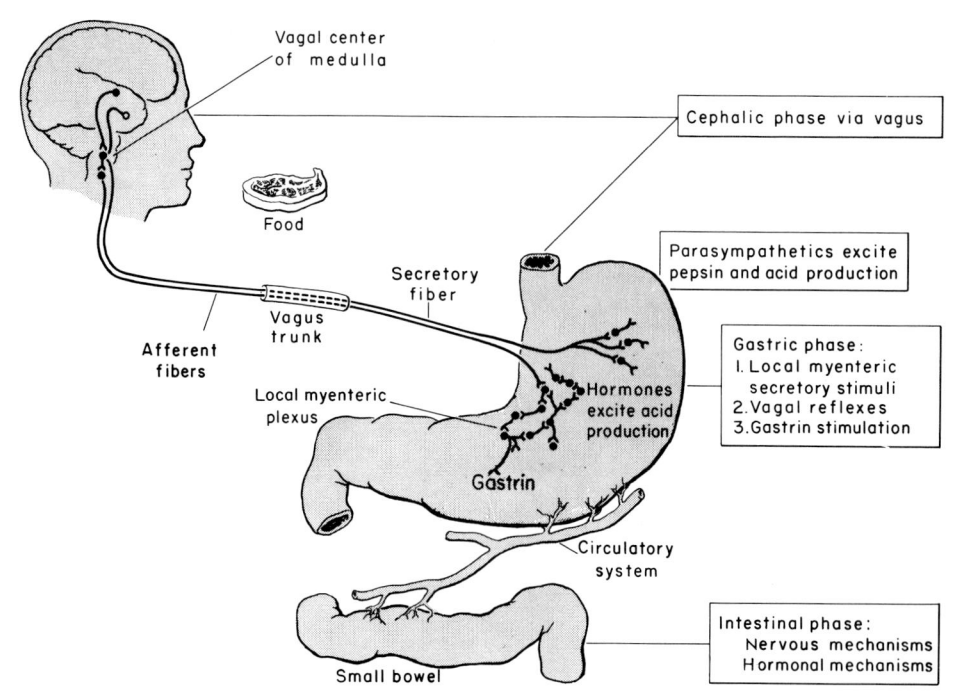

Figure 1–16. The phases of gastric secretion and their regulation. (From Guyton, A. C.: Textbook of Medical Physiology. Philadelphia, W. B. Saunders Company, 1981.)

INTESTINAL PHASE. The presence of food in the upper portion of the small intestine, particularly in the duodenum, also causes the stomach to secrete small amounts of gastric juice. This stimulation is probably mediated by small amounts of a chemical substance identical with or closely resembling gastrin in its activity, called enteric gastrin. This is also released by the duodenal mucosa in response to distention or chemical stimuli of the same type as those that stimulate the stomach gastrin mechanism (Dragstedt, 1967; Guyton, 1981). Gastrin may be extracted from the duodenal mucosa. However, the stimuli responsible for this phase of gastric secretion are not completely known. It is possible that several other hormones released by the upper small intestinal mucosa, such as secretin or cholecystokinin, also play minor roles in causing gastric juice secretion under certain conditions.

Dragstedt (1967) commented, "Considering the meager amount of gastric stimulation resulting from the introduction of neutral food into the duodenum, together with the inhibitory effect of the introduction of acid into the dudodenum on gastric secretion, it becomes exceedingly doubtful that under normal conditions the passage of the partially digested chyme from the stomach into the intestine has any significant stimulating action on gastric secretion. It may well be that the intestinal phase of secretion represents an auxiliary mechanism which becomes operative only when there is an insufficient secretion of gastric juice in the stomach, and as a consequence the food which enters the duodenum is neutral or only slightly acid."

Inhibition of Gastric Secretion

Without mechanisms to limit gastric secretion, unchecked acid production could become intolerable. Several mechanisms inhibit gastric secretion:

VAGAL-ANTRAL PHASE INHIBITORS. After completion of a meal, absence of further intake of food deprives the vagi of continued stimuli so vagal activity and gastric secretion decrease. Also, antral distention, an important stimulus to gastrin release from the antrum, subsides with gastric emptying.

Another inhibition factor is that when the acidity of the antral contents increases to a pH of 2.0 the gastric mechanism for stimulating gastric secretion becomes totally blocked, regardless of the stimulus. It is thought that this effect "probably results from two different factors: First, greatly enhanced acidity depresses or blocks the extraction of gastrin itself from the antral mucosa. Second, the acid seems to extract an inhibitory hormone from the gastric mucosa or to cause an inhibitory reflex that inhibits gastric acid secretion" (Guyton, 1981). The existence of this inhibitory hormone remains unproved.

INTESTINAL PHASE INHIBITORS. Although chyme stimulates gastric secretion during the intestinal phase, paradoxically it often partially inhibits secretion during the gastric phase.

The presence of food in the small intestine initiates an *enterogastric reflex* transmitted through the myenteric plexus, the sympathetic nerves, and the vagus nerves that inhibits gastric secretion and motility. This reflex can be initiated by distention of the small bowel, the presence of acid in the upper intestine, the presence of protein breakdown products, or irritation of the mucosa.

The entrance of acid gastric chyme into the duodenum lowers duodenal pH. Acidification of the duodenum inhibits both gastric secretion and motility via neural and humoral pathways.

The presence of acid, fat, protein breakdown products, hyper- or hypo-osmotic fluids, or irritation in the small intestine causes release of several intestinal hormones. Two of these, which have been identified in pure form, are secretin and cholecystokinin, both important for control of pancreatic secretion; cholecystokinin is particularly important in promoting emptying of the gallbladder. In addition, both these hormones, under some conditions, can cause increased gastric secretion, though under usual conditions they have a moderate inhibitory effect on gastric secretion.

Ward and Bloom (1975) have presented evidence that gastric inhibition by intraduodenal acid more closely depends on a vagal reflex than on secretin release in human beings.

Alday and Goldsmith (1973) demonstrated, by experiments on dogs, that if the pH level of material within the small intestine remains within a neutral range of 6 to 7, no gastric secretory activity occurs. However, gastric activity is stimulated if the pH of material within the small intestine is outside this neutral range in either the acid or alkaline zone. The proximal portion of the upper part of the small intestine was found to be the most sensitive to pH variation. Performance of truncal vagotomy interrupted this intestinal-gastric relationship.

Dragstedt (1969), to whom all of us are deeply indebted for what is known about gastric secretion and the selection of appropriate operations on the stomach, has shown, by his own studies and collected reports of others correlated and arranged in temporal and logical sequence, that

". . . the passage of the acid gastric contents into the duodenum . . . inhibits . . . gastric secretion. This inhibition is mediated in part at least by hormones. Pancreatic secretin and cholecystokinin have both been found to cause inhibition of food-stimulated secretion. . . . Extirpation of the duodenum in whole or in part causes an increase in gastric secretion. Experimental operations such as the Exalto and Mann-Williamson procedures [Figs. 1–17, 1–18, and 1–19], which prevent the acid gastric content from entering the duodenum, cause an increase in gastric secretion through removal of the normal brake on gastric secretion exerted by the duodenum. The experimental ulcers produced by these operations are in part due to this hypersecretion. . . . Inadequacy of the duodenal brake on gastric secretion should be considered in relation to the cause of the hypersecretion of gastric juice in patients with ulcers. Clinical procedures such as gastroenterostomy with closure of the pylorus deviate the gastric acid from the duodenum and this is probably responsible for the disastrous results of this operation. The superiority of the Billroth I over the Bilroth II operation is probably chiefly due to better preservation of the duodenal inhibition of gastric secretion."

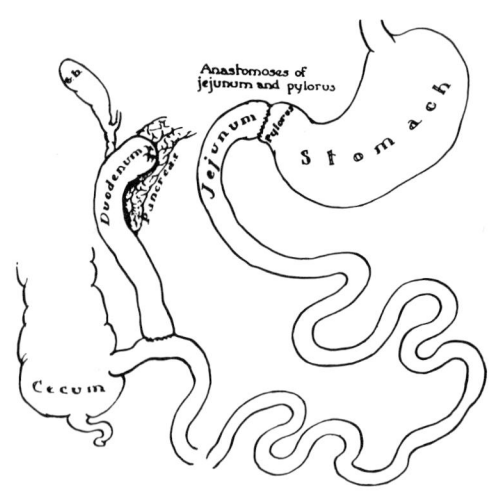

Figure 1–18. The Mann-Williamson procedure. Gastric acid is completely excluded from the duodenum. (From Dragstedt, cited in previous figure.)

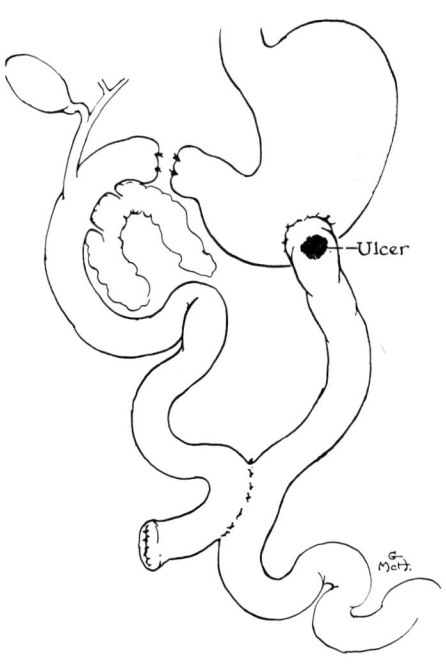

Figure 1–17. The Exalto procedure for the production of experimental peptic ulcers. Gastric acid is excluded from the duodenum except for a small amount which could regurgitate from the upper jejunum. (From Dragstedt, L. R.: Duodenal inhibition of gastric secretion. Am. J. Surg. 117:845, 1969.)

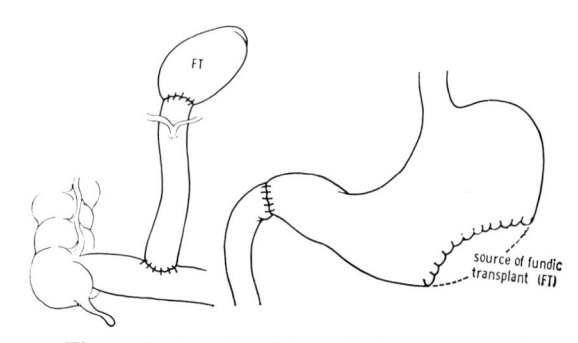

Figure 1–19. The Mann-Williamson procedure modified by the attachment of a fundic pouch to the excluded duodenum. The entrance of acid into the duodenum abolished the hypersecretion caused by the operation and delayed the appearance of the usual experimental ulcer. (From Dragstedt, cited in Figure 1–17.)

Summary of Gastric Secretory Response to Feeding

Menguy's (1976) clear and concise summary will be quoted. "The main factor responsible for stimulation of acid secretion incidental to a meal is direct vagal stimulation of the acid-secreting cells. In addition, vagal stimuli cause a prompt and abundant release of gastrin (evidenced by an increased serum gastrin level). This vagally induced release of gastrin by the antrum is further stimulated by food distending the antrum, by an alkaline antral pH, and by the action of specific secretagogues on the antral mucosa. Gastrin and cholinergic stimulation interact at the level of the acid-secreting cells and potentiate each other in the stimulation of acid secretion.

"Inhibition of gastric secretion is effected by a cut-off in vagal drive related to satiety. At the same time, gastrin release from the antrum diminishes as antral distention subsides and as secretagogues are evacuated into the proximal small intestine. An important factor in the cessation of gastrin release is the fall in antral pH. As gastric chyme enters the proximal small intestine, feedback inhibitory mechanisms of a neural and humoral nature, originating in the small intestine, are triggered."

Rivilis and associates (1974) have shown, by experiments on dogs, that an elemental diet markedly decreases the volume of gastric secretions and their acidity, which leads to a reduction of all the other alimentary exocrine secretions, especially pancreatic secretion. The volume ingested was not related to the gastric juice produced. Because of these widespread effects, an elemental diet can be valuable in a variety of surgical conditions while retaining an adequate nutritional capability.

Pharmacologic Stimulants of Gastric Secretion

Histamine and its analogues are the most commonly used stimulants of gastric secretion (see Gastric Analysis, p. 29). Large amounts of histamine are present in the mast cells of the gastric mucosa, along with serotonin. Histamine has been proposed as the final common mediator of gastric acid secretion (Blair, 1966). Recently Code (1977) analyzed what is known about this subject.

Pentagastrin, the synthetic analogue of gastrin, evokes a response similar to that of histamine and may be preferred, as described later in the section on the Kay augmented histamine test.

Insulin may be used as a stimulant, as described later in the section on the Hollander insulin gastric analysis.

Acetylcholine administered systemically evokes a gastric secretory response similar to that resulting from direct or indirect vagal stimulation of the stomach. When directly applied to the antral mucosa, acetylcholine produces a strong secretory response which is believed to be due to cholinergic stimulation of the release of gastrin. "As a general rule, it may be said that all synthetic cholinergic agents are capable of eliciting gastric acid secretion" (Menguy, 1976).

Intravenous injection of calcium stimulates gastric secretion in human beings, as was reported by Sereghy and Von Gyurkovich in 1927. Induction of hypercalcemia by administration of calcium is followed by an increase in volume, hydrogen ion concentration, and pepsin content of the gastric secretion. The stimulatory effect of intravenous calcium on gastric secretion is nearly abolished by atropine as well as by ganglionic blocking agents.

In normal subjects and in patients with duodenal ulcer, calcium is a relatively weak stimulant of acid secretion. Although basal secretion may increase during calcium infusion (Reeder, Becker, and Thompson, 1974) the response is only about one third of the maximal Histalog response (Barreros and Donaldson, 1966). In contrast to this is the marked response of acid secretion with calcium infusion in patients with Zollinger-Ellison syndrome. A response of 75 per cent or more of the maximal Histalog response has been reported (Passaro, 1970).

Gastrin seems to be an important mediator of calcium-induced gastric acid secretion though direct stimulation of the parietal cells also occurs (Christiansen, Rehfeld, and Stadil, 1975).

Normal subjects and patients with duodenal ulcer have moderate gastric response to calcium infusion; however, the gastrin response will rarely exceed 300 pg./ml. (Reeder, Becker, and Thompson, 1974). If the basal gastrin levels are already markedly elevated, smaller increases will occur (Trudeau and McGuigan, 1969).

Inhibitors of Gastric Secretion

ATROPINE. Atropine is the most potent available inhibitor of gastric secretion. It and its analogues are used widely in the treatment of patients with duodenal ulcer. Atropine acts on the direct cholinergic stimulation of the acid-secreting cells and on the cholinergic stimulation of the cells releasing gastrin. It has been shown experimentally that although atropine completely suppresses gastric acid secretion to both feeding and sham feeding, its blocking of vagally mediated gastrin release is less potent. However, even though small amounts of gastrin may be released, the parietal cell becomes less responsive to stimulation by gastrin during atropinization.

H-2 RECEPTOR ANTAGONISTS. Certain effects of histamine are blocked by conventional antihistaminic compounds such as atropine. These effects are mediated by the H-1 receptor. Recently another receptor of histamine has been described, the H-2 receptor. H-2 receptor antagonists that effectively inhibit gastric acid secretion have been developed. Metiamide and cimetidine are two such compounds. Agranulocytosis is a serious side effect of metiamide (Feldman and Isenberg, 1976) and is due to the thiourea part of this compound (Fleischer and Samloff, 1977). Cimetidine has a cyanoguanidino group in place of the thiourea group, and this has eliminated agranulocytosis. Cimetidine effectively reduces acid secretion, and the degree of inhibition is dose related (Henn and associates, 1975). Stimulated acid secretion can be reduced by 67 per cent after 300 mg. of cimetidine. Since serum gastrin levels are not affected by H-2 receptor antagonists, they probably act directly on the parietal cell.

Most of the short-term studies with cimetidine have demonstrated that it significantly decreases acid secretion in patients with duodenal ulcer disease and does not have any significant side effects. It has also been successfully used in patients with Zollinger-Ellison (Z-E) syndrome. Cimetidine (Tagamet) is now available for short term use in these two groups of patients. Whether cimetidine can be used as a definitive treatment for the Zollinger-Ellison syndrome has not been established. Tumor regression has been reported in patients with the Z-E syndrome following total gastrectomy (Friesen, 1967); however, it is not known whether this is attributable to the gastrectomy or is a part of the natural history of gastrinoma tumors. Until more information has accumulated from current controlled trials, total gastrectomy remains the treatment of choice for the Z-E syndrome. Cimetidine is recommended for short-term use, especially when severe electrolyte imbalance occurs because of large volumes of gastric secretion. It also may be indicated in highly selected patients in whom the risks of operation are prohibitive.

Wallace and colleagues (1977) reported having observed perforation of chronic peptic ulcers within two weeks after stopping a 6-week course of cimetidine in 3 patients, 2 with duodenal ulcers and 1 with prepyloric ulcer. Hence some would recommend a maintenance course of cimetidine — 400 mg. at night for up to 3 months following a 6-week course — to prevent both this complication and also recurrence of the peptic ulcers. The reports of "cimetidine rebound," however, have not been confirmed by others.

The use of cimetidine has been suggested for other conditions, especially in patients who have a damaged gastric mucosal barrier. The H-2 receptor antagonists may not only inhibit acid secretion but also preserve the integrity of the gastric mucosal barrier (Ivey, Baskin, and Jeffrey, 1975). Cimetidine may prove to be a very useful drug in the prevention and treatment of stress ulceration.

PROSTAGLANDIN ANALOGUES. Prostaglandins are long-chain cyclic fatty acids. Those of the E and A class inhibit gastric acid secretion; however, the naturally occurring ones are inactivated by gastric juice. This can be prevented by the synthesis of analogues in which the C-15 or C-16 positions are methylated (Konturek, 1976). These synthetic analogues can inhibit basal and stimulated gastric secretion by 80 per cent. The exact mechanism of inhibition is unknown; however, they probably act directly on the parietal cell and also on the gastrin cell. Unlike the H-2 receptor antagonists, prostaglandins also decrease gastrin release (Ippoliti, 1976). Diarrhea is a significant side effect, especially at higher doses. Other problems include the successful formulation of a stable compound and evaluation of toxic effects with chronic use.

At the present time, the prostaglandins are experimental drugs and are not available for general use.

MEASUREMENT OF GASTRIC ACIDITY

The assessment of gastric secretory function is often helpful in the clinical management of patients. The main points of information sought are "(1) whether or not the gastric mucosa is capable of secreting acid and/or pepsinogen; (2) if it is capable of secreting acid, what is the basal acid output (BAO), the peak acid output (PAO), or the maximum acid output (MAO) per specific unit of time, and what is the ratio of BAO to PAO or MAO; (3) what is the simplest and most accurate means of obtaining this information; and (4) what is its clinical significance" (Segal, 1969).

The simplest method of determining whether or not the gastric mucosa can secrete acid during a basal period or after stimulation with Histalog or histamine is by use of the azure A resin tubeless technique developed by Segal, Miller, and Plumb in 1955. The patient is fed an acidic ion exchange resin which has been combined with the base quinine or the basic blue dye azure A. At pH below 3.5, hydrogen ions displace the base from the resin and the free base is absorbed and excreted in the urine, where its presence (blue color) indicates acid in the stomach. "Judged by comparison with results of maximal histamine stimulation and sampling of gastric contents by intubation, the diagnosis of achlorhydria made by the tubeless method is incorrect in 4 of 10 instances. On the other hand, the tubeless test indicates secretion of acid by persons who are otherwise found to be achlorhydric in 2 of 100 cases. On account of its unreliability, the tubeless test is suitable only for mass screening, not for individual diagnosis" (Davenport, 1971). Its value, therefore, is doubtful.

If the initial tubeless gastric analysis denotes achlorhydria, the test can be repeated with Histalog as the gastric stimulant. If the result is unchanged, further investigation is necessary to establish that true achlorhydria is present. For this, the augmented histamine intubation method is the most reliable.

Tubeless gastric analysis is sometimes used by physicians as a qualitative screening test, but it is not reliable enough for quantitative measurement of gastric acid secretion.

Segal stated that "this test" is contraindicated in individuals with subtotal gastrectomy, gastroenterostomy or pyloroplasty, pyloric obstruction, severe malabsorption, liver or renal disease, or urinary obstruction. In the latter and in patients in whom the urine collection may be unreliable, measurement of the blood azure A level can be substituted for that of the urinary azure A determination.

Surgeons often want to know whether or not a patient is a "hypersecretor" before subjecting the person to a gastric operation; therefore they need to determine the concentration of hydrochloric acid in the gastric juice. This requires sampling of gastric contents by intubation.

The amount of acid secreted is estimated by titration with a standard base. A sample of gastric juice collected in a given interval may not contain all the acid secreted in the collection period, because acid may be lost by the flow of gastric contents through the pylorus, by back-diffusion of acid into the mucosa, and by neutralization by bicarbonate contained in nonacid secretions. Loss through the pylorus can be minimized by good collection technique or estimated by indicator dilution methods, but acid lost through back-diffusion or by bicarbonate neutralization can be estimated only by calculations that are of doubtful validity. Acid in gastric contents may also be buffered by proteins and by other buffers contained in nonacid secretions. This moiety of acid can be recovered if the titration with a standard base is carried to the correct endpoint, which in most instances is between the pH of plasma, 7.4, and about 8.3. Since the latter pH is the one attained in the routine titration of gastric contents with phenolphthalein as the indicator, the usual estimation of total acidity is reasonably accurate (Davenport, 1971).

The long-standing practice has been to titrate a sample of gastric contents with standard NaOH, first to an approximate pH of 3.5, judged by the color change of diaminobenzene (Topfer's reagent) used as an indicator. The quantity of acid thus determined is arbitrarily termed "free acid."

Then the titration is continued to pH 8, judged by the color change of phenolphthalein used as an indicator, and the difference between total and free acid is called "combined acid." The free and combined acids are often reported in terms of clinical units, which are the number of ml. of 0.1 N NaOH required to neutralize 100 ml. of gastric juice. By happenstance, clinical units of HCl are identical with "milliequivalents per liter." Davenport (1971) recommended that "the acid of gastric juice, determined by titration, should always be expressed in milliequivalents secreted in a given time or as milliequivalents per liter (mN) and the terms "clinical unit" or its alternative "milligrams of HCl" should be avoided. This is generally agreed. Menguy (1976) also commented that "both the meaningless concept of 'free acid' and the use of 'Topfer's reagent' should be discarded. Most workers in the field, as well as most modern clinical laboratories, measure H^+ in the gastric juice by titration to pH 7.4 (using phenol red as an indicator). The amount of HCl in a sample of gastric juice is calculated by multiplying the volume (liters) by the HCl concentration (mEq./L)."

Gastric Analysis

After determining that the stomach can secrete HCl, a more detailed intubation gastric analysis "can provide additional useful information and should be performed (1) when the Zollinger-Ellison syndrome is clinically suspected; (2) in patients with peptic ulcer disease that has been difficult to control medically and who are being considered for operation; (3) in patients who have persistent symptoms after operation for peptic ulcer; and (4) in all patients with gastric ulcer" (Dunphy, Way, and associates, 1973).

Several methods of gastric analysis are available.

The simplest way to determine the basal acid output is to measure the acid output of the secretion obtained by tube aspiration during a 45- to 60-minute morning fasting period.

However, this and additional information can be obtained by a standard gastric analysis. This consists of (1) Measurement of acid production by the unstimulated stomach under basal fasting conditions. The result is expressed as H^+ secretion in mEq./hr. and is termed the basal acid output (BOA). (2) Measurement of acid production during stimulation by histamine, betazole (Histalog), or pentagastrin giving in a maximally stimulating dose. The result is expressed as H^+ secretion in mEq./hr. and is termed the maximal acid output (MAO).

Standard gastric analysis is performed as follows: for 12 hours before the test the patient fasts, except for intake of water. Antacids, anticholinergic drugs, or other agents known to affect gastric secretion, such as some tranquilizers like Valium, must be withheld.

A nasogastric sump tube is passed into the stomach and preferably placed halfway down the greater curvature under fluoroscopic verification, though this precise placement is optional (Hall and Hodges, 1976). The stomach is emptied of its contents, which are discarded; subsequent secretions are to be preserved.

With the patient kept in the left oblique reclining position, the gastric juice is aspirated continuously by hand suction with a syringe or by using a low-power suction pump. Frequently a small amount of air is injected through the tube to ensure its continued patency. Thus the basal acid secretion is continuously collected for 60 minutes in divided 15-minute aliquots. The total volume collected during this hour may be measured for "free" and "total" hydrochloric acid outputs in milliequivalents or, preferably, only for gastric acid output (pH of 7.0 to 7.4).

Most surgeons prefer to measure only for gastric acid output and have discontinued use of the terms "free" acid, "combined" acid, and "degrees" of acidity, as just discussed, because they were confusing and without pathophysiologic significance.

At the end of the basal hour collection, the gastric stimulant is given by hypodermic injection. If histamine is used for the stimulant, histamine acid phosphate (0.04 mg. per kg. of body weight) is injected subcutaneously, but more recently the analogue betazole hydrochloride (Histalog) has largely replaced histamine because its side effects are much fewer. When this is done Histalog (1.7 mg. per kg. of body weight) is injected intramuscularly.

Regardless of which stimulant is used, gastric juice is collected for 1.5 hours, again in 15-minute aliquots, after its administration. Acid concentration in each 15-minute specimen is then titrated to pH 7.0 (endpoint determined with either a pH meter or phenol red indicator). The output (in mEq.) is obtained as the product of concentration and volume of the specimen. BAO is determined as the sum of the four 15-minute periods before the stimulant was injected. The generally accepted upper limit of normal basal acid secretion is 5 mEq./hr.

MAO is calculated by adding the four highest consecutive periods after stimulation. Its accepted upper limit of normal is 30 mEq./hr.

The term achlorhydria denotes no acid (pH>6.0) after maximal stimulation.

Although still used, the formerly favored method of collecting gastric secretions during a 12-hour fasting overnight period for clinical analysis is now considered to be no more accurate than the basal one-hour collection, so it has lost favor.

"The *Kay augmented histamine test* provides the best means of measuring either the peak acid output (PAO) during two successive 15-minute periods or the MAO during the 0 to 60 minutes after the subcutaneous injection of the augmented dose of histamine diphosphate" (Segal, 1969). The performance of this test is identical to that of the standard gastric analysis just described through the measurement of BAO. It differs in the method of measuring MAO.

In the augmented histamine test, at the end of the basal hour collection:

1. A dose of 100 mg. of mepyramine hydrogen maleate (Neo-antergan), or a comparable antihistamine, is injected intramuscularly.

2. The gastric juice is now aspirated for the next 30 minutes and discarded.

3. Histamine acid phosphate (0.04 mg. per kg. of body weight) is injected subcutaneously, following which the gastric secretion is continuously collected for 60 minutes in divided 15-minute periods.

4. The 60-minute volume is measured for milliequivalents of acid output as described for BAO. This is the MAO. "Peak (PAO) and maximal (MAO) outputs of acid are the same" (Davenport, 1971).

Pentagastrin, the analogue of gastrin, in a dose of 6 μg. per kg. of body weight, evokes a response similar to that with 0.04 mg. of histamine acid phosphate per kg. and does not require medication to cover side effects, so, when available, it may be preferred as the stimulant.

"The augmented histamine test is now used in many hospitals and the results obtained in normal subjects are remarkably uniform. The response to the augmented histamine test is reduced to about half the normal value in superficial gastritis and almost to zero in gastric atrophy. On the other hand, it is raised in patients with duodenal ulcer, and one such unfortunate person holds the world's record for secreting 91.7 mEq. of acid in 60 minutes" (Davenport, 1971).

The *Hollander insulin gastric analysis* is a method of measuring gastric acid secretion to determine the status of the vagal innervation of the stomach. It is used principally in postvagotomy patients to evaluate the completeness of the vagotomy and is particularly helpful in patients who have recurrent ulcer after a previous operation.

The test is performed as follows: first the BAO is measured for 1 hour as described above for a standard gastric analysis. Then regular insulin, 0.2 units per kg. of body weight, is rapidly injected intravenously. A blood sample is taken just before the insulin is given and again 30 and 60 minutes afterward. Gastric juice is aspirated continuously for 2 hours after the insulin is given, and each 15-minute aliquot is titrated to pH 7.0. This dose of insulin should lower blood glucose below 50 mg./dl. The hypoglycemia activates cortical centers, thus increasing vagal activity and stimulating gastric secretion if gastric innervation has not been interrupted.

The concentration of acid in the gastric juice rather than the quantity in milliequivalents is used to interpret the Hollander test. The criterion for a positive test indicating persisting significant vagal innervation is: If the basal secretion contained no acid, a level of 10 mEq./L. after insulin is positive; if the basal secretion contained acid, an elevation of its concentration by 20 mEq./L. over basal, after insulin injection, is positive.

The Hollander test carries the potential danger of rapidly producing extreme hypoglycemia (less than 15 mg./dl.) with its associated unpleasant symptoms. To produce hypoglycemia more gradually and to a lesser degree, Carter, Dozois and Kirkpatrick

(1973) introduced the *insulin infusion test* for determining the gastric secretory response in vagotomized patients. This test is performed as follows: After a 12-hour overnight fast, a nasogastric tube is passed and positioned in the stomach. Basal gastric secretions are collected for 30 minutes before commencing insulin infusion (0.04 U/kg./hr.). Gastric juice is then collected at 15-minute intervals during the 3-hour infusion.

The investigators performed the insulin infusion test in 50 patients 2 months or more after vagotomy and a drainage procedure. Twenty-five of these 50 patients were also subjected to the conventional Hollander test at least 2 months after vagotomy and within 2 months of the insulin infusion test. The results were compared in the 25 patients subjected to the two tests.

The magnitude of acid response to both tests was almost identical in individual subjects, despite the fact that less profound hypoglycemia followed insulin infusion. Carter and associates concluded that "with the present criteria for interpretation the insulin infusion test may be no better than the Hollander test for defining patients at risk of recurrent dyspepsia. However, the small amounts of insulin used, the gradual lowering of blood glucose, and the reduced incidence of profound hypoglycemia which attend the insulin infusion test suggest that this technique should be adopted for the assessment of vagotomy in preference to the potentially dangerous Hollander test."

CLINICAL SIGNIFICANCE OF GASTRIC ANALYSIS. It may be advisable for each laboratory to establish its normal ranges (by age and sex) for basal and maximal acid outputs in order to provide a basis for the diagnosis of the causes of various gastric secretory disorders.

Although of limited value, gastric analysis can provide information valuable not only for the diagnosis of certain disorders but also for selecting the type and magnitude of the operation when surgery is indicated.

Some generalized diagnostic interpretations: The finding of hypochlorhydria during the interdigestive phase or after maximal stimulation has no significance in the diagnosis of cancer or in distinguishing between a benign gastric ulcer and cancer (Davenport, 1971).

The acid secretion tends to fall with progression from superficial to atrophic gastritis.

True achlorhydria after maximum stimulation is incompatible with the diagnosis of peptic ulcer and can be valuable for ruling out the diagnosis of duodenal ulcer in a patient with suggestive ulcer symptoms and equivocal radiologic findings. The finding of achlorhydria suggests further investigation for the early detection of gastric carcinoma and, when present in a patient whose x-ray studies have demonstrated gastric ulcer, this finding would indicate the presence of an underlying gastric cancer and the advisability of a surgical operation. The finding of hyperchlorhydria does not rule out a gastric malignant lesion.

Gilbertson and Knatterud (1967) reported that the use of gastric analysis as the sole screening measure for the early detection of gastric cancer is impractical because it may result in overlooking most of the younger, potentially curable patients. However, the results of gastric analyses did appear to have substantial prognostic value, as patients who have cancer of the stomach with demonstrable free acid show a significantly better rate of survival than those found to be achlorhydric.

The finding of achlorhydria is also helpful in diagnosing gastritis, pernicious anemia, and pellagra. It is commonly present following a high gastrectomy or a thorough vagotomy. With rare exceptions, the diagnosis of pernicious anemia in an adult can be discounted as the cause of anemia if free hydrochloric acid is detected (Segal, 1969).

When the basal secretion is 5 mEq./hr. or more, or maximally stimulated gastric output is higher than normal, the patient has hyperchlorhydria which is commonly associated with a duodenal ulcer.

The constancy of this association is debatable. Some free acid is present in the basal secretion of every patient with duodenal ulcer, and absence of basal acid secretion indicates that the patient has no duodenal ulcer. In one series, 21 per cent of 238 patients with duodenal ulcer and 7 per cent of 137 patients without duodenal ulcer had hyperchlorhydria (Segal, 1969). Bockus (1974) measured the basal acid output in 194 cases of duodenal ulcer and found that 57.5 per cent had definite hyperchlorhydria. The average BAO for this group was almost twice that of the BAO in a large series of normal persons. Some patients with normal acid secretory values may have active duodenal ulcer and vice versa.

In patients with gastric ulcers, hyperchlorhydria is not as common. In many of these patients the BAO is normal or hypochlorhydric. Indeed hyperchlorhydria in the presence of a demonstrable gastric ulcer raises the suspicion of an associated duodenal ulcer. Achlorhydria after stimulation with histamine strongly suggests that the gastric ulcer is malignant, but hyperchlorhydria does not rule out malignancy. Bernardo, Soderberg, and Migliaccio (1958) studied 519 cases of gastric ulcer; 90 per cent were benign. Fourteen per cent of the patients with benign ulcers had achlorhydria and 24 per cent of those with malignant ulcers had hyperchlorhydria. A gastric analysis is not reliable in differentiating between benign and malignant gastric lesions.

Patients with Zollinger-Ellison syndrome have elevated levels of gastrin (a powerful stimulant of gastric acid secretion) in their serum. As a result, their parietal cells are subject to maximal or near maximal stimulation even under the basal conditions of gastric analysis. Basal acid secretion is often greater than 15 mEq./hr. Although there may be overlapping of the BAO or MAO between patients with uncomplicated duodenal ulcer and those with Z-E syndrome, the measurement of BAO and MAO and their ratio will usually differentiate between these conditions. The basal output of more than 200 ml. of gastric secretion or 20 mEq. of acid per hour usually occurs only in the Z-E syndrome. Furthermore, in a hydrated patient, a ratio of BAO to MAO of 43 to 60 per cent is suggestive, and of more than 60 per cent is said to be pathognomonic, of the Z-E syndrome. It is advisable to confirm the diagnosis by measurement of the serum gastrin level, which is elevated in the Z-E syndrome.

It should be remembered that in a patient whose gastric antrum has been retained and excluded from acid secretions, the gastric analysis can simulate that obtained in patients with Z-E syndrome. Van Heerden, Bernatz, and Rovelstad (1971) reported 17 cases wherein portions of gastric antra excluded from gastric secretions were retained inadvertently after Polya gastrectomy with gastrojejunostomy. It is well known that the gastric antrum releases the hormone gastrin (a parietal cell stimulant) in response to both local and vagal stimuli, but the release can be inhibited by mucosal acidification. In the excluded gastric antrum, where the acid inhibition mechanism cannot operate, gastrin is released continuously. Hence gastric analyses in these 17 patients closely resembled those considered characteristic for Z-E syndrome. Gastrojejunal ulceration occurred in all these cases. In 11 of the 17 patients, adequate gastric analyses were done, and in 6 of the 11 at least one of the criteria proposed for the diagnosis of Z-E syndrome was met. The proposed criteria are an hourly BAO greater than 15 mEq. in the intact stomach or greater than 5 mEq. after partial gastrectomy; BAO more than 60 per cent of MAO; 12-hour nocturnal secretion in excess of 1000 ml. or 100 mEq.; and a ratio of basal acid concentration to maximal acid concentration (BAC/MAC) greater than 0.6, or 60 per cent.

In 6 of the 11 adequate gastric analyses, at least one of the criteria proposed for the diagnosis of the Z-E syndrome was met in patients with postoperative retention of the antrum. In 5 of the 6 patients, it was the BAC/MAC criterion; in only one case were both the BAO/MAO and BAO criteria satisfied, but in that case the BAC/MAC standard was not met. BAO criteria were satisfied in three cases. If either the BAO/MAO or BAO criterion had been required, only 3 of the 6 cases would have been recognized. Equally noteworthy is the finding that among the 11 patients with satisfactory gastric analyses, in 5 the data did not have the Z-E pattern permitting recognition of the antral retention.

Kajiwara, Tamura, and Suzuki (1977) pointed out that "hypersecretion of gastric acid after massive intestinal resection has been widely documented in both clinical and experimental studies but its mechanism is still a matter of speculation."

Gastric analysis is of predictive value in patients with upper gastrointestinal symptoms in whom normal findings are seen on roentgenograms. Harrison, Wechsler, and Elliott (1972) reported a retrospective evaluation of 80 patients with upper gastrointestinal complaints who had negative findings on x-ray evaluation. All these patients had gastric analysis, and 59 had hyperacidity by the investigators' criteria. After a mean follow-up period of only 55 months, the data indicated that (1) eventual morbidity due to peptic ulcer disease increases as maximal free acid concentration increases. (2) Eventual significant morbidity can be expected in 61 per cent, major morbidity can be expected in 20 per cent, and surgical intervention will be required in 17 per cent of the patients with hyperacidity.

Furthermore, these workers pointed out the value of gastric analysis in selecting the appropriate operation for those hypersecreting patients requiring elective surgery for peptic ulcer disease. They arbitrarily chose an output of 25 mEq./hr. in response to maximal histamine stimulation as a cut-off point. Any patient with a higher rate of secretion was treated with vagotomy and hemigastrectomy. Those with a lower rate of secretion were treated with vagotomy and pyloroplasty.

This policy was used in the elective surgical treatment of 153 patients with peptic ulcer during a 7-year period. A 100 per cent follow-up of these patients revealed that only 3 of the 153 patients had recurrence of their ulcer, in contrast to a 25 per cent recurrence rate in their patients treated with routine vagotomy and pyloroplasty. All the operations were elective procedures.

The authors concluded that a patient with a high secretory level probably should undergo a more extensive operation than vagotomy and pyloroplasty in order to remove the major stimulatory mechanisms.

Kothe and associates (1971) emphasized the importance of a carefully performed and interpreted gastric analysis in preoperative and postoperative evaluation of ulcer patients, and the necessity of tests of stimulated secretion in addition to the standard overnight and base line values. For this they administer both the submaximal histamine and the insulin tests and use the difference between the base line and the stimulated values for the same period of time as the value for stimulated acid. They consider a positive insulin test to be evidence of increased vagal activity and an indication for vagotomy. A positive histamine test implies an increased antral phase, which they consider an indication for resection. These guidelines are altered by such factors as age and general condition of the patient and findings at operation. The investigators feel that this approach affords a better rationale for operations than does location of the ulcer alone.

We agree that preoperative gastric analysis may be an important guideline in selecting an appropriate operation for patients who require elective surgery for peptic ulcer disease, provided the factors of patient age, history of previous gastrointestinal bleeding, degree of operative risk of the patient, location of the ulcer, and ease of dissection found at operation are also considered in the choice.

DIGESTIVE FUNCTION OF THE STOMACH

Although important, the digestive role of the stomach is not essential.

Ingested food is mixed with salivary amylase before it reaches the stomach. When well chewed, carbohydrates exposed to the salivary amylase are hydrolyzed as long as the gastric pH remains elevated; as gastric pH falls, amylase is inactivated. Less than 40 per cent of the ingested carbohydrates are digested in the stomach.

Gastric juice contains a lipolytic enzyme, but gastric lipolysis is negligible.

Only 10 to 15 per cent of dietary protein is reduced to peptones in the stomach. Although gastric pepsin is a powerful proteolytic enzyme, it can initiate only the hydrolysis of ingested protein. Pepsin also disperses intracellular contents by digesting cell walls. The acidity of gastric chyme plays an important role by denaturing protein. This facilitates the action of other proteolytic enzymes of pancreatic and intestinal origin.

In summary: "The stomach decreases the particulate size of ingested foods, denatures alimentary protein by acidification, and brings ingested materials to levels of temperature and osmolarity which will be tolerated by the mucosa of the proximal small intestine" (Menguy, 1976).

"The gastric contents are delivered to the duodenum at a rate that is determined by the texture of the meal, its osmolarity and acidity, and its contents of fat. A meal of lean meat, potatoes, and vegetables leaves the stomach within 3 hours. A meal with very high fat content may remain in the stomach for 6 to 12 hours" (Way and Richards in Dunphy and Way, 1973).

Gastric Motility

The muscular coat of the stomach differs from that of the remainder of gut by having three layers instead of two. It has an outer layer of longitudinal muscle fibers which is continuous with the longitudinal muscle layer of the esophagus and is thickest along the two curvatures; a middle circular layer which is continuous with the circular muscle layer of the esophagus and is thickest in the antrum; and a deep layer of oblique muscle fibers which originates from the left side of the cardia and fans out toward the greater curvature. "A particularly important feature of the muscular coat of the stomach is *its greater thickness in the prepyloric antrum*" (Menguy, 1976). "There is no functional division between antrum and pylorus as the pylorus is simply the terminal part of the antral muscle" (Davenport, 1971).

The stomach musculature acts as a unit. The myenteric and submucous plexuses are continuous throughout the stomach. The extrinsic innervation — sympathetic via the celiac plexus, and parasympathetic via the vagus nerves — is distributed to the whole of the human stomach. Sympathetic stimulation depresses all movement of the stomach and vagal stimulation enhances it. Both act through the intrinsic plexuses to reduce or enhance contraction of gastric muscle. Nervous influences, mediated through either branch of the autonomic nervous system, have the same effects on the pylorus as on the rest of the stomach muscle (Davenport, 1971).

The motor functions of the stomach include (1) storage of large quantities of food until it can be accommodated in the intestines; (2) mixing this food with gastric secretions until it forms chyme, and (3) slow emptying of the food from the stomach into the small intestine at a rate suitable for optimal digestion and absorption by the small intestine.

A cyclic change in electrical potential, the pacesetter potential (slow wave or control potential), is present in the wall of the human stomach. The cycles, which are omnipresent, have a regular rhythm and a frequency of about 3 per minute. They were thought to arise from a pacemaker located somewhere in the proximal stomach and to spread aborally from the pacemaker through the distal stomach to the pylorus, phasing the onset of action potentials and peristaltic contractions as they go. The exact location of the gastric pacemaker and the pattern of spread of the pacesetter potentials were unknown until recently.

In 1977, Hinder and Kelly of the Mayo Clinic reported their studies of the human pacesetter potential: its site of origin, spread, and response to gastric transection and proximal gastric vagotomy.

Gastric electrical activity was recorded from 26 patients at celiotomy. The human gastric pacemaker was localized to an area in the midcorpus along the greater curve. Pacesetter potentials were generated regularly by the pacemaker at a mean frequency of 3.2 cycles/min. and were propagated circumferentially and aborally from the pacemaker, increasing in amplitude and velocity as they approached the pylorus. The pattern of pacesetter potentials in patients with gastric ulcer, gastric cancer, and duodenal ulcer was similar to that of patients without such diseases. Complete transection of the gastric corpus isolated the distal stomach from the natural pacemaker and resulted in the appearance of a new pacemaker in the distal stomach with a slower frequency. The fact that proximal gastric vagotomy did not greatly alter the frequency of generation or the pattern of propagation of the pacesetter potential provided further evidence that both are myogenic phenomena.

Storage Function of the Stomach

The empty stomach is small and relaxed. Its motor activity comprises transient 5–10-minute phases of nonpropulsive motor activity separated by 15–20-minute periods of quiescence. These feeble contractions have negligible effects on intragastric pressure. "When a man is hungry, vigorous contractions may occur at a frequency of 3 per minute and occasionally pressure in the empty stomach rises briefly" (Davenport, 1971).

When food enters the stomach, motor

activity gradually increases. The characteristic manifestation of gastric motor activity is a *peristaltic wave* originating near the cardia and moving toward the pylorus.

As food enters the stomach, it resides in layers, determined by the sequence of arrival but with fat floating to the top, in the body of the stomach. Gastric contents are well mixed with gastric secretions only in the antrum.

As the stomach fills, its wall relaxes, allowing its volume to increase without significant increase in intragastric pressure, despite marked distention, until volume greater than 1500 ml. is reached. Stretch of the stomach causes a vagal reflex that inhibits muscle activity in the body of the stomach. After the stomach is filled, its peristaltic waves diminish in force.

Mixing in the Stomach

After the ingested food is layered in the stomach, the portion lying against the mucosal surface of the stomach is in immediate contact with the gastric digestive juices, but the deeper layers are not.

When the stomach is filled, weak *constrictor waves*, also called *mixing waves*, move along the stomach wall about once every 20 seconds. These waves begin most often near the midpoint of the stomach, but originate farther back up the stomach wall as the stomach empties. Generally, they become more intense as they approach the antral portion of the stomach.

The mixing waves tend to move the gastric secretions and the outermost layer of food gradually toward the antrum where gastric digestion occurs. On entering the antrum the waves become stronger, and the food and gastric secretions become progressively mixed to greater degrees of fluidity.

In addition to the mixing caused by the waves in the body of the stomach, mixing is also caused by intense peristaltic movements in the antral portion of the stomach.

The resulting mixture of food and gastric secretions is called chyme and is passed on down the gut. The degree of fluidity of chyme depends on the relative amounts of food and gastric secretions and on the degree of digestion that has occurred. Chyme has the appearance of a murky, milky semifluid or paste.

Propulsion of Food Through the Stomach

During the height of digestion, strong peristaltic waves occurring at a rhythmic rate of about 4 per minute push stored food down to add it to the chyme in the antrum. "The peristaltic waves often exert as much as 50 to 70 cm. of water pressure which is about six times as powerful as the usual mixing waves (Guyton, 1981).

Hunger contractions are a third type of intense contractions which often occur when the stomach has been empty for a long time. These are usually rhythmic peristaltic contractions in the body of the stomach. However, when they become extremely strong, they often coalesce to cause a continuing tetanic contraction lasting for as long as two to three minutes. They are greatly increased by hypoglycemia. Gastric hunger contractions sometimes cause pain in the pit of the stomach, termed *hunger pangs*, and are often associated with a feeling of hunger. Hunger pangs usually do not begin until 12 to 24 hours after the last ingestion of food; in starvation they reach their greatest intensity in three to four days, and then gradually weaken in succeeding days.

Distention of the stomach by food initiates vagal afferent signals that pass to the medulla oblongata and reflexly inhibit the tone in the storage area of the stomach and simultaneously increase the rate of gastric secretions and the intensity of both the mixing and peristaltic waves. Thus the rate of digestion and removal of the stored food are accelerated.

Emptying of the Stomach

Stomach emptying is promoted by peristaltic waves in the gastric antrum and is opposed by resistance of the pylorus to the passage of food.

At rest, the pylorus normally remains almost, but not completely, closed by mild tonic contraction. Normally the pressure exerted by the pyloric sphincter on the lumen of the pylorus is about 5 cm. of water (Guyton, 1981). Since at rest there is no pressure gradient between the stomach and the duodenum, this very weak closing force is usually sufficient to prevent flow of chyme into the duodenum except when a peristaltic wave in the antrum forces it through.

DIGESTIVE FUNCTION OF THE STOMACH

Hence the rate of emptying of the stomach is determined principally by the degree of activity of the antral peristaltic waves.

When active, the antral peristaltic waves characteristically occur at a rhythmic rate of about three times a minute. The waves become very strong near the incisura angularis. As the wave approaches the pylorus its strength and speed increases so that the antrum contracts almost as a unit (antral systole) and, simultaneously, the pyloric sphincter and proximal portion of the duodenum receptively relax. In addition, the gastric peristaltic wave creates a positive pressure gradient from the stomach to the duodenum. With each peristaltic wave, several (2 to 6) ml. of chyme are forced into the duodenum.

This pumping action of the antral part of the stomach is sometimes called the "pyloric pump."

"At the end of the cycle the peristaltic wave passes over the pylorus, closing it, and gastric emptying ends for that cycle. The chyme evacuated into the duodenum is propelled distally by contraction of the duodenum and is prevented from refluxing into the stomach by closure of the pylorus" (Menguy, 1976) (Fig. 1–20).

The *rate* of emptying of the stomach is controlled by a number of factors.

The degree of activity of the pyloric pump is regulated by signals from both the stomach and the duodenum. Those from the stomach are (1) the degree of distention of the stomach by food, and (2) the presence of gastrin released from the antrum in response to stretch and to the presence of certain types of food in the stomach, particularly meat. Gastrin is a potent stimulant of gastric motility, especially of the activity of the pyloric pump, while at the same time relaxing the pylorus itself. Thus, gastrin strongly promotes gastric emptying. It also has a constrictor effect on the gastroesophageal sphincter in preventing reflux of gastric contents into the esophagus during the enhanced gastric secretory and motility activity.

Both these signals from the stomach increase the pyloric pump force and therefore promote gastric emptying.

A greatly increased volume of food in the stomach does not promote increased gastric emptying by increased intragastric pressure because in the usual normal range of volume, the increase in volume does not increase the pressure significantly, as noted earlier. Instead, the increased gastric emptying is because the stretch of the gastric wall elicits vagal and local myenteric reflexes in the wall of the stomach that in-

Figure 1–20. Schematic illustration of gastric propulsive motor activity. *A*, A shallow wave originates in the proximal corpus. *B*, The wave becomes stronger and deeper as it sweeps toward the antrum. *C*, The wave sweeps over the antrum. *D*, As the wave approaches the pylorus, the sphincter relaxes. *E*, The wave passes down to the duodenum; the pylorus is now closed, preventing gastric reflux of the bolus. *F*, Another wave begins. (From Menguy, R.: Surgery of Peptic Ulcer. Philadelphia, W. B. Saunders Company, 1976.)

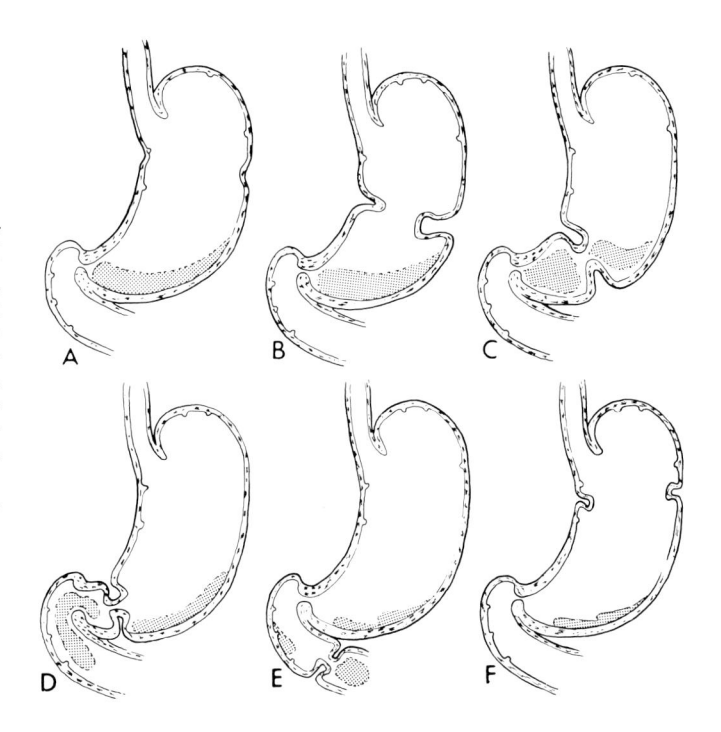

crease the activity of the pyloric pump. "In general, the rate of gastric emptying is approximately proportional to the square root of the volume of food remaining in the stomach at any given time" (Guyton, 1981).

The more liquid the stomach chyme, the greater the ease of emptying. Therefore, pure fluids ingested into the stomach pass rapidly into the duodenum, while more solid foods must await mixing with the gastric secretions and beginning fluidization of the solids by gastric digestion.

Signals from the duodenum depress pyloric pump activity. Normally, when excesses of volume or of certain types of chyme have entered the duodenum, strong feedback signals, both nervous and hormonal, are transmitted to the stomach to depress the pyloric pump. Thus chyme is allowed to enter the duodenum only as rapidly as it can be processed by the small intestine.

The mechanism of this inhibitory effect from the duodenum on pyloric activity is termed the *enterogastric reflex*. It acts as follows: Strong nervous signals are transmitted from the duodenum back to the stomach most of the time, especially when the stomach is emptying food into the duodenum. These signals probably play the most important role of all in determining the activity of the pyloric pump and, thereby, also the rate of gastric emptying. The nervous reflexes are mediated mainly via vagal afferents to the brain stem and thence by vagal efferents back to the stomach. Some of these signals are probably transmitted directly by the myenteric plexus as well.

The types of factors that are continually monitored in the duodenum and that can activate the enterogastric reflex include:

1. The degree of distention of the duodenum.
2. Any degree of irritation of the duodenal mucosa.
3. The degree of acidity of the duodenal chyme. The enterogastric reflex is especially sensitive to the presence of irritants and acids in the duodenal chyme. Whenever the pH of the chyme in the duodenum falls below about 3.5 to 4, the enterogastric reflex is activated. It inhibits the pyloric pump and reduces, or even blocks, further release of acidic gastric contents into the duodenum until the duodenal chyme can be neutralized by pancreatic and other secretions.
4. The degree of osmolality of the chyme.
5. The presence in the chyme of breakdown products of protein digestion. Thus, by slowing the rate of gastric emptying, sufficient time is gained for adequate protein digestion in the upper portion of the small intestine.
6. The presence of either hypo- or hypertonic (especially the latter) fluids in the stomach. This prevents too rapid flow of nonisotonic fluids into the small intestine, thereby avoiding rapid changes in electrolyte balance during absorption of the intestinal contents.
7. The presence of fatty foods, especially fatty acids, in the chyme that enters the duodenum. This depresses the activity of the pyloric pump, and gastric emptying is correspondingly slowed. This is important because it allows slow digestion of the fats before they proceed farther down the small intestine. The precise mechanism by which fats cause this effect of slowing gastric emptying is not known. A hormone called enterogastrone has been suggested as the specific cause but has never been identified as such. Another hormone, secretin, has also been suggested, but not proven, to be a cause.
8. Contraction of the pyloric sphincter has a role in regulating gastric emptying. Ordinarily the degree of pyloric sphincter contraction is weak, and the contraction that does occur is usually blocked as the pyloric pump peristaltic wave approaches the pylorus. However, many of the same duodenal factors that inhibit gastric contraction can simultaneously increase the degree of contraction of the pyloric sphincter. This factor, added to the diminished gastric contractions, therefore enhances control over the emptying process. For example, the presence of excess acid or excess irritation in the duodenal bulb promotes a moderate degree of pyloric contraction.

In summary, gastric emptying is controlled to a moderate degree by stomach factors, such as the degree of gastric filling and of gastric paristaltic activity. However, probably the more important control of gastric emptying is by feedback signals from the duodenum, including especially the enterogastric reflex and, to a lesser extent, hormonal feedback. These two feedback signals work together to slow the rate of emptying when too much fluid is already in the small intestine, or the chyme is excessively acid, contains too much protein or fat, is hypotonic or hypertonic, or is irritating. Thus the rate of gastric emptying is limited to the amount of chyme that the small intestine can process.

Hancock and associates (1974) studied the effect of posture on gastric emptying of solid meals in 10 healthy volunteers, 5 patients within 3 months of truncal vagotomy and pyloroplasty, and 5 patients within 3 months of highly selective vagotomy. In each subject the rate of gastric emptying was studied on two occasions, once while lying down and once while standing. The stomach of normal subjects emptied at the same rate whether they were standing up or lying down. Patients tested less than 3 months after truncal vagotomy and pyloroplasty and also after highly selective vagotomy had significantly faster gastric emptying when standing than when lying down. After truncal vagotomy and pyloroplasty, emptying was significantly slower than normal when patients were lying down but normal when they were standing. After highly selective vagotomy, emptying was normal when patients were lying down but significantly faster than normal when they were standing up.

Disruption of the pylorus by pyloroplasty, by bypass with gastroenterostomy, or by distal gastrectomy is associated with rapid gastric emptying. In distal gastrectomy, the antrum is gone so that gastric emptying is largely by gravity.

Vagotomy without a drainage procedure has been associated with delayed gastric emptying.

Chapter 2

ANATOMY AND PHYSIOLOGY OF THE DUODENUM

SURGICAL ANATOMY OF THE DUODENUM

The duodenum is the first portion of the small intestine and may be defined as the tubular musculocutaneous continuation of the alimentary canal which begins at the pyloric end of the stomach and forms a C-shaped bend (Fig. 2–1) as it curves around the head of the pancreas in its descent to connect with the jejunum at the duodenojejunal flexure. In its course it receives the external secretions from the bile and pancreatic ducts which enter its descending portion (Fig. 2–2).

The anterior wall of the duodenum is made up of four coats: an outer *peritoneal* or *serous* coat; a muscular coat made up of longitudinal and circular fibers, the *muscularis*; a submucous coat, the *submucosa*; and the *mucous coat* which forms its inner lining. Portions of the posterior and lateral walls of the duodenum are retroperitoneal and therefore lack a peritoneal or serosal coat.

The histology of the superficial duodenal mucosa resembles that of the remainder of the small intestine. The characteristic histologic feature of the mammalian duodenum is the presence in its proximal portion of the *glands of Brunner* which are situated in the submucosa and empty into the crypts of Lieberkühn via small secretory ducts. Their viscous, mucoid, alkaline secretion probably contributes to protection of the duodenal mucosa against corrosive action of gastric juice.

The duodenum was so named because it is about 12 fingerbreadths in length. That portion which is proximal to the ampulla of Vater is called the protoduodenum or super- or preampullary portion, while that which is distal to the ampulla is called the metaduodenum or sub- or postampullary portion.

The duodenum begins just to the right of the spine at the level of the first lumbar vertebra and extends from the pyloric ring 25 to 30 cm. to the duodenojejunal flexure. Its lumen is larger than that of the jejunum.

DIVISIONS

For convenience of description the duodenum is divided arbitrarily into four divisions, differentiated by the alteration in direction that the duodenum takes (Fig. 2–2).

The *superior* or *first portion* of the duodenum (duodenal cap) passes backward and upward toward the neck of the gallbladder and is about 5 cm. in length. Its proximal half is freely movable and surrounded by peritoneum. Its intimate relations with the gallbladder explain the adhesions between these structures and the frequency of spontaneous passage of gallstones into the duodenum. The distal 2.5-cm. portion is covered only in front by peritoneum. Its range of movement depends upon the elasticity of the peritoneal coat. The most common site of ulcer is upon its anterior or anterolateral surface.

The *descending (vertical) second divi-*

38

SURGICAL ANATOMY OF THE DUODENUM

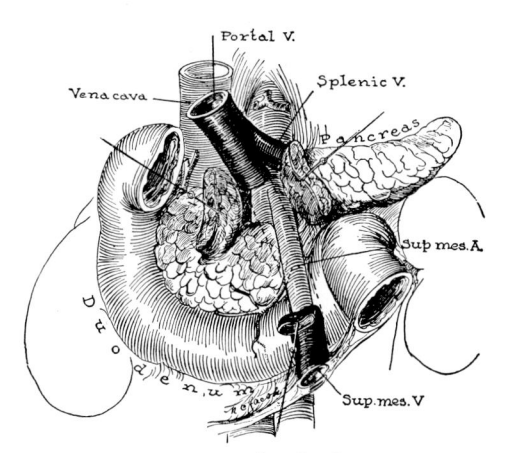

Figure 2-1. The duodenum.

sion forms an acute angle with the first division and descends 7.5 cm. to the inferior duodenal flexure. It is crossed by the transverse colon which, at this point, may or may not possess a mesocolon. The common opening of the bile and pancreatic ducts is upon the summit of a papilla (Fig. 2-2) about halfway down the posteromedial surface of this segment. The superior pancreaticoduodenal branch of the gastroduodenal artery runs in the anterior groove between the head of the pancreas and the descending duodenum (Fig. 1-11).

The descending portion of the duodenum is fixed definitely in position by fusion of its lateral visceral peritoneum to the parietal peritoneum of the lateral abdominal wall. By dividing the peritoneum at the right lateral edge of the upper half of the segment (Kocher's maneuver) (Fig. 2-3), the descending duodenum can be mobilized medially so as to render surgically accessible the retroduodenal, intrapancreatic, and intraduodenal portions of the common duct. After mobilization, the duodenum can be turned forward, downward, and to the left to bring it into position for anastomosis with the part of the stomach left after partial gastrectomy (see Billroth I Principle of Partial Gastrectomy with Gastroduodenostomy, p. 296) or Finney pyloroplasty (p. 357).

The *third* or *transverse division* of the duodenum, 12.5 cm. in length, runs horizontally to the left in front of the ureter, inferior vena cava, lumbar column, and aorta and ends at the left of the third lumbar vertebra. Near its termination, it is crossed by the root of the mesentery of the jejunoileum. The superior mesenteric artery runs downward over the anterior surface of the transverse duodenum to enter the root of the mesentery. Tight stretching of the artery over this segment may cause duodenal obstruction. The pancreas is separated

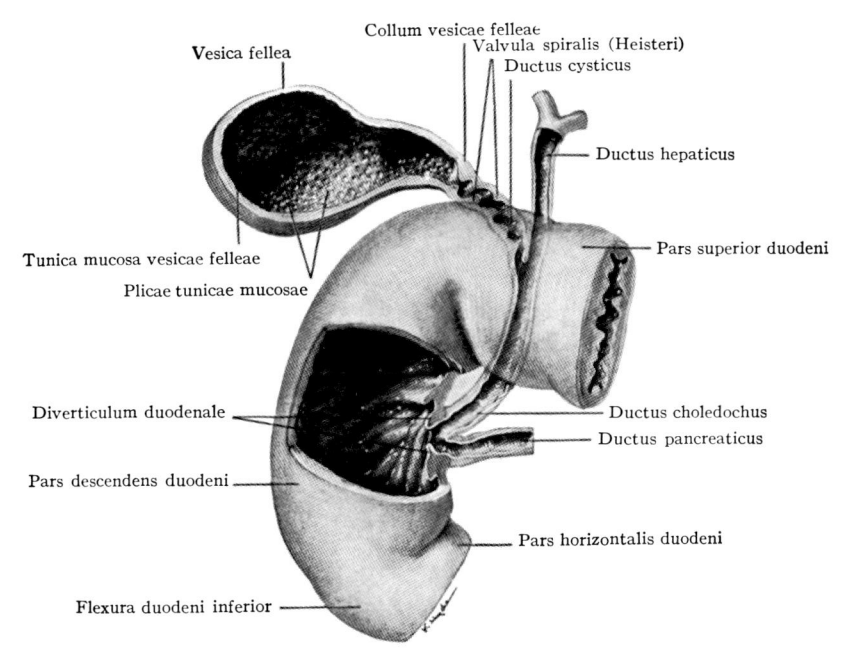

Figure 2-2. The duodenum, showing the superior, descending, and transverse portions with the relationship to the gallbladder and bile ducts.

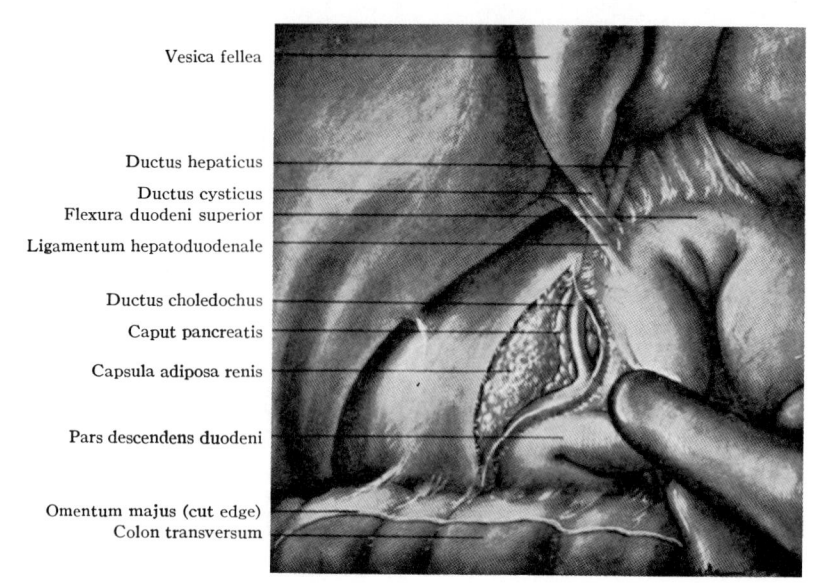

Figure 2-3. Surgical mobilization of the descending duodenum completed. Kocher's maneuver.

from the upper border of the segement by a groove in which lies the inferior pancreaticoduodenal artery (see Fig. 1-11).

The *fourth* or *ascending part* of the duodenum runs upward and slightly to the left for 2.5 cm. along the left side of the spine to the duodenojejunal angle at the root of the transverse mesocolon. At the left of the second lumbar vertebra, the terminal part of the duodenum bends sharply downward, forward, and to the left to form the *duodenojejunal flexure*.

At this point the suspensory ligament of the duodenum (Treitz's ligament) attaches to the duodenum. This ligament is a small triangular band of muscular and fibrous tissue which extends retroperitoneally, behind the pancreas and splenic vein and in front of the left renal vein, from the left or right crus of the diaphragm to attach retroperitoneally to the upper margin of the terminal duodenum and sometimes to the adjacent jejunum (Figs. 2-4 and 2-5).

Treitz's ligament is usually tenuous and not invariably present. The superior fold of the peritoneum above the paraduodenal fossa is often mistakenly termed Treitz's ligament.

The *duodenojejunal flexure* is a readily recognized landmark to guide the search for obstruction in the small bowel and to locate a loop of upper jejunum for gastrojejunostomy. It is found by passing the hand backward to the posterior abdominal wall behind the greater omentum and palpating upward along the left of the spine until the flexure is identified by its fixation. The bend is in contact with the inferior margin of the pancreas through the root of the transverse mesocolon.

FIXATION

In human beings, all of the duodenum except part of the first portion ultimately is anchored to the primitive posterior parietal peritoneum. Variations in its fusion to the posterior abdominal wall account for variations in mobility.

The right colic flexure and the fixed portion of the transverse mesocolon anchor the duodenum still more firmly and render it doubly retroperitoneal. In its deep position, the duodenum appears to be well protected from injury; yet it sometimes is crushed and even torn against the spine in severe abdominal contusions, partly because of its rigid peritoneal fixation.

The cap or first portion of the duodenum is covered entirely by peritoneum and is quite mobile, which facilitates plastic operations upon the pylorus and duodenum. Pyloroplasties and gastroduodenal resections are performed with greater ease and safety when the pylorus and adjoining duodenum can be mobilized forward into the abdominal cavity by Kocher's maneuver (Fig. 2-3).

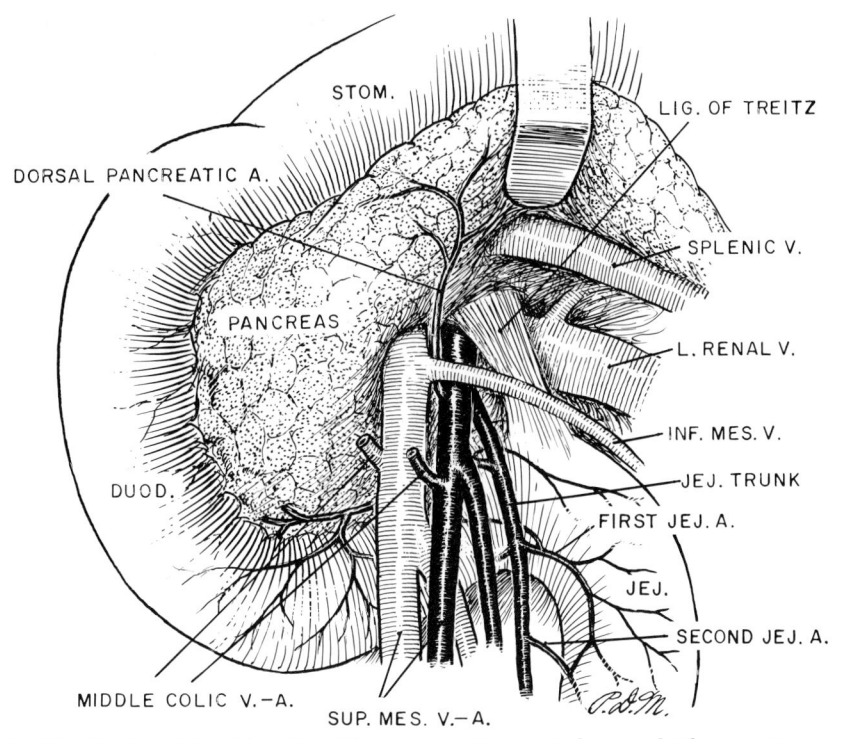

Figure 2–4. The duodenojejunal junction. The pancreas is retracted upward. The superior mesenteric vein is formed by two trunks and is joined by the inferior mesenteric vein. (From Edwards, E. A., Malone, P. D., and MacArthur, J. D.: Operative Anatomy of Abdomen and Pelvis. Philadelphia, Lea and Febiger, 1975.)

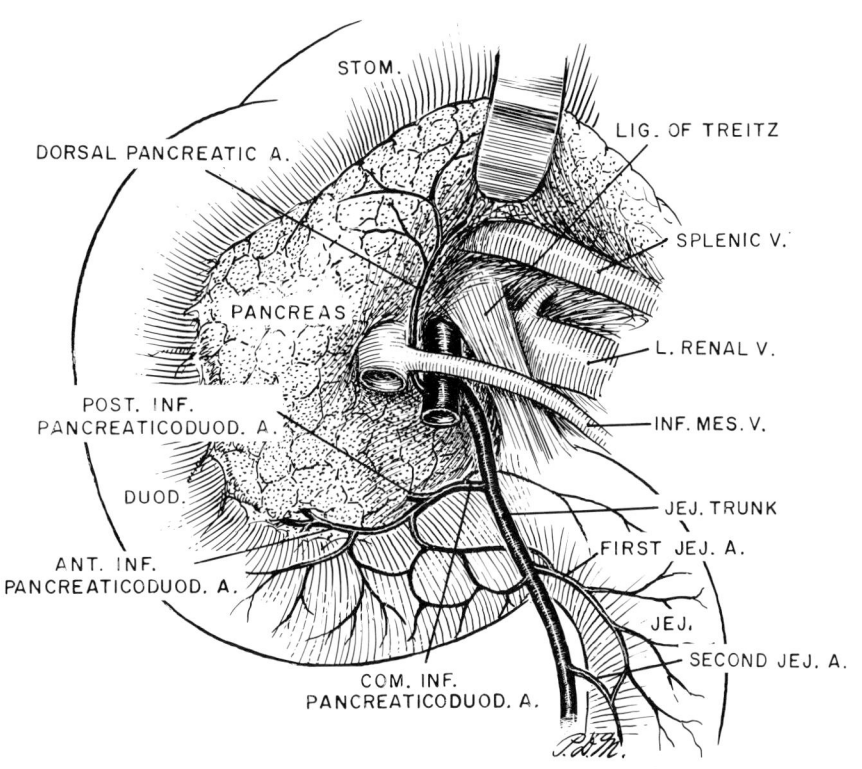

Figure 2–5. The duodenojejunal junction. The superior mesenteric vein and artery have been removed to show the detail of arterial supply to the bowel. The artery gives off an anomalous branch to the pancreas and a special jejunal trunk. (From Edwards, Malone, and MacArthur, cited in previous figure.)

CIRCULATION

The arterial supply of the duodenum is derived from the *pancreaticoduodenal* arteries. The *superior* pancreaticoduodenal artery is a branch of the hepatic artery, and the *inferior* pancreaticoduodenal artery is a branch of the superior mesenteric artery. These two arteries run in a groove between the descending and transverse portions of the duodenum and the head of the pancreas (see Fig. 1–11), anastomosing to form a continuous marginal artery.

The *veins* paralleling the pancreaticoduodenal arteries are arranged in anterior and posterior pancreaticoduodenal arcades accompanying the arteries. "The posterior arcade ends in the portal vein above, and the superior mesenteric below. The posterior superior pancreaticoduodenal vein may follow its companion artery anterior to the bile duct or it may run behind the duct. The inferior vein terminates on the left border of the superior mesenteric vein. Here it may be joined by a jejunal vein, or by the anterior inferior pancreaticoduodenal vein. Most of the anterior arcade is drained by the gastrocolic trunk" (Edwards, 1975).

Preduodenal Portal Vein

"Although variations in the tributaries of the portal vein are numerous, the course of the portal vein itself, behind the duodenum, and its relationship to the porta hepatis are quite constant." (Braun and associates, 1974).

A preduodenal portal vein is a rare congenital anomaly in which the portal vein passes anteriorly to the duodenum rather than in its normal posterior location (Fig. 2–6A). The anomaly is due to abnormal development of the vitelline veins. Bower and Ternberg (1972) made an excellent diagram of the embryology of the portal vein, showing a possible explanation of how a preduodenal portal vein may develop (Fig. 2–6B).

The first description of a preduodenal portal vein was published in 1912 by Begg, who found this anomaly in a 10-mm. pig embryo. The first report of a preduodenal portal vein in a human being was published in 1921 by Knight, who found the anomaly in a dissecting-room cadaver of an adult. He pointed out that the anomaly is of special interest to surgeons because of its unusual and exposed position, which may cause difficulties in operations involving the gallbladder, bile ducts, and duodenum. It must be recognized and protected. Tearing the vein could result in serious hemorrhage; excessive handling could result in thrombosis; and ligation of the vein could be catastrophic. Furthermore, since a preduodenal portal vein passes anteriorly to the duodenum rather than in its normal posterior location, it can compress, and thus obstruct, the duodenum, though it does not in all cases.

In 1926 Schnitzler was the first to operate successfully on an adult patient with this anomaly. The patient was a 41-year-old man with duodenal obstruction due to a preduodenal portal vein.

Since Knight's report at least 46 patients with a preduodenal portal vein have been recorded in the literature (Braun and Cuendet, 1971; Braun, Collin, and Ducharme, 1974; Davis, 1976). The majority of these were infants or children. There was a very high association with additional congenital anomalies. In the 32 cases analyzed by Bower and Ternberg (1972), 23 of which were pediatric, the most commonly associated anomaly was "malrotation" (23 patients). Partial or complete situs inversus was another frequent finding (9 patients), as were pancreatic and duodenal anomalies. There were 16 cardiovascular lesions in 11 patients, but only dextrocardia and dextroposition of the aorta occurred three or more times.

The preduodenal portal vein was discovered at operation in 22 of the 32 cases. The other 10 cases were anatomic descriptions of necropsy findings.

Nineteen patients presented acute or chronic intestinal obstruction originating above the ligament of Treitz. Four were adults with long histories of epigastric complaints secondary to chronic gastric outlet obstruction. The cause of the obstruction was the preduodenal portal vein in 10 cases. Other causes of obstruction included duodenal atresia, duodenal stenosis, duodenal web, annular pancreas, malrotation, or a combination of these anomalies.

Of the ten patients in whom the preduodenal portal vein was considered to have caused the obstruction, four had an

SURGICAL ANATOMY OF THE DUODENUM

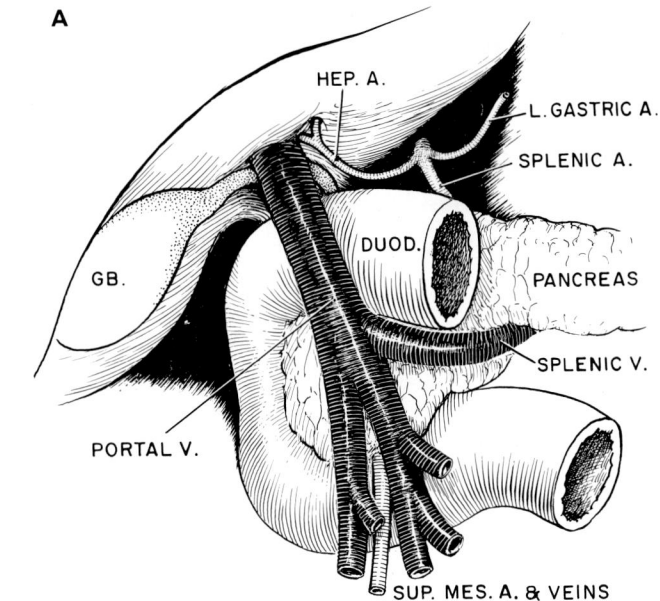

Figure 2–6. *A*, Anomalous preduodenal portal vein. (From Edwards, E. A., Malone, P. D., and MacArthur, J. D.: Operative Anatomy of Abdomen and Pelvis. Philadelphia, Lea and Febiger, 1975.)

B, (A), Normal development of portal vein. (B), Possible explanation of preduodenal portal vein. (From Bower, R. J., and Ternberg, J. L.: Preduodenal portal vein. J. Pediat. Surg. 7:579, 1972.)

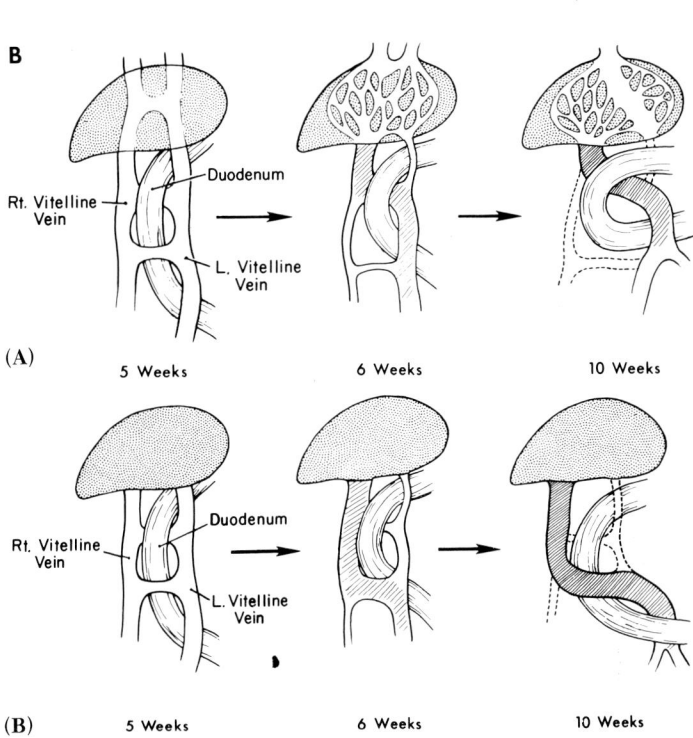

associated anomaly that could also be a possible cause of obstruction. Bower and Ternberg warned that "it is important, therefore, after recognizing and treating the more common causes of duodenal obstruction, to be sure that the preduodenal portal vein is not also contributing to the obstruction."

Davis (1976) reported a 38-year-old woman with a 1-year history of right upper quadrant pain. Cholecystography showed numerous medium-sized stones in an hourglass-shaped gallbladder. At operation a preduodenal portal vein was found, associated with a bilobed gallbladder containing numerous stones. Since there had been no symptoms, nor was there any evidence, of duodenal obstruction, a routine cholecystectomy was performed, and the anomalous vein was left undisturbed. The patient was discharged 12 days postoperatively.

The diagnosis of a preduodenal portal vein was not made preoperatively in any of the 23 cases collected from the literature plus two of their own reported by Braun and Cuendet (1971). In the majority the portal vein anomaly was unexpectedly discovered at operation for abdominal pain or evidence of duodenal obstruction thought to be due to some other cause.

At operation, when the duodenum is found to be obstructed and a preduodenal portal vein and associated anomalies are present, it is extremely important to determine accurately whether obstruction is caused by the anomalous vein, or by the associated anomalies, or by both.

Connehaye and associates (1975) reported two newborn infants with high intestinal obstruction associated with a preduodenal portal vein. In one infant there was also malrotation, and in the other there was also situs inversus. The portal vein was not causing obstruction in either case.

Surgical treatment of patients who have a preduodenal portal vein is directed primarily to the associated anomalies. If the anomalous vein is not causing obstruction, it is left undisturbed. Its mere presence is innocuous, as demonstrated by those patients in whom no sequelae developed when the nonoffending vein was not disturbed, and by the discovery of these veins in autopsies of older persons who died from unrelated conditions without ever having had symptoms of duodenal obstruction.

If the preduodenal vein causes duodenal obstruction, relief can be obtained by either of two surgical procedures: (1) transecting the proximal duodenum and performing an end-to-end duodenoduodenostomy, placing the portal vein dorsal to the duodenum. Bower and Ternberg successfully treated two of their three cases by this procedure. Or (2) using a bypass procedure to perform a duodenojejunostomy or gastroenteric anatomosis. This also has been used successfully (Braun and Cuendet, 1971).

Block and Zikria (1961) reported a 10-year-old patient with duodenal obstruction caused by a preduodenal vein and associated pneumatosis cystoides intestinalis of the lower ileum. The duodenal obstruction was relieved by a duodenoduodenostomy and the pneumatosis cystoides intestinalis disappeared following relief of the duodenal obstruction.

Braun and associates (1974) reported their experience with the treatment of two newborn infants with a preduodenal portal vein. In both instances the malformation was discovered during surgical exploration for duodenal obstruction. In one the obstruction was due to an associated complete atresia at the junction of the second and third portions of the duodenum. A side-to-side duodenoduodenal anastomosis was performed. The postoperative course was uneventful. In the other a malrotation with obstructing Ladd bands and also an intraluminal diaphragm (windsock type with a small, eccentrically located aperture) was found to be causing obstruction. The Ladd procedure was performed, the anterior portion of the diaphragm was excised through a duodenotomy, and a tube gastrostomy was established. The postoperative course was smooth. The preduodenal portal vein was not causing obstruction in either of these cases, so was left undisturbed in both.

Braun and coworkers tabulated the 39 cases of preduodenal portal vein they found in the literature, plus their own 2 cases. Analysis of these 41 patients revealed that 34 (83 per cent) had other associated malformations, often multiple. The most frequent of these were intestinal malrotation (30 patients), situs inversus (12 patients), anomalies of the duodenum (stenosis in 1, atresia in 3, and intrinsic diaphragm in 7 patients), anomalies of the pancreas (10 patients), biliary atresia (4 patients), duodenal malformations (II patients), and congenital duodenal bands (8 patients).

The sex distribution was equal — 19 female patients and 18 male patients, with four cases not recorded. Of the 39 patients whose ages were recorded, 29 (71.8 per cent) were infants and children, 8 (20.5 per cent) were adults, and 2 (5.2 per cent) were adolescent.

Duodenal obstruction due to the preduodenal portal vein was recorded as present in 13 and absent in 27 patients. Duodenal obstruction due to other causes was recorded as present in 14 and absent in 26 patients.

The researchers stated, "A detailed analysis of these 41 cases has not convinced us that in the anterior position the portal vein can obstruct the duodenum. It seems difficult to believe that a low venous pressure within a thin-walled vessel can cause such an obstruction. It is more likely that the reverse is true, that the duodenum obstructs the portal vein and creates portal hypertension. Yet this has never been reported. Furthermore, in most cases (83 per cent) the associated malformations can adequately explain the symptoms. Finally, many of the cases were treated by performing a short-circuiting anastomosis around the portal vein without making any real attempt to exclude intrinsic stenosis of the duodenum. The fact that many cases of preduodenal portal vein have been reported in adults does not rule out an intrinsic diaphragm as the real cause of obstruction. Smiley, Perry, and McCleland (1967) reviewed 20 cases of congenital diaphragm in adults and stated that 29 per cent of these patients first developed symptoms after the age of 24 years."

In conclusion, Braun and associates believe that associated anomalies, and not the preduodenal portal vein, produce the clinical picture of duodenal obstruction, and these anomalies lead to discovery of the abnormal position of the vessel. They believe the preduodenal portal vein is probably never responsible for duodenal obstruction, and, when it is found in association with some degree of duodenal obstruction, the duodenum should be explored. The presence or absence of a diaphragm can be determined by inserting a Foley catheter into the duodenum, inflating the balloon, and then withdrawing it. If there is a diaphragm, it can be excised through a duodenotomy. "The main, surgical implication of a preduodenal portal vein is the recognition of this anomaly and avoidance of its injury during operations on the biliary tract and the duodenum."

PHYSIOLOGY OF THE DUODENUM

The duodenum normally is the site at which food passed from the stomach in a partially digested and acid state has its acidity neutralized by alkaline secretions. In addition to the effects of these alkaline secretions of the duodenum, the digestion of the food is implemented also by trypsin (pancreatic protease), amylopsin (pancreatic amylase), steapsin (pancreatic lipase), and rennin secreted by the pancreas into the duodenum where it is activated by enterokinase produced by the duodenal glands.

The duodenum is also the site at which normally the food is brought into contact with bile, which aids in the digestion of fats by the emulsification of fatty materials and by rendering soluble the fatty acids liberated during fat digestion. Bile salts also serve as specific activators of pancreatic lipase.

It is important for the surgeon to know that all or part of the duodenum may be removed with little recognized disturbance to the patient, as its functions apparently can be taken over by the remaining small intestine. However, provision must be made for the entry of bile and should, but not necessarily must, be made for the re-entry of pancreatic juice into the intestinal tract. Furthermore, as mentioned, when selecting such an operation, consideration should be given to the fact that extirpation of the duodenum in whole or in part, or operations that bypass the gastric acid around the duodenum, impair or eliminate the normal duodenal brake on gastric secretion and, therefore, are followed by increased gastric secretion.

Chapter 3

INTUBATION

Gastrointestinal intubation is usually limited to four indications: gastric drainage, small bowel decompression, for feeding tubes, and in gastrointestinal bleeding.

Gastric Drainage

The primary use of gastrointestinal intubation is to empty gastric and upper intestinal contents, either by suction or by straight drainage. It is a popular misconception that straight drainage is achieved by siphonage alone. Straight drainage by a gastrointestinal tube from the stomach is achieved not only by siphonage but also by increased intra-abdominal pressure during a Valsalva maneuver, coughing, or deep inspiration. Increased intra-abdominal pressure forces the fluid into the tube and then into the collecting bottle. Since siphonage is an open system, this method is not usually the most important.

Suction, on the other hand, can be either intermittent or continuous. Intermittent suction has the theoretic advantage of not obstructing the lumen or holes of the tube with gastric mucosa, although this does occur periodically. In an attempt to overcome this problem, sump nasogastric tubes have been developed. These double-lumen polyethylene tubes have one lumen for suction and the other as an air entrance (air port). The tubes are placed on continuous suction, and air is constantly circulated through the stomach so that accumulated fluid is sucked out the patent orifices. These tubes are fairly effective but also can be occluded by the loose gastric mucosa. All nasogastric tubes, whether conventional or sump, need periodic flushing or repositioning to ensure patency. Standard practice is periodic lavage with 20 to 30 ml. of air or saline to unclog a tube and maintain patency, but moving the tube at intervals is more effective.

Long Intestinal Tubes for Small Bowel Decompression

The use of long intestinal tubes for the early management of bowel obstruction or partial ileus has remained popular over the years. The two tubes used most often for this purpose are the Cantor tube, a long intestinal tube with a single lumen and a mercury-filled bag at the tip, or the Miller-Abbott tube, a double-lumen, balloon-tipped tube with one lumen used to distend the balloon with air or fluid. These tubes are best used in the initial management of patients with possible small bowel obstruction, or in the postoperative period when small bowel obstruction may occur on the basis of filmy adhesions. Occasionally, the partial small bowel obstruction resolves by decompressing the upper intestinal tract with a long tube. We do not recommend the use of long intestinal tubes as the primary treatment of small bowel obstruction. These tubes are usually connected to intermittent suction or dependent drainage. Frequently they will not pass down the intestines when decompression is most urgently needed—that is, in patients with the most marked distention due to longstanding intestinal obstruction or paralytic ileus. However, they are sometimes successful and their use is a valuable adjunct in the treatment of such cases.

Getting a tube to pass through the pylorus is the most difficult part of the passage of the long intestinal tube. Under fluoroscopic control, with the injection of Gastrografin as a contrast media, the passage of the tube through the pylorus often can be assisted by a radiologist. Once in the duodenum, the tube will usually migrate on its own by peristalsis. There has also been some recent enthusiasm by endoscopists to help move the tube through the pylorus by the use of the flexible gastroduodenoscope. Sophisticated sidearm equipment has been developed which can be used to grasp the tube and help pass it through the pylorus. Both these aids can help shorten the time necessary to advance the long intestinal tubes.

Complications of long intestinal tubes are rare. These usually consist of erosion of the intestinal tract or rupture of the mercury-filled bag. Luminal metallic mercury is innocuous, and there is little evidence that mercury toxicity can occur. However, the presence of metallic mercury in the peritoneal cavity via intestinal tract perforation can be followed by such sequelae as intraabdominal granulomas and additional adhesion formation though this is very rare. Occasionally, knotting or overdistention of the bag occurs, requiring operative intervention to remove the tube. This also is a very rare occurrence.

The removal of long intestinal tubes is usually not a problem. Suction must be discontinued to eliminate the tube's adherence to the mucosa. With the Miller-Abbott tube, the balloon is deflated, and steady gentle traction is applied. With the Cantor tube, steady gentle traction is applied to remove it slowly so as not to intussuscept the bowel. Occasionally an intestinal tube may pass the ileocecal junction, making its removal very difficult or impossible without laparotomy. See the section on Complications later in this chapter.

Feeding Tubes

Conventional polyethylene No. 16 F. or 18 F. tubes can be used for feeding purposes, but recently developed Silastic No. 8 F. to 12 F. mercury-weighted tubes have been useful for this purpose. The tubes are small and pliable, have a heavy tip which makes them easy to pass, and are well tolerated by the patient. Many of these are now commercially available. These tubes are passed by the conventional nasogastric route and can be taped to the side of the cheek with no discomfort. This allows continuous infusion of many of the commercially available enteral diets. This form of enteral alimentation or enteral hyperalimentation is particularly useful in the malnourished patient with an intact gastrointestinal tract. These diets usually begin with a continuous infusion of 30 to 50 ml. per hour of a dilute diet (usually quarter-strength). The volume and concentration are then slowly increased over a few days in order for the patient's gastrointestinal tract to adapt to the volume load as well as the increased osmolarity. This prevents the associated diarrhea upon too-rapid infusion of these hyperosmolar solutions.

If a commercially available mercury-filled feeding tube cannot be obtained, one can be fashioned from a No. 8 F. pediatric feeding tube with a mercury-filled finger cot sewn to the tip. A very small amount of mercury, less than 0.5 ml., is necessary to aid in placement.

During continuous feeding, care must be taken not to overdistend the stomach and cause regurgitation and aspiration. In addition, patients should not be fed through a nasogastric tube while supine but instead the head of the bed should be elevated or they should sit.

Intubation in Gastrointestinal Bleeding

For the management of significant upper gastrointestinal bleeding, we prefer the use of the Ewald tube for irrigation of gastric contents. This tube is larger than the conventional No. 16 F. to 18 F. nasogastric Levin tube, and ranges in size from No. 22 F. to 32 F. By cutting side holes in the tube we are able to clear the stomach more effectively. By clearing the stomach of most residual blood, endoscopists have a better opportunity to identify the site of bleeding. These tubes are more effective than standard Levin tubes for removing blood and large quantities of fluid from the stomach. They are also more effective for introducing iced saline or iced water lavage in attempting to control upper gastrointestinal hemorrhage. The large-size tube lumen makes the clots easier to withdraw, and iced water makes the clots lyse more easily.

Because the tube is considerably larger than the standard nasogastric tube, we do not recommend it for conventional use. There is some reservation about passing a tube of this size in a patient with known esophageal varices. However, we feel that the benefits gained by appropriate irrigation and endoscopic confirmation of bleeding sites outweighs the potential danger of irritating an esophageal or gastric varix. We recommend that this tube be withdrawn after no longer than 48 hours for it will cause erosions of the esophagus, esophageal-gastric junction, and nares.

The use of the Blakemore-Sengstaken tube for the control of esophageal varices is discussed in the section on the esophagus and esophageal varices, p. 663 of Volume 1.

PERORAL GASTRIC INTUBATION

Indications

Gastric intubation by the peroral route is utilized mainly for gastric lavage: (1) to wash out toxic substances such as alcohol, mercurial poisons, acids, alkalis, barbiturates, or other potentially lethal materials that have been swallowed accidentally or with suicidal intent; (2) in the days before postoperative decompression of the stomach was used, to treat acute dilation of the stomach or paralytic ileus or both which occurred so commonly after intra-abdominal operations. This complication is now uncommon; (3) to empty a stomach of contents retained because of pyloric obstruction or other cause; (4) to empty a recently filled stomach just prior to performance of an emergency operation; and (5) using ice water or saline, to attempt to control massive hemorrhage from bleeding esophageal varices (see p. 658 in Vol. 1).

Usually the gastric (stomach) tube is employed in these procedures. Compared with the nasal tube, its larger caliber permits more rapid evacuation of the stomach contents and faster introduction and withdrawal of water or other solutions used to wash out the stomach. Its large lumen also permits the passage of small particles of food without obstruction of the tube.

Its disadvantages in comparison with the nasal tube are that its larger size makes it less comfortable for the patient, the necessity of passing it through the mouth makes it possible for an uncooperative patient to bite it unless prevented from doing so with a gag, and the relative rigidity of its walls permits the use of a certain degree of force to push it down the esophagus with some danger of perforation of that structure. Furthermore, its size and relative rigidity prohibit its routine passage beyond the pylorus. It is too uncomfortable to leave in place for any length of time. For these reasons, the smaller nasal tubes are preferable except as indicated above, when haste or volume lavage is required.

Technic

Preferably the patient sits upright with his or her head thrown backward and mouth open. If the patient must remain recumbent the tube can still be passed with ease if he is placed flat on his back with a small pillow under his shoulder but not under his head, so that his head drops backward, with the chin up. The oral cavity is then placed more nearly in line with the esophagus.

A peroral large-bore rubber stomach tube is soaked in ice water until thoroughly cold, and its tip is lubricated with glycerin or white oil. These two steps are not essential but lessen to some degree the unpleasantness caused by the passage of the tube. If the patient has an unusually active gag reflex an anesthetizing solution may be applied to the uvula and palatal arches. This is rarely necessary, however.

The tube is held in pen-fashion in the operator's right hand about 15 cm. from its tip. In the conscious, cooperative patient the tip of the tube is placed on top of the tongue and passed backward until the posterior wall of the pharynx is contacted. The patient is then told to swallow repeatedly, until the tip is engaged in the esophagus, after which gentle and continuous force applied by the operator's hand above will pass the tube down into the stomach as shown by the white mark on the tube. During this part of the procedure it is important that the patient be instructed to *breathe through his mouth* for if he closes his mouth he will clamp his teeth on the tube and prevent its further passage.

In uncooperative, hysterical, psychotic, unconscious, or very young patients more positive steps may be necessary. In these patients a gag should be placed between the teeth to prevent the operator's finger or the tube from being bitten. The tongue is pulled forward by an assistant whose fingers are covered with gauze to prevent slipping. The operator's left index finger is inserted into the widely opened mouth to depress the base of the tongue and hook it forward. The tube is passed steadily and firmly backward to contact the posterior pharyngeal wall, along which it is guided until the tip is well engaged in the esophagus. When these maneuvers are employed the patient's cooperation in swallowing is not required. The tube is then passed deftly and continuously down the esophagus into the stomach, thus minimizing the gagging which occurs when the tube passes from the pharynx into the esophagus.

When the tube has entered the stomach, obvious gastric contents usually begin to drain immediately from the outside end of the tube. Such drainage indicates that the tip of the tube is in its sought-for location. If such confirmatory drainage does not occur then the open end of the tube should be placed below the level of water in a glass. If the tube has been misplaced and is lying within the trachea instead of the esophagus, as can easily occur, bubbles of air will appear with each expiration or cough. If such is the case the tube must be completely withdrawn and reinserted into the esophagus. *No fluid should be passed into the tube until the operator is positive it is within the esophageal lumen and not within the trachea.* Many cases of aspiration pneumonia have been caused by this serious mistake.

In the average adult, the distance from the upper incisor teeth to the upper end of the esophagus is 14 cm.; from the same point to the arch of the aorta it is 23 cm.; and to the esophageal opening in the diaphragm it is 37 cm. Pouches and diverticula of the esophagus must be avoided.

Lavage

If the stomach content is fairly liquid, it may be siphoned; if it is thick, tepid ordinary tap water, weak bicarbonate of soda solution, or normal saline may be used for lavage. For each washing, about 10 to 12 ounces of fluid are introduced through a funnel attached to the tube. The funnel is held just enough higher than the level of the stomach to enable the liquid to flow. As soon as the fluid is introduced or if the patient complains of discomfort, the funnel is lowered below the level of the stomach for siphonage.

The lavage is continued until the fluid is returned clear. At the end of the procedure, the tube is pinched off and withdrawn carefully.

A large peroral gastric tube is unsuitable for leaving in place as a retention tube. It is too large for comfort, it necessitates the mouth remaining constantly open with the consequent drying of the tongue and oral mucous membranes, and its rigid walls may cause esophageal ulceration and even perforation. After the stomach has been satisfactorily lavaged, the stomach tube should be replaced by a nasal catheter if an indwelling tube is then desirable.

NASOGASTRIC, GASTRODUODENAL, AND LOWER GASTROINTESTINAL INTUBATION

For nasal intubation, several types of tubes are used. The most common are the Levin single-lumen duodenal tube, the bilumen gastrojejunostomy tube, the bilumen gastroduodenal tube, and long intestinal tubes, such as the Cantor or the Miller-Abbott tube (Fig. 3–1). These tubes may be made of rubber or plastic material. Tubes made of plastic are better tolerated than those made of rubber.

LEVIN TUBE

In 1921, A. L. Levin, of New Orleans, described his smooth, catheter-tipped, duodenal tube for use in adults. Its advantages over most other duodenal tubes were that it could be passed through the nares and it was made of one solid piece of rubber.

The Levin tube is now probably the most frequently used type of indwelling gastric tube. It is a single-lumen catheter long enough for passage from the nares to

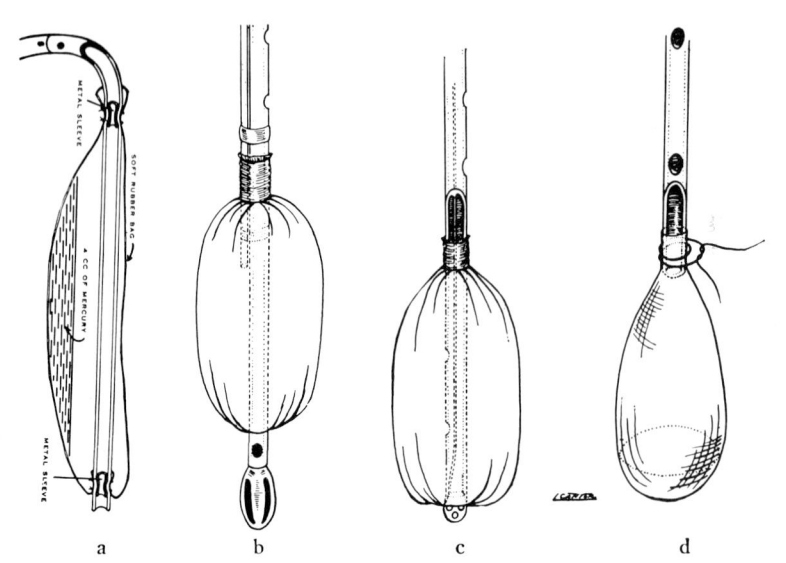

Figure 3–1. Tube heads of the most commonly used intestinal decompression tubes. *a*, Harris tube. *b*, Johnston tube. *c*, Miller-Abbott tube. *d*, Cantor tube. The Johnston tube and the Miller-Abbott tube are double-lumen tubes. Note position of balloon along the shaft of the tube. These tubes were designed for inflation of the balloon with air to propel the tube. The construction of the Harris tube head is exactly the same as that of the Miller-Abbott and Johnston tubes. It is a single-lumen tube and uses mercury as a weight. In the Cantor tube, the loose balloon at the tip of the tube permits an unrestricted free flow of the mercury.

the pylorus and into the duodenum. Its tip is rounded and has an eye opening into the lumen at the side. The tube is soft but radiopaque; its radiopacity permits the location of the tip to be confirmed by x-ray examination. It is made in several sizes; a 14 F. caliber is most often used. Markings indicate the length of tubing required for the tip to be (1) within the stomach and (2) within the duodenum (at 47.5 cm., nares to cardia; at 75 cm., nares to pylorus; at 90 cm., nares to 15 cm. within the duodenum).

There is no propulsive mechanism in this type of tube.

Technic

The Levin tube is usually prepared in the same manner as is the stomach tube, namely, by chilling in ice water and lubricating its tip with glycerin. The patient's position should be the same as that for passing the gastric tube.

A local anesthetic applied to the nostril to be used is helpful but not necessary.

Although the insertion of a Levin tube is facilitated by a patient who is conscious and will cooperate by swallowing the tip of the tube, this tube can be inserted in an unconscious or uncooperative patient.

In the conscious and cooperative patient, the subject's head is held backward and the tip of his or her nose is slightly elevated by the operator's left index finger. This places the nostril, pharynx and esophagus in an almost straight line. The patient should breathe through the mouth. The tube is passed slowly through the nostril into the pharynx. The patient is instructed to swallow repeatedly and when the tip of the tube engages in the esophagus the remaining part of the tube is fed through the nostril with downward pressure to speed its passage into the stomach. This pressure must be slight, however, for the progress of the tube is due mainly to the patient's act of swallowing and since the tube is quite soft too much pressure will cause it to curl up in the pharynx instead of moving down the esophagus. If the tube curls it should be withdrawn and reinserted.

In an unconscious or uncooperative patient, a mouth gag is placed between the subject's teeth to prevent his closing them on the operator's finger. Then, as the operator passes the tube through the nostril with the right hand, the index finger of the operator's left hand can be placed in the back of the patient's open mouth and the tip of the tube guided into the esophagus, after which it can be pushed down into the stomach.

Usually, when the tube enters the stomach gastric contents will drain from its open end, indicating its proper location. If gastric drainage does not occur the external open end of the tube should be held under water. If the tube is mistakenly within the trachea, air will bubble up with each expiration. No fluid should be introduced into the tube until one is *certain* that the tube is *not within the respiratory tree.*

Confused elderly patients and patients

who are delirious, psychotic, uncooperative, or combative frequently frustrate their treatment by pulling out a nasogastric tube despite its being taped to their nose. Carr and Heimlich (1972) described a maneuver of encirclement that prevents dislodgement of a nasogastric tube (Levin or long intestinal tube) by the patient, performed as follows:

The Levin tube is introduced through the nose, passed into the stomach in the usual manner, and the stomach is aspirated. The physician then places a hand or a right angle clamp in the gagged open mouth of the patient, hooks the index finger or the clamp around the tube where it is accessible in the oropharynx, and draws a loop of the tube out though the mouth. A short length of umbilical tape is tied around the tube at the point intended to lie in the pharynx. For a Levin tube this will usually be near the first mark, about 18 inches from the distal end. The shorter end of the tied cord tape is cut close to the knot. The loop of tube is then returned through the mouth to its proper position in the pharynx. The long, free end of the tape is left protruding from the mouth. It may be necessary to withdraw the tube slightly where it enters the nose to straighten the tube.

After another check of the oropharynx to be certain that the knot around the tube is in the correct position, the free end of the tape is tied to the tube beneath the external naris. The nasogastric tube and the cord tape now form a complete circle around the palate and maxilla (Fig. 3–2). The security of the tie is then tested by pulling on the tube at any point beneath the nose. The cord tape will draw tight under the tension, preventing any significant movement of the tube.

The nasogastric tube is then taped to the nose in the usual manner, with the tape covering the outside cord tape knot. Although not mandatory, the taping serves several purposes. The adhesive tape protects the knot from the patient and helps prevent the outside knot from slipping. Also, anyone seeing the tape detached from the nose or tube is warned that the patient has attempted to remove the tube.

Long intestinal tubes are secured in a slightly different way that enables them to be passed gradually into the small intestine. The inside knot is tied as a loose loop around the tube, which can then slip

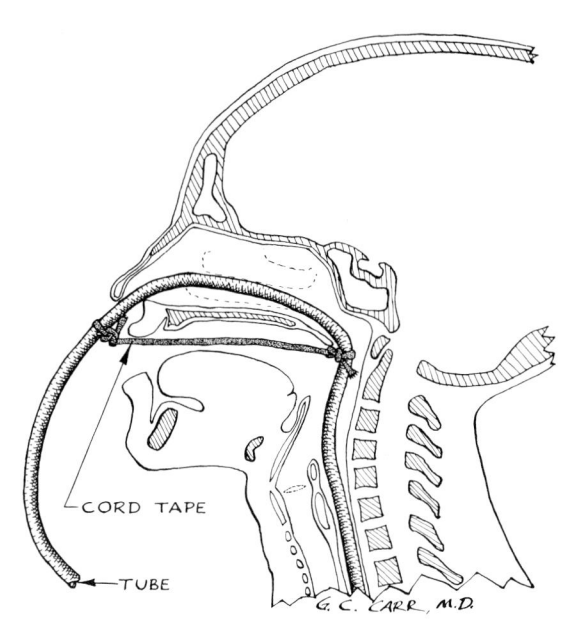

Figure 3–2. The cord tape and nasogastric tube form a complete circle around the palate and maxilla; this prevents the patient from pulling out the tube.

through it. A bowline knot with a short loop works well, but a square knot is adequate. When the tube is advanced, only the outside knot need be untied to permit the tube to be lubricated and advanced. The outside knot is then retied to the tube. The loose loop formed by the inside knot does not compromise the security of the tube.

Carr and Heimlich reported 10 patients with nasogastric tubes that required management by this method. There was no morbidity. The tubes functioned well and were not dislodged. While this technic may be of help in dealing with the occasional patient, it is unusual to have to resort to such measures.

BILUMEN GASTROJEJUNOSTOMY TUBE

This round tube is bisected by a central longitudinal partition which gives it a double semicircular lumen (Fig. 3–3). Each lumen can be used independently because it has separate openings at each end. The catheter tip is of solid rubber impregnated with lead which gives the tube the necessary weight for smooth and easy passage. Next to the tip are the openings for the longer-lumen jejunal segment of the tube. The shorter or stomach lumen has its slotted

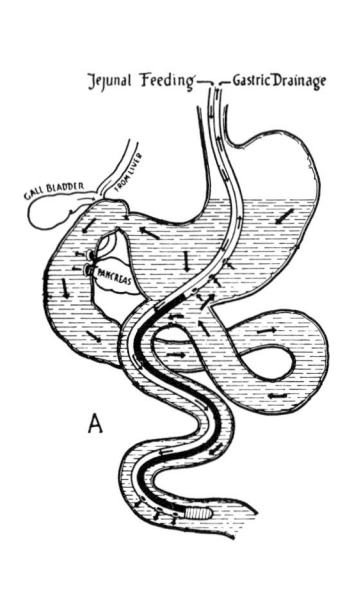

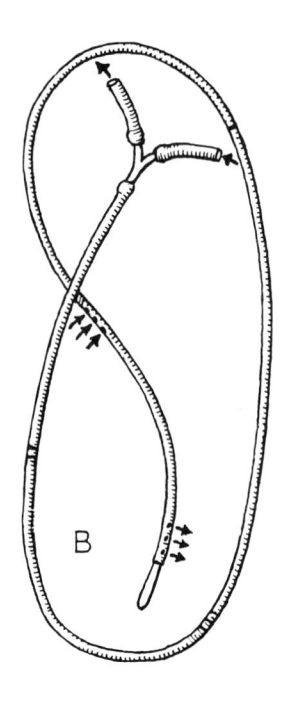

Figure 3-3. Simultaneous jejunal feeding and gastric drainage with a bilumen gastrojejunostomy tube. *A*, Diagrammed tube in place. *B*, The inlets and outlets of the tube are indicated. (Courtesy of Moses Einhorn.)

openings 36.2 cm. proximal to the end of the tube.

Before a gastrojejunal operation, this tube may be passed through the patient's nose and swallowed until the tube is at the single or 75-cm. mark. This indicates that about 27.5 cm. of the tube is in the patient's stomach.

Before the gastrojejunal anastomosis is completed, the tube is located within the stomach and is slipped into the distal limb of the anastomosing jejunal loop as far as the double, or 92-cm., mark. With the tube in this position, jejunal feeding and drainage and gastric drainage can be carried out independently or simultaneously.

BILUMEN GASTRODUODENAL TUBE

This tube has the same specifications as the gastrojejunostomy tube except that it is shorter (Fig. 3–4). The openings for the gastric lumen are 23.7 cm. from the terminal end of the tube, and the duodenal openings are at the end of the tube. The tube has markings at 47.5 cm. (nares to cardia), 75 cm. (nares to pylorus) and 82.5 cm. (nares to 12.5 cm. within the duodenum).

Gastroduodenal intubation may be used preoperatively and postoperatively in gastrointestinal and other abdominal operations in which the upper gastrointestinal tract must be kept decompressed. It may be used in any form of vomiting when duodenal lavage, duodenal feeding, and gastric drainage are indicated. Theoretically it permits simultaneous gastric drainage and duodenal feeding but practically the two opposing procedures can rarely be successfully performed simultaneously.

One of the alleged advantages of the double-lumen (sump) nasogastric tube at-

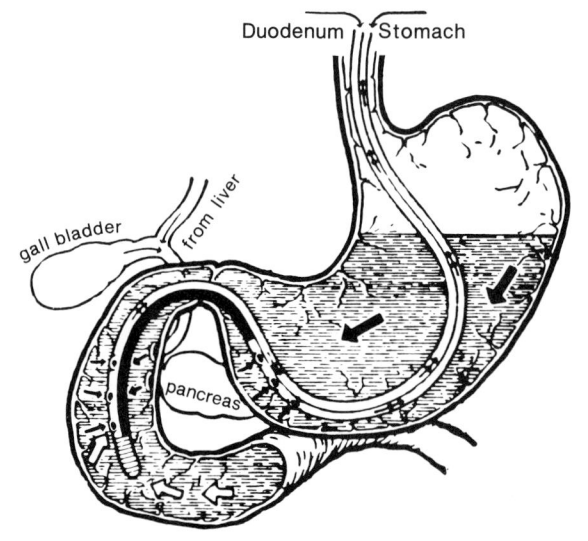

Figure 3-4. Simultaneous drainage from the stomach and duodenum with a nasal bilumen tube. (Courtesy of Moses Einhorn.)

tached to suction and used for gastric decompression is that its double-lumen design prevents gastric mucosa from being sucked into the sucking ports, thereby becoming ulcerated and also obstructing the ports. However, Greene, Sawicki, and Doyle (1973) reported four patients, treated with the double-lumen nasogastric tube, in whom multiple gastric ulcers had been seen at autopsy. The location and uniform size of the ulcers accurately reproduced the arrangement and size of the sucking ports on the tube. They warned that double-lumen nasogastric tubes on suction, therefore, should be used with as much caution as single-lumen tubes.

MILLER-ABBOTT TUBE

The Miller-Abbott tube is double channeled (Fig. 3–5). It serves the special purpose of decompressing the bowel in small bowel obstruction, no matter how low the obstructing lesion may be. In addition, the patient can be fed and the excess of food or the bowel secretion proximal to the obstruction can be removed rapidly.

The small lumen of the tube is used to inflate the balloon which may be attached proximal or distal to the perforated metal tip on the end of the tube. The larger lumen, independent of the first, is the feeding or aspirating part of the tube. Care must be taken to correctly identify the proper lumen. When inflated, the balloon stimulates peristalsis, which propels the balloon and the attached tube through the whole normal small intestine in from 3 to 4 hours. The balloon passes more slowly when the small bowel is obstructed. Suction applied to the tip in the larger lumen empties the normal or obstructed bowel. Barium sulfate in suspension, or some other contrast medium, can be injected down the aspirating lumen of the tube for x-ray studies of lesions of the small intestine.

The diameter of the standard Miller-Abbott tube is 16 F.; 14 F.- and 18 F.-diameter tubes are available. A 12 F.-diameter tube, 90 cm. long, is used for infants.

Indications

The indications for decompression by suction are:
1. Obstruction of the small intestine by adhesions in which the distention is moderate and one can be certain that there is *no strangulation*. If relief of the obstruction does not occur after 24 hours of suction then operation should be performed. Relief of obstruction should be determined by radiologic evidence of gas distal to the obstruction.
2. Obstruction of small intestine due to inflammatory lesions.
3. Obstruction of small intestine due to paralytic or spastic ileus.
4. Prophylactically after major abdominal operations to prevent postoperative paralytic ileus.
5. Abdominal distention from other than obstructive causes, such as in pneumonia or other acute infections, or after injuries to the spinal cord or major fractures of bones.
6. Pre- and postoperatively in perforations of the stomach or duodenum.

Contraindications

The contraindications to suction tube drainage are:
1. Strangulating obstruction with compromise of the blood supply.
2. Acute obstruction of the colon with distention of the proximal colon. In these cases it may be used in conjunction with surgery, but operation should not be delayed for a trial of treatment by intestinal intubation and suction.

It obviously cannot be used when there is obstruction of the esophagus.

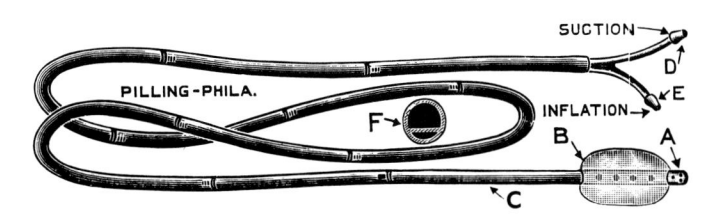

Figure 3–5. Miller-Abbott double-lumen small intestine intubation tube. *A*, Perforated metal tip; *B*, balloon; *C*, double-lumen tube; *D*, tip on suction lumen of the tube; *E*, tip on balloon-inflation lumen of the tube; *F*, cross section of tube showing the larger suction lumen and the smaller inflating lumen. (Courtesy of G. P. Pilling Company.)

Technic

To pass the tube properly, the air should be withdrawn from the balloon, the tube should be lubricated with a nonoily substance, and the tip passed through the patient's nose. When the first (45-cm.) mark disappears, the tip has entered the stomach. Continuous suction is begun and is maintained thereafter. The patient is supported on the right side and the tube is advanced inch by inch, in the same manner as a duodenal tube is passed, until the mark (75 cm.) is at the level of the nose. Sufficient length of tube now has been passed to allow the tip to engage the duodenum. A syringe then is attached to the inflating tip which leads to the balloon, and 10 cc. of air are injected. If a sensation of rhythmically recurring resistance is imparted to the plunger of the syringe, the tube is in the duodenum; the rhythmic resistance is caused by duodenal contraction. The air is left in the balloon for 20 minutes. If the duodenal contraction can be felt at the end of that interval, an additional 15 cc. of air are injected into the balloon and the inflation lumen is clamped. Thenceforth the patient swallows 15 cm. of tube each half hour. If no resistance is felt when the syringe is applied, a half hour should be allowed to pass, and the procedure should be tried again. When no sensation of duodenal contraction can be felt after a considerable time, the tube will have to be guided into the duodenum under the fluoroscope.

It has been our unhappy experience that frequently these tubes will not pass down the intestine in cases in which they are most urgently needed; that is, in patients with the most marked distention due to longstanding intestinal obstruction or paralytic ileus secondary to peritonitis or other causes. However it is sometimes successful and a valuable adjunct in the treatment of such patients. One must be cautious lest operative treatment be delayed while prolonged attempts are made to pass the tube.

HARRIS AND CANTOR SINGLE-LUMEN MERCURY-WEIGHTED TUBES

These tubes are illustrated in Figure 3-1 (a and d). They are used in the same manner and for the same purpose as the Miller-Abbott tube.

However, the balloons in Harris and Cantor tubes are filled with mercury, instead of air, so that the greater weight of the metal will help the tube advance down the intestinal tract. This it may do. However, a mercury-containing balloon of a nasogastric tube may rupture and spill the metallic mercury into the bowel lumen.

Spillage of mercury into the bowel generally has been considered inconsequential since, in the past, metallic mercury frequently was given orally as a cathartic, apparently without complications. Although swallowed metallic mercury usually passes down an intact alimentary tract and out in the feces, in an exceptional case it may cause severe or even fatal poisoning (Greenberg, 1972).

Hanselman and Meyer (1962) collected the reports of six such cases. "There was no evidence of mercury toxicity, the mercury passing in small globules within 8 days." Recently we had a similar experience with such a case. However, "Krais (1955) reported a case of fatal mercury poisoning following rupture of a mercury-weighted balloon of a nasogastric tube" (Greenberg, 1972).

The presence of metallic mercury in a nonintact intestinal tract is more likely to be followed by sequelae. Metallic mercury produces granulomas whenever it gets into interstitial tissue. As Greenberg (1972) stated, "This can occur when the mercury-containing balloon of a nasogastric tube ruptures and spills the metallic mercury into the bowel lumen. If there is a recent anastomosis, the mercury can leak through the suture line and produce an intra-abdominal granuloma with its accompanying sinuses and massive adhesions."

Zimmerman (1969) reported a death from the aspiration of metallic mercury when a nasogastric tube balloon ruptured in the nasopharynx as it was being removed.

Complications Attending Use of Indwelling Gastrointestinal Tubes

Hanselman and Meyer (1962) have published a collective review of this subject which includes a valuable bibliography and full discussion of the various complications and the ways in which they have been managed.

Complications that may attend use of indwelling gastrointestinal tubes in some cases include the following:

Knotting may occur in any tube passed into the intestinal tract. This may cause difficulty in its removal and rarely may require operation for the removal of the tube.

Too great pressure within the balloon of the Miller-Abbott tube may arrest its migration down the intestinal tract, and protracted delay at one place in the bowel may injure that point in the bowel. This can be avoided by periodically deflating and then reinflating the balloon. Twenty to 30 cc of air have usually been found to be a satisfactory amount in the balloon.

In some instances in which a balloon-tipped tube has been permitted to remain in the gastrointestinal tract for longer than 5 days the balloon has absorbed gas from the bowel and become more inflated than was intended. An x-ray examination will reveal this increase in the size of the balloon and it can be appropriately deflated.

Fricke and Niewodowski (1976) recently reported three patients in whom a gastrointestinal tube balloon had unintentionally become overdistended by gas absorbed from the intestinal tract and caused intestinal obstruction. They pointed out that although it has long been known that gas can dissolve in, diffuse through, and evaporate from the surface of rubber, this hazard's association with the use of gastrointestinal balloons has been infrequently mentioned in the literature. Hence physicians are unaware of the potential problem. Using only vented small-intestinal balloons or prophylactically venting the unvented balloon by puncturing it with a 21-gauge needle to allow spontaneous decompression as pressure increases inside the balloon should prevent this problem. "If a balloon inflates, proximal decompression should be attempted before laparotomy is considered."

Infants may develop otitis media owing to obstruction of the eustachian canal if the tube is left too long in place. In one reported case, "this occurred after a Miller-Abbott tube was used for two days and necessitated myringotomy on two occasions before complete recovery" (Hanselman and Meyer, 1962). This apparently is not likely to occur in adults.

Laryngeal edema, cricoid and arytenoid chondritis, vocal chord paralysis, and laryngeal stenosis have each been reported as complications that had occurred occasionally after protracted use of an indwelling gastrointestinal tube. "In practically all of the reported cases, there was evidence that one or more of the following factors were present: diabetes, uremia, advanced cancer, and prolonged use of the tube" (Hanselman and Meyer, 1962).

Laryngeal involvement is a rare but serious complication. Dyspnea develops gradually over a period of days and finally may require tracheostomy. In most instances, signs of laryngeal involvement become manifest after removal of the tube. A number of investigators who have had a large experience with gastrointestinal intubation mention not encountering laryngeal involvement in any of their patients.

Partial or complete intestinal obstruction may occasionally be caused by an inflated balloon. An overdistended intestinal tube balloon or a balloon-induced intussusception has been the most frequent cause of this complication. Coiling, folding, and doubling back do not usually cause serious trouble unless they occur above an already present obstruction or interfere with deflation of the balloon.

If an inflated balloon-tipped tube has passed beyond the stoma of an intestinal anastomosis, it should be deflated before attempting to withdraw it as otherwise traction upon it may tear apart the anastomotic suture line.

Other complications have occasionally developed with the use of the Miller-Abbott tube. In some instances it has passed through the entire length of the intestinal tract, and the tip has extruded from the rectum. On occasions it has progressed through so many coils of intestine that it has been impossible to withdraw it through the nose. In such cases it is advisable to let it continue to progress by intestinal peristalsis and be extruded through the rectum. In a few instances in which this had been intended, the tube did not pass and had to be removed by laparotomy.

Acute angulation of the tube where it emerges from the nostril may produce enough pressure to cause ulceration. Most of these ulcers heal spontaneously, but, in some, septal abscesses with destruction of a portion of the nasal cartilage have occurred.

Deviation of the nasal septum may be a factor in this complication and should be considered before inserting a tube through the nose.

Esophageal damage has been infrequently reported as a significant complication of gastrointestinal intubation. Postmortem findings have shown that small longitudinal superficial ulcerations that had been clinically insignificant are all that usually occur in the esophagus after gastrointestinal intubation with use of the conventional tubes just described. Postmortem ulcerative esophagitis has been an uncommon finding.

Benign esophagitic stricture in the lower third of the esophagus has been reported to occur following prolonged use of an indwelling nasogastric tube. However, many such cases have also had persistent vomiting or a hiatus hernia or both, which may also have been factors in causing reflux esophagitis and the strictures.

Rupture of esophageal varices by gastrointestinal intubation has occurred infrequently, but "the two most frequent causes of gastrointestinal hemorrhage associated with intubation are esophageal varices and stress ulcers" (Hanselman and Meyer, 1962). Rupture of the esophagus is a rare complication of conventional gastrointestinal intubation but has occurred more often with compression tamponade of esophageal varices by a Blakemore-Sengstaken tube. The complications associated with the use of this type of tube are discussed on page 666 of Volume 1.

Some surgeons avoid using a nasogastric tube after esophagogastric anastomosis because of the occasional postmortem finding of an erosion at the site of anastomosis. By substituting gastrostomy in such cases they report an increased recovery rate, greater patient comfort, and decrease in pulmonary complications. Others, however, have experienced major complications with the use of gastrostomy and prefer the use of a nasogastric tube in these cases.

Perforation of a normal stomach by an indwelling nasogastric tube has not been reported, to our knowledge, but in one reported case the tip of a Levin tube was found protruding through a small perforation of an ulcerating carcinoma of the stomach.

Perforations of the small intestine have been reported (Hanselman and Meyer, 1962) under varying circumstances of intubation. In two cases the metal tip of a Miller-Abbott tube perforated the ileum just proximal to a constricting band. In another case, the terminal ileum was perforated at the site of a Miller-Abbott tube balloon in a patient with ulcerative colitis. Pleating of the intestine over a tube may cause ulceration of the mucosa and perforation, particularly if the tube is taped in place with the balloon inflated, or if prolonged traction is applied (12 ounces of traction for 24 hours in one case) in an effort to remove the tube. The presence of a tube in a segment of bowel adjacent to an abscess has also been reported to be a factor in the production of intestinal perforation. It is important to discontinue suction before attempting to remove the tube. Pulling on the tube while suction is being applied has been known to cause perforation of the small bowel.

The tube can double back on itself at any level along the course of upper gastrointestinal tract, and this is most often discovered when radiographic control is used during the intubation process. Obviously, this will prevent advancement of the tube, and kinks, coiling, and folding of the tube in the stomach will prevent its functioning.

Inability to withdraw the tube may be due to knotting of the tube, making it so bulky as to seriously impede or prevent this maneuver. Another cause of this complication is gaseous distention of the balloon. Once an intestinal tube passes the ileocecal junction, its removal may be difficult or impossible without laparotomy, should it fail to pass per rectum. In one case an hourglass constriction of the balloon at the ileocecal junction prevented removal of the tube until its distal portion was ruptured.

In another case, a tear in the bowel with production of a local abscess resulted from trying to remove a tube when the mercury-filled balloon had passed the ileocecal junction. Similar difficulties may occur when a mercury- or air-filled balloon descends below an anastomotic suture line. Passage of a tube around a gastroenterostomy circuit after a Billroth II subtotal gastrectomy has been described in four patients in two of whom operative removal of the tube was necessary.

Inability to remove a tube at the first attempt is seldom a cause for undue concern. Radiographic studies may demonstrate the cause and the necessary corrective procedure. Fluids given orally with the tube clamped may increase intraluminal fluid and facilitate removal of the tube. If removal is still difficult, delay withdrawal for several hours. Repositioning the patient and intermittent gentle traction rather than prolonged steady traction may dislodge the tube with less danger of ischemic necrosis of the bowel wall that might result from the pressure of prolonged steady traction. Giving mineral oil by mouth or through the tube may be helpful by serving as a lubricant.

Cutting the tube in the hope that it will pass through the intestinal tract is occasionally indicated, provided no appreciable degree of intestinal obstruction is present. On the other hand, even if laparotomy should be necessary, there are definite advantages to having control of the proximal end of the tube. Knots may be untied, a bag may be manipulated, or, if distended with gas, it can be decompressed transmurally with a small-caliber needle so that the tube can be removed. Rupture of a distended bag by squeezing the intestine between the surgeon's palms is risky.

Most tubes will eventually pass through a normal intestinal tract. The length of time to allow for a released tube to pass varies with the individual patient, the type of tube, the location of its distal end, and the degree of partial obstruction present. The development of abdominal pain or tenderness may indicate ulceration from the presence of the tube or underlying disease.

Removal of a tube that has descended below a recent anastomosis is a special problem. With the degree of narrowing and the progress of healing of the anastomosis in doubt, even removal of a tube with a completely deflated balloon may be dangerous. Laparotomy is indicated if the tube is not passed per rectum within a reasonable time.

Intestinal tubes have been lost down the gastrointestinal tract inadvertently because of accidental detachment of the metal Y adapter from a Miller-Abbott tube. One patient misinterpreted instructions and swallowed the proximal end of the tube before the distal end appeared at the anus. When obstruction was not present, tubes passed in 4 hours to 18 days, but operative removal has been necessary in some cases.

Fluid and electrolyte imbalance due to loss via the indwelling tube may occur as a complication of gastrointestinal intubation. The two most common deficiencies have been hypokalemia and hyponatremia. Nasogastric suction removes about 11 grams of sodium chloride per 24 hours. If water is permitted by mouth during the nasogastric suction, there is an added loss of one-third to one-half more than when no water is allowed orally. The potential electrolyte depletion varies with the level of the gastrointestinal tract which is being drained most effectively. Fluid and electrolyte requirements of the patient while suction is being used can ordinarily be covered by intravenous administration.

Intussusception caused by the inflated bag acting like a leading point is a rare but serious complication of gastrointestinal intubation. The isoperistaltic type has been far more common than the retrograde type. "Of 20 reported cases of intussusception associated with intubation, death occurred in 3" (Hanselman and Meyer, 1962).

The extent to which the passage and presence of a gastrointestinal tube contribute to serious pulmonary complications is difficult to evaluate. It frequently interferes with ventilation. The presence of such a tube increases the secretion of mucus and, if this is not coughed up, some may be aspirated into the lung and produce atelectasis and bronchopneumonia.

Pulmonary complications directly attributed to intestinal intubation have occurred uncommonly. At least two patients have been reported in whom a mercury-filled intubation bag ruptured, and mercury aspirated into the lungs was demonstrated by chest radiographs. Postural drainage resulted in the passage of large quantities of mercury mixed with mucus. At late follow-up (4 years in one patient) only minute quantities of mercury were revealed by x-ray, and no serious residual effect was noted in either case.

Plugging of the lumen of the tube by gastrointestinal contents or by mucosa sucked into the lumen occurs in almost all cases of suction intubation. This must be checked periodically lest the patient derive no benefits while being subjected to possible complications of intubation.

Hanselman and Meyer's collective review of the literature on complications of gastrointestinal intubation disclosed 530 cases of all degrees of severity beyond the most trivial. There were 43 deaths, a mortality rate of 8 per cent, in patients who had significant complications. Since uncomplicated cases and those with the most trivial complications were not included, the incidence of complications associated with these procedures cannot be stated. In our experience, the incidence of serious complications related to intubation, when all cases in which the procedure was used are considered, is low.

Hanselman and Meyer "were impressed with the relatively few fatal cases, even when other extensive complications were playing a role, and with the effectiveness of surgical intervention in the more serious complications of intestinal intubation." They concluded that "with informed management, intubation is a relatively safe procedure."

It is important to point out that the major complications recorded here have nearly all been related to the use of long gastrointestinal tubes, usually those with balloon tips.

Use of a nasogastric tube for the short period of postoperative gastric decompression has been associated with minor complications of questionable relationship, but rarely with a major complication. When used for a prolonged period, reflux esophagitis with stricture formation may occur as a serious complication.

Comment on Use of Indwelling Gastrointestinal Tubes

Indwelling gastric or gastrointestinal tubes are commonly used before and after gastric or intestinal operations, other abdominal operations, and in intestinal obstruction. After insertion to the appropriate level in the alimentary tract, the indwelling tube may be connected to a suction apparatus for continuous or intermittent suction or its open end may be placed below a water trap to act only as a siphon. Suction is used when obstruction, abdominal distention, or both are present.

Continuous or intermittent suction removes large quantities of fluid and electrolytes from the patient, so care should be taken to replace sufficient fluids and electrolytes, parenterally if necessary, to cover the loss. This is particularly true of chloride and potassium salts. For this reason, for routine postoperative gastric decompression many surgeons prefer to use the indwelling tube for suction only for the first 18 hours after operation, and thereafter as a siphon below a water trap unless obstruction or marked abdominal distention occurs, in which case suction is continued or resumed. (At present, routine use of postoperative gastric decompression is a somewhat controversial subject that will be discussed in a following section.)

Indwelling gastrointestinal tubes have been left in place for varying lengths of time. Ulcers of the esophagus, reflux esophagitis with lower esophageal strictures, and perforations of the intestinal tract have been reported in association with prolonged use of the tubes. Exactly how long it is safe to leave such a tube in place is unknown and probably varies with individual patients. Arbitrarily, it seems advisable not to leave a tube in place for longer than 5 days. If necessary, it may be reinserted. However, tubes left in place for 8 weeks and longer without the occurrence of ulceration or other complications have been reported.

1. Some general guidelines for the use of tubes include: It is important to avoid gastrointestinal intubation if possible in patients with upper respiratory tract infection.

2. Avoid introducing a nasogastric tube through a nostril that is partially obstructed by septal deviation or some other cause.

3. When introducing a gastrointestinal tube, advancing it too rapidly may cause coiling, kinking, knotting, or doubling back. Radiographic observation can be helpful for avoiding or correcting this problem.

4. When a nasally passed tube has been appropriately placed and is taped in position, ensure that the tube is not sharply angulated at its point of exit from the naris. This is uncomfortable for the patient and may erode the nostril.

5. Avoid prolonged use of nasogastric intubation in patients with esophageal varices as the varices may become eroded by pressure and friction from the tube or by reflux of gastric contents.

6. And most importantly, in patients with mechanical and strangulating obstruction, when the blood supply to the bowel is compromised, in tubation must be limited to rapid preparation of the patient for operation and not used for definitive treatment. A tube may relieve symptoms and give a false sense of security. When the blood supply is impaired, delay of operation may be catastrophic.

POSTOPERATIVE GASTRIC DECOMPRESSION

At present there is controversy about whether or not postoperative gastric decompression is a necessary routine after abdominal operations, and whether nasogastric intubation or tube gastrostomy is the better method for establishing postoperative gastric decompression.

These subjects can be discussed with better perspective and sounder reasoning if the experience before postoperative gastric decompression came into use is described, along with an account of its development and mention of the parallel improvement in management of other factors that influence the occurrence of postoperative gastric dilatation and paralytic ileus.

The purpose of postoperative gastric decompression is to evacuate fluid and gas from the upper gastrointestinal tract and thus relieve or prevent its distention. This reduces tension on recent suture lines in the bowel and the abdominal incision, benefits the vascularity and nutrition of the bowel wall, and minimizes elevation of the diaphragm and embarrassment of cardiac and pulmonary function.

Tinckler (1972) has shown that after abdominal operations, gastric tone and motility either decrease or disappear for approximately 24 to 48 hours postoperatively, depending on the nature of the operation, while small bowel tone and movement persist.

Surgeons who were house officers before postoperative gastric decompression came into general use have vivid recollections of acute dilatation of the stomach and paralytic ileus as a common, and also the most lethal, postoperative complication of major abdominal operations. Once it occurred it was usually fatal, as there was no reliably effective treatment. Preventive measures were neither recognized nor available.

During this period the gastrointestinal tube employed by surgeons was the Ewald stomach tube which was inserted through the mouth and was too large to be left indwelling. Surgeons used it most often to lave an acutely dilated stomach with or without associated paralytic ileus. This complication most often became manifest on the second or third day following a major intra-abdominal operation, most commonly one on the biliary tract. Lavage was successful in treating some cases of acute gastric dilation alone but was futile when paralytic ileus was present.

During this period of time, the importance of administering fluids postoperatively was recognized, but little was known about electrolyte balance, and intravenous infusion of fluids and electrolytes was not yet in general use. Postoperative fluids consisted of normal saline or 5 per cent glucose in water or in normal saline, given painfully, less effectively, and in smaller amounts than now, by continuous drip infusion into the subpectoral tissues.

Blood was transfused directly from a vein of the donor into the vein of the recipient, the two people lay side-to-side. The procedure was a major one, performed in a special room, and the volume of blood transfused would be considered useless, or even malpractice, by present-day standards. Blood transfusions were performed infrequently.

Anesthesia was administered by the open drop method; ether was the usual anesthetic.

During this period the mortality rate following operations on the biliary tract was about 15 per cent. The most frequent cause of death was complication by paralytic ileus with or without acute gastric dilatation.

During the same period the mortality rate following resections of the stomach was 25 per cent. In these cases the most frequent cause of death was complication by hemorrhage or leakage from the anastomotic suture line (closed "aseptic" anastomoses were being used then). Acute gastric dilatation and paralytic ileus rarely occurred as a postoperative complication following resections of the stomach.

Differences in postoperative care between these two types of operation probably contributed to the difference in the incidence of postoperative gastric dilatation and paralytic ileus, and in the types of postoperative complications that were the most frequent cause of death.

At that period of time, patients who had undergone operations on the biliary tract, or other abdominal operations in which no alimentary tract anastomosis was performed, were permitted water by mouth as soon after operation as they were fully conscious and postanesthetic nausea and vomiting had ceased. If the patients were free of nausea and vomiting on the morning after operation, fruit juices, hot chocolate, and tea and coffee with or without cream and sugar were added to their oral intake.

On the second postoperative morning, the resident surgeons on their rounds often found the patient apathetic and lying in bed with the tell-tale brown stain of regurgitated stomach contents soiling the pillow in the area nearest to the patient's mouth. There was no active vomiting, abdominal cramps, nor audible peristaltic sounds heard on auscultation, but there was visible upper abdominal fullness and distention.

The customary routine was to pass an Ewald tube into the stomach. This usually evacuated more than a liter of brown gastric contents, indicating the presence of a dilated stomach. The tube was left in place and through it the stomach was lavaged by alternately filling it with and siphoning off tap water or normal saline until the siphonage was clear and colorless. This often required an hour and a half of continuous lavage. Then 2 ounces of castor oil were injected through the tube into the stomach and left to stimulate peristalsis. The tube was then removed (indwelling nasogastric tubes were not available then). Often the castor oil was vomited without having had the desired effect. This method of treatment was frequently successful in patients with only gastric dilatation but failed when paralytic ileus was present. The latter condition was almost invariably fatal as there was no effective method for its treatment.

On the other hand, patients who had undergone resections of the stomach or other operations that required gastrointestinal anastomoses were forbidden oral ingestion of water or any other fluid or food for the first 3 to 5 postoperative days. Fluids and some calories were provided by subpectoral infusions, as noted. Occasionally, additional amounts of glucose and saline were instilled into the rectum through an indwelling rectal tube (proctoclysis).

On the fourth or fifth postoperative day the patient was first permitted to drink water, beginning in amounts of 1 teaspoonful an hour, increasing very slowly on a meticulously planned and rigidly enforced schedule over a period of 14 days. Nutrient fluids were permitted about the sixth postoperative day and then, in restricted amounts, soft diet about the 10th day and selected solids about the 14th postoperative day. During this period infusions of saline and glucose into the subpectoral tissues or the soft tissues in the thigh were continued until the oral intake seemed adequate.

Patients on this regimen seldom developed gastric dilatation or paralytic ileus unless intestinal obstruction or peritonitis occurred. This difference between the two groups was striking.

Levin introduced his nasoduodenal tube in 1921, but for the first 10 years it was used almost exclusively by physicians for examining and analyzing duodenal secretions as a diagnostic procedure. In 1924 Matas, of New Orleans, advocated general use of siphonage drainage of the stomach in postoperative treatment and in any condition accompanied by gastric and intestinal paresis. In 1925 Ward, of San Francisco, originated continuous suction aspiration of duodenal tubes. In 1932 Paine and Wangensteen introduced gastric suction by nasal catheter as an adjunct in postoperative treatment and showed the excellent prophylaxis it affords against distention of the gastrointestinal tract, provided it is instituted before the distention has progressed to an extreme degree.

During subsequent years postoperative gastric decompression by use of a nasogastric tube has been used extensively after major abdominal operations. Many surgeons use it routinely after all operations on the gastrointestinal and biliary tracts, some use it routinely after all major abdominal operations, and others use it as a postoperative prophylactic routine only in cases selected because of certain anticipated postoperative abdominal complications and as a method of therapy in patients who have developed certain postoperative abdominal complications.

The method has proved extremely useful and generally its use is simple and safe. Certainly any deaths or major complications directly related to the use of the nasogastric tube for postoperative gastric decompression must be very rare. The presence of a nasogastric tube does cause patients to complain of some subjective discomfort, the degree of which varies in different patients. Complications such as pharyngitis, irritation of the nasal septum, sinusitis, otitis media, and pneumonitis have occurred occasionally but usually cleared up rapidly after removal of the tube. However several reports by others have pointed out the disadvantages of nasogastric suction as a method for postoperative gastric decompression and listed the frequent minor and occasional major complications associated with its use. For these reasons, the decision about in which circumstances to use a nasogastric tube is highly variable.

In 1956 Farris and Smith recommended the use of temporary tube gastrostomy as a substitute for nasogastric suction in providing postoperative gastric decompression. Its claimed advantages were that it obviated the disadvantages and complications of nasogastric suction. Tube gastrostomy became widely used and has proved to be effective for postoperative gastric decompression with the primary advantage of eliminating the need for an indwelling nasogastric tube. However, its use has also been associated with frequent minor and sometimes major or even fatal complications.

Sawyers commented, "We had four fatalities in the Nashville area that have occurred following a tube gastrostomy.... Three of these patients died of peritonitis from leaks around the tube and one patient died of cardiac arrest following reoperation to suture the gastrostomy opening which had failed to close spontaneously." Other similar examples of deaths following use of a tube gastrostomy for routine postoperative gastric decompression have been reported, the principal cause being death from peritonitis, due to leaks around the tube.

Herrington (1965) wrote, "Indeed, the significant complication rate [of tube gastrostomy] has been shown to exceed that of simple nasogastric suction. Complications such as persistent fistula, abdominal abscess, massive bleeding, intraperitoneal leakage with peritonitis or obstruction, wound infection, and nonfunction of the tube have been recorded frequently. Several reports have cited a nonfatal complication rate varying from 5 to 15 per cent with temporary gastrostomy, and the fatality rate due directly to complications after gastrostomy has been recorded as high as 6 per cent . . . at least one death has occurred in practically every institution that has practiced the method." The high incidence of major and fatal complications occurred regardless of the technique used for constructing the tube gastrostomy, so the procedure itself, rather than the method used in its construction, was at fault.

As a result of these experiences, the former enthusiasm for the tube gastrostomy method of postoperative gastric decompression has waned, and it is no longer widely used routinely for this purpose. Nasogastric intubation is simpler, safer, and preferable for postoperative gastric decompression in routine cases.

However, temporary tube gastrostomy can be valuable and may be indicated in some cases such as in the postoperative patient requiring gastric decompression who has esophageal or respiratory problems; also in selected cases of severe thoracoabdominal trauma, in certain major pediatric surgical problems, and in patients requiring prolonged intubation.

In 1955, 1958, and 1963, Gerber and his associates published reports that opposed the then prevailing concept that the routine use of postoperative gastric decompression was essential for patient recovery following operations on the upper gastrointestinal tract. The method had been overused, they stated and its routine use was not only unnecessary but also contributed complications of its own, some of which were of significant degree. They argued that paralytic ileus should not be considered a complication or a disease but rather a physiologic response to operative trauma and that a nasogastric tube did nothing to stimulate peristalsis, which usually does not resume until 48 to 72 hours postoperatively. Also, they pointed out that although nasogastric suction did remove the swallowed salivary secretions and gastric juice, which was beneficial in a patient with gastric outlet obstruction, the removal of these contents was detrimental to patients with a properly functioning gastric outlet because it complicated the postoperative maintenance of fluid and electrolyte balance.

Nasogastric and gastrostomy suction were devised to prevent or alleviate abdominal distention. Gerber (1963) believes that suction tubes accomplish this chiefly by removal of swallowed air from the stomach. He pointed out that "it has been shown that important amounts of air are swallowed only with deglutition. Thus gaseous distention is most easily prevented by maintaining parenteral feedings postoperatively and administering nothing orally. If oral intake is withheld until the patient is hungry or passing flatus and peristalsis is audible, suction decompression will not be necessary. This statement is based upon a series of more than 2000 operations, personally observed, in which no form of gastrointestinal decompression was utilized postoperatively." The stated advantages of treating postoperative patients without using gastric suction were that such patients will require less house staff and nursing care, will need 1000 ml. less fluid intravenously per day, will have fewer pulmonary complications, and will be immeasurably more comfortable.

Other surgeons have also questioned the value of any form of gastrointestinal decompression following abdominal operations.

Eade, Metheny, and Lundmark (1955) pointed out some of the more serious complications of nasogastric suction. In 143 consecutive cases of major abdominal surgery, they had not used suction at all in 130. (No mention was made as to whether or not a nasogastric tube was used for prophylactic siphonage.) "These patients were instructed not to swallow anything and were given nothing by mouth until flatus was passed by rectum. There was no mortality. No adverse effects were seen. The tube was inserted without hesitation if indications appeared. This happened in two of the 143 cases."

They concluded that postoperative nasogastric suction after gastrointestinal surgery should be used only when specific indications exist.

In 1962 Hendry, in England, presented evidence that postoperative gastric decompression was unnecessary following partial gastric resection or vagotomy with a drainage procedure. He reported two series of patients who were operated upon between 1947 and 1962. One series comprised 114 cases of Billroth I partial gastrectomy for duodenal and/or lesser curvature ulceration. The other series comprised 118 cases of vagotomy and Finney pyloroplasty for similar lesions.

The postoperative regimen was the same in both series of cases. (I) No nasogastric intubation and no intravenous or other parenteral fluid was used. (2) No antibiotic therapy was used except for special indications. (3) After full recovery from anesthesia, the following strict progressive fluid regimen was begun: 28 ml. of water orally per hour in the first 24 hours, and double the quantity of water per oram each succeeding 24 hour period until the fifth, when a soft diet was commenced.

The regimen failed in four patients who developed temporary gastric discomfort and moderate distention, which necessitated the insertion of a nasogastric tube.

In 1964 and thereafter (1965, 1967a and b, 1972), Herrington and his colleagues published a series of reports on their experience with the omission of routine use of postoperative gastric decompression following operations on the stomach. The most recent report was on their accumulated 8-year experience with a personal series of 904 patients who underwent vagotomy-pyloroplasty for gastroduodenal ulcer in which routine postoperative nasogastric suction was not employed.

Of these, 815 patients had an elective operation and 89 had an emergency operation. Among the 815 elective cases, 62 patients (7.6 per cent) required postoperative suction. Among the 89 emergency cases, 56 patients (63 per cent) required decompression during the postoperative period.

The 62 patients who required decompression after elective operation were those who presented difficult technical problems that suggested the possible development of postoperative anastomotic leakage or duodenal stump blowout. Also, a few in this group developed postoperative abdominal distention or nausea and vomiting which required reinsertion of the nasogastric tube.

Of the 89 emergency cases, over half required postoperative gastric decompression. Most of these patients initially presented bleeding or acute perforation, and the gastrointestinal tract was filled with blood, or the peritoneal cavity was flooded with gastric contents. Such patients invariably develop profound ileus with abdominal distention as a complication if suction is omitted. This is also more likely to occur in large obese individuals who have undergone a rather long period of anesthesia and a difficult technical procedure. In some of the emergency procedures, the findings at operation and the technical maneuvers posed no particular problem, so postoperative decompression was deemed unnecessary. A few patients bled from suture lines while still in the recovery room, and this complication postponed early removal of the nasogastric tube.

Herrington (1972) stated that "if the operation is uncomplicated and progresses smoothly, the nasogastric tube may be removed 8 to 12 hours following operation. The patient is then maintained on parenteral fluids with no oral intake for 72 hours. We have not elected to start oral alimentation after the first 24 postoperative hours as advocated by some surgeons. . . . We have not been impressed by the shorter hospital stay among patients in whom we have omitted postoperative decompression" as has been reported by others.

Herrington concluded that "postoperative decompression was unnecessary as a routine measure and that definite indications should exist to justify its use. . . . There are circumstances, however, in which nasogastric suction is both necessary and vital, and it should not be withheld. The use or non-use of the nasogastric tube should be governed by the judgment and experience of the surgeon. The aphorism of David Sprong regarding use of the nasogastric tube should be cited: Avoid routinely using decompression and avoid routinely not using decompression."

It should be pointed out that Herrington and associates did not advocate omitting use of a nasogastric tube entirely. In these operations (vagotomy with pyloroplasty), they routinely inserted a nasogastric tube at operation and left it in place on suction for the first 12 hours, more or less, and then if the indications were satisfactory the tube was removed. If indicated, the tube was left in as long as seemed desirable. They disagree with those who advocate routinely leaving the nasogastric tube in place for 5 to 10 days just because vagotomy has been performed and despite absence of indications for its prolonged use (1976).

They (1972) also emphasized that "it is imperative that patients managed postoperatively without decompression be examined frequently by a competent observer. Should abdominal complications occur, for they are inevitable in a few cases, nasogastric suction should be instituted immediately. In hospitals where a competent house staff is not available, it is much safer to leave the indwelling nasogastric tube in place for 48 to 72 hours following operation."

In summary, it is generally agreed that postoperative gastric decompression is unnecessary in many patients who have undergone major abdominal operations, but that in some of these patients it is both necessary and vital. Even at conclusion of the operation it is impossible always to predict accurately in which cases it will be, or become, essential and in which it will not.

Past experience has shown that the postoperative complications of acute gastric dilatation or abdominal distention are easier to prevent than to treat after they have developed.

There are differences of opinion about (1) whether or not it is advisable to use postoperative gastric decompression routinely for prophylaxis after major abdominal operations; (2) the choice of method (nasogastric tube or tube gastrostomy) for gastric decompression; and (3) the technic and management of each of these methods.

Some surgeons advocate and use postoperative gastric decompression, at least temporarily, as a routine after practically all major abdominal operations, particularly operations on the alimentary tract, the biliary tract, obese patients, and patients with intra-abdominal injury and/or hemorrhage, and after repairs of large hernias when it is important to prevent abdominal distention.

It is generally agreed that nasogastric intubation is simpler, safer, and preferable for postoperative gastric decompression in routine cases than tube gastrostomy, which is reserved for selected cases.

Routine Postoperative Nasogastric Intubation

Surgeons who use nasogastric intubation as a rule in routine cases usually have the anesthesiologist insert the tube during the operation while the patient is under anesthesia. The tube can be guided into the stomach and appropriately placed under direct observation. This minimizes kinking or doubling back on the tube, or damage to an anastomosis through which it may be passed and permits placement of its tip at the site of election. The tube can be inserted more easily and satisfactorily at this time than later when the patient is conscious, and it spares an already miserable, conscious patient the additional misery of undergoing blind insertion of a nasogastric tube, which may require repeated attempts before success is attained.

"It is vastly preferable to insert a nasogastric tube under controlled conditions in the operating room in anticipation of its need than to insert it in the early postoperative period after the patient has become distended and is vomiting" (Sanders, 1963). Furthermore, it is far easier to remove a tube found to be unnecessary than to insert one when a need for it has arisen.

When a nasogastric tube has been left indwelling following operation many surgeons leave it in place, attached to suction, until the following day, in order to remove salivary and gastric secretions and old blood that may have resulted from the operative manipulations, and to detect the presence of fresh blood should postoperative hemorrhage occur. Then, if conditions are satisfactory, some remove the tube. On the first postoperative day we prefer to discontinue the suction if there is no distention but to leave the tube in place as a siphon for another 24 hours. If evidence of abdominal distention occurs, suction is resumed. Fluids and electrolytes are given intravenously as long as the nasogastric tube remains in place.

When no distention is present the tube is left in place without suction, as a siphon, until the siphonage is watery, clear, and scant and until peristalsis is audible or flatus has been passed spontaneously. This usually occurs between the second and fifth postoperative day. Then the tube is removed, and oral intake is commenced, beginning with small amounts of water and progressing as tolerated. Use of a nasogastric tube for this short period of time has rarely caused any serious complication.

Many of us have used this or a similar regimen for many years without having encountered any serious complications related to use of the nasogastric tube.

The presence of a nasogastric tube is uncomfortable to the patient, but not intolerably so, and is not as distressing as the vomiting and distention which may occur in the absence of a tube. Patients have requested return of the tube when vomiting or distention has occurred following its premature removal. Omitting use of a nasogastric tube or removing it too early has been regretted more often than has use of the tube until audible peristalses or passing of flatus occurs.

OMISSION OF ROUTINE POSTOPERATIVE GASTRIC INTUBATION

Recently a number of surgeons have advocated and are practicing omission of routine gastric decompression following most major abdominal operations. They have demonstrated that after most such procedures done electively the patients have recovered uneventfully without gastric decompression having been required. In those who developed complications a nasogastric tube was inserted then with satisfactory results.

When the operations were emergencies, more than half of such patients required gastric intubation.

Hence, these surgeons advocate utilizing postoperative nasogastric intubation not as a postoperative routine, but only when faced with certain real or anticipated postoperative abdominal complications.

"The omission of routine postoperative gastric decompression is based on the concept that paralytic ileus is a physiologic response and gastric siphonage accomplishes little in recovering the normal 8 liters of fluid that traverse the gastrointestinal tract every 24 hours. If nausea, vomiting, or abdominal distention occurs, a normal physiologic response is not represented and suction is immediately indicated in such circumstances.... The success of the method of eliminating postoperative decompression *depends upon permitting absolutely nothing by mouth for the first 72 hours* postoperatively. After this time peristalsis is usually audible, and some patients will have passed flatus" (Herrington, 1965).

It is important to point out again that at least some surgeons who advocate omission of routine postoperative gastric decompression do insert a nasogastric tube more or less routinely, during the operation and leave it in place on trial for the first 8 to 12 postoperative hours and then remove it if gastric decompression seems unnecessary.

It is important also that patients managed postoperatively without decompression be examined frequently by a competent observer. Should abdominal complications occur, nasogastric suction should be started immediately. "In hospitals where a competent house staff is not available, it is much safer to leave the indwelling nasogastric tube in place for 48 to 72 hours following operation" (Herrington, 1972).

A summary of these arguments seems to justify the conclusions that:

1. Routine postoperative gastric decompression has been overused.

2. Its use is not vitally necessary after all major abdominal operations.

3. Many such cases will do well without its use.

4. It is impossible to predict always in which cases it will be required and in which it will not.

5. Patients managed postoperatively without decompression must be examined frequently. Should complications occur, nasogastric suction should be started immediately.

6. In hospitals where a competent house staff is not available it is safer to leave an indwelling nasogastric tube in place for 48 to 72 hours following operation.

7. The only benefits to the patient of omitting postoperative decompression are fewer minor respiratory complications and less patient discomfort.

8. David Sprong's aphorism — "Avoid routinely using postoperative decompression and avoid routinely not using it" — is sound advice.

Chapter 4

GASTROSCOPY AND PERITONEOSCOPY

PERORAL GASTROSCOPY

Gastroscopy is the direct examination of the interior of the stomach through a gastroscope. The procedure was first attempted in 1868 by Kussmaul, who introduced an open tube into the gullet, using as illumination the reflected light of a gasoline lamp. It was first performed successfully by Mikulicz in 1881. The early gastroscopes were rigid, open-end metal tubes with a light at either end, which were passed down the esophagus into the stomach where, by awkward manipulations, they could be passed distally far enough to visualize the pylorus and a short distance of the duodenum. However, the visual field was restricted, establishment of a diagnosis was not dependable, and the incidence of perforation of a viscus was higher than desirable.

The rigid gastroscopes were superseded by the "flexible" gastroscope (Wolf-Schindler type), which is a closed tube containing 48 to 51 lenses. The proximal part of the instrument is rigid, and the distal part is flexible. The essential difference between this gastroscope and its predecessors is that it can be bent to a considerable degree in any direction without interfering with the visual field because of its series of convex lenses so arranged that the image is not distorted on moderate flexion of the tube. This permitted wider visualization of the lining of the stomach, but still only four-fifths of the stomach could be seen. The lesser curvature near the cardia and above the pylorus, the fornix above the cardia, and the pylorus were difficult or impossible to visualize. However, this instrument made gastroscopy more reliable for diagnosis and a safer procedure.

Schindler (1935) found that in 22,351 examinations with this gastroscope there was one fatal perforation of the esophagus, eight perforations of the stomach (all recovered), and one perforation of the jejunum in a patient whose stomach had been resected (this patient recovered). The chief dangers of gastroscopy in experienced hands were those attending anesthesia. The chief difficulties encountered were due to physical deformities or congenital anomalies. Gastrophotographic examination had not come into extensive use because adequate methods had not been developed.

Gastroscopy increased in popularity with gastroenterologists, but surgeons remained skeptical of its value as a diagnostic procedure because of its potential hazards and the frequency of its failure to establish the diagnosis.

In 1958 Hirschowitz and associates introduced the fiberscope for upper gastrointestinal endoscopic examination. The lumen is coated with glass or plastic fibers having special optical properties. Subsequent technical advances and increased experience have made it possible now to use the fiberscope diagnostically or therapeutically in the esophagus (see Chapter 3, Esophagoscopy, in Vol. 1), stomach, duodenum, biliary tree, and pancreatic duct. All these can be examined at one sitting by use of a flexible fiberoptic esophagogastroduodenoscope. Several models are available, but the instrument which is now widely used for endoscoping the upper gastrointestinal tract is the end-viewing, closed, 100-cm. Olympus esophagogastroduodenoscope (model GIF-D) which is equipped with channels for biopsy and irrigation, suction, air inflation, and lens washing. It also has four-directional controls by which its flexible tip can be moved 150 degrees up or down, as well as 100 degrees to either the right or left. Illumination is by a cold light supply which provides a magnified, well-illuminated field of vision without transmission of heat. A 35-mm. medical camera linked with the light supply permits direct viewing with automatic exposure when it is attached to the eyepiece of the fiberscope. Attachment of a fiberoptic side-arm viewing endoscope allows an additional person to observe equally well without interrupting the procedure.

Flexible fiberoptic upper gastrointestinal endoscopes have superseded the Wolf-Schindler type of "flexible" gastroscope because they have made the procedure much simpler, safer, and easier for both the examiner and the patient. The illumination is far brighter, color photography can be done through the endoscope at will and without interrupting the procedure, and visualization is magnified. Perforation of a viscus is less likely. The technic is simpler. It causes little discomfort so requires less anesthesia and is better tolerated by the patient who is therefore more willing to undergo repeated gastroscopies when they are indicated. The fiberoptic endoscope is flexible enough to negotiate the length of a tortuous esophagus that is too curvaceous for passage of a rigid endoscope, and it can be passed the full length of the stomach into the duodenum. Biopsies of suspected areas can be made, polypoid lesions can be removed, the ampulla of Vater can be catheterized, and irrigation and insufflation can be performed through an esophagogastroduodenoscope.

An esophageal stricture can be dilated by passing the Eder-Puestow spring-tipped wire through the strictured area via the biopsy channel of the endoscope with or without the help of fluoroscopy. The endoscope is then withdrawn so that serially graded, olive-shaped metal dilators can be passed over the wire to dilate the stricture. Chung and associates (1976) prefer to dilate esophageal strictures by inserting a fiberoptic endoscope into the esophagus and then passing woven silk bougies alongside the endoscope under direct observation so that the process can be observed in detail. The technic provides a better view of the procedure, and splitting of the mucosa covering the entrance of the stricture can be seen as a warning against attempting further dilation at this time. They reported 16 patients whose esophageal strictures were successfully dilated by this method.

As a result of these advantages, and its demonstrated value in the diagnosis and treatment of gastric disorders, fiberoptic gastroscopy is now widely accepted and used.

Dent (1973) published a timely commentary, "The Surgeon and Fiberoptic Endoscopy," that merits being called to your attention.

"Much of the development and use of these diagnostic instruments has been by nonsurgeons. Busy gastrointestinal surgeons have welcomed and encouraged the use of these instruments by internists and gastroenterologists seeking to make more accurate diagnoses of gastrointestinal lesions.

The emphasis in the use of gastrointestinal fibroscopes is now shifting from diagnosis to therapy. Electrocautery is being used through these instruments to remove polyps and to coagulate bleeding areas.

The increasing importance of fiberoptic endoscopy in the diagnosis and ... treatment of many gastrointestinal diseases behooves surgeons operating upon the gastrointestinal tract to become more interested in and familiar with the use of these instruments. He may ultimately be required to operate on these patients and first-hand knowledge of the appearance of the lesion, pliability of the tissue, and source of the biopsy may be critical in the operative management of patients with these lesions. . . .

As fiberoptic endoscopic capabilities widen to include therapeutic as well as diagnostic measures, the need for involvement of the gastrointestinal surgeon is increased. The timid biopsy, the overzealous electrocoagulation, and the inevitable time lost in the recognition and treatment of endoscopic complications can be avoided or diminished by participation of a gastrointestinal surgeon in fiberoptic endoscopic procedures of the gastrointestinal tract."

Except for use in diagnosis of acute upper gastrointestinal hemorrhage, gastroscopy should not be done until after a radiologic study of the esophagus, stomach, and duodenum has been made with the aid of a barium swallow. It is important to know whether the status of the esophagus will permit a gastroscope to pass through uneventfully and safely, or whether abnormalities may be present, which alert the endoscopist to take special precautions. It is helpful to have information as to what specifically to look for during the examination, or what situations might contraindicate endoscopy.

The x-ray study of the stomach may discover abnormalities that might be missed if the endoscopist were not alerted to their presence. Study of the duodenum may reveal an unsuspected abnormality which makes desirable advancing the gastroscope into the duodenum for direct inspection.

Abnormalities of the esophagus that require special precautions when passing an endoscope are diverticula, the lumen of which may be confused with that of the esophagus and entered into by the endoscope, thus perforating the diverticulum. Carcinoma or stricture of the esophagus may obstruct the lumen of that organ too much to permit passage of the gastroscope, but esophagoscopy to determine its nature by inspection and biopsy is indicated in either case.

The history and presence of varices that have bled but presently are not bleeding call for special precautions during gastroscopy and, in some cases, are a contraindication for the procedure because of the danger of restarting the bleeding. The presence of an aneurysm of the aortic arch adjacent to the esophagus contraindicates gastroscopy. Severe cardiac decompensation is another contraindication unless an endotracheal tube is in place to secure an airway. Furthermore, gastroscopy may be contraindicated in an uncooperative, combative, or psychotic patient, unless it is performed under general anesthesia, for fear of damage to both the patient and the expensive, delicate instrument by the patient's violent movements.

Esophagogastroduodenoscopy (EGD)

INDICATIONS AND CONTRAINDICATIONS

Fiberoptic esophagogastroduodenoscopy is an effective method for evaluating the mucosal surface in three-dimensional anatomy of the upper gastrointestinal tract to the level of the third portion of the duodenum. This procedure can be performed with few contraindications, all of which are relative. The list in Table 4–1 is to be used as a set of guidelines and not as a simple checklist for exclusion.

Indications *for* upper gastrointestinal endoscopy, given in Table 4–2, are divided into emergency and elective, each of which is subdivided into diagnostic and therapeutic needs. These indications can be considered as exemplary and not exhaustive.

With the use of the upper gastrointestinal tract endoscope the physician can inspect the esophagus, stomach and duodenum; aspirate secretions for study; biopsy and brush the mucosa; coagulate bleeding sites, using electrocautery or topical anticoagulants; pass cannulas into the biliary tree and pancreatic duct for purposes of radiographic visualization; and perform endoscopic sphincterotomy of the ampulla of Vater. The use of upper tract endoscopy results in clinically accurate assessment of the upper gastrointestinal tract in 95 per cent of studies. This figure has been repeatedly documented (Belber, 1971; Allen, Block, and Schuman, 1973; Cotton, 1975). A recent report (Martin and associates, 1980) suggests not only that endoscopy is diagnostically superior to contrast radiology of the upper gastrointestinal tract but also that the accuracy of endoscopy is not influenced by prior knowledge of the radiographic studies. Furthermore, interobserver discordance among experienced endoscopists has been found to be only 2 to 4 per cent.

PREPARATION AND PROCEDURE

For upper tract endoscopy, the patient should have nothing by mouth for at least

Table 4–1. Relative Contraindications for Gastrointestinal Tract Endoscopy

Subluxation of atlanto-occipital joint
Hypopharyngeal or esophageal diverticula
Perforated esophagus, stomach, or duodenum
Recent upper abdominal surgery
Recent or concurrent myocardial infarction
Severe bleeding diathesis
Critically ill patients for whom no therapeutic use is intended and increased diagnostic information will not have clinical use
Extremely uncooperative patients

PERORAL GASTROSCOPY

Table 4-2. Indications for Upper Gastrointestinal Tract Endoscopy

Emergency
Diagnostic
   Acute upper gastrointestinal bleeding
   Esophageal pain in immunosuppressed patients
Therapeutic
   Treatment of upper gastrointestinal bleeding
      Electrocautery
      Topical coagulants
      Laser
   Removal of foreign bodies
   Cautery of Mallory-Weiss lesion
   Sclerosis of esophageal varices

Elective
Diagnostic
   Evaluation of chronic gastrointestinal blood loss
   Evaluation of abdominal and chest pain
   Evaluation of esophageal and gastric lesions found by contrast studies
   Evaluation of upper gastrointestinal symptoms preceding and/or following upper tract surgery
   Evaluation of the mucosa by histologic and cytopathologic studies
   Evaluation of pancreatic and biliary tract disease
Therapeutic
   Removal of polyps
   Removal of foreign bodies
   Removal of surgical sutures
   Dilatation of esophageal strictures
   Enlargement of the stoma in postoperative gastroenterostomy patients
   Mechanical dissolution of gastric bezoars
   Endoscopic sphincterotomy and common duct stone removal

6 to 8 hours prior to the procedure, except for those with achalasia, gastric bezoar, gastric outlet obstruction, or acute upper gastrointestinal hemorrhage in whom a longer period of fasting or lavage with a nasogastric tube or both is necessary to clear the stomach or esophagus. Patients for elective study are given meperidine, 50 to 100 mg. intramuscularly, and atropine, 0.3 to 1 mg. intramuscularly, 1 hour prior to the procedure. Just prior to the procedure the patient drinks 30 ml. of Mylicon. Following this, the oropharynx is topically anesthetized using 4 per cent Xylocaine or Cetacaine spray. At this point the patient is placed in the left lateral decubitus position with the knees flexed (Fig. 4-1). Five to 40 mg. of diazepam are administered intravenously to bring the patient almost to sleep. Additional amounts of diazepam may be given during the procedure to maintain sedation. The total dose of diazepam should not exceed 50 mg.

The tip of the endoscope is lubricated with warm water, and the endoscopist places the endoscope in the patient's mouth, holding the endoscope tip with the first and second fingers. Using these fingers as a guide, the endoscopist advances the endoscope into the posterior pharynx and directs the tip downward toward the esophagus.

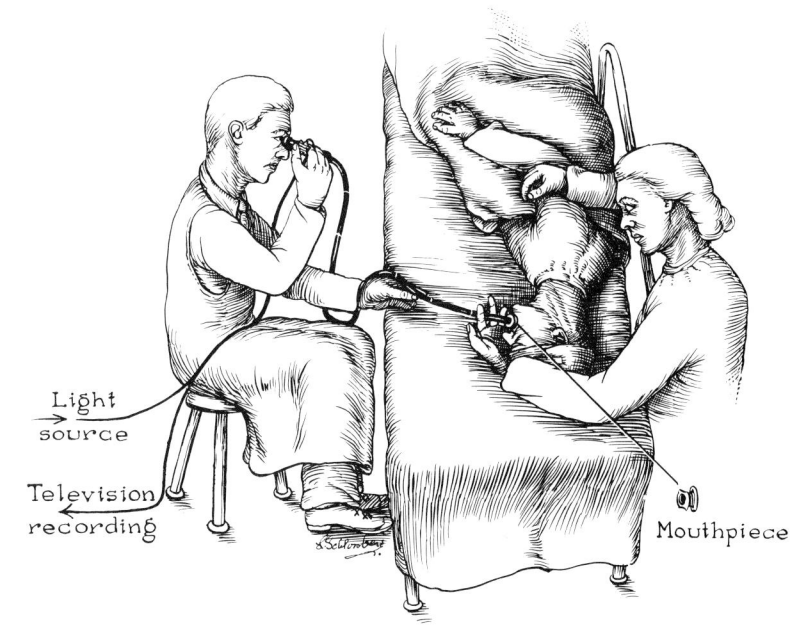

Figure 4-1. Upper gastrointestinal fiberendoscopic examination. Illustrated are positions of patient on table and of endoscopist and assistant in the technic.

The patient is asked to swallow, and, with the act of swallowing, the endoscope is gently advanced beyond the upper esophageal sphincter into the upper esophagus. If the patient is unable to swallow, the endoscope may be passed with direct visualization. This is accomplished by first placing a bite piece into the patient's mouth and then passing the tip of the endoscope through the aperture in the bite piece. The esophageal opening is located anterior to the epiglottis and with gentle insufflation of air can be readily visualized. The endoscope is passed into the upper esophagus when the cricopharyngeus muscle relaxes. In certain instances, when the patient will not swallow the endoscope and when the endoscope cannot be passed with direct visualization, a No. 48 F. Maloney dilator is lubricated and passed into the esophagus. The endoscope is then placed into the posterior pharynx, and the dilator is slowly withdrawn as the endoscope is advanced over it into the esophagus.

Once into the esophagus, the endoscope can be passed readily into the stomach, which is then expanded using insufflated air. The endoscope's flexibility will allow it to move easily along the floor of the greater curvature into the antrum. The pylorus appears as a small hole in the distal antrum with sphincteric motion. By means of the controls, the endoscope can be directed toward and through this opening into the duodenal bulb. Once in the duodenal bulb the endoscope is directed downward and sharply to the right, which carries it naturally into the first portion of the duodenum. There only modest air insufflation is used as duodenal expansion causes a degree of patient discomfort. The entire upper tract can be inspected carefully during the withdrawal, which usually results in visualization superior to that obtained during the passage of the endoscope. When the tip of the endoscope is at the level of the incisura angularis, the endoscope may be retroflexed to provide a view of the fundus, cardia, and gastroesophageal junction. At any time during the procedure brushing, biopsy, electrocautery, polypectomy, or foreign body removal can be accomplished. Examples of the types of lesions seen on upper tract endoscopy are included in Figure 4–2 for reference.

Upon removal of the endoscope the patient's vital signs are checked and he or she is allowed to sleep comfortably until the effect of the diazepam wears off. This usually takes 60 to 90 minutes. Patients usually report no ill effects other than mild sore throat.

Duodenoscopy

The duodenum may be inspected using either the end-viewing (Olympus GIF-D) or side-viewing (Olympus JF-B) endoscopes (Fig. 4–3). The end-viewing instrument presents a greater depth of field to the endoscopist and provides greater maneuverability in performing biopsies and polypectomies; the lens is less likely to become obscured by blood. Therefore, it is most helpful in identifying bleeding sites and in performing biopsies of tumors or polyps in the duodenum.

The side-viewing instrument was designed specifically to visualize the papilla of Vater, but it also allows more careful inspection of the mucosa, including villous detail, and can be retroflexed within the duodenum for inspection of the proximal bulb. To detect the papilla of Vater, the endoscope is passed into the second portion of the duodenum, and the lumen is adequately distended with air. The patient should receive glucagon, 1 to 2 mg. intravenously, to reduce peristalsis in the duodenum. The papilla is usually identified at about 9 o'clock in the viewing field and appears as a moundlike structure often at the distal end of a fold called the plica longitudinalis, which runs at right angles to the usual circular pattern of the valvulae conniventes. In about 20 per cent of patients, the papilla is flat and can be difficult to identify. Once the papilla has been identified, the instrument is positioned so that it lies at 90 degrees to the opening of the papilla.

The cannula is then carefully advanced into the ampulla, using both the distal tip directional lever and the rising lever of the cannula for control. Once the tip of the cannula is engaged in the ampulla, it can be advanced perpendicularly into the pancreatic duct or in a cephalad direction into the common bile duct. After the cannula is in place, Renografin-60 is injected into its proximal end via a 30-ml. syringe, using

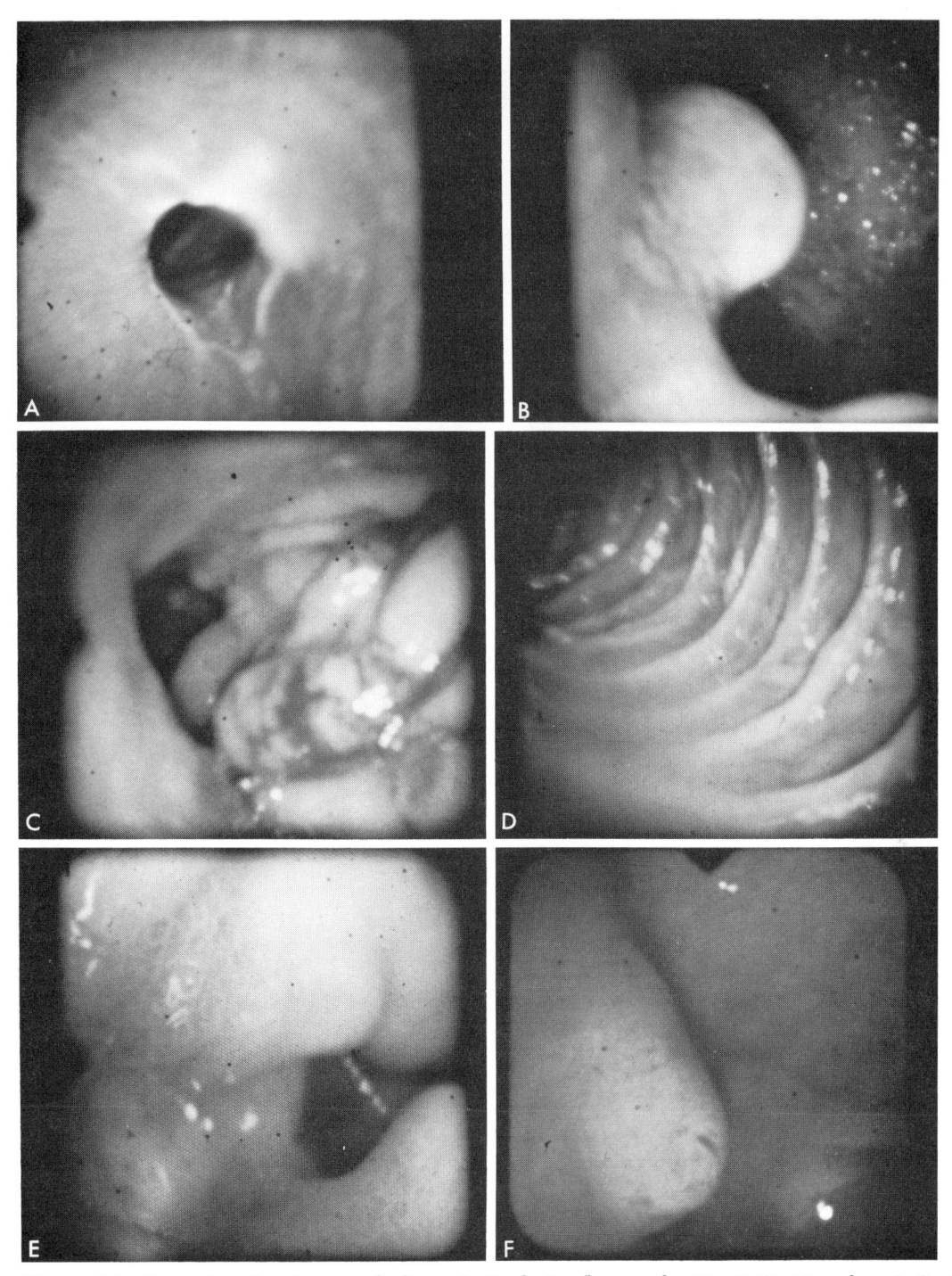

Figure 4–2. Examples of endoscopic findings. *A*, Grade 2 reflux esophagitis. *B*, Gastric polyp. *C*, Gastric cancer. *D*, Normal duodenum. *E*, Duodenal ulcer. *F*, Normal-appearing ampulla of Vater.

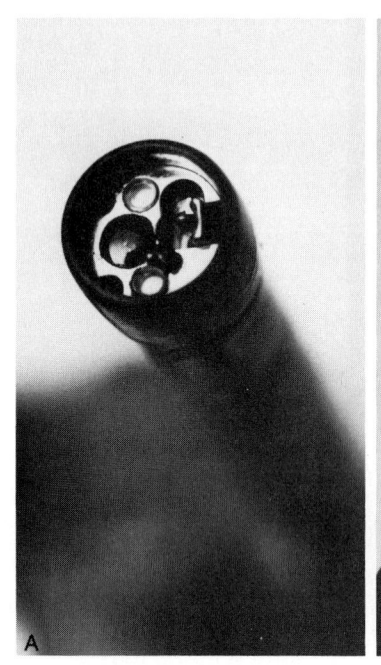

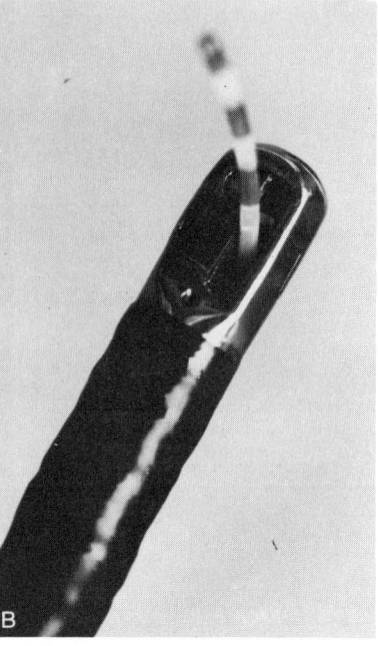

Figure 4–3. *A*, End-viewing duodenoscope, with viewpoints of the port, 2 light ports, and the opening for passage of biopsy forceps (Olympus GIF-D2.) *B*, Side-viewing OD duodenoscope, with cannula for injecting the pancreatic and common bile ducts (Olympus JF-B.)

manual pressure. Fluoroscopy should be used to demonstrate filling of the pancreatic duct or biliary tree or both, and appropriate x-ray exposures can be made. In slightly less than 50 per cent of cases, both ducts will fill from a single injection. If the desired duct does not fill, the cannula should be repositioned and another injection made. In approximately 20 per cent of cases, the common bile duct and pancreatic duct have separate openings, and this requires careful inspection of the papilla to identify separate orifices.

In the 5-year period of 1971–1976 at The Johns Hopkins Hospital the following procedures were performed:

Esophagoscopy	3630
Gastroscopy	3293
Duodenoscopy	2770
Dilatation	368
Biopsy	2266

During this time only 5 perforations occurred, and these were all in patients undergoing esophageal dilatation for benign stricture. Four of the five patients were treated with open drainage and one with no oral feeding and antibiotics. All patients did extremely well postoperatively. There were no complications associated with passage of the endoscope and no perforation of malignant lesions, although biopsies were done in 2266 patients.

Endoscopic Retrograde Cholangiopancreatography (ERCP)

The discussion of upper tract endoscopic methodology would not be complete without including a section on endoscopic retrograde cholangiopancreatography (ERCP). The purpose of this study is to visualize the biliary tree and pancreatic duct radiographically by injecting contrast material via a cannula inserted into the ampulla of Vater. While the principal product of this study is radiographic, skilled endoscopists can obtain reasonable endoscopic information about the remainder of the upper gastrointestinal tract during the procedure. The passage of this instrument is more difficult because the lens is side-viewing, but this provides a frontal view of the medial wall of the duodenum, and hence a frontal view of the ampulla of Vater, which appears as a small mound with a punctate opening.

Glucagon, 0.3 mg., is given intravenously to reduce gastrointestinal motility. Additional increments of glucagon, 0.3 mg., can be given throughout the procedure, with a maximal dose of 1.5 mg. The cannula is advanced through an independent channel with special controls that permit up-down motion of the cannula independent of the endoscope's own tip movement. With the combination of endoscopic tip control and cannula tip control, the cannula is inserted directly into the ampullary opening. Renografin 60, which has been heated to reduce viscosity, is then injected with manual pressure, using a 30 ml. syringe. The entire process is observed under fluoroscopy, and appropriate radiographs are taken when the duct systems have been adequately filled. The success rate of visualization of both duct systems approaches 85 to 95 per cent in skilled hands.

This procedure has been modified to pass an electrocautery microtome encased in a Teflon cannula for the purpose of doing microsurgery on the ampulla. Using this microtome, endoscopic sphincterotomy and removal of common duct stones can be accomplished. Figure 4–4 is ERCP radiographs, demonstrating normal findings; Figure 4–5 contains examples of abnormal studies in patients with pancreatic or biliary tract disease, or both.

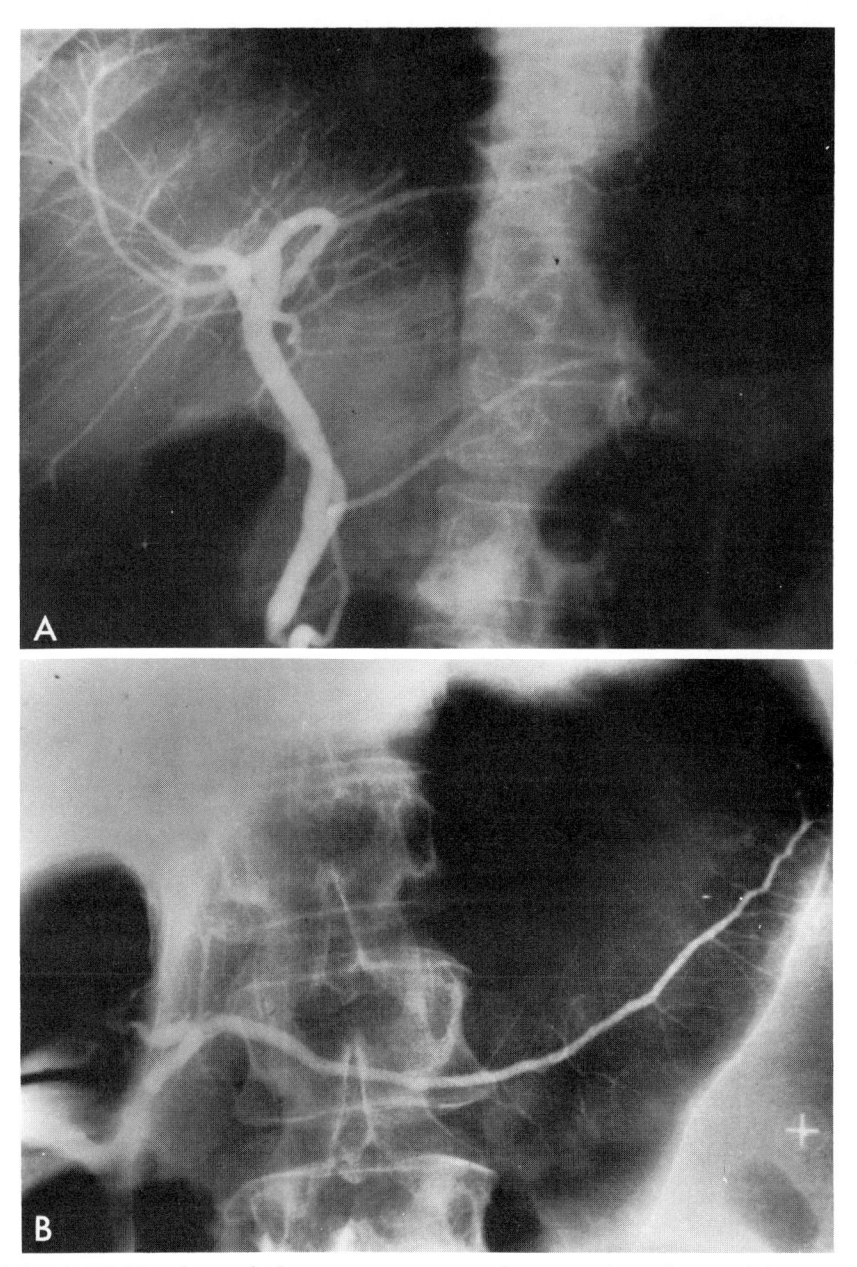

Figure 4–4. *A*, ERCP radiograph demonstrating a normal extra- and intrahepatic biliary tree and a normal pancreatic duct. *B*, ERCP radiograph demonstrating a normal pancreatic duct system.

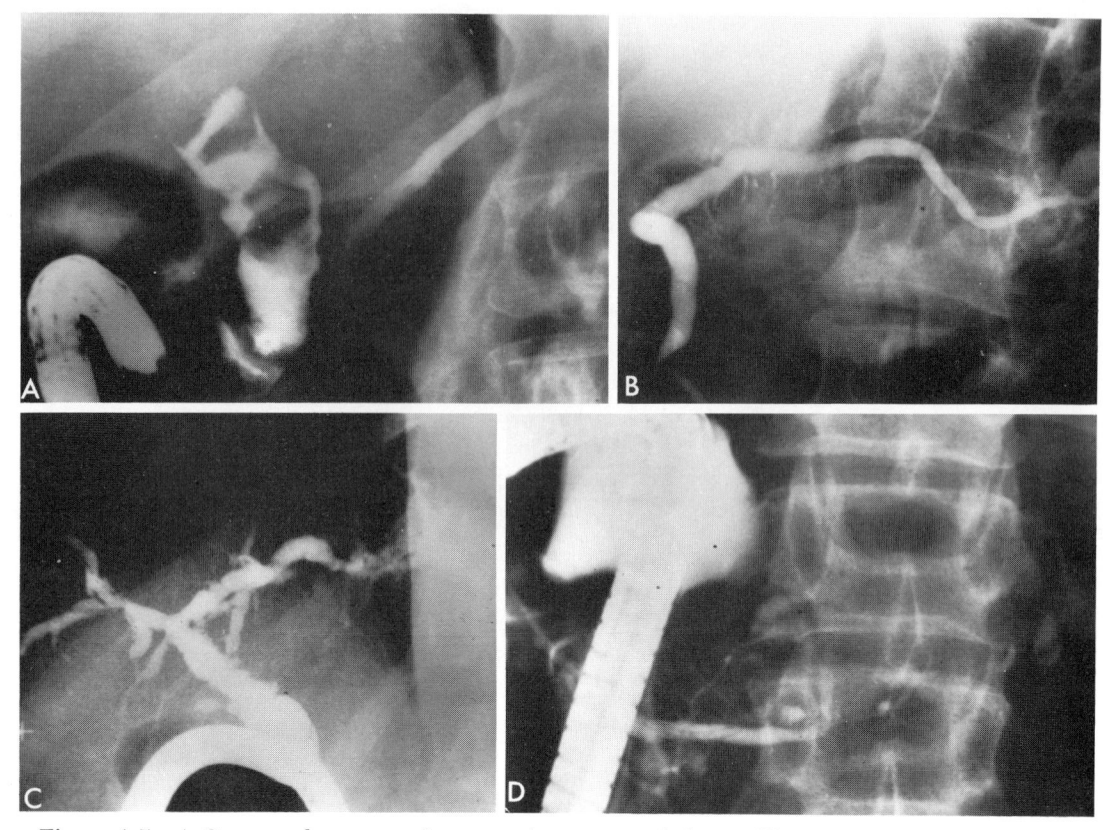

Figure 4–5. *A*, Common duct stones. Stones can be seen as radiolucent filling defects in the greatly enlarged common duct. *B*, Chronic pancreatitis. Dilatation of the pancreatic duct, beading, loss of smaller order radicals, and small sacculations of the first order radicals can be seen. *C*, Sclerosing cholangitis. A great degree of irregularity of the duct diameter in association with loss of the smaller radicals is readily apparent. *D*, Cancer of the pancreas. Typical complete obstruction of the distal duct with "rat-tail" appearance of the proximal duct.

Although septic complications such as ascending cholangitis or pancreatic abscesses may occur following endoscopic retrograde cholangiopancreatography (ERCP), they usually occur in patients with obstructed duct systems. Therefore, care should be taken not to force radiocontrast material beyond a narrowed area or into a pseudocyst unless surgery is contemplated within the near future. It has been our policy at The Johns Hopkins Hospital to tentatively schedule such patients for surgery within 24 hours of cholangiopancreatography. However, antibiotic therapy beginning just prior to or immediately following ERCP in cases of biliary or pancreatic obstruction has obviated the necessity for surgery in many instances and is now used routinely in these patients.

In over 50 per cent of patients, a significant hyperamylasemia will occur within 24 hours of an ERCP study, but frank pancreatitis is extremely rare, occurring in less than 1 per cent of cases in our experience. No treatment is given to the patients with hyperamylasemia, and those with pancreatitis have responded well to the usual medical regimen of nothing by mouth, atropine, and pethidine. The following figures indicate our success and the associated complications with endoscopic retrograde cholangiopancreatography:

Attempts	350
Success	307 (88%)
Desired duct	263 (78%)
Pancreatitis	2
Cholangitis	7
Pseudocyst abscess	2

Other Reported Experiences With Upper GI Endoscopy

In 1975 Knutson reported his experience with 200 consecutive fiberoptic endoscopic examinations of the upper gastrointestinal tract in patients whose ages ranged from 11 to 97 years. The majority of examinations were performed in a special endoscopy room, but a significant number were done at the bedside, in the intensive care unit, or in treatment rooms. The examination was definitive in 190 (95 per cent) of the 200 procedures. Ten examinations (5 per cent) were inadequate or inconclusive because of retained gastric contents, mechanical problems in passing the endoscope, or questionable significance of the endoscopic findings. Specific disease was noted endoscopically in 133 patients (67 per cent). No pathologic changes were seen in 57 patients (29 per cent).

In this experience with flexible fiberendoscopic diagnostic endoscopy there was no mortality and minimal morbidity. In one patient, repeated unsuccessful attempts to pass the endoscope through the cricopharyngeus mechanically traumatized the area, resulting in extreme supralaryngeal edema and hoarseness but no evidence of perforation. The symptoms completely cleared after medication and antibiotic therapy for 5 days.

After the procedure patients commonly had a sore throat for 8 to 12 hours, but this was easily relieved by gargling with lidocaine (Xylocaine viscous solution). There were no reactions to the Cetacaine used for hypopharyngeal anesthesia and no cases of aspiration or esophageal perforation.

The practical results obtained in these 200 endoscopic examinations were listed as follows:

1. The clinical diagnosis was changed in 44 patients (22 per cent).
2. It was the ultimate means of establishing the diagnosis, clarified questionable radiologic findings, and was the only effective method used for these purposes in 54 patients (27 per cent).
3. The clinical diagnosis was confirmed in 74 patients (37 per cent).
4. The examination was normal in 18 patients (9 per cent).
5. The examination was inadequate or inconclusive in 10 patients (5 per cent).

Knutson pointed out that early endoscopy of the upper gastrointestinal tract is safe for both young and elderly patients. In this series the youngest was an 11-year-old patient with a foreign body in the stomach. General anesthesia was recommended for children, owing to their unpredictable behavior. The oldest patient was 97 and had iron deficiency anemia. Endoscopy revealed atrophic hemorrhagic gastritis. Twenty-seven of the patients were 70 years of age or older.

The high rate of diagnostic accuracy (74 per cent) for endoscopic detection of the specific site or sites of acute upper gastrointestinal hemorrhage was due to the incidence of superficial lesions that are missed by routine standard radiographic contrast technics.

The fact that endoscopic examination can be done in any physical setting is important for the patient who, for various reasons, cannot easily or safely be transported to the radiology department for barium or angiographic study.

In 35 patients (18 per cent), upper gastrointestinal endoscopy prevented a needless operation when the endoscopic diagnosis altered the initial clinical impression, clarified questionable radiographic findings, demonstrated none of the reported radiographic findings, or revealed specific sources of upper gastrointestinal loss of blood that, when documented, were best treated by nonoperative methods.

Knutson concluded that endoscopic examination with the flexible fiberoptic instruments is the most accurate method of diagnosing any upper gastrointestinal tract disease.

Comparison of Diagnostic Accuracy Between Upper GI Tract Endoscopy and Roentgenography

Renner and associates (1974) studied 450 patients with disorders of the stomach and duodenum by both roentgenography and endoscopy and compared the two methods for diagnostic accuracy and correlation with the final diagnosis. Patients included those with neoplasms and ulcers of the stomach and duodenum, gastritis, duodenitis, erosions, polyps, hiatal hernias, diverticula, and cicatricial contractures. Gastritis was a difficult diagnosis to make with either method. Endoscopy was superior for neoplasms, ulcers, polyps, and erosions. Roentgenography was better for hiatal hernias, diverticula, and duodenal scarring. With use of both methods combined, the diagnostic accuracy for ulcers and neoplasms ranged from 92 to 96 per cent.

Endoscopy for Upper GI Hemorrhage

Allen, Block, and Schuman (1973), at the Henry Ford Hospital in Detroit, reported 101 patients with acute upper gastrointestinal tract hemorrhage who were gastroduodenoscoped for diagnosis.

In 77 patients, x-ray studies and endoscopy were performed within 48 hours of admission for bleeding. The combination established a positive diagnosis in 69 (90 per cent) of these patients. A positive diagnosis was established in only 8 (33 per cent) of the 24 patients not endoscoped until more than 48 hours after onset of the bleeding.

Radiologic studies with barium swallow showed a possible cause for bleeding in 54 per cent of the 71 patients studied within 48 hours but correctly identified the actual cause of hemorrhage in only 23 (32 per cent). Endoscopy gave only one false-positive diagnosis. A previous diagnosis or the patient's history suggested a cause of bleeding in 61 of the 101 patients but was correct in only 35 (57 per cent). Massive bleeding prevented endoscopy in two patients, and technical factors limited the examination in four.

The investigators concluded that "early endoscopy in acute upper gastrointestinal tract hemorrhage permits a high incidence of accurate identification of the bleeding lesion, elimination of other incidental abnormalities as the cause of bleeding, improved direction of medical and surgical management, and an assessment of the severity of the bleeding."

Weill and associates (1975) reported 210 emergency esophagoscopies, gastroscopies and duodenoscopies performed with the panendoscope for bleeding in the upper gastrointestinal tract. An accurate diagnosis of the cause of hemorrhage was made in 91.4 per cent of these patients by emergency endoscopy. An interesting finding was that the bleeding was from varices in fewer than half of the patients with cirrhosis.

Sugawa and associates (1973) published a detailed report of the experience of Detroit General Hospital's surgical endoscopy unit with the use of endoscopy in 183 patients who had acute upper gastrointestinal hemorrhage. All the examinations were made with an esophagogastroduodenoscope. Most patients (160) were examined within 48 hours of admission. Successful visualization of the esophagogastroduodenal area, with identification of one or more specific sites of bleeding, was accomplished in 178 of the 183 patients (97 per cent). Seventy-six patients had multiple bleeding sites.

The specific lesions identified as the cause of bleeding were, in decreasing order of frequency, acute erosive gastritis, 75 (42 per cent); gastric ulcer, 32 (18 per cent); Mallory-Weiss syndrome, 27 (15 per cent); duodenal ulcer, 20 (11 per cent); esophageal varices, 8 (5 per cent); gastric cancer, 6 (3 per cent); hemorrhagic esophagitis, 3 (2 per cent); hemorrhagic duodenitis, 2 (1 per cent); esophageal cancer, 2 (1 per cent); gastric leiomyosarcoma, 1 (1 per cent), gastric renal cell cancer, 1 (1 per cent), and gastric varices, 1 (1 per cent).

Barium x-ray studies revealed the lesion in only 34 per cent of the patients

Although esophageal varices were endoscopically demonstrated in 21 patients, the varices were the cause of bleeding in only 8. Concomitant lesions in the stomach or duodenum caused the bleeding in the other 13 patients.

Preoperative endoscopy identified the specific sites of bleeding in 40 of the 42 patients who underwent emergency or elective operation. Thirteen of the 26 patients requiring emergency operation could not be endoscoped preoperatively because of continued active bleeding and unstable vital signs. These patients were endoscoped during laparotomy. This technic circumvented the need for exploratory gastrotomy in all but one patient, whose stomach was full of clots that could not be removed by gastric lavage. The information obtained in these 12 patients permitted a definitive surgical procedure to be performed in a relatively uncontaminated field, shortened the operating time, and eliminated the frustration frequently attendant on searching for the bleeding site among the gastric folds. There were no deaths or significant complications due to endoscopy.

The investigators pointed out that intraoperative endoscopy is particularly helpful in patients in whom preoperative endoscopy has not been feasible as it will usually reveal the bleeding site. Endoscopy during laparotomy also has the advantages of being safe and simple to perform, and it is quick and accurate: "With the abdomen open, the proximal jejunum is occluded with a noncrushing clamp to prevent small bowel distention by the instilled air. The endotracheal tube is deflated, and the endoscope is passsed. After visualizing the esophagus and passing the endoscope into the stomach, the cuff on the endotracheal tube is reinflated to prevent regurgitation and aspiration during air insufflation. Although usually unnecessary, if desired the surgeon can help the endoscopist view the proximal portion of the stomach by manually flexing the fiberoptic endoscope toward the cardia. He may also lead the endoscope through the pylorus to examine the duodenum." When there is special urgency in establishing an early diagnosis in the patient with persistent bleeding, endoscopy under general anesthesia with an endotracheal tube in place and the operating room prepared may be invaluable in determining whether or not operation is necessary.

The data from this series confirmed observations made by others: that more than 40 per cent of patients with bleeding in the upper gastrointestinal tract have multiple sites of potential bleeding and that 60 per cent of patients have lesions so superficial that radiologic examination is unsatisfactory. Consequently, the presumption that a previously demonstrated lesion such as a duodenal ulcer or esophageal varices is the source of the current bleeding episode is frequently incorrect.

The investigators state, "In experienced hands, the endoscope is a safe and highly accurate instrument which produces little patient discomfort and provides invaluable information in about 10 minutes." In our experience at The Johns Hopkins Hospital, however, the examination has usually taken longer.

Intraoperative Endoscopy of the Digestive Tract

Sugawa and associates (1973), cited in the previous section, mentioned their use of, and described their technic for, intraoperative endoscopy in patients with acute hemorrhage in the upper gastrointestinal tract. To my knowledge intraoperative endoscopy has not been widely used in the United States; apparently it is used more frequently abroad.

Doutre and associates (1974) in France reported successful gastroscopies during laparotomy in nine patients with bleeding in the upper gastrointestinal tract in whom diagnoses were not established preoperatively. Duodenoscopy and visualization or retrograde cannulation of the ampulla of Vater was used in eight patients.

A bleeding adenoma of the ampulla in one patient and an "ampulloma" in another were diagnosed by this method. In three patients with pancreatic injury, a pancreatogram of the duct indicated the extent of pancreatectomy needed in one patient and in two patients demonstrated resection to be unnecessary. In three other patients intraoperative endoscopy helped in determining how to drain a pancreatic pseudocyst.

These workers reported also having used intraoperative colonoscopy in 30 patients. After the instrument is introduced through the anus and rectum by the endoscopist, its progression is facilitated by the surgeon from within the abdomen. Manipulation of the instrument and air insufflation permit easy and rapid visualization. This method eliminates the necessity for making openings in the intestine to inspect its interior and allows detection of a small lesion within the intestinal folds.

Doutre and associates stated that "by performing endoscopy of the digestive tract as a complementary method during laparotomy, the inconveniences and drawbacks of both methods have been overcome. This combined approach yielded more accurate diagnoses as well as the precise localization of the pathologic process, such as bleeding, ulceration, and neoplasm, in those patients in whom endoscopy could not or did not result in a preoperative answer to the problem."

Endoscopy in Symptomatic Patients Following Gastric Operations

Endoscopy is often helpful in evaluating patients who have symptoms following gastric operation. Cotton and associates (1973) reported their experience with 212 fiberendoscopic examinations performed in 177 patients who were symptomatic following a variety of operations for peptic ulceration (Table 4–3). The time intervals from the original operation to endoscopy ranged from 2 months to 42 years.

Five symptom groups were distinguished: 48 patients had dyspepsia (discomfort related to food relieved by alkalis); 75 patients had vague abdominal discomfort including atypical pain and vomiting; 18 patients complained of heartburn; 17 patients presented acute gastrointestinal bleeding; 19 patients had iron deficiency anemia.

All the examinations were satisfactory and there were no complications. A diagnosis of a condition other than gastritis was made in 83 patients, including 46 ulcers. Five ulcers were not seen, four because of an inadequate instrument early in the series. Radiology detected only 60 per cent of the ulcers and occasioned many false-positive diagnoses. Retained sutures were seen by endoscopy in 13 patients. Gastric mucosal congestion and gastritis were a common finding but their clinical significance was uncertain.

The diagnoses were listed anatomically as follows:

Esophagus: esophagitis (12 patients); varices, web, and cancer, 1 case each.

Stomach: cancer (5 patients), ulcer (7 patients), erosions (4 patients), metaplastic polyp (3 patients), bezoar (1 patient).

Anastomosis: ulcer, (12 patients); retained sutures were seen 1 to 16 years after operation in 13 patients, in 8 of whom the sutures were closely associated with ulcers at the suture line. In 6 of these patients the sutures were successfully removed with biopsy forceps. Two ulcers healed following removal of the sutures. Of the 7 other patients with retained sutures, 3 underwent suture-line resection and further ulcer surgery with apparent cure. In one patient the suture material disappeared spontaneously before repeat endoscopy.

Gastric mucosal congestion and gastritis were common in the operated stomach but its clinical significance was uncertain. No diagnosis other than gastritis was made at endoscopy in the remaining 94 patients. In this group 7 lesions missed by endoscopy were subsequently discovered: 3 recurrent duodenal ulcers after pyloroplasty (while no duodenoscope was available), 2 gastric cancers (1 beyond a midgastric stenosis, and 1 diagnosed visually and on biopsy as a benign gastric ulcer), 1 anastomotic ulcer (bleeding profusely), and 1 gastric ulcer in a deep pit near a gastrectomy stoma.

Forty-six of the 51 ulcers known by radiology were visualized by endoscopy; five were not. Of the 39 known ulcer patients who underwent barium meal x-ray examination within 3 weeks of endoscopy, ulcers were diagnosed in only 23 (40 per cent were missed.) The investigators pointed out that endoscopy may occasionally be useful in the early postoperative period. "While radiology is usually adequate in detecting hold-up at an anastomosis, endoscopy can often distinguish between its different causes (ulceration, edema, sutures, etc.)." They concluded that "investigation of symptomatic patients is incomplete, and may be inadequate, without properly performed endoscopy."

Venables (1973) studied 69 patients

Table 4–3. Previous Operations Performed in the Patients Examined

Previous Operation	Number of Examinations	Number of Patients
Partial gastrectomy		
Polya	83	72
Billroth I	16	14
Vagotomy and pyloroplasty	69	61
Vagotomy and		
gastroenterostomy	28	17
Other	16	13
Total	212	177

with recurrent symptoms who had undergone a previous ulcer operation. X-ray studies failed to reveal the cause of symptoms in these patients, but fiberoptic endoscopy demonstrated recurrent ulcers. Bowden (1977) compared the use of upper gastrointestinal fiberoptic endoscopy with barium contrast x-ray studies in 50 patients who had complaints after a variety of gastric operations. Endoscopic examination demonstrated definite abnormalities in 36 (72 per cent) of these patients. Of the 36 patients with positive endoscopic findings only 12 patients had abnormal x-ray films, an accuracy index of only 33 per cent.

Alkaline reflux gastritis was diagnosed by endoscopy in 13 (26 per cent) of the other 50 patients. All 13 had x-ray examinations reported to be within normal limits. The diagnosis of alkaline reflux gastritis cannot be made without gastroscopic examination and biopsy. Six (12 per cent) of the 50 patients were found to have one or more intraluminal nonabsorbable sutures at either a pyloroplasty site or a stoma, causing varying degrees of gastric outlet obstruction from reactive edema and inflammation, confirmed by biopsy. Of the 6 patients, 5 were found on x-ray examination to have partial outlet obstruction with delayed emptying and stasis. The sixth patient had an anastomotic ulcer demonstrated by the upper gastrointestinal x-ray series but the nonabsorbable suture in the center of the ulcer crater was seen only by endoscopy. In five of the patients, all the sutures were removed through the endoscope, using the biopsy forceps. In the sixth patient, equipment difficulties prevented removal of the sutures, and he was subsequently lost to follow-up. In those patients whose sutures were removed, gastric emptying improved and all have been free of symptoms for over one year.

Bowden concluded that patients with gastrectomy complaints cannot be completely evaluated until fiberoptic endoscopy and x-ray study have been done since these two diagnostic procedures are complementary and necessary for the most complete evaluation.

Endoscopic Diagnosis of Aortoduodenal Fistula

Baker and associates (1976) reported the case of a 49-year-old woman who was brought to an emergency room in shock, with a blood pressure of 70 mm. Hg and hematocrit of 15.8 per cent. Prior to admission she had vomited coffee-ground material and had passed bright red, bloody stools. She had undergone an aortofemoral bypass graft six months previously.

On the day of admission upper gastrointestinal x-ray studies with barium were unremarkable, and that evening upper gastrointestinal endoscopy showed multiple punctate hemorrhagic lesions of the stomach and esophagus. A falling hematocrit was evidence of continued blood loss, so endoscopy was repeated. This showed a vascular graft protruding into the duodenal lumen and oozing bright red blood. Exploratory laparotomy was performed that evening and showed an aortofemoral graft that had eroded into the duodenum and was slowly leaking blood. An axillofemoral bypass graft and femorofemoral crossover were performed to maintain circulation to the lower extremities. The aortofemoral graft was then removed and the duodenal defect was closed. The patient recovered and is currently well with no symptoms of vascular insufficiency in the lower extremities.

The investigators pointed out that the cardinal sign of development of an aortoduodenal fistula is gastrointestinal hemorrhage manifested by hematemesis, hematochezia, or melena, and that this complication should be strongly suspected when gastrointestinal bleeding occurs in a patient who has had aortic reconstructive surgery. They urged the early and aggressive use of upper gastrointestinal endoscopy as a diagnostic adjunct in upper gastrointestinal hemorrhage. When endoscopy demonstrates (1) arterial bleeding in the second or third part of the duodenum, (2) a pulsatile structure in the wall or lumen, (3) a suture line, or (4) a bile-stained structure in a patient who has had aortic reconstructive surgery, the diagnosis of aortoduodenal fistula should be considered.

Endoscopy in Patients with Malignant Conditions of the GI Tract

Yamada and associates (1975) reported their experience with the use of fiberoptic esophagogastroduodenoscopy in 215 patients with suspected cancer of the upper gastrointestinal tract who were examined at the Roswell Park Memorial Institute. Their ages ranged from 23 to 83 years, with a mean of 60 years. In each patient an attempt was made to visualize from the upper esophagus to the second part of the duodenum and as far distally as possible. This included visualization of the papilla of Vater and any area suspected by symptoms or by radiologic study.

All endoscopic diagnoses in patients with malignant lesions or suspected malignant disease were established by visualization and by direct biopsy of the lesion. At least three biopsy specimens were taken from each lesion examined.

The major indications for endoscopy were postoperative follow-up after surgery for gastric cancer in 36 patients; acute gastrointestinal hemorrhage in 29 patients; unknown primary malignant tumor in 23 patients; and negative upper gastrointestinal x-ray studies in 12 patients. The remaining 115 patients were endoscoped for future evaluation of positive, negative, or questionable results of upper gastrointestinal x-ray studies prior to surgical exploration and for cholangiopancreatography.

In this series, endoscopic biopsy examination was accurate in 83 per cent of patients with malignant tumors of the stomach detected by endoscopic examination. False-negative biopsy examinations from infiltrating diffuse lesions occurred in 13 per cent. The investigators found that biopsy specimens, in such lesions as linitis plastica or in possible submucosal infiltration, should be taken from that surface most eroded or having tiny ulcerations, when possible. For these cancers the combination of brush cytologic examinations, washing the lesion under direct vision through the fiberscope, and biopsy may be more fruitful than biopsy alone. Endoscopy established the diagnosis of carcinoma of the stomach in one-third of the patients with metastatic adenocarcinoma of unknown primary source.

Significant complications attributed to endoscopy occurred in two patients: One, with carcinoma of the stomach, had aspiration pneumonia following esophagoscopy, which responded to antibiotic therapy; another, with sarcoma of the stomach, had bronchospasm when the endoscope was inserted into the esophagus following an intravenous single injection of 10 mg. of diazepam but recovered with endotracheal intubation and oxygen therapy.

Hatfield and colleagues (1975) studied 20 freshly resected specimens, each with an ulcerated carcinoma, to determine the best site for gastric biopsy. With an endoscopic biopsy forceps they obtained multiple biopsy specimens from various sites around the ulcer. Carcinoma was detected with equal frequency in specimens from the slough and from the rim of the ulcer, but in some it was positive from the slough but not from the rim and vice versa. The positive biopsy rate increased to 95 per cent when specimens were biopsied from both the slough and the rim, which is the procedure they recommend.

Fiberoptic Endoscopic Palliative Intubation of Inoperable Esophagogastric Neoplasms

Atkinson and Ferguson (1977) reported that they had performed palliative intubation for inoperable malignant structures of the cardia on 16 occasions in 13 patients, using preliminary endoscopic dilation with a Puestow-Eder dilator and then passing a Celestin tube mounted on an introducer over a guide wire inserted at fiberoptic endoscopy. Only one death resulted from the procedure, and all except one patient left the hospital swallowing satisfactorily. "The method provided a simple and relatively safe means of relieving dysphagia and improving nutrition."

FIBEROPTIC ENDOSCOPIC THERAPEUTIC PROCEDURES IN UPPER GI TRACT

A number of therapeutic procedures have been performed with the use of fiberoptic endoscopes, which may be the procedure of choice in many cases.

Endoscopic Electrocoagulation in Upper GI Hemorrhage

Papp (1974) reported seven actively bleeding patients in whom emergency upper gastrointestinal endoscopy was performed with a flexible end-viewing endoscopy. The site of bleeding was found and electrocoagulated with a flexible suction coagulator electrode (Cameron-Miller) passed through the endoscope, resulting in cessation of bleeding in all the cases. This technic allowed time both to stabilize the patient and to determine further therapy.

The lesions coagulated were four benign gastric ulcers, one duodenal ulcer, one area of hemorrhagic gastritis, and one gastric varix. No morbidity or death resulted from the coagulation. The patient with the gastric varix died because of esophageal bleeding; no further bleeding occurred until 12 hours after the coagulation, and then repeat endoscopy showed active esophageal variceal bleeding. The coagulated site was not bleeding. Despite use of a Sengstaken-Blakemore tube, the patient continued to bleed and died. The remaining six patients were treated medically and discharged from the hospital.

Papp warned that this method has potentially serious complications if it is not performed by an endoscopist experienced with electrocoagulation. Reported complications have been increased hemorrhage and transmural coagulation with ulceration and subsequent perforation. "Proper grounding of the patient and the instrument is necessary to avoid electrical injury."

In 1976 Papp updated his experience with this procedure. He reported that endoscopic electrocoagulation had been performed on 40 occasions for 38 patients with bleeding gastrointestinal lesions. Cessation of bleeding was achieved in 95 per cent. Fifteen gastric ulcers, 14 duodenal ulcers, 6 Mallory-Weiss tears, 1 gastric varix, 1 case of hemorrhagic gastritis, and 1 esophageal ulcer were successfully electrocoagulated. Three duodenal and three gastric ulcers re-bled. One duodenal and one gastric ulcer were successfully re-electrocoagulated. Electrocoagulation failed to stop bleeding in one Mallory-Weiss tear and one duodenal ulcer. No morbidity nor mortality was attributed to endoscopic electrocoagulation. The duration and cost of hospitalization were less for patients treated by electrocoagulation than for patients with bleeding upper gastrointestinal lesions who were treated by the usual medical and surgical methods.

Papp pointed out that it is important to understand that electrocoagulation of bleeding upper gastrointestinal lesions is not definitive therapy but a therapeutic tool to stop hemorrhage. Electrocoagulation hemostasis permits stabilization of the patient's condition and election of a program of treatment on a less emergent basis.

Yellin and associates (1976) used an argon-ion laser, coupled to a flexible fiberoptic endoscope, to coagulate experimentally produced bleeding gastric ulcers in dogs. Argon-ion laser phototherapy rapidly and effectively achieved hemostasis in all bleeding ulcers. Bleeding arteries up to 2 mm. in diameter were photocoagulated. Healed laser-treated ulcers could not be differentiated from nontreated control ulcers or normal stomach one month after injury.

The investigators pointed out that the argon-ion laser may be a useful adjunct in the control of certain types of bleeding gastric lesions. Superficial lesions and hemorrhaging vessels less than 2 mm. in diameter can be effectively photocoagulated. Such therapy can be instituted simultaneously with diagnostic endoscopy and adds but a few additional minutes to the total procedure.

Later, the same investigators (Dwyer and associates, 1976) reported their use of argon-ion laser phototherapy for the treatment of acute upper gastrointestinal bleeding in two patients. One was a 50-year-old woman with a history of chronic alcoholism who had hematemesis. Endoscopy showed nonbleeding esophageal varices and hemorrhagic gastritis. An actively bleeding area high on the lesser curvature of the stomach was treated. Ninety seconds of exposure were required to obtain hemostasis. There was no clinical evidence of recurrent bleeding during the hospital course.

The other patient was a 42-year-old alcoholic man who came to the hospital with a two-day history of epigastric pain, hematemesis, and melena. Twenty years previously he had had a 70 per cent subtotal gastrectomy and Billroth 2 gastrojejunostomy for peptic ulcer. Shortly after admission he passed a large black stool and became diaphoretic. Iced saline gastric lavage for two hours did not stop the bleeding. Emergency endoscopy showed esophageal varices, a Billroth 2 gastrojejunostomy, and a 2- by 3-cm. bleeding anastomotic ulcer. Blood transfusions and intragastric levarterenol bitartrate did not stop the bleeding. After four hours, at endoscopy the bleeding gastric ulcer was treated for several minutes by moving the visible laser light beam back and forth across the ulcer until bleeding stopped. Twelve hours later bleeding recurred, and operation was performed. The bleeding vessel in this ulcer was suture-ligated. Biopsy of the ulcer showed adenocarcinoma. Ten days later radical subtotal gastrectomy and gastrojejunostomy were performed.

Fruhmorgen and coworkers (1976) reported the use of endoscopic laser coagulation 94 times in 14 patients to stop gastrointestinal bleeding or coagulate potential bleeding sources during nonbleeding intervals. Lasting hemostasis was accomplished in three cases of incomplete gastric erosion, one of gastric ulcer, one of duodenal ulcer, and one bleeding after antral rugectomy. It failed to stop severe arterial bleeding in a patient with gastric carcinoma. Lasting hemostasis was achieved in 6 patients with hemangioma of the colon, one with angiomatosis of the antrum in 62 individual sites, and two with angiodysplasia of the colon, and in 17 lesions in Osler's disease of the esophagus (2 patients), stomach (10 patients), and duodenum (5 patients). The procedure was performed during diagnostic endoscopy with an argon-ion laser developed by the writers. No complications have been observed so far.

The mechanism by which laser irradiation causes hemostasis is related to the heating of the absorptive tissues. This method of treatment and its instrumentation are awaiting further experimentation and development.

Endoscopic Removal of Gastric and Duodenal Polyps

Gaisford (1973) reported ten gastric polypectomies performed via a fiberendoscope, using an electrosurgical-snare technic, without significant complications. Four of these polyps were situated in the body of the stomach and six were in the antrum. They ranged in size from 1.2 to 3.5 cm. Histologically, all were benign: six were adenomatous polyps, two were interpreted as "atypical cellular changes," and two were leiomyomas.

Gaisford emphasized that the risk of bleeding from the divided pedicle of the polyp and perforation of the viscus is minimized by accurately positioning the snare around the pedicle so that the snare is clearly visualized during all coagulating and cutting current applications, and by using a combination of alternating and cutting currents to divide the pedicle without undue tension on the snare, which might cause premature separation of the polyp and pedicle bleeding. He also modified the distal end of the endoscope by covering both metal bands with latex rubber sheaths to insulate the gastric mucosa from potential electric current transmitted from the cautery probe tip through electrolyte solution.

Appel (1976) reported six patients in whom polyps were removed by fiberoptic endoscopy — from the stomach in three cases and from the duodenum in three cases. The gastric polyps were all in the antrum. Two were adenomatous polyps and the third was not recovered for histologic identification. One of the duodenal polyps was Brunner's gland hyperplasia, another was a lipoma, and the third was not recovered for histologic identification.

Precise positioning of the snare wire was carefully individualized for each polyp. To be certain that all polyp tissue was being removed, the wire was positioned at the halfway point on the stalk. This provided an adequate specimen for the pathologist and also protected the true gastric wall from potential perforation. A mixed cutting and coagulating current was applied in approximately half-second bursts at a level that averaged 25 to 40 watts per second, individualized for each polyp. After the polyp had dropped off its pedicle, the pedicle was inspected to assure hemostasis. Then the polyp was picked up in the tip of the endoscope with suction, and the endoscope and polyp were removed.

The patients were observed overnight in the hospital or on an outpatient basis if they lived nearby. The only complication that occurred was a minor bleed in one patient.

Appel pointed out that the advantages of endoscopic gastric and duodenal polypectomy included minimal morbidity, very low mortality, and large savings in both time and money, as well as avoiding the risks of abdominal surgery and potential postsurgical complications. However, endoscopy may also be followed by complications.

Endoscopic Removal of Foreign Bodies from the Stomach

Although many foreign bodies have been removed from the esophagus with a rigid or a fiber esophagoscope, most foreign bodies in the stomach that did not pass spontaneously required surgery for removal. Maimon and Milligan, in 1972, were the first to remove a foreign body from the stomach by means of a fiberendoscope. Their patient was a 66-year-old man admitted to The Johns Hopkins Hospital with a spontaneous pneumothorax. He subsequently developed pneumonia which was treated successfully with antibiotics. While in the hospital the patient inadvertently swallowed a 15.5-inch rubber tube intended for tracheal aspiration. The tube caused no symptoms but x-ray films showed it to be curled upon itself within the stomach with no distal progression during a 4-day period (Fig. 4–6). An attempt to remove it by endoscopy was elected.

The patient was premedicated with Demerol, 75 mg. IM; atropine, 0.6 mg. IM, and Xylocaine pharyngeal anesthetic locally. The esophagoscope was easily passed into the stomach, where the rubber catheter was seen (Fig. 4–7). The margin of the eye of the catheter's rubber tip was grasped with the biopsy forceps of the fiberesophagoscope under direct vision, and both were gradually withdrawn together.

This case demonstrated that the fiberendoscope may be used for removing certain foreign bodies from the stomach without the use of general anesthesia or surgery and with minimal discomfort to the patient. However, extraction of foreign bodies was limited to objects capable of being removed with the small-mouthed biopsy forceps then supplied with the fiberendoscopes, such as needles, rubber catheters, and safety pins.

Brady and Johnson (1977) reported that they had successfully removed three foreign bodies from the upper gastrointestinal tract with a fiberoptic endoscope: a food bolus lodged above an esophageal stricture, a metallic nebulizer tip impacted in the mid-esophagus, and a spoon lodged in the stomach. A razor blade could not be removed from the duodenum in a fourth case.

Subsequently, larger and sturdier grasping forceps for use with fiberendoscopes were developed and are now available (Fig. 4–8). These permit direct visualization, manipulation, and firm grasping of foreign bodies, so what can be removed from the stomach by fiberendoscopy has been enlarged considerably.

Larkworthy and associates (1974) re-

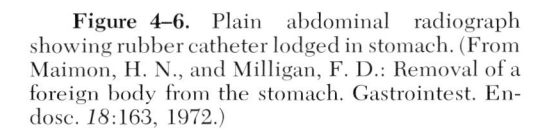

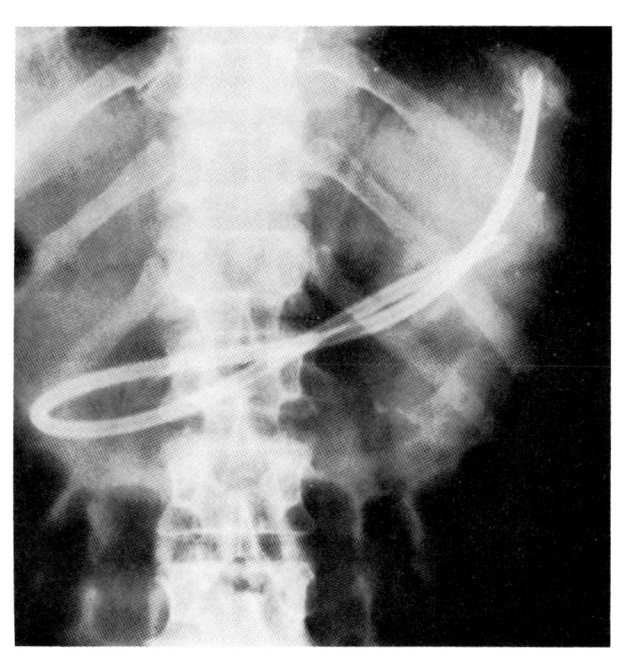

Figure 4–6. Plain abdominal radiograph showing rubber catheter lodged in stomach. (From Maimon, H. N., and Milligan, F. D.: Removal of a foreign body from the stomach. Gastrointest. Endosc. *18*:163, 1972.)

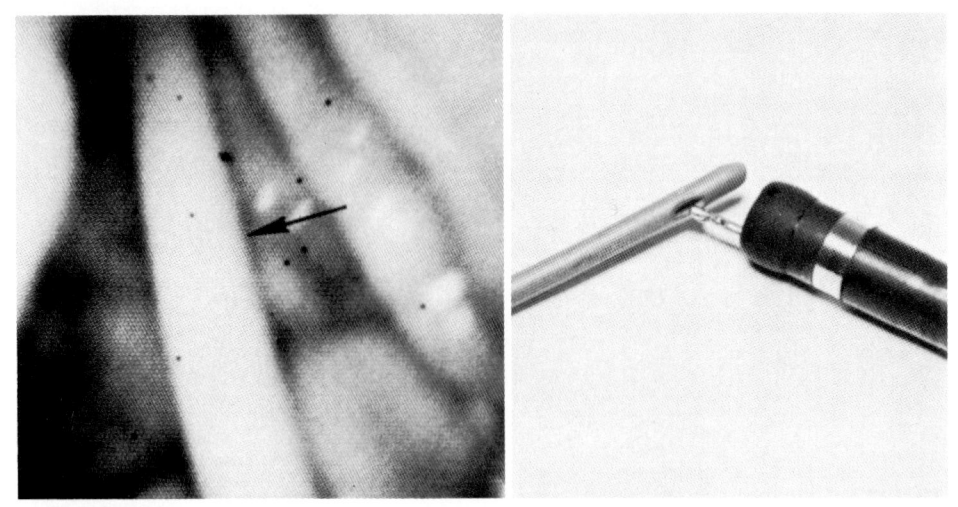

Figure 4–7. Endoscopic view (left) of swallowed catheter and (right) the means by which it was retrieved by the fiberesophagoscope. (From Maimon and Milligan, cited in previous figure.)

ported two such cases. In the first, a 36-year-old serviceman was admitted to the surgical division with a history of accidentally swallowing a coin while drinking beer, 8 weeks prior to admission. X-ray films showed the coin in the stomach. Surgery was contraindicated because of severe nasal sinusitis.

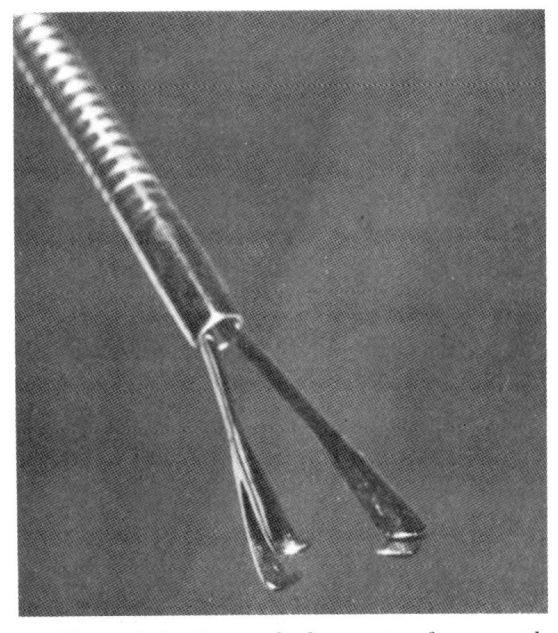

Figure 4–8. Foreign body–grasping forceps with jaws partly opened. (From Larkworthy, W., Jones, R. T., Mahoney, M., et al.: Removal of ingested coins utilizing fibre-endoscopy and special forceps. Br. J. Surg. 61:750–752, 1974.)

Since fiberendoscopy does not require general anesthesia and a specially designed retrieval forceps was available, this method of removing the foreign body was elected.

After premedication with pethidine, 100 mg. IM, atropine, 0.6 mg., and local anesthesia to the pharynx, the patient was sedated with intravenous diazepam given slowly to a total dose of 25 mg. A fiberendoscope was passed into the stomach. On the first attempt the coin, lying in the antrum, was easily found and with little difficulty was grasped with the forceps. It was easily drawn up through the stomach and esophagus but twisted out of the forceps nearing the pharyngeal opening of the esophagus.

At a second attempt the coin was rotated into the coronal plane and easily withdrawn under visualization (Fig. 4–9). There were no sequelae. The patient left the hospital the following day to return to duty.

The second patient was a 76-year-old man with severe arthritis and an 8-year history of repeated attacks of vomiting lasting up to 48 hours, associated with epigastric discomfort and, on numerous occasions, the vomiting of jet-black, offensive liquid. Barium swallow x-ray study showed the pyloric antrum to be dilated and containing a coin. There was some narrowing of the distal stomach. The patient could not recall swallowing a coin but said it had been a family custom to hide new silver coins in Christmas puddings.

In 1973 the patient was premedicated,

sedated, and fiberendoscoped, as described for the first patient. A blackened coin was identified (Fig. 4–10). The pylorus was narrowed and encircled by inflammation, with a small ulcer lying inferiorly in the pyloric canal. The duodenal mucosa had prolapsed through the pylorus into the stomach. The duodenal bulb could not be entered. The coin was grasped with the retrieval forceps, rotated into the coronal plane, and easily removed under direct vision with continuous esophageal insufflation. It was a sixpence, dated 1953.

The investigators advised that withdrawal should be done with care, and the endoscope forceps with the grasped foreign body trailing should be slowly removed as a single entity (Fig. 4–8). Foreign bodies should be rotated to lie with their long axis in the coronal plane to avoid excessive traction or relinquishment at the regions of anatomic narrowing of the esophagus. Splayed or sharp objects such as safety pins or hairpins, which are likely to have their points facing upward, should be gently pushed into the stomach and turned prior to withdrawal. Alternatively, they suggested that a sheath could be fixed to the distal end of the fiberendoscope and safety pins withdrawn into it, effecting either closure or additional protection. During withdrawal the foreign body should be kept under constant observation, and continuous gentle esophageal inflation should be maintained.

Larkworthy and colleagues pointed out the considerable advantage of foreign body removal by the method described in these two patients, in whom surgical operation would have been specially hazardous because of the severe sinusitis in one and the advanced age and severe arthritis in the other.

Endoscopic Removal of Bleeding Brunner Gland Adenoma

Appel and Bentlif (1976) reported what they believed to be the first endoscopic

Figure 4–9. Coin removed from Case 1, showing the distal end of the fiberendoscope, forceps, and coin withdrawn as a single entity. (From Larkworthy, et al., cited in Figure 4–8.)

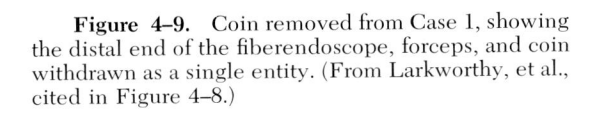

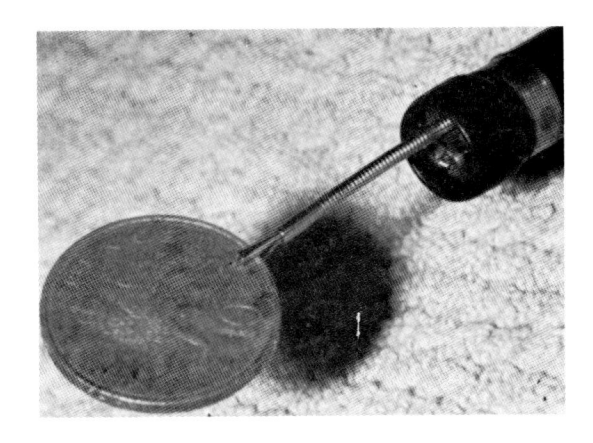

Figure 4–10. Sixpence removed from Case 2. (From Larkworthy, et al., cited in Figure 4–8.)

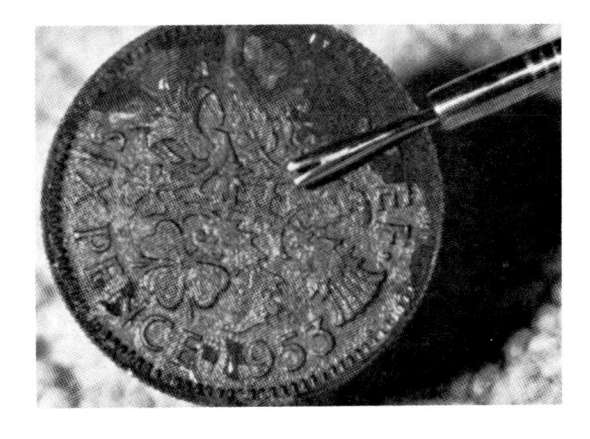

removal of a bleeding Brunner gland adenoma. The patient was a 36-year-old man who developed hematemesis with no preceding gastrointestinal symptoms. Gastroduodenoscopy showed a polyp in the postbulbar portion of the duodenum. It was excised with the snare and cautery technic. Histologic analysis confirmed the presence of a Brunner gland adenoma. At this time there was no evidence of ulceration or inflammation elsewhere in the stomach or duodenum. The patient made an uneventful recovery and remained asymptomatic at follow-up 6 months later.

The investigators emphasized that the ampulla of Vater must be carefully identified prior to endoscopically excising the polyp. After identification, the small size of the snare wire and careful avoidance of other than the minimal amount of cauterizing current that might overheat the surrounding tissues make it safe to excise a polyp that lies any appreciable distance from the ampulla. However, they cautioned that upper gastrointestinal polypectomy can be expected to be accompanied by a higher incidence of bleeding than colonic polypectomy because the stomach and duodenum are more vascular than the colon, and because acid peptic juices will bathe the polypectomy site. For that reason they suggested that these procedures be done on inpatients or when very close outpatient follow-up is available.

Duodenoscopic Papillotomy and Gallstone Removal

Cotton and colleagues (1976) pointed out that "the routine use of operative cholangiography during cholecystectomy has reduced, but not abolished, the incidence of residual common bile duct stones. When detected on a postoperative T-tube cholangiogram, some stones may be released by nonoperative technics. However, residual stones may not be suspected or detected for months or years after cholecystectomy, in which case re-exploration has, until now, provided the only method of treatment. Using modified experimental fiberscopes, it is now possible to make a diathermy incision in the roof of the papilla, allowing spontaneous passage of the stones or their extraction from below using a Dormia-type basket" (Figs. 4–11, 4–12, and 4–13). They

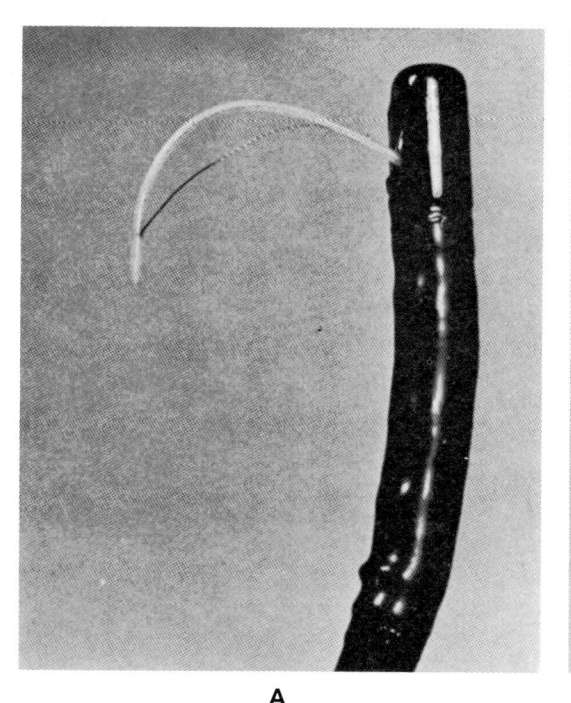

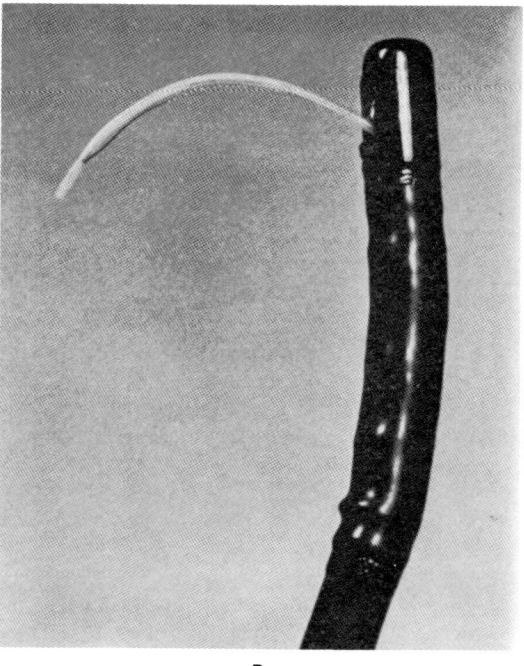

Figure 4–11. Tip of experimental insulated endoscope, with diathermy catheter closed (A) and open (B). (From Cotton, P. B., Chapman, M., Whiteside, C. G., and Le Quesne, L. P.: Duodenoscopic papillotomy and gallstone removal. Br. J. Surg. 63:711, 1976.)

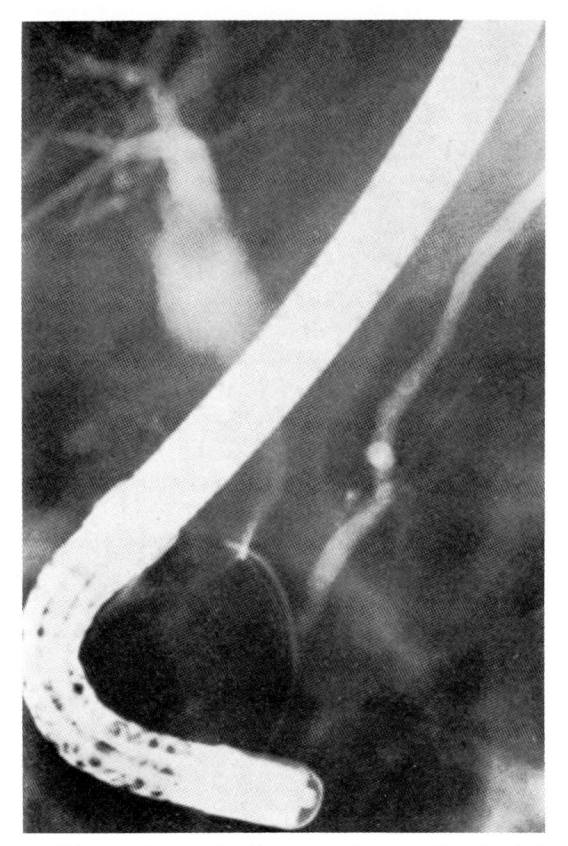

Figure 4-12. Diathermy catheter within the bile duct, with the bare wire oriented away from the pancreas. (From Cotton, et al., cited in previous figure.)

cited the reports of Classen and Demling (1974), Classen and Safrany (1975), Koch (1975), and Kawai and associates (1974), which had demonstrated the effectiveness and relative safety of endoscopic papillotomy both in animals and in human beings. They also reported their own experience with endoscopic papillotomy.

Using an experimental insulated duodenoscope and a diathermy wire, Cotton and associates performed papillotomy on 10 patients under diazepam sedation. Seven patients had common bile duct stones (6 following cholecystectomy), and three had papillary stenosis. Nine of the patients had severe medical or surgical contraindications to further operative treatment. Papillotomy was successful in all patients, with no significant bleeding or other complications. Repeat endoscopy 6 to 14 days after papillotomy demonstrated a healed biliary orifice 7 to 10 mm. in diameter. Stones had already passed in three of the seven patients; in two others, stones were extracted using balloon catheters or Dormia-type baskets. Two larger stones could not be removed; in one of these patients, the stone and basket became impacted at the papilla and had to be removed surgically 2 days later.

These investigators concluded that endoscopic papillotomy is an acceptable alternative to surgery in high-risk patients, particularly in the treatment of retained common bile duct stones. In their small series endoscopic diathermy papillotomy proved to be safe. They cited Rosch (1975), who reviewed the German experience with 130 cases and reported 4 episodes of hemorrhage, 4 of perforation (2 deaths), and 1 of pancreatitis. This complication rate seemed acceptable since most patients had been selected because of contraindication to further surgery. Also, surgical papillotomy is not without difficulty and risk.

The main indication for endoscopic papillotomy has been for release or removal of retained stones. This was accomplished in 5 of Cotton and colleagues' patients and in 33 of the 39 patients in Classen and Sa-

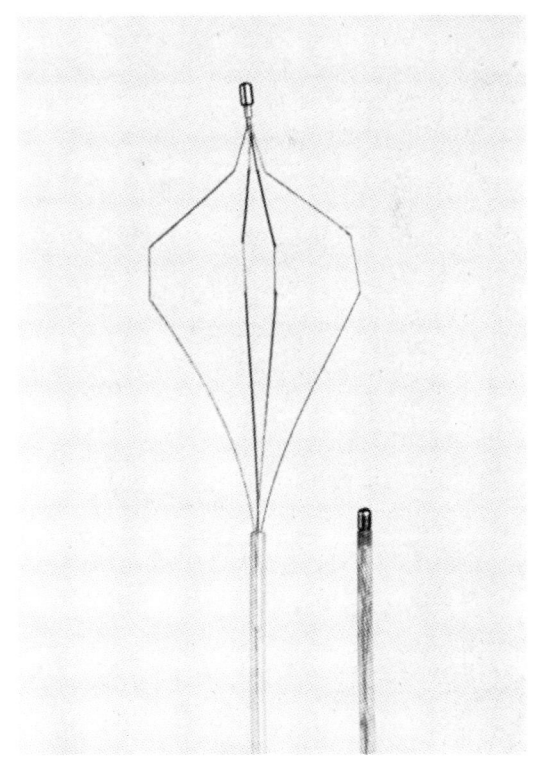

Figure 4-13. Dormia-type basket. (From Cotton, et al., cited in Figure 4-11.)

frany's (1975) combined series. Failures occurred with large stones. Full evaluation of the procedure awaits greater experience with, and longer-term results following, its use.

FIBERENDOSCOPIC COMPLICATIONS

There is extravagant enthusiasm for, and widespread usage of, fiberendoscopy for the diagnosis and treatment of disorders of the gastrointestinal tract. Much has been written about such virtues as its clinical efficacy, excellent patient acceptance, simplicity and safety of performance, and its versatility. The fact that the procedures may be associated with complications is often overlooked. However, when performed by experienced endoscopists, the incidence of these complications and their morbidity and mortality justify its use.

The American Society for Gastrointestinal Endoscopy conducted a survey of the complications of endoscopic procedures performed during the years 1972 and 1973. Silvis and associates (1976) reported the results, which is the source of the following discussion.

The types of examinations, the number of cases in which each was performed, and the incidences of complications with each type were listed as follows:

Esophagogastroduodenoscopy: Of 211,410 examinations, the complication rate was 1.3 per 1000 cases. The complications were 70 perforations, 63 cases of bleeding, 129 cases of cardiopulmonary symptoms, 17 infections, and 228 minor miscellaneous events such as medication reactions (hives, and so on).

The complications of esophagoscopy alone were slightly higher (2.3 per 1000 cases) than for gastroscopy (1.2 per 1000 cases) or duodenoscopy (1.4 per 1000 cases).

Duodenoscopy with cannulation was performed 3884 times, with a complication rate of 21.6 per 1000 examinations. The complications were 3 perforations, 2 cases of bleeding, 4 cases of cardiopulmonary symptoms, 25 cases of cholangitis, 51 cases of pancreatitis, and 8 miscellaneous minor events.

This procedure had a high complication rate. The most common complications were cholangitis, which occurred only in patients with obstruction of the common duct, and pancreatitis. The cause of pancreatitis following cholangiopancreatography is not known. It is thought to be related to the extent of filling of the pancreatic duct. In this survey its incidence was related to the experience of the examiner. The researchers commented, "the risks of this procedure must be weighed against its diagnostic benefit. It should be used only in patients who are candidates for surgery."

Diagnostic coloscopy was performed 25,298 times, with a complication rate of 3.4 per 1000 examinations. The complications listed were 50 perforations, 23 cases of bleeding, 10 cases of cardiopulmonary symptoms, 3 infections, and 15 miscellaneous minor events.

Coloscopy with polypectomy was performed in 6,124 cases, with a complication rate of 23.3 per 1000 cases. The complications listed were 20 perforations, 106 cases of bleeding, 1 case of cardiopulmonary symptoms, 4 infections, and 6 miscellaneous minor events.

The complication rate of coloscopy with polypectomy was higher than in diagnostic coloscopy because the most frequent complication associated with polypectomy is bleeding. The perforation rate is only slightly higher than with diagnostic coloscopy (2 versus 3.3 perforations per 1000 cases).

Esophageal dilations were performed with mercury bougies in 13,139 cases with a complication rate of 4.25 per 1000. The complications listed were 12 perforations, 45 cases of bleeding, and 1 case of cardiopulmonary symptoms.

Dilations with metal olives in 9,431 cases had a complication rate of 6.1 per 1000 treatments. The complications listed were 33 perforations, 8 cases of bleeding, 5 cases of cardiopulmonary symptoms, 2 infections, and 3 miscellaneous minor events.

Pneumatic or mechanical dilation for achalasia was performed in 1224 patients, with a complication rate of 18.4 per 1000 procedures. The complications listed were 14 perforations, 4 cases of bleeding, and 1 case of cardiopulmonary symptoms.

The complications for dilations varied with the technic used. Mercury-filled rubber bougies (Hurst or Maloney dilators) had the lowest complication rate (4.3 per 1000 cases), with the metal olive dilators having a slightly higher rate of complications (6.1 per 1000 cases). Pneumatic or mechanical dilators were associated with the highest complication rate (6.1 per 1000 cases) but there were insufficient data to distinguish between these two types.

Peritoneoscopy (4404 reported examinations) had a complication rate of 5.4 per 1000 patients. The complications were 6 perforations of the bowel, 1 gallbladder perforation, 1 ovarian cyst perforation, 10 cases of bleeding, 3 cases of cardiopulmonary symptoms, 4 infections, and 6 other problems consisting of mild medication reactions and emphysema from CO_2 injection. Its complication rate is similar to that of diagnostic coloscopy.

In this series of over 240,000 examinations there were 17 deaths, 1 for each 1411 examinations. The fatal complications:

Perforation of the cervical esophagus	3
Cardiac arrest during procedure (one during esophagoscopy, one during cannulation)	5
Myocardial infarction during procedure	1
Postbiopsy bleeding	1
Cholangitis	2
Aspiration during emergency endoscopy, with respiratory arrest	1
Pancreatic sepsis after endoscopic pancreatograms	2
Perforation of colon	1
Unexplained sudden death after peritoneoscopy	1
Total	17

It can be concluded that "the value of these diagnostic and therapeutic procedures is now well established but must be weighed against a potential risk of complications" (Silvis and associates, 1976).

Compared with previous surveys of upper gastrointestinal endoscopic complications, the risk of perforation with modern instruments appears to have been slightly reduced, to 0.3 per 1000 cases compared with 0.4 to 1.2 per 1000 cases, but this decrease in perforation has been offset by a serious complication rate from bleeding (0.3 per 1000 cases) related to the introduction of biopsy techniques. If bleeding and perforation are combined, the complication rates remain about the same, at 0.6 per 1000 cases. However, the mortality from perforations has been greatly reduced, to 0.6 per cent, compared with that in previous surveys (15 per cent and 43 per cent). The majority of patients with bleeding did not require surgery, and only a single death resulted from postbiopsy bleeding.

Bloom and colleagues (1976) reported two patients who developed a focal mass in the head of the pancreas presumably following attempted endoscopic retrograde cholangiopancreatography (ERCP). These lesions grossly mimicked carcinoma of the pancreas. In one patient a radical pancreatoduodenectomy was performed because of the misleading gross findings. Although successful cannulation was not achieved in either case, manipulations around the ampulla presumably produced focal inflammatory reaction in the head of the pancreas. Neither patient had had signs nor symptoms consistent with clinical pancreatitis, even though one patient had histologic confirmation of, and the other had strong presumptive evidence for, the diagnosis. The importance of focal pancreatitis occurring after retrograde cannulation is that it may be grossly indistinguishable from carcinoma of the head of the pancreas and be mistakenly treated as such.

A word about overmedication is in order. While the procedure has documented efficacy and safety in the aged, small doses of diazepam in this group, often as little as 2 mg., can lead to pernicious apnea. This underscores the value of meperidine in the anesthetizing method. Larger doses of meperidine with smaller doses of diazepam are recommended because of the reversibility of meperidine with Narcan.

A potential risk for endoscopy is the transmission of type B hepatitis. There have been no reported cases of this although there is a negative study (McDonald and Silverstein, 1976) in which four patients were followed after being endoscoped with an instrument that had been used on a jaundiced hepatitis B–positive patient. None developed signs of hepatitis after 6 months of follow-up. This continues to be a potential risk, and thorough cleaning and sterilizing of the endoscope following use in HBsAg-positive patients is recommended.

ANTERIOR GASTROSCOPY AND DUODENOSCOPY THROUGH A GASTROTOMY OR GASTROSTOMY STOMA

Examination of the interior of the stomach may be made through a gastrostomy wound. The stomach can be partially filled with water (holding the stomach wound uppermost to prevent spilling) and its interior then examined with a cystoscope.

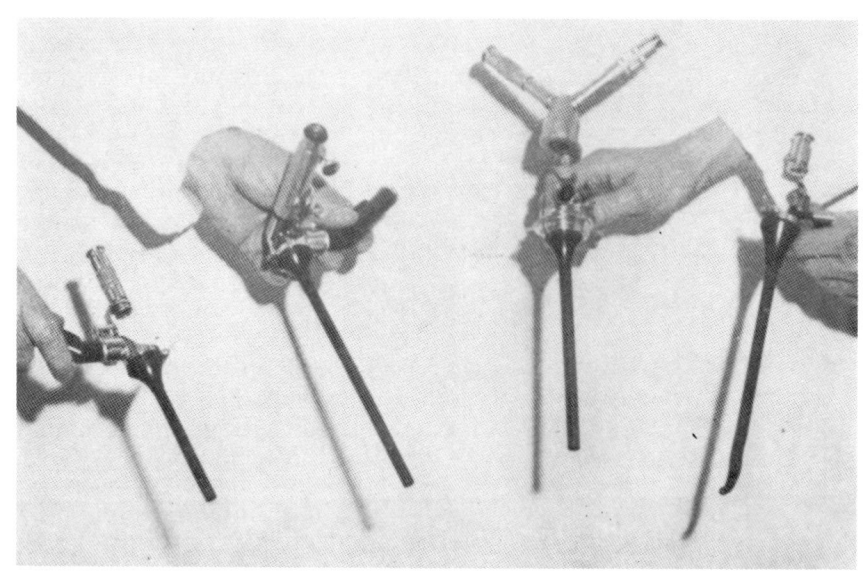

Figure 4–14. The operating televentroscope. A form of anterior gastroscope provided with a telescopic and focusing lens system combined with open endoscopic tubes for intragastric instrumentation. From left to right: (1) The monoplane vision telescope; (2) the periscopic vision telescope; (3) the double vision or teaching telescope; (4) the intragastric resectoscope with monoplane telescopic vision. (From Livingston, E. M., and Pack, G. T.: Surgical aids to intracavitary treatment and study of cancer of stomach. Am. J. Surg. 51:453, 1941.)

The stomach sometimes is examined through a gastrostomy stoma with a rigid-tube or with a flexible-tube gastroscope. The rigid-tube gastroscope is superior to the flexible oval gastroscope for use through a gastrostomy opening in that it may serve as an operating as well as an observation instrument. The instrument illustrated (Fig. 4–14) is called a televentroscope. This is an electrically lighted endoscope with a telescopic lens system.

Grasping forceps, punch biopsy tools, and electrosurgical snares or endoscopic resectoscopes can be used through a variety of open endoscopic tubes. A camera can be attached.

This method of examination is useful only in exceptional cases. It is particularly useful for antegrade and retrograde dilation of stricture in a patient with severe esophageal stricture who has a gastrostomy. The patient swallows a string, the lower end of which can be retrieved in the stomach by passing a televentroscope or its equivalent and a grasping forceps through the gastrostomy. A chain of bougies then can be attached to the string and the stricture thus dilated.

PERITONEOSCOPY, OR LAPAROSCOPY*

Peritoneoscopy and laparoscopy are synonymous. The procedure is the examination of the peritoneal cavity and its contents by using an optical instrument called a peritoneoscope or laparoscope. It is used after creating a pneumoperitoneum by injecting air or carbon dioxide into the peritoneal cavity to form an empty space within which the peritoneoscope can be maneuvered. The examiner can see clearly certain intraperitoneal structures through a small abdominal puncture wound and, if desired, may obtain a biopsy specimen of a lesion not on a hollow viscus. In some carefully selected disorders, the examiner may perform a therapeutic operation.

Peritoneoscopy (laparoscopy) was introduced in 1901 by Kelling, a German physician, but attracted little notice except in Germany until Ruddock (1937) of Califor-

―――――――――
*Portions of this section are adapted from Shackelford, R. T.: Peritoneoscopy. *In* Practice of Medicine, Vol. II. Hagerstown, Md., Harper & Row, 1975.

nia, also a physician, published the report of a large series of cases examined with his instrument, which had been specially designed for this purpose. Subsequently peritoneoscopy attained only moderate popularity in the United States, where it was used most often by internists and seldom by surgeons, although it led to the introduction of culdoscopy, which is now widely used by gynecologists.

About 1970, fiberoptic peritoneoscopes became available that had a source of light outside the instrument, providing bright illumination sufficient to permit intra-abdominal photography and offering other advantages. Since then, interest in peritoneoscopy has increased enormously.

The most prolific use of the new 'scopes has been by gynecologists, for diagnosis and for surgical procedures such as tubal interruption; by internists; and to a lesser extent by surgeons, for diagnosis of intra-abdominal conditions that had defied diagnosis by clinical, laboratory, or radiologic methods.

Advantages and Limitations

Peritoneoscopy is a minor procedure which can be performed with either local or general anesthesia in cooperative adults; general anesthesia is used for infants, for children, and for adults who are uncooperative or psychotic. It causes minimal discomfort, morbidity, and mortality. Although peritoneoscopy provides less information than laparotomy, the associated mortality, morbidity, and hospital expenses are lower.

The reported accuracy of peritoneoscopy in diagnosis varies from 87 to 95 per cent, the mortality rate from 0.001 to 0.02 per cent, and the complication rate from 0.002 to 2.4 per cent. In our experience with more than 1500 procedures done for diagnosis with or without biopsy, the diagnostic accuracy has been 89 per cent (Shackelford, 1975). The diagnostic failures were due to unsatisfactory examination because of adhesions in 7 per cent and false-negative findings in 4 per cent. Peritoneoscopy is most reliable for what is seen rather than for what is apparently absent. Our mortality rate in this group has been 0.001 per cent, and the complication rate, 0.006 per cent.

The structures and tissues that can be seen in most peritoneoscopic examinations are the anterior and part of the posterior surfaces of the liver; the dome of the gallbladder; the anterior walls of the stomach and colon; the lower portion of an enlarged (but not of a normal) spleen; the peritoneal surface of the urinary bladder; the surface and surface vessels of the omentum, parietal peritoneum, and short segments of small bowel; and intraperitoneal fluid or adhesions or both. Hernial orifices (inguinal and femoral) can usually be seen. Hence the procedure is particularly useful for diagnosing lesions of the liver, uterus, fallopian tubes, and ovaries; for differentiating the causes of hepatomegaly or ascites or both; and in determining the presence of metastases or tubercles in the liver, in the omentum, or on the surface of the peritoneum.

However, the posterior surfaces or intraluminal or intramesenteric abnormalities of structures cannot be seen, nor can the kidneys, aorta, or retroperitoneal structures. Except in children, the spleen cannot be visualized unless it is enlarged; hence visualization of the spleen in an adult indicates splenomegaly. The spleen should not be biopsied at peritoneoscopy because of the danger of uncontrollable hemorrhage. Occasionally an abnormality in the usually invisible areas may appear as a visible mass bulging into the peritoneal cavity, but its specific origin and nature are not usually revealed. Rarely, usually hidden lesions such as a mucocele of the appendix or diverticulum of the bowel are seen through the peritoneoscope, but this is not to be expected.

Peritoneoscopy is indicated in patients with a suspected intra-abdominal lesion in whom laboratory studies, clinical findings, and technical procedures have failed to provide a satisfactory diagnosis, and there is reason to believe that direct inspection or biopsy of the surface of a specific organ may determine its nature. The procedure should be used only for a specific purpose, e.g., to make a differential diagnosis, to confirm a clinical impression, or to determine the nature and extent of an abdominal tumor, and then only after the simpler laboratory and technical procedures have failed to supply the information desired. It should not be used as a short cut to a rapid diagnosis or for a general inspection of the peritoneal cavity without a specific differential diagnosis in mind; if it is so used, the operator will often be disappointed. Peritoneoscopy is suitable only for recognizing lesions on the surfaces of organs; except in rare instances, it does not provide the information gained by palpation; nor can one explore the depths of the peritoneal cavity. When correctly used it is approximately 90 per cent accurate in establishing the diagnosis. It is an established method of diagnosis in patients for whom it is indicated.

Peritoneoscopy cannot entirely replace exploratory laparotomy because the latter (1) provides added information gained by palpation, (2) gives access to deep structures inaccessible to the former, and (3) often provides opportunity for a therapeutic or palliative operation. On the other hand, peritoneoscopy often avoids the necessity of laparotomy by demonstrating the absence of a suspected lesion, or the presence of a lesion that is nonsurgical or inoperable.

The method is more accurate in certain lesions than in others. It is particularly accurate in diagnosing cirrhosis, primary and secondary carcinoma of the liver, hepatitis, metastases to the omentum or peritoneum, ectopic pregnancy, tumors and cysts of the ovaries and tubes, chronic pelvic inflammatory disease, and fibroids of the uterus; it seems especially valuable in cases of ascites. Some physicians and surgeons have found it useful in determining operability of cancer of the stomach, and some advocate its use in management of carcinoma of the esophagus to determine whether or not the liver is involved by metastases and if so, how extensively. However, the information to be gained by peritoneoscopy in all cases with these lesions is insufficient to justify its routine use. About 5 per cent of peritoneoscopies fail to accomplish their purpose because adhesions prevent or limit visualization of the free peritoneal cavity. An additional 3 to 5 per cent obtain false-negative diagnoses.

Indications and Contraindications for Diagnostic Peritoneoscopy

Peritoneoscopy is a valuable diagnostic tool when reserved for a small group of highly selected patients in whom one is attempting to determine a specific disorder in the organs accessible to the peritoneoscope. It is not satisfactory for a general exploration within the abdomen and should not be expected to accomplish more than the purpose for which it is used. When this previously set purpose is accomplished, the procedure should be considered successful and should be terminated.

Based on our experience, the indications for peritoneoscopy are as follows:

1. In any undiagnosed patient about to undergo paracentesis for known or suspected ascites. Peritoneoscopy is similar to paracentesis, but it establishes the presence or absence of ascites with greater certainty. Ascitic fluid can be removed with equal facility by both procedures. Additional information is provided by visualization of the intraperitoneal organs and peritoneal surfaces, and suspicious lesions may be biopsied.

2. In any undiagnosed case of hepatomegaly. In these cases peritoneoscopy has an advantage over needle biopsy of the liver because it permits visualization of the surface of that organ, permits biopsy under direct vision of an abnormal-appearing area with arrest of bleeding by electrocoagulation of the biopsy wound, and permits taking a larger biopsy specimen.

3. To differentiate primary or secondary malignancy of the liver, hepatitis, cirrhosis, and obstructive jaundice.

4. To differentiate tuberculous peritonitis and peritoneal carcinomatosis.

5. To differentiate myomatous uterus, ovarian cysts, and carcinoma of the ovary, and to determine ectopic pregnancy.

6. To determine the operability of some tumors.

7. To corroborate a clinical diagnosis in selected cases.

8. To obtain a biopsy in known liver disease for study of its progress under therapy.

9. To diagnose endometriosis and other pelvic disorders in women.

10. Bagley and associates (1973), at the National Cancer Institute in Bethesda, reported that peritoneoscopy with liver biopsy is useful in staging Hodgkin's disease, and in the post-therapy follow-up of patients with Hodgkin's disease and non-Hodgkin's lymphomas. It is limited, however, in that access to retroperitoneal lymph nodes is not possible.

11. Emergency peritoneoscopy for suspected traumatic bleeding or peritonitis after blunt trauma to the abdomen has been used widely with gratifying results in significant numbers of patients in France and Germany and reported frequently in their literature. This use of peritoneoscopy has been mentioned only scantily in the English language literature.

Although our experience is not extensive, two examples will demonstrate the value of emergency peritoneoscopy in two patients with multiple injuries, including blunt abdominal trauma, seen recently in the emergency ward (Shackelford, 1975).

One was an unconscious child with fractures of all four extremities, blunt abdominal trauma, and head injury. Attempts to determine the presence of intra-abdominal bleeding were unsuccessful because after each of 3 peritoneal lavages of 500 ml. of saline was injected into the abdomen, no fluid could be withdrawn through the tube. The abdomen became distended — whether because of bleeding or because of the 1500 ml. of saline injected was uncertain. While the neurosurgeons and orthopedists worked on the other injuries, emergency peritoneoscopy was performed, and a ruptured and bleeding spleen was visualized. Immediate laparotomy and splenectomy were performed.

Another patient was an inebriated woman with multiple injuries, including blunt abdominal trauma. Abdominal lavage recovered the injected saline, which was slightly tinged with blood. This finding was equivocal. Because of the multiple injuries, avoiding an unnecessary laparotomy was essential. Since the patient was inebriated, her symptoms and signs were obscure, so prolonged observation was risky. Emergency peritoneoscopy was performed. No evidence of ruptured viscus or of hemorrhage was seen. Laparotomy was avoided. Both patients did well.

These two cases are offered as examples that emergency peritoneoscopy can be valuable for determining whether or not exploratory laparotomy is indicated in patients with multiple injuries that include blunt abdominal trauma.

Fahrländer (1969) in Germany reported 107 patients in whom emergency peritoneoscopy was performed for suspected bleeding or peritonitis after blunt trauma to the abdomen. The correct diagnosis was established in the 65 cases of suspected bleeding. There was one false-negative diagnosis in the 34 patients with suspected peritonitis, and the procedure was of limited value in the 8 patients with suspected pancreatitis. No untoward results related to the procedure were mentioned.

Llanio and associates (1973), in France, reported 1265 emergency peritoneoscopies for acute abdominal conditions. The diagnostic accuracy was 97.5 per cent. Gynecologic disorders, including 230 ectopic pregnancies, accounted for 54 per cent of the cases. The second most common diagnosis was gallbladder disorder (17 per cent), and the remainder comprised miscellaneous intra-abdominal conditions.

Poor selection of patients is the greatest cause of failure to make a diagnosis by peritoneoscopy.

Contraindications for peritoneoscopy are:

1. Acute inflammatory disease within the abdomen. In these patients there is danger that introduction of the instrument may perforate an abscess or wall of a viscus made more friable by inflammation, or that introduction of carbon dioxide or air under pressure to create a pneumoperitoneum may separate a newly formed wall of protective adhesions and thus spread the infection.

Contrary to this statement, some gynecologists believe that acute inflammatory disease within the abdomen does not always contraindicate peritoneoscopy. A significant number of women appear with pain in the right lower quadrant in whom the differential diagnosis among acute appendicitis, salpingitis, and tubal pregnancy could not be established by conventional clinical and laboratory methods. Emergency peritoneoscopy has provided the diagnosis in some of these cases. Those with visualized acute appendicitis and tubal pregnancy are admitted to the hospital for prompt operation. Those with visualized salpingitis need not be hospitalized but can be treated by immediate administration of appropriate antibiotics, observed overnight, and returned to their homes, thus saving days of unnecessary hospitalization. Our surgical service does not use peritoneoscopy for this differential diagnosis.

2. Suspected dense intra-abdominal

adhesions in patients who have had multiple abdominal operations. Most of the reported perforations of the bowel have occurred in patients with intra-abdominal adhesions because adhesions prevent the intestine from slipping away from the advancing blunt trocar; thus the intestine is perforated. By selecting the site of puncture away from the scar of a previous operation, a satisfactory and safe examination can often be made. Another contraindication for peritoneoscopy in this type of case is that even if the instrument is introduced safely into the peritoneal cavity, its range of examination is limited by the presence of adhesions, which may make the region to be examined inaccessible. In some instances, however, the knowledge of adhesions may be all that is needed to establish the diagnosis.

3. Abdominal distention. To my knowledge there have been no reports of complications following peritoneoscopic examination of patients with abdominal distention due to gas and we have had none; however, it would seem that a markedly distended intestine, with its wall thin and tense from intraluminal pressure, would be vulnerable to an advancing trocar and might perforate whether or not adhesions limited its mobility. Furthermore, the increased area occupied by a dilated gastrointestinal tract would limit the air space necessary for a satisfactory peritoneoscopic examination.

4. Serious cardiac or pulmonary disease. In these patients the peritoneal insufflation with air or carbon dioxide may embarrass the circulation and diaphragmatic movements enough to cause serious trouble. Peritoneoscopy can be used in patients with cardiac or pulmonary disease in whom these ailments are not severe enough to cause cyanosis or orthopnea.

5. Hemorrhagic disorders are a contraindication. Their possible presence should be investigated before peritoneoscopy.

Technic

Instruments

The rigid Ruddock peritoneoscope with its Foroblique lens and a light at the tip of both the telescope and the biopsy forceps has been superseded by the newer fiberoptic peritoneoscopes with a source of light outside the instrument, providing much better illumination that permits clearer views of the visualized intra-abdominal structures and/or lesions and also permits intra-abdominal photography. These instruments have accessories for obtaining surface bite and/or needle puncture biopsies, for pushing structures out of the line of vision, for grasping objects or structures, for electrocoagulating visualized areas, and for performing various minor operative procedures. However, these more sophisticated instruments are expensive. A variety of fiberoptic peritoneoscopes made by different companies is available. Each has its advocates.

Preparation

The electric circuit of the peritoneoscope should be tested before each use.

All equipment except the light source is sterilized.

The patient is given no breakfast and is asked to empty the bladder by voiding before being brought to the operating room.

Preferably, peritoneoscopy is performed with the patient on an all-position table in an operating room or an adequately equipped endoscopic room that can be darkened. Aseptic precautions and draping are the same as for an exploratory laparotomy.

Anesthesia

For infants, children, and adults who are uncooperative or psychotic, general anesthesia through an endotracheal tube is used. For other adults, general or local anesthesia may be used. There is divided opinion about which is preferable. Our preference is for local anesthesia. We have routinely used premedication with 10 to 16 mg. of morphine given hypodermically about 30 minutes before the appointed time, and local infiltration anesthesia with 1 per cent lidocaine (Xylocaine) during the procedure. This method was used in more than 2000 cases with satisfaction and without untoward incident. Rarely was supplementary general anesthesia required. The gynecologic service routinely uses local anesthesia with preoperation medication consisting of 50 mg. of meperidine (Demerol) and 10 mg. of diazepam (Valium). The medical endoscopists use local anesthesia with premedication by intravenous injection of diazepam (Valium Injectable).

Local anesthesia has the advantages that the patient is conscious, can breathe and swallow normally, and can cooperate by tensing the abdominal wall during insertion of the needle to create a pneumoperitoneum, thus facilitating that maneuver. Following completion of the procedure there are no postanesthetic sequelae.

Others prefer general anesthesia. This involves insertion of an endotracheal tube, which has its own postextubation sequelae and makes peritoneoscopy a procedure of greater magnitude than when local anesthesia is used. Other disadvantages are that the abdominal wall is flaccid during insertion of the pneumoperitoneum needle, and this increases the possibility that the needle may not enter the abdominal cavity but instead remain in the extraperitoneal tissues. Also, if the needle should enter the peritoneal cavity, the flaccid abdominal wall would increase the hazard of the closely underlying bowel being punctured before there is a pneumoperitoneal space between the intestine and the abdominal wall. These two mishaps can be avoided by grasping the anesthetized abdominal skin with a towel clip at the intended site of puncture and tenting the flaccid abdominal wall anteriorly to create a space between it and the underlying bowel during insertion of the pneumoperitoneal needle at right angles to the skin surface and into the peritoneal cavity.

Advantages with general anesthesia and relaxants are that the rise in intra-abdominal pressure induced by pneumoperitoneum is not as marked as with local anesthesia, and that it permits creating a larger air space. This facilitates the examination without respiratory and hemodynamic effects. However, it should be pointed out that with local anesthesia the patient is fully conscious and breathing normally, so that excessive pressure is manifested by the patient's complaints and by clinically recognized signs of respiratory distress which can be promptly relieved by removing the excessive amount of intraperitoneal gas. Another advantage of general anesthesia is that the patient cannot move and therefore, if the electrocautery is used the danger of it inadvertently contacting and burning a loop of intestine is minimized.

In earlier days, with use of the Ruddock peritoneoscope, pneumoperitoneum was created by manually pumping air into the peritoneal cavity with an ordinary Baumanometer air bulb attached to the pneumoperitoneum needle. This increased intra-abdominal pressure slowly. There was ample time for the patient to warn of intolerable pressure. Excessive pressure never became a problem, nor did air embolism occur in our experience with more than 1000 cases. Only 3 cases of air embolism, resulting from the use of air for this purpose, are reported in the literature.

With the newer fiberoptic instruments, pneumoperitoneum is created with carbon dioxide delivered from high-pressure tanks by a mechanized CO_2 insufflator. A pressure-reduction valve monitors intra-abdominal pressure and the flow of carbon dioxide into the abdomen. Intra-abdominal pressure should be kept at 10 mm. Hg. Unless carefully regulated, this machine can distend the abdomen too rapidly. Furthermore, absorption of carbon dioxide from the peritoneal cavity in anesthetized patients can raise the arterial PCO_2 value and cause a significant fall in arterial pH. Since a large amount of the insufflated carbon dioxide is eventually excreted through the lungs, the patient who is undervenilating because of the Trendelenburg position and the diaphragm splinted by increased intra-abdominal pressure may be unable to eliminate the carbon dioxide adequately when breathing spontaneously. Hence some anesthetists condemn spontaneous breathing and recommend increased positive airway pressure during all peritoneoscopies performed under general anesthesia. We have not experienced that problem in our patients in whom local anesthesia was employed.

In our experience, acidosis developed in patients in whom the procedure was done under general anesthesia and whose spontaneous breathing was inadequate. It did not occur in those under general anesthesia with positive pressure through an endotracheal tube, nor in those under local anesthesia who breathed and swallowed normally; nor did aspiration occur in the locally anesthetized group. Furthermore, acidosis did not occur if the intra-abdominal pressure of carbon dioxide was kept below 20 mm Hg.

Site of Puncture

After sterilizing the skin of the abdomen in the usual way, a site of puncture is carefully selected. The vicinity of operative scars should be avoided because of the possibility of adherent intestines at that point. The puncture is most satisfactory if it is not immediately over the greatest convexity of a palpable intra-abdominal mass, because that would bring the instrument too close to the tumor to inspect it and would prevent the proper perspective. Any point on the abdominal wall may be selected; usually the most satisfactory site, when not contraindicated, is the lower midline, about 4 cm. below the umbilicus (Fig. 4–15). From this point the length of the instrument permits visualization and biopsy of all the intra-abdominal organs in a patient of average size. If the site selected is to either side of the midline, care should be taken to avoid the deep epigastric artery.

Another site, particularly useful in an obese abdomen, is the midline of the inferior margin of the umbilicus. At this point the layer of fat is thinnest. While the locally anesthetized skin is raised with two towel clips, one placed on either side of the umbilicus, the pneumoperitoneum needle can be inserted through the thin abdominal wall directly into the peritoneal cavity with minimal opportunity for it to be misplaced in the extraperitoneal tissues.

From either of these points, the length of the instrument permits visualization and biopsy of all the intra-abdominal organs in a patient of average size. However, in a few large and obese patients, it has been necessary to make a second incision in the right upper quadrant to obtain a biopsy of the liver because the forceps could not reach this organ from the original wound. To avoid this inconvenience in obese patients, before the incision is made the operator may place the instrument on the abdominal wall with its eyepiece at the planned site of puncture to see whether the instrument reaches the estimated area of the lesion to be viewed and biopsied. If the distance is too great, a right upper quadrant incision can be made initially. An upper midline incision is less satisfactory because from this site the instrument must pass through the voluminous fatty tissue in the folds of the falciform ligament.

Other locations have been selected for examining special areas.

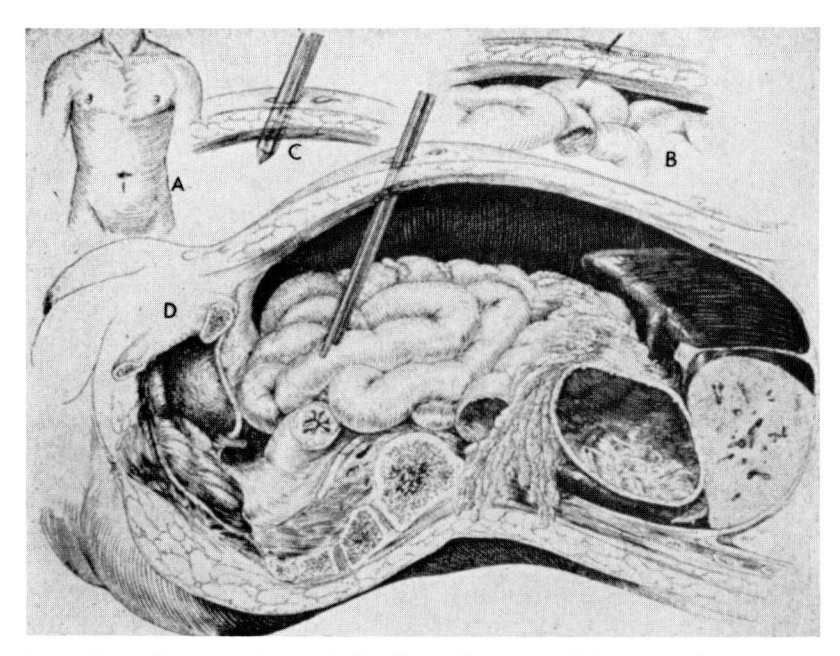

Figure 4–15. Technic of peritoneoscopy. *A*, Usual site of puncture. *B*, Insertion of pneumoperitoneum needle. *C*, Insertion of trocar. *D*, Visualization of peritoneal contents with peritoneoscope.

Insertion of Needle

After the proper site has been selected, and if local anesthesia is to be used, the skin is infiltrated with 1 per cent Xylocaine or its equivalent in a vertical line about 4 cm. in length. (Fig. 4–16). The hypodermic needle is then inserted entirely through the skin at the lower end of the infiltrated area and passed subcutaneously in a line obliquely (45°) upward to the right and again obliquely (45°) upward to the left; about 5 ml. of the anesthetic are injected in each direction. The process is repeated downward at the upper end of the infiltrated area, thus blocking off a diamond-shaped subcutaneous area around the planned incision. Puncture wounds completely through the skin, subcutaneous tissue, and fascia are then made at 1-cm. intervals around the periphery of this area, and 2 ml. of solution are injected at each point. This should result in a completely anesthetized region about the size of a 50-cent piece. If general anesthesia is used, local infiltration is omitted.

A 2-cm. vertical incision through the entire thickness of the skin is made with a No. 11 Bard-Parker knife; this is deepened through the subcutaneous fat until resistance by the deeper fascia is felt. The fascia is then nicked with the point of the knife. The pneumoperitoneum needle, with its stylet in place, is then dipped in sterile liquid petrolatum or glycerin to lubricate its passage through the tissues. It is inserted gently through the wound into the free peritoneal cavity, which it enters with a sudden cessation of resistance to its progress. The needle is then moved so that its point describes an arc within the peritoneal cavity. If the needle moves freely, almost certainly it is in the free peritoneal cavity. If, however, its mobility is limited by the point catching upon some intra-abdominal object, one should investigate whether this is due to having penetrated the lumen of the bowel, to adhesions, or to not having penetrated the peritoneum at all because the needle point is caught in the preperitoneal tissue.

Information about its position may be obtained by withdrawing the stylet and observing the lumen of the needle. Escape of ascitic fluid indicates it is in the free peritoneal cavity. Malodorous gas or recognizable intestinal contents are a sign that the bowel has been perforated. If no gas or fluid escapes, the three possible positions are neither excluded nor confirmed.

In the latter case, information can be obtained by attaching the insufflator and insufflating carbon dioxide or air through the needle. If the point of the needle is in the free peritoneal cavity, the abdomen will be seen to distend gradually and symmetrically with the insufflated air. If the needle is in the lumen of the bowel, abdominal distention is usually localized or absent but rumbling sounds may be heard or air may escape from the rectum. If the needle has remained extraperitoneal, palpation of the abdominal wall may reveal crepitus in the tissues as carbon dioxide is pumped through the needle.

When the needle is found to have perforated the bowel, it is best to leave the needle in place while exposing the perforation and to place a pursestring in the bowel wall around the perforation and the in situ needle. The purse string is drawn tight and

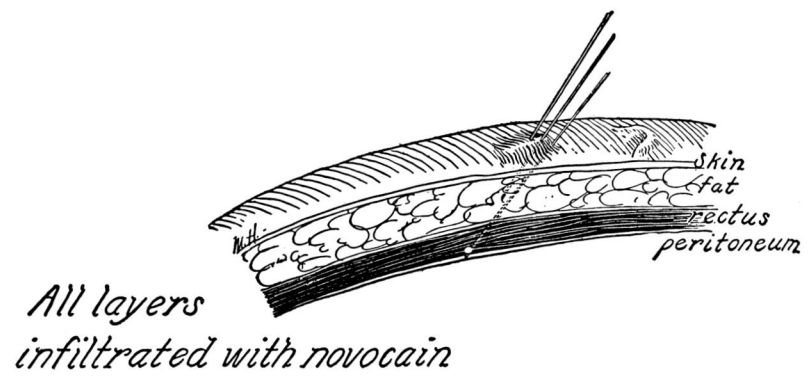

Figure 4–16. Infiltration of the layers of skin and peritoneum with Novocain.

tied as the needle is withdrawn. Usually no further repair is necessary, but the examination is discontinued.

When the needle point is found to have remained extraperitoneal, the point is withdrawn to the level of the fascial layer and reinserted more perpendicular to the contour of the abdominal wall until it has penetrated into the peritoneal cavity. If its mobility is then limited, the needle should be withdrawn and another site selected for puncture.

Inflation of the Abdomen

When the operator is satisfied with the puncture, the stylet is withdrawn and the abdomen is inflated. Formerly this was done by attaching a sterile Baumanometer bulb with its rubber connection to the open end of the needle and manually inflating the abdomen with ordinary unfiltered air to the limit of the patient's tolerance. Peritonitis due to use of unfiltered air has not been reported, nor have any explosions occurred during use of the cautery.

When manual inflation with air is used in a patient under local anesthesia, the quantity of air introduced is not measured. The degree of distention of the abdomen and the conscious patient's complaint of a feeling of fullness or difficulty in breathing indicates that sufficient air has been insufflated. In unconscious patients under general anesthesia, this warning is absent.

The former method of inflating the abdomen has been superseded by the use of carbon dioxide instead of air. Carbon dioxide has the advantages of rapid absorption by the tissues, noninflammability during the use of a cautery; and elimination of the possibility of air embolism. However, a few instances of suspected CO_2 embolism have been reported. The disadvantage of carbon dioxide is that its rapid absorption from the peritoneal cavity may elevate the arterial PCO_2 and lower the arterial pH.

The advantages of the CO_2 insufflator are that the amount of carbon dioxide insufflated and the intra-abdominal pressure are measured and can be monitored. When the patient is under general anesthesia, careful monitoring is important to avoid overdistention and cardiorespiratory embarrassment. The machine also can maintain a constant optimum pneumoperitoneum by replacing gas that escapes during the various maneuvers. In addition, it is physically less fatiguing and tedious than the former method of creating and maintaining an optimum pneumoperitoneum.

We insufflate 2 to 3 liters of carbon dioxide at a flow rate of 1 liter per minute and carefully avoid letting the intra-abdominal pressure exceed 15 mm. Hg. During inflation it is advisable to note whether or not the abdomen progressively distends and, if so, whether it distends symmetrically. If the needle point is placed properly within the free peritoneal cavity, the abdomen distends symmetrically and without pain even in the conscious patient under local anesthesia.

If the needle inadvertently enters the intestinal lumen, distention will be localized, and a conscious patient may complain of pain. The complaint of pain during this phase of the procedure suggests making sure that a complication has not developed. If the abdomen does not distend at all, the needle point is probably misplaced in the extraperitoneal tissue. This can be confirmed by palpating crepitus of subcutaneous emphysema in the abdominal wall.

The intraperitoneal gas creates a space between the abdominal wall and the intestines, providing a margin of safety for insertion of the trocar cannula.

Insertion of Trocar Cannula

The pneumoperitoneum needle is withdrawn and replaced by the cannula with its trocar through the same wound (Fig. 4–17). The tip of this instrument is dipped in sterile liquid petrolatum or sterile glycerin to permit its penetrating more smoothly through the tissues. It is advanced slowly through the abdominal wall with the instrument pointed slightly downward and to one side of the midline so that if it should enter the cavity too suddenly and too deeply, a viscus will not be impaled between its point of entry and the vertebral column. There is a popping sound as the peritoneum gives way. If the abdomen is adequately distended there is no difficulty in inserting the trocar cannula. Insertion is more difficult, painful, and hazardous when the abdomen is not adequately distended. This is the most uncomfortable phase of peritoneoscopy for the conscious patient because of the

PERITONEOSCOPY, OR LAPAROSCOPY

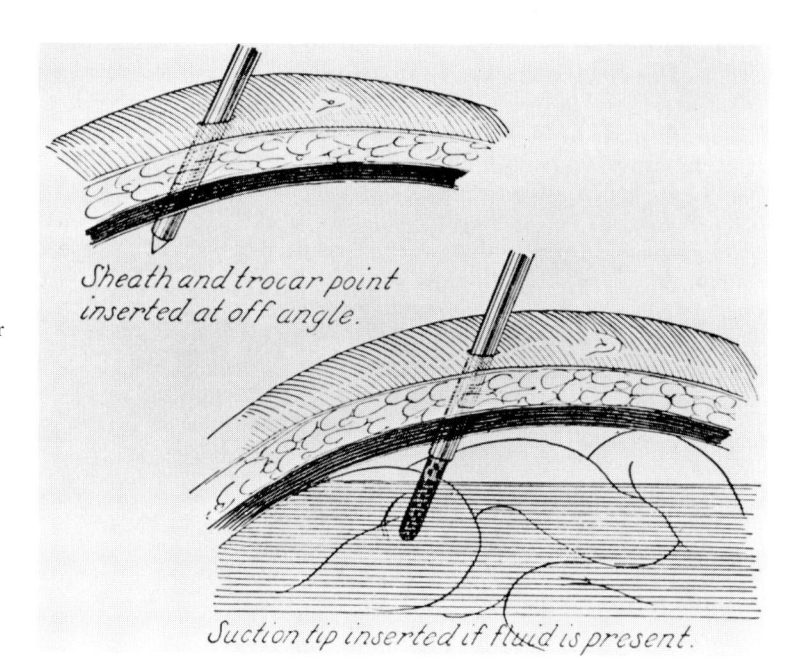

Figure 4–17. Sheath and trocar inserted at off angle.

pressure necessary to force the entrance of the trocar. The patient complains of a sense of pressure, not of pain; this is not severe and persists only during the few moments of application of pressure.

After the instrument has penetrated the peritoneum, its point is moved around in an arc, as described for introduction of the pneumoperitoneum needle. Unrestricted movement indicates it is in the free peritoneal cavity. Restricted movement suggests adhesions or penetration into a loop of bowel. When the operator is satisfied with the instrument's position, the trocar is withdrawn, leaving the cannula in place. If ascites is present the aspirator is inserted and the fluid is removed by suction. The aspirator is replaced by the observation telescope (after retesting the light to be sure that it is in working order). The gas that escapes during this change is then replaced until the abdomen is again distended and the gas space maximal in size. The greater the dimension of this space, within the limits of comfort, the more room there is for maneuvering the instrument and the more satisfactory is the examination.

Visualization

The telescope, with its light turned on, is advanced through its sliding cuff until it projects beyond the open end of the cannula. Before starting the examination, the operator looks through the telescope to make certain of clear visualization. At the beginning of the examination the lens within the peritoneal cavity may become clouded from moisture condensed on its surface as the cold instrument or gas is introduced into the warm body cavity. This disappears spontaneously in a few minutes. During the examination the examiner's eye should not touch the eyepiece, not only for the sake of asepsis, but also because heat radiating from the observer will cause the lens to become misted, interfering with sharp vision. When this occurs, clarity can be regained by wiping the lens of the eyepiece with a dry, sterile, gauze sponge. The distal lens may become blurred by contact with intraperitoneal fat or blood. This can be corrected by withdrawing the lens from the cannula, cleaning it with dry gauze, and reinserting it. When this is done, the gas lost during the maneuver must be replaced.

A clear view of the peritoneal cavity within the range of the lens should be obtained. Different areas can be viewed by rotating the telescope around its long axis or moving the entire instrument transversely or vertically in the desired direction.

The undersurfaces of the diaphragm and the parietal peritoneum are the only sensitive areas encountered within the abdominal cavity during the examination.

Free movement of the instrument causes no discomfort if these areas are not touched. In most cases the telescope is long enough for the entire abdominal cavity to be explored from a single puncture point.

The examination should be made with a fixed plan in mind. The plan should vary only in relation to the purpose of the examination. A general complete and systemic examination of the abdominal cavity with identification of organs and landmarks should be done first. A useful routine is to locate first the falciform ligament and the liver as a starting point and proceed from these in a clockwise direction. The anteroinferior surfaces of the liver are examined first from a distance and then in detail by approximating the instrument to the liver's surface. The dome of the gallbladder can usually be seen. The parietal peritoneum in this region can be inspected by rotating the lens. The anterior surface of the pylorus, the anterior wall of the stomach, and the undersurface of the diaphragm are then visualized. The splenic region is then viewed but the spleen is usually not visible in adults unless it is enlarged. In children its tip can be seen, and when the table is tilted to elevate the left side a considerable portion of its surface comes into view. The omentum and the anterior wall of the transverse colon are examined. As the 'scope is moved down the left side of the abdominal cavity, numerous loops of small intestine and portions of the descending and sigmoid colon come into view. The patient is then placed in the Trendelenburg position and the uterus, ovaries, tubes, peritoneal surfaces of the urinary bladder, and parietal peritoneum are inspected. The patient is returned to the original position and the instrument is passed up the right side of the anterior wall of the cecum. Often, but unreliably, a portion of the appendix may be seen.

A general examination is completed when the liver again comes into view. The examiner then returns to study in more detail any abnormalities noted during the general examination, obtain any biopsy material indicated, or perform whatever surgical procedure is intended. The appearance of normal and abnormal tissue seen through a peritoneoscope is similar to that seen an exploratory laparotomy.

Biopsy

Biopsies should not be done in the spleen or a hollow viscus. In many cases a visualized lesion can be confidently identified by inspection alone. With the fiberoptic peritoneoscopes they also can be photographed for a permanent record. However, it is usually desirable to obtain tissue, particularly when there is some doubt about the nature of the lesion. On such occasions biopsies may be obtained under direct vision through the peritoneoscope by one or both of two methods.

For superficial biopsy of an organ, such as the liver (see Fig. 4–18), the telescope is replaced by the biopsy forceps. The coagulating current is connected to its proper receptable. While the examiner is looking through the lens, the jaws of the instrument are opened and approximated to the tissue in question. The jaws are pressed into the tissue to be biopsied and then closed, biting off the desired section. The instrument is left in place with the jaws closed for use as an electrode and, while it is pressed against the wound in the organ, the coagulating current is turned on, thus coagulating the area thoroughly until all bleeding has been stopped. The area is inspected for a few moments to be sure that bleeding does not recur, and then the biopsy forceps is withdrawn from the cannula. The specimen contained within the closed jaws is about the size of a pea and is not damaged by the electrocoagulation.

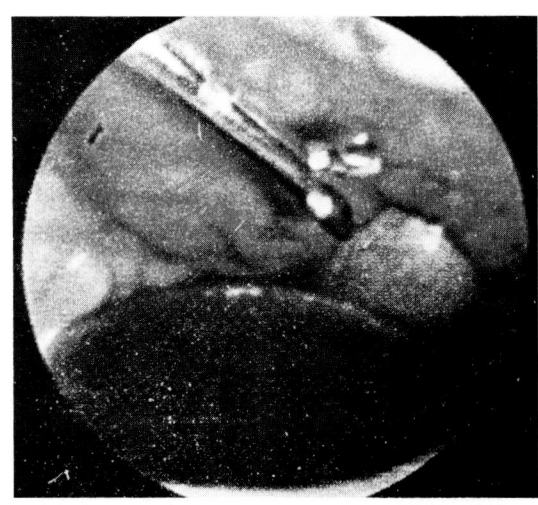

Figure 4–18. Forceps taking a biopsy of a hepatic lesion.

Deep biopsy of the liver may be made by selecting a site over the liver and percutaneously inserting a Vim-Silverman needle through the abdominal wall into the peritoneal cavity where, under peritoneoscopic visualization, it is guided into the desired area in the liver. If bleeding occurs, it can be controlled by electrocoagulation through the peritoneoscope.

All specimens removed are sent immediately to the laboratory, where half is used for immediate frozen sections and half is placed in fixing fluid for later permanent sections.

It has been suggested that biopsy specimens obtained from the depth of the liver by needle biopsy are more informative than specimens of relatively superficial liver tissue, such as obtained by peritoneoscopy. As a result, needle biopsy of the liver (with some morbidity and a mortality of about 1 per cent) became popular. Needle biopsies are blind procedures; although they are helpful in diffuse liver disease, they cannot be depended upon to find and obtain tissue from localized, discrete lesions in that organ. When hepatic metastases are scattered, the needle may be inserted between metastases and obtain normal liver tissue, missing the malignant tissue altogether.

To obviate this it has become a common practice first to perform a peritoneoscopy on the patient and, with the endoscope in place, to perform a needle puncture of the liver through another puncture site, guiding the needle by direct vision through the telescope so that the needle enters the area suspected to be abnormal. Tumors on the surface of the liver can be biopsied by the peritoneoscope alone, but those deep in the liver cannot. By combining the two methods, a deeply situated lesion can be biopsied, and any bleeding that occurs can be controlled by electrocoagulation with the peritoneoscopic biopsy forceps.

Brühl in 1967 surveyed the experience of 67 peritoneoscopists with this procedure. Their combined series totalled 63,845 peritoneoscopies (48,766 of these were combined with needle puncture of the liver). There were 1594 complications (2.49 per cent); 19 patients died (mortality 0.029 per cent). Eight of the deaths were due to biliary peritonitis and seven to bleeding. Less severe complications were pneumo- omentum (803), subcutaneous emphysema (366), and circulatory collapse (166); mediastinal emphysema and perforation of the gut occurred less often.

Special Examinations

Peritoneoscopic cholangiography has been used for the differential diagnosis of jaundice. Two different technics have been reported.

Lee (1942) introduced cholangiography by a technique that combined needle puncture of the abdomen and peritoneoscopy, the point of the needle being guided into the dome of the gallbladder under direct vision through the telescope. When bile is obtained, the contrast medium is injected into the gallbladder, followed by radiographs of the area. Excellent visualization of the gallbladder, the cystic duct, and the common duct is said to have been obtained. This method appears to present the hazard of a bile leak into the peritoneal cavity, but Keil and Landis (1951) reported the procedure to be safe and reliable. They enthusiastically recommended its use when oral and intravenous cholangiography failed. Despite this strong recommendation, the procedure apparently is not widely used.

The other method, described by Berci and associates (1973), is more complicated and requires more sophisticated equipment. It is doubtful that either technique will be used widely. Duodenoscopic cholangiography (ERCP) seems simpler, safer, and more informative.

Yamamoto and Reynolds (1964) reported a peritoneoscopic method for measuring portal venous pressure and making portal venograms. Omentum is manipulated with the peritoneoscope so that when the instrument is withdrawn some omentum extrudes through the small opening in the abdominal wall. A suitable vein is intubated with a suitable catheter, and portal pressure is measured with a saline manometer. This is followed by immediate portography with 30 ml. of contrast medium. Afterward the omentum is easily reduced. Successful visualization was obtained in four of seven patients, but the three failures developed complications.

Berci and associates (1973) performed peritoneoscopy in two patients in whom the diagnosis of mesenteric vascular insufficiency or intestinal infarction was strongly suspected. Visualization of the surface of the intestine excluded mesenteric vascular insufficiency in one case, while in the second case an area of localized gangrene was seen, and prompt laparotomy was performed. For this condition, diagnostic findings are more likely to be serendipitous than expected. We are unaware of the use of peritoneoscopy for this purpose by others.

With the patient in the Trendelenburg position, the orifices of inguinal and femoral hernias are usually dilated by the pneumoperitoneum and are readily visible.

Examination of abdominal masses or viscera often can be improved by tilting the table up and down or from side to side. Gallstones within the gallbladder have been palpated by the instrument by several examiners.

Operative Procedures

Performance of minor operative procedures during peritoneoscopy has been reported. Adhesive bands have been successfully severed in the abdominal cavity. According to Ruddock (1957), who has performed this procedure, the electric tip (knife and coagulator) should be constantly under direct vision. No attempt should be made to sever adhesions that are situated between loops of bowel, and only those adhesions attached to the parietal peritoneum or the liver should be separated. The blood vessels in adhesive bands can be visualized. These should be slowly coagulated before being cut. A point of severance should be selected so that the cutting electrode is not in close proximity to a loop of bowel or hollow viscus.

Benedict (1951) aspirated a large ovarian cyst in an elderly, poor-risk patient by inserting a peritoneoscope with its observation lens and then passing an aspirating trocar and cannula through a separate puncture wound in the abdominal wall. While guiding it by direct vision through the peritoneoscope, he plunged the aspirator into the cyst and evacuated its contents. One surgeon reported having incised simple follicular cysts of the ovary in the same manner. Some have performed uterine suspensions by using a special needle, and others have reported repair of a patent inguinal hernia ring. Some liver abscesses have been drained successfully by inserting a needle or small trocar through a separate puncture wound directly into the abscess under vision through the peritoneoscope. Siegler (1973) reported successful use of peritoneoscopy to remove ectopic intrauterine contraceptive devices from the abdominal cavity in 8 cases, with varying degrees of difficulty.

In our opinion, these operative procedures are more effective, reliable, and safe if performed by conventional surgical methods.

Sterilization of women is the most frequent indication for peritoneoscopy. It is performed by gynecologists, and the details of its technics are beyond the scope of this book. Wheeless and Thompson (1973) reported 3600 such procedures. Complications were uncommon; the most serious were inadvertent burning of the intestine during use of the cautery. This occurred in ten patients, of whom six required exploratory laparotomy and repair of the bowel. The remainder were treated conservatively and did well. Immediate hemorrhage occurred in 58 patients but was controlled by coagulation through the peritoneoscope.

Regional Examination from the Usual Site of Puncture

In Figures 4–19 through 4–28, lesions are depicted in photographs and drawings as they appear through the peritoneoscope.

Liver

The liver can easily be seen from the usual site of puncture in the lower midline; when its size is normal, the entire anteroinferior surface and part of the dome can be visualized. If it is greatly enlarged, a smaller proportion of the surface can be explored. A normal liver is smooth and homogeneous and has a deep mahogany color. If jaundiced, it is grayish green. If biliary cirrhosis is beginning, the surface is marked with yellowish trabeculations. When cirrhosis of the liver has developed, the organ has a symmetrically nodular, hobnail appearance (see Fig. 4–19). The symmetry and equality of the nodules are important for distinguishing this lesion from metastatic nodules (see Fig. 4–20). In the latter condition, the whole liver may be nodular and of a color similar to the cirrhotic organ, but inspection will show that the nodules vary in size and shape. Metastatic involvement in the liver substance may also result in other appearances (see Fig. 4–21). The organ may have dull reddish, raised nodules with concave, depressed centers. Metastases on the surface of the liver are seen as chalk-white nodules.

Tuberculomas and syphilomas sometimes appear as raised, concave, nodular metastases. However they are not as numerous or diffuse. Biopsy may be necessary to establish the diagnosis. Primary carcinoma of the liver may be suspected when a tissue of different color and somewhat raised above the surface is seen. Biopsy is necessary to confirm the visual impression. Abscess may be recognized by the raised, edematous appearance of the affected area, occasionally with overlying fibrin.

When enlargement of the liver is due to chronic passive congestion, it is dark red in color, with a smooth surface and rounded edge. If the congestion has been longstanding, as in Pick's disease, the capsule is thickened, and the liver appears pale. In far-advanced disease, it may appear to be coated with sugar. This thickened, tough capsule may make biopsy difficult.

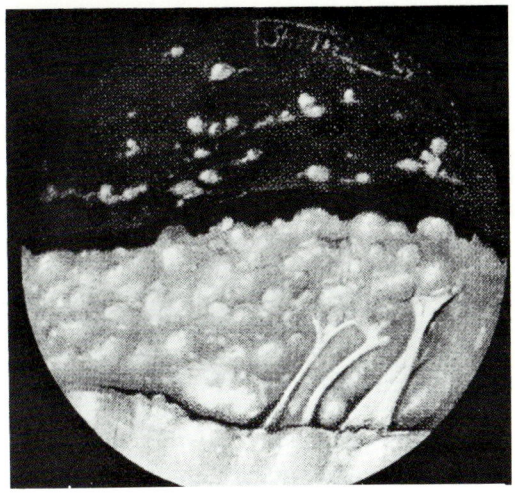

Figure 4–20. Tubercles on liver.

When alcoholic hepatitis is present, the liver is swollen, smooth, and reddish brown with rounded edges. Ascites is often, but not always, present. In von Gierke's disease in infants the liver is markedly enlarged, smooth, very pale, and edematous. Biopsy is necessary to establish the diagnosis. In polycystic disease of the liver, multiple clear cysts appear throughout the organ. In amyloidosis, the liver is greatly enlarged, with rounded edges and a pale brown color. Biopsy is necessary. In acute yellow atrophy, the liver is small, wrinkled, and dark brown in color.

Extra lobes of the liver and adhesions between the liver and other structures are usually unmistakable.

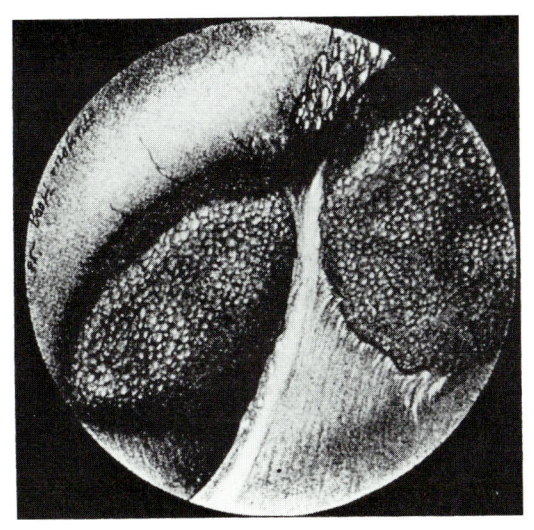

Figure 4–19. Cirrhosis of liver.

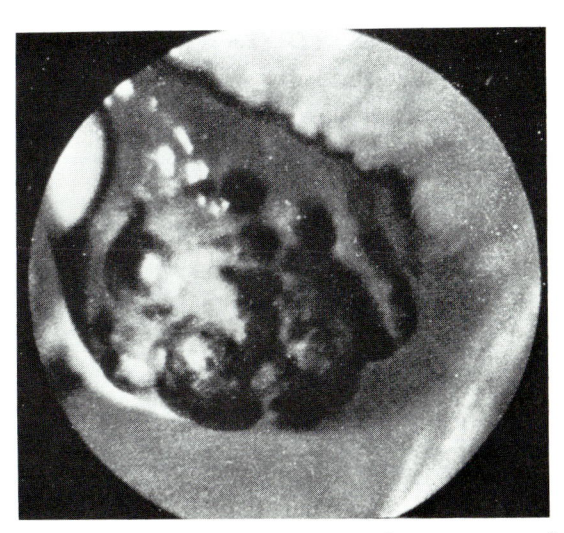

Figure 4–21. Liver metastases from carcinoma of the pancreas.

Gallbladder (See Fig. 4-22)

The fundus of the normal gallbladder is usually visible. It is bluish in color and nonadherent. If previous infection has occurred, the wall appears pale white. If hydrops is present, the gallbladder is white, distended, and easily seen. If empyema is present, the viscus is usually covered by an adherent omentum. A small and contracted gallbladder cannot be visualized. In a few cases gallstones have been palpated, but this is not to be expected. Primary carcinoma of the gallbladder, if it involves the fundus, can be seen as an indurated whitish lesion that may extend out along adherent omentum as nodules (see Fig. 4-23). Biopsy of one of these nodules may establish the diagnosis.

Biliary Ducts

The cystic, hepatic, and common ducts cannot be seen. Obstruction of one of these ducts may be suggested by a distended gallbladder and, if longstanding, by an enlarged, jaundiced liver showing some degree of biliary cirrhosis. The nature of the obstruction will not be found, however, unless accessible metastases are present and biopsy of one of these reveals the tumor.

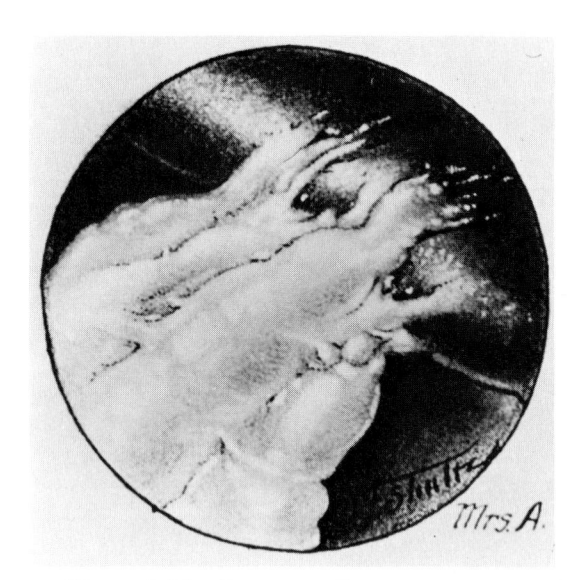

Figure 4-23. Omentum adherent to carcinoma of gallbladder and containing metastatic nodules. Biopsy specimen showed carcinoma of gallbladder.

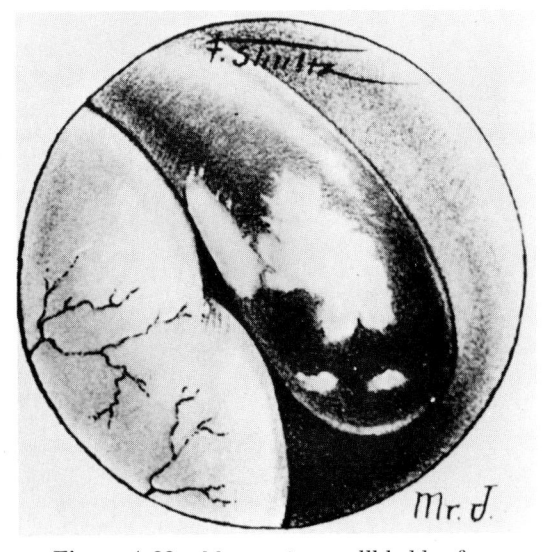

Figure 4-22. Metastasis to gallbladder from unsuspected carcinoma of prostate.

Stomach

The surface of the anterior wall and the greater curvature of the stomach from the pylorus to just below the cardia can be seen. In a few cases, edema, fibrin, and puckering on the anterior wall near the pylorus or adherence of omentum to that area has led to the discovery of peptic ulcer. However, these are exceptions; peritoneoscopy has not been of much value in diagnosing peptic ulcer. It has been used in the past to evaluate the operability of carcinoma of the stomach but is also unreliable for this purpose. Gastroscopy provides more information about the stomach than does peritoneoscopy.

Spleen

In adults, the normal spleen cannot be seen in the dorsal recumbent position. It is visible only if it is enlarged. In children the tip of a normal spleen can be examined in the dorsal recumbent position; by tilting the table to the right so the patient's left side is up, a large portion of its surface can be seen. There is nothing pathognomonic about its appearance. The spleen *should not be biopsied*.

Omentum

The surface of the omentum can be examined throughout. Whether it is smooth and glistening or nodular, and whether it is adherent, and if so, where, should be noted. Malignant metastases occur as nodules in the fatty tissue (see Figs. 4–23 and 4–24). Some of these are slightly redder than the normal fat, while others have a whitish, glistening appearance. Although they can usually be recognized grossly, they may be mistaken for the tubercles seen in tuberculous peritonitis or for the white, opaque areas of "fat necrosis" scattered over the surface of the omentum and parietal and visceral peritoneum, often seen in patients who have injury or disease of the pancreas. Biopsy should be performed. This can be done easily, and often the nature of the parent growth may be determined by microscopic study of the specimen.

Tuberculous peritonitis is usually seen as a number of small, pinpoint white specks or nodules distributed over the entire omentum, parietal peritoneum, and surface of the various organs. When it arises from tuberculous salpingitis, the amount of involvement seen is much greater in the pelvis than elsewhere.

Retroperitoneal tumors can be recognized only as masses beneath the omentum that apparently are not attached to it but raise its surface.

Occasionally, the site of adherence of the omentum may indicate an inflammatory process at that point. Some edema and fibrin may be present, and, although the actual lesion cannot be identified, the findings are strongly suggestive.

Colon

The anterior walls of the cecum and of the ascending, transverse, descending, and sigmoid colons can be seen quite easily. It is difficult to trace their course in continuity, as other structures may temporarily obscure them and disorient the examiner as to the exact part being examined. The hepatic and splenic flexures usually are not seen satisfactorily. Normally they are whiter in color than the small intestine. Primary or secondary carcinoma of the colon may be visualized. The former is usually seen as an encircling, constricting, rigid mass puckering the otherwise pliable gut. A metastasis usually appears as an isolated nodule, sometimes with a concave center puckering the bowel wall.

Tuberculous implants are seen as white flecks or nodules scattered on the surface of the bowel. Adhesions are common. Biopsy should not be taken from the surface of any of the hollow viscera because of the danger of perforation by either the biopsy forceps or the coagulation current.

The appendix often may be seen when it lies freely in the abdominal cavity or, occasionally, when its tip projects upward like a pole (see Fig. 4–25).

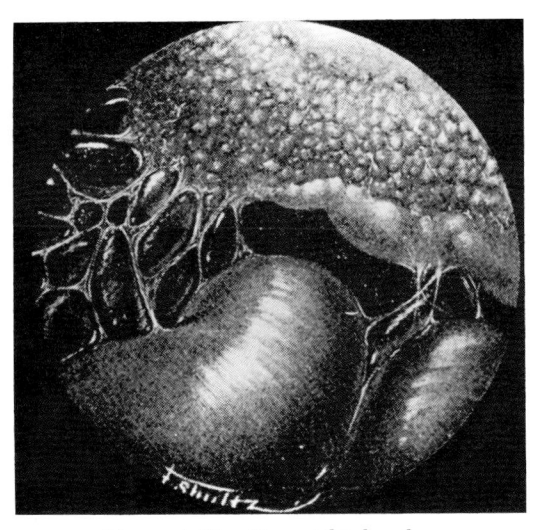

Figure 4–24. Omental tubercles.

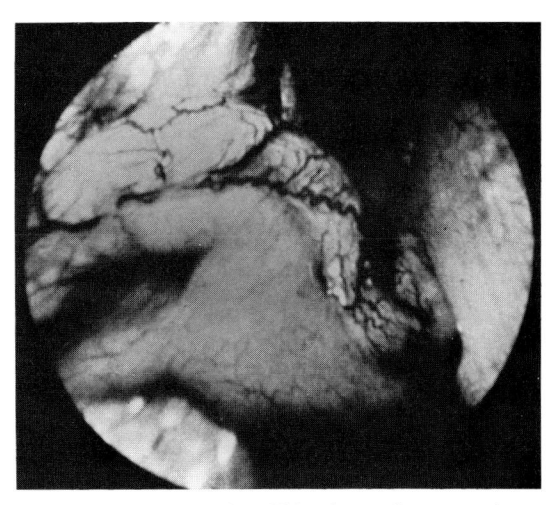

Figure 4–25. Dilated blood vessels on acutely inflamed appendix.

Peritoneoscopy obviously does not visualize intraluminal abnormalities. Colonoscopy and barium enema x-ray studies are more informative for examining the colon.

Small Intestine

The surface of many loops of small intestine can be visualized. They are normally reddish brown in color, and peristaltic waves can be seen. Very few lesions in which the peritoneoscope would be of any value occur in the small bowel. Adhesions between loops or between loops and the abdominal wall or other structures are often seen. However, cases in which there is intestinal distention are not suitable for peritoneoscopy because of the very real danger of perforation. Malignant or tuberculous implants may be seen on the intestine; they look the same here as elsewhere. *These should not be biopsied.*

Pelvic Organs

Both ovaries can be easily seen when the patient is placed in the Trendelenburg position, provided adhesions of the omentum or the sigmoid or some pelvic mass does not completely cover them. It may be helpful to have an assistant place a finger in the vagina and manipulate these organs to expose various surfaces. Normally the ovaries have a whitish appearance flecked with reddish follicles. Small follicular cysts may be seen, or the entire ovary may be recognized as a large, glistening cyst. Corpora hemorrhagica and corpora lutea may be seen. The ovary may be bound down by adhesions from old pelvic inflammatory disease, or some edema or fibrin indicating a subacute stage may be present.

Carcinoma of the ovary appears as a hard, glistening, edematous mass. Papillary cystadenocarcinoma has a characteristic picture of multiple cystic masses in the ovary and scattered over neighboring organs as implants (see Fig. 4–26).

The size and shape of the tubes can be seen easily. If a tubal pregnancy is present, the tube will bulge at the site of the fetus, and possibly a small amount of blood will exude from the fimbriated end. If the ectopic pregnancy has ruptured recently, the abdomen will be filled with blood, and visualization of the various structures will be impossible. However, if the rupture occurred some time previously, old hemolyzed blood may be in the cavity, which can be removed by a suction so the the encysted lesion can be visualized.

Hydrosalpinx and myomas of the uterus are readily recognizable (see Fig. 4–27). Tuberculous salpingitis is seen as an edematous, swollen tube associated with multiple tuberculous implants on the neighboring organs. The implants can be biopsied and the visual impression confirmed.

Intrauterine pregnancy may be recognized by the dusky color and soft appearance of the uterus.

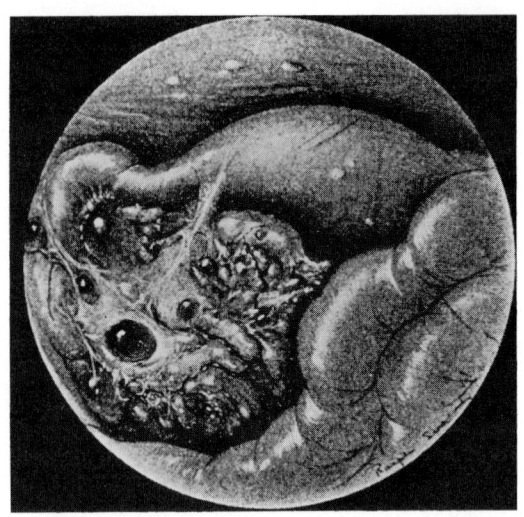

Figure 4–26. Papillary cystadenocarcinoma.

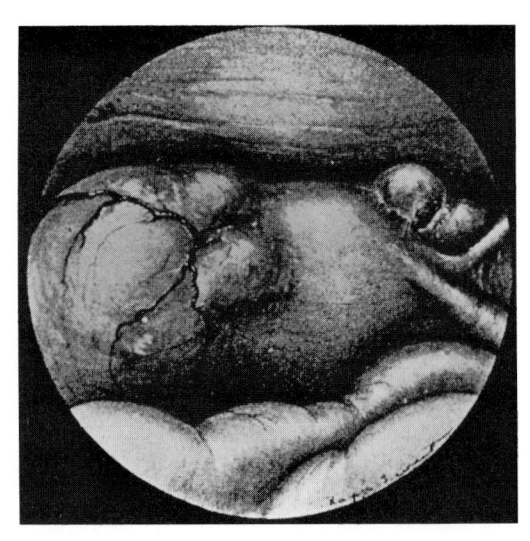

Figure 4–27. Harmless uterine myoma in a woman past the menopause in whom this palpable mass necessitated ruling out carcinoma of the ovary.

Urinary Bladder

Peritoneoscopy is not helpful in the diagnosis of lesions within the bladder cavity.

Peritoneum (Fig. 4–28)

The inner surface of the parietal peritoneum is easily seen by peritoneoscopic examination. Tuberculous peritonitis is identified by multiple, whitish, tuberculous implants over the surface of the peritoneum and various organs. The peritoneum likewise has a reddened, chronically inflamed appearance. In carcinomatosis, the peritoneum is studded with whitish implants of various sizes; often biopsy is necessary to distinguish them from tuberculosis.

Adhesions between the abdominal wall and intestine are often seen as either thin bands or dense masses. Inguinal hernias can be recognized either by seeing the omentum or intestine wedged into the internal inguinal ring or by visualizing this empty, but patent, opening. The cul-de-sac of Douglas, with its contents, can be seen when the patient is placed in the Trendelenburg position. Often in patients with cirrhosis of the liver, the blood vessels of the parietal peritoneum are greatly dilated.

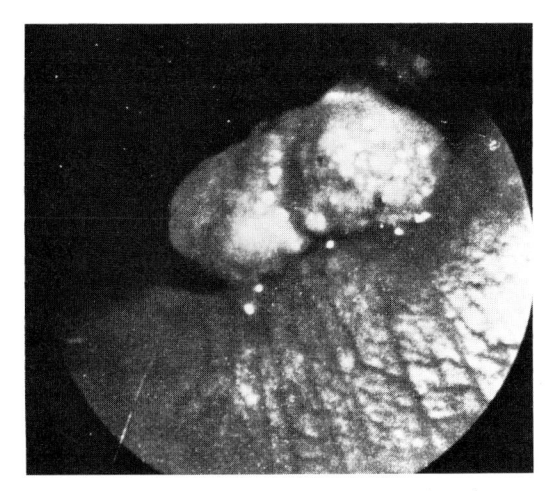

Figure 4–28. Pancreatic carcinoma implant on bowel peritoneum.

Wound Closure

When the examination has been completed, the telescope or biopsy forceps, as the case may be, is withdrawn from the cannula. The air or carbon dioxide within the abdomen is allowed to escape, aided by pressure applied to the sides of the abdominal wall. The cannula is withdrawn and the wound is closed by two silk sutures through the skin only. X-ray examinations made serially after peritoneoscopy in some patients have shown that all of the air does not escape immediately; that which remains is absorbed, or at least disappears, within 3 or 4 days and causes no symptoms. We have not studied how long carbon dioxide remains. Subcutaneous emphysema has developed in some patients following the procedure. It is probable that this was due to air or carbon dioxide which escaped through the unclosed opening in the peritoneum, was trapped by the closure of the skin, and hence traveled along the subcutaneous fascial pathway. It has not caused serious inconvenience in any of these patients.

In patients without ascites the wound heals promptly without drainage. In those with ascites a small amount of reaccumulating fluid may drain through the wound for 2 or 3 days, but in none of our cases has a fistula persisted permanently. Berggren (1964) reported that in one case a Littre's hernia occurred at the site of a peritoneoscopy performed the previous day. To avoid this complication the insufflated air or carbon dioxide should be thoroughly expelled at the conclusion of the examination and the instrument withdrawn slowly. We know of no other herniation into the wound or of any instance of intestinal obstruction due to adhesions at the site of the incision.

Examination in Children

Examination in children is performed with the same instruments and the same techniques, except that general anesthesia is substituted for local anesthesia, and the site of puncture is usually the belly of the rectus muscle to safeguard against producing a hernia. Infants as well as children have been successfully examined with the peritoneoscope. Their abdominal organs are easily visualized because of the virtual absence of omentum. Transillumination of an infant's abdomen is particularly striking and may, in itself, be valuable in diagnosing liver disease.

Precautions

Certain warnings apply to the performance of peritoneoscopy.

1. The abdomen must not be entered at a point at or adjacent to previous operative scars, since the intestine may be adherent at that point.

2. The patient must not have a full stomach or a full bladder, for either might be perforated if distended.

3. The abdomen must be distended with carbon dioxide or air insufflated through the pneumoperitoneum needle before the trocar cannula is inserted.

Postoperative Care

In some institutions peritoneoscopy is an outpatient procedure and the patient returns home after several hours of observation. This is the routine of gynecologists for patients in whom the procedure, including tubal interruption, was uneventful. It is also the routine for medical and surgical peritoneoscopists when the examination has been uneventful and no biopsy or other procedure was performed. When a biopsy has been done, it is advisable that the patient remain in the hospital overnight for observation of possible complications, such as hemorrhage or infection. The patient's normal diet is resumed after the procedure.

Complications

Complications have occurred in 0.002 to 2.4 per cent of patients in 29 reported series totalling over 75,000 peritoneoscopies. The complications included hemorrhage, biliary peritonitis, subcutaneous emphysema, pneumo-omentum, mediastinal emphysema, bowel perforation or damage, pneumothorax, air or CO_2 embolism, diaphragmatic or other hernia, cardiac arrest, electrical burns of the peritoneoscopist's face and/or hand, and rectus sheath hematoma. The majority of these complications either required no treatment or were treated successfully. Very few were followed by sequelae or were fatal.

The American Society for Gastrointestinal Endoscopy conducted a survey of the complications of endoscopic procedures performed during 1972 and 1973. The findings were reported by Silvis and associates in 1976.

In the 4404 peritoneoscopy examinations reported, a complication rate of 5.4 per 1000 patients was found, similar to that for diagnostic colonoscopy. The peritoneoscopy complications were 6 perforations of the bowel, 1 gallbladder perforation, 1 ovarian cyst perforation, 10 with bleeding, 3 cardiopulmonary complications, 4 infections, and 6 other problems consisting of mild medication reactions. The only death after peritoneoscopy was sudden and unexplained.

McDonald, Rich, and Collins (1978) pointed out that injury to the intra-abdominal vessels by percutaneously introduced instruments may result in significant blood loss because of delayed recognition and treatment. They reported their experience with two cases of major vascular injury caused by laparoscopy and reviewed the literature on this problem. The first case was a 32-year-old woman who underwent laparoscopy for elective sterilization by tubal cautery. The pneumoperitoneum needle was inserted, but when rocked to and fro it did not move freely; the tip was fixed. It was withdrawn and reinserted. Blood oozed from the needle, and it was again withdrawn. The vital signs were stable for 5 minutes, but the systolic blood pressure, which had been 120 mm. Hg, precipitously fell to unmeasurable levels, and abdominal expansion was noted. Ringer's lactate solution, albumin, and 2 units of packed cells were infused rapidly, increasing the systolic blood pressure to 90 mm. Hg. When the abdomen was hastily opened in the midline, approximately 3 units of clotted blood were present in the peritoneal cavity. Digital pressure on the aorta partially controlled bleeding and permitted indentification and repair of a 3-mm. hole in the aorta. Bilateral partial salpingectomies were performed. A total of 3 units of packed red blood cells and 2 units of whole blood was required during the operation. Delayed primary wound closure was done on the fourth postoperative day. There were no postoperative complications. One year after operation, the peripheral pulses remained normal.

The other case was a 21-year-old nulliparous woman admitted to the hospital for evaluation of infertility, with a suspected diagnosis of polycystic ovaries. Peritoneoscopy was performed under general anesthesia. The pneumoperitoneum needle was inserted for insufflation of carbon dioxide. As in the first case, a drop of blood returned through the needle when the obturator was removed. The needle was withdrawn and vital signs observed for several minutes. Then a second insertion was made with the needle tip directed more caudally. Blood spontaneously returned from the needle. It was withdrawn and vital signs observed. The blood pressure remained normal for 3 minutes, then drifted from 120 to 90 mm Hg. After one minute the blood pressure was unobtainable, but a thready pulse was maintained. Rapid infusion of Ringer's lactate solution, albumin, and blood over 2 minutes raised the blood pressure to 50 mm Hg. When the abdomen was opened, approximately 3 units of clotted blood were noted in the peritoneal cavity. An expanding retroperitoneal hematoma was centered over the terminal aorta. Upon opening the peritoneum, a through-and-through perforation of the right side of the aorta and a small tear in the vena cava were noted. In addition, there was a through-and-through perforation of the right common iliac artery and a 1.5 cm. rent in the left iliac vein as it passed under the right iliac artery. The arterial injuries were sequentially repaired by lateral suture technic with 5-0 Prolene. The venous injuries were likewise repaired. The diagnosis of bilateral polycystic ovaries was confirmed, and bilateral wedge biopsies were obtained. Four units of blood were given to replace the estimated blood loss of 3000 ml. There were no postoperative complications. Delayed primary closure of the wound was done on the fourth postoperative day. Six months after operation, the peripheral pulses were normal.

The writers commented that the importance of inserting the needle at a 45-degree angle to the abdominal wall has been emphasized. If the angle of insertion is too steep, injury to retroperitoneal structures may result. In both of their patients, the operators thought they had inserted the needle correctly. However, the locations of the injuries indicate that the needles may have been inserted nearly perpendicular to the abdomen since the injuries were almost directly posterior to the umbilicus.

McDonald, Rich, and Collins reviewed the English language literature and noted that laparoscopy is a commonly used diagnostic and therapeutic procedure with low morbidity and mortality. They found only 2 deaths in 10,193 gynecologic laparoscopies. There were 34 deaths in 72,029 nongynecologic laparoscopies, 30 of which were associated with significant intraperitoneal hemorrhage or bile peritonitis due to liver injury.

Results

The diagnostic accuracy of peritoneoscopy has averaged 88 per cent. Six per cent of the failures have been due to inability to carry out the procedure because of adhesions or other reasons. The remaining 5 per cent have been false-negative diagnoses due to overlooking, or inability to visualize, obscure lesions, particularly metastatic malignancy. False-positive diagnoses are rare. Poor selection of patients is the greatest cause of failure to make a diagnosis by peritoneoscopy. The practical results have been that the procedure has avoided laparotomy in 25 per cent, indicated laparotomy in 25 per cent, and indicated medical therapy in 25 per cent of the patients undergoing peritoneoscopy for diagnosis. Management was unchanged in 25 per cent. Its use has reduced the length and expense of hospitalization in these cases.

Friedman and Wolff (1978) reported that peritoneoscopy was successful in 94 per cent of 140 consecutive procedures performed on patients with nongynecologic diseases for the purpose of evaluating hepatic status, metastatic intraperitoneal carcinoma, abdominal masses, and miscellaneous conditions, and for staging lymphomatous disease. There were no deaths. The therapeutic management of 80 per cent of these patients was significantly altered, and the morbidity was low.

Wolfe, Behn and Jackson (1979) reported a series of 11 patients with tuberculous peritonitis. In eight, a definite diagnosis was made by laparoscopy with target biopsy, thus avoiding laparotomy. They recommended laparoscopy as a safe and effective method for obtaining an early diagnosis in patients with suspected tuberculous peritonitis.

Coleman and associates (1976) reported their use of peritoneoscopy to evaluate the liver in 35 previously untreated patients with Hodgkin's disease. Four were found to have hepatic involvement. Of the 31 patients with normal peritoneoscopies, only 1 had liver disease demonstrated at confirmatory exploratory laparotomy. The diagnostic accuracy for peritoneoscopy was 93 per cent for patients at high risk for hepatic disease, and 97 per cent for all patients studied. Morbidity from the procedure was minimal. There was no mortality. They concluded that peritoneoscopy is a highly accurate staging procedure that should be considered as an antecedent or as an alternative to laparotomy in patients with Hodgkin's disease. Its accuracy and minimal morbidity should be considered in the critical selection process of determining which patients should undergo laparotomy.

Conclusions

We agree with Friedman and Wolff's (1978) statement that "peritoneoscopy is a safe, readily available, and accurate diagnostic tool which should be used more widely by abdominal surgeons." It is often definitive in evaluating intra-abdominal disease and may make more hazardous diagnostic or therapeutic procedures unnecessary, as well as shorten hospital stays.

Compared with exploratory laparotomy, which exposes patients to unnecessary hazards of general anesthesia and procedural complications, peritoneoscopy provides information and valuable tissue specimens, and possibly offers earlier definitive management in situations where surgery would otherwise be delayed until a diagnosis could be confirmed by indirect means.

Contraindications of laparoscopy are few: extreme obesity, intestinal obstruction, acute peritonitis, large hiatus hernias, and hemorrhagic disorders. Caution should be exercised in patients with previous abdominal surgery if adhesions are present.

Peritoneoscopy is widely used by gynecologists for diagnosis and minor operative procedures, and by physicians both for diagnosis and for following the results of medical treatment. It is not widely used by surgeons, although in many instances it could be most helpful.

Chapter 5

OBSTRUCTIVE DISORDERS

ACUTE DILATATION OF THE STOMACH

Acute dilatation of the stomach was formerly a common and dangerous complication of abdominal operations. (See Postoperative Gastric Decompression on page 59.) In 1933, Henry wrote, "Two grim specters look over the shoulder of every operating surgeon. One is called pulmonary embolus and the other is acute dilatation of the stomach."

This condition is characterized by a rapid enlargement of the stomach and duodenum without actual organic obstruction. It is associated with a marked accumulation of the gastric and intestinal juices, which are not resorbed.

When Henry wrote, the mortality of acute dilatation of the stomach was reported to be 75 per cent. Its occurrence has been markedly reduced by the frequent use of nasogastric tubes left in the stomach postoperatively for gastric decompression by siphonage or suction, and now mortality from this condition is almost negligible.

Etiology

Acute dilatation of the stomach occurs most frequently following a surgical operation. It may follow any operative procedure but is more common when a general anesthetic has been used. It is seen most frequently after vagotomy and operations upon the stomach, gallbladder, and pelvic organs but may be noted after minor operative procedures, trauma, or even the application of a body cast. "The condition develops occasionally in patients with bowel obstruction who are being treated with a long intestinal (Miller-Abbott) tube, and the presence of the tube often contributes to the delay in diagnosis as attending physicians are apt to assume mistakenly that the tube is acting to keep the stomach decompressed" (Thompson, 1977). Emergency resuscitative measures in patients with respiratory arrests and administration of inhalation anesthesia or oxygen often distend the stomach with gas.

Acute gastric dilatation also may occur in nonsurgical conditions, which include pneumonia, typhoid fever, bulbar poliomyelitis, arteriosclerotic heart disease, parturition, overeating, and wasting diseases like tuberculosis and debilitating chronic illness.

Jennings and Klidjian (1974) reported the cases of two young women with diagnosed anorexia nervosa who were admitted to the hospital surgical service as emergencies. Both were dehydrated, were vomiting profusely, and had obvious extreme gastric dilatation. They were treated conservatively by intubation and responded well. Radiologic examination showed extreme gastric dilatation but no other disease process. The investigators commented, "The condition of these patients is analogous to that of prisoners of war being fed too rapidly on their release."

Acute gastric dilatation *does not occur in patients having constant gastric siphonage or suction after operation.*

111

No general agreement exists about the cause of postoperative acute gastric dilatation of the stomach. The following theories have been suggested:

1. It is paralytic ileus involving the gastric wall, as evidenced by its frequent occurrence, both clinically and experimentally, after vagotomy.

2. It is caused by mechanical obstruction from compression of the third portion of the duodenum by the overlying mesenteric vessels as the duodenum crosses the spine. Clinical, autopsy, and experimental evidence has shown that factors other than mechanical obstruction must be present for dilatation of the stomach to occur.

3. Aerophagic swallowing of air distends the stomach and with distention there is an outpouring of gastric juice, which increases the distention. The fluid retained in such stomachs is composed of gastric, pancreatic, and duodenal secretions and bile. The secretions do not pass into the intestine where they can be resorbed.

4. Disproportionate potassium and chloride electrolyte losses inhibit gastric motility.

Probably several of the above factors, in various combinations, are important in initiating acute gastric dilatation.

Clinical Manifestations and Diagnosis

The onset of acute gastric dilatation is usually gradual and its recognition is delayed. Vomiting and upper abdominal distention are the most constant symptoms and signs. The early symptoms may be only nausea, apathy, and a sense of fullness in the epigastrium, without pain. Usually on the second or third postoperative day characteristic manifestations appear. Among these are the apathetic, though not distressed, appearance of the patient; emesis, which may be copious, though the stomach is rarely emptied completely by the act of vomiting; or, more characteristically, frequent, painless, and effortless regurgitation of small amounts of brown- or black-stained fluid. A tell-tale brown or black stain at the angle of the mouth or on the pillow in a postoperative patient should arouse suspicion of this complication. Pain is absent or only moderate. Symptoms of dehydration and electrolyte imbalance usually appear.

The characteristic physical findings are rapidly increasing asymmetric distention of the abdomen, with the left hypochondrium fuller than the right; an audible splashing sound when the distended portion of the abdomen is manipulated; and the presence of a uniformly tympanitic note on percussion over the distended area when the patient lies supine.

A plain x-ray film of the abdomen characteristically demonstrates a fluid level in the greatly distended stomach, shown best by an upright film of the abdomen or a lateral decubitus film (Fig. 5–1).

The laboratory findings are those of dehydration and electrolyte imbalance. Acid-base balance may be little disturbed, because the loss of carbonates in the succus entericus parallels the hydrogen ion loss from the stomach, but either acidosis or alkalosis may occur in individual cases.

As distention of the stomach increases, there may be bleeding. Massive hemorrhage or rupture of the stomach may occur and require immediate operative repair. Acute gastric dilatation may be fatal in a short time if not recognized and corrected.

The diagnosis of acute gastric dilatation is confirmed by the recovery of an enormous residue of gastric contents after a tube is passed into the stomach.

Treatment

The treatment of acute dilatation of the stomach is *nonsurgical* and is most efficacious. If a nasogastric tube is not already in the stomach one should be passed at once. If the amount and nature of the gastric contents obtained through the tube are characteristic of gastroduodenal ileus, the tube should be left in the stomach and connected with a suction apparatus until the return fluid is normal in appearance. Frequent changing of the patient's position is important and a prone position with the hips or foot of the bed elevated may help in the relief of any arteriomesenteric ileus that may be present.

Electrolyte, fluid, and nutritional requirements and a normal output of urine are maintained by intravenous injections.

The indwelling gastric tube usually can be removed as soon as the gastric contents are normal in appearance and there is evidence of normal peristaltic activity.

GASTROLYSIS AND DUODENOLYSIS (FREEING OF ADHESIONS)

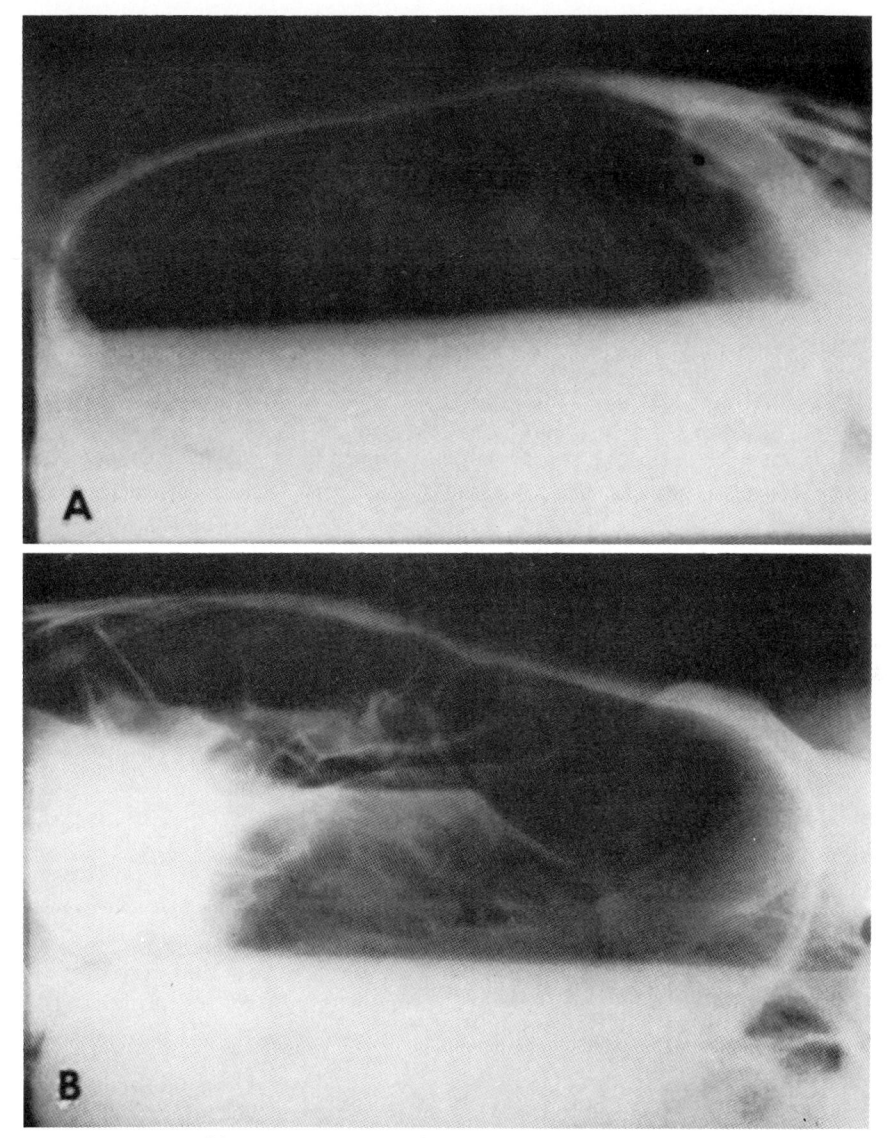

Figure 5-1. Acute gastric dilatation. *A*, Supine decubitus and *B*, right lateral decubitus adequately demonstrate an air fluid level in the stomach. (From Gillesby, W. J., and Wheeler, J. R.: Acute gastric dilatation. Am. Surg. 22:1154, 1956.)

In some instances following vagotomy, chronic dilatation of the stomach due to atony has persisted and required later gastrojejunostomy.

Practically, "the most important treatment is prophylactic. Any patient who has ileus should have a functioning nasogastric tube. If a nasogastric tube is removed from a postoperative debilitated or elderly patient whose bowel function is still questionable, it is wise to check the gastric residual in 6 to 8 hours to be sure that the stomach has not dilated" (Thompson, 1977).

GASTROLYSIS AND DUODENOLYSIS (FREEING OF ADHESIONS)

Adhesions affecting the stomach or duodenum may be congenital in origin or may result from an inflammatory or malignant lesion of the stomach, duodenum, gallbladder, pancreas, appendix, or female reproductive organs or may be due to a previous operation. Division of these adhesions, whether as an operation in itself or in the course of any surgical procedure, is known as gastrolysis or duodenolysis, according to the viscus freed.

Gastric adhesions seldom cause symptoms and gastrolysis alone is rarely, if ever, indicated.

Duodenal adhesions occasionally cause symptoms but duodenolysis is not indicated unless there are definite symptoms and signs of mechanical obstruction positively confirmed by x-ray study, made following a barium swallow, showing evidence of such an obstruction. Operations for vague symptoms without objective evidence of obstruction will usually be disappointing in their results.

Technic

General anesthesia is used.

An upper midline or upper right paramedian incision gives equally satisfactory exposure. After the abdomen is entered the exact site of obstruction should be identified by seeing a sharply constricted ring, with a dilated lumen proximal to the point of obstruction and a relatively small, collapsed duodenum distal to the obstruction. It is important that this point be identified before it is disturbed as otherwise the surgeon will not be satisfied that the cause of the condition has been found and corrected.

Limited, filamentous adhesions usually are separated by blunt dissection with a gauze-covered finger.

Cordlike or bandlike adhesions are divided between double ligatures.

Extensive, dense, and firm adhesions may require dissection, followed by repair of the wall of the viscus or structure from which they are dissected. In some patients with extensive adhesions it may be preferable to perform a shunting operation around the obstruction, such as a gastrojejunostomy, a gastroduodenostomy, or a duodenoduodenostomy or duodenojejunostomy, whichever is suitable for the particular case.

Surfaces left raw by the freeing of adhesions should be covered in such a way as to minimize the reformation of these adhesions. Raw areas are protected by suturing adjoining serous surfaces together or by placing omental grafts.

Intraperitoneal adhesions are considered in detail in the section on Intestinal Obstruction in Volume 4, The Small Intestine.

ATRESIA AND STENOSIS OF THE STOMACH (Neonatal Gastric Outlet Obstruction)

"Congenital atresia is less common in the stomach than in other portions of the alimentary tract and, when present, is limited to the antrum and pyloric region" (Gray and Skandalakis, 1972). Atresia occurs somewhere in the entire gastrointestinal tract approximately once in every 10,000 births. Pyloric and prepyloric atresia account for less than 1 per cent of these atresias (Parrish and associates, 1968).

Gastric atresia is seen most often as a membranous diaphragm composed of only mucosa and submucosa (Fig. 5–2A and B). The diaphragm may be complete, or it may be incomplete with a small opening about 3 to 10 mm. in size situated centrally or eccentrically. The muscular wall of the stomach has no part in the formation of the diaphragm.

In fewer cases there has been more extensive obliteration of the lumen (Fig. 5–2C and D), but the muscle layer was not involved.

Complete atresia of all parts of the pyloric region (Fig. 5–2E) has been reported (Wuensche, 1875; Neale, 1884; Holladay, 1946 — all cited in Gray and Skandalakis, 1972). There may or may not be a fibrous cord connecting the proximal and distal segments across the atresia.

One patient had a double complete web with a cyst between the two membranes, which were not far apart (Metz, Householder, and De Pree, 1941).

Congenital atresias or membranes that occur at the pylorus are termed pyloric, while those that occur 1 centimeter or more proximal to the pylorus are termed prepyloric or antral (Fig. 5–3).

Gerber and Aberdeen (1965) proposed a simple classification of neonatal gastric outlet obstructions that is widely used:

STOMACH ATRESIA AND STENOSIS (NEONATAL GASTRIC OUTLET OBSTRUCTION)

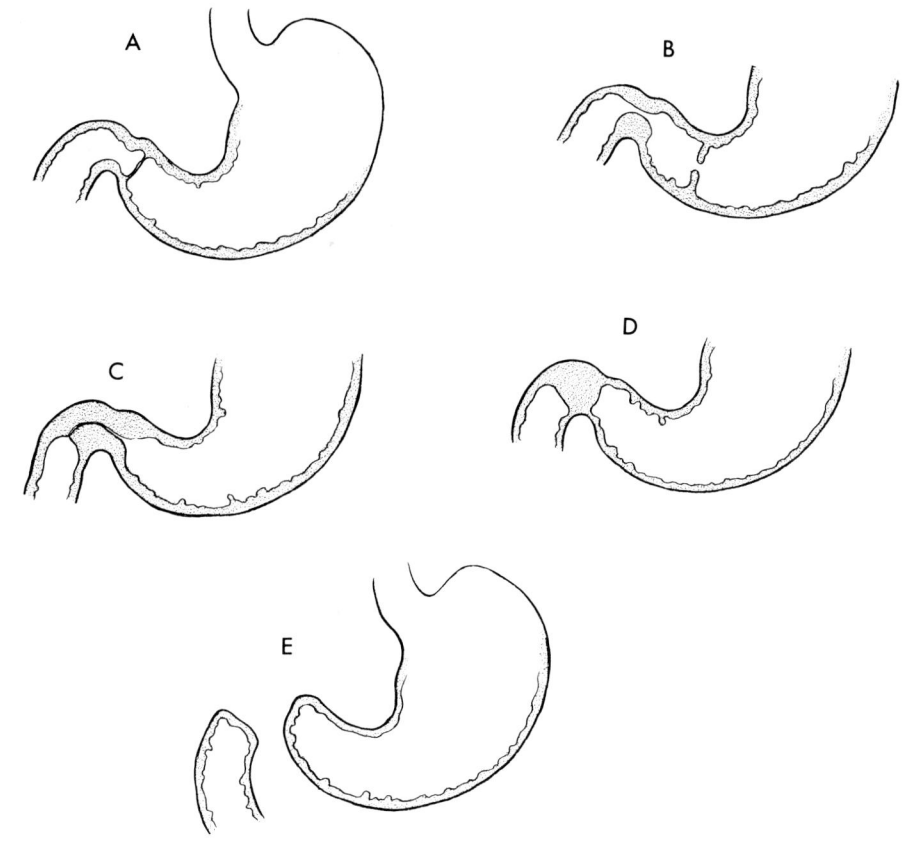

Figure 5–2. Five types of gastric atresia. *A*, Membranous atresia; *B*, perforated membrane (stenosis); *C*, luminal atresia with a microscopic endodermal canal; *D*, complete, solid atresia; and *E*, complete atresia with discontinuity. (From Gray, S. W., and Skandalakis, J. E.: Embryology for Surgeons. Philadelphia, W. B. Saunders Company, 1972.)

1. Pyloric
   A. Membrane
   B. Atresia
2. Antral (1 cm. or more proximal to pylorus).
   A. Membrane
   B. Atresia

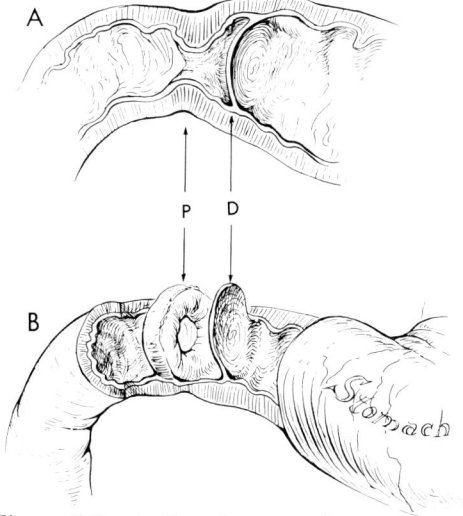

Figure 5–3. *A*, Prepyloric membrane; *B*, antral diaphragm. P, pylorus; D, diaphragm. (From Benson, C. D.: Prepyloric and pyloric obstruction. *In* Mustard, W. T., et al.: Pediatric Surgery. Vol. 2. 2nd ed. Chicago, Year Book Medical Publishers, 1969.)

"The septum has never been reported proximal to the antrum" (Rowling, 1959).

If an occluding membrane is thin, it may perforate soon after birth, from pressure of the gastric contents, and leave only a mild stenosis, which will not cause symptoms until later in life. An incomplete prephyloric membrane is rare in the neonate. Such stenoses in older infants and adults are not all of congenital origin. In some the perforation results from ulcers. When ulcer scarring is present, the stenoses are probably acquired.

Tan and Murugasu (1973) were the first to report the occurrence of complete pyloric atresia in siblings. One, a male, and the other, a female, were born to a German mother and an English father who had one other child. The *first* pregnancy was complicated by hydramnios, and two days after birth the male infant died from peritonitis after operation to close a gastric perforation. Autopsy revealed complete obstruction at the pylorus by a thick membrane (atresia), generalized peritonitis, and right subphrenic abscess. The *second* pregnancy progressed normally without hydramnios and resulted in a normal female infant who has developed normally.

The *third* pregnancy was complicated by severe hydraminos. A female infant was delivered by cesarean section at 36 weeks' gestation. High gastrointestinal obstruction was diagnosed and she was operated upon. The stomach was found to be grossly distended by air, and the intestines were completely collapsed. No abnormality was detected externally along the whole gastrointestinal tract. Gastrotomy and duodenotomy revealed a thick membrane causing complete obstruction at the pyloroduodenal junction. A side-to-side gastroduodenostomy was performed. The infant progressed satisfactorily and when last seen at 11 weeks of age appeared normal.

The investigators pointed out that although the report of congenital pyloric atresia in two siblings suggests that this anomaly is a genetically determined condition, their review of the world literature on complete pyloric or prepyloric atresia revealed no other case in which it has occurred in siblings.

History

According to Gray and Skandalakis (1972), "the first reported case of luminal occlusion was that of Crooks in 1828. Wuensche, in 1875, and Neale, in 1884, described complete segmental atresia. The complete diaphragmatic form of [gastric] atresia was first described by Bennett in 1937," in a 4-day-old infant who underwent pyloroplasty for pyloric stenosis and died 36 hours later. Autopsy revealed the cause of obstruction to be an imperforate prepyloric diaphragm.

The first successfully treated patient with prepyloric membranous obstruction was recorded by Touroff and Sussman in 1940. The patient was a 1-day-old infant who was treated by multiple incisions in the prepyloric septum and pyloroplasty.

In 1941 Metz, Householder, and De Pree reported a 3-day-old infant who had a double septum at the pylorus with cyst formation between the two membranes, which were a short distance apart. Incision of both diaphragms resulted in recovery.

In 1951, Benson and Coury reported the third successful operation, and in 1959 Brown and Hertzler reported successful treatment of two premature infants 10 and 7 days old.

In 1963 Wolf and Zwymüller reported that 28 cases of complete gastric atresia had been recorded in the literature up to that date. The membranous form of atresia was the most common. Segmental atresia had been reported in two patients and complete aplasia in four.

Since the incidence of mongolism among patients with esophageal atresia is about 11 per cent (Gray and Skandalakis, 1972) and among patients with duodenal atresia from 4 to 35 per cent in different series, it is surprising that gastric atresia and mongolism are not more frequently associated. We found no reports in which this association had occurred; but Dineen and Redo (1963) mentioned the subsequent detection of mongolism in some of these infants born of hydramniotic mothers.

Incomplete prepyloric membranes (antral webs) are rare in the newborn. This lesion is thought to represent a membranous atresia which has undergone perforation in utero. DeSpirito and Guthorn in 1957 reported the first case, in a 21-day-old infant. In 1967, Cremin reported two infants, 3 and 4 days old, respectively, who had this anomaly. He made the diagnosis preoperatively by radiologic studies in one and was the first to describe the radiologic features that suggest the diagnosis of congenital incomplete prepyloric membrane. Bell and associates (1978) reported a series of 28 children with a radiographic diagnosis of antral web during a 26-month period. Twenty-four of the patients were diagnosed in the first 6 months of life. Vomiting, described as both projectile and bilious in some cases, was the predominant presenting symptom.

The typical radiographic appearance of an antral web in an infant is as a thin, membranous septum projecting into the antral lumen perpendicular to its longitudinal axis, 1 to 2 cm. proximal to the pylorus. It is thought necessary also to observe the degree of gastric outlet obstruction during fluoroscopic study of the stomach. Histologically, the webs were described as having two mucosal surfaces supported by muscularis mucosae and submucosa without a muscular layer.

The treatment recommended was pyloroplasty with excision or incision of the web. Four of 20 patients, all less than 2 months of age, were not treated surgically because the web was not felt to be obstructive. Of 19 surviving infants who were treated with pyloroplasty, all remained asymptomatic during follow up periods of 8 to 34 months.

Subsequent analysis by Tunell and Smith (1980) of 11 patients presenting radiographic evidence of antral web places the need for surgical treatment of this lesion in question. The 11 patients were followed from 1 to 6 years after diagnosis. Seven had excision of the web and pyloroplasty. Four were treated nonoperatively with antispasmodics and small-curd formula. Five of the seven operated infants had persistent vomiting postoperatively. *All* patients in both the operated and nonoperated groups were free of vomiting 6 months post-treatment. The investigators conclude that antral web in infancy is a self-limited disease and that surgical correction is indicated only for severe clinical illness.

Symptoms and Diagnosis

The onset of bile-free vomiting in infants immediately after birth distinguishes prepyloric atresia from hypertrophic pyloric stenosis, which rarely begins before the second week (Fig. 5–4).

A catheter passed successfully into the stomach rules out esophageal atresia. The presence of meconium in the stool, and its absence in the vomitus, places the obstruction above the papilla of Vater.

Polyhydramnios was present in at least 50 per cent of reported cases of infants with prepyloric atresia; these infants frequently were premature. As in esophageal atresia, normal swallowing and absorption of amniotic fluid are prevented by the obstruction.

The three cardinal signs of gastric atresia in infants are (1) persistent bile-free vomiting after the first feeding; (2) distention of the upper but not the lower abdomen; and (3) stools decreasing in quantity.

A plain x-ray film of the abdomen, without the use of barium, shows air and fluid levels in the stomach, but no air is seen in the intestines when the occlusion is complete.

Cremin (1967) was the first to describe the radiologic features of incomplete membrane in newborn infants with prepyloric atresia. His classic description:

A plain film will show a distended stomach with limited gas in the intestine. This is not, however, diagnostic as similar appearances may be seen in hypertrophic pyloric stenosis, pylorospasm, and in peptic ulceration of the newborn. A barium meal, using limited amounts of dilute barium via an intra-gastric tube, is safe and necessary to make the diagnosis. At a barium meal examination there is marked delay in emptying, vigorous peristalsis occurs, and there is a smooth, blunt, pyloric region [Fig. 5–5A]. Eventually a thin, central streak of contrast is seen when emptying occurs [Fig. 5–5B].

The condition must be differentiated from hypertrophic pyloric stenosis which commonly occurs between 2 and 6 weeks after birth. It is uncommon before 2 weeks, but so are membranes. Delay in emptying occurs in both conditions. There are not enough cases to see if this is more consistent with incomplete membranes. However, comparing the signs of incomplete membrane with those of hypertrophic stenosis, the differences are shown in [Figure 5–6].

Incomplete pyloric-prepyloric diaphragm is a rare lesion in infants and children. The degree of obstruction is related to the size of the aperture in the diaphragm. Such lesions have been reported in a 5-week-old infant (Wurtenberger, 1961); in a 2-year-old child (Berman and Ballenger, 1948); in another 2 year old (Gerber and Aberdeen, 1965); in a 4-year-old child (Liechti, Mikkelson, and Snyder, 1963); and in an 11-year-old patient operated upon by Benson (1969). All recovered. They were managed by excision of the diaphragm or excision of the diaphragm and a Heineke-Mikulicz type of pyloroplasty.

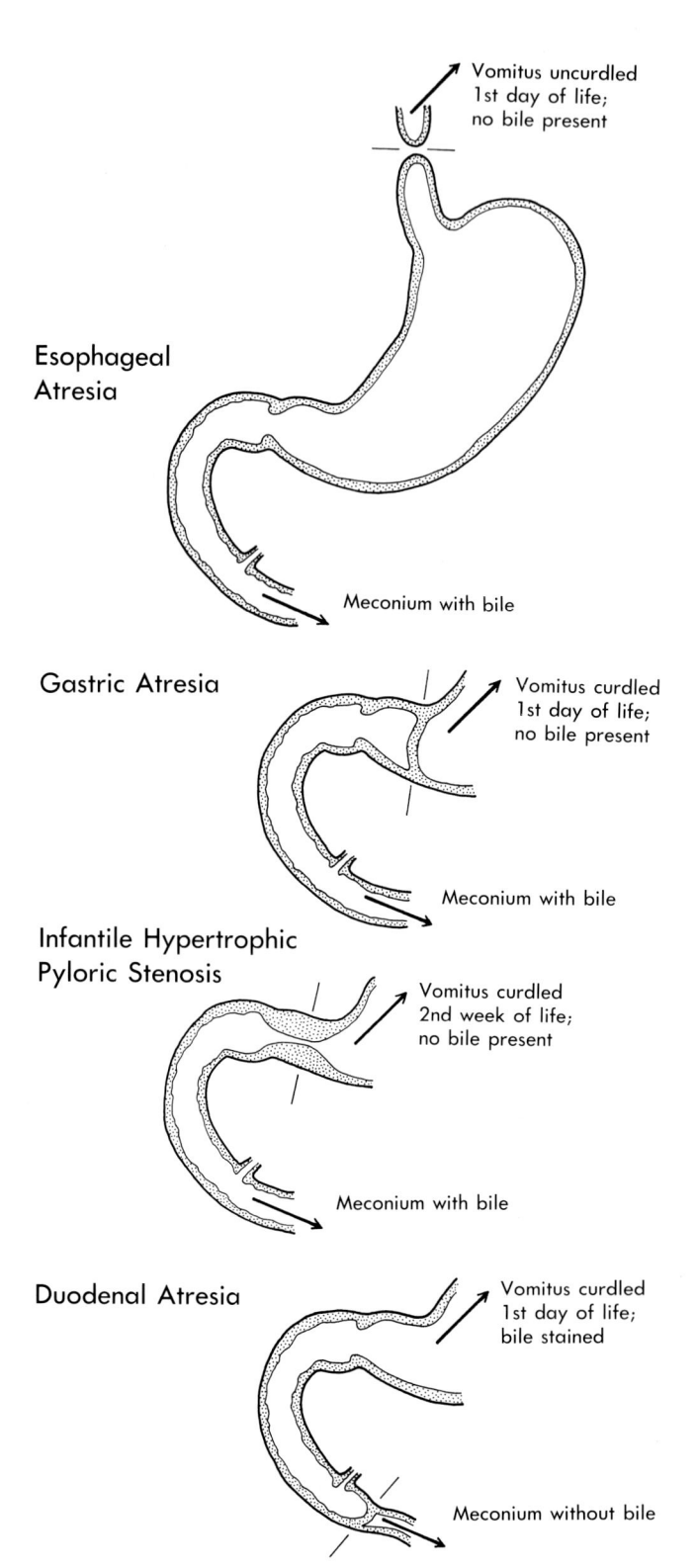

Figure 5-4. The differential diagnosis of high alimentary tract obstruction. Observation of both vomitus and feces is necessary. (From Gray, S. W., and Skandalakis, J. E.: Embryology for Surgeons. Philadelphia, W. B. Saunders Company, 1972.)

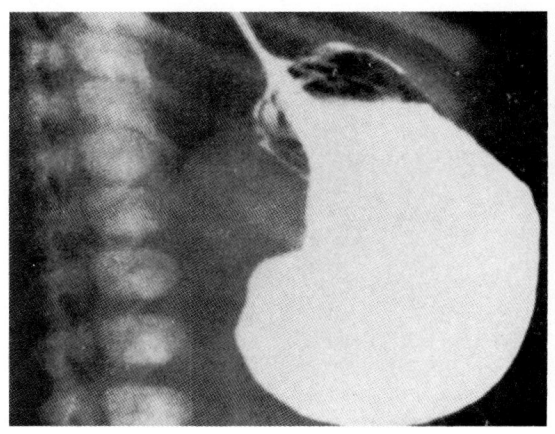

STOMACH ATRESIA AND STENOSIS (NEONATAL GASTRIC OUTLET OBSTRUCTION)

Figure 5–5. Barium meal. *A*, In the early stages there is complete obstruction of the pylorus which is round and blunt. *B*, After 1 hour, barium has passed the membrane. The pyloric canal and duodenum are outlined. (From Cremin, R. J.: Neonatal prepyloric membrane. South Afr. Med. J., *41*:1077, 1967.)

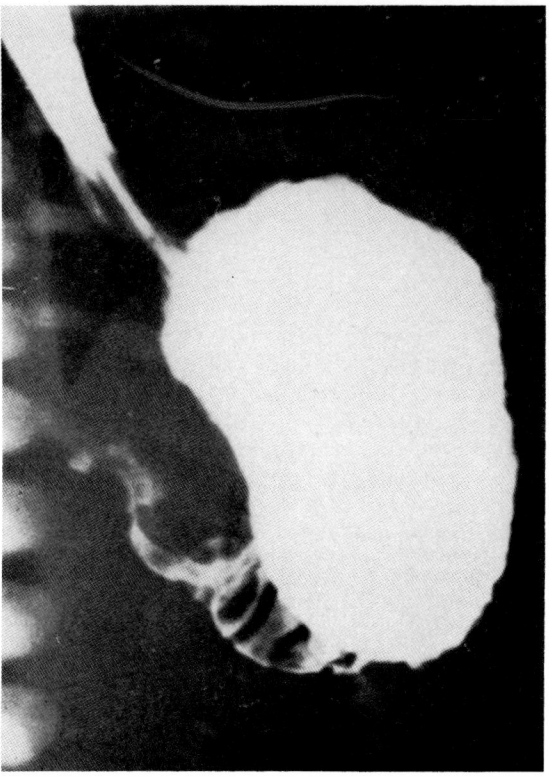

Treatment

Prompt surgical intervention is indicated for treating a neonate with atresia of the stomach. In the newborn infant with a complete diaphragm or a diaphragm with an aperture, local excision or incision of the diaphragm with a Heineke-Mikulicz pyloroplasty is effective. In infants who have a segmental atresia, the atretic segment is resected along with the diaphragmatic mucous membrane pouch, and an end-to-end gastroduodenostomy is performed, closing the anterior wall as in a Heineke-Mikulicz pyloroplasty.

At operation there may be no external evidence of an abnormality at the gastroduodenal junction, and the obstruction can be detected only by gastrotomy. This is especially true of the diaphragmatic obstructions. Complete atresia usually can be recognized from a fibrous cord which connects the proximal and distal portions of the stomach across the atresia, although not in all cases. Because it is difficult to diagnose true pyloric atresia at laparotomy, it is always advisable to make an opening in the distended proximal bowel in cases of neonatal obstruction.

When obstruction is caused by a membrane, excision of the membrane is the treatment of choice. However, among six patients so treated, four required reoperation because of postoperative obstruction due to edema (Davis and Douglas, 1961). "All four patients who were treated by inci-

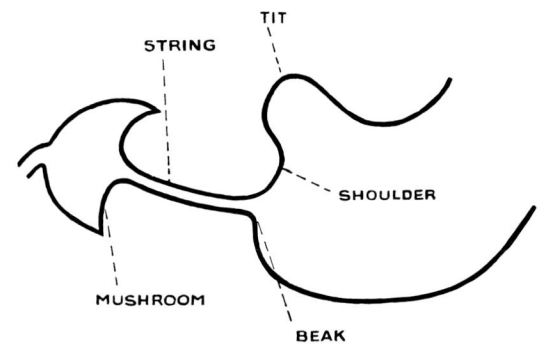

Figure 5–6. Signs of hypertrophic pyloric stenosis. Compare this diagram with signs of incomplete membrane shown in Figure 5–5*A* and *B*. In incomplete membrane, there are (1) no tit, that is, a wave of peristalsis seen on the lower lesser curvature; (2) no shoulder — in fact the reverse is true, a convex round border; (3) no beak, the rounded convexity at the pylorus; (4) no string sign, the lumen of the pyloric canal is not narrowed; and (5) no mushrooming or indentation of the duodenal cap. (From Cremin, cited in previous figure.)

sion or excision of the membrane and the addition of a feeding tube introduced through the gastrotomy and passed distal to the site of surgery through the duodenum into the jejunum, in order to ensure patency, survived with a single operation."

Alternatives to excision or incision of the membrane are gastrojejunostomy or a Finney or Heineke-Mikulicz pyloroplasty. Gastrojejunostomy is undesirable in infants because of the possibility of marginal ulceration. Vagotomy should not be done in children.

All the successful operations have been performed before the tenth day of life. In several cases, a second or third operation was required (Wurtenberger, 1961).

Regardless of the procedure employed, the surgeon should be careful to inspect the remainder of the gut, to be certain no other areas of obstruction exist in the upper gastrointestinal tract.

Prognosis

With early diagnosis and surgical treatment, the prognosis is excellent. Benson, in 1969, reported that a total of 25 patients with some form of gastric atresia had been treated surgically in the newborn period, with 20 recoveries.

Combined Congenital Gastric and Duodenal Obstruction

Congenital obstruction of the duodenum is fairly common in the neonate, but gastric obstruction, due to either pyloric atresia or a membranous mucosal diaphragm, is a rare finding. A combination of the two is even rarer and is harder to diagnose both preoperatively and at operation.

The first, and to our knowledge still the only, case of congenital prepyloric mucosal diaphragm in association with duodenal atresia was reported by Haller and Cahill in 1968. The patient was a female infant born after a full-term pregnancy, which was complicated by maternal hydramnios. The delivery was spontaneous, and the baby weighed 3025 grams at birth. A plain film of the abdomen at 30 hours of age revealed gastric dilation and what was thought to be air in the first portion of the dilated duodenum. The remainder of the intestine was air-free. Repeat x-ray examination after injecting air into the stomach showed a greatly distended stomach with a gas bubble apparently in the first portion of the duodenum (Fig. 5–7).

Duodenal atresia proximal to the ampulla of Vater was diagnosed. Exploratory laparotomy revealed a greatly distended stomach with a normal pylorus. The first portion of the duodenum was slightly dilated. The remainder of the duodenum and the small intestine were collapsed. There was no evidence of malrotation of the cecum or abnormal mesenteric attachment (Fig. 5–8A). A proximal segment of jejunum was isolated and its patency confirmed by injecting saline. The colon contained meconium and appeared normal. A side-to-side isoperistaltic duodenojejunostomy was performed (Fig. 5–8B).

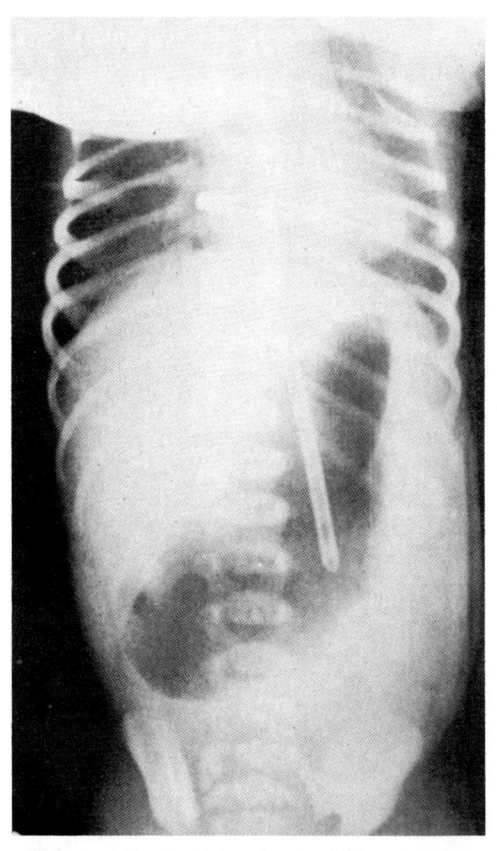

Figure 5–7. Initial abdominal film at 30 hours of age, showing distended stomach and gas bubble apparently in first portion of duodenum. (From Haller, J. A., Jr., and Cahill, J. L.: Combined congenital gastric and duodenal obstruction; Pitfalls in diagnosis and treatment. Surgery 63:504, 1968.)

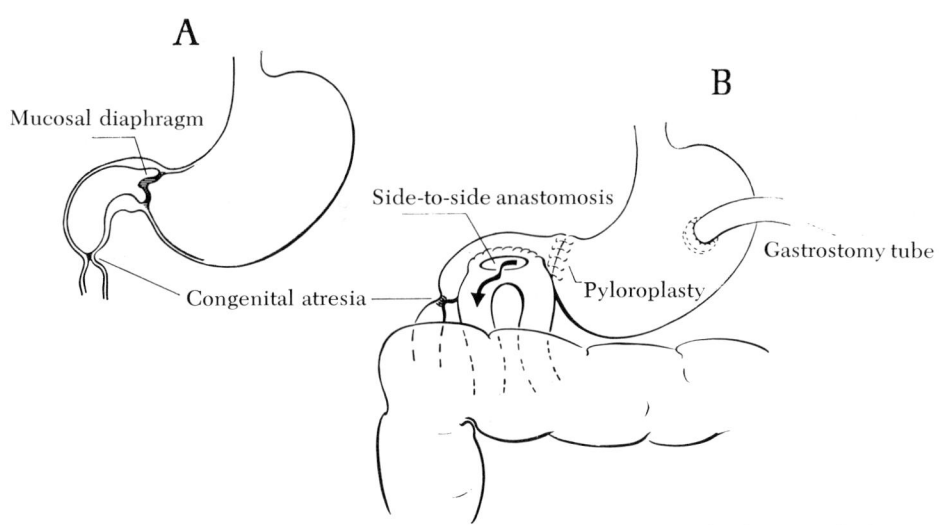

STOMACH ATRESIA AND STENOSIS (NEONATAL GASTRIC OUTLET OBSTRUCTION)

Figure 5-8. *A*, Double obstruction due to duodenal atresia and pyloric diaphragm, which were ultimately identified. *B*, Initial operative procedure was side-to-side duodenojejunostomy and gastrostomy; second operation was excision of pyloric diaphragm and pyloroplasty. (From Haller and Cahill, cited in previous figure.)

A catheter was passed distally through the duodenotomy; it would not pass beyond the second portion of the duodenum. A curved instrument was passed proximally and thought to enter the stomach. A Stamm type of gastrostomy was then performed. The gastrostomy tube was placed on suction for 48 hours and the patient was given intravenous feedings of glucose in water and saline. On the first postoperative day the baby passed a normal-appearing meconium stool. Gastrostomy aspiration, following feedings of small amounts of glucose and water, revealed an abnormally large volume of residual gastric content. Feedings were discontinued for the next 2 days and then resumed, and again large volumes of gastric contents were obtained. Another plain film again revealed an airless abdomen, except for a moderate amount of gas in the stomach. A dilute solution of Gastrografin was given orally and was swallowed normally under fluoroscopic observation. However there was complete obstruction at the level of the pylorus with no emptying of the stomach after several hours (Fig. 5-9).

A second exploration was then performed and a gastrotomy made in the prepyloric region. A complete pyloric mucosa diaphragm was found. The pyloric channel and musculature appeared to be normally developed distal to this point and the pre-

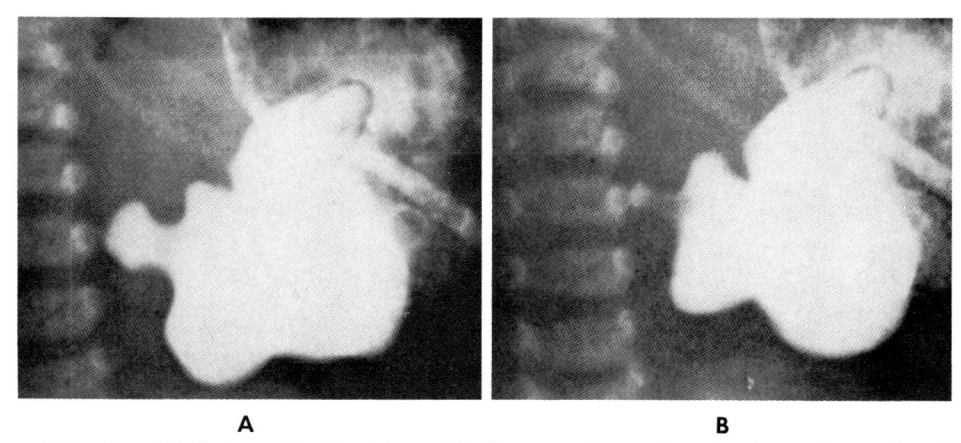

Figure 5-9. *A* and *B*, Gastrografin-filled stomach before second operation, showing prolapse of gastric mucosal diaphragm through the pylorus. (From Haller and Cahill, cited in Figure 5-7.)

viously made duodenojejunostomy was patent. The pyloric diaphragm was longitudinally incised along its anterior border and a wide Heineke-Mikulicz pyloroplasty was constructed. Again a catheter could not be passed beyond the second portion of the duodenum. A small feeding tube was placed through the duodenojejunostomy (Fig. 5–8). Immediately after operation jejunal feedings were instituted and appeared well-tolerated. Oral feedings were resumed on the fifth postoperative day and the diet advanced. Convalescence was uneventful and the baby was discharged 24 days after the first operation.

One month after discharge she was gaining weight normally. Three months postoperatively, a follow-up gastrointestinal series showed a normal-sized stomach, a blind duodenal segment, and a patent jejunoduodenostomy (Fig. 5–10). At 18 months she was a vigorous, happy child with normal growth and development.

In discussing this case, the physicians pointed out pitfalls in its diagnosis and treatment. The absence of bile-stained vomitus in the newborn infant suggested obstruction proximal to the ampulla. The plain film of the abdomen was interpreted as a "double bubble," which confirmed the clinical impression. The apparent demonstration of patency of the pyloric canal at the time of duodenal exploration, by retrograde passage of an instrument into the stomach, was also misleading. The false impression of air in the first portion of the duodenum was probably due to prolapse of the greatly distended mucosal diaphragm into the first portion of the duodenum, producing a distal gas bubble (Fig. 5–9). This error could have been prevented by passing a catheter in an antegrade manner via the eventual gastrostomy, but the presence of duodenal atresia seemed adequate to explain the findings. Furthermore, complete obstruction of the duodenum is a relatively common cause of intestinal obstruction in the newborn. It may or may not be heralded by bile in the vomitus, depending upon the level of obstruction. If obstruction is intrinsic, the established treatment of choice is a side-to-side bypassing duodenojejunostomy. Obviously the exact nature of the obstruction will remain unknown since definitive, inquisitive dissection in this C loop of the duodenum is unwise. The management of this component of the double anomaly was standard.

Failure to recognize the dual nature of the obstruction necessitated a second operation. A wide gastrotomy is necessary to recognize a prepyloric mucosal diaphragm. Pyloroplasty with incision of the diaphragm is the treatment of choice in infants.

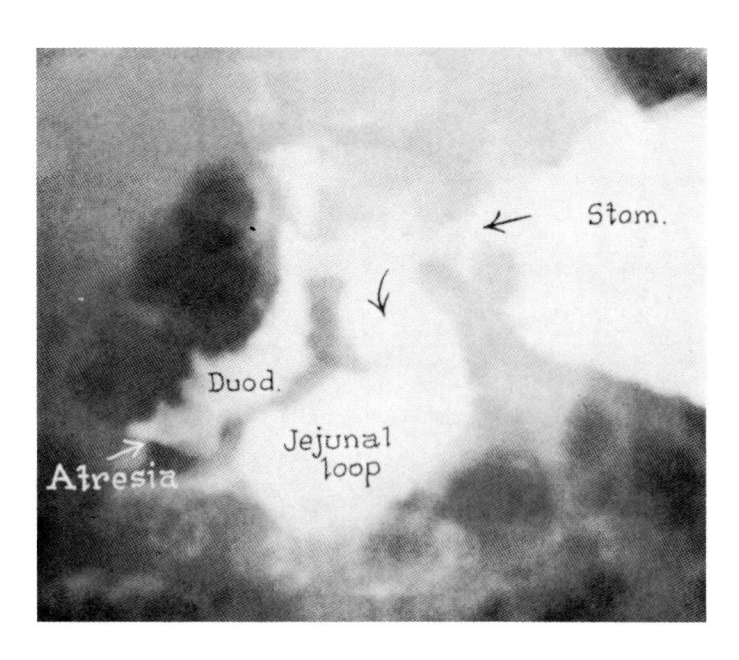

Figure 5–10. Follow-up Gastrografin study at 4 months of age showing blind duodenal pouch and functioning duodenojejunostomy. (From Haller and Cahill, cited in Figure 5–7.)

Congenital Antral Membrane in Older Children and Adults

As noted earlier, a congenital pyloric or prepyloric membrane may be asymptomatic until childhood or adulthood.

The first adult case of prepyloric membrane or septum was reported by Sames, in 1949, in a 40-year-old woman with a history consistent with peptic ulcer disease of 6 years' duration. Barium x-ray studies of the stomach revealed an ulcer of the lesser curvature, a prepyloric diaphragm, and no evidence of obstruction. Subtotal gastrectomy was performed, and the specimen revealed the diaphragm 1.5 cm. proximal to the pylorus. It consisted of only mucosa and submucosa.

In 1953 Rota reported a prepyloric membrane in a 74-year-old woman who had had obstructive symptoms for 8 years. Partial gastrectomy was performed. The removed specimen contained a diaphragm similar to that in Sames' patient and also showed chronic antral gastritis. Recovery was complete, and no recurrence was seen during the period of follow-up.

A similar case was reported later in 1953 by Gross and Durham. The antral membrane was demonstrated by preoperative barium study of the stomach, and at surgery the membrane was incised and a Finney pyloroplasty done with a successful outcome.

In 1955, Albot and Magnier reported a 32-year-old man operated upon in 1946 for an antral membrane recognized by x-ray examination.

In 1959, Rowling recorded two additional cases in the literature. Both were adult men with symptoms suggestive of peptic ulcer disease. In one the antral membrane was recognized at surgery and excised. The other patient was thought to have antral peptic disease and was treated by partial gastrectomy; examination of the specimen showed an antral membrane — inflammation and ulceration were absent. Both patients recovered uneventfully.

Although at least two neonates with incomplete antral membrane have been reported, this lesion is seen most commonly in middle-aged patients and there is no predominance of either sex.

In 1968 Parrish and associates reviewed the literature and reported that a perforated mucosal diaphragm located in the gastric antrum and causing obstruction had been recorded in 14 adults, including one reported by them in 1966. Since then they had treated three more adults and a 6-year-old child with obstructing antral diaphragm. Their additions increased the number of cases of incomplete antral mucosal diaphragm reported as of 1968 to a total of 22: 17 in adults and 5 in children.

The gross and microscopic findings were constant. In every case the abnormality was a thin diaphragm situated about 2 cm. proximal to the pylorus and composed only of the mucosa and submucosa. The 2- to 3-mm. orifice in the septum was eccentric or central in location, soft, and free from fibrosis but resisted dilation. Microscopically, loose connective tissue was seen to form the septum between the layers of mucosa. The muscular wall of the stomach took no part in formation of the diaphragm. In none was there ulcerative scarring at the site of the perforated membrane. The gross and microscopic characteristics of the membranes seemed typical of a congenital anomaly and incompatible with an acquired lesion.

The youngest patient having an antral diaphragm with an aperture was a 2-year-old male, reported by Berman and Ballenger in 1942.

After study of this combined collected and personal series of 22 cases, Parrish and coworkers pointed out that the similarity of cases of congenital antral membranes that cause symptoms in older children and adults is so constant that the condition warrants recognition as a specific entity.

Symptoms

In adults with perforate diaphragms the symptoms are usually mild, and their onset is late. The most constant symptoms of congenital antral membrane in these older children and adults were a feeling of fullness associated with episodes of nausea and vomiting, occurring usually shortly after eating.

Other symptoms, such as epigastric pain, anorexia, weight loss, and temporary relief by ingestion of antacids, were highly variable and not helpful in the differential diagnosis. Likewise, physical examination revealed nothing of diagnostic value.

There was remarkable similarity in the

barium x-ray studies of the stomach in all the reported cases. The antral membrane or septum appeared as a thin, constant, knife-like filling defect approximately 2 cm. proximal to the pyloric channel; barium passed beyond the defect and filled the distal portion of the antrum, the pylorus, and the duodenum (Fig. 5–11). Although emptying time of the barium-filled stomach was highly variable, no evidence of complete obstruction was seen in any patient.

In adults the clinical picture may resemble carcinoma, cicatricial scarring secondary to peptic ulceration, prolapse of the antral mucosa, benign ulcer, or gastritis with pylorospasm. The late onset of acute symptoms in these adult patients is difficult to explain.

"One patient, aged 52, had complete loss of appetite, dyspepsia and vomiting for only four months [Bariety, Poulet, and Courtois-Suffit, 1957]. Another patient, aged 74, had a membrane with an aperture of 4 mm. yet his symptoms had been present for only eight years. Barium retention was much higher [Rota, 1953]. An even smaller aperture was found in a 53-year-old woman whose gastric symptoms dated from only a few months [Young, 1961]. Death from inanition was barely averted by surgical intervention" (Gray and Skandalakis, 1972).

Swartz and Shepard (1956) suggested that the late onset of acute symptoms in these adult patients is due to a generalized decrease in gastric tone that occurs with aging and theorized that the stomach has hypertrophied and forced food through the membrane for many years, but, like the urinary bladder, it finally loses tone and becomes distended and decompensated. "The frequently observed thickening and dilatation of the stomach in the reported patients tends to support this theory" (Parrish and associates, 1968).

However, Gray and Skandalakis (1972) pointed out that "the accepted belief is that membranous atresia in the stomach and in the intestine may perforate soon after birth, leaving only a mild stenosis. Therefore the presence of very small perforations in adults who had had obstructive symptoms for only a few months suggests that the perforation may become progressively smaller with age. It is difficult to believe that these small apertures sufficed for more or less normal functioning for many years. If they represent perforation of congenital diaphragmatic atresias, a subsequent stenosis must have occurred. Hence, in the absence of scarring, increasing stenosis by either local proliferation or concrescent slipping of the mucosa must be postulated."

The explanation for the late onset of acute symptoms in these adult patients remains uncertain.

Feliciano and Van Heerden (1977) reported seven adults aged from 32 to 80 years of age with pyloric antral mucosal webs, who were seen and treated at the Mayo Clinic, and concluded, "Whether these adult patients are the late symptomatic form of this congenital anomaly, or whether an acquired lesion from the healing of acid peptic ulcer is present, or both, is presently unknown."

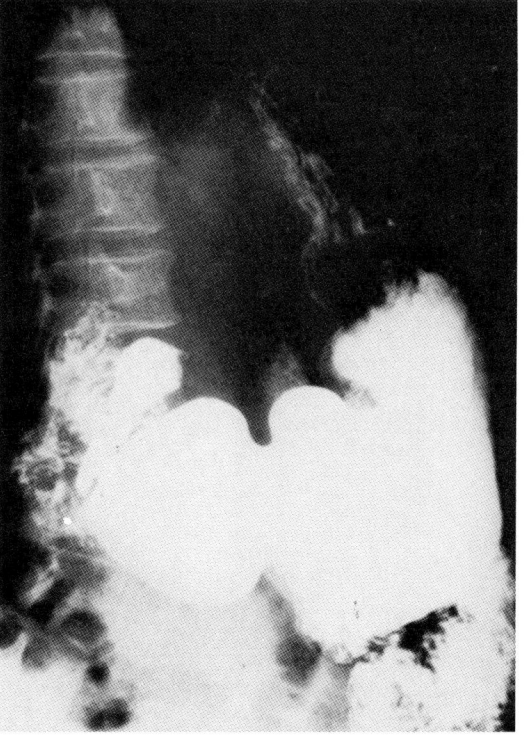

Figure 5–11. Selected roentgenogram from upper gastrointestinal barium study reveals partial obstruction at gastric outlet. The diagnosis of an antral membrane is clearly evident as a filling defect on this film. The barium-filled pylorus and incompletely filled duodenal bulb beyond the membrane are evident. (From Parrish, R. A., Kavanage, C. B., Wells, J. A., et al.: Congenital antral membrane. Surg. Gynecol. Obstet. *127*:1003, 1968.)

STOMACH ATRESIA AND STENOSIS (NEONATAL GASTRIC OUTLET OBSTRUCTION)

Diagnosis

Because these findings have to be differentiated from those of more common entities, the preoperative diagnosis of antral membrane may be easily overlooked. However, if the possibility is thought of, diagnosis can be made preoperatively by plain and barium x-ray studies or endoscopy. In two reported cases (Sames, 1949; Rowling, 1959), preoperative gastroscopic examination gave negative results because the membrane consists of normal mucosa and was difficult to identify. However, the radiologic and endoscopic findings were positive in all seven cases reported more recently by Feliciano and Van Heerden (1977).

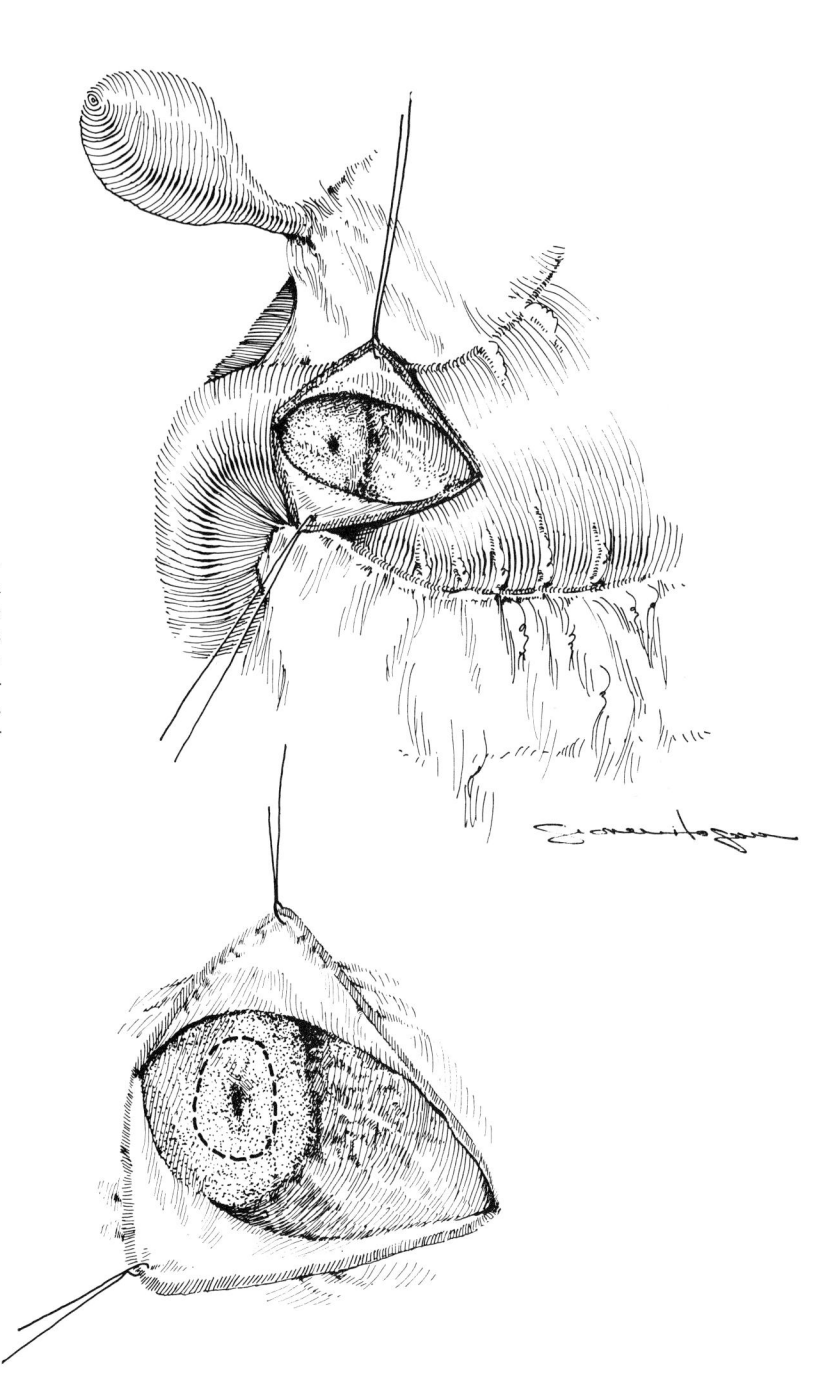

Figure 5–12. Artist's conception of operative findings in a patient. *Top*, antral membrane with small central aperture, as seen through gastrotomy. *Bottom*, the dotted line outlines excision of the mucosal membrane. (From Parrish, et al., cited in previous figure.)

As noted, antral membrane may also be difficult to diagnose at operation because, in most cases, no external evidence of an abnormality at the gastroduodenal junction can be seen. In only one adult (Sames, 1949) was there any evidence, in the external gastric wall, of the presence of an obstructing membrane.

A gastrotomy is necessary to examine the interior of the gastroduodenal area and be most certain of determining the presence or absence of a membrane. Retrograde examination through a duodenotomy has been unreliable for this purpose.

"Approximately 50 per cent of the adult patients had an accompanying gastric ulcer proximal to the membrane, presumably due to excessive antral stimulation as a result of chronic gastric stasis" (Parrish and colleagues, 1968).

Treatment

The treatment of symptomatic congenital antral membrane in older children and adults is surgical.

In the past, some form of partial gastrectomy has been used most frequently for this purpose. This operation was done without first ascertaining the pathology present via a preliminary exploratory gastrotomy. As a result, many of these gastrectomies were unnecessary.

Experience has shown that it is a mistake to perform a gastrectomy without first opening the stomach to ascertain the pathology, because when an antral membrane is recognized at surgery without associated peptic disease, a lesser procedure that promotes gastric emptying is preferable.

In a child with an antral membrane, incision or excision of the membrane seems to be the procedure of choice. The addition of a pyloroplasty seems necessary only in those patients in whom an adequate gastric outlet is not otherwise assured. Likewise, unless an adult has associated peptic disease requiring operative therapy, subtotal gastrectomy should not be necessary for this simple congenital deformity. The procedure of choice for these patients is simple excision of the membrane (Fig. 5–12). Follow-up examination of patients undergoing this procedure tends to support this opinion.

Preliminary exploratory gastrotomy should eliminate the unnecessary gastrectomies performed for this simple lesion.

Prognosis

The prognosis for these patients is excellent, provided the obstruction is completely relieved.

In 1972, Gray and Skandalakis reported that of 22 patients operated upon for an antral membrane, only 5 failed to survive. In addition, only one adult has died following operation for a perforated diaphragm.

In 1967, Sloop and Montague collected from the world literature reports of 41 patients with perforate antral diaphragms and added one of their own. Two of the reported patients died without any surgery. One was a 44-year-old male whose perforate prepyloric membrane was an incidental finding at autopsy. The other was a stillborn infant whose autopsy showed a pyloric membrane and multiple other anomalies. The 40 patients who underwent surgical treatment ranged in age from 1 month to 74 years, with a median age of 52 years. Thirty-eight (95 per cent) of these operated patients survived, and only 2 died, following the operation. Both deaths followed performance of a gastrojejunostomy; one patient was a 1-month-old child and the other was a 59-year-old man.

ANTRAL MUCOSAL DIAPHRAGM ASSOCIATED WITH ESOPHAGEAL HIATAL HERNIA

Diethrich and Regan (1965) reported a 64-year-old woman with a lifelong history of intermittent epigastric discomfort who was referred to the surgical service because of recent additional complaints of weight loss and postprandial vomiting. An upper gastrointestinal radiographic study revealed a sizable hiatal hernia and also a prepyloric antral diaphragm which, in retrospect, was present but not recognized in radiographic studies made five years previously (Fig. 5–13). Figure 5–14 is the preoperative upper gastrointestinal study made on the current admission to the hospital. Note the narrowing of the opening in the diaphragm, compared with the study five years earlier.

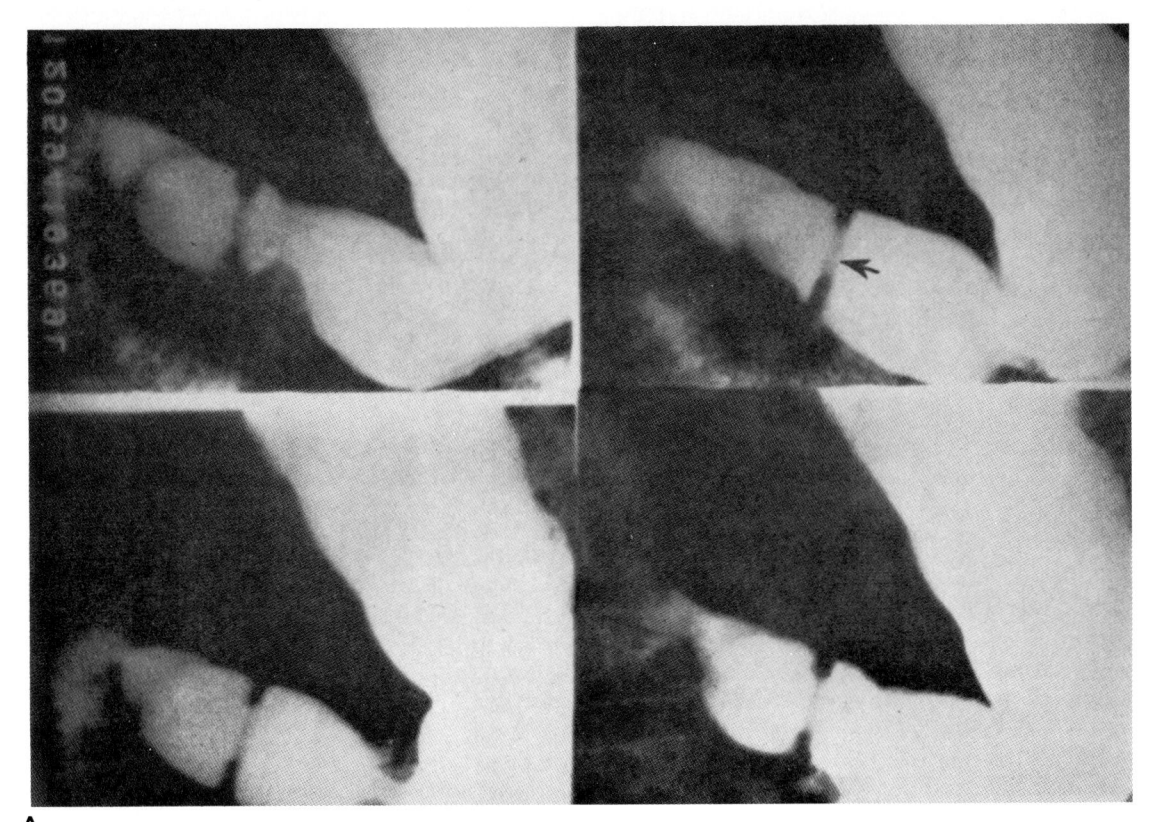

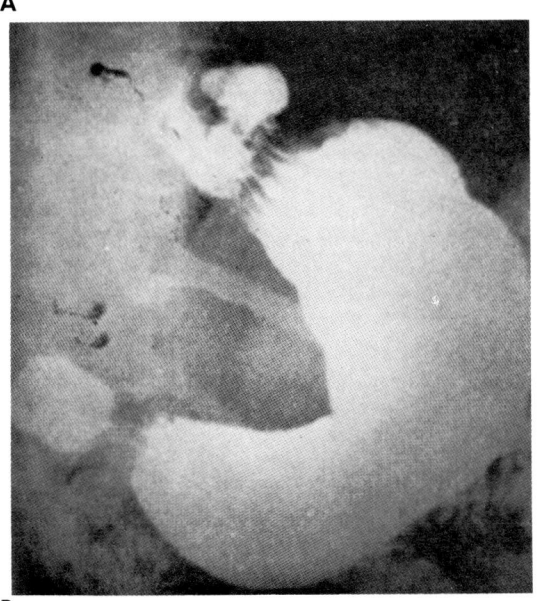

Figure 5-13. Upper gastrointestinal study 5 years prior to operation; *A*, prepyloric antral deformity and *B*, hiatus hernia. The mucosal diaphragm (arrow) was interpreted as pyloric channel, the pathologic condition not being recognized on this study. Note the persistence of the diaphragm in the four spot films. (From Diethrich, E. B., and Regan, W. J.: Antral mucosal diaphragm associated with esophageal hiatus hernia: Case report and review of the literature. Am. J. Surg. *110*:483, 1965.)

The authors pointed out that this progressive narrowing probably accounted for the gradual increase in the patient's symptoms.

The patient was treated surgically with a subdiaphragmatic hiatal herniorrhaphy, bilateral vagectomy, and 40 per cent gastric resection with a Billroth I reconstruction. Her postoperative recovery was uneventful except for a transient pneumonitis. The postoperative upper gastrointestinal study showed an adequate repair of the hiatal

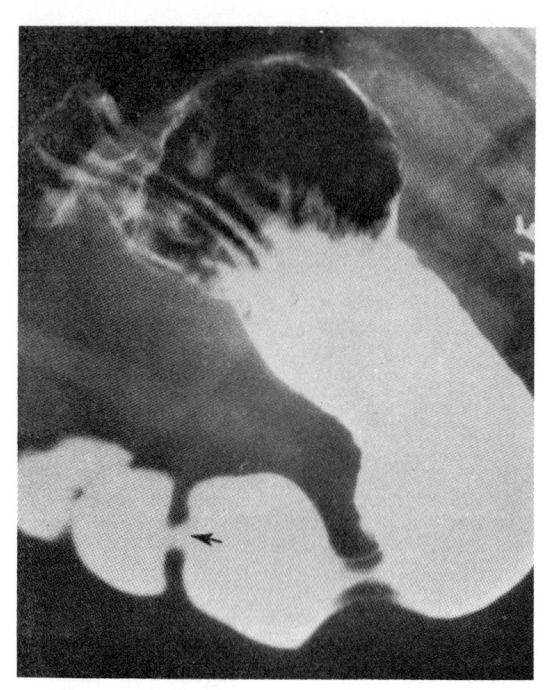

Figure 5-14. Preoperative upper gastrointestinal study again demonstrating the mucosal diaphragm. Note the narrowing of the opening in the diaphragm as compared with the study 5 years earlier (Fig. 5-13). This progressive narrowing probably accounted for the gradual increase in the patient's symptoms. (From Diethrich and Regan, cited in previous figure.)

hernia and elimination of the mucosal diaphragm (Fig. 5-15).

Examination of the distal 40 per cent of the stomach including the pylorus revealed a mucosal diaphragm situated 2.5 cm. proximal to the pylorus and having a centrally located perforation 4 by 6 mm. in size. An index finger placed through the pylorus could not be advanced through the smaller unyielding opening in the pyloric diaphragm. Microscopic examination of the diaphragm showed mucosa, beneath which only muscularis mucosa was present.

The investigators reviewed the literature and reported this to be the fourteenth case report of antral mucosal diaphragm that has been described, and the first case recorded in association with an esophageal hiatal hernia. In the reported cases, gastroenterostomy, pyloroplasty, incision and excision of the diaphragm, and subtotal gastrectomy had yielded equally satisfactory results. In this patient, vagectomy and repair of the hiatal hernia accompanied partial gastric resection.

Except for concomitant gastric ulcer in several cases and perforation of the stomach proximal to the obstructing membrane in at least two infants, associated gastrointestinal disorders in these patients have not been recorded.

CONGENITAL DUODENAL ATRESIA

Congenital intrinsic obstruction of the duodenum is the third most common cause of gastrointestinal tract obstruction in the neonate, following imperforate anus and esophageal atresia. The obstruction results from a complete occlusion in approximately 90 per cent of patients, with a significant stenosis in the remaining 10 per cent. The level of atresia will occur at or within a centimeter of the ampulla of Vater in 80 to 90 per cent of patients; in the remainder it usually occurs in the third portion of the duodenum. Nonbilious vomiting may occur when the atretic level is above the ampulla of Vater. This has been reported in as many as one-third of patients. The more common bile-stained vomiting indicates obstruction below the ampulla of Vater. If untreated, the obstruction results in dehydration and a metabolic hypochloremic alkalosis and hypokalemia, causing death in the first 8 to 12 days of life.

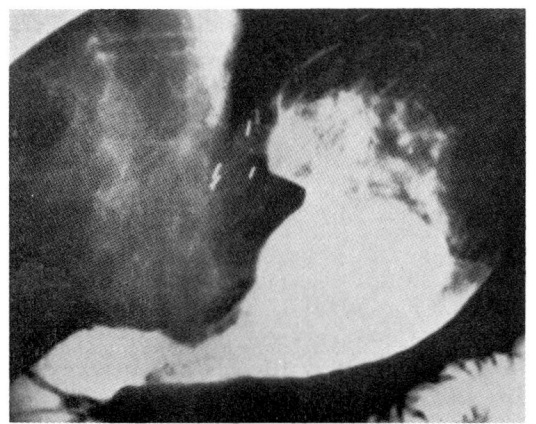

Figure 5-15. Postoperative upper gastrointestinal study after vagectomy, repair of hiatal hernia, and 40 per cent Billroth I gastric resection. (From Diethrich and Regan, cited in Figure 5-13.)

Congenital obstruction of the duodenum was first reported by Calder in 1733, and the first successful operative correction was reported in 1916 by Ernst. Evans reported, in 1951, that only 139 patients had survived surgical correction up to that time. Since that time, survival is the rule rather than the exception. Although decreasing, the mortality rate remains higher than the relatively simple surgical treatment currently employed would be expected to yield. In the series reported from The Children's Hospital of Los Angeles (Wesley and Mahour, 1977), the overall survival for the period 1951 through 1975 was 67 per cent; for the 10-year period of 1965 to 1975, the survival rate was 88 per cent.

Factors felt to be important in the current improvement in survival include (1) early diagnosis and complete preoperative preparation of the infant; (2) expert anesthesia; (3) improved surgical awareness of associated gastrointestinal anomalies, such as duodenal diaphragm and distal bowel atresia; (4) proper use of effective postoperative gastric decompression; (5) parenteral hyperalimentation; and (6) improved intensive care nursing.

Factors considered to be responsible for the continuing morbidity associated with duodenal atresia are (1) prematurity, seen in approximately 40 per cent of such infants; (2) associated congenital anomalies, such as Down's syndrome, severe congenital cardiac anomalies, genitourinary tract anomalies, esophageal atresia, and tracheoesophageal fistula; and (3) sepsis.

The factors that combine to maintain a significant mortality in the infant with duodenal atresia will reappear as significant factors in many of the congenital anomalies to be discussed.

Embryology

No single theory so far proposed adequately explains the pathogenesis of all cases of duodenal atresia and stenosis. The one most widely accepted is the following:

Up to the fifth week of fetal life the intestine is a patent tube lined with epithelium. In the fifth to sixth weeks the epithelial mucosa proliferates and obliterates the duodenum, so that the intestinal lumen changes from a hollow tube to a solid cord (Fig. 5–16). Shortly thereafter, vacuoles appear in the previously solid cord and coalesce to re-establish a patent intestinal lumen. This recanalization of the duodenal lumen is completed by the eighth to tenth week. Failure of recanalization could produce an atretic or stenotic area.

Duodenal atresia is due to persistence of one or more of the septa following the solid stage, and stenosis is due to a remaining but partially perforated septum. Atresia and stenosis are different degrees of the same defective process. (Congenital stenosis is discussed on page 141.)

Congenital duodenal obstruction may be classified into three broad categories: (1) *intrinsic obstruction,* which includes atresia, stenosis, webs, diaphragms, congenital

Figure 5–16. Sketches of the duodenum from the normal embryo, illustrating the solid stage which normally exists in embryos between the 7-mm. and 30-mm. stages. *Above:* longitudinal section of intestine showing coalescence of the walls and the formation of multiple cystic spaces. *Below: A,* Solid stage showing concrescence of epithelial surfaces. *B,* Later stage with development of isolated pockets. *C,* Final attainment of a continuous intestinal lumen.

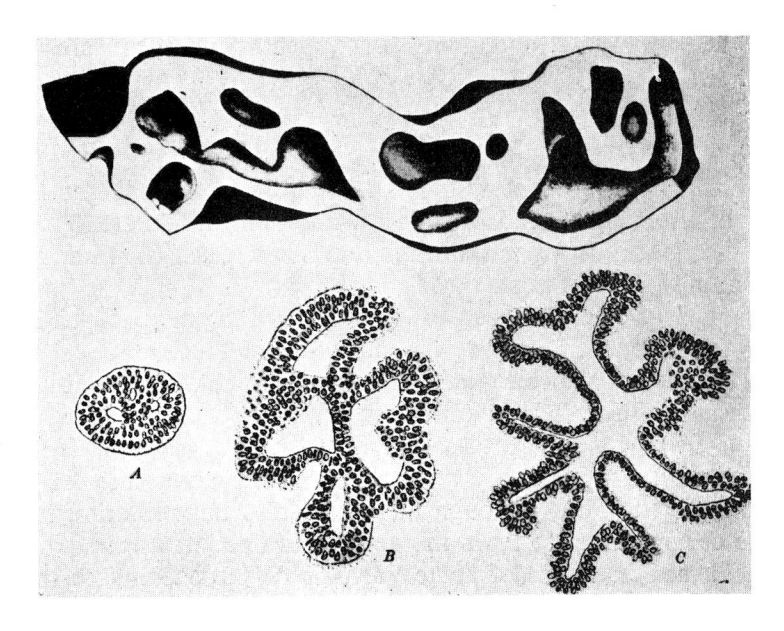

absence of duodenal musculature, and congenital absence of Auerbach's plexus; (2) *extrinsic obstruction*, which includes annular pancreas and congenital constricting bands other than those associated with malrotation, such as obstruction of the duodenojejunal junction by congenital extrinsic bands; and (3) *anomalies of rotation and fixation*, including malrotation with paraduodenal bands.

Boyden, Cape, and Bill (1967) examined human fetuses of from five to eight weeks of gestation with regard to duodenal occlusion. They noted that as the epithelial plug begins to break up, vacuoles coalesce to form two channels, and two communications arise from the duodenum to the hepatopancreatic duct. The two openings enter separately into the two duodenal channels. This state is usually transitory, but persistence of the two channels is substantiated by cases reported in which atresia has occurred at the site of the papilla of Vater, leaving a forked common bile duct entering both proximal and distal segments of the duodenum. Failure of absorption of the two channels may lead to a membranous atresia with an intraluminal diverticulum, as described by Heilbrun and Boyden (1964).

Maternal hydramnios is present in about 50 per cent of the infants born with duodenal atresia. An obstetric history of maternal hydramnios should alert one to the possibility of a congenital high-intestinal obstruction.

Premature birth was noted in 25 per cent and additional congenital malformation in 41 per cent of the 32 cases of congenital intrinsic duodenal obstruction (atresia or stenosis) reported by Moore (1956).

Pathology

Duodenal atresia occurs in a variety of forms (Fig. 5–17). According to Gray and Skandalakis (1972):

1. In the commonest form of atresia, obstruction is by a diaphragm or membrane formed of mucosa and submucosa; the muscularis is not interrupted [Fig. 5–17A]. The diaphragm may be intact or perforated. Whether perforated or not, it forms an inverted dome across the duodenal lumen. Pressure upon it may produce a slight external indentation at its site of attachment. The perforation, when present, is usually off-center and may be 2 to 10 mm. in diameter. Because of its shape under proximal pressure, the dia-

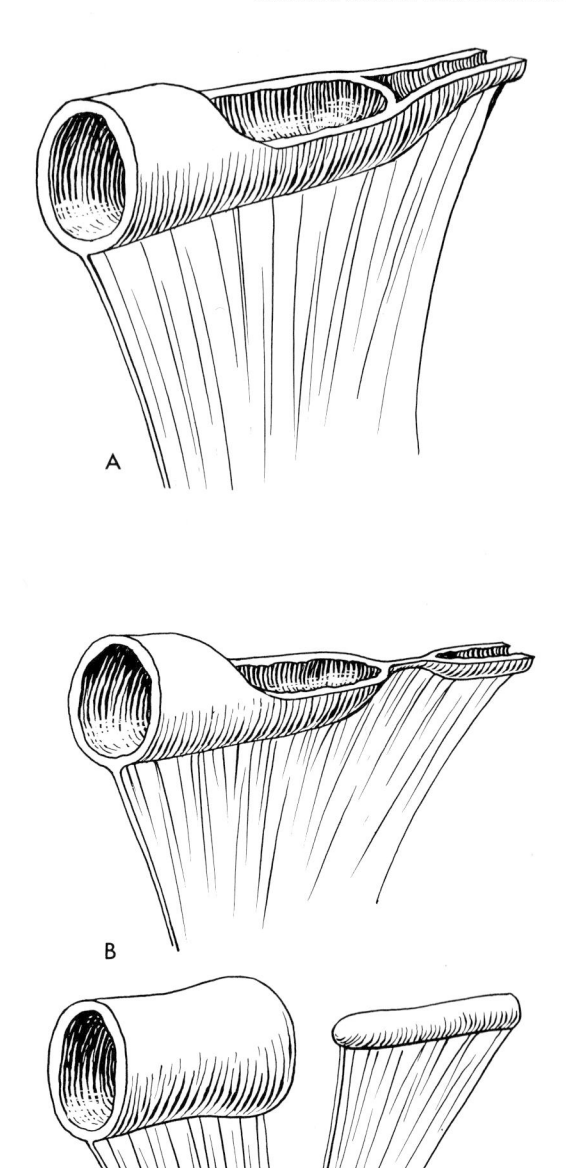

Figure 5–17. Three types of intestinal atresia. *A*, Closure by a diaphragm of mucosa. *B*, A segment of the intestine is reduced to a solid cord without a lumen. *C*, Complete segmental absence of a portion of the intestine and of the associated mesentery. In all types, the proximal normal segment is dilated and the distal normal segment is unexpanded. (From Gray, S. W., and Skandalakis, J. E.: Embryology for Surgeons. Philadelphia, W. B. Saunders Company, 1972.)

phragm usually appears to be situated more distally than is actually the case. When the perforation is not central, an intraluminal diverticulum, resembling an airport windsock, may form the fundus of the diaphragm [Fig. 5–18]. In a few cases the duodenal lumen is obliterated over an

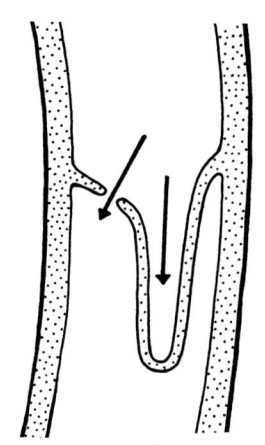

Figure 5–18. An internal intestinal diverticulum formed in a perforated membranous atresia. Such a mucosal pocket will continue to enlarge until it forms an obstruction. (From Gray and Skandalakis, cited in previous figure.)

appreciable distance, forming a plug rather than a diaphragm. The muscle coats are unaffected.

2. The blind end of the dilated proximal duodenal segment may be connected by a short solid cord running, along the edge of the intact mesentery, to the distal undilated segment of intestine [Fig. 5–17B].

3. There is complete absence of a segment of the duodenum with its mesentery so that the duodenum ends blindly, both proximal and distal to the atresia. There is no connecting fibrous cord and the mesentery between the blind ends is absent [Fig. 5–17C]. In all the above types, the proximal normal segment above the atresia is dilated and the distal normal segment is collapsed.

4. There may be a membranous ring within the duodenum with little effect on the lumen other than loss of distensibility.

"Ninety-five per cent of the atretic lesions are distal to the ampulla of Vater" (Benson and Lloyd, 1961). Atresia proximal to the ampulla is rare.

Atresias may be multiple and involve more than one segment of the intestinal tract. This occurs in about 15 per cent of the infants with duodenal atresia. Five of the ten neonates with duodenal atresia reported by Rowe, Buckner, and Clatworthy (1968) had a second source of mechanical intestinal obstruction. One patient had a second duodenal web, three had imperforate anus, and one had Hirschsprung's disease.

Associated Anomalies

For reasons unexplained, a high incidence of Down's syndrome (mongolism) is associated with duodenal atresia and stenosis, especially the former. The incidence has ranged from 4 to 35 per cent in different reported series.

Esophageal atresia has been an associated malformation in about 1 per cent of the duodenal atresias. Annular pancreas, atresia or other malformations of the bile ducts, and imperforate anus are among the various other anomalies that have also been associated with duodenal atresia or stenosis. In some cases, two or more associated anomalies were seen. Malrotations in association with duodenal atresia have been reported.

Clinical Characteristics

The most consistent symptom is vomiting. Some vomiting usually occurs on the first day of life. An occasional newborn infant may not vomit until after the first feeding, but this is rare. Since two-thirds of duodenal atretic lesions are distal to the ampulla, these infants uniformly vomit bile. When the atresia is proximal to the ampulla, there is no bile in the vomitus. In such cases prepyloric atresia and pyloric stenosis (see Neonatal Gastric Outlet Obstruction, p. 120) must be considered in the differential diagnosis. Although the onset of symptoms of hypertrophic pyloric stenosis is usually later, some patients with this disorder had had some vomiting since birth.

Little or no abdominal distention is noted, because of the high level of the atresia. The infants decompress themselves by their persistent vomiting. Abdominal distention, when present, is confined to the upper abdomen. The lower abdomen may be scaphoid.

The infant who has radiographic documentation of a high duodenal obstruction and has undergone nasogastric decompression of the stomach should have a scaphoid abdomen. If the abdomen remains distended, one must consider another gastrointestinal anomaly, such as midgut volvulus, and a barium enema should be performed to evaluate this possibility.

Diagnosis

Lloyd and Clatworthy (1958) found that over two-thirds of infants with congenital obstructive lesions proximal to the first 15 to 20 cm. of the jejunum are born of mothers with polyhydramnios. Benson and Lloyd (1961) emphasized that "although there are other causes of polyhydramnios, every physician responsible for the care of newborn infants should be alert to the possibility that any otherwise normal baby born of a polyhydramnios mother may have proximal high-grade intestinal obstruction."

The clinical characteristics alone are usually sufficient to indicate the absence of a high intestinal obstruction. The diagnosis can be established and the site of the atresia localized by a plain x-ray film of the abdomen, without the use of barium, taken in the upright position.

Wasch and Marck (1948) demonstrated by radiographic studies that in the normal newborn infant air reaches the stomach on the first breath, the duodenum within a few minutes, and the cecum in 3 to 8 hours. When duodenal atresia is present, the characteristic radiographic sign is a double bubble (Fig. 5–19) representing a large collection of air in the distended stomach and first portion of the duodenum. This contrasts strikingly with the rest of the abdomen, in which other gas-filled intestinal loops are absent, thus indicating duodenal obstruction.

The use of radiopaque material is unnecessary and contraindicated. If the plain films are equivocal, a catheter may be passed into the infant's stomach and 50 to 60 ml. of air injected to distend the stomach and provide better contrast (Benson and Lloyd, 1961).

If air is present in the intestinal tract, a barium enema may be required to rule out malrotation and distinguish low small intestinal obstruction from colonic obstruction. Rowe, Buckner, and Clatworthy (1968) pointed out that in the presence of incomplete rotation, a markedly dilated duodenum suggests an intrinsic lesion.

Because another atresia frequently may be found distal to the primary obstruction, many investigators recommend routine use of barium enemas.

Clinical Course

Although duodenal atresia is surprisingly well tolerated by the neonate, dehydration and weight loss develop and eventually complete constipation occurs. The fluid and electrolyte imbalances are generally less severe than in cases of lower gastrointestinal obstruction. All infants with duodenal atresia will die if surgical relief is not afforded.

Evans (1951) found that untreated patients lived an average of 5 to 6 days. However, Lynn (1969) reported one patient "who survived for 17 days with no treatment other than sugar water by mouth. Autopsy revealed complete atresia with loss of continuity in the third portion of the duodenum."

Treatment

Duodenal atresia is treated by a surgical procedure that restores the continuity of the gastrointestinal tract in a manner that is least likely to disturb the delicate structures in the area of the congenital obstruction, and at the same time preserves the simple continuity and function of the gut. Because of the significant incidence of associated congenital lesions, such as cardiac malformations, and improved management in intravenous manipulation of electrolyte abnormalities and nutritional needs, it is

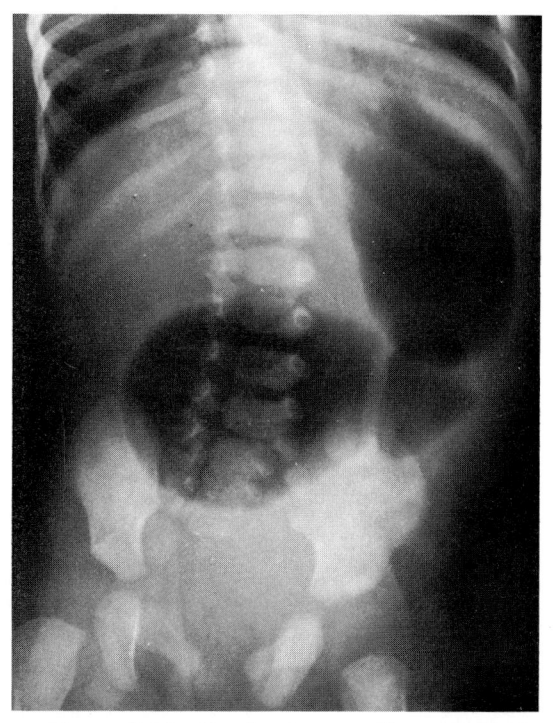

Figure 5–19. Duodenal atresia. The markedly dilated stomach and duodenal cap are filled with air. The absence of other gas-filled intestinal loops indicates a duodenal obstruction. (From Gray and Skandalakis, cited in Figure 5–17.)

possible to complete a thorough evaluation of the infant's cardiovascular, pulmonary, and renal systems before undertaking surgical correction.

This examination may be expeditiously carried out in the first day of life with the following tests: A simple chest x-ray film will usually provide considerable information about cardiovascular anomalies as well as about significant pulmonary pathology. When an arterial or capillary blood gas analysis is added, one is capable of predicting many operative or postoperative problems, and often such knowledge will significantly aid the pediatric anesthesiologist in providing optimal ventilation. Normal urination usually occurs by the second day of life, and analysis of the urine along with serum UREA nitrogen and creatinine provides a good means of assessing renal function. If these factors are found acceptable, the infant may be safely scheduled to undergo the surgical correction of the duodenal atresia.

Preoperative Care

A nasogastric tube is inserted into the stomach and intermittent suction applied to avoid the aspiration of vomitus and subsequent pneumonia, which may cause death in these patients. Replacement of fluid and electrolytes through a peripheral intravenous catheter is initiated. Vitamin K is given to reduce the danger of postoperative bleeding from hemorrhagic disease of the neonate.

Since over 50 per cent of children with duodenal obstruction are premature, the consideration of preoperative or intraoperative antibiotic administration is reasonable.

The length of time that can be spent profitably in preparation for surgery varies considerably, depending upon the initial weight of the infant and the degree of metabolic abnormality present. The presence of duodenal atresia itself no longer represents an indication for prompt, emergency surgery. Time spent in the preoperative evaluation of potential associated anomalies, once the distended stomach is decompressed, may make a significant difference in the eventual recovery of the infant. The surgical relief of the duodenal atresia is intended to provide problem-free gastrointestinal alimentation for many years and its accomplishment should await optimal condition of the infant as well as the expertise of the pediatric anesthesiologist, appropriately cross-matched blood, and optimal operating room conditions.

Anesthesia

Currently, choice of anesthesia and anesthetic agents depends upon the degree of prematurity and associated cardiovascular and pulmonary abnormalities. All infants undergoing an exploratory laparotomy for the evaluation of a duodenal obstruction are managed with controlled ventilation through an endotracheal tube.

The first step in the preanesthetic period is to ascertain the infant's temperature in the operating room and take steps to maintain a temperature between 36 and 37° C throughout the operative procedure. These include a suitably warmed operating room, a heating blanket, overhead heating or infrared lights, the means to warm both infused blood and anesthetic gases, and preheated irrigating solutions. We have employed a double layer of Steri-Drape, the first containing a preformed hole exposing the operative site and adjacent abdominal wall, the second applied after the operative site has been prepared with organically bound iodine solution. This prevents the pooling of the surgical prep solution and subsequent irrigating fluids beneath the infant.

With normothermia assured, the stomach of the infant is completely evacuated and the nasogastric tube removed, to allow for several minutes of oxygenation of the infant with 100 per cent oxygen. If the infant is premature or has any potential upper airway pathology, an "awake" endotracheal intubation is carried out by the senior pediatric anesthesiologist. The endotracheal tube is carefully placed just beyond the vocal cords of the infant, equal bilateral ventilation is assessed, and the endotracheal tube is firmly anchored to the infant's face. If the infant is full-term and active, the intubation may be carried out rapidly with cricoid pressure after administration of a muscle-paralyzing agent. Continuous anesthesia through the operative period is maintained with a mixture of oxygen, air, and Fluothane if tolerated, which is an agent felt to be safe in the pediatric population and associated with a minimum of cardiovascular effects in the well-controlled setting.

Insertion of a radial artery catheter at the beginning of the operation allows the anesthesiologist to control accurately the degree of oxygenation — an important consideration in cases in which the operative time may exceed several hours.

Intraoperative fluid and blood administration are calculated prior to surgery on the basis of the infant's weight and updated on the basis of frequent evaluation of blood loss by weighing all surgical sponges and measuring blood evacuated by means of suction. Blood replacement begins when blood loss reaches an estimated 10 per cent of total blood volume, and is continued at an even rate throughout the period of surgery.

At the completion of the operative procedure the decision to allow the infant to return to normal, unassisted ventilation will depend on a vaiety of factors, including degree of prematurity, length of operation, and effective lung gas exchange as assessed by blood gas measurement. The concept of "weaning" the infant from controlled endotracheal ventilation, especially in the small, premature infant, often has proved advantageous. This allows time for the complete elimination of anesthetic agents while simultaneously preventing significant postoperative metabolic changes secondary to shunting in areas of lung which become atelectatic.

In summary, the current concept of anesthesia for the neonate involves a very close interaction between the surgeon and anesthesiologist, emphasizing steps that are prophylactic in preventing complications during the surgical correction of any gastrointestinal anomaly.

Technic of Surgical Treatment

The patient is positioned supine on the operating table. The abdomen is prepared in the manner previously described, with a double layer of Steri-Drape. After the anesthesia is complete, a nasogastric tube should be passed through the nose to decompress the stomach. The one incision chosen should provide an adequate and rapid exposure for a limited dissection of the lesion, followed by a thorough running of the entire small bowel and a simple shunting operation, and then permit easy closure with good wound healing.

A right upper quadrant transverse incision placed 1 or 2 cm. above the umbilicus is satisfactory for operations on atresia at any level of the duodenum. Initially, the incision is made only through the right rectus sheath, transecting the muscle. This provides adequate exposure for exploration and confirmation of the diagnosis and usually is significant for the definitive procedure. If more exposure is needed, the incision may be extended laterally to the right or across the left rectus muscle as indicated.

After the peritoneal cavity is opened, the entire length of the small intestine is examined for the site or sites of obstruction (Fig. 5–20). The duodenum proximal to the obstruction is usually greatly dilated but should be in a flaccid, empty state. The intestine distal to the obstruction is collapsed and smaller than normal. It contains no gas and usually little or no meconium.

If the point of obstruction remains un-

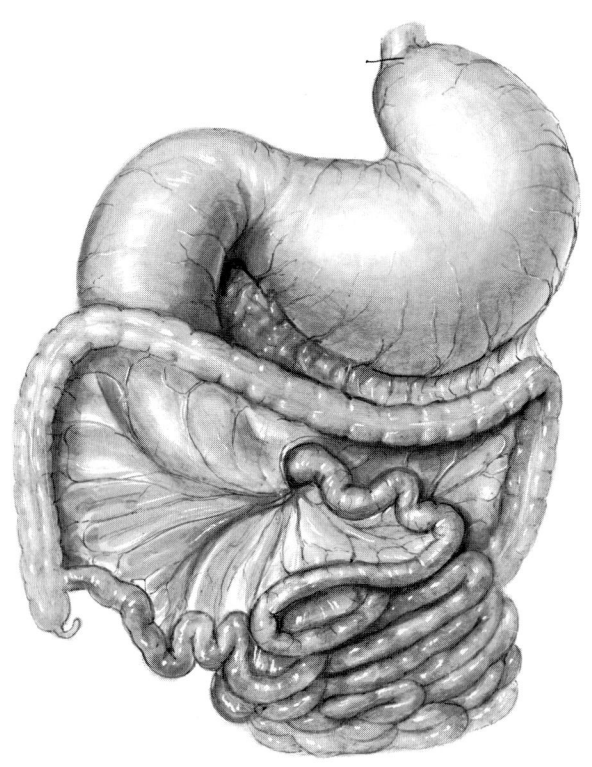

Figure 5–20. Atresia of duodenum. (From Gross, R. E.: An Atlas of Children's Surgery. Philadelphia, W. B. Saunders Company, 1970, p. 15.)

Figure 5–21. Identifying a duodenal web is readily accomplished by passing a stiff catheter through a gastrostomy and into the duodenum. Pressure on such a catheter causes invagination of the duodenal wall at the point of origin of the web (arrow). (From Rowe, M. I., Buckner, D., and Clatworthy, H. W., Jr.: Wind sock web of the duodenum. Am. J. Surg. *116*:448, 1968.)

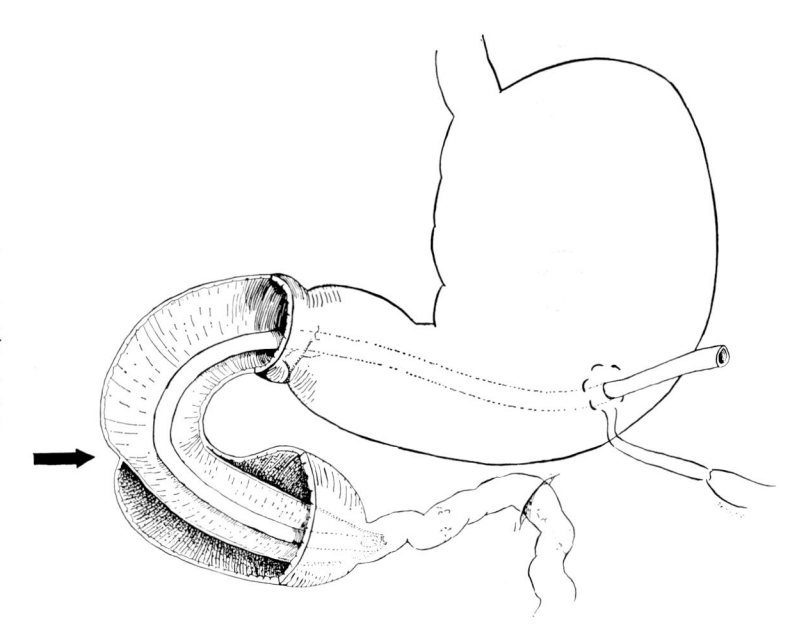

clear, it can be positively identified by placing a purse-string suture in the anterior wall of the stomach, making a small gastrotomy at its center, and passing a stiff catheter into the stomach, then through the pylorus and down the duodenum to the point of obstruction (Fig. 5–21). If a web is present, further pressure on the catheter will cause invagination of the dilated bowel at the level of origin of the web. A stitch may be placed in this area of indentation as a marker. After the site has been identified, it is important to determine whether there is more than one site of atresia, before deciding upon the type of operation to be performed. "The incidence of multiple atresia of the intestine is too common (15 per cent) to warrant any definitive operation until the entire bowel has been carefully examined for additional sites of obstruction" (Lynn, 1969).

Experience has shown that it is far wiser to treat duodenal atresia with a bypassing procedure to relieve the obstruction than to attempt to correct or revamp the local obstructing lesion. When the obstruction is in the form of a diaphragm there is a strong temptation simply to open the duodenum just above or below the block, excise the diaphragm, and then close the duodenotomy. Richardson and Martin (1969) have reported their improved management of duodenal diaphragms by employing increased preoperative diagnosis, with use of contrast studies of the colon and upper gastrointestinal tract, use of a Foley catheter or appropriate instrument to help locate and calibrate intrinsic obstructions throughout the length of the gastrointestinal tract, and preference for excision of the diaphragm with protection of the bile ducts.

The surgical procedure of choice currently employed most successfully is the side-to-side duodenoduodenostomy as modified by Weitzman and Brennan (Fig. 5–22). The importance of this modification lies in the exposure provided by the mobilization of the cecum and right colon to the left abdomen and rotation of the small bowel to the right side of the abdomen by bringing the distal duodenum and jejunum out from under the superior mesenteric ar-

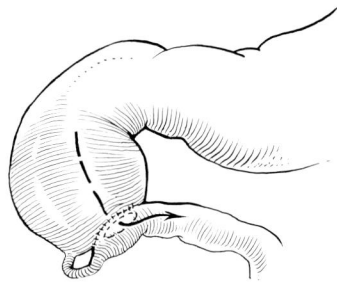

Figure 5–22. Duodenoduodenostomy, frequently the simplest and most satisfactory shunt. (From Lynn, H. B.: Duodenal obstruction: Atresia, stenosis and annular pancreas. *In* Mustard, W. T., et al. (eds.): Pediatric Surgery, 2nd ed. Vol. 2. Chicago, Year Book Medical Publishers, 1969.)

tery. This maneuver should provide total access to the dilated proximal duodenum and the smaller distal duodenum.

After passing a catheter through a small purse-string gastrotomy to assure proximal patency and definitively pinpoint the level of obstruction, a transverse incision is made in the anterior surface of the duodenum beyond the obstruction. Passage of a Foley balloon catheter or saline should be performed the entire length of the small bowel, assuming patency of the colon had been established by preoperative barium enema. With distal patency assured, a similar transverse duodenotomy is made in the proximal duodenum just above the obstruction. The lower lip of the proximal duodenotomy is then sutured to the upper lip of the distal duodenotomy with full thickness 5-0 Dexon sutures on atraumatic needles. The incisions are then joined by suturing the superior lip of the proximal transverse duodenotomy to the inferior lip of the distal duodenotomy, again with full thickness 5-0 Dexon suture material. A second layer may be added to bolster the outer suture line. A decompressing gastrostomy may be performed to protect the anastomosis. The colon is placed in the left abdomen and the proximal jejunum in the right side. An inversion type of appendectomy may be performed to protect against subsequent errors in diagnosis of appendicitis in the left abdomen.

Survival of infants with duodenal atresia now is reported to be between 80 and 90 per cent. Postoperative complications following duodenoduodenostomy are rare and consist of either complications arising from associated congenital anomalies, or sepsis. Sepsis is usually related to minor wound infections. Significant systemic sepsis may be associated with indwelling venous catheters used in parenteral hyperalimentation. The recovery of gastrointestinal tract function is usually complete within a week of the surgical repair of duodenal atresia. It may be advantageous, therefore, to rely on modified peripheral venous administration, with slightly less caloric input but potentially less likelihood of septic complications.

Long-term function of duodenoduodenostomy has been proved effective without late sequelae of obstruction or malabsorption problems.

BILIARY TRACT ABNORMALITIES ASSOCIATED WITH DUODENAL ATRESIA

The diaphragmatic form of duodenal atresia or stenosis is commonest in the ampullary region (75 per cent), but when all forms of neonatal duodenal obstruction are considered, only 7 per cent occur at the ampulla. Duodenal occlusion due to a diaphragm rarely may block the ampulla and produce secondary biliary obstruction (MacKenzie and associates, 1960).

Duplication, stenosis, and atresia of the distal common bile duct are frequently associated with duodenal stenosis or atresia in the region of the ampulla.

Reid (1973) examined the records of patients with intrinsic duodenal obstructions at the Royal Children's Hospital in Melbourne (88 cases), and the Royal Alexander Hospital for Children in Sydney (79 cases) — a total of 167 patients. Autopsy reports were available for 81 of the 95 children who died. In 9 of the 81 necropsies, anomalies of the distal common bile duct were associated with duodenal atresia or stenosis at the level of the ampulla. Three patients in the series had agenesis of the gallbladder in association with duodenal atresia, an association not previously recognized.

Symptoms and Signs

If the occluded segment involves or is proximal to the ampulla, the vomitus will not contain bile unless an aberrant biliary duct is present. Infants with duodenal obstruction are frequently jaundiced, but occlusion of the biliary tree rarely is present, even when the duodenal block is in the ampullary region.

Jaundice is extremely common in neonates. If biliary atresia is suspected, delaying operation for 4 to 6 weeks to establish the diagnosis and exclude other causes of neonatal icterus is recommended.

Duodenal occlusions demand early operation. If jaundice is also present, the detection of bile in the vomitus or the stools is the only preoperative method of excluding biliary tract obstruction. Some infants with biliary atresia may have small quantities of bile pigment in the stools, presumably by re-excretion from the blood in the lower intestinal tract.

Treatment

Biliary obstruction without treatment in the neonate is not fatal for months or a few years, therefore operation may be delayed for a short time in order to establish the diagnosis. However, duodenal atresia will be fatal in 1 to 2 weeks unless promptly diagnosed and treated surgically. Hence in neonates with both disorders, early operation is urgently needed.

The operative procedure has two main purposes. One is to relieve the obstruction of the duodenum. This is accomplished by one of the bypass procedures used for treating duodenal stenosis described in the next section: duodenojejunostomy if the obstruction is distal to the ampulla, and gastrojejunostomy if the obstruction is proximal to the ampulla.

In rare cases duodenal occlusion by a diaphragm may block the ampulla and cause secondary biliary obstruction. "Duodenotomy with excision of the diaphragm has been recommended for relief of this form of duodenal occlusion" (MacKenzie and associates, 1960).

The second purpose is to relieve the biliary obstruction. When this is due to biliary atresia, "anastomosis of the common duct to the duodenum is preferred whenever possible." MacKenzie and coworkers suggest that "if obstruction of the biliary tract at the distal end of the common duct is suspected, an operative cholangiogram through the gallbladder is a simple technique which may obviate extensive dissection in the ampullary area."

Reid (1973) warned against unnecessary dissection at operation to define the nature of bile duct anomalies because operative edema may precipitate complete obstruction in a stenotic distal common bile duct, which occurred in three of his reported cases. He also warned against excision of a septum at the site of entrance of the bile duct. The possibility of the ampulla of Vater opening between the leaves of the web must be borne in mind, according to Hudson (1961).

In 1960, MacKenzie and coworkers reported the first successful surgical survival of an infant with atresia of the second portion of the duodenum associated with complete biliary obstruction:

> The patient was a premature white male, weighing 3 pounds and 10 ounces, who regurgitated all oral feedings; the vomitus contained no bile. Bowel movements were scanty and acholic. The skin was moderately icteric.
>
> Flat films of the abdomen showed marked gaseous distention of the stomach and absence of gas in the remainder of the bowel. A Lipiodol swallow demonstrated obstruction at the junction of the first and second portions of the duodenum.
>
> Laparotomy was performed through a right paramedian incision. The stomach and first part of the duodenum were grossly distended, while the remaining small bowel and colon were collapsed.
>
> The second portion of the duodenum, for a length of 2 cm., was represented only by a strand of fibrous tissue (Fig. 5-23). The distal end of the common bile duct also terminated in fibrous tissue. The proximal common duct measured 2 cm. in length and was markedly distended, as were the cystic duct and the gallbladder. There was no other abnormality of the biliary tree or remainder of the bowel and the pancreas was grossly normal.
>
> A loop of jejunum distal to the ligament of Treitz was distended with air and saline, and a

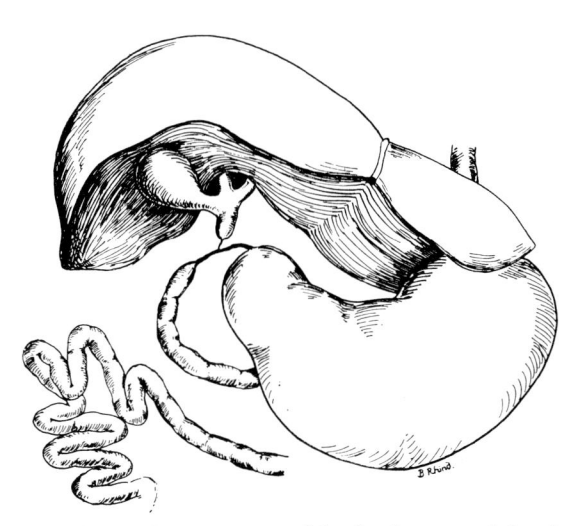

Figure 5–23. Atresia of the duodenum and distal common bile duct. (From MacKenzie, W. C., Lang, A., Friedman, M. H. W., et al.: Congenital atresia of second portion of duodenum. Surg. Gynecol. Obstet. *110*:755, 1960.)

two-layer antecolic gastrojejunostomy was performed. Then the fundus of the gallbladder was anastomosed to a proximal segment of the jejunal loop (Fig. 5–24) to drain the biliary tract. The abdomen was closed in layers.

The postoperative course was stormy but the baby recovered and was discharged from the hospital 47 days after the operation. His weight was 4 pounds and 3 ounces, jaundice had disappeared, feedings were being taken well, and bowel movements were normal. At age 7, he was small for his age; weighed only 48 pounds; and was alert, cooperative, intelligent, in excellent health, and asymptomatic. A barium meal x-ray examination demonstrated that the gastroenterostomy functioned satisfactorily. Fortunately, mongolism was not present.

Jona and Belin (1976) pointed out that the descending portion of the duodenum, at the confluence of the biliary and pancreatic ducts, is a site of major embryonic developments. Serious congenital defects in this region are commonly manifested by partial or complete obstruction of the duodenum. Because of the intimate relationships between the termination of the pancreatic and the common bile ducts with these duodenal anomalies, extensive dissection and exposure of these structures at the time of repair should be avoided. However, precise identification of the ampulla of Vater and the terminal part of the common bile duct is important to prevent surgical damage to these vital structures. They reported six patients with duodenal anomalies that demonstrated this close relationship (Fig. 5–25).

The first patient was a premature boy with duodenal atresia and bifid common bile ducts (Fig. 5–25A). This was treated successfully by surgery in two stages. A gastrostomy for decompression and jejunostomy for feeding were the first stage. Four months later the second stage comprised a duodenoduodenostomy with minimal mobilization of the duodenum to prevent injury to the aberrant ducts. Partial nonrotation of the colon was also found and corrected.

The second patient was a full-term newborn boy with a complete duodenal diaphragm and bifid common bile ducts, Ladd's bands, and nonrotation of the proximal part of the intestine (Fig. 5–25B). Operative treatment comprised division of heavy adhesive peritoneal bands that coursed over the duodenum, and duodenoduodenostomy. Bile was noted above and below the web and was attributed to bifid biliary drainage. After restoration of duodenal continuity, the colon was mobilized to the patient's left and fixed in this position. An incidental appendectomy was also performed. Recovery was prompt.

The third patient was a full-term boy with a complete duodenal web and bifid biliary tract. He was 14 days old and cachectic when admitted. After 5 days of intensive preoperative preparation, only a gastrostomy for decompression and a jejunostomy for feeding were performed. Bile was noted on both sides of the atresia.

At 6 weeks of age, reoperation confirmed the presence of a complete diaphragmatic obstruction of the second part of the duodenum and associated bifid common bile ducts (Fig. 5–25C). A side-to-side duodenoduodenostomy was performed, with care taken not to injure the adjacent biliary channels. He appeared to be normal in size and development at 3 years of age.

The fourth patient was an 8-month-old girl with a fenestrated duodenal diaphragm and insertion of the ampulla of Vater on the diaphragm (Fig. 5–25D). At operation, the diaphragm with its eccentric aperture was exposed through a longitudinal duodenotomy. The ampulla of Vater, situated on the medial aspect of the aperture, was easily identified and cannulated. The diaphragm was partially excised, preserving its medial wall, and the duodenotomy was closed transversely. Her postoperative recovery was uneventful.

The fifth patient was a 30-month-old girl with a fenestrated duodenal diaphragm (Fig. 5–25D). The central portion of the diaphragm was elongated and prolapsed distally, simulating

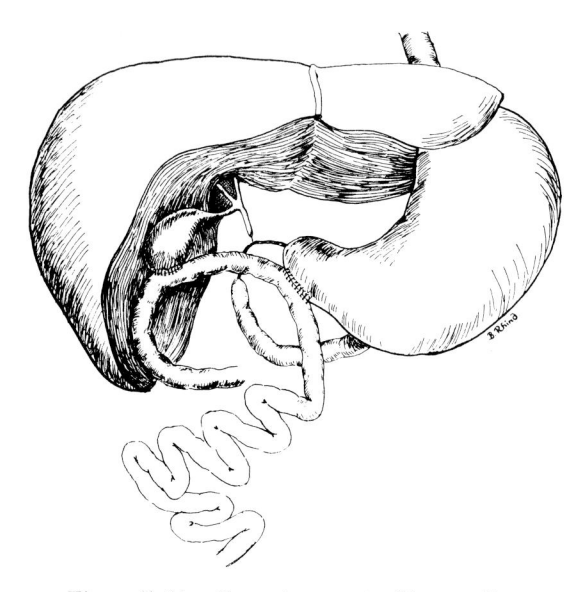

Figure 5–24. Operative repair of lesion illustrated in Figure 5–23. This consisted of cholecystojejunostomy and gastrojejunostomy. (From MacKenzie, et al., cited in previous figure.)

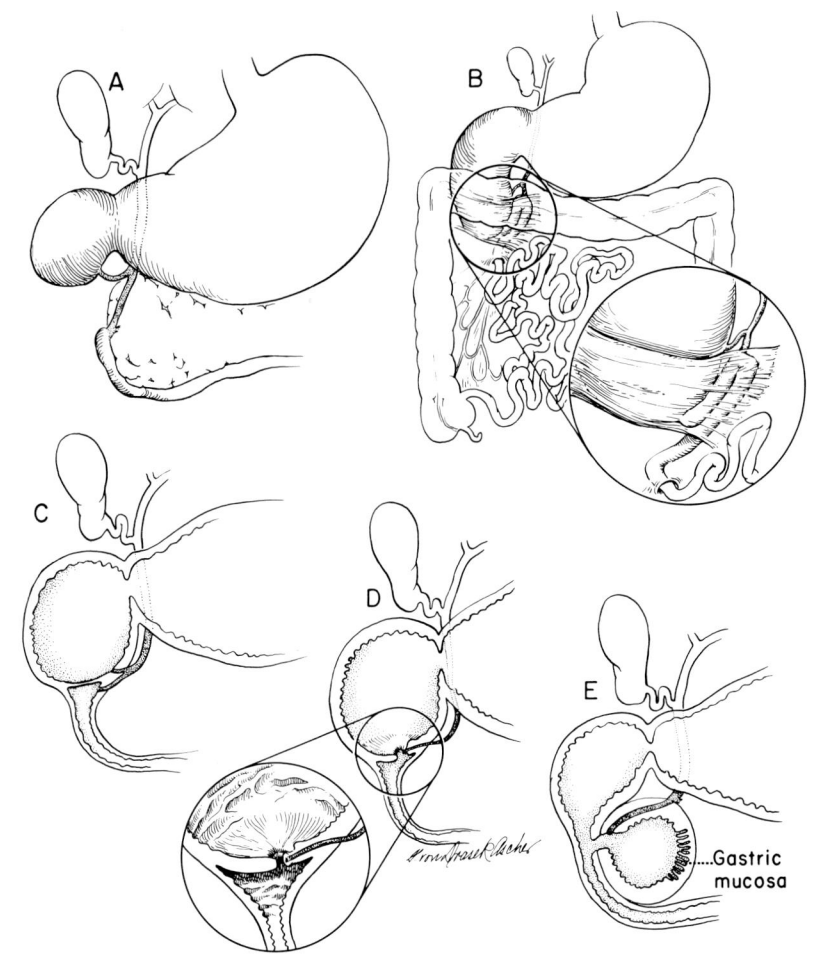

Figure 5–25. Composite of duodenal and biliary anomalies. *A*, Patient 1. Duodenal atresia with bifid biliary ducts. *B*, Patient 2. Duodenal atresia with bifid biliary duct, Ladd's bands, and malrotation of the proximal midgut. *C*, Patient 3. Complete duodenal diaphragm with bifid biliary ducts. *D*, Patients 4 and 5. Duodenal diaphragm with ampulla of Vater inserting on its medial wall. *E*, Patient 6. Duplication cyst of the duodenum with incorporation of the terminal portion of the common bile ducts into the superior wall of the cyst. (From Jona, J. Z., and Belin, R. P.: Duodenal anomalies and the ampulla of Vater. Surg. Gynecol. Obstet. *143*:566, 1976.)

Figure 5–26. *A*, The surgical findings. The bulk of the diaphragm prolapsed distally, simulating a diverticulum with food particles entrapped in it. Note the eccentric, medial aperture in the diaphragm. *B*, Proximal longitudinal duodenotomy was performed, through which the contents were evacuated. The diaphragm was then everted with the aid of an inflated Foley catheter. *C*, The ampulla of Vater inserted on the medial wall of the diaphragm was easily cannulated. To preserve the ampulla, subtotal resection of the diaphragm — dotted line — was performed. (From Jona and Belin, cited in previous figure.)

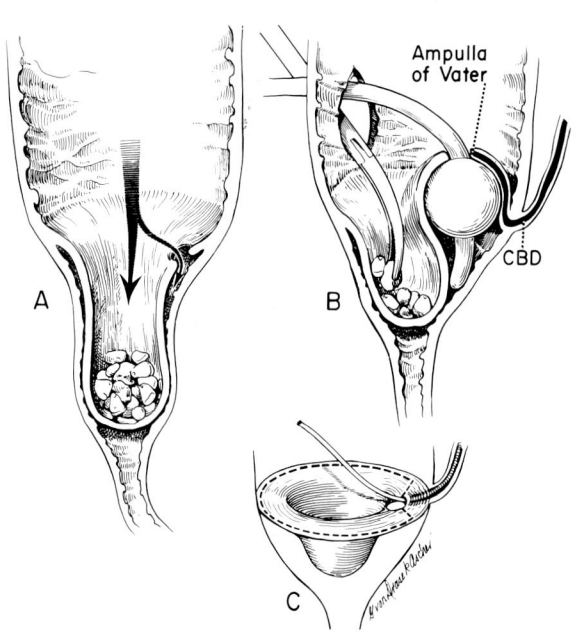

an intraluminal diverticulum. At operation a proximal duodenotomy was made, and food particles were removed from the distally pouching diaphragm (Fig. 5–26). With an inflated Foley catheter, the diaphragm was everted toward the duodenotomy. On the medial wall of the diaphragmatic aperture, the ampulla of Vater could easily be identified. The diaphragm was resected, preserving its medial portion which contained the terminal common bile ducts. The postoperative course was smooth and the patient has remained totally asymptomatic.

The sixth patient was an 8-year old boy who had a duodenal duplication cyst, with the distal part of the common bile ducts incorporated into the wall of the cyst. Exploratory laparotomy was performed. Duodenotomy revealed a golfball-sized mass pressing on the medial wall of the duodenum. Bile was exiting through a small opening at the cephalad portion of this mass. The common wall between the cyst and the duodenum was incised, revealing gastric mucosa lining the interior of the cyst. The ampulla was located at the junction of the wall of the cyst with the duodenum and was easily cannulated with a soft catheter. This demonstrated the intramural course of the common bile ducts within the superior wall of duplication cyst (Fig. 5–25E) for a distance of more than 2 cm. Care was taken not to injure the ductal system while marsupializing the cyst into the main lumen of the duodenum. The patient's recovery was uneventful and no gastrointestinal disturbances occurred in the subsequent 6 years.

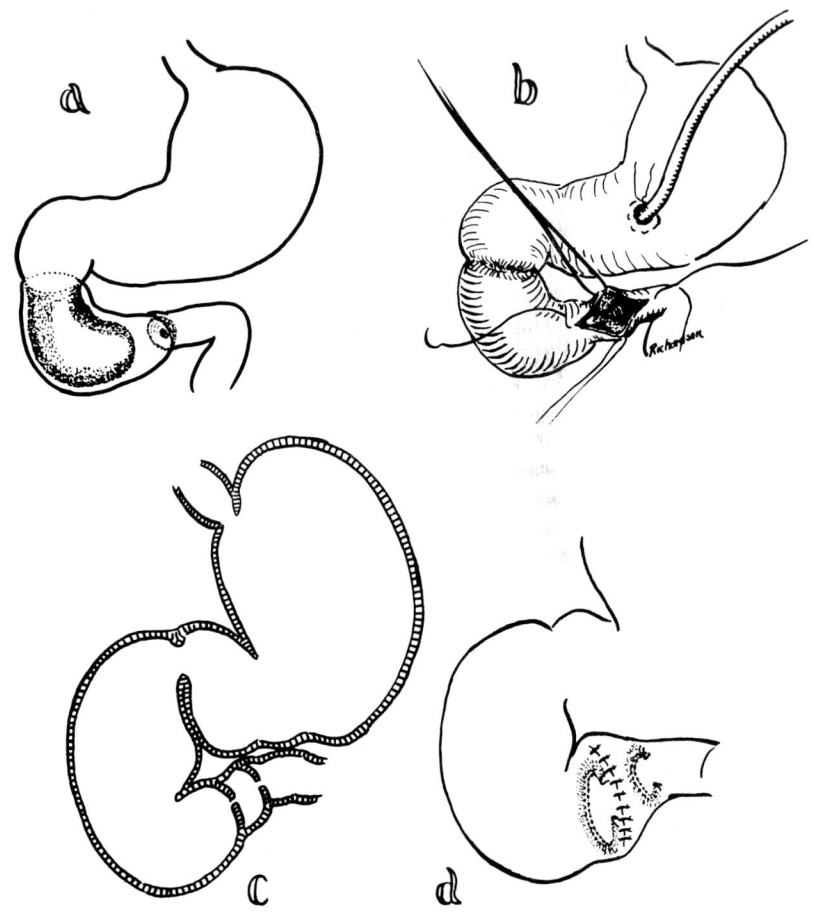

Figure 5–27. Some features of two patients encountered with double diaphragms. *A*, Proximal septum was prolapsing and had an eccentric aperture, but the external constriction shown here was not present. Distal septum was at the sudden caliber change in the fourth portion of the duodenum after complete mobilization of the duodenum and division of the ligament of Treitz. *B*, Longitudinal duodenotomy at the taper allowed the septum to be divided through its central aperture. Transverse closure allowed proximal duodenal content to be milked through easily, but continued obstruction, both clinically and radiologically, led to re-exploration and successful excision of the elongated upper septum. *C* and *D* indicate the nature of the other double diaphragm in the series. The cross-section shows two septa with small, central perforations, separated by about 2 cm. of the distal second part of the duodenum into which the common bile duct was found to drain. After both were subtotally excised through the single duodenotomy, transverse closure provided an ample lumen. (From Richardson, W. R., and Martin, L. W.: Pitfalls in the surgical management of the incomplete duodenal diaphragm. J. Pediatr. Surg. *4*:306, 1969.)

Jona and Belin also pointed out that inadvertent surgical injuries to the major ductal systems are possible when operating on patients with congenital anomalies of the duodenum. Cholangiography may demonstrate intrinsic biliary malformations, and surgical exploration may reveal them; however, both of these technics are difficult and hazardous in infants. When encountering a duodenal diaphragm, they advised an intense search to identify and preserve the ampulla of Vater, which is frequently found on the medial aspect of the diaphragmatic aperture. Partial excision of the diaphragm should spare the segment that contains the terminal part of the common bile ducts.

Resection of the blind ends of atretic duodenum, as is done in jejunoileal atresia, is inadvisable, partly because of the risk of transecting the common bile ducts. When air, bile, or barium is noted distal to an atresia in the duodenum, bifid biliary drainage is likely to be present, and great care should be exercised during the mobilization and the construction of the duodenal anastomosis. Excision of duodenal duplication cysts is hazardous because of their tendency to be located within the head of the pancreas. It is preferable to marsupialize the common wall between the duodenum and the adjacent cyst. The ampulla of Vater should be carefully identified prior to excision of the common wall so as to avoid serious injury to the common bile ducts.

Richardson and Martin (1969) reported two patients with double diaphragm who were treated successfully by duodenotomy and excision of the diaphragm, as shown in Figure 5–27.

CONGENITAL DUODENAL STENOSIS

Congenital stenosis occurs more commonly in the duodenum than elsewhere in the gastrointestinal tract; about 50 per cent of stenoses are found here (MacKenzie and associates, 1960). The stenosis may be in one of three types suggested by Walker, Dewar, and Stephen (1958) (Fig. 5–28): Type A in which the duodenal lumen is obstructed by a perforated diaphragm, Type B in which the obstruction is by mural stenosis, and Type C in which obstruction is by a possible combined form. In the literature, Type A is the most common lesion.

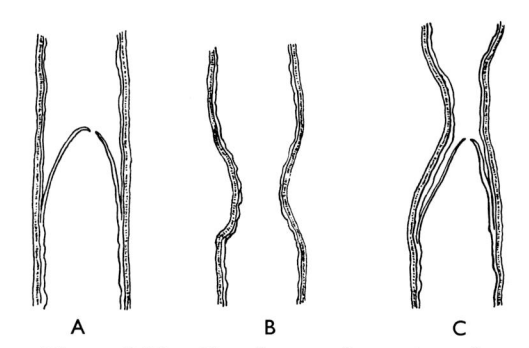

Figure 5–28. Classification of type. *A*, Perforated septum. *B*, Mural stenosis. *C*, Possible combined form. (From Walker, W. F., Dewar, D. A. E., and Stephen, S. A.: Congenital intrinsic duodenal stenosis presenting after infancy. Br. J. Surg. 46:30, 1958.)

Congenital duodenal stenosis closely resembles congenital duodenal atresia embryologically and pathologically but differs somewhat in its symptoms, methods of treatment, and prognosis. The frequent association with maternal hydramnios and other anomalies is similar to that of atresia. See Congenital Duodenal Atresia, page 128.

Pathology

Congenital stenosis may occur at any level of the intestinal tract from the pylorus to the rectum (Fig. 5–29) but is found most commonly in the duodenum. The present discussion is limited to duodenal stenosis; stenoses in other parts of the intestine are discussed in the chapter on the small intestine.

The duodenal lumen at the narrowed zone is of variable size (2 mm. to almost the full diameter of the duodenum). Examined microscopically, the narrowed zone shows heaped-up mucosa supported by smooth muscle and connective tissue. *The portion of duodenum proximal to the obstruction is always dilated* and the pylorus may be patulous. Although the distention in some of these patients may be great, it is not as tense as may occur in atresia; while perforation is less likely, it can occur. Also in contrast with atresia, more than one site of stenosis is rare, though two patients in Richardson's and Martin's series (1969) had two separate duodenal diaphragms.

The degree of collapse of the intestine distal to the stenosis varies with the degree of obstruction caused by the stenosis.

STENOSES

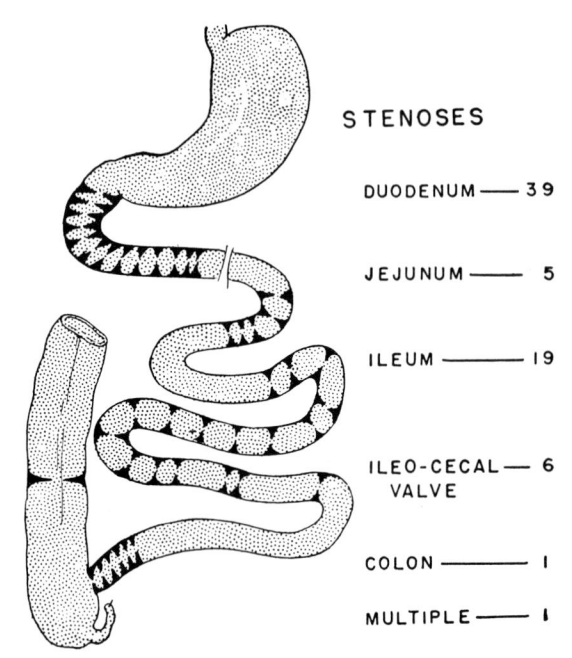

DUODENUM —— 39
JEJUNUM —— 5
ILEUM —— 19
ILEO-CECAL —— 6
VALVE
COLON —— 1
MULTIPLE —— 1

Figure 5–29. Positions of stenoses of intestinal tract in 71 patients. (From Gross, R. E.: Surgery of Infancy and Childhood. Philadelphia, W. B. Saunders, 1953.)

Symptoms and Diagnosis

These vary according to the degree of obstruction. Early, severe cases are difficult or impossible to distinguish from cases of intestinal atresia because they exhibit the signs of obstruction during the first week of life.

The most important symptom is *persistent vomiting.* If the vomitus does not contain bile (absence of green color), the stenosis is probably proximal to the ampulla of Vater, which is uncommon. In most cases the vomitus is green (indicating presence of bile), and the stenosis is distal to the ampulla. There is little or no abdominal distention.

Loss of weight or failure to gain weight usually occurs. *The stools are usually diminished in size and number.* The finding of milk curds or cornified epithelial cells in the stools is positive evidence that the obstruction is incomplete.

In the usual case of stenosis in the neonate, the symptoms increase gradually to the point at which it is impossible to differentiate it from complete atresia except by the history.

In a significant number of cases the symptoms are so mild that the patient is not brought to a surgeon until later in life. Lynn (1969) reported a child who had a relatively severe stenosis but went untreated until 13 months of age because she had a reasonable weight gain. Another child was 5 years old before the symptoms seemed to warrant consultation with a surgeon. Hase, Shaw, and Gould (1967) reported a 13-year-old girl with a congenital duodenal stenosis causing enormous dilatation and hypertrophy of the first portion of the duodenum, and coexisting pneumoperitoneum, without peritonitis. At operation no perforation could be found. A retrocolic, side-to-side, isoperistaltic duodenojejunostomy and a tube gastrostomy for decompression were performed. Her postoperative course was stormy, but 18 months after operation she had gained 20 pounds, had grown 5 inches, and was asymptomatic.

Richardson and Martin (1969) reported that "the hugely dilated proximal duodenum in a 3-year-old child mimicked pneumoperitoneum, and another child's roentgenograms demonstrated gastric intramural gas without gangrene or perforation."

A number of patients have been reported with congenital duodenal stenosis who did not require surgical treatment until they reached adulthood — some not until they were in their sixties or seventies!

In patients with suspected congenital stenosis, an x-ray plate of the abdomen should be taken in the upright position without the use of contrast media. If the obstruction is severe, the film will usually show the stomach filled with gas and the duodenum dilated. Such a finding, with the history and physical findings, eliminates the necessity for further x-ray examination, and the patient should be prepared for prompt operation.

If the x-ray findings by this method are inconclusive in demonstrating an obstruction, then a thin barium mixture can be introduced into the stomach and another x-ray study made. In very young, acutely ill babies this procedure entails some risk, but in older children and adults with milder symptoms it is relatively safe. Such a study in congenital duodenal stenosis will usually demonstrate a dilatation of the duodenum, abruptly ending at the point of obstruction, and a small amount of barium that has passed into the intestine beyond the point of obstruction. After completing this x-ray study, it is advisable to remove the barium by gastric lavage and suction through a tube inserted into the stomach before proceeding with the operation.

Treatment

Congenital duodenal stenosis is treated by prompt operation. Even if the obstruction is only partial there is little point in delaying operation, as the child will not gain normally and, indeed, will probably lose ground, so that operation at a later date will be required under less favorable circumstances. Once the diagnosis is made or considered most likely, operation is delayed only until the patient can be prepared.

Preoperative Care

This is similar to that described for congenital atresia (p. 133). Fluid and electrolyte balance are restored by parenteral administration. The stomach and duodenum are decompressed by suction through a nasogastric tube, as this facilitates the operative procedures and lessens the chances of vomiting and aspiration. It is advisable to leave this tube in the stomach during the operation and for use in the postoperative period for gastric decompression.

Surgical Treatment

General inhalation anesthesia is preferred, as described for atresia (p. 133). Also see Surgical Technic for atresia.

If the stenosis is in the duodenum proximal to the ampulla of Vater (which is rare), an antecolic gastrojejunostomy (Fig. 5–30) should be performed (see page 344).

If the stenosis is situated in the duodenum distal to the ampulla or is located in the upper jejunum, a side-to-side duodenojejunostomy is usually the procedure of choice. This can be done easily by holding the transverse colon and mesocolon up, making an opening in the mesocolon to expose the underlying distended duodenum, and then performing a retrocolic, side-to-side, two-layer anastomosis of the lowest point of the distended duodenum to the highest point of jejunum that is below obstruction and permits placement without kinking or angulation (Fig. 5–31). In some cases it may be technically more feasible to

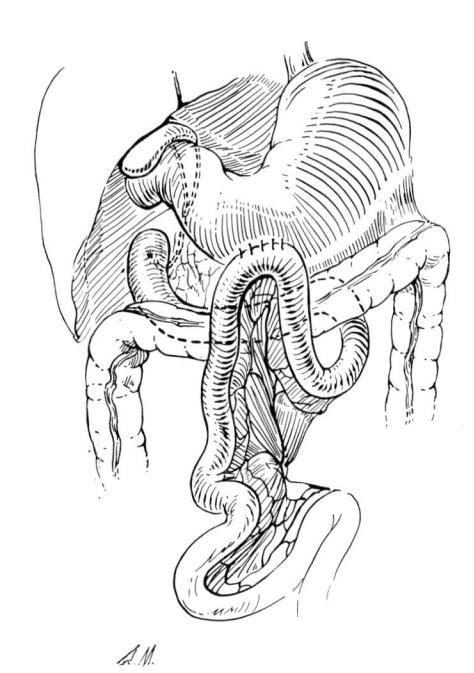

Figure 5–30. An antecolic anastomosis, which is the preferred procedure for alleviating obstruction caused by atresia in the first portion of the duodenum. (From Benson, C. D., and Lloyd, J. R.: Duodenal obstruction of congenital origin. Am. J. Surg. 101:610, 1961.)

perform an antecolic duodenojejunostomy (Fig. 5–32).

When these procedures are used, the lengths of bowel apposed should be sufficient to permit forming an anastomotic stoma at least 3 cm. long. The anastomosis may be made either isoperistaltic or antiperistaltic, although the former is usually preferred. The technic of forming an anastomosis in congenital stenosis is similar to but easier than that in atresia because, although the distal segment is somewhat collapsed, it is always larger than is the distal segment in atresia. A two-layer suture line anastomosis should be performed as described in detail for atresia on page 136. The outer layer is made with No. 5-0 atraumatic silk suture, which may be interrupted, or with a continuous Lembert or Cushing suture. The inner layer is made with No. 5-0 atraumatic continuous catgut suture placed as an over-and-over stitch on the posterior wall and continued as a Connell stitch on the anterior wall.

When the duodenojejunostomy is retrocolic, following completion of the anastomosis, the margins of the opening in the mesocolon are sutured to the duodenum to prevent the weight of the colon from pulling

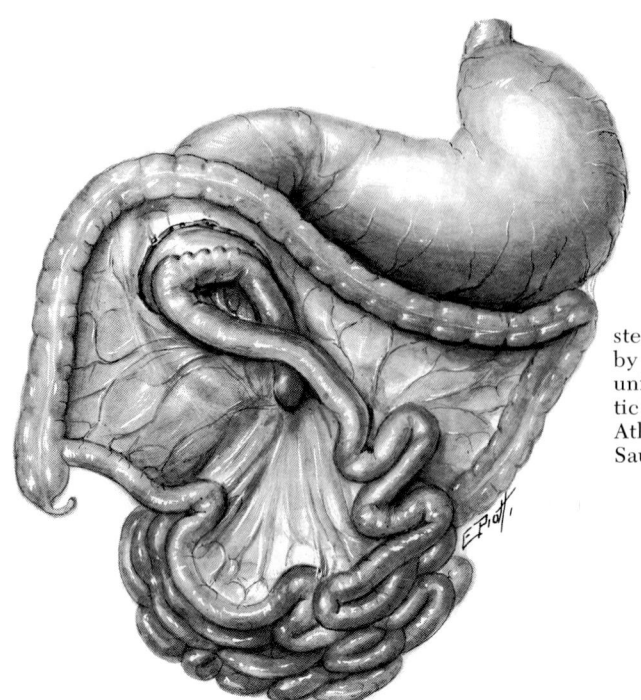

Figure 5-31. Preferred method in treatment of stenosis of the *second or third part of the duodenum* by retrocolic duodenojejunostomy. Antiperistaltic unions have given as satisfactory results as isoperistaltic anastomoses. (Illustration from Gross, R. E.: An Atlas of Children's Surgery. Philadelphia, W. B. Saunders Company, 1970, p. 15.)

down the mesocolon and producing a jejunal spur or angulation which might cause obstruction.

When operation has been completed, the abdominal incision is closed with nonabsorbable sutures, gastric decompression is provided, and postoperative care is the same as that described for atresia.

CONGENITAL INTRINSIC DUODENAL STENOSIS PRESENTING AFTER INFANCY

As mentioned, some neonates with congenital duodenal stenosis have symptoms so mild that no surgery is required until childhood or even adulthood. Congenital duodenal diaphragm in the adult is rare. Smiley, Perry, and McClelland, in 1967, reported a 60-year-old woman with this condition and could find only 20 such cases recorded in the literature. Of the 17 patients whose sex was recorded, 9 were men and 8 were women. The distribution of the 18 for whom age was reported was:

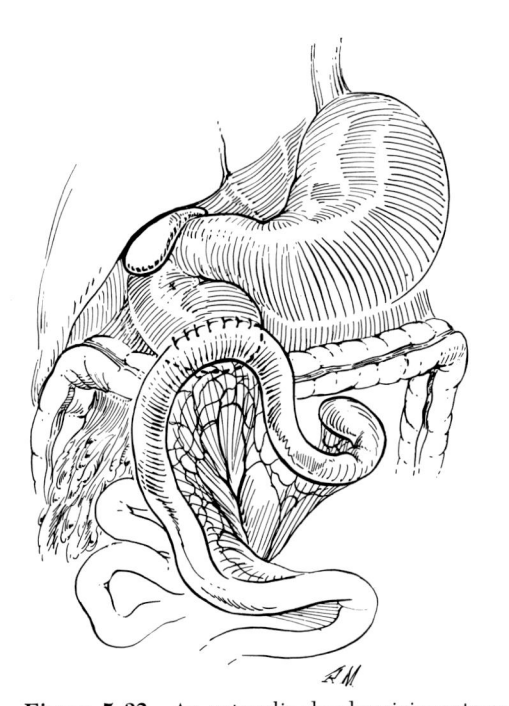

Figure 5-32. An antecolic duodenojejunostomy. (From Benson, C. D., and Lloyd, J. R.: Duodenal obstruction of congenital origin. Am. J. Surg. *101*:610, 1961.)

5 to 9	2
10 to 19	0
20 to 29	3
30 to 39	3
40 to 49	3
50 to 59	0
60 to 69	5
70 to 76	2

"It has been stated that 29 per cent of congenital duodenal diaphragms become symptomatic after age 24 and that this incomplete septum may account for 0.8 to 25 per cent of all duodenal obstructions" (Kreig, 1937).

"The symptoms of congenital duodenal web in children and adults are postprandial fullness, cramping, nausea, and vomiting. These complaints often develop slowly and insidiously in the early adult years" (Smiley, Perry, and McClelland, 1967). The rapidity of development depends upon the size of the opening in the web.

There may be weight loss or the patient may be obese; mild upper right quadrant abdominal tenderness is often the only abdominal finding. Laboratory tests are usually normal except for an occasional result indicating a patient with hypochloremic alkalosis secondary to recurrent vomiting.

The rare occurrence and the nonspecific clinical manifestations of this disorder in adults make its diagnosis difficult. The most characteristic finding is a very large, dilated proximal duodenum seen on barium swallow x-ray studies. The difficulty in establishing a preoperative diagnosis, even by roentgenograms, is demonstrated by the fact that in Smiley's collected series of patients only 2 of the 13 operated upon were diagnosed before operation.

Walker, Dewar, and Stephen (1958) reported a 45-year-old male in whom duodenohepatic reflux was visualized at preoperative barium meal x-ray examination. A retrocolic gastrojejunostomy relieved the duodenal obstruction, but reflux of barium and air into the biliary tract persisted without causing symptoms during the 2 years of follow-up.

Surgical Treatment

Surgical treatment for congenital duodenal stenosis in the adult is quite different from that in the infant.

Threadgill and Hagelstein (1961) pointed out that in the infant the obstruction is recent and acute. Dilatation and fibrosis of the duodenum have not become irreversible, so it is capable of emptying when obstruction is relieved. Hence duodenojejunostomy that bypasses the obstructing diaphragm works well and is the treatment of choice. In the adult the obstruction is long-standing and is associated with proximal dilatation and hypertrophy of the duodenum, which will persist and remain symptomatic if the obstruction is only bypassed. In addition, pylorospasm, pyloric stenosis, or a patulous pylorus is present; also, there may be associated peptic ulcer and duodenal pseudodiverticula.

Although successes have been reported with the use of duodenojejunostomy for treating adults with congenital duodenal stenosis, the overall results have been disappointing. Usually the duodenum has not decreased in size postoperatively, and frequently subsequent operations have been necessary. Threadgill believes that "the poor results obtained from duodenojejunostomy in adults are due to the failure of this operation to occlude the duodenum and relieve the continuing stress of the dietary stream on the dilated and diseased or paralyzed duodenum and pylorus. To effect permanent relief, the pylorus as well as the dilated duodenum and the duodenal diaphragm or other obstructive cause should be bypassed by a Billroth II operation or similar operative procedure. Obviously, prior to beginning a formal subtotal gastrectomy it will be necessary to explore the duodenum in these adult cases to make an exact diagnosis and to remove any detritus such as the pebbles and buttons found in my second case."

In support of this view he reported on two men, 23 and 45 years old, respectively, with congenital duodenal stenosis. Both underwent duodenojejunostomy. Following operation the duodenum remained dilated and the preoperative symptoms persisted in both cases. When the first patient was last seen 1 year after operation his condition was unchanged. The second patient underwent a gastrojejunostomy 2 months after the duodenojejunostomy. Three months after the second operation x-ray examination showed marked duodenal dilatation and a functioning duodenojejunostomy as well as a functioning gastrojejunostomy, but antral and duodenal stasis was evidenced by barium retention and symptoms of obstruction, with intermittent vomiting of large amounts of fluids. Repeat x-ray studies demonstrated a functioning gastroenterostomy with a markedly dilated duodenum that showed a churning effect on fluoroscopy. Reoperation was performed; the stomach distal to the gastrojejunostomy, the pylorus, and the first portion of the duodenum were removed. Recovery was uneventful. The patient suffered no further indigestion or vomiting and gained weight. X-ray films taken 5 months after this operation showed a well-functioning gastrojejunostomy and only a trace of residual barium in the stomach after 3 hours. He felt well and when last seen was eating three solid meals a day.

Gastrojejunostomy to bypass the obstruction has been used successfully for treating congenital duodenal stenosis in adults but has several theoretic disadvantages. "A blind loop may be created in the dilated proximal duodenum, which leads to recurrent abdominal pain and macrocytic anemia. Also, poor mixing of food with pancreatobiliary secretions may lead to steatorrhea and malnutrition. Finally, marginal ulceration and dumping symptoms may occur after gastroenterostomy" (Smiley, Perry, and McClelland, 1967).

DUODENOTOMY AND EXCISION OF THE DIAPHRAGM WITH ADEQUATE POSTOPERATIVE DUODENAL DECOMPRESSION. This procedure has been used frequently for treating congenital duodenal stenosis in older children and adults. It is the most physiologic operation for this purpose since the obstructing septum is completely removed and normal anatomic relationships are restored. Injuries to the biliary and pancreatic ducts are hazards. These can be avoided by identifying the ducts and by carefully inspecting the web and its opening. A duct may open at the exact site of obstruction or just above or below it. At least three cases have been reported in which an unsuspected terminal bile duct was injured during local excision of the web or duodenum. In some cases it may be advisable to insert a polyethylene tube in the ampulla of Vater as a safeguard, because of its proximity to the web.

Another hazard is postoperative leakage at the closed duodenotomy suture line, a complication that can be minimized by careful closure and adequate postoperative decompression.

Six of the 20 reported cases of congenital duodenal stenosis in adults collected by Smiley, Perry, and McClelland (1967) were treated by duodenotomy and excision of the web. There was no mortality. Complications were fewer than in those treated by gastroenterostomy. Furthermore, although the site of the diaphragm is usually indicated by a slight indentation in the duodenal wall, the web cannot be palpated externally and may be missed unless the bowel is opened.

These investigators reported treating an adult patient with congenital duodenal stenosis by this operation, and described their operative technic:

A 60-year-old woman was hospitalized in 1962, complaining of epigastric and right upper quadrant abdominal pain and nausea and vomiting of 40 years' duration. The symptoms had intensified. Cholecystography showed several radiolucent gallstones. Cholecystectomy was performed. Common duct exploration and an operative cholangiogram were negative; contrast medium flowed freely into the duodenum. The duodenum was unusually large but was not explored. Recovery was uneventful. A postoperative T-tube cholangiogram showed no stones, but free flow of dye into the duodenum was never seen. The patient remained asymptomatic and the T-tube was later removed.

In 1963, she complained of recurrent postprandial pain without vomiting. In 1964, postprandial discomfort and abdominal bloating were followed by vomiting. Upper gastrointestinal x-ray studies showed barium retention in what was thought to be a grossly dilated duodenum or duodenal diverticulum, but no obstruction was seen. Her symptoms gradually worsened and were only partially relieved by antacids and by induced vomiting, which often revealed food eaten the previous day.

In 1966, the patient was readmitted with the above complaints. She was obese (166 pounds) and in no distress. The only positive physical findings were a moderately distended abdomen with minimal tenderness in the right upper quadrant. Laboratory findings were all within normal limits. A 12-hour overnight gastric aspirate contained 3.6 mEq. of free HCl, but the presence of partially digested food invalidated this finding. A preoperative diagnosis of duodenal diverticulum was made and laparotomy was performed.

Operative Technic. On entering the abdomen, a greatly dilated duodenum was found. The stomach was slightly enlarged, and the pylorus was wide and patulous. The preoperative diagnosis of duodenal diverticulum was not confirmed, and further exploration showed that the dilation was limited to the first and second portions of the duodenum. A duodenotomy was made and distal obstruction was encountered. Dissection from the ligament of Treitz proximally demonstrated the site of transition from dilated to normal-sized duodenum. There was no indentation or constriction in the wall of the duodenum at the point of transition. Another duodenotomy was made over this area. An incomplete diaphragm about 2 mm.

thick was found, partially obstructing the duodenum. There was an eccentrically placed, 6-mm. opening in the diaphragm. At the medial portion of this opening the ampulla of Vater was identified, and, just proximal and anterior to the ampulla, the pancreatic duct was found.

The web was entirely resected to the region of the entrance of the two ducts. The mucosal edges of the web were oversewn with a continuous 3-0 chromic catgut suture. Both longitudinal duodenotomies were closed transversely. To insure adequate duodenal drainage and decompression, a tube gastrostomy, duodenostomy (with a No. 10 Foley catheter), and retrograde jejunostomy were performed and constant suction was maintained until bowel activity returned.

The postoperative course was uneventful. Abdominal distention with fever occurred on the fourth postoperative day, but there was no abdominal pain or tenderness. The three decompression tubes were reattached to suction and all symptoms quickly disappeared. All decompression tubes were removed by the 12th day, and she ate normally and has continued to do so.

Gastrointestinal x-ray films 14 days postoperatively showed a much smaller duodenum, with no obstruction. Fluoroscopy showed duodenal peristalsis to be sluggish, but functional. The patient has continued to be asymptomatic.

The surgeons commented that "the extensive gastrointestinal decompression used in this case may be questioned but the decompensated, thin-walled duodenum in these patients would be especially prone to leak if duodenal distention occurred even briefly. Also, the prolonged *complete* decompression and delay in alimentation allows time for more adequate reestablishment of muscle tone in the thin-walled proximal duodenum with perhaps better expectation of good duodenal peristaltic activity and normal gastric emptying.... Such gastroduodenal decompression may provide additional safeguard against duodenal malfunction following excision of the web, as well as against duodenal leak." They recommended this method for surgically treating an incomplete congenital duodenal diaphragm in an adult patient.

MEGADUODENUM

As suggested by Melchior (1924), this term is reserved for those cases of functional duodenal obstruction without mechanical obstruction of the lumen. The causes may be functional — dilatation associated with ulcer, syphilis, duodenal ileus, idiopathic, Chagas' disease due to infestation by *Trypanosoma cruzi* which produces a neurotoxin that damages the ganglion cells of the duodenal myenteric plexus — or congenital, due to congenital absence of myenteric ganglion cells of the duodenum or duodenal musculature.

The congenital types will be discussed here.

CONGENITAL AGANGLIONIC MEGADUODENUM

Congenital absence of myenteric ganglion cells of the duodenum is uncommonly the cause of megaduodenum, and proof of aganglionosis has seldom been obtained.

In 1955, Barnett and Wall reported a proven case of their own and collected from the world literature 35 cases of aganglionosis of the duodenal myenteric plexus with megaduodenum. Thirty-two of these cases were reported in sufficient detail to permit analysis. The average age in 31 patients was 40 years, with a range from 5 to 74 years. An additional case was reported in a stillborn infant. Seventeen were men, 13 were women, and the sex was not given in two patients.

Several investigators have called attention to the fact that many cases of congenital megaduodenum have been misdiagnosed and reported as examples of superior mesenteric ileus. This is not surprising since congenital megaduodenum often terminates abruptly just proximal to the crossing of the superior mesenteric vessels. Nine cases of megaduodenum have been reported in which the dilatation extended to involve the proximal portion of the jejunum.

A number of investigators have been impressed by the similarity between aganglionic megaduodenum and the megacolon that is associated with Hirschsprung's disease. The two conditions have occurred in the same patient in at least four reported cases. Also, megacystis is often associated with both of these disorders.

In 1924, Melchior suggested that megaduodenum was a congenital, neurogenic abnormality. Its hereditary nature has been documented by Weiss (1938), who described megaduodenum alone in six members of three generations of a German family, and later by Law and Ten Eyck (1962), who reported the association of megaduodenum and megacystis in nine members of an Italian family. Newton (1968) reported two Negro brothers with megaduodenum.

"Megaduodenum is most commonly seen in children. Most adults with the condition relate their symptoms back to childhood. The functional status has been likened to that in heart disease, namely, a compensated and a decompensated stage. With a normal work load the duodenal musculature is able to hypertrophy and maintain a state of compensation, but with age and dietary indiscretion a decompensated state is reached, with resulting dilatation and failure. This would explain the appearance of megaduodenum in later years of life" (Barnett and Wall, 1955).

Pathology

Functional obstruction, produced by the aganglionic segment of bowel, increases the workload of the proximal duodenum. This causes marked hypertrophy of the muscle layer, thus thickening the bowel wall. Dilatation and elongation appear with the increasing inability to overcome the obstruction. Inflammation due to stasis causes periduodenal adhesions and enlarged lymph nodes. Ulceration is prone to occur in this dilated, stagnant bowel, which explains the common complaints of melena and hematemesis. Diverticula occasionally result from the increased intraluminal pressure. Microscopically, diminution of ganglion cells, profusion of neural sheath cells, thickened layers of bowel wall, and infiltration by inflammatory cells are seen.

Symptoms and Signs

The symptoms and physical findings were described in 31 of the reported cases of congenital aganglionic megaduodenum collected by Barnett and Wall. The symptoms and the number of patients in whom each occurred were listed as follows: epigastric pain (23 patients), right upper quadrant pain (3), nausea (10), vomiting (21), weight loss (15), belching (6), anorexia (5), melena (5), and hematemesis (3).

The physical signs were epigastric tenderness (8 patients), right upper quadrant tenderness (2), epigastric distention (4), right upper quadrant mass (1) and negative physical examination (19).

Diagnosis

The most common symptoms are epigastric discomfort, nausea, vomiting, and weight loss, which are also frequently associated with other upper gastrointestinal tract lesions much more common than megaduodenum. Physical signs are often absent or not diagnostically suggestive when present. The diagnosis is usually first suspected following radiologic examination by a plain flat x-ray film of the abdomen followed by a barium enema x-ray study to rule out malrotation, and an upper gastrointestinal x-ray series.

"The enlarged, dilated, elongated, coiled duodenum presents an unmistakable and striking finding on radiologic examination. Hyperperistalsis and reverse peristalsis are frequently seen. The absence of demonstrable intraluminal masses by radiologic examination is in favor of the diagnosis of megaduodenum" (Barnett and Wall, 1955). However, the diagnosis cannot be established until exploratory laparotomy has confirmed the absence of mechanical obstruction, and biopsy of a portion of the duodenal wall has determined the status of its myenteric plexuses.

Treatment

Medical methods used have included ptosis belts, the knee-chest position, sleeping with head of the bed elevated, and abdominal exercises. The end results of such treatment are uniformly poor, according to Barnett and Wall (1955).

Surgical Methods

A great majority of patients with congenital megaduodenum require surgical intervention. The primary purpose of the operation is to decompress mechanically the functionally obstructed bowel.

Many operative procedures have been used for treating congenital megaduodenum. The series of 31 patients with this disorder collected by Barnett and Wall (1955) had the following operations: duodenojejunostomy was the primary surgical procedure in ten patients and a secondary procedure in two cases — one following gastrectomy and one following gastroenterostomy. One of the 12 patients died from pulmonary embolism, and in one the duodenojejunal stoma became obstructed. The others were reported to have had good results, with subsidence of symptoms and rapid weight gain. Gastrectomy was the primary treatment in 11 cases, with one death (jejunal volvulus), and one required reoperation because of persistent vomiting. Enteroenterostomy was used in addition to gastrectomy in 4 of these 11 cases. Four patients were treated by gastroenterostomy, with two requiring reoperation because of persistent symptoms: two were treated by exclusion operations, and four had only exploratory laparotomy.

Analysis of these surgical procedures showed that only after duodenojejunostomy is the dilated duodenum adequately drained. Because the stoma is located between the dilated segment and the first portion of the jejunum, this segment can be evacuated into the jejunum, while in all the other methods it continues to be necessary for the failing duodenal musculature to propel the voluminous biliary, pancreatic, and duodenal secretions along the original route. Gastroenterostomy is a notoriously poor method for dealing with megaduodenum. Antral exclusion is undesirable because it is ulcerogenic. The results of gastrectomy have been acceptable, but it is of much greater magnitude than duodenojejunostomy with no better result, so the latter seems to be preferable.

The patient reported by Barnett and Wall (1955) was a 30-year-old housewife with a history of frequent vomiting since birth. She had been a premature baby. The family history was negative, except for one brother who complained of symptoms compatible with duodenal ulcer. One hour before admission to the hospital she vomited a quart of blood. On admission she was in hypovolemic shock and required transfusion. Barium enema x-ray study was negative. Upper gastrointestinal x-ray examination showed the duodenum to be markedly dilated from its cap down to the middle of its third portion, where the dilation stopped abruptly. The 4-hour film showed most of the barium still in the duodenum and a small amount in the small intestine.

Laparotomy was performed through an upper right rectus incision. There was no mechanical obstruction. An inframesocolic duodenojejunostomy (Fig. 5–33) was performed. The duodenum, the jejunum, and a lymph node were biopsied. The pathologic report was "normal lymph node; normal jejunum with normal myenteric plexus; duodenum shows hypertrophy of its muscular wall and replacement of its myenteric plexus by neural sheath cells, compatible with the diagnosis of megaduodenum."

The patient's recovery from operation was uneventful and she was discharged from the hospital on her eighth postoperative day. Five days later she was readmitted because of abdominal swelling and vomiting. In-hospital treatment was by Levin tube drainage, no oral intake, and intravenous fluids for one week, then a liquid diet gradually increasing to normal diet. She returned to her home 18 days after this admission. She gained 19 pounds in 4 months. Seven months later x-ray films showed the duodenum still dilated, the anastomosis functioning, and only a small amount of duodenal and gastric retention. In September, 1976, 24 years after her operation, Wall (1976) informed us that the patient was then 54 years old and in excellent health with no gastrointestinal complaints.

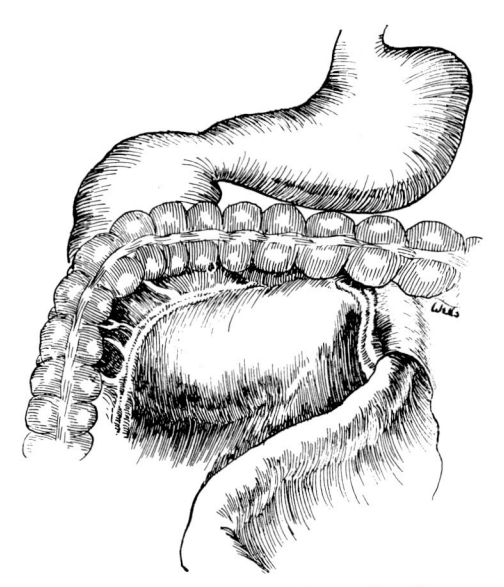

Figure 5–33. Dilated duodenum found at operation. (From Barnett, W. O., and Wall, L.: Megaduodenum resulting from absence of the parasympathetic ganglion cells in Auerbach's plexus. Ann. Surg. *141*:529, 1955.)

In 1965, when their report was published, Barnett and Wall concluded, on the basis of their experience with this patient and their review of the literature, that duodenojejunostomy is the procedure of choice for treating congenital megaduodenum. Subsequent experiences of Handelsman and associates (1965) and of Newton (1968) indicate that this is not true in all cases of congenital megaduodenum.

MEGADUODENUM DUE TO CONGENITAL ABSENCE OF DUODENAL MUSCULATURE

This anomaly is a rare cause of neonatal intrinsic duodenal obstruction. The literature discloses (1) A newborn infant with intestinal obstruction due to absence of the musculature in five separate segments of the intestine (Emanuel, Gault, and Sanson, 1967); (2) 34 cases of gastric perforation in neonates with gastric musculature deficits (Inouye and Evans, 1963); and (3) sporadic reports of intestinal perforation in neonates with comparable anomalies (Bender, 1964). In all these cases, except the first, the area of muscular absence has been sharply circumscribed and small. In some cases multiple absences have been reported.

Handelsman and associates (1965) reported the only patient, to our knowledge, in whom congenital absence of the intestinal musculature involved only the duodenum. Obstruction was the presenting symptom. The child required multiple operations, and ultimately was left with a stomach essentially anastomosed to the jejunum which passed inferiorly, with a flap of duodenum permitting entrance of bile and pancreatic secretions into this newly created juncture. Apparently the procedure was successful. Her recovery was slow and it was necessary for her to be in the semi-erect position for feeding. When discharged from the hospital at 6 weeks of age she was feeding well and gaining weight. At 2 months of age a gastrointestinal x-ray study demonstrated an adequate lumen and satisfactory continuity. Her weight and height were well within normal limits for her age. In September, 1976, Handelsman reported that the child was 11 years old, had never had any further trouble, and was a healthy, normal child for her age.

These surgeons were unable to explain the lesion precisely on an embryologic basis but pointed out that in this case the absence of scarring, perfect approximation of mucosa to the serosal layer, concurrent abnormal vascularization of the segment, and failure to demonstrate thrombosis or other destructive mechanical influences in this segment indicated that this was a congenital rather than an acquired aberration.

They also commented that functionally the lesion caused mechanical intestinal obstruction, which was not relieved by a bypass procedure because the muscular segment was unable to propel its contents onward, hence there was an ever-present threat of distention with perforation and disaster. Apparently "only resection provides a means of coping with the difficulty. In the case reported, resection of the duodenum was accomplished economically by preserving that minimal portion necessary to spare the patient extensive surgery in order to transplant the ductal system."

HEREDITARY MEGADUODENUM WITHOUT ANATOMIC EXPLANATION

In 1968, Newton reported two American Negro brothers who were afflicted with congenital megaduodenum and in whom no anatomic defect was found to explain the atonic duodenum.

The father of the two brothers had a gastric operation in his third decade, for persistent abdominal pain, but the hospital records have been destroyed. The mother, a sister, another brother, and five children are asymptomatic. The status of deceased relatives is unknown.

Both brothers, in contrast to their relatives, were tall and thin, with long, tapered fingers but no other stigmata of Marfan's syndrome. Both brothers had intermittent bilateral parotid swelling before their operations, as described in some patients with intestinal atrophy due to Chagas' disease, but their sera were inactive in a hemagglutination inhibition test and a complement-fixation test for Chagas' disease. Newton pointed out that "although the family history is not as clear-cut as in the families described by Weiss [1938] and by Law and Ten Eyck [1962], it seems reasonable that the atonic megaduodenum in these brothers is another example of a hereditary defect. The defect is distinct from congenital aganglionosis... and Chagas' disease, in that no microscopic abnormality of the myenteric plexus has been demonstrated." It also differs from congenital absence of the duodenal musculature described earlier by Handelsman and colleagues (1965).

Newton reported his two patients as follows:

A 31-year-old man was admitted for the third time to a veterans hospital in June, 1961, complaining of vomiting blood. Because of repeated episodes of vomiting, he had had an operation at age 11. A distended duodenum was found and the jejunum was mobilized at the ligament of Treitz. Intermittent episodes of vomiting continued throughout his adolescence. Late in adolescence he noted that suprapubic hand pressure was necessary to empty his urinary bladder. He was discharged from the Army after gastrointestinal x-ray studies showed "obstruction of the duodenum." At age 23 he underwent a partial gastrectomy with retrocolic gastrojejunostomy to bypass an enormously dilated duodenum. A side-to-side duodenojejunostomy also was performed, using the afferent loop of the jejunum. The patient's complaints of intermittent vomiting, foul eructations, and episodes of dull right quadrant and epigastric pain were only partially relieved. At age 25 transurethral resection of the bladder neck was performed because of increased difficulty in emptying his urinary bladder. Radiologic studies demonstrated megaureter and megacystis. One year later a barium swallow x-ray study showed regurgitation of barium into the dilated duodenal sac.

Three weeks after this x-ray study the patient returned to the hospital with a partial small intestinal obstruction which was relieved by tube decompression. At this time plain films of the abdomen showed the enormous duodenum outlined by retained barium from the study done three weeks before. During the year before the current admission the patient had been admitted to the hospital twice complaining of epigastric pain and vomiting. On both occasions the vomitus contained occult blood. The morning of his current admission the patient vomited bloody fluid and passed a tarry stool. Examination showed a very thin man with bilateral enlarged but nontender parotid glands. The epigastrium was full and tender. A nasogastric tube was passed and drained grossly bloody fluid. Gastric irrigation showed the bleeding which continued intermittently for the next 48 hours. A barium meal x-ray demonstrated a marginal ulcer.

Laparotomy was performed. There were multiple marginal ulcers, one of which had perforated posteriorly into the duodenal sac. Since the megaduodenum had obviously not been drained by the earlier operations, the greater portion of the duodenum was excised, preserving the ampulla of Vater. Subdiaphragmatic vagectomy and partial gastrectomy also were performed. Gastrointestinal continuity was restored by a new antecolic gastrojejunostomy. A tube jejunostomy was created in the jejunal afferent loop, with the tube placed retrograde so as to decompress the duodenal pouch (Fig. 5–34). The patient's postoperative recovery was satisfactory. Pathologic examination of the specimen showed the duodenal wall to be thin, but ganglion cells were normal throughout. The patient gained 44 pounds in three months following operation. He has had no vomiting nor abdominal pain in the six years since operation and works fulltime as a chef. Intermittent parotid swelling occurred during the first year after operation but not thereafter. He continues to require suprapubic pressure to empty his bladder.

The 25-year-old brother of this patient presented complaints of increasingly frequent episodes of dull right upper quadrant and epigastric pain, vomiting, foul eructation, and a 20-pound weight loss over a 2-year period, and occasional episodes of enlarged, nontender parotid glands. Barium swallow cineradiographic studies showed distention of the duodenum extending beyond the superior mesenteric artery and regurgitation of the barium back into the stomach on relaxation of the pylorus. There was no evidence of duodenal muscular contraction during the examination. Approximately one-third of the barium remained in the stomach 48 hours later.

A duodenal resection, partial gastrectomy, and vagectomy similar to those performed on his brother were repeated in this patient. Only the median wall of the duodenum, 5 cm. above and

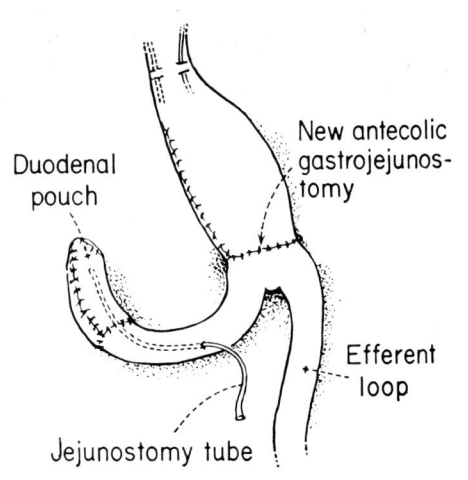

Figure 5–34. Diagram of procedure used in first patient. (From Newton, W. T.: Radical enterectomy for hereditary megaduodenum. Arch. Surg. 96:551, 1968.)

below the ampulla of Vater, was left for anastomosis to the jejunal loop. Again, microscopic examination of the entire length of resected duodenum and jejunum failed to show any abnormalities.

The patient gained 23 pounds in 3 months after the operation and held a fulltime job. He had occasional episodes of diarrhea but no vomiting or abdominal pain following recovery from his operation.

Comment

As Newton pointed out, some patients with atonic megaduodenum can be treated without operation; only one of the nine cases reported by Law and Ten Eyck (1962) required operation and all nine are now asymptomatic. However, in other reported series, patients have had progressive disability requiring an attempt for relief by surgery.

Also note that bypass procedures alone have been unreliable for treating atonic megaduodenum. Weiss' (1938) cases were uncontrolled by gastrojejunostomy or by duodenojejunostomy. Newton cited a series of 12 Brazilian patients with surgically treated megaduodenum; duodenojejunostomy was satisfactory in 8 patients, but 4 required an enterectomy. Newton's first case, described above, had been treated unsuccessfully elsewhere by gastrojejunostomy and duodenostomy. Both of his cases were treated successfully by resection of the greater part of the atonic duodenum. The same sequence of failure with treatment by duodenojejunostomy and eventual success by use of subtotal resection of the duodenum in a case of megaduodenum due to absence of duodenal musculature had been reported earlier by Handelsman and coworkers (1965) (see p. 150).

On the other hand, Barnett and Wall (1955) (see p. 150) reported duodenojunostomy to be the procedure of choice for treating congenital aganglionic megaduodenum.

This disparity in the effectiveness of duodenojejunostomy for treating megaduodenum appears to depend upon the muscular activity of the abnormal duodenum. In the patient with aganglionic megaduodenum of Barnett and Wall, although the duodenum was dilated its walls were thickened by hypertrophy of their muscular layer, indicating muscular activity. Hence, when the obstruction was bypassed, the duodenum could propel its contents down the intestine. But in Handelsman's patient with absence of duodenal musculature, and in Newton's two patients with an atonic duodenum, the walls of the dilated duodenum were very thin and there was no evidence of any muscular activity, so, even when the obstruction was bypassed, duodenal contents could not be propelled down the bowel.

Newton (1968) commented, "Since the normal junction between the duodenum and jejunum is patent and unobstructed in these patients, it is difficult to see how another duodenojejunostomy could benefit the patient, particularly if the entire duodenum is atonic. If nonoperative measures fail in a patient who is an otherwise good surgical risk, resection of the greater portion of the atonic duodenum with anastomosis to the proximal end of the jejunum would seem to be the procedure of choice."

Experience with this procedure is still too meager for it to be fully evaluated as a procedure of choice, but it has proved its value as a last resort.

CONGENITAL EXTRINSIC OBSTRUCTION OF DUODENOJEJUNAL JUNCTION

Soper and Selke (1970) pointed out that "persistent neonatal vomiting, generally bile-stained, is the hallmark of congenital obstruction of the duodenum" and that, in descending order of the frequency of their occurrence, atresia and stenosis of the duodenum, malrotation with Ladd's bands compressing the duodenum, and annular pancreas are well-documented and understood causes. They called attention to a less well-recognized cause: obstruction of the duodenojejunal junction by congenital extrinsic adhesive bands other than the Ladd's bands mentioned above.

Soper and Selke (1970) referred to the reports of Haley and associates (1943, 1949) who had made detailed anatomic dissections of the ligament of Treitz in 141 cadavers in order to study its method of attachment to the bowel. They found that in 5 per cent of the cadavers there was a narrow insertion of the ligament at the duodenojejunal junction; in 80 per cent the ligament was attached over a broad area to the duodenum and jejunum; and the ligament of Treitz could not be identified in 15 per cent (Fig. 5-35; also see Figs. 2-4 and 2-5, page 41).

Haley and Peden (1943) suggested that a broad attachment of the ligament of Treitz makes a smooth, obtuse angle at the duodenojejunum, whereas a narrower insertion creates an acute angle that predisposes to obstruction by kinking the bowel. This observation has escaped wide attention. In the pediatric surgical literature much has been written about congenital obstruction of the duodenum, but there is scant reference to this type of extrinsic obstruction of the duodenojejunal junction; most imply that all extrinsic duodenal obstructions are associated with malrotation or volvulus. Soper and Selke (1970) disagree with this thesis. They reported three infants with congenital extrinsic obstruction of the duodenojejunal junction unassociated with malrotation or volvulus and outlined the anatomy of this anomaly, emphasizing its clinical and radiographic features and describing a surgical approach to the duodenum that permits its accurate recognition and safe treatment. Their report is the source of the following discussion.

In congenital extrinsic obstruction of the duodenojejunal junction, the duodenum is normally rotated. This distinguishes it from incomplete midgut rotation in which the duodenum does not cross the midline behind the superior mesenteric vessels, and the duodenum is generally obstructed in its second or third portion by extrinsic adhesions passing from the right posterior parietes to the high-riding cecum.

A second type of congenital duodenal obstruction that must be distinguished from extrinsic duodenojejunal obstruction is atresia or stenosis of the distal duodenum.

Diagnosis

The salient clinical manifestation is persistent or recurrent vomiting, generally bile-stained. The anomaly usually causes complete or partial obstruction in the neo-

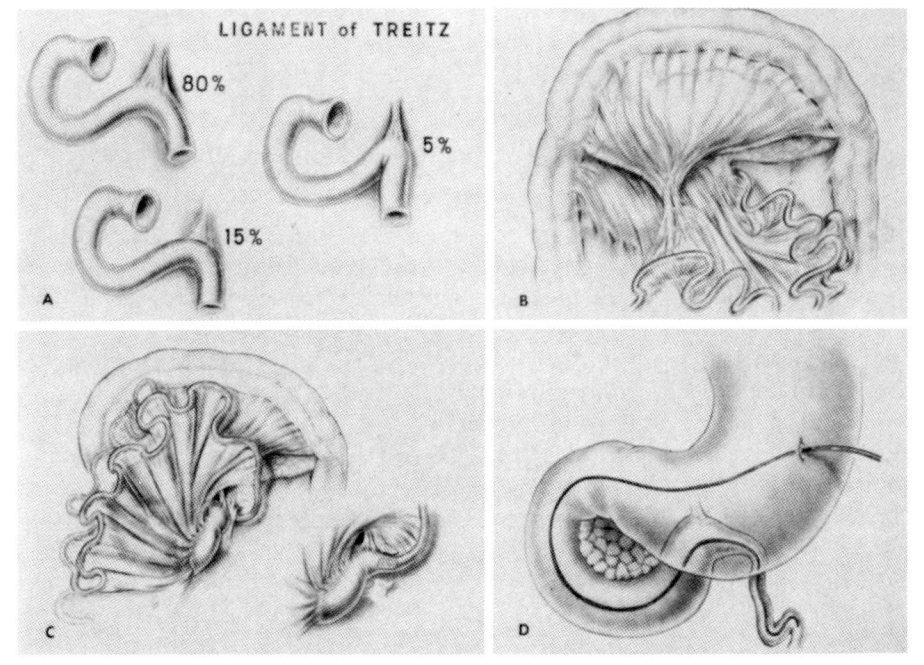

Figure 5-35. A, Different anatomic insertions of the ligament of Treitz. A narrow attachment, found in 5 per cent of cadavers, angulates the duodenojejunal junction to favor obstruction. B, Obstructed duodenum as seen from the conventional anterior approach. The superior mesenteric vessels and the mesocolon obscure the distal duodenum and its junction with the jejunum. C, Congenital extrinsic obstruction of the duodenojejunal junction as seen from the caudad position, with the small bowel elevated and exteriorized cephalad onto the anterior abdominal wall. Inset shows division of the adhesions. D, The completed operation. An indwelling plastic catheter splints the area of obstruction and serves as a feeding vehicle. (From Soper, R. T., and Selke, A. C., Jr.: Congenital extrinsic obstruction of the duodenojejunal junction. J. Pediatr. Surg. 5:437, 1970.)

natal period of life, but can cause partial intermittent obstruction throughout infancy or childhood. The abdomen is generally either normal or scaphoid in contour, but, occasionally, mild epigastric distention may be seen on close scrutiny. Gastric hyperperistaltic waves have not been described with this entity but could occur in patients beyond the neonatal age. Bilious vomiting and no palpable "olive" is evidence against hypertrophic pyloric stenosis.

In Soper's and Selke's three patients, the radiographic findings were not specifically diagnostic, although strikingly similar. The plain abdominal films showed gaseous dilatation of the stomach and proximal duodenum, prior to suction decompression, with fluid levels in the upright films. The amount of gas more distal in the intestine varied inversely with the completeness of the obstruction.

The clinical features and plain abdominal x-rays suggested incomplete midgut rotation, with duodenal obstruction by Ladd's bands. Therefore barium enema examinations were performed in all three cases. These showed the cecum to be in a normal anatomic position in two and in the right upper abdominal quadrant in one. The latter patient proved to have only a failure of cecal descent, with normal midgut rotation. One of the patients had a contrast study of the upper gastrointestinal tract at a previous hospital, which revealed an obstructing lesion of the distal duodenum. Soper and Selke do not believe that upper gastrointestinal study is routinely necessary; the plain radiographs clearly indicated the need for laparotomy in their three cases. They note, however, that Lewis (1966) recommends an upper gastrointestinal contrast study with special attention directed to cinefluoroscopy to demonstrate the to-and-fro peristaltic pattern at the point of obstruction.

The preoperative diagnosis generally is partial or complete obstruction of the third or fourth portion of the duodenum, of unknown cause. To establish the diagnosis of congenital extrinsic obstruction of the duodenojejunal junction, laparotomy is essential.

Surgical Treatment

Soper and Selke pointed out that in the conventional "anterior" surgical approach to the duodenum through the mesocolon (Fig. 5–35B), the interposed mesocolon and mesenteric vessels obscure the distal duodenum, making its exposure hazardous and difficult. In the past, most surgeons simply bypassed obstructions of the distal duodenum by side-to-side duodenojejunostomy. The nature of the obstruction was seldom identified but most were assumed probably to be due to an intrinsic diaphragm, a concept Soper and Selke now believe to be false.

Recently a method has been described of exposing the duodenum from the "posterior" or caudad aspect after evisceration of the midgut onto the upper anterior abdominal wall (Fig. 5–35C). This has the advantage of displacing the vessels and mesocolon out of the way, permitting safe and complete exposure of the distal duodenum and the duodenojejunal junction. Obstructing extrinsic bands can then be identified and lysed. Passage of a Foley catheter, with its bag inflated, through a gastrotomy and down the duodenum past the obstruction rules out intrinsic obstruction. This avoids unnecessary opening of the bowel. Since the morbidity-mortality rate is much higher when bowel has to be opened, accurate distinction between intrinsic and extrinsic obstruction is desirable. Furthermore, if an intrinsic membrane is discovered, this approach provides ample exposure for its correction.

Operative Technic

General inhalation anesthesia via an endotracheal tube is used. The patient is positioned supine on the operating table. There is a choice of incision. Soper and Selke preferred a right transverse supraumbilical incision. A right paramedian or upper midline incision of adequate length also seems to be satisfactory.

After entering the abdomen, obstruction of the duodenum is verified by inspection and palpation. The entire small bowel is examined to rule out malrotation, volvulus, atresia, and stenosis.

The midgut is then exteriorized onto the upper anterior abdominal wall (Fig. 5–35C). This brings into view the duodenum crossing the midline at the ligament of Treitz, without the interposed superior mesenteric vessels or mesocolon obscuring the visual field or making the exposure dangerous. The parietal peritoneum is then dissected away, directly exposing the second, third, and fourth portions of the duodenum.

The dilated and hypertrophied duodenum is seen to be narrowed abruptly at the duodenojejunal angle, where extrinsic adhesions, which are continuous with the ligament of Treitz, cross the bowel. These adhesions are divided above and below the bowel on its antimesenteric surface (Fig. 5–35C, inset) as in the Cattell-Braasch method of mobilizing the distal duodenum. After division of the adhesions, gas and liquid flow from the dilated duodenum downward into the jejunum and downstream.

To rule out a partial intrinsic membrane, a small Foley catheter is inserted through an anterior gastrotomy into the gastric lumen whence it is threaded through the pylorus and down the duodenum into the proximal jejunum (Fig. 5–35D). The bag on the Foley catheter is then inflated with 1 to 2 ml. of air and the catheter is gently withdrawn; if there is no holdup at the duodenojejunal junction, one can be confident of intrinsic patency. Soper and Selke then "prefer to replace the Foley catheter with a soft plastic feeding catheter threaded through the gastrotomy and into the jejunum in a gentle curve during the first few postoperative days while adhesions reform in the area. Early postoperative feedings are given through the indwelling splinting catheter to obviate lengthy parenteral feeding and to improve the caloric and protein intake. Some surgeons prefer not to use this catheter for splinting and feeding. A gastrostomy tube is brought out through a separate stab wound for postoperative gastric decompression. The effluent fluid from the gastrostomy tube is re-fed through the feeding tube to further simplify the postoperative fluid and electrolyte management."

All three infants with congenital extrinsic obstruction of the duodenojejunal junction, who were treated in this way by Soper and Selke, recovered uneventfully and were reported to be doing well 10 to 12 months after the operation.

Other causes of congenital extrinsic obstruction of the duodenum are annular pancreas, described in the chapter on the pancreas in Volume 4, and constricting bands associated with congenital malrotation of the intestine, described in the chapter on the small intestine, Volume 4.

SUPERIOR MESENTERIC ARTERY (SMA) SYNDROME

This condition has also been termed arteriomesenteric duodenal compression syndrome, duodenal ileus or stasis, vascular compression of the duodenum, duodenal compression, arteriomesenteric occlusion, and Wilkie's syndrome. It is a symptom complex resulting from obstruction of the duodenum due to its compression by the superior mesenteric artery or one of its branches where this vessel crosses over the third (transverse) portion of the duodenum as it descends from the aorta. The duodenum is compressed against the aorta and the vertebral column at the level of the second or third lumbar vertebra. The resulting obstruction may be chronic or acute, intermittent, partial, or complete.

According to Gray and Skandalakis (1972), the first description of this condition appears to be that of Boener in 1754, but Rokitansky in 1861 was the first to suggest its etiology. Bloodgood in 1907 first suggested duodenojejunostomy for its treatment, and Stavely (1908) has been credited with performing the first successful duodenojejunostomy for the condition in 1908. In 1921 Wilkie made the most thorough study published up to that time, hence the eponym Wilkie's syndrome.

Since then the diagnosis of vascular compression of the duodenum has had alternating periods of being in vogue and being in disrepute. Some have claimed that it is often overdiagnosed, particularly by being mistakenly diagnosed in some cases of congenital megaduodenum. Others have doubted existence of the syndrome. However, in 1963, Barnes and Sherman published a collective review of the 281 cases considered to be adequately documented in the world literature. In 1976, Akin, Gray, and Skandalakis reported 10 cases of their own and reviewed 125 cases recorded in the literature since 1962. Since more than 400 well-documented cases have been reported, the

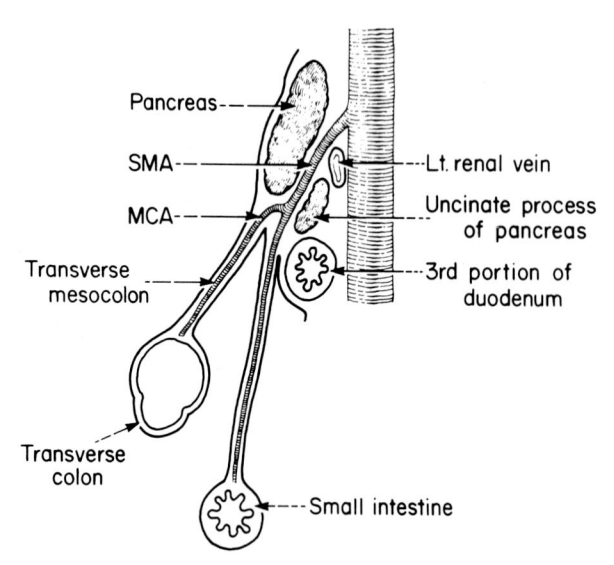

Figure 5-36. Sagittal section through the neck of the pancreas showing the relation of the third portion of the duodenum to the superior mesenteric artery (SMA), the middle colic artery (MCA), the aorta, and the mesentery. (From Akin, J. T., Jr., Gray, S. W., and Skandalakis, J. E.: Vascular compression of the duodenum: Presentation of ten cases and review of the literature. Surgery 79:518, 1976.)

current consensus is that this syndrome is a clinical entity that does occur occasionally.

The anatomy of vascular compression of the duodenum has been described and diagrammed by Akin, Gray, and Skandalakis (1976). "A consequence of man's erect posture is that the superior mesenteric artery leaves the aorta at a more acute angle than it does in quadrupeds. Through this vascular angle the third or fourth part of the duodenum passes, held in place by the suspensory muscle of Treitz. The posterior limb of the angle is formed by the vertebrae and the paravertebral muscles, as well as by the aorta; the anterior limb is formed by the superior mesenteric artery, and sometimes by one of its first two branches in the transverse mesocolon, the middle and right colic arteries. The narrowest part of the angle, above the duodenum, contains the uncinate process of the pancreas and the left renal vein. These relationships are shown in sagittal section [Fig. 5–36] and in anterior view [Fig. 5–37]. The position of the duodenum beneath the superior mesenteric artery is the result of normal intestinal rotation."

They pointed out three important anatomic variables:

1. *Variations in the length and attachment of the suspensory muscle.* When this muscle is short, the duodenum may be pulled higher into the vascular angle, but only the flexure may be raised, increasing the angulation of the fourth part and leaving the third part at the usual level.

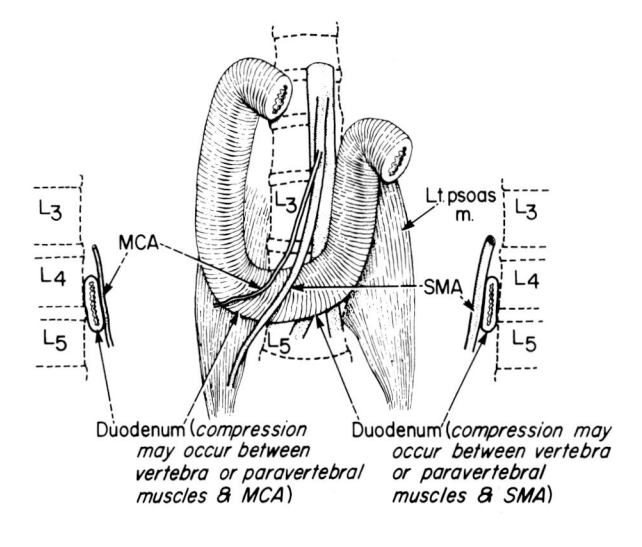

Figure 5-37. Anterior view of the duodenum, superior mesenteric artery (SMA), middle colic artery (MCA), and the vertebral column. (From Akin, Gray, and Skandalakis, cited in previous figure.)

The suspensory muscle of the duodenum (ligament of Treitz) connects the right crus of the diaphragm with the duodenojejunal flexure. Variations of its insertion are shown in Figure 5–38. Although the type shown in Figure 5–38B is the most common, multiple separate divisions (Fig. 5–38D) are not unusual. There were three divisions in one of Akin's and colleagues' 10 patients and four in another.

2. *The level at which the duodenum crosses the vertebral column.* The duodenum usually crosses the vertebral column at the level of the third lumbar vertebra, but, particularly in women, it may cross at a lower level. In a few patients the crossing may be as high as at the second lumbar vertebra. Either the third or the fourth portion of the duodenum may lie over the vertebral column.

A lower crossing might seem to allow more room for the duodenum, but the lumbar curve of the spine reaches the most anterior position at the fourth lumbar vertebra so the space between the limbs of the angle does not increase. Usually, this lumbar curvature is more pronounced in women than in men.

3. *The level of origin of the superior mesenteric artery.* This vessel arises from the aorta at a level between the upper third of the first lumbar vertebra and the disc

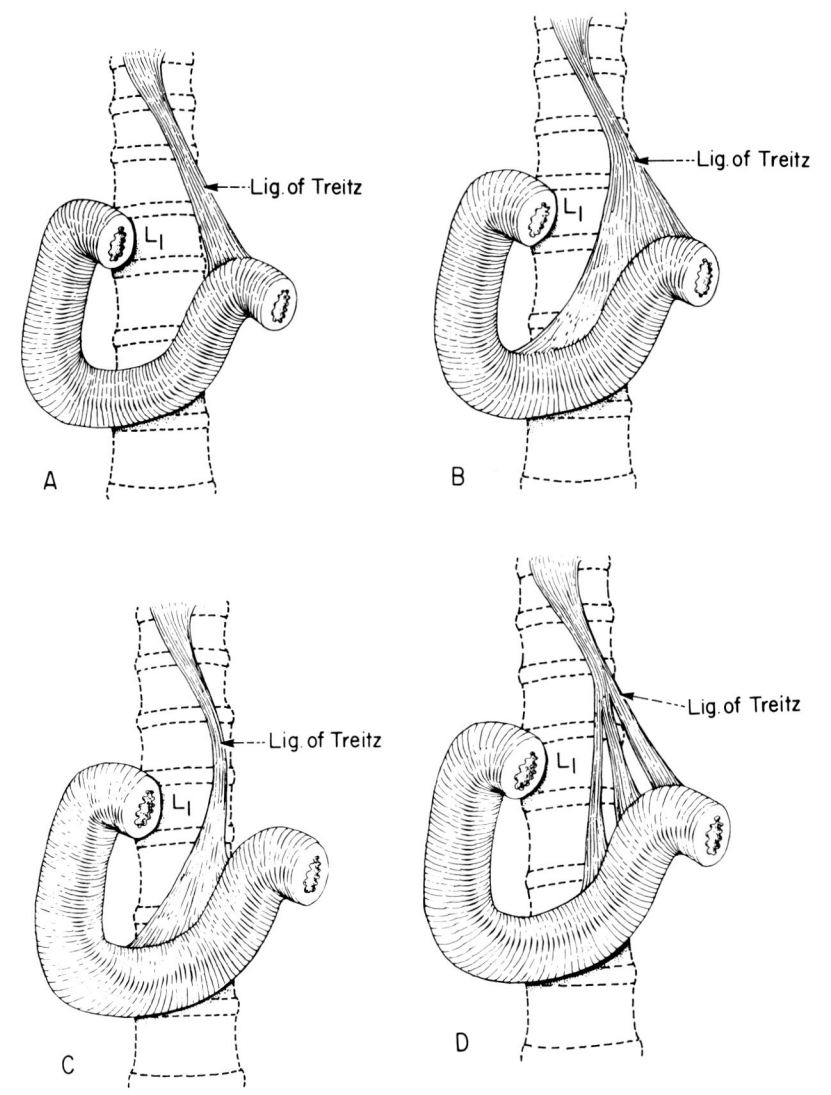

Figure 5–38. Variations in the attachment of the suspensory muscle (ligament) of Treitz. B is the most common type. (From Akin, Gray, and Skandalakis, cited in Figure 5–36.)

between the first and second lumbar vertebrae in 75 per cent of individuals (Cauldwell and Anson, 1943). The artery frequently produces a groove on the anterior surface of the duodenum. Its course and relations to structures posterior to it are shown in Figure 5–36.

Occasionally, compression is caused by the middle colic artery which arises from the superior mesenteric artery at the inferior border of the pancreas, lies in the transverse mesocolon, and crosses the third part of the duodenum.

"Branches of the inferior pancreaticoduodenal artery supply the duodenum in this region. These short vessels limit caudal displacement of the distal part of the duodenum beneath the superior mesenteric artery [Fig. 5–39]. They assume particular importance when treating patients with vascular compression of the duodenum" (Thompson and Stanley, 1974).

The normal angle made by the superior mesenteric artery and the aorta has been measured in 95 cadavers (Derrick and Fahdi, 1965; Mansberger and associates, 1968). It averaged about 35 degrees, with a range from 18 to 70 degrees. Hearn (1966) measured this angle by radiography in seven living patients. In the five normal persons, the average measurement was 56 degrees ranging between 45 and 65 degrees, while in the two with operatively confirmed superior mesenteric artery syndrome the average measurement of the angle was 11 degrees, with a range between 10 and 12 degrees.

Mansberger and colleagues (1968), using biplanar angiography, reported that in five normal persons the superior mesenteric

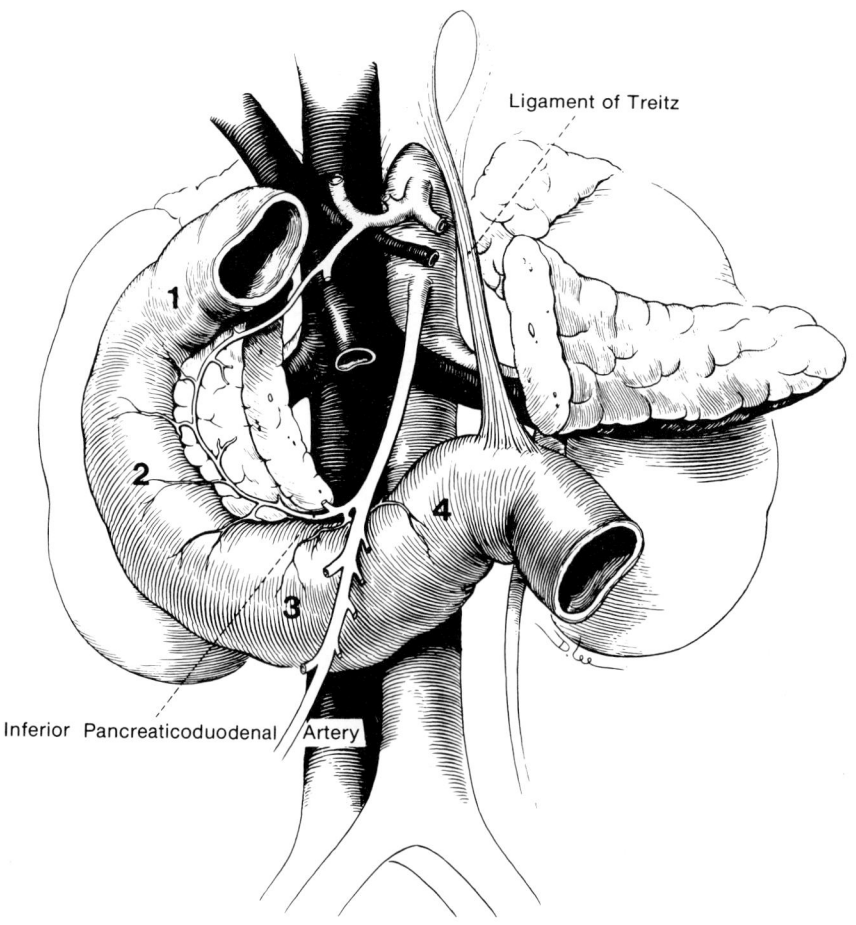

Figure 5–39. Anatomic structures involved in vascular compression of duodenum. Numerals refer to duodenum's four portions. (From Thompson, N. W., and Stanley, J. C.: Vascular compression of the duodenum and peptic ulcer disease. Arch. Surg. *108*:674, 1974.)

artery–aortic angle varied between 45 and 60 degrees, and the distance from the superior mesenteric artery to the anterior surface of the aorta at the point of duodenal crossing varied from 7 to 20 mm.

In the three patients with vascular compression the angle measured 10, 12, and 22 degrees, respectively, and the distance from the superior mesenteric artery to the anterior surface of the aorta at the point of duodenal crossing measured 2, 2, and 3 cm., respectively.

Etiology

The mechanics of the obstruction are obvious. The compression is caused by a viselike effect produced as a result of the angle formed by the superior mesenteric vessels with the aorta. However, the factors that contribute to causing the obstruction are moot.

A number of congenital factors that predispose the patient to duodenal compression have been suggested. These include congenital short mesentery of the intestine, aberrant mesenteric artery or anomalous branches, excessive mobility of the right colon, malrotation of the intestines, and abnormally high fixation of the suspensory muscle of the duodenum.

"The last two of these are easily recognized, but they are not present in many cases of the syndrome. The first three are difficult to evaluate anatomically and impossible to prove embryologically. In very few cases can a specific anomaly be demonstrated. All degrees of duodenal compression may be found, and clinical obstruction may appear only when other factors, minor in themselves, are added" (Gray and Skandalakis, 1972).

Akin, Gray, and Skandalakis (1976) analyzed the etiologic factors reported in 94 patients with vascular compression of the duodenum. In 24 patients (25.5 per cent) the probable cause of the disorder could be identified. In nine patients, including four with extensive burns, immobilization in the supine position produced symptoms in a few hours or days. Eight other patients had been placed in a body cast. One of these had symptoms immediately, others only after a few days — a syndrome first termed "cast syndrome" by Dorph (1950). In one young woman, a new girdle provided the equivalent of a body cast.

In seven cases a large and rapid weight loss from illness or dieting preceded the onset of symptoms. One case (Vanatta, Cagas, and Cramer, 1976) was associated with anorexia nervosa. In eight other patients, malrotation (2), arteriosclerosis (1), paraduodenal hernia (1), abdominal aortic aneurysm (1), and psychogenic factors (3) were considered to be possible but entirely speculative etiologic factors. In 24 cases (25.5 per cent) weight loss after the onset of symptoms was considered to be an aggravating factor. In 38 cases (40.4 per cent) the condition was idiopathic.

No patients with vascular compression of the duodenum have been described as obese. The absence of mesenteric fat, to act as a cushion to protect the duodenum from the relatively nonyielding arteries, is an important etiologic factor in vascular compression of the duodenum. In obese cadavers the duodenum could not be compressed by pulling on the mesentery until the fat was removed from the mesenteric root. An arteriosclerotic artery is more prone to compress the duodenum (Akin, Gray, and Skandalakis, 1976).

In summary, "the duodenum is immobilized by its retroperitoneal attachments and lies wedged within the mouth of an anatomic scissors. The hinge is the origin of the superior mesenteric artery from the aorta. The anterior jaw is the superior mesenteric artery. The posterior jaw is the aorta and the vertebral bodies (L2, L3). Normally the jaws of this scissors are kept open by a generous fatpad providing a wide angle between the aorta and the superior mesenteric artery. A loss of body fat changes the supports of the artery from a bulky band to a linear structure. This causes the superior mesenteric artery to fall in a dorsal direction, thereby decreasing the angle between it and the aorta. Hence emaciated bedridden persons tend to have a more acute superior mesenteric artery-aortic angle. Standing erect, leaning forward, going about on all fours, or lying in the prone position opens the jaws of the scissors, relieving compression of the duodenum. Recumbency in the supine position closes the jaws of the scissors, increases the compression on the transverse portion of the duodenum, and may obstruct it" (Wayne, Miller, and Eiseman, 1971).

It appears that the common denominator in vascular compression of the duodenum is a thin patient with little mesenteric and retroperitoneal fat. Contributing factors are mesenteric tautness and an accentuated lordosis. Whether a high- or low-lying duodenum is more vulnerable, or whether the level of origin of the superior mesenteric artery is significant remains undecided.

Clinical Characteristics

"Statistical analysis of the cases of vascular compression of the duodenum reported in the literature reveals a predominance in females at a ratio of about 3:1 with a peak incidence in the second and third decades of life" (Hall, 1974). It tends to occur in young adults, chiefly females, though no age is immune to the disorder. In one series of 116 patients (Akin, Gray, and Skandalakis, 1976), 75 per cent were between 10 and 39 years old, few patients were very young or very old (the age range was from infancy to 99 years), and, although over 60 per cent of all patients were female, fewer women than men were affected in the third decade of life — the child-bearing years.

The chief symptoms of vascular compression of the duodenum are intermittent episodes of vomiting and postprandial epigastric pain. The pain is seldom severe enough to cause the patient to double up. Vomiting usually produces immediate relief. Eructation with foul breath is common. At first, not all meals cause an episode, but the disorder is often progressive, and both the frequency and severity of the episodes increase. A feeling of fullness after meals is usually present for some months before pain occurs. Abdominal tenderness is present between episodes in many patients. The tenderness is usually epigastric but may occur elsewhere in the abdomen.

In one series of 74 patients, "half of those in whom symptoms were described had suffered for 6 months or less. Among the remainder one patient reported 23 years of misery" (Akin, Gray and Skandalakis, 1976).

Since these patients regurgitate their food or become afraid to eat, weight loss frequently occurs after the onset of symptoms and exacerbates the symptoms. Gastric dilatation with delayed gastric emptying may make ingestion of sufficient food impossible. In the series of 74 patients, such dilatation was present in 17, and in 13 patients gastric or duodenal ulcers were present.

Frequently the patient's discomfort is greatest when standing or when lying supine, and it is relieved by lying on the left side or by assuming the knee-chest position. Although the presence of postural relief is diagnostically significant, its absence does not exclude the diagnosis, as in some cases postural relief has been specifically denied.

Patients may be grouped according to their symptoms in the following manner:

1. *Pediatric patients.* Seventeen of the 31 pediatric patients with this disorder who were recorded in Barner's and Sherman's collective review (1963) had onset of their symptoms with commencement of feeding, and 9 were seen and treated in the neonatal period. A newborn infant may have acute obstruction; a neonate, repeated attacks of vomiting; or a child, a syndrome similar to that of an adult. Characteristically, the emesis contains bile. Several investigators have mentioned the occurrence of gastromegaly in pediatric patients with duodenal compression.

2. *Chronic cases* with a history beginning in childhood of right upper quadrant fullness, flatulence, malnutrition, and vomiting. If the pylorus maintains its tone, a closed-loop type of obstruction may occur, resulting in severe pain relieved when the pylorus opens to permit vomiting. In other obstructions, chronic dilatation of the stomach and duodenum, relieved by occasional voluminous but effortless vomiting, may occur. These patients are usually poorly nourished, of asthemic build, and seldom dynamic. Such patients may endure this ill health for years and be labeled psychoneurotic.

Wilkie found an incidence of ulcer in 25 per cent of this group. The peptic ulcer did not respond to treatment until duodenal stasis was relieved (Thieme and Postmus, 1961).

3. *Chronic patients who suddenly become acutely obstructed* and present as a surgical emergency. There may be no inciting factor, or there may be an emotional crisis or illness, producing weight loss or trauma. In some, prolonged bed rest may contribute. Autopsies of such patients show tremendous dilatation of the stomach and duodenum, as mentioned in the original description of this syndrome.

4. Patients with *acute obstruction* without a previous history of gastrointestinal complaints. These cases may be due to trauma or an acute illness or may be without a known precipitating cause.

Diagnosis

The diagnosis of the syndrome of vascular compression of the duodenum is suggested by the onset of intermittent episodes of vomiting and abdominal discomfort and other clinical manifestations of duodenal obstruction. A plain, flat, x-ray film of the abdomen that shows a dilated duodenum with or without associated dilatation of the stomach supports the possible presence of this disorder.

The diagnosis is established by an x-ray study of the stomach and duodenum, using barium. This may not demonstrate the condition in mild or early cases, but in those that are severe or long-standing a dilated duodenum obstructed near the ligament of Treitz is usually revealed. Hartenstein, Ziperman, and Smith (1961) pointed out that an x-ray film showing a sharp, linear, straight obstructing line in this area, which points toward the right iliac fossa, is characteristic of vascular compression of the duodenum. However, this diagnosis should not be made unless significant dilation of the duodenum and obstructive symptoms are also present.

In some patients evidence of concomitant peptic ulceration of the duodenum or stomach or both may also be seen in the roentgenograms. Gastric dilatation may or may not also be present. Cinefluoroscopy may show an abnormal, churning, to-and-fro motion of the barium column.

When the upper gastrointestinal x-ray study shows duodenal obstruction, it is advisable to place the patient in the prone and left lateral decubitus positions to observe whether the obstruction is relieved, as seen by barium passing beyond the point of obstruction. If it does, a trial with nonoperative treatment may be elected.

Lateral angiography provides the most definitive criterion for diagnosis but is not often necessary. Mansberger and associates (1968) and Wayne, Miller, and Eiseman (1971) reported a narrowed superior mesenteric artery–aortic angle and a markedly reduced distance from the artery to the aorta at the point of duodenal crossing. Anderson and associates (1973) recommended the following diagnostic criteria: (1) visualization of intermittent obstruction to the passage of barium in the third portion of the duodenum; (2) leading bolus of barium shows straight line cut off at point of obstruction; (3) dilatation of duodenum proximal to the obstruction; (4) on fluoroscopy, evidence of reverse peristalsis proximal to the obstruction; and (5) one cinefluorography, relief of obstruction in the prone position and its accentuation in upright and supine positions.

"In 95 per cent of 81 patients for whom information was available, the diagnosis was by radiology. In the remainder, the compression was diagnosed only at operation. Among the 66 patients for whom a preoperative diagnosis was reported, it was correct in 52 (79 per cent). In another ten patients 'obstruction' was the diagnosis" (Akin, Gray, and Skandalakis, 1976).

A factor that may complicate the diagnosis is the mental instability of many of these patients whose disorder has escaped diagnosis for years and who have been considered to be neurotic. This has been attributed to the chronicity of the illness and the patient's inability to get relief (Thieme and Postmus, 1961).

A normal upper gastrointestinal tract has often been observed during asymptomatic periods and does not exclude the presence of this disorder (Thompson and Stanley, 1974). Upper gastrointestinal x-ray study during actual episodes of obstruction may be required to establish a diagnosis.

Vascular compression of the duodenum may not be suspected until surgical exploration. At operation duodenal dilatation proximal to the superior mesenteric vessels, relieved by elevation of the mesenteric root, shows that the obstruction is mechanical. The presence or absence of this type of obstruction usually cannot be determined merely by palpation within or alongside the duodenum as it passes through the aortovertebral-mesenteric space.

A simple procedure, suggested by Wilkie (1921) over 50 years ago, to facilitate intraoperative diagnoses is gastroduodenal insufflation of 150 to 300 ml. of air through a nasogastric tube. An increase in the duodenal diameter of more than 3 or 4 cm. indicates critical distal obstruction. Thompson and Stanley (1974) reported that "the inadequacy of ligament of Treitz transection in our first patient, the importance of the redundant duodenum in our second patient, and the mechanical basis of obstruction in our third patient all might have been discovered earlier had this simple intraoperative test been utilized." Its usefulness has also been confirmed by others.

Natural Course

Untreated vascular compression of the duodenum may be chronic or may become acute with fatal results. Chronic cases are usually slowly progressive in the severity of symptoms. Acute cases may cause serious electrolyte imbalance, dehydration, alkalosis, and occasionally tetany and may be fatal unless the obstruction is relieved by surgical intervention.

Treatment

It is generally agreed that patients with vascular compression of the duodenum should be treated first by a trial with *medical methods*. In nonacute cases this comprises frequent small feedings and positioning of the patient in the knee-chest, prone, or left lateral position, and removing the body cast in those with the "cast syndrome."

"In view of the fact that vascular compression is unknown in fat patients, it is possible that a diet producing a gain in weight might alleviate or even remove symptoms in patients who are not yet suffering acutely" (Akin, Gray, and Skandalakis, 1976).

In acute obstruction, gastroduodenal suction, correction of electrolyte and fluid imbalance, and supportive measures are indicated. Medical methods have frequently been successful in relieving the patients' discomfort and making surgery unnecessary.

Surgical treatment is used for those patients in whom conservative methods have been unsuccessful and the symptoms are severe enough to interfere with the patient's health, or for those who have associated severe peptic ulcer disease.

The operation of choice depends on whether there is concomitant peptic ulcer disease, which is present in about 25 per cent of these patients and is probably due to longstanding antral stasis. If the peptic ulcer problem is severe, it may also require surgical treatment.

SMA SYNDROME WITHOUT ASSOCIATED PEPTIC ULCER DISEASE

A duodenojejunostomy to shunt around the obstruction was first used successfully by Stavely in 1908, to treat vascular compression of the duodenum without peptic ulcer disease. It has been the operation most frequently used for this disorder and has proved satisfactory. The operation involves an anastomosis of dilated, atonic bowel, hence the anastomosis may not function until the duodenum regains normal size and tone, a process that frequently takes several weeks (Wayne and Burrington, 1972).

In 1958, Strong reported a new procedure that releases the duodenum at the ligament of Treitz, allowing it to be displaced downward, thus eliminating the angulation of the bowel at this point and moving the duodenum out from the sharp angle formed at this level by the superior mesenteric artery and aorta. He reported a case with dramatic cure by this simple technic. In 1960, Major, Ottenheimer, and Whalen reported a similar case, cured equally dramatically by Strong's operation. The technic was described and illustrated as follows:

At laparotomy the diagnosis was confirmed by finding the duodenum to be dilated and sharply angulated at the ligament of Treitz. The attachment was so firm that the duodenum could not be displaced caudally by manual traction. There was compression of the duodenum behind the superior mesenteric artery so that it was difficult to pass even the tip of one finger behind the artery at this level [Fig. 5–40].

The distal duodenum was easily freed from the ligament of Treitz and other ligamentous attachments to the pancreas and retroperitoneal tissues and moved downward 3 or 4 cm. The retroperitoneal tissues and peritoneum were then closed longitudinally to eliminate raw surfaces and to fix the duodenojejunal junction in its new location [Fig. 5–41].

The patient made a rapid recovery. She was tolerating liquids within 24 hours and enjoying a regular diet with no distress within 1 week. She has gained 15 pounds in weight and is asymptomatic. Three months after operation an upper gastrointestinal x-ray study showed a normal

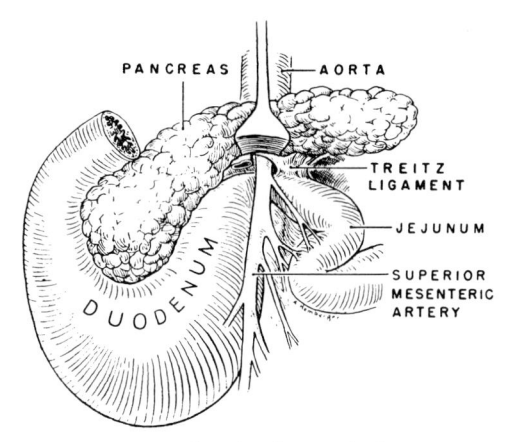

Figure 5-40. The duodenum before operation. (From Major, J. W., Ottenheimer, E. J., and Whalen, W. A., Jr.: Duodenal obstruction at the ligament of Treitz: Report of a case treated by a plastic procedure. N. Engl. J. Med. 262:444, 1960.)

duodenum except for its new position in relation to the ligament of Treitz and superior mesenteric artery.

Strong's operation does not require an anastomosis and seems to be simpler, more physiologic, and less hazardous than duodenojejunostomy and is equally effective. Several others have reported satisfactory experiences with its use and recommend it as the procedure of choice for the surgical treatment of vascular compression of the duodenum. However, in some cases the duodenum is not freed by division of Treitz's ligament and duodenojejunostomy is required.

Akin, Gray, and Skandalakis (1976) reported the results of treatment in 104 patients: 94 collected from the literature and 10 of their own. Over 75 per cent of these patients were treated surgically. Ten required a second operation to relieve their symptoms. The results of conservative treatment alone were poor.

In the collected series, duodenojejunostomy was performed in 47 per cent of the surgically treated and Strong's operation was performed in 15 per cent. All patients treated by the latter method only were relieved of their symptoms. Duodenojejunostomy alone was nearly as effective, with 82 per cent relieved.

In their own series of ten patients, division of the ligament of Treitz was sufficient to release the duodenum in seven. In two patients, the duodenum was not freed by division of Treitz's ligament and duodenojejunostomy was required. They concluded that most of these patients can be relieved by division of the ligament of Treitz and relocation of the duodenojejunal junction. A few will require duodenojejunostomy. This can be determined only at operation. Many patients with less severe compression live in discomfort, more or less palliated by a medical regimen.

The mobilization procedure has very little morbidity, does not involve an intestinal anastomosis, and has a significantly shorter convalescence than that necessary after duodenojejunostomy, according to Wayne and Burrington (1972).

SMA SYNDROME WITH ASSOCIATED SEVERE PEPTIC ULCER DISEASE

The association of peptic ulcer disease with vascular compression of the duodenum syndrome appears to be more than coincidental.

Thompson and Stanley (1974) analyzed 291 patients with this disorder described in 65 reports since 1960. Peptic ulcer disease was present in 31.8 per cent of the 182 patients with chronic duodenal compression. In this group duodenal ulcers were present in 44 patients, gastric ulcers were present in 11, and both types of ulcer occurred in two patients. Ulcer disease was not described among the 109 patients with the acute form of this syndrome except for acute ulcers in 8 of 28 patients with severe injuries, including extensive thermal burns. Here other factors probably played a role.

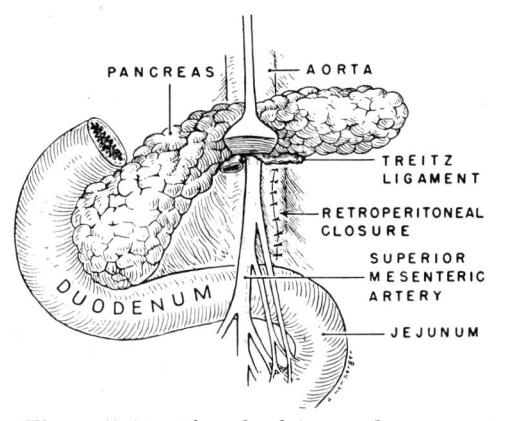

Figure 5-41. The duodenum after operation. (From Major, Ottenheimer, and Whalen, cited in previous figure.)

The incidence of peptic ulcer disease in various other reported series (Barner and Sherman, 1963; Anderson and associates, 1973; Appel, Bentlif, and Dickson, 1976) has ranged from 8.4 to 60 per cent. The cause or causes of this frequent association remain the subject of much speculation. It has been hypothesized that chronic duodenal obstruction predisposes to peptic ulcer by causing hyperchlorhydria. The evidence for this, however, is conflicting.

It has been difficult to establish the temporal sequence of duodenal compression and ulcer disease, but speculations can be made, based on established physiologic observations. Factors that contribute to duodenal or antral stasis, or both, result in gastric hypersecretion presumably caused by prolonged antral stimulation and increased production of gastrin. On this basis one would suspect that the intermittent duodenal obstruction preceded peptic ulceration. However, this cannot be proved because of the difficulty in correlating the various symptoms with findings of x-ray examinations.

The possibility that peptic ulcer contributes to the arteriomesenteric duodenal compression syndrome seems less tenable. The frequent occurrence of peptic ulcer and the rarity of vascular compression of the duodenum syndrome suggest that ulcers play little, if any, etiologic role in this syndrome.

Some surgical procedures used for treatment of peptic ulcer disease may contribute to the development of compression of the duodenum. Vagotomy has been implicated. Impaired duodenal motility and postvagotomy gastric atony may exacerbate pre-existing partial obstruction. Whenever persistent gastric atony follows vagotomy, secondary duodenal obstruction should be considered a possible cause. "Despite the roentgenographic appearance suggestive of severe gastric atony in two of our patients, prompt gastric emptying and normal motility occurred immediately following operative decompression of the obstructive duodenum" (Thompson and Stanley, 1974).

Other surgical procedures directly involving the stomach and duodenum may also be followed by the development of this duodenal compression syndrome. This complication has occurred most commonly after operations requiring extensive mobilization of the duodenum, which may displace the second and third portions of the duodenum superiorly, causing its entrapment in the aortovertebral-mesenteric angle. Duodenal compression has been reported after Billroth I and II operations and certain types of pyloroplasties. The first patient developing vascular compression of the duodenum after pyloroplasty was described by Finney in 1906. The altered anatomic arrangements created by these operations, which are used so commonly for treating peptic ulcer disease, may explain partly the frequent association of vascular duodenal compression and peptic ulcer disease.

Treatment

When concomitant severe peptic ulcer disease is present, the ulcer will not respond to treatment until duodenal stasis is relieved. In these cases primary surgical intervention is indicated. Treatment should be individualized as no one method is consistently effective. All methods of treatment may occasionally fail, usually because of severe associated disease such as continued alcoholism, injury to the spinal cord, or scleroderma.

When peptic ulcer surgery is contemplated the surgeon should check for the possible presence of intermittent duodenal obstruction and, if present, also give consideration to its relief. If stasis in the duodenum contributes significantly to the ulcer diathesis, alleviation of the stasis may be curative but is unreliable as a definitive procedure. Gastrojejunostomy alone has been used but has proved unsatisfactory, because bile and pancreatic juices must still potentially flow across the area of obstruction or be regurgitated back into the stomach. If gastrojejunostomy is performed, vagotomy must be added for protection against marginal ulceration.

When the ulcer has been discovered preoperatively, the ulcer and the obstruction should be treated as two independent lesions. The procedure of choice to accomplish these purposes appears to be vagotomy and antrectomy with a Billroth I or II anastomosis combined with a duodenojejunostomy or with division of the ligament of Treitz. These choices are made at operation. The presence of a gastric ulcer is an indication for the gastrectomy to include the ulcer-bearing portion of the stomach, if possible.

CONGENITAL DUODENAL DIAPHRAGM PLUS SMA SYNDROME

Sutherland, Miller, and Najarian (1972) reported the occurrence of both a congenital duodenal diaphragm and vascular compression of the duodenum in an elderly patient — the first and, to our knowledge, the only such case recorded in the literature. The uniqueness of the case, difficulties in its diagnosis, and the custom-made surgical methods for its treatment are informative:

The patient was a 70-year-old woman who was admitted to the University of Minnesota Hospital in 1970. Since early adulthood she had experienced weight loss, diarrhea, and postprandial, crampy, upper abdominal pain incompletely relieved by the vomiting of partially digested food. In 1948 a diagnosis of superior mesenteric artery compression of the duodenum was made at exploratory laparotomy, and gastrojejunostomy was performed. Although partially relieved, the patient's symptoms continued and were unaltered by cholecystectomy in 1960. In 1969 an upper gastrointestinal x-ray study showed a chronically dilated duodenum retaining food and barium. The symptoms were attributed to a malfunctioning gastrojejunostomy, so operation was performed. At operation the gastrojejunostomy was taken down and, just distal to the superior mesenteric artery crossover, the fourth portion of the duodenum was utilized for a gastroduodenostomy.

The patient remained symptomatic even though an upper gastrointestinal x-ray study 1 year later showed the gastroduodenostomy to be functioning well. She passed loose, light-colored stools up to 12 times daily, could not gain weight, and vomiting became more frequent, often containing food ingested the previous day.

In 1970, examination in hospital showed a spry, elderly woman weighing 77 pounds. Except for extreme thinness, physical examination showed nothing abnormal.

An upper gastrointestinal x-ray study showed an enormously dilated duodenum with considerable peristaltic activity, which filled only to the second portion where there was an abrupt cutoff. The gastroduodenostomy allowed free passage of barium into the efferent loop but almost no filling of the afferent loop. The small bowel follow-through was normal.

Gastroscopy showed a widely patent gastroduodenostomy stoma and a normal-appearing pylorus. The duodenum was visualized through the pylorus and was filled with fluid and food particles.

Preoperatively it was assumed that the patient had compression of the duodenum by the superior mesenteric vessels; that the gastroenterostomy distal to the obstruction did not permit adequate drainage of pancreatic, biliary, and duodenal secretions; and that megaduodenum acted as a reservoir for food which would have to be regurgitated. A procedure to allow emptying of duodenal contents directly into the jejunum was planned.

At exploratory operation the duodenum was massively enlarged, not only in the first and second portions as shown on the upper gastrointestinal series but also in the third portion to the level of the superior mesenteric vessels. The dudodenum was held snugly in the angle between the origin of the superior mesenteric artery and aorta due to cephalad tension exerted by the gastroduodenostomy, ligament of Treitz, and surrounding scar tissue.

It was decided not to disturb the gastroduodenostomy, but rather to perform a bypass from the dilated portion of the duodenum to the proximal jejunum, utilizing an isolated segment of jejunum. In preparation for the bypass a duodenotomy was made proximal to the mesenteric vessel crossover; large amounts of bile were aspirated from the duodenum. An attempt was made to grasp the nasogastric tube to bring it through the anastomosis, but it was impossible to enter the stomach from this duodenotomy. Even with the aid of a distal gastrotomy the nasogastric tube could not be passed down to the duodenotomy.

A second and more proximal duodenotomy revealed the presence of a thin mucosal diaphragm extending completely across the duodenum just proximal to the ampulla of Vater. With care not to injure the ampulla, the web, which contained a minute, eccentric perforation, was excised and the remaining raw mucosal edges oversewn. The proximal duodenotomy was extended to the gastrotomy and then closed transversely, creating a large pyloroplasty.

Attention was then redirected toward the more distal obstruction. An 18-cm. segment of jejunum was isolated approximately 30 cm. distal to the ligament of Treitz and an end-to-end jejunojejunostomy performed between the remaining proximal and distal limbs of jejunum. With use of end-to-side anastomoses, the isolated segment of jejunum was interposed isoperistaltically from the distal duodenotomy to the jejunum, just distal to the previous jejunojejunostomy. Bilateral truncal vagotomies completed the operation.

The pathology as it existed is illustrated in Figure 5-42, and Figure 5-43 illustrates the operation performed.

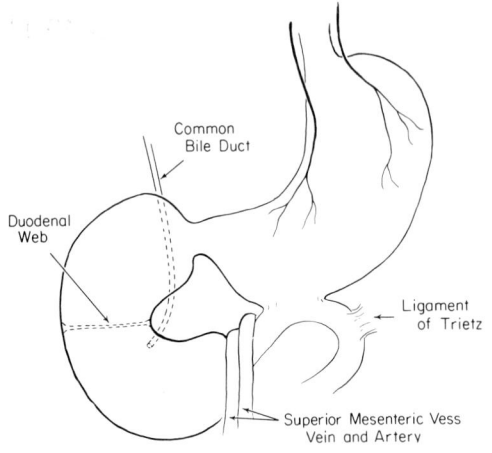

Figure 5–42. Pathology as it was encountered at operation. The duodenal web is located proximal to the ampulla of Vater. The second obstruction from the external compression occurs where the superior mesenteric vessels cross over the duodenum. (From Sutherland, D. E. R., Miller, I. D., and Najarian, J. S.: Occurrence of both congenital duodenal diaphragm and vascular compression of the duodenum in an elderly patient. Am. J. Surg. 123:352, 1972.)

The patient's recovery was uneventful. In 10 days she was eating an unrestricted diet. Two weeks after operation an upper gastrointestinal x-ray study showed the duodenum still enlarged but significantly decompressed compared with the preoperative study. Barium flowed easily from the duodenum through the interposed segment of jejunum. When last seen 6 months after surgery the patient was gaining weight, had no diarrhea, and had not experienced abdominal pain or any episode of vomiting.

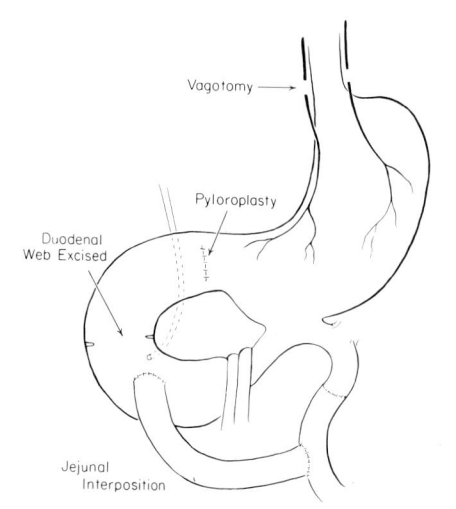

Figure 5–43. An operation was performed to relieve obstruction from both lesions. (From Sutherland, Miller, and Najarian, cited in previous figure.)

Comment

This case demonstrated that the diagnosis of both a congenital web and vascular compression of the duodenum may be difficult. As Sutherland and colleagues pointed out, cramps or pain after eating, a sense of fullness, nausea, vomiting, and weight loss occur in both conditions, and these symptoms are often vague and intermittent and develop slowly. In an upper gastrointestinal series an obstruction itself may not be demonstrated; a widely dilated duodenum may be the only finding. In cases of vascular compression of the duodenum, dilatation will include the third portion of the duodenum, with a vertical flattening sometimes demonstrated at this level.

Furthermore, a duodenal web is so rarely encountered in elderly persons that its possible presence is seldom thought of. This case also demonstrated that surgical treatment of duodenal obstruction distal to the pylorus, whether due to an intrinsic cause (such as duodenal diaphragm) or an extrinsic cause (such as vascular compression of the duodenum), should establish duodenal drainage without the necessity for duodenal contents to reflux retrograde through the pylorus.

Gastroenterostomy, even with vagotomy to prevent stomal ulceration, results in a blind loop and has been unsatisfactory in many reported cases. In either vascular compression of the duodenum or a duodenal web situated distal to the ampulla, pancreatic, biliary, and duodenal secretions along with any food that enters the duodenum will regurgitate into the stomach.

This patient "experienced all the difficulties expected after gastroenterostomy for either duodenal web or vascular compression of the duodenum" (she had both). It can be concluded that in such cases gastroenterostomy should not be used. Instead, it appears preferable to explore the lumen of the duodenum with a bagged tube passed down through a small gastrotomy. When a duodenal diaphragm is found, duodenotomy with excision of the web seems to be the procedure of choice, if injury to the entrance of the common and pancreatic ducts can be avoided, and then relief of obstruction due to vascular compression of the duodenum, preferably by dividing the ligament of Treitz or, if necessary, by duodenojejunostomy.

PEDIATRIC PATIENTS

Wayne and Burrington (1972) reported seven previously healthy children who developed vascular compression of the duodenum. Two were 3 and 10 weeks old, respectively, and in good health except for symptoms related to their duodenal obstruction. In these children the obstruction was considered to be congenital. The other five children were aged 13 to 16 years and were of strikingly similar asthenic body builds. Four of the five had experienced a recent adolescent growth spurt without commensurate weight gain. One patient developed the syndrome while hospitalized for an esophageal burn. The diagnosis of vascular duodenal compression in each case was established by radiological studies.

Four of these patients were treated by complete lysis of the ligament of Treitz and mobilization of the right colon and the second, third, and fourth portions of the duodenum (Fig. 5–44). The duodenum and several feet of proximal jejunum were moved from beneath the widely mobilized superior mesenteric artery and placed in the right lateral gutter, thus removing the duodenum entirely from passing beneath the superior mesenteric artery (Fig. 5–45). The four patients treated by this procedure experienced prompt and complete relief of symptoms, with an average hospital stay of 5 days after surgery. All four subsequently gained an average of 1 pound per week.

Another patient was treated by a duodenojejunostomy to bypass the area compressed by the superior mesenteric artery. He could not tolerate clear liquids until the eighth postoperative day. The diet was then rapidly advanced and he was discharged on the 12th postoperative day, feeling entirely well.

The remaining two patients were treated nonoperatively. One was a 15-year-old boy who had swallowed a commercial cleansing agent, which caused severe corrosive esophagitis with inability to swallow and necessitated a feeding gastrostomy. Feeding via the gastrostomy caused abdominal distention and pain. The patient lost 22 pounds during the 13 days following admission. Barium study showed almost complete obstruction of the third portion of the duodenum by the superior mesenteric artery. Placement of the patient in the prone and left lateral decubitus positions after feeding enabled him to tolerate full gastrostomy feedings without difficulty. On discharge from the hospital he had regained 10 pounds, and he subsequently regained his preadmission weight.

The other nonoperatively treated patient was a 16-year-old boy who entered the hospital with a 2-day history of postprandial fullness, epigastric pain, and repeated episodes of nausea and vomiting. He had intentionally lost 15 pounds during the previous 3 weeks in order to qualify for a 105-pound interscholastic wrestling competition.

On admission he weighed 105 pounds; the upper abdomen was distended and slightly tender. Initial aspiration of the stomach obtained 2 liters of gastric contents.

Figure 5–44. Duodenal mobilization. (From Wayne, E. R., and Burrington, J. D.: Duodenal obstruction by the superior mesenteric artery in children. Surgery 72:765, 1972.)

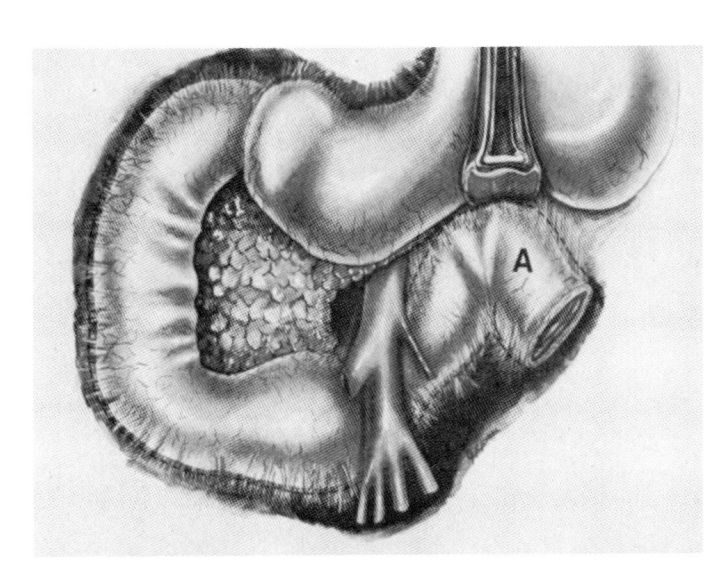

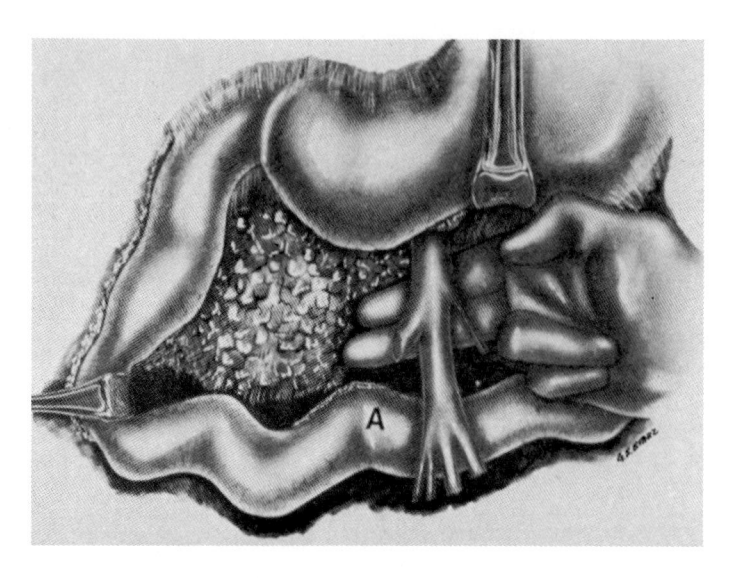

Figure 5–45. Transposition of duodenojejunum. (From Wayne and Burrington, cited in previous figure.)

An upper gastrointestinal x-ray study showed obstruction at the third portion of the duodenum which, however, could be relieved by turning the patient into the prone position. Hence, it was elected to treat this episode of duodenal obstruction by having him lie prone for 30 to 60 minutes after each feeding. After repeated early failures this treatment was ultimately successful, and he began to gain weight. After a weight gain of 15 pounds, a repeat upper gastrointestinal x-ray study was normal, and he was discharged. The total time from diagnosis to discharge was 17 days.

In summary, three different modes of treatment were used for the seven patients, and all are now asymptomatic since diagnosis was established and specific therapy initiated.

BURNED CHILDREN

Ogbuokiri, Law, and MacMillan (1972) reported that 4 of 390 children with acute burns developed superior mesenteric artery syndrome. All four were of slender or average physique. Vomiting was the first symptom. It appeared during the first postburn week in two patients and during the second week in the other two patients. The burns ranged from 45 to 86 per cent of the body surface and were mostly third degree.

The investigators emphasized that all patients with extensive burns tend to lose weight. The feeding difficulties created by the superior mesenteric artery syndrome further complicate the problem of maintaining adequate nutrition. By the time the diagnosis was established, all four patients had lost between 8 and 14 per cent of their weight on admission. Weight loss aggravates the syndrome in a vicious circle. Diagnosis of the syndrome is suggested by the occurrence of postprandial bilious vomiting in the presence of active bowel sounds. It should be confirmed by an upper gastrointestinal series which, the authors stated, can be performed safely in patients with extensive burns if special precautions are taken. If obstruction is present, most of the barium must be removed from the patient's stomach and a large-bore Levin tube must be left in place at the termination of the procedure to avoid aspiration of gastric contents. They have performed 98 upper gastrointestinal series in 74 patients without complications. The radiographic appearance is characteristic. The stomach and duodenum may be dilated. The site of obstruction in the third portion of the duodenum is clearly demonstrated. Some barium usually passes through the partial obstruction. Cinefluoroscopy shows duodenal dilatation and reflux of barium within the duodenum and into the stomach.

When the diagnosis is established, conservative management is promptly begun. This consists of nasogastric suction drainage to decompress the dilated stomach. Thereafter, various positional changes should be tried for feeding. The knee-chest position cannot be used in burned patients. Although the prone position has often been recommended for treating superior mesenteric artery syndrome, Ogbuokiri, Law, and MacMillan reported that in their four burned children (aged 5 to 15 years) the prone position on a Stryker frame was associated with vomiting. A semi-sitting position with the head elevated 45 degrees was found to give symptomatic relief. They recommended that duodenojejunostomy be considered if conservative measures fail. In two of their cases conservative therapy proved adequate, but one of the other patients was terminal and too ill to undergo surgery, and the extent of the burn contraindicated surgery in the remaining patient. These contraindications to intra-abdominal surgical treatment seem likely to be present in many patients with extensive, severe burns of the trunk.

"The most effective method to prevent this syndrome in patients with extensive burns is to control the initial severe weight loss by giving a supplementary high caloric–high protein diet throughout their hospital stay. In those who cannot tolerate oral feedings, intravenous hyperalimentation, despite its risks, may be lifesaving," according to Ogbuokiri, Law, and MacMillan (1972).

Pruitt (1971) reported his experience with 17 severely burned patients who developed superior mesenteric artery syndrome and commented that at fluoroscopic examination the majority had maximum passage of barium in the left lateral decubitus, rather than in the prone, position. He emphasized nonoperative treatment and intravenous hyperalimentation as a preference, but when supervening complications, associated injuries, or a geographic distribution of the burn prevents placement in the prone or lateral position, he and associates do not hesitate to relieve the obstruction operatively.

BEDRIDDEN COMBAT CASUALTIES

Wayne, Miller, and Eiseman (1971) reported on five combat casualties from the Vietnam War with superior mesenteric artery syndrome who were seen at the Fitzsimons General Army Hospital in 1969 and 1970. Each underwent initial operation in Vietnam and frequently again elsewhere prior to treatment at Fitzsimons. Four patients had severe skeletal injuries requiring prolonged immobilization. Two had severe intra-abdominal injuries that did not involve the stomach or duodenum but required prolonged bed care. All, therefore, were in body casts or otherwise confined to bed for the entire period of hospitalization.

The initial symptoms of the syndrome occurred 8 to 12 weeks following injury, by which time the average weight loss was 65 pounds. Each patient had extensive contrast radiographic studies of the gastrointestinal tract. In two of these patients, abdominal aortic and superior mesenteric artery angiograms in both lateral and posteroanterior planes were also performed.

In all five patients the x-ray studies showed gastroduodenal dilatation and obstruction to passage of contrast material past the third portion of the duodenum. Relief of the radiographic signs of obstruction by moving the patient onto his side or his abdomen confirms this diagnosis, but such rotation of the patient is not always easy in the presence of unstable fractures or interfering orthopedic accoutrements. However, the investigators believe it should be done.

"Biplanar arteriographic visualization of the aorta and superior mesenteric artery is ideal but unnecessary in most cases. It is advisable to use double contrast with opaque material in the duodenum simultaneously with angiographic visualization. Three features should be sought: (1) duodenal obstruction; (2) the superior mesenteric artery–aortic angle; and (3) distance from the superior mesenteric artery at the point of duodenal crossing to the anterior border of the aorta."

Wayne and colleagues pointed out that delay in the diagnosis may be caused by ascribing weight loss solely to metabolic deficit associated with injury or sepsis. Clinical suspicion may be supported by a plain radiograph of the abdomen showing a huge air bubble in the distended stomach and right half of the duodenum that characteristically stops abruptly where the superior mesenteric artery overlies and obstructs the duodenum. This can be confirmed by contrast visualization.

Four of the five patients were treated successfully by nonoperative methods, consisting of first correcting gastroduodenal distention and acute dehydration by nasogastric suction and fluid and electrolyte replacement. Later, the patients were fed orally on a Stryker frame rolled into the face-down position, thus relieving the obstruction.

The fifth patient, after nasogastric decompression and rehydration, did not respond to three attempts at oral feeding in the prone position over a 2.5-week period. A duodenojejunostomy was then performed. Postoperatively, the patient did well and regained his pre-injury weight within 5 months.

From this experience the authors concluded that "by the conservative treatment just described the vicious circle of obstruction and weight loss can be broken. Ultimately, as fat stores are replenished, the superior mesenteric artery will be lifted off the duodenum by the normal gasket of fat that surrounds the origin of this vessel from the aorta. Only after several failures of this type of conservative management should operative therapy be implemented." They advocate the use of duodenojejunostomy in the occasional patient in whom operation is required.

CAST SYNDROME

When the superior mesenteric artery syndrome occurs after the application of a body cast, it is termed the cast syndrome, which was first described by Willett in 1878. In 1950, Dorph reported a case of his own, reviewed the literature, and named it.

In 1975, Bisla and Louis presented three cases and reported that the "cast syndrome is a rare but serious condition which, if not diagnosed and treated early, can lead to death. A complete survey of the literature revealed only 40 documented instances of cast syndrome."

Analysis of these cases showed the cast syndrome to be most common in the second decade of life, with a range in age from 13 to 67 years. Eighty per cent of patients were between 13 and 20 years of age, and only eight patients were older than 20 years.

The disorder usually is manifested by intermittent or continuous nausea, vomiting, and abdominal distention, leading to dehydration, prostration, metabolic alkalosis, shock, and oliguria. It can be fatal if not recognized and appropriately treated soon after its onset. Six of the 40 reported cases died. In these the condition was either recognized late or treatment was begun too late.

Twenty-six of the 40 reported patients had some type of disease of the spinal column. One had a shoulder fusion. In all the others, there was disease of the hip or fracture of the pelvis or femur. The onset of symptoms varies from immediately after casting to 12 weeks thereafter. In 28 patients initial symptoms occurred less than 2 weeks after cast application, and in 11 patients the symptoms began between 3 and 12 weeks after casting. Bisla and Louis stated that only those with onset of symptoms within 2 weeks after casting should be classified as having a cast syndrome, because the mere presence of a cast does not necessarily implicate it as the cause. Other factors, such as weight loss with loss of fat in the mesentery, accompanied by prolonged bedrest in the supine position, and accentuated lumbar lordosis, may be the cause, as has been mentioned by others (Wayne, Miller, and Eiseman, 1971; Bunch and Delaney, 1970). In some patients in whom the cast syndrome followed weight loss, the symptoms disappeared after the lost weight was regained, despite the presence of a cast. The cast syndrome should be suspected in any patient in whom nausea and vomiting occur within 2 weeks after application of a body cast. This suspicion can and should be investigated by a plain, flat x-ray film of the abdomen. It is supported if the film shows dilatation of the duodenum and stomach.

When the patient's condition permits, an upper gastrointestinal fluoroscopic and x-ray film study is indicated to confirm the diagnosis. An aortogram to show the acuteness of the angle and the decreased distance between the superior mesenteric artery and the aorta is the most accurate diagnostic method (Mansberger and associates, 1968) but is seldom required to establish the diagnosis.

When the diagnosis is established, prompt treatment is begun by restoring fluid and electrolyte balance. A nasogastric tube is inserted and attached to suction in order to decompress the stomach and duodenum. If symptoms persist for more than 24 hours, the cast should be removed. "Simple windowing of the cast is insufficient. This was done in five patients and resulted in two deaths and delayed function in three. Conservative treatment should be continued following removal of the cast, using change of position for stomach drainage. If there is no evidence of recovery with conservative treatment, surgical intervention is indicated. Among the 40 reported patients, conservative treatment was successful in only 14 patients. Operation was performed in 20 patients, duodenojejunostomy in 18, and mobilization of the duodenum with division of the ligament of Treitz in 2. Operation also should be considered in those patients for whom cast removal is not advisable" (Bisla and Louis, 1975). Of the three patients, two were treated by conservative methods, but the third required duodenojejunostomy after removal of the cast and conservative therapy had been unsuccessful. All were successful.

ASSOCIATION WITH SCOLIOSIS

The treatment of *scoliosis, lordosis,* or *scoliolordosis* is occasionally associated with acute obstructive vascular compression of the duodenum. Evarts, Winters and Hall (1971) reported a total of 30 such cases collected from the literature and from their own experience. Eighteen were associated with correction of spinal curvature and 12 with the application of a body jacket. "Traction on the spine in patients with scoliosis, with significant correction of the spinal curvature (21 to 61 degrees in this series) may increase the acuteness of the angle of departure of the superior mesenteric artery sufficiently to cause duodenal obstruction. Abrupt correction of a spinal curvature by internal spinal fixation, halo-femoral traction, a localizer cast, or Milwaukee brace may apply the requisite traction."

Other factors that contribute to the association of vascular compression of the duodenum and operative treatment of scoliosis are immobilization in bed, prolonged supine position, and weight loss. The term "cast syndrome" is a misnomer when used to describe the vascular duodenal obstruction that may develop as a complication of the treatment of scoliosis without the application of a corrective cast.

Although the incidence of this complication in surgery for scoliosis is low, it seems advisable that all patients undergoing surgery for scoliosis have prophylactic nasogastric suction in the immediate postoperative period until bowel function returns, as suggested by Puranik, Keiser, and Gilbert (1972).

VOLVULUS OF THE STOMACH

Gastric volvulus or torsion is a rare condition. It has been recognized as an entity since 1866 when Berti first described the lesion found at necropsy. During the following 103 years approximately 265 cases were reported in the medical literature (Camblos, 1969). The condition may occur at any age; the age range is from 3 days to 87 years in the literature, with the majority between the ages of 45 and 75 years. Gastric volvulus is rare in infants and children (Cole and Dickinson, 1971). Only 10 of Dalgaard's (1952) 150 patients were in the pediatric age group. The sex incidence is about equal at all ages.

Volvulus is defined as "intestinal obstruction due to a knotting and twisting of the bowel;" hence, as pointed out by Cole and Dickinson (1971), "the use of the term *volvulus* should be restricted to those instances in which a hollow organ undergoes a rotation that results in complete obstruction of its lumen. If such obstruction does not occur, then torsion is the only accurate terminology. True volvulus, as defined above, cannot be partial or chronic." This strict semantic distinction is so frequently violated in the literature that for convenience it also will be violated here.

To understand the mechanism of torsion of the stomach it is important to remember that the stomach is held firmly only at the cardia and that the pylorus is not so firmly fixed. The four suspensory ligaments of the stomach are the hepatic, splenic, colic, and phrenic.

Three types of volvulus, depending upon the axis of rotation, have been described:

1. *Mesenterioaxial volvulus* in which the rotation occurs from right to left or, less frequently, left to right, and the rotating part may pass either forward or backward around

the axis of the gastric mesenteries, which is roughly a vertical line at right angles to the cardiopyloric line (Fig. 5–46A and B). It tends to approximate the fixed cardioesophageal and pyloric portions of the stomach. This type is more likely to be chronic or intermittent.

2. *Organoaxial volvulus* (Fig. 5–46C) consists of rotation of the stomach around an axis of a line connecting the cardia and the pylorus. The rotation is usually from right to left but may be from left to right and the rotating part may pass either backward or forward. Usually the colon and spleen are also displaced.

This type is most often seen as the "upside-down stomach" in patients with large paraesophageal hernias (see page 358 in Volume 1). It tends to cause obstruction at the cardia and at the pylorus. Thus the stomach becomes a closed loop, distends rapidly, produces acute symptoms, and requires rapid decompression.

3. A *combined type of volvulus*. The stomach can twist in a combination of the mesenterioaxial and the organoaxial directions, usually with one of the major axial rotations predominating — for example, a primary mesenterioaxial rotation with a secondary organoaxial rotation of the fundus.

"Patients with the combined type usually give a long history of vague symptoms, occasionally with acute, severe episodes. This occurs because mesenterioaxial volvulus tends to cause approximation of the fixed cardioesophageal and pyloric portions of the stomach and in doing so predisposes to further twisting in an organoaxial direction" (Gosin and Ballinger, 1965).

The combined type is the least common of the three. The relative frequency of the mesenterioaxial and organoaxial types has varied in different reported series.

Volvulus may be partial or complete, or more than one turn may occur. Even a 180-degree, organoaxial rotation of the stomach can completely occlude both pylorus and cardia and lead to gastric gangrene. Complete twists usually lead to disturbances of the blood supply with obstruction of the lumen and present an acute surgical emergency. Rotation may be in either direction.

The severity of the volvulus accounts for either acute or chronic symptoms. Volvulus up to 180 degrees may be without obstruction and may undergo spontaneous resolution or reduction. Rotation beyond 180 degrees presents a picture of an acute abdominal catastrophe and acute obstruction.

The initial effect of rotation is to close the pyloric end of the stomach by combined kinking and twisting. As the amount of rotation increases, the mobile pylorus approximates the immobile cardiac end of the stomach and the two orifices may form one pivot around which further twisting of the viscus occurs. In these cases death may occur if the volvulus is not reduced surgically.

Wastell and Ellis, in 1971, collected from the literature the reports of 198 cases of gastric volvulus, added 8 cases of their own, and tabulated their analyses of the total. Not all reports contained all details for each category of information, therefore the number of patients in each group varies, as seen in Table 5–1. Item 3 shows that "occasionally, only part of the stomach is involved in the volvulus. This happens more often in an acute volvulus, 9 of the 11 cases of partial organoaxial volvulus being of an acute type. Even though a volvulus is partial in nature, necrosis of the stomach wall may still occur."

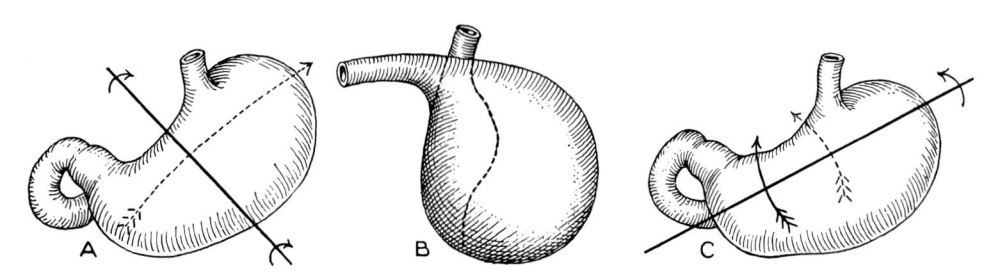

Figure 5–46. *A* and *B*, Mesenterioaxial volvulus. *C*, Organoaxial volvulus. (From Buchanan, J.: Volvulus of the stomach. Br. J. Surg. *18*:99, 1930.)

Table 5-1. Gastric Volvulus: Type, Sex, Extent, Direction, and Severity

1. The Type of Gastric Volvulus Found in 206 Patients

Mesenterioaxial	60	(29%)
Organoaxial	122	(59%)
Combined	5	(2%)
Not classified	19	(10%)
Total	206	

2. The Type of Volvulus Found in Men and Women

	Men	Women
Mesenterioaxial	29	27
Organoaxial	48	66
Combined	2	1
Total	79 (46%)	94 (54%)

3. The Extent of the Volvulus in Each Type

	Total	Partial
Mesenterioaxial	57	3
Organoaxial	111	11
Mixed	5	0
Total	173	14

4. The Direction of the Volvulus in Each Type

	Anterior	Posterior
Mesenterioaxial	37	10
Organoaxial	85	8
Total	122	18

5. The Occurrence of Primary and Secondary Volvulus in Each Type

	Primary	Secondary
Mesenterioaxial	22	38
Organoaxial	32	90
Total	54 (30%)	128 (70%)

6. The Severity of Volvulus in Each Type

	Acute	Chronic
Mesenterioaxial	36	24
Organoaxial	73	49
Total	109	73

From Wastell, C., and Ellis, H.: Volvulus of the stomach; A review with a report of 8 cases. Br. J. Surg. 58:557, 1971.

In Item 4 of Table 5-1, an organoaxial volvulus, in which the transverse colon lies in front of the stomach, and a mesenterioaxial volvulus, in which the pylorus passes in front of the stomach, are both termed "anterior." Anterior rotation is much more common than posterior rotation, as would be expected for anatomic reasons. For posterior rotation to occur in the organoaxial type of volvulus, the transverse colon must pass behind the stomach, elongating or tearing the mesocolon as it passes.

Etiology

An essential predisposing cause of gastric volvulus is marked relaxation or abnormality of the four suspensory ligaments of the stomach. The anatomic abnormalities associated with gastric volvulus have been summarized by Tanner (1968): With extreme laxity of the ligaments, volvulus may occur merely because a heavy food bolus lies in the central axis around which rotation takes place. Abnormal elongation of the ligaments of the stomach may be an accompaniment of gastric ptosis or chronic pyloric obstruction. Congenital absence of one or more of these ligaments is another predisposing cause of volvulus. Gastric volvulus may be caused by abnormal bands and adhesion produced by a gastric ulcer or tumor. Other etiologic factors include failure of attachment of the greater omentum, permitting increased mobility of the stomach.

The commonest of these types are caused by herniation into abnormal spaces. The best example is (1) a large sliding hiatal or paraesophageal hernia. Because the cardia and pylorus are relatively fixed, the body of the stomach (with or without the transverse colon) is drawn into the posterior mediastinal space by negative intrathoracic pressure to form an organoaxial volvulus. These usually can be treated surgically by withdrawing the stomach and sac to below the diaphragm and repairing the hernial orifice. This type of hernia is illustrated on page 358 of Volume 1.

(2) Other forms of diaphragmatic hernia, either congenital or acquired—most often acquired and traumatic—are far less frequently the cause of gastric volvulus. Tanner (1968) reported a 65-year-old woman who had fallen from a height 30 years previously and now needed treatment. At operation, a traumatic defect in the posterior diaphragm was seen, and the most mobile part of the stomach, the greater curvature, had entered the chest, followed by all but the cardia and antrum, to form a 180-degree volvulus. It was easy to reposition

the stomach and repair the diaphragmatic defect with sutures.

A number of cases have been reported in which a surgical diaphragmatic incision, made to enter the abdomen through a thoracotomy, was repaired and then dehisced postoperatively, creating a defect in the diaphragm through which a gastric volvulus developed.

(3) Gastric volvulus is frequently associated with abnormalities of the diaphragm, such as congenital or acquired diaphragmatic eventration. Eventration may be congenital in origin, be of unknown cause, or occur after disease or accidental or operative division of the phrenic nerve. Eventration is seen much more commonly on the left side. Acquired eventration has frequently resulted from a previous left phrenicotomy for the treatment of tuberculosis. It has also been reported following a right phrenicotomy. Acquired eventration following surgical phrenicotomy was the etiologic factor in 21 of the 27 cases with gastric volvulus reported by Tanner (1968), and also in a significant number of patients with gastric volvulus reported by others.

In an elevated diaphragm, the increased subphrenic space invites being filled with abdominal viscera, thus leading to an organoaxial volvulus. The negative intrathoracic pressure and paradoxic movement of the diaphragm will continue to increase the eventration, hence the gastric volvulus tends to increase with time (Tanner, 1968).

Other conditions reported with an associated gastric volvulus are hour-glass stomach, tears in the gastrohepatic and gastrocolic omenta, and intrinsic and extrinsic pressure on the stomach by tumors which may act as leading or precipitating factors. Included among the exciting causes are phrenicotomy, acute dilatation of the stomach, intractable vomiting, and excessive antiperistaltic movements. Ruckley and Fraser (1968) described a case of gastric volvulus associated with leukemic splenomegaly.

In two of the seven cases of gastric volvulus reported by Sawyer, Hammer, and Fenton (1956), obstructing organoaxial volvulus occurred as acute postoperative complications 3 weeks after cholecystectomy. In both cases an associated large hiatal hernia apparently was neither recognized nor repaired at the time of the cholecystectomy, and the stomach volvulated into it 3 weeks later. This demonstrated that gastric volvulus is a potential postoperative complication following an intra-abdominal operation for some other disorder, particularly if there is a concomitant esophageal hiatal hernia or other diaphragmatic defect. It also suggests that if a large concomitant esophageal hiatal hernia or other diaphragmatic defect is found in an upper abdominal operation it may be advisable to repair the diaphragmatic defect at this time, provided the patient's condition is satisfactory and it can be done without increasing the surgical hazards and magnitude. If repair proves inadvisable, the defect is an alert for the possible occurrence of gastric volvulus as a postoperative complication.

Some investigators have considered distention of the adjacent colon to be an etiologic factor in gastric volvulus. Colonic distention frequently accompanies chronic intermittent volvulus, but its etiologic role is disputed. Stremple (1973) reported a 21-year-old female patient who presented chronic intermittent gastric volvulus and concomitant splenic flexure syndrome. It was believed that the distended colon had contributed to the patient's obstipation and chronic intermittent gastric volvulus. Operation was performed because of intractable symptoms. At laparotomy through a midline incision the transverse colon and the splenic flexure were seen to be distended with gas. There was no attachment between the stomach and colon. The greater omentum and gastrocolic and gastrolienal ligaments were absent. The stomach remained in situ on delivery of the colon. Both the descending and ascending colons had long mesenteries.

Approximately 4 feet of dilated colon, corresponding to the transverse colon and splenic flexure, were resected, and end-to-end anastomosis was performed. The greater curvature of the stomach was fixed to the newly positioned transverse mesocolon with interrupted sutures, forming a new gastrocolic ligament. The remainder of the greater curvature of the stomach was fixed to the posterior parietal peritoneum up to the esophagocardiac junction as a posterior gastropexy (Fig. 5–47). The patient was discharged 16 days postoperatively and 12 months later was satisfactory on follow-up.

VOLVULUS OF THE STOMACH

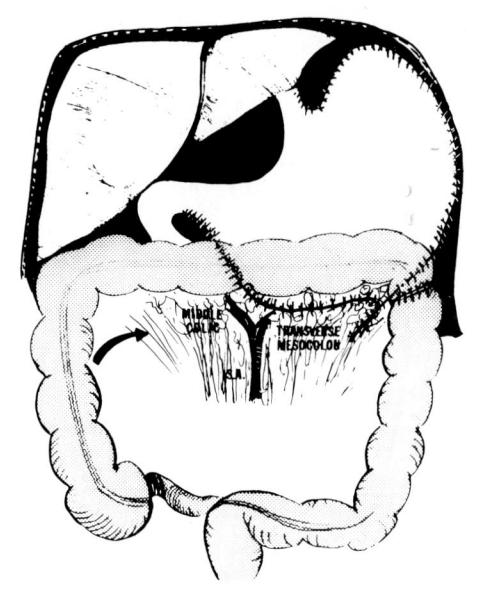

Figure 5–47. Operative procedure used to correct anatomic and functional abnormalities. (From Stremple, J. F.: A new operation for the anatomic correction of chronic intermittent gastric volvulus. Am. J. Surg. 125:362, 1973.)

Any volvulus that occurs in the presence of intra-abdominal disease or abnormality which is directly related to that condition is termed *secondary*, such as when the stomach herniates through a congenital or acquired defect in the diaphragm. When there is no associated intra-abdominal disease or abnormality, or when disease or abnormality is present but no specific cause and effect relationship can be established, the volvulus is termed *idiopathic*. In the world literature on gastric volvulus, 30 per cent of the reported cases occurred idiopathically, and the remainder were related to anatomic defects (Wastell and Ellis, 1971). Dalgaard (1952) pointed out that before an idiopathic volvulus can occur there must be considerable lengthening or even rupture of the gastrosplenic and gastrocolic ligaments which fix the stomach.

The volvulus is called *primary* when rotation occurs solely because of laxity of the fixed points around the stomach; i.e., laxity of the gastric vessels, the gastrosplenic ligament, and the second part of the duodenum must be present.

Sixty cases of mesenterioaxial volvulus for which data were available were collected by Wastell and Ellis. Thirty-eight (63 per cent) were of the secondary type. Ninety (74 per cent) of a total of 122 cases of organoaxial volvulus were secondary (see Item 5 in Table 5–1). The severity of the volvulus in each type is shown in Item 6 of Table 5–1. The researchers commented that they had not seen an acute gastric volvulus despite the fact that 60 per cent of the mesenterioaxial and 64 per cent of the organoaxial cases of volvulus collected from the literature were recorded as acute. This discrepancy was believed to be due to bias, in that cases of acute volvulus, with its often dire consequences, were considered worth reporting more often than cases of asymptomatic chronic volvulus. In actual practice an acute gastric volvulus is encountered relatively rarely. An acute volvulus has a much graver prognosis. In this collected series, 20 (56 per cent) of 36 patients with an acute mesenterioaxial volvulus and 31 (42 per cent) of 73 patients with an acute organoaxial volvulus died. Only 3 (13 per cent) of 24 patients with chronic mesenterioaxial volvulus and 4 (10 per cent) of 41 patients with chronic organoaxial volvulus died.

Symptoms

"Gastric volvulus may present as an acute emergency, produce long-standing symptoms, or produce no symptoms at all" (Tanner, 1968). The symptomatology of gastric volvulus varies according to whether the volvulus is acute with complete obstruction or chronic with partial obstruction and with or without intermittent episodes of acute obstruction.

Acute complete volvulus is rare. The onset of symptoms follows, with striking frequency, the ingestion of a heavy meal. The disorder is usually manifested by the unheralded sudden onset of severe epigastric pain which often radiates into the back or left chest or both. This is accompanied by vomiting, followed by intractable retching without the production of appreciable vomitus and without bile in the vomitus. The upper abdomen becomes distended, with little if any abdominal tenderness. The lower abdomen remains flat. Shock is not an initial symptom, as strangulation of the blood supply does not occur until later. If the volvulus remains untreated, pyloric occlusion causes incessant retching; obstruction of the cardia causes inability to vomit or to have a tube passed into the stomach; and the resulting closed-loop type of obstruction causes the stomach to become rapidly distended with gas and fluid. "Acute gastric volvulus is a surgical emergency of the first magnitude" (Guernsey and Conolly, 1963). If not relieved, vascular occlusion with subsequent necrosis of part of or the entire gastric wall occurs, accompanied by shock and eventual death.

Many patients with a gastric volvulus secondary to a large sliding hiatal or paraesophageal hernia are almost symptom-free or have only isolated attacks of epigastric pain, sometimes radiating into the back, with retching that mimics biliary colic. At times Borchardt's triad is present, indicating obstruction of the cardia. Abdominal physical signs are usually absent. X-ray examination usually shows an upside-down stomach in a hiatal hernia. Such patients rarely have heartburn because in the rolling hernia the esophagogastric angle is increased.

Diagnosis

Borchardt, in 1904, described a triad of criteria he considered must be present to diagnose acute gastric volvulus: (1) sudden onset of severe epigastric pain, accompanied by (2) early vomiting, followed by intractable retching and inability to vomit, and (3) inability to pass a nasogastric tube into the stomach. The test of time has proved its value.

The diagnosis of acute gastric volvulus is suggested by the presence of Borchardt's triad and usually can be confirmed by a plain x-ray film of the abdomen, taken in the upright position, which shows tremendous distention of the stomach with two fluid levels. In some cases the correct diagnosis is not established until laparotomy.

A barium swallow x-ray is unlikely to be helpful in diagnosing acute complete gastric volvulus, because the barium is unable to enter the stomach, or, if it does, it cannot be retained. The barium swallow x-ray will demonstrate only the area of the upper twist and the relative inability of the barium to enter the stomach (Guernsey and Conolly, 1963).

A few of the more important conditions confused with acute gastric volvulus are ruptured peptic ulcer, intestinal obstruction, abdominal apoplexy, acute pancreatitis, and mesenteric embolism (Sawyer, Hammer, and Fenton, 1956).

Ascherman, Bednarz, and Olix (1958) pointed out that the x-ray picture may not be diagnostic but may show gas between the liver and the diaphragm and pose the differential diagnosis among (1) free air from a perforated viscus or induced pneumoperitoneum; (2) encapsulated subdiaphragmatic abscess; and (3) a segment of large (more common) or small bowel interposed between the diaphragm and the liver. The haustral markings of gas-filled distended colon traversing the radiolucent area beneath the right hemidiaphragm identify large bowel. Also, gaseous distention of the transverse colon (aerocoly) can be recognized by the fact that the left half of the transverse colon can produce a filling defect by compressing the greater curvature of the stomach, resulting in a biloculate-appearing stomach. Often absence of the falciform ligament permits the transverse colon to travel upward in the front of the stomach and be insinuated under the diaphragm between the anterior surface of the liver and the diaphragm, they report.

X-ray differentiation from simple cascade stomach, which is said to be found fluoroscopically in obese persons (Stremple, 1973), may also be difficult. Helpful hints are (1) there is one fluid level in cascade stomach, whereas there may be two fluid levels in gastric volvulus; (2) the greater curvature of the stomach is uppermost in volvulus and is in normal position in cascade stomach; and (3) the esophageal orifice is in the usual normal anatomic position in cascade stomach and is in a lower position in volvulus.

Chronic gastric volvulus is more common than the acute type. It is more difficult to diagnose and more likely to be overlooked because its symptoms are less striking and less characteristic, or may even be absent. In partial volvulus without complete obstruction, the symptoms may be mild. Gastrointestinal symptoms associated with chronic intermittent gastric volvulus are not as well defined as are Borchardt's triad of symptoms in acute gastric volvulus. Pain or even severe discomfort is not necessarily a feature of chronic gastric volvulus.

The symptoms associated with chronic intermittent gastric volvulus are frequently those of a mild continuous or intermittent dyspepsia. Some patients complain of distress or bloating during or shortly after the intake of food, while others repeatedly suffer from short or prolonged attacks of recurrent cramping epigastric pains accompanied by vomiting or retching. Since these symptoms can occur with many different upper abdominal conditions, both functional and organic, "the true diagnosis is often unsuspected and may be made only after upper gastrointestinal x-ray studies are obtained (Gosin and Ballinger, 1965). Plain films of the abdomen usually show a large gas bubble in the epigastrium. If the patient is placed in the lateral or erect position, an air-fluid level within this bubble may be demonstrated. In partial or chronic volvulus, a barium swallow upper gastrointestinal x-ray series will visualize the abnormal placement of the stomach. The diagnosis of chronic intermittent gastric volvulus is made by combination of the symptoms and x-ray studies. Since the episodes are intermittent "the x-ray is not always diagnostic when taken between episodes" (Guernsey and Conolly, 1963).

"The secondary forms of gastric volvulus may present the picture of the basic disorder, e.g., of hiatal hernia or of pyloric obstruction. During the attacks, abdominal examination is usually uninformative, but there may be some epigastric distention. Plain radiographs of the upper abdomen may show eventration of the diaphragm, a large hiatal hernia or a dilated gas- and fluid-filled stomach. Barium meal examination between attacks of discomfort may show hiatal hernia, peptic ulcer, or some other primary or associated lesion. The volvulus may present a confusing picture, but usually it can be recognized. It may be difficult to pass a nasogastric tube during an attack. However, if the tube is placed in the stomach, the volvulus may correct itself after gastric decompression alone" (Tanner, 1968).

It has been suggested that if the volvulus can be corrected by nasogastric aspiration of the stomach, it will not recur, so definitive surgical correction of the disorder is unnecessary. However, Gosin and Ballinger (1965) and others have shown that a gastric volvulus which has been reduced spontaneously or at operation is likely to recur unless the factors that caused the volvulus are corrected surgically.

Complications

Metcalfe-Gibson (1975) reported that "volvulus of the stomach is a rare condition, and complications of gastric volvulus are even more uncommon." He described a 60-year-old man with volvulus of the gastric fundus that was complicated by hemorrhage. The predisposing cause of the gastric volvulus was eventration of the left diaphragm due to a left phrenic nerve crush for tuberculosis at age 19.

At laparotomy the stomach was seen to be enlarged and lying more anteriorly than usual. There was no external evidence of peptic ulceration. When opened, the lesser peritoneal sac revealed the gastric fundus rotated posteriorly and occupying the lesser sac, pushing the stomach anteriorly (Figs. 5–48 and 5–49). Through a gastrotomy the bleeding could be seen coming from the opening into the retroverted fundus. In order to gain access to the fundus, the duodenum was transected and the stomach mobilized as far as the esophagus on the lesser curvature and to above the short gastric vessels on the greater curvature. By elevating the stomach vertically the fundus could be mobilized from the posterior abdominal wall by blunt dissection and invaginated up through the gastrotomy. Multiple erosions of its mucosa were seen. The invaginated

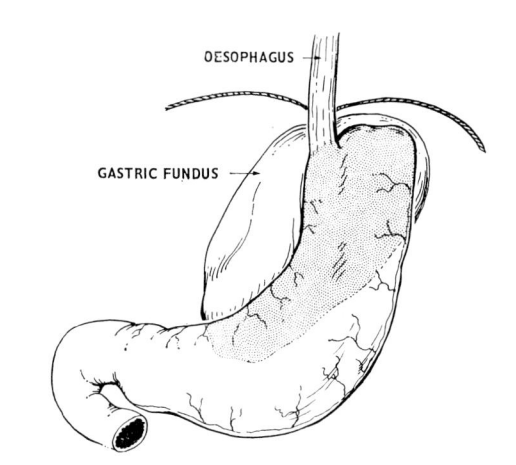

Figure 5–48. Anterior aspect of stomach and gastric fundus. (From Metcalfe-Gibson, C.: A case of haemorrhage from volvulus of the gastric fundus. Br. J. Surg. 62:225, 1975.)

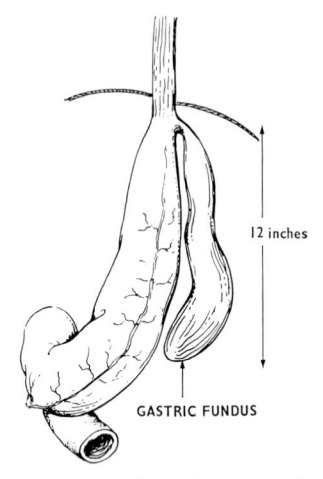

Figure 5–49. Left lateral aspect of stomach and empty gastric fundus. (From Metcalfe-Gibson, cited in previous figure.)

fundus was excised level with the esophageal opening and, since the antral region of the gastric remnant appeared ischemic, Polya gastrectomy was also performed. The completed anatomy is depicted in Figure 5–50.

The postoperative course was complicated by transient jaundice and prolonged left basal pneumonia, but the patient was asymptomatic and back at work at the 5-month follow-up.

Gastric volvulus associated with paraesophageal hernias commonly develops one or more of the following complications: (1) ulceration of the herniated stomach; (2) hemorrhage; (3) complete obstruction; (4) strangulation with gangrene requiring partial or, rarely, total gastrectomy; (5) occasionally perforation with resulting peritonitis; and/or (6) pulmonary complications. These are discussed in the section on paraesophageal hernia on pp. 358 to 372 in Volume 1.

An occasional complication of gastric volvulus has been rupture of the spleen. Hudspeth and McWhorter (1971) reported such a case. The patient was a 61-year-old woman with a history of intermittent episodes of epigastric pain and vomiting and retching, recurring about once a year during the past 15 years. She was admitted to the hospital in acute distress, with abdominal pain and distention and nausea and retching without vomiting, which had begun shortly after she ate a large meal four hours previously. Laparotomy was performed after rapid preoperative preparation. At operation, a mesenterioaxial type of gastric volvulus twisted 180 degrees in a counterclockwise direction was found. Other findings included congenital absence of the gastrocolic ligament and great redundancy of the gastrohepatic ligament. Also, a large quantity of blood was noted free in the peritoneal cavity. "Further exploration showed the source of the bleeding to be a ruptured spleen which literally had been torn from its peritoneal attachments by the pull of the greater curvature of the stomach on the gastrosplenic ligament as it was forced anteriorly and to the right. No other abnormalities were noted in the abdominal cavity."

Treatment consisted of reduction of the volvulus, construction of a gastrocolic ligament, plication of the gastrohepatic ligament, and splenectomy. The mesentery of the ascending colon was redundant so it also was plicated. The patient had an uneventful recovery and was well 5 years later.

Treatment

Methods of treating gastric volvulus can be divided into nonoperative and operative.

NONOPERATIVE TREATMENT. This depends primarily upon passing a nasogastric tube into the stomach for decompression of that distended organ. This method cannot be used in cases of acute complete gastric volvulus because one of the diagnostic characteristics of such cases is the fact

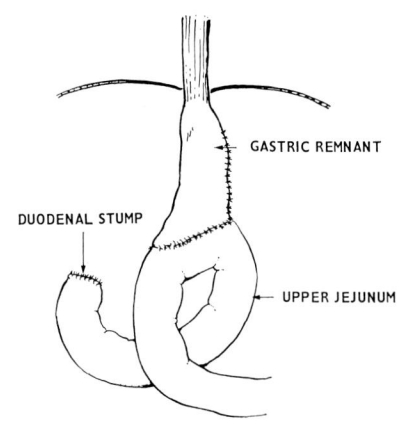

Figure 5–50. Completed anatomy after fundectomy and gastrectomy. (From Metcalfe-Gibson, cited in Figure 5–48.)

that a tube cannot be passed into the stomach. In patients with chronic or intermittent gastric volvulus, it may be difficult to pass a nasogastric tube during an episode of discomfort. Furthermore, Cole and Dickinson (1971) warned that in patients with gastric volvulus, particularly children, attempts to pass a nasogastric tube into the stomach are fraught with the danger of perforating that organ, and they cited cases in which this mishap occurred.

When a tube is passed successfully into the stomach and decompresses that viscus, spontaneous detorsion of the volvulus may occur once the stomach is completely emptied. Although some have recommended that simple decompression is sufficient treatment, Gosin and Ballinger (1965) have shown that decompression alone without operative fixation of the stomach provides no protection against recurrence of the volvulus. They believe that it should be considered only as a preoperative measure, not as a definitive procedure, and that operative inspection and appropriate surgical measures are necessary to prevent recurrences.

Some patients with recurring partial obstruction due to incomplete volvulus have been controlled on a medical program without resort to surgery. Sawyer, Hammer, and Fenton (1956) reported such a case. However in patients whose symptoms persist and are unbearable, and in all patients with acute gastric volvulus, some type of operative intervention is imperative.

SURGICAL TREATMENT. According to Gosin and Ballinger (1965), Berg reported the first operation for gastric volvulus in 1897. Since then over 200 cases have been described in the world literature. Experience has shown that surgical treatment is indicated in all cases of acute complete gastric volvulus. Such cases usually are acute surgical emergencies, requiring stabilization of the patient's condition by IV fluids and often by adjunctive therapy, followed by prompt operation. Although the mortality of operations for acute total gastric volvulus in the past has been 40 per cent (Wastell and Ellis, 1971), patients not operated upon have invariably died. In recent years the operative mortality rate has notably decreased.

Surgical treatment is not as universally indicated for chronic or recurrent gastric volvulus. Tanner (1968) warned that "care must be taken in the selection of these cases for surgery and their symptoms differentiated from those of nervous, gastritic, and biliary dyspepsia, peptic ulcer, or hiatal hernia."

Operations for treating gastric volvulus include decompression and detorsion of the stomach as well as methods to prevent recurrence by repair of its causative anatomic defect. Furthermore, when it seems necessary, the stomach should be fixed in place after reduction of the volvulus and any related concomitant pathology should be removed or corrected. This would include any associated tumor, hiatal hernia, diaphragmatic eventration or hernia, or absence or relaxation of ligaments.

A variety of surgical procedures for treating gastric volvulus have been suggested and performed by various surgeons and commented upon by Tanner (1968) in his classic paper on gastric volvulus given as the Philip B. Price Lecture at the University of Utah on October 6, 1966. The choice of operation depends upon the etiology of the volvulus and the condition of the stomach, the contiguous structures, and the patient at the time of operation.

Surgical Technics

For operations on patients with gastric volvulus, general inhalation anesthesia, using an endotracheal tube, is the method of choice. The patient is placed supine on the operating table, and the abdominal cavity is entered through an upper midline or right or left paramedian incision. Tanner (1968) advised a long upper abdominal incision in all patients with *chronic* volvulus who require surgery; because there is often some doubt about the true cause of the symptoms a generous exposure is needed. Before manipulating the stomach one can then carefully inspect the anatomy; note any bands, obstruction, ulcers, tumors, or abnormal ligamentous laxity; and, by palpation, search for gallstones, a diaphragmatic hernia, or eventration of the diaphragm. An eventrated diaphragm is felt to be thinned, and, in extreme cases, one can palpate the chest wall through it to as high as the inner surface of the second rib.

When the abdominal cavity has been entered, the surgeon may have difficulty recognizing the exact anatomy of the disorder. In acute cases, and in some chronic cases, at opening of the abdomen the greatly distended stomach presents immediately into the wound and is so distended, and its walls so dangerously thinned, by trapped gas and fluid that even with an extensive incision it is often impossible to untwist the volvulus without first emptying its contents. If the volvulus cannot be reduced, the gas and fluid trapped in the twisted stomach can be evacuated by passing an aspirating trochar through its wall. This opening in the stomach wall should be closed by suture before the volvulus is reduced, since the gastric opening may migrate to an inaccessible location when normal anatomic relations are restored.

An alternative method for decompressing the stomach, after the peritoneal cavity has been opened at operation, is by direct aspiration with a needle, instead of a trochar, passed through the gastric wall. This partially reduces the dilatation and volvulus so that the anesthesiologist can then pass a nasogastric tube which the surgeon may guide manually through the gastroesophageal junction to complete the decompression after the needle has been withdrawn and the puncture closed by suture. The trochar method seems simpler, quicker, and preferable.

After most of the gastric contents have been evacuated, the volvulus can be promptly reduced, returning the stomach to its normal position with rapid return of its vascular supply. Guernsey and Conolly (1963) pointed out that rotation of the stomach is not completely corrected until the coronary vessels have been returned to their normal position.

After decompression and detorsion of the stomach, exploration of the abdomen, and return of the stomach to its normal position, two additional major procedures must be considered: (1) correcting the abnormality causing the volvulus in the secondary type; and (2) deciding whether or not gastropexy is needed, and, if it is, performing the gastropexy that is most appropriate for the patient.

SECONDARY VOLVULUS

If the volvulus is secondary in type, and other organic lesions or abnormalities, such as ulcers, adhesions, tumors, herniation, eventrated diaphragm, and absent or deficient gastrocolic or some other ligament, are also present as a significant causative factor, it is essential that the operation be designed to correct the abnormality causing the volvulus. This may require repair of a hiatal or diaphragmatic hernia, plication of an eventrated diaphragm, closure or plication of a deficient gastrocolic or some other ligament, or partial gastrectomy for a benign or malignant lesion in the stomach or proximal duodenum.

In some cases, such as eventration of the diaphragm, it may be too difficult or risky to repair the primary cause. However, when feasible, satisfactory repair of the causative factor usually obviates the need for gastropexy, as exemplified by the following types of cases.

REPAIR OF A DIAPHRAGMATIC HERNIA. The commonest type of mild volvulus or upside-down stomach is that synonymous with paraesophageal hiatal hernia. Tanner (1968) reported 26 such cases as well as 2 cases of gastric volvulus associated with traumatic diaphragmatic hernia, treated successfully by reduction of the hernia and simple repair of the diaphragm via the abdominal route but omitting gastropexy.

Others (Wastell and Ellis, 1971) have reported similar successes in treating these types of secondary gastric volvulus by the same technic, without recurrence of the volvulus during follow-up for various periods of time.

REPAIR OF EVENTRATION OF THE DIAPHRAGM. Tanner (1968) called attention to the fact that some patients with gastric volvulus associated with eventration of the diaphragm have dyspnea on exertion as their primary complaint. Postprandial discomfort and fullness is a secondary consideration. In these cases it seems desirable to restore the diaphragm to its normal shape by an operation directly upon it. He warned that such a procedure is a major one and may be unsuitable for some elderly patients. Also, it is not known how well the often paper-thin diaphragm will retain its normal shape. However, in a 43-year-old woman with these manifestations, Tanner reconstructed the diaphragm as follows: Through a left transthoracic approach, the diaphragm was reduced in size by inverting folds of the eventrated diaphragm into the abdomen and suturing the edges together, making a keel-like projection into the peri-

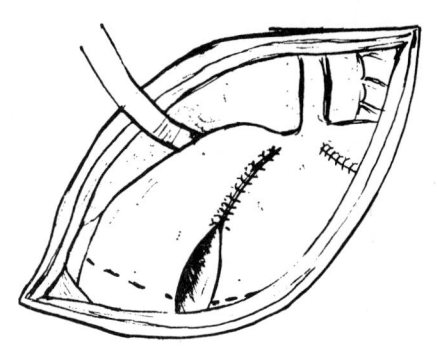

Figure 5-51. Tanner's method of direct repair of the eventrated diaphragm. Three radial keel-like inversions of the diaphragm and then a circumferential keel are made to project into the peritoneal cavity, and finally the diaphragm is carefully darned over with monofilament nylon to help maintain the new shape. (From Tanner, N. C.: Chronic and recurrent volvulus of the stomach. Am. J. Surg. *115*:505, 1968.)

toneal cavity. Three keels were made in a radial direction (Fig. 5–51). To retain this new shape, the diaphragm was extensively darned with monofilament nylon on an atraumatic needle. On examination three years later, her symptoms had disappeared and roentgenograms showed that the diaphragm remained much as it was after operation.

In two other patients treated by colonic displacement, respiratory embarassassment remained a problem and Tanner was considering phrenicorrhaphy for them.

DIVISION OF BANDS. Simple division of the bands that obstruct or sling up the stomach was adequate in two such cases reported by Tanner (1968), but partial gastrectomy was necessary in a third, and gastropexy with colonic displacement was also performed in two additional cases. Cole and Dickinson (1971) reported that of five pediatric patients with gastric volvulus associated with bands, one was treated successfully by division of the bands alone and the remaining four were treated successfully by division of the bands plus gastropexy.

In some cases fixation of the stomach in place may also be indicated even though the cause of the volvulus has been corrected. Although in many cases fixation of the stomach occurs naturally by development of postoperative adhesions between the stomach and anterior abdominal wall, this cannot be relied upon. If fixation is indicated, it is more reliable to perform gastropexy by suturing the anterior gastric wall to the anterior abdominal wall.

IDIOPATHIC OR PRIMARY VOLVULUS

When no causative factor is found, treatment for idiopathic or primary cases consists of detorsion and emptying of the stomach and some type of gastropexy to fix the stomach in place and prevent recurrence of the volvulus.

Although some investigators have reported that in many cases of primary volvulus all that needs to be done at operation is to guide a nasogastric tube into the stomach, decompress that organ, untwist the volvulus, and reposition the stomach to normal, experience has shown that decompression and detorsion alone are likely to be followed by recurrence. Therefore, after the volvulus has been untwisted and the stomach repositioned normally, the stomach should be anchored in some way to prevent recurrence of the volvulus.

Methods that have been advocated for fixing the stomach in place include *suturing the greater curvature of the stomach to the wall of the transverse colon.* This could be ineffective and dangerous if the colon is extremely redundant, dilated, and thin-walled and its ligaments greatly relaxed so that it is free to rotate on a long mesentery.

PARTIAL GASTRECTOMY. This has been widely advocated in the past as a method for preventing recurrence, after a gastric volvulus has been decompressed and detorsed. Tanner (1968) stated that the main objective of his paper was to deprecate the universal use of gastrectomy for gastric volvulus because this procedure is too severe to be used for minor degrees of dyspepsia or for recurring crises. He noted that if gastrectomy is performed for discomfort caused by nonulcer dyspepsia, dumping and other postcibal disabilities are more likely to occur than when the operation is performed for ulcer. He cited cases that supported this observation.

However, partial gastrectomy is imperative occasionally in acute cases with gangrene and is the procedure of choice in those cases of gastric volvulus that are complicated by peptic ulcer or other benign or malignant lesions in the stomach or first portion of the duodenum. Its use is reserved for these cases. Tanner reported two patients with an active gastric ulcer and one with an active duodenal ulcer present in addition to gastric volvulus and eventration of the diaphragm. In all three, a Billroth I partial gastrectomy was performed with satisfactory results.

SIMPLE GASTROPEXY. In the past, simple fixation of the stomach was done by suturing it in the desired position, often to the anterior abdominal wall. Tanner (1968) pointed out that "the defect in this operation which usually leads to recurrence is that the original force causing the gastric rotation was not dealt with, so the suturing would eventually slacken or tear out and the volvulus recur."

Cole and Dickinson (1971) pointed out that gastropexy alone does not guarantee nonrecurrence. They cited a case in which the initial volvulus was treated by suturing the gastrocolic ligament to the anterior abdominal wall. When volvulus recurred 13 months later, no evidence of fixation could be found, and the greater curvature of the stomach lay free within the peritoneal cavity.

Another objection to this type of gastropexy is that the anterior parietal peritoneum has an abundant sensory innervation. The tug of the attached stomach on the anterior parietal peritoneum has caused pain, requiring a second operation and release of the anterior gastropexy (Stremple, 1973).

ANTERIOR OR POSTERIOR GASTROENTEROSTOMY. This has been advocated for gastric fixation and used with various degrees of success. Tanner (1968) stated that gastroenterostomy will not relieve gastric volvulus due to eventration of the diaphragm and reported a case in which it had failed.

GASTROSTOMY. This alone will anchor the stomach to the anterior abdominal wall and also can be used for postoperative gastric decompression and for early supplementation of oral intake (Guernsey and Conolly, 1963). Stremple (1973) pointed out that a theoretic objection to its use is the possibility of its creating an additional axis for rotation. I am unaware of this complication having occurred. Cole and Dickinson (1971) state that in infants the surgical treatment of gastric volvulus should include gastrostomy.

MAINGOT'S METHOD. Maingot (1969) believes that the simplest, safest, and most satisfactory method of obtaining permanent fixation of the stomach is by suturing the entire gastrocolic ligament and the gastrosplenic ligament to the peritoneum of the anterior abdominal wall so as to anchor these ligaments along a wide arc from the lower pole of the spleen toward the pylorus. Care must be taken to avoid gaps between the sutures to minimize the possibility of later herniation of the intestine with obstruction. In his experience with the use of this method of gastropexy in six patients with gastric volvulus, there was no recurrence, and x-ray studies showed the stomach and duodenum to be normal in shape, position, and function. Stremple (1973) reported a patient in whom this method could not be used because the gastrocolic and gastrosplenic ligaments were absent.

GASTROPEXY WITH COLONIC DISPLACEMENT. Because of the tendency for gastric volvulus to recur if simple gastropexy is performed, Tanner, in 1948, devised the following procedure for treating patients with gastric volvulus associated with eventration of the left diaphragm: The stomach is separated from the transverse colon by dividing the gastrocolic omentum from the duodenum to the gastric fundus (Fig. 5–52). Any adhesions of the ascending colon or the hepatic and splenic flexures of the colon are divided. When this is completed, and provided there is an average length of mesocolon, the whole mobilized transverse colon and greater omentum can now be made to rise and fill the left subphrenic area without tension. A simple gastropexy will now give a far greater chance of success (Fig. 5–53). The anterior lesser curve of the stomach is usually sutured to the free edge of the liver and of the ligamentum teres, which allows reasonable mobility; and, as the subphrenic space is now filled with colon, the upward pulling force and the direct drag on the greater curve of the stom-

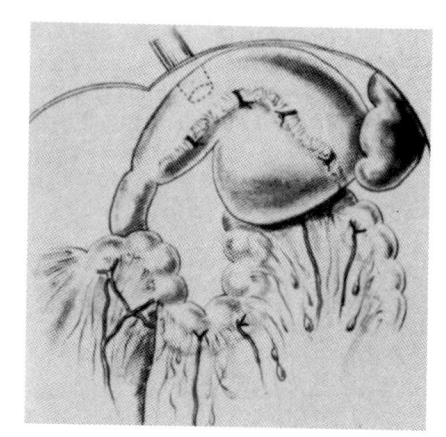

Figure 5–52. Colon separated from the rotated stomach. (From Tanner, cited in previous figure.)

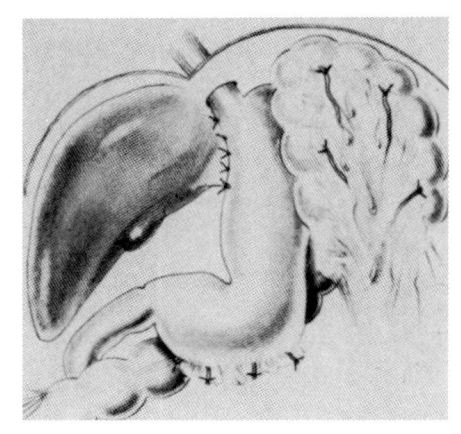

Figure 5-53. After the gastropexy is completed, the colon fills the subphrenic space. (From Tanner, cited in Figure 5-51.)

ach are eliminated so there is a greatly reduced chance of recurrent volvulus.

Tanner reported that this operation was the major procedure for 15 patients. In addition, it has twice been added after division of a band. Furthermore, in patients with eventration in whom gastrectomy has been carried out for coincident peptic ulcer, he has found it wise to mobilize the colon very freely in order to reduce the upward forces on the gastrectomized stomach.

The treatment performed in 21 patients for gastric volvulus associated with eventration of the diaphragm has been: gastropexy with colonic replacement, 15 patients; partial gastrectomy, 4 patients; repair of eventration, 1 patient; and no operation, 1 patient.

Results of Colonic Displacement Operation. "This procedure was the primary operation performed on 15 patients with gastric volvulus whose ages ranged from 35 to 74 years. There was no mortality and no recurrence of the volvulus during a 2- to 12-year follow-up" (Tanner, 1968).

OPOLZER'S OPERATION. In 1957, Opolzer suggested that for severe gastric volvulus due to eventration of the diaphragm, a short circuit should be made by a side-to-side anastomosis between the rotated gastric fundus and antrum. Tanner (1968) pointed out that the operation cannot be recommended because risk of strangulation still exists and if the volvulus causes obstruction, it will occur in the pyloric and cardiac regions rather than the mid-part of the stomach. This will not be bypassed by this procedure, which therefore seems illogical. I am unaware of any recent reports of its use.

GASTRIC VOLVULUS IN PEDIATRIC PATIENTS

Volvulus of the stomach is an extremely rare occurrence in the pediatric population. Campbell and Davis (1976) reviewed a total of 48 cases of gastric volvulus in the neonate. They concluded that volvulus was related to associated anatomic abnormalities, including diaphragmatic defects, such as paraesophageal hernia or eventration, and failure of fixation of the stomach with insufficient gastrosplenic or gastrocolic ligaments. However, one-third of the cases had no associated anatomic defects.

Clinical signs and symptoms occurred acutely, with sudden, severe upper abdominal pain, distention, and retching with little vomiting; or chronically, with intermittent upper abdominal pain usually occurring immediately following meals. A barium meal may reproduce symptoms and demonstrate the pathologic state. In the acute type of volvulus, inability to decompress the stomach by insertion of a nasogastric tube should prompt early surgical intervention to prevent ischemic insult or perforation. The two types of gastric volvulus which have been described are the mesenterioaxial and the organoaxial gastric volvulus, as in the adult. Surgical correction consists of insertion of a gastrostomy tube with anterior gastropexy. Partial gastrectomy may be necessary if irreversible ischemic necrosis has occurred.

Cohen (1970) reported five cases of intrathoracic gastric volvulus in children. In each case the repair was done through a right lateral thoracotomy. Two cases were associated with absent hemi-diaphragm and another case was associated with a paraesophageal hernia.

The review by Cole and Dickinson (1971) of all cases of acute volvulus of the stomach in infants and children to 1971 revealed 43 patients. It emphasized the need for complete obstruction of the lumen of the stomach to fulfill the criteria for volvulus. Associated diaphragmatic defects were seen in 25 (65 per cent) of these patients. Vomiting associated with abdominal distention and inability to pass a nasogastric tube is the usual clinical setting. The recommended treatment is transabdominal reduction of the volvulus and fixation of the stomach by gastropexy. Overall mortality has been 68 per cent; however, since 1950 only 2 of 26 cases have died.

Chapter 6

OBSTRUCTION-LIKE DISORDERS

GASTROPEXY

Gastropexy is surgical fixation of the stomach to prevent displacement.

In former years, gastropexy was employed frequently for the treatment of gastroptosis, but now surgical therapy of that condition has been abandoned. Now gastropexy is used as part of some operative procedures for hiatal hernia and also in some operative procedures for gastric volvulus (p. 180). (The types of gastropexy or hiatal hernia are described in Volume 1: Hill, page 412; Nissen I, page 417; Boerema, page 421; and Waterston, page 453.)

A number of other methods of gastropexy have also been devised for fixing the stomach in a desired position in unusual cases. Usually the operation is performed incidental to a more important surgical procedure that determines the type of anesthesia and incision to be used.

When performing any of these procedures, care should be taken that the stomach is fixed in a functional position, so that it will not be angulated by changes in the patient's position. Other risks include leakage due to penetration of fixation sutures into the lumen; leaving openings in its fixation into which bowel can herniate; or having its vascular supply impaired. Some of the less commonly used methods of gastropexy will be illustrated, as occasionally they have been applicable for unusual circumstances.

BEYEA'S METHOD (Fig. 6–1). In this procedure the lesser omentum is shortened by plicating it with interrupted silk sutures.

COFFEY'S METHOD (Fig. 6–2). In this method, after the gastrohepatic omentum has been shortened by pleating, the stomach and transverse colon are further suspended anteriorly by pleating and suturing the gastrocolic and greater omentum to the anterior abdominal wall with nonabsorbable sutures.

PERTHES' METHOD. This procedure is illustrated in Figure 6–3.

DURET'S METHOD (Fig. 6–4). In the Duret technic, the anterior wall of the stomach along the lesser curvature is sutured directly to the anterior abdominal wall at the desired level, using a continuous silk mattress suture that includes the anterior stomach wall and rectus muscle but not the anterior rectus sheath.

ROSVING'S METHOD (Fig. 6–5). The anterior wall of the stomach is secured to the anterior abdominal wall by interrupted silk sutures. Each suture passes through the entire thickness of the anterior abdominal wall on the right, includes the seromuscular coats of the anterior gastric wall which is

GASTRIC PLICATION

Figure 6–1. Gastropexy, by suspension, through shortening the lesser omentum.

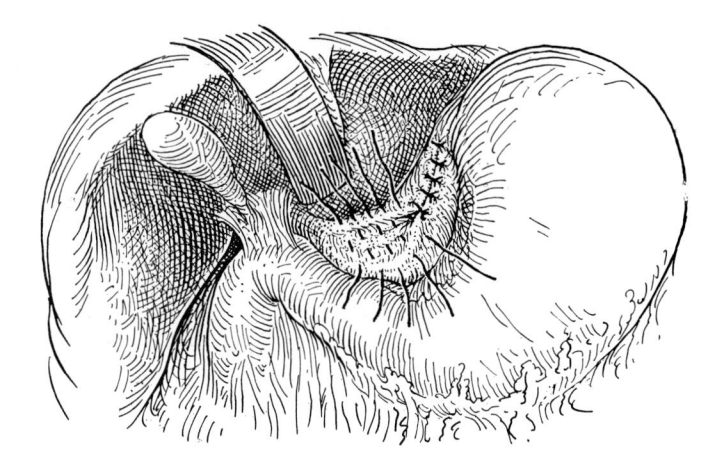

scarified, and passes out through the entire thickness of the left abdominal wall. These sutures are pulled taut to approximate the stomach to the anterior abdominal wall while the abdominal incision is being closed. After closure, the two ends of the silk sutures forming the gastropexy are tied over a glass rod or gauze roll. Four weeks later these sutures are cut and removed.

GASTRIC PLICATION

Gastric plication is the operation for reduction in size of the gastric lumen by infolding the stomach walls by suture. It formerly was employed for the treatment of a dilated stomach but has been abandoned for that purpose. It is rarely, if ever, indicated as an operation per se but at present it is occasionally used to reduce the bulk of the stomach so it can be pulled up through the esophageal hiatus or via the retrosternal or antethoracic subcutaneous route to form a high esophagogastrostomy for esophageal replacement or bypass.

TECHNICS

WEIR'S MODIFICATION OF BIRCHER'S METHOD (Fig. 6–6). In this method, the anterior wall of the stomach is plicated in its long axis by securing it over a urethral sound with two layers of interrupted Lembert sutures of silk.

MOYNIHAN'S MODIFICATION OF BIRCHER'S METHOD. A series of vertical, interrupted, seromuscular sutures of silk are

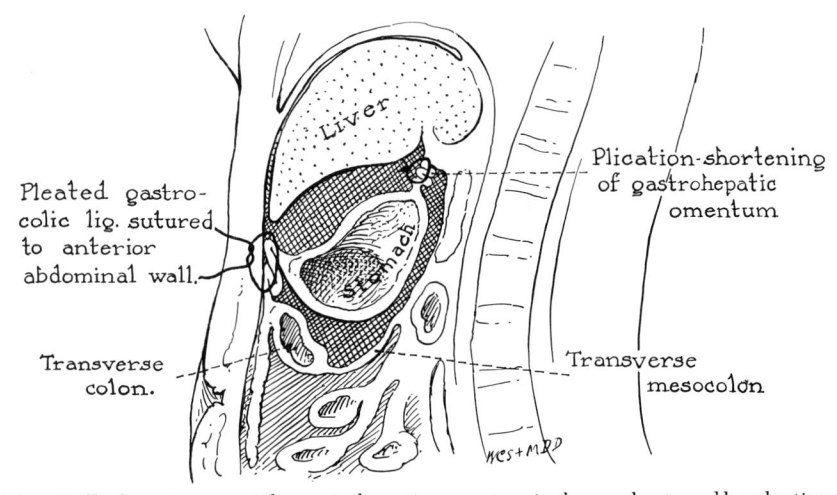

Figure 6–2. Coffey's gastropexy. The gastrohepatic omentum is shown shortened by pleating, and the stomach and transverse colon are suspended anteriorly by pleating and suturing the gastrocolic and greater omentum to the anterior abdominal wall.

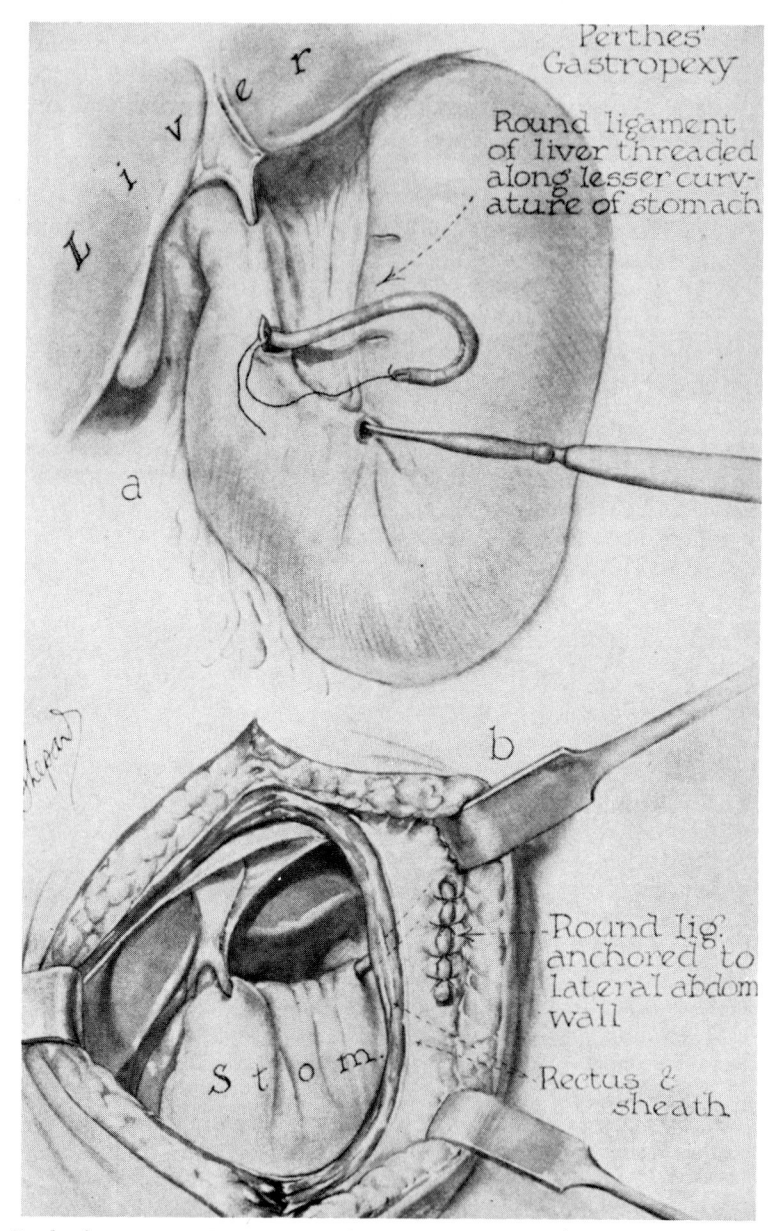

Figure 6–3. Perthes' gastropexy. Note course of round ligament of the liver along course of lesser curvature of stomach, through the abdominal wall to the point of anchorage to the costal margin and fascia of the transversus abdominis muscle. (Thorek: Modern Surgical Technic. Vol. III. J. B. Lippincott Company.)

GASTRIC PLICATION 187

Figure 6-4. Duret's gastropexy. Exposed through a left rectus incision, the anterior stomach along the lesser curvature is sutured directly to the abdominal wall, using a continuous suture which includes the seromuscular coats of the stomach, the peritoneum, the posterior sheath, and rectus muscle but not the anterior sheath.

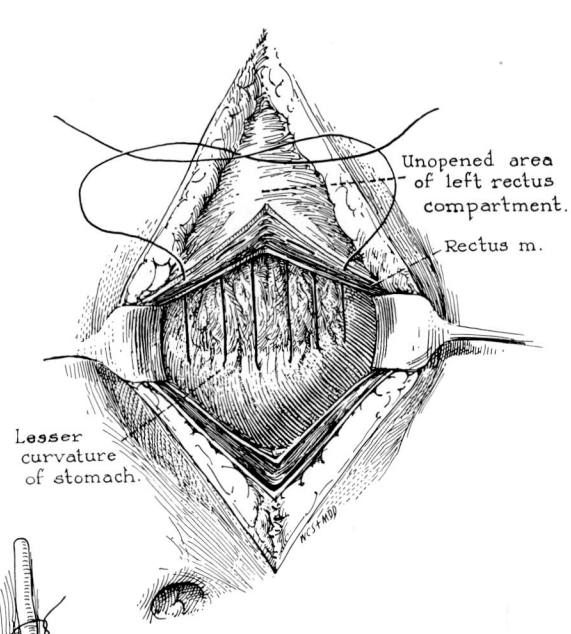

Figure 6-5. Rosving's gastropexy. The anterior aspect of the stomach is sutured directly to the anterior abdominal wall.

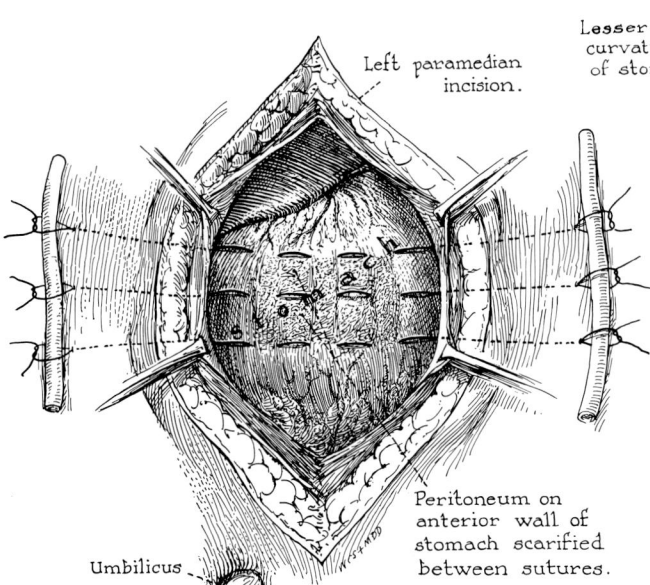

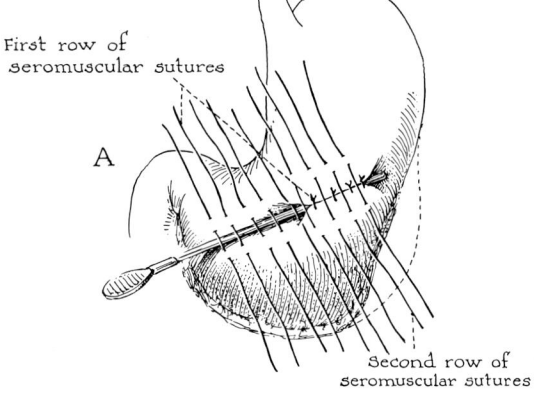

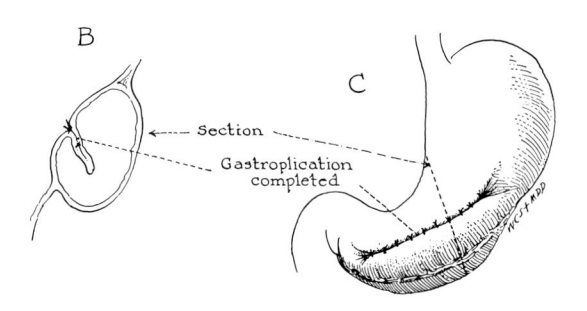

Figure 6-6. Gastroplication (Weir's modification of Bircher's method). *A*, Plication, over a urethral sound, of the anterior stomach wall in its long axis with two layers of Lembert sutures. *B* and *C*, Sectional view and the completed operation.

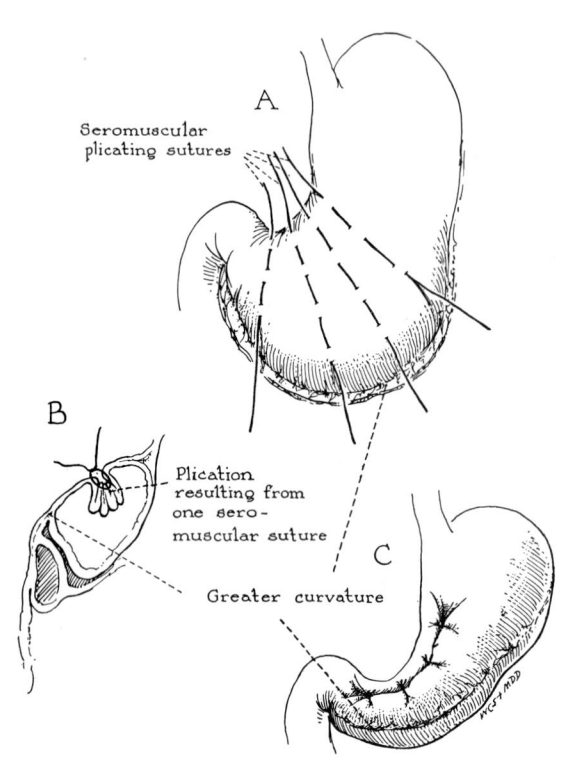

Figure 6–7. Gastroplication (Moynihan's modification of Bircher's method). *A*, A series of vertical, interrupted seromuscular sutures is placed in the anterior abdominal wall. *B* and *C*, Sectional and external views of the plicated stomach wall.

placed in the anterior wall of the stomach, as shown in Figure 6–7. Each stitch passes through the seromuscular coats of the stomach several times. When these sutures are drawn tight, the wall of the stomach is folded into as many ridges as there are bites in each suture.

In plicating the stomach, great care should be taken that the seromuscular sutures do not inadvertently penetrate the entire thickness of the gastric wall into the gastric lumen to become a site of leakage. It is also important not to strangulate the blood supply so as to cause local ischemia of the gastric wall, or to cause suture cut-through because of being tied too tightly.

BILOCULAR STOMACH OR HOURGLASS CONTRACTION OF STOMACH

In this uncommon condition, the stomach is divided into two cavities that are connected by a narrow channel, usually located in the middle portion of that viscus. Rare cases have been reported in which the stomach has been divided into more than two cavities by multiple constrictions.

The communication between the cavities of the stomach is usually located nearer the lesser curvature. The proximal gastric cavity hypertrophies and enlarges to a varying degree.

ETIOLOGY

In 1851, Struther suggested that in at least some cases hourglass stomach was a congenital deformity. In 1895, Hirsch reviewed the literature and concluded that all cases were congenital. Moynihan, in 1904, was the first to state that all these cases are sequelae to gastric ulcer, an opinion that was restated by Rowlands in 1931.

In 1949, Schroeder reported a case of hourglass stomach caused by annular muscular hypertrophy without evidence of ulceration or scarring and revived the question of their congenital origin. In 1962, Gandhi and Robarts called attention to the occurrence of hourglass stricture of the stomach and pyloric stenosis due to ferrous sulfate poisoning.

In 1973, Filpi and colleagues reported the case of an 18-month-old baby who swallowed ferrous sulfate tablets and was treated by gastric lavage, intravenous fluids, isoproterenol drip, cathartics, and exchange transfusion. She recovered and was discharged from the hospital 2 weeks after admission. Five weeks after the ingestion a routine barium swallow x-ray study revealed a stricture involving the fundus of the stomach without obstruction to the flow of contrast material. Six months after ingestion a repeat upper gastrointestinal x-ray series was normal. The patient continued to do well and to be asymptomatic. These physicians found 12 cases of gastric stricture following iron poisoning in the English literature. All had involved the body, antrum, or pylorus, and 11 of the 12 patients had required surgery. The only patient not operated upon had died. Their patient is the first in whom only the proximal portion of the stomach was involved and also the first in whom spontaneous resolution of a stricture had been demonstrated.

Current opinion is that hourglass stomach is due most often to annular constriction that usually has resulted from (1) an *intrinsic* ulcerative process such as chronic gastric ulcer (over 90 per cent), gastric cancer, gastric syphilis, large stomal ulcer, or stenosing hypertrophy resulting from corrosive poisoning; or (2) *extrinsic* causes such as perigastric adhesions, pressure from a colon distended with gas, or spasmodic hourglass contraction due to reflex causes. Occasionally, an hourglass stomach showing no trace of ulceration or ulcer scarring is reported and raises the question of its congenital origin. Maingot (1969) doubts whether hourglass stomach is ever a congenital condition. The development of hourglass stomach depends upon the size, position, form, and chronicity of the ulcer. A saddle-shaped ulcer of the body of the stomach is often a precursor.

PATHOLOGY

According to Palmer (1969), "It is exceptional to find malignant change develop in hourglass deformity of the stomach that is secondary to peptic ulceration. External adhesions rarely cause the deformity, and when they do the degree of obstruction is not high. Inexplicably, hourglass contraction is seen more often in females than in males, the ratio being 8 or 9 to 1." Maingot (1969) reported that "this complication occurs in 8 per cent of all cases of chronic gastric ulcer occurring in women. It rarely occurs in men — probably less than 2 per cent of all those with gastric ulcer." The lesion may be located at any point along the lesser curvature of the stomach. The contracture involves a corresponding point on the greater curvature.

Haubrich (1976) pointed out that active peptic ulcers situated along the saddle area of the gastric lesser curvature are often associated with a more or less persistent incisura in the greater curve opposite or somewhat distal to the level of the ulcer crater. This "opposite incisura" is produced by segmental spasm in the gastric wall. Hence, he suggested that it is probably this unrelenting spasm, plus an extending inflammatory process, that eventually may lead to an unyielding segmental cicatrix in the body of the stomach and produce a bilocular or a trilocular stomach. A true hourglass contracture is almost always cicatricial, not spastic, but may be accentuated by spasm. It may involve chiefly the mucosa, hence its extent may not be apparent from the external appearance of the stomach. Furthermore, it is much less pronounced in the contracted empty stomach than in the distended full stomach.

Hurst and Stewart (1929) found that 90 per cent of a collected series of 335 cases of hourglass stomach were in women, and that about 25 per cent of these patients had an associated pyloric stenosis caused by duodenal ulcer. When these two complications coexist, the distal pouch may be greatly distended while the proximal pouch may be small. At operation the ulcer causing the constriction is found to be completely healed in 50 per cent of the cases. Perforation and hemorrhage are relatively rare complications of hourglass stomach.

SYMPTOMS

The symptoms of hourglass stomach vary with the degree of gastric constriction, the caliber of the channel connecting the two cavities, and the activity of the ulcer that caused the constriction. There is usually a long history of active peptic ulcer disease. A well-developed hourglass stomach produces symptoms of pyloric obstruction: cramplike epigastric pain, nausea, and vomiting or regurgitation. Because in most instances the deformity is associated with an open ulcer crater, the symptoms include the distress or pain of active ulcer disease.

"Because of a diminished gastric reservoir, uncomfortable fullness may be felt immediately after eating only small quantities. Nausea and vomiting or regurgitation almost invariably occur" (Haubrich, 1976).

DIAGNOSIS

Physical examination rarely contributes to the diagnosis of hourglass stomach because the limited distensibility of the proximal stomach cavity is unlikely to be a visible or palpable physical sign.

Gastric analysis of the acid secretions in a bilocular stomach is usually similar to the findings in cases of uncomplicated gastric ulcer, that is, essentially normal levels

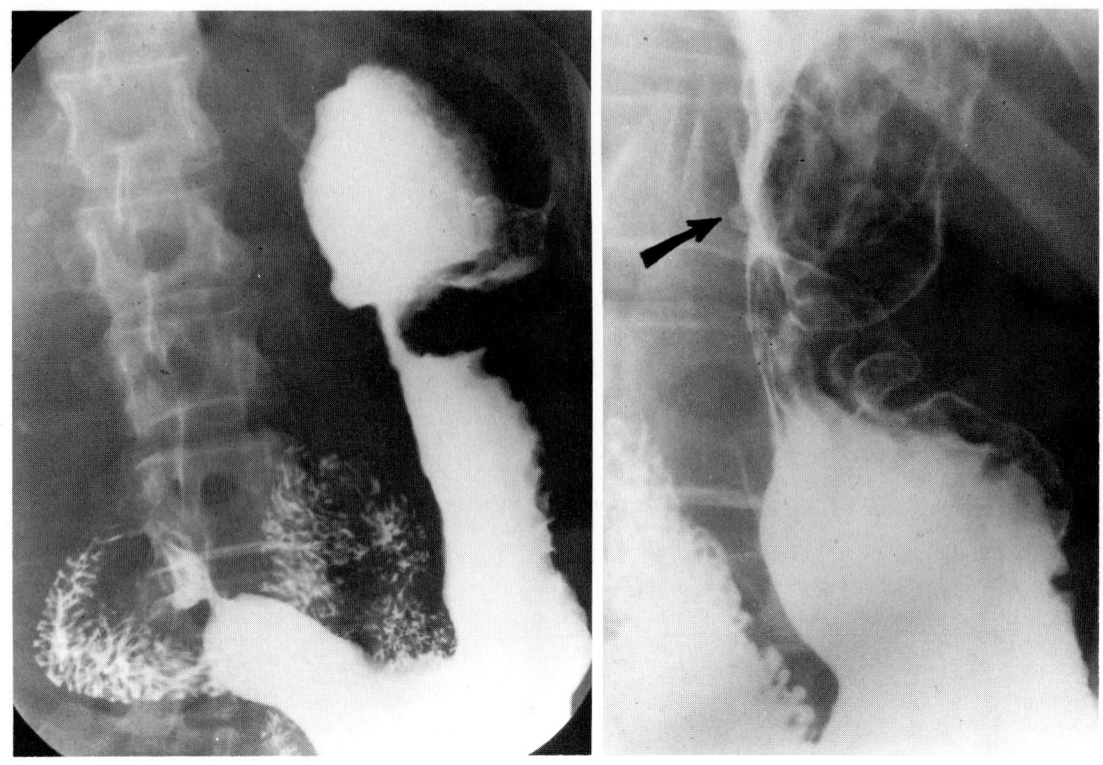

Figure 6–8. Bilocular stomach as demonstrated in a 69-year-old woman who had had episodic epigastric distress for 10 years. Only a narrow channel separates the smaller fundic sac and a larger sac consisting of the body and antrum of the stomach. The arrow in the exposure at the right points to a benign peptic ulcer niche along the lesser curve toward which the greater curve is drawn. (From Bockus, H. L.: Gastroenterology. 3rd Ed. Philadelphia, W. B. Saunders Company, 1974, p. 758.)

(Haubrich, 1976). Achlorhydria should make one suspect a misplacement of the aspirating tube, a constricting cicatrix in the absence of an active ulcer crater, or a disease other than a peptic ulcer deforming the stomach, particularly a gastric cancer. Whether or not there is acid secretion, cytologic examination of aspirated fluid after lavage is advisable.

The diagnosis of a bilocular stomach is made by a barium swallow x-ray study (Fig. 6–8). The demonstrated presence of an ulcer niche projecting from the lesser curve of the constricted area suggests that it is nonmalignant. "An additive ulcer niche associated with the characteristic hourglass deformity is rarely produced by a malignant lesion" (Haubrich, 1976). The most reliable method for ruling out malignancy is by endoscopic biopsy. If benign, there may be doubt as to whether the contraction is due to cicatricial fibrosis or to concomitant spasm. A trial period of strict stomach rest will demonstrate slow disappearance of that portion of the deformity caused by the spasm. Segmental hypertonicity or spasm may mimic an organic hourglass contracture and may occur rarely with inflammatory disease elsewhere in the abdomen, such as cholecystitis or appendicitis. Gastric syphilis may also produce an hourglass deformity.

The radiologic appearance of a cascade stomach (see Fig. 6–16, p. 196) may closely simulate that of an organic hourglass contracture. However, oblique and lateral films will make the differentiation by showing the typical appearance termed "cup and spill" by the British that is characteristic of cascade stomach, which is discussed in the last section of this chapter.

TREATMENT

The recommended primary treatment for cases of nonmalignant hourglass stomach associated with an active penetrating ulcer niche is medical because, until the active ulcer has healed, it is impossible to gauge the extent of fibrosis, since part of the deformity may be due to concomitant spasm and edema.

Medical Treatment

This consists of the usual dietary regimen for gastric ulcer. Many patients with hourglass stomach have responded to medical treatment and have not required surgery. However, if the symptoms and evidence of obstruction are not relieved after a fair trial with medical therapy or if the associated gastric ulcer does not heal, surgical intervention is advisable.

Hourglass stomach due to gastric syphilis has been treated successfully by medical antiluetic therapy, which resulted in complete disappearance, or marked dilatation, of the stricture in two cases reported by Haubrich (1976). Penicillin is the treatment of choice for gastric syphilis in any of its stages.

Medical management is also recommended for primary treatment of patients with hourglass stomach without active ulcer if the obstruction is not complete and if cancer can be excluded. Haubrich (1976) noted that many patients with cicatricial hourglass deformity may remain relatively comfortable on a modified ulcer regimen. If not relieved of their symptoms by medical management, surgical treatment of patients may be indicated.

Maingot's (1969) recommendations are somewhat different. Although medical management may keep patients moderately nourished, he noted that when the ulcer heals and leaves a small but adequate channel for food, such patients are chronic invalids and sooner or later require an operation to relieve the obstruction. Hence he regards hourglass deformity an indication for surgical treatment, at any age.

Operations

Hourglass deformity is rare and those operated upon are even rarer. During the senior author's surgical residency training, 1929 to 1934, five cases of hourglass stomach were seen. All were operated upon, three by Dr. J. M. T. Finney and two by the chief resident. All survived but have been lost to long-time follow-up. Since then we have not seen another patient with this disorder.

An attempt was made to determine the incidence of hourglass stomach in our hospitals in recent years. A search of the medical and radiologic records from 1970 to the present at Johns Hopkins and Union Memorial hospitals in Baltimore disclosed no recorded case of hourglass stomach. This could be misleading because there is no longer a separate coding for hourglass stomach, and these cases are now indexed according to their etiology and included among the cases of gastric ulcer, gastric syphilis, and so on.

The Loch Raven Veterans Administration hospital recorded one case in 1972. This case was associated with a gastric ulcer and was treated medically with apparent success, but there was no post-hospitalization follow-up.

Apparently hourglass deformity of the stomach is even rarer now than in former years and fewer of those that do occur require operation. A probable explanation of this decreased incidence is that improved radiologic and endoscopic methods have made it possible to recognize and treat definitively such etiologic lesions as gastric ulcer and carcinoma earlier, before they have progressed to form an hourglass deformity; and also because now penicillin is available for more effective treatment of gastric syphilis.

Since there is a paucity of reports in the recent surgical literature on the operative treatment of this rare condition, the operations that have been used in the past will be described and their indications updated.

The object of all operations for hourglass stomach is the enlargement of the opening between the two pouches to permit satisfactory emptying of the viscus unless, as is the usual present-day procedure, the isthmus and the distal pouch are excised by partial gastrectomy. A large number of technical procedures have been devised, the chief of which are mentioned here even though several of them are only of historic interest.

Usually partial gastrectomy is the most suitable procedure for this condition, as plastic operations may present technical difficulties because of lack of available normal stomach wall. For this reason a careful estimate of the difficulties should be made before deciding upon the type of operation to be used. If in doubt, a partial gastrectomy will usually prove to be the more satisfactory procedure.

Some of the operations employed, including plastic and shunting procedures, do not remove the lesion underlying the stenosis, which in most cases is a scarred indurated ulcer, frequently still active. Objections can be raised to any operation for hourglass stomach that does not remove the constriction or its cause, as does a partial gastrectomy with removal of the lesion. Moreover, the mortality rate of a carefully done partial gastrectomy will be no higher than that for the other procedures if the stomach can be easily mobilized. In some instances, however, the stomach may be so bound down by adhesions or the patient's general condition so poor that another type of operation will be preferable.

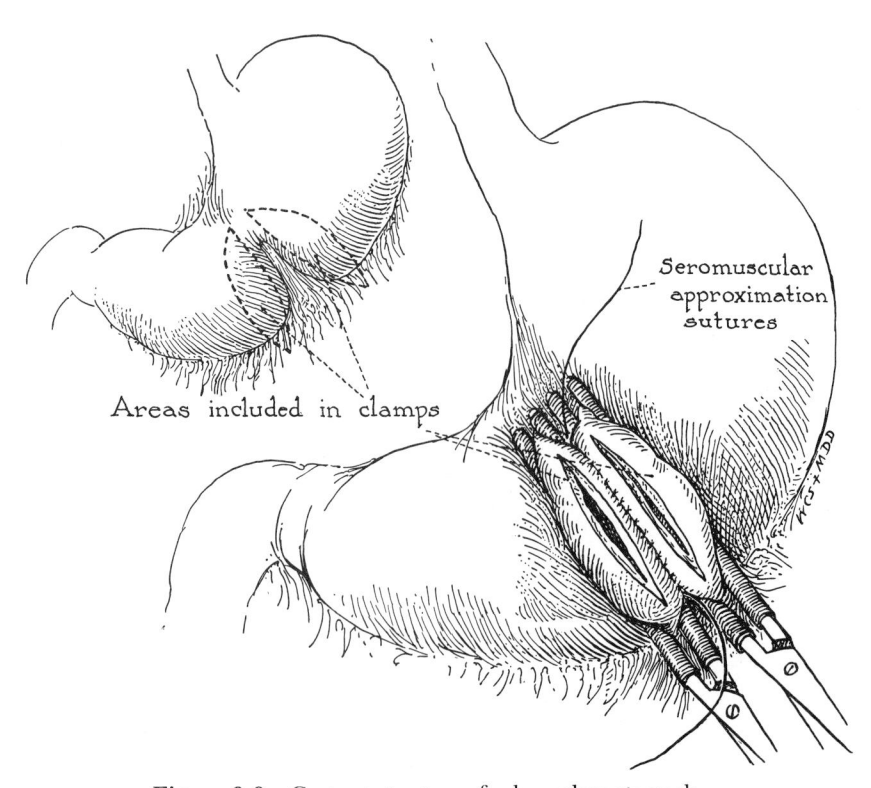

LATERAL GASTROGASTROSTOMY FOR HOURGLASS STOMACH. As illustrated in Figure 6–9, this procedure is simply a side-to-side anastomosis of the two pouches of the hourglass stomach. It may be used when the two pouches are of nearly equal size. It is one of the simplest procedures but does not remove the lesion causing the stenosis. Hurst and Stewart (1929) reported 25 such operations without a single death or recurrence despite the presence of a large active ulcer in many of these cases. Others have found it unsatisfactory when an active gastric or concomitant duodenal ulcer is present. In such cases a partial gastrectomy is the operation of choice if the gastric ulcer is not located too near the cardia. However, in elderly, undernourished patients with completely healed ulcers and a stricture situated high up in the stomach, lateral gastrogastrostomy is recommended. A gastrojejunostomy may be simultaneously peformed if pyloric obstruction coexists.

KAMMERER-FINNEY GASTROPLASTY FOR HOURGLASS STOMACH. This procedure, illustrated in Figure 6–10, is performed exactly like a Finney pyloroplasty (p. 357). The method is particularly applicable in cases in which it is difficult to free the posterior wall of the stomach.

HEINEKE-MIKULICZ GASTROPLASTY FOR HOURGLASS STOMACH. This procedure (Fig. 6–11) is performed like the Heineke-Mikulicz pyloroplasty. The opera-

Figure 6–9. Gastrogastrostomy for hourglass stomach.

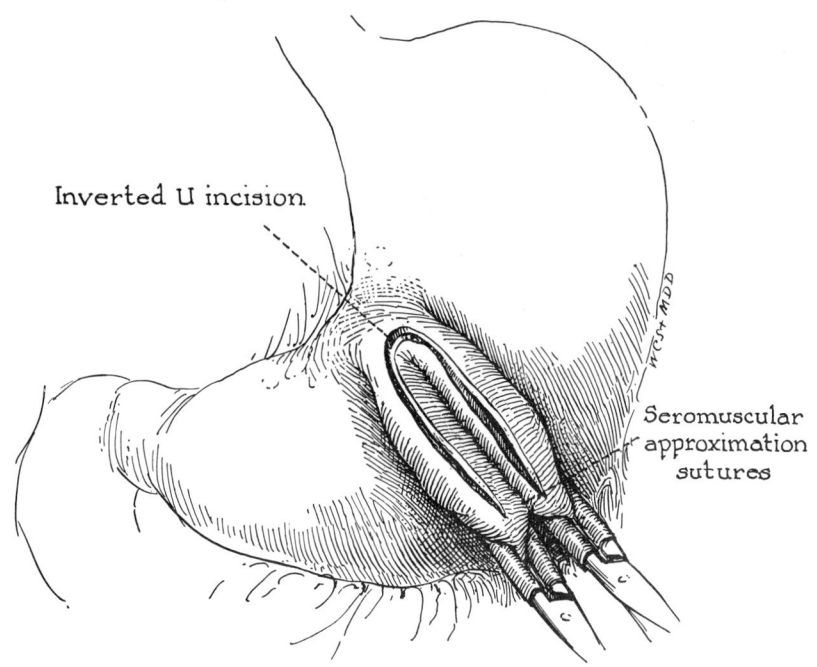

Figure 6–10. Kammerer-Finney method of gastrogastrostomy for hourglass stomach.

tion is not applicable if the constriction is marked, as the lumen cannot be widened to any great degree by this method.

WEDGE-SHAPED EXCISION FOR HOURGLASS STOMACH. To carry out this procedure it is necessary that the posterior wall of the stomach be mobilized. This technic is particularly appropriate when the sulcus between the pouches is not deep. The line for the wedge-shaped excision is shown in Figure 6–12A. The stomach after the excision and anastomosis is shown in Figure 6–12B. The steps of this operation do not differ materially from those for Wedge-Shaped Excision of Ulcer on the Lesser Curvature of the Stomach (p. 000).

SLEEVE RESECTION FOR HOURGLASS STOMACH. The chief indication for band excision of the middle portion of the stomach is the presence of an obstinate progressive ulcer. Ability to mobilize the stomach for the needed manipulations is essential.

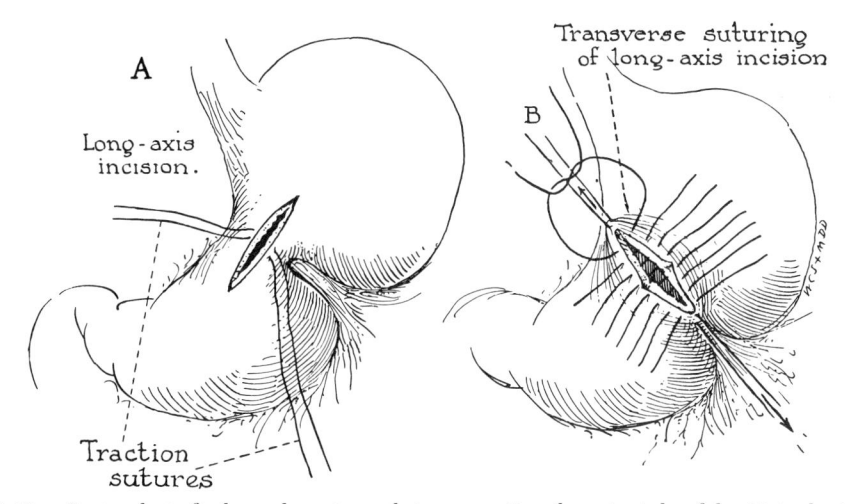

Figure 6–11. Gastroplasty for hourglass stomach incorporating the principle of the Heineke-Mikulicz operations.

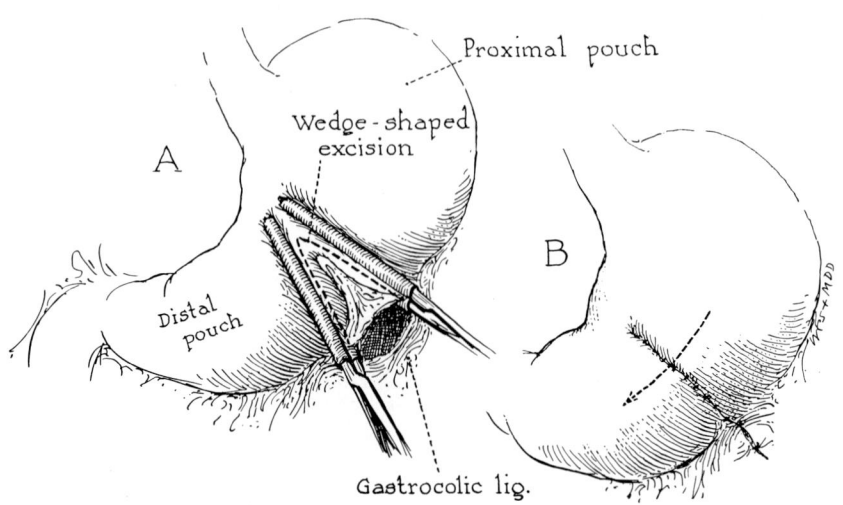

Figure 6–12. Operation for hourglass stomach by wedge-shaped excision of the contiguous aspects of the cardiac and pyloric pouches, followed by union of the divided parts of the stomach. *A*, Area of excision between clamps. *B*, The union completed.

The involved region, including the ulcer-bearing area, is clamped off and excised. The free edges of the remaining portion are united end-to-end (Fig. 6–13), performing the gastrogastrostomy. Preferably the whole distal segment is removed, as in a standard partial gastrectomy (Fig. 6–14).

This operation is rarely performed at present, as other types of partial gastrectomy are preferred. Many surgeons have found sleeve resection of the stomach unsatisfactory because of the increased danger of anastomotic stricture following the operation and because of recurrent gastric ulcer.

ANTERIOR OR POSTERIOR GASTROJEJUNOSTOMY WITH THE PROXIMAL POUCH FOR HOURGLASS STOMACH. The anastomosis is made between the first part of the jejunum and the proximal stomach pouch (Fig. 6–15). This procedure is indicated if the proximal pouch is very large (sometimes it is even larger than a normal stomach), the pyloric pouch is small, and the pyloric outlet is not obstructed. The operative steps are those of an ordinary posterior or anterior gastrojejunostomy. A jejunojejunostomy (enteroentero anastomosis) also may be performed if an anterior gastrojejunostomy is

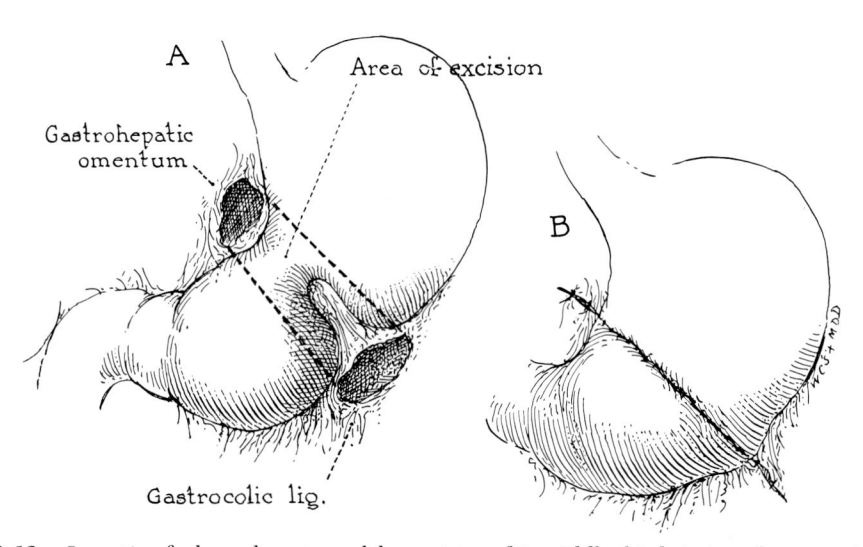

Figure 6–13. Operation for hourglass stomach by excision of its middle third. *A*, Area (between dotted lines) of excision. *B*, The cardiac and pyloric ends are anastomosed.

CASCADE STOMACH

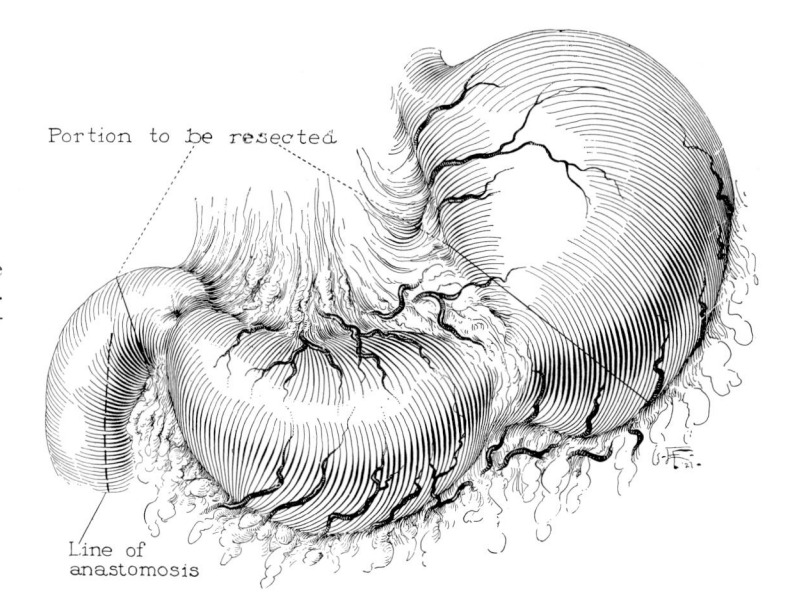

Figure 6–14. Resection of the stomach for hourglass contraction. (Eusterman and Balfour: The Stomach and Duodenum.)

used but is usually unnecessary and may carry with it the risk of stomal ulceration. Gastrojejunostomy to drain the upper segment is "unphysiologic because of the necessity for making a high anastomosis and the danger of subsequent jejunal ulcer" (Haubrich, 1976).

CASCADE STOMACH

Cascade stomach is described frequently in the medical literature but seldom in the surgical literature. It is included here because its radiologic appearance may closely resemble and be confused with an hourglass stomach or gastric volvulus.

According to Niessen (1976), cascade stomach is generally regarded as a variant of the normal gastric contour. It has been called the physiologic hourglass stomach; the English use the term "cup and spill" stomach. In a cascade stomach the fundus droops posteriorly over the body of the stomach, forming a pouch into which food or barium gravitates when the patient is erect. When sufficient barium is drunk to fill

Figure 6–15. Operation for hourglass stomach by posterior gastrojejunostomy with the cardiac pouch.

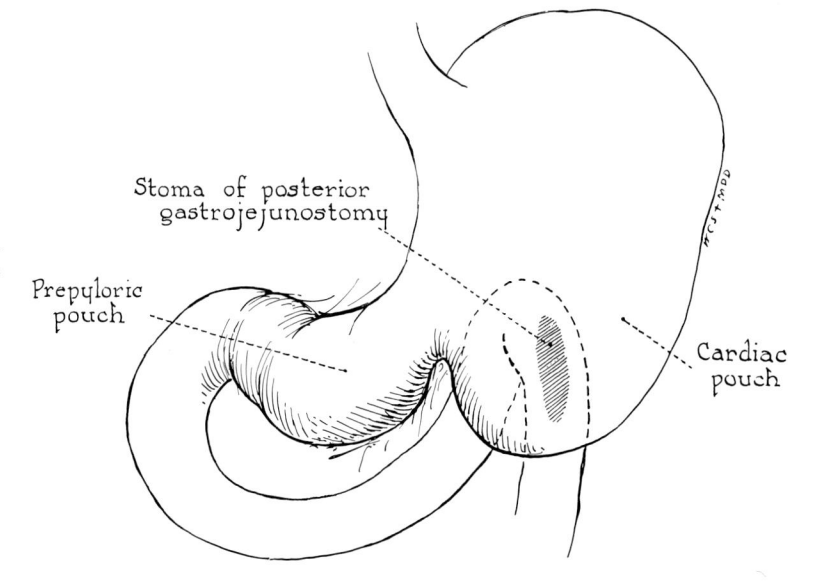

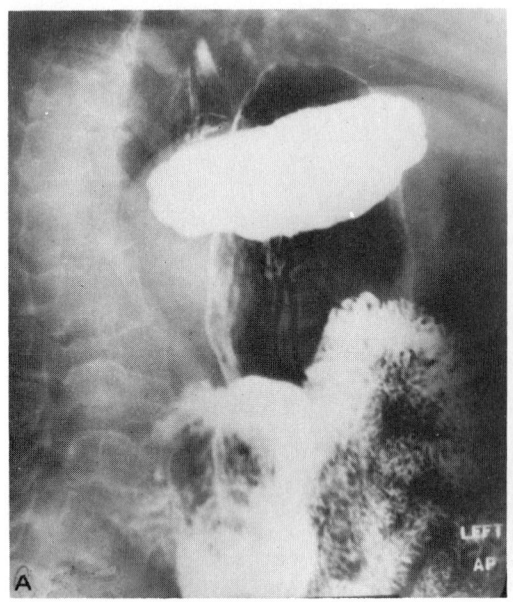

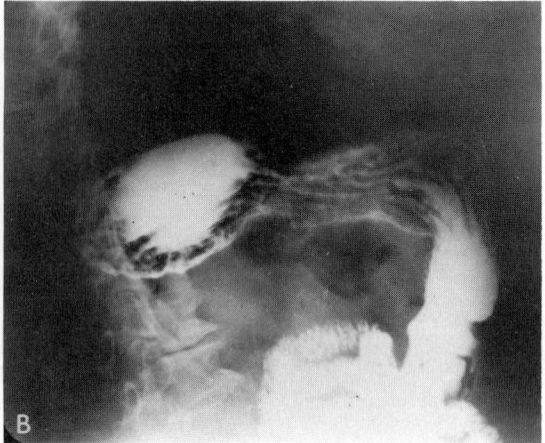

Figure 6–16. Cascade stomach. *A*, Erect posture with barium loculated in the upper segment and gas trapped in the body of the stomach below the angle of cascade. *B*, Lateral projection showing the extremely high infradiaphragmatic position of the upper stomach. (From Bockus, H. L.: Gastroenterology. 3rd Ed. Philadelphia, W. B. Saunders Company, 1974, p. 1104.)

the pouch, it will then cascade or spill into the dependent portion of the stomach. The condition is best demonstrated radiologically with the patient in the lateral or oblique position (Fig. 6–16). This usually shows barium loculated in the dilated upper segment and gas trapped in the body of the stomach. The left dome of the diaphragm may be elevated and the heart tilted upward by the high infradiaphragmatic position of the dilated upper portion of the stomach.

Cascade stomach may be congenital, or there may be an organic cause for the deformity, such as external pressure of a tumor which produces a concave defect on the greater curvature that superficially resembles the appearance of a congenital cascade stomach. Cascade stomach per se causes no symptoms but does predispose toward gastric dysfunction when that organ is adversely affected by various circumstances.

The treatment of cascade stomach is medical. Surgery may be considered in severely ill patients only when medical treatment fails and then only when the mechanism of the complaint is clearly established. Niessen (1976) mentions two patients with cascade stomach who were seen by Bockus and were treated by partial gastrectomy. The first was a man who had distressing symptoms of epigastric distention, pain, inability to eructate, and respiratory embarrassment, which occurred intermittently for years. Eventually he developed a duodenal ulcer with localized perforation. A 75-percent gastrectomy was performed, after which his episodes of severe symptoms never returned.

The second patient had severe symptoms resembling angina pectoris associated with his cascade stomach and underwent gastric resection with complete disappearance of the anginal attacks. Niessen (1976) emphasized that "these cases are cited not to recommend such radical treatment for the ordinary magenblase syndrome in association with cascade stomach but merely to point out that surgery may be considered" in some of these patients.

Chapter 7

INJURIES OF THE STOMACH

Gastric or duodenal injuries may be caused by blunt or penetrating trauma of the abdomen or chest; by ingestion of corrosive substances or of foreign bodies that remain within the lumen and perforate these viscera; by iatrogenic injury during instrumentation or inadvertent hyperdistention of the stomach during administration of inhalation anesthesia; or by spontaneous rupture or perforation caused by excessive distention of the viscus with gas or by disease of its wall. Stomach injuries are discussed in this chapter and duodenal injuries, in Chapter 8.

GASTRIC INJURIES BY BLUNT TRAUMA

The stomach is thick-walled, very mobile, and usually high in the abdomen and protected by the rib cage, so it is unusual for it to be damaged by blunt trauma unless it is distended by a recent meal. Duodenal injuries are more common. However, the stomach is frequently injured by penetrating trauma. Perry (1970) reported that in 235 patients with blunt abdominal trauma the stomach had been injured in only 2 (0.008 per cent), while in 131 patients with penetrating trauma, the stomach had been injured in 14 (10.6 per cent).

Harrison and Debas (1972) reported 18 cases of gastroduodenal injuries by blunt trauma and reviewed the literature on the subject. They found that high-speed motor accidents account for the rising incidence of injuries to the upper gastrointestinal tract by blunt abdominal trauma. Seat-belt injuries cause trauma distal to the ligament of Treitz, but impact against the steering wheel is the main cause of injury proximal to the duodenojejunal flexure.

Siemens and Fulton (1977) reported six patients with gastric rupture caused by blunt trauma and also reviewed the literature. They found that gastric rupture due to blunt trauma is uncommon, having occurred in only 0.9 to 1.7 per cent of hollow viscus injuries. When it did occur, associated injuries to other viscera and gross contamination of the peritoneal cavity by escaped gastric contents were common. A history of a recent meal with a full stomach just before injury was found in 59 per cent of the cases reviewed. Fifty per cent (15 of 30) of the patients whose mode of injury was described underwent rapid deceleration during a fall or an automobile accident often associated with direct injury from the steering wheel. Various types of direct trauma were the second most common cause (11 of 31), with cardiopulmonary resuscitation (5 of 30) the third most common.

Inertia and rapid deceleration cause the

full stomach to move forward, while the lesser curvature remains fixed. The resulting shearing force causes tearing along the anterior wall or the lesser curvature. The greater curvature is freely mobile and less vulnerable. The rupture in the gastric wall in these cases was anterior in 15, in the lesser curvature in 7, in the greater curvature in 5, and in a transection of the stomach in 1.

The severity of the injury was demonstrated by the number of patients in shock on admission (18 of 21), those with multiple systems injured (19 of 28), and the combined mortality rate of 50 per cent. The most common cause of death was sepsis, resulting from massive contamination. This caused intra-abdominal abscesses that were often inadequately drained.

The trauma necessary to rupture the stomach may be severe or trivial. Of the four cases in the series of Harrison and Debas (1972), two were due to motor vehicle accidents in which the patient sustained multiple trauma. In two patients the injury was isolated and was caused by relatively minor trauma. One of these was a 25-year-old woman who, after "10 pushups," developed left upper quadrant and left shoulder tip pain. This was associated with extensive pneumoperitoneum from a small perforation of the anterior gastric wall. The other was a 77-year-old man who, in an alcoholic stupor, fell down a stairs and developed massive upper gastrointestinal bleeding from a 5-cm. mucosal and submucosal laceration of the greater curvature of the body of the stomach.

Lundberg and associates (1967) reported 5 cases of acute upper gastrointestinal hemorrhage due to gastroesophageal lacerations found in autopsies of 50 patients who had received closed chest cardiac massage. In these cases, positive pressure ventilation during cardiopulmonary resuscitation had caused acute gastric dilatation, and the external compression probably contributed to the injury. Two types of injury may occur: one is laceration of the mucosa and submucosa of the gastric wall, which causes bleeding and presents the clinical manifestations of the Mallory-Weiss syndrome (see p. 81 in Vol. 1). The other type of injury is transmural perforation, which usually presents in a manner similar to a perforated peptic ulcer. Occasionally the perforation may be confined and not manifested clinically until a walled-off abscess is found some time later. To prevent these complications, Lundberg and associates advised prompt decompression of acute gastric distention occurring during cardiopulmonary resuscitation.

DIAGNOSIS

The diagnostic work-up of a patient who has suffered blunt abdominal trauma is directed first to evaluating the patient's general condition, assuring an open airway, controlling massive hemorrhage or replacing blood, and treating shock. When the patient's general condition permits, the following basic diagnostic studies are made for determining the presence or absence of injury to the intra-abdominal viscera.

History

A history of the mode of injury provides information about the potential force, extent, and severity of the injury; whether or not the stomach was full; and the patient's present complaints.

Physical Examination

Physical examinations repeated at frequent intervals by the same examiner permit evaluation of the patient's general condition; the presence or absence of shock and additional extra-abdominal injuries; the degree of the patient's consciousness; the presence or absence of abdominal guarding or rigidity; and the changes, for better or worse, found on successive examinations. Abdominal rigidity warrants exploration in most cases of blunt trauma.

Auscultation of the abdomen is important, as the presence or absence of peristaltic sounds has some diagnostic significance. Although these sounds are usually thought to be absent in patients with injuries to the intra-abdominal viscera, Ballinger, Rutherford, and Zuidema (1979) pointed out that "the *presence* of peristaltic sounds is not a reliable sign since it has been demonstrated that normal peristaltic sounds can be heard both in the presence of active intraperitoneal bleeding and following rupture of hollow abdominal organs. Thus reliance upon the presence of peristalsis as assurance that no intra-abdominal injury exists is fallacious and dangerous. However, the *absence* of peristaltic sounds, when carefully sought, should be given serious consideration. Abnormal location of peristaltic sounds has diagnostic importance; e.g., peristaltic sounds heard in the chest in this setting are diagnostic of traumatic diaphragmatic hernia."

Monitoring of the blood pressure, central venous pressure, and urinary output also is important in these patients.

Nasogastric Tube

Bloody aspirate can usually be obtained from a nasogastric tube when the stomach has been injured, but the absence of blood does not exclude the presence of a gastric injury. Hematemesis and the presence of blood escaping from the nasogastric tube suggest laceration of the gastric mucosa and submucosa (Mallory-Weiss syndrome) and the need for injecting Gastrografin via the tube followed by an x-ray study of the stomach and duodenum, to determine the absence, or presence and location, of a perforation of these viscera. If no evidence of perforation is found, fiberoptic gastroduodenoscopy is performed to exclude sites of bleeding proximal to the cardia and to confirm the diagnosis of Mallory-Weiss syndrome by visualizing the area of bleeding in the stomach.

Insertion of a nasogastric tube is both an important diagnostic and therapeutic aid in the care of patients who have suffered severe abdominal trauma. In addition to the valuable diagnostic clues it provides, as just described, it permits decompression of the stomach, removal of gastric contents, and prevention of further accumulation of gastrointestinal air or gas.

Roentgenologic Studies

Plain x-ray films of the upright chest, supine abdomen, and decubitus abdomen with the right side up should be obtained in patients who have been subjected to severe blunt abdominal trauma. The chest film is an integral part of the abdominal examination, because thoracic injuries are frequently associated with abdominal trauma, and knowledge of supradiaphragmatic or diaphragmatic injury is valuable for interpreting abdominal findings. These radiographic studies provide valuable diagnostic information about the chest and abdomen by detecting injuries to bones, pneumothorax, hemothorax, intrapulmonary contusion, diaphragmatic rupture with herniation, and free subdiaphragmatic gas. The latter finding is characteristic of a ruptured or perforated intra-abdominal hollow viscus, but it was absent in two of the six patients with gastric rupture by blunt abdominal trauma reported by Siemens and Fulton (1977).

Urinalysis

When the patient is unable to void voluntarily, insertion of a Foley catheter into the urinary bladder will provide an immediate specimen of urine, which is examined for blood. A positive test suggests injury to a kidney or the urinary tract or both and indicates the need for a cystogram and intravenous pyelogram. Renal injury is common in patients with blunt abdominal trauma, and preoperative knowledge that the kidneys and urinary tract are uninjured may avoid the need for operative exposure of these structures. Should a renal injury be discovered, the preoperative status of the other kidney becomes critically important. Urinalysis will also determine the presence or absence of diabetes mellitus or severe underlying renal disease. Aside from its diagnostic value, the use of a Foley catheter enables monitoring of urine output, which is essential in the management of severely injured patients.

Other Laboratory Tests

Additional laboratory tests helpful for evaluating a patient with abdominal trauma include a *hematocrit* and a *leukocyte count*. "The diagnosis of massive hemorrhage is usually fairly obvious and the hematocrit merely confirmatory. Massive hemorrhages of more than 20 per cent of blood volumes are associated with rapid plasma refill rates and consequently early decreases in the hematocrit level. Hence a low hematocrit early in the treatment of the patient may be significant" (Ballinger, Rutherford, and Zuidema, 1979).

Leukocytosis is associated with all types of trauma, with up to 15,000 cells per cubic millimeter commonly being seen shortly after the injury. Hence it has little significance early in blunt abdominal trauma evaluation but may be significant later.

Creatinine, glucose, and *electrolyte* determinations are usually obtained for baseline values.

Serum amylase values are important because injury of the pancreas is often associated with gastroduodenal injuries by blunt or penetrating abdomen trauma. According to Ballinger, Rutherford, and Zuidema (1979), "Serum amylase values can be normal in patients with major pancreatic trauma, but elevated values give important information. The serum amylase values are elevated in 48 to 91 per cent of patients with blunt pancreatic trauma, and in 9 to 40 per cent of patients with penetrating trauma to the pancreas. Elevated serum amylase is more commonly associated with injury of the head of the pancreas than with injury of its tail. Elevated serum amylase values usually return to normal within 48 hours after injury. Elevated amylase values can also occur in patients with perforation of the gastrointestinal tract, particularly retroperitoneal ruptures of the duodenum."

Some have found the amylase value in a 2-hour urine collection to be the most reliable index of pancreatic injury. Increased concentrations of amylase in the peritoneal fluid following pancreatic injury have been noted. Perry (1970) reported that a concentration of amylase greater than 100 Somogyi units/dl. in the peritoneal fluid obtained by peritoneal lavage has been uniformly diagnostic of injury to the pancreas or upper small bowel in patients with blunt abdominal trauma.

Peritoneal Lavage

Perry reported that in his group's experience, diagnostic peritoneal lavage is more accurate than four-quadrant tap for diagnos-

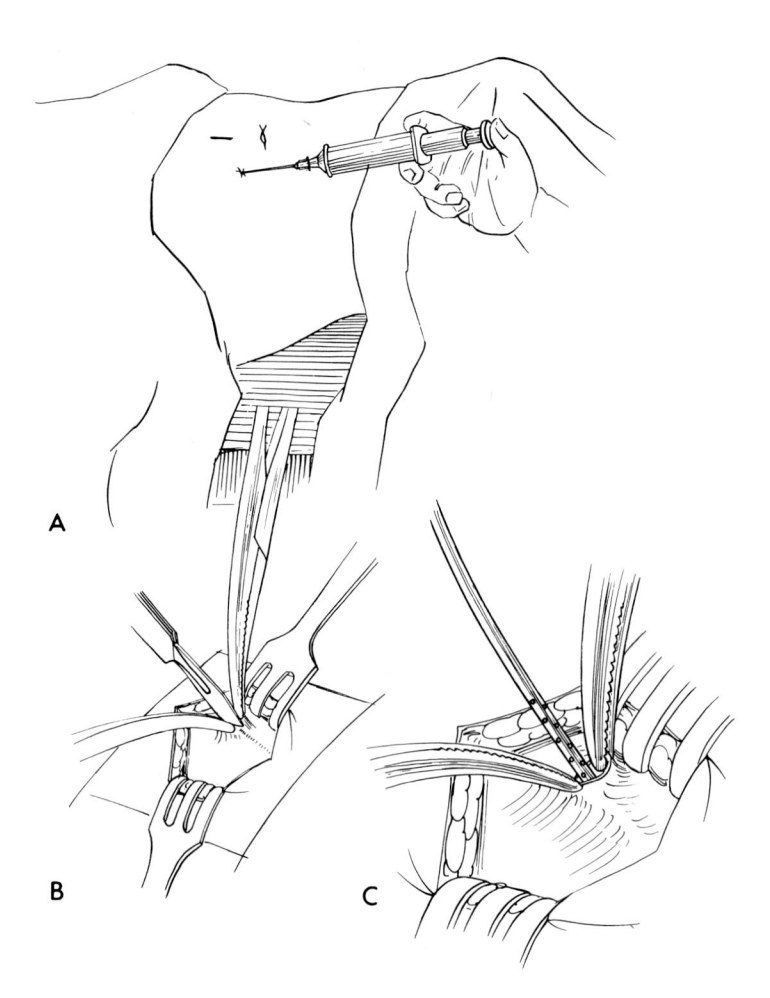

Figure 7–1. Diagnostic peritoneal lavage. The urinary bladder is first emptied by catheter. *A*, The abdominal wall is prepared, draped, and infiltrated with a local anesthetic agent containing epinephrine. A small incision is made in the midline just below the umbilicus, with careful hemostasis. *B*, The fascia of the abdominal wall is incised in the midline and the peritoneum visualized and opened. *C*, A peritoneal dialysis catheter is then inserted into the peritoneal cavity. (From Perry, J. F., Jr.: Blunt and penetrating abdominal injuries. Curr. Prob. Surg., May, 1970, p. 8.)

ing abdominal trauma and is the most rapid means they have found to determine whether intraperitoneal bleeding or other manifestations of visceral injury are present in patients with blunt abdominal trauma. He stated that the simplicity and accuracy of the test are such that it has become a most important part of the diagnostic work-up in such patients. Figures 7–1 through 7–4 illustrate the procedure.

Perry's group used the peritoneal lavage test in 304 patients with blunt abdominal trauma (Table 7–1). Of these, 160 (52 per cent) had a true positive test with operative confirmation of visceral injury, and 132 (44 per cent) had a true negative test as evidenced in most by the subsequent clinical course and in one patient by negative laparotomy. There were 3 (1 per cent) false-positive tests and 9 (3 per cent) false-negative tests. In two patients, complications resulted from diagnostic peritoneal lavage. One had an injury to small bowel mesentery, and another suffered a puncture of the small bowel. Perry found that "diagnostic peritoneal lavage is especially helpful in blunt abdominal trauma patients with multiple injuries, shock, or unconsciousness. If positive, laparotomy can be performed without delay. If negative, the patient can be treated for any other injuries with reasonable assurance that an abdominal visceral injury is not being overlooked."

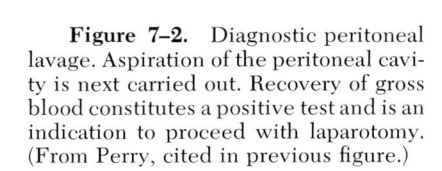

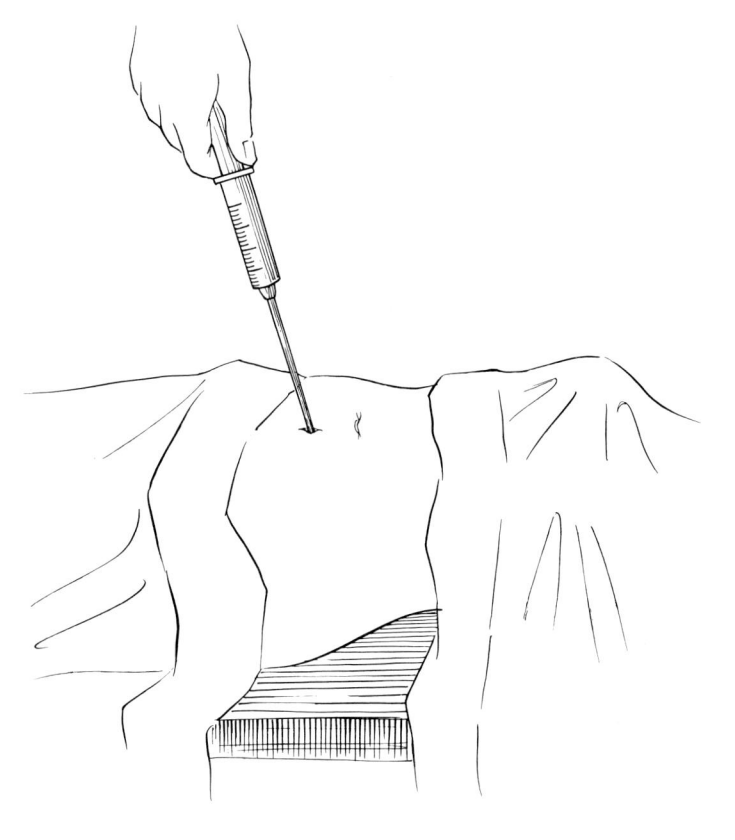

Table 7–1. Interpretation of Results of Diagnostic Peritoneal Lavage

	Test Result
Blood in catheter	Positive
Aspiration of blood	Positive
Clear or pink lavage fluid	Negative*
Grossly bloody lavage fluid	Positive
Many white blood cells in lavage fluid (>500 WBC/cu. mm.)	Positive
High amylase activity (>100 U./dl.)	Positive
Many red blood cells (>100,000 RBC/cu. mm.)	Positive
Bile or intestinal content in lavage fluid	Positive
Bacteria in lavage fluid	Positive

*Presumed negative pending microscopic study. (From Perry, J. F., Jr.: Blunt and penetrating abdominal injuries. Curr. Prob. Surg., May, 1970.)

Figure 7–2. Diagnostic peritoneal lavage. Aspiration of the peritoneal cavity is next carried out. Recovery of gross blood constitutes a positive test and is an indication to proceed with laparotomy. (From Perry, cited in previous figure.)

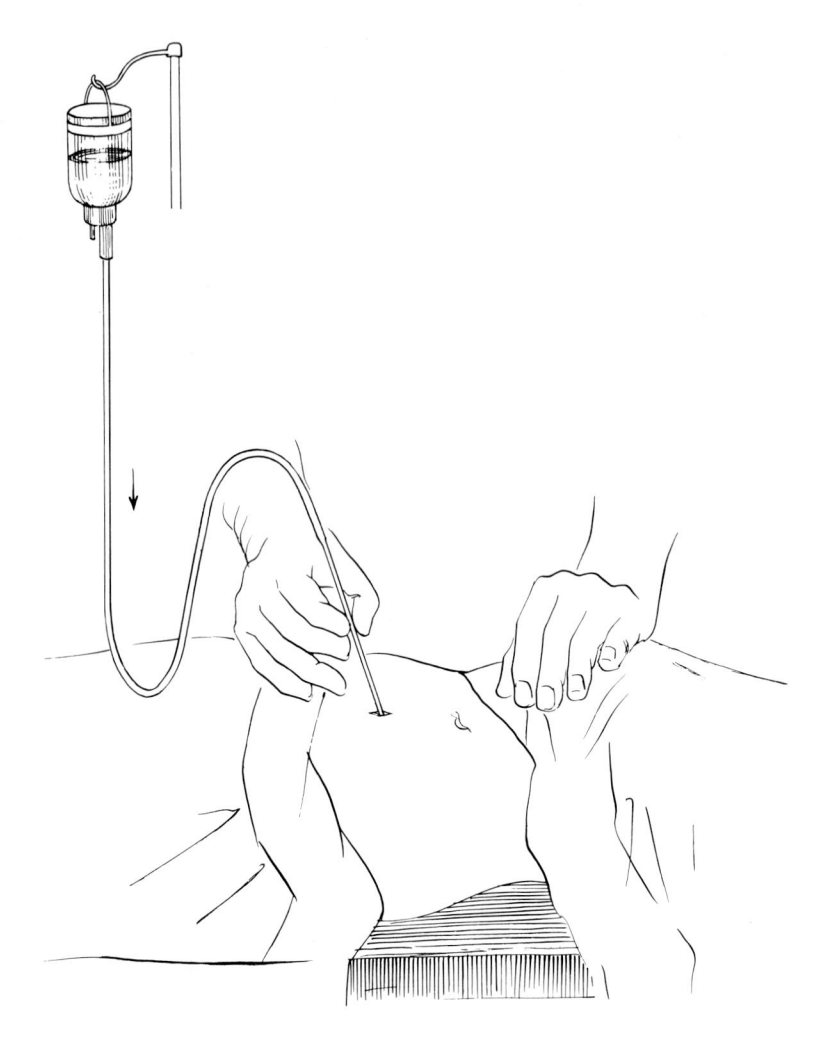

Figure 7-3. Diagnostic peritoneal lavage. If no blood is recovered by aspiration through the dialysis catheter, it is attached to a tubing and 1 liter of saline or balanced salt solution is allowed to run into the peritoneal cavity. (From Perry, cited in Fig. 7-1.)

Bivins and colleagues (1978) reported a prospective comparative study of the diagnostic accuracy of peritoneal lavage versus clinical diagnosis in 142 patients with blunt abdominal trauma. The clinical diagnosis was correct in only 59 per cent; peritoneal lavage was correct in 90 per cent. "There were one false-negative, ten false-positives, and three indeterminate lavages. This technique was especially useful in children and in patients with multiple injuries."

Paracentesis

Four-quadrant abdominal paracentesis is another useful diagnostic procedure in patients with nonpenetrating abdominal injury, especially those with associated craniocerebral or other serious injuries. It is contraindicated when the peritoneal space is suspected of being extensively involved with adhesions. The patient's bladder is emptied by voiding or catheterization before the test is begun.

TECHNIC. The procedure is performed with the aid of local infiltration anesthesia. The left lower quadrant is tapped first at a point lateral to the rectus sheath, in order to avoid injury to the inferior epigastric artery. A wheal is made in the skin, and the underlying tissue is infiltrated down to the peritoneal layer with 1 per cent Xylocaine, using a 25-gauge needle. An 18- or 20-gauge spinal needle with a short bevel, attached to a 10-ml. syringe, is gently inserted through the abdominal wall and peritoneum (Fig. 7-5). When it enters the peritoneal cavity, the operator applies gentle suction as the needle is slowly advanced in a lateral direction toward the

GASTRIC INJURIES BY BLUNT TRAUMA

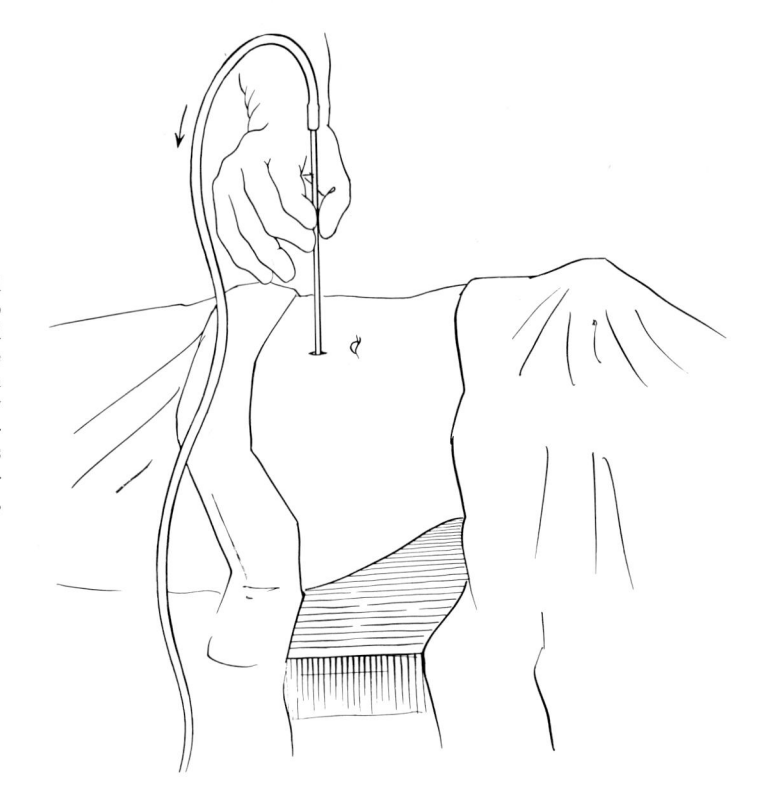

Figure 7-4. The bottle is placed on the floor and the fluid now returns to the bottle. The patient can be turned from side to side prior to removing the peritoneal fluid if his or her condition permits. The fluid is examined grossly and microscopically, and amylase concentration is determined. Characteristics of the returned fluid and their interpretation are given in Table 7-1. (From Perry, cited in Fig. 7-1.)

gutters. Gentle repositioning of the needle within the peritoneal space may permit withdrawal of a small quantity of fluid. As little as 0.1 ml. of nonclotting blood is sufficient evidence of intraperitoneal bleeding. Any nonbloody fluid obtained should be cultured and smeared immediately. If the first tap is negative, it is repeated in the other quadrants. Aspiration of nonclotting blood, air, or bile-stained fluid into the syringe is a positive test and is considered to be strong evidence of intraperitoneal injury. Only positive taps are accorded any value. A negative abdominal tap has no diagnostic significance.

The diagnostic accuracy of abdominal

Figure 7-5. Diagnostic peritoneal tap. (From Ballinger, W. F., Rutherford, R. B., and Zuidema, G. D.: The Management of Trauma. 3rd Ed. Philadelphia, W. B. Saunders Company, 1978, p. 416.)

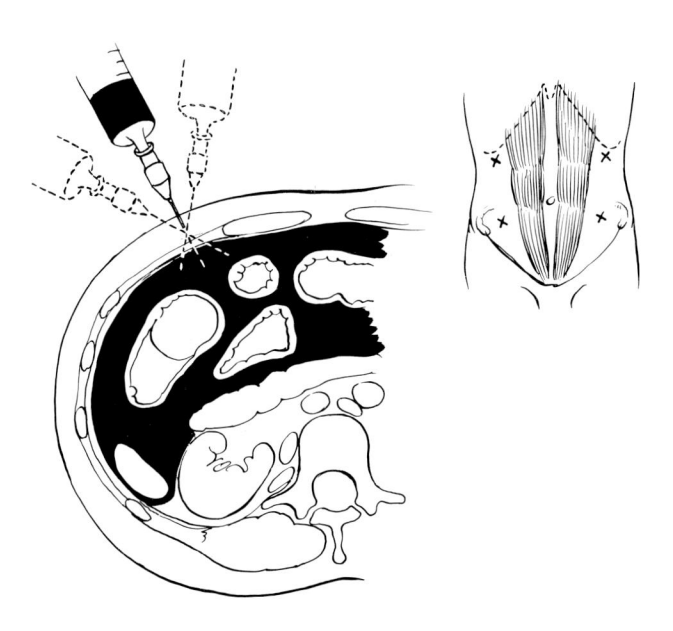

paracentesis has varied in different reports. Yurko and Williams (1966) indicated it could be 90 per cent when properly performed. Olsen and Hildreth (1971), in a comparative study of abdominal paracentesis versus peritoneal lavage on the same patients, reported that abdominal paracentesis was accurate in showing hemoperitoneum in only 21 per cent of cases while peritoneal lavage was accurate in 100 per cent. As previously mentioned, Perry also reported diagnostic peritoneal lavage to be more accurate than four-quadrant tap.

Laceration of the Gastric Mucosa

This is one type of gastric injury that may result from blunt abdominal trauma. Another, transmural perforation of the gastric wall, will be discussed later.

Laceration of the gastric mucosa and submucosa causes hemorrhage and presents with hematemesis. The injury, clinical characteristics, diagnosis, and management are similar to that of the Mallory-Weiss syndrome (pp. 81 to 87, Vol. 1).

The diagnosis of this injury is suggested by the patient's vomiting and hematemesis without associated abdominal pain and rigidity, and by persistent presence of blood in the nasogastric tube passed into the stomach. It is difficult to diagnose clinically, as it must be differentiated from other causes of upper gastrointestinal hemorrhage. Also, it is important to determine whether or not there is perforation of the gastric or duodenal wall. Gastrografin injected through the nasogastric tube, followed by radiographic study of the stomach and duodenum, will demonstrate the presence or absence of perforation. Absence of perforation further suggests, but does not establish, the diagnosis of laceration of the gastric mucosa and submucosa with bleeding. If the patient's condition permits, fiberoptic gastroduodenoscopy can exclude sites of bleeding proximal to the cardia and may establish the diagnosis by visualizing areas of bleeding in the stomach. In a few cases, selective celiac arteriography has been used successfully to diagnose and treat this injury. Operative treatment is indicated when the lesion is not located, the bleeding is massive, and trial of nonoperative treatment has failed to stop the bleeding, or if the injury was severe and there are clinical manifestations of additional intra-abdominal injuries.

The operative treatment is the same as that described for the Mallory-Weiss syndrome.

Transmural Perforation

Transmural perforation presents as a perforated peptic ulcer, but occasionally the perforation may be confined and not manifest until later development of a walled-off lesser sac abscess. The diagnosis is difficult when transmural perforation of the stomach is associated with other injuries. In two of Harrison's and Debas' (1972) patients, the gastric rupture was unsuspected until autopsy, because the predominant clinical signs were those of a severe central nervous system injury. When a patient with multiple trauma is comatose, a nasogastric tube should be inserted and plain films of the abdomen obtained. Whenever gastric or duodenal injury is suspected, but the diagnosis is in doubt, Gastrografin studies of the upper gastrointestinal tract should be obtained. Plain x-ray films of the abdomen showed free air within the peritoneal cavity in four of Siemen and Fulton's (1977) six gastric rupture cases, but no air was seen in the other two.

When perforation or rupture is diagnosed or strongly suspected, prompt operation is indicated. A vertical midline incision is recommended because it can be extended from the xiphoid to the pubis if necessary. A complete abdominal exploration to exclude injury to other viscera is mandatory. The entire surface of the stomach should be inspected. Anterior perforations are easily found, but posterior perforations will be missed unless the entire posterior surface is visualized by entering the lesser peritoneal sac through either the gastrocolic or the hepatogastric omentum. It is important to debride damaged margins of the defect back to normal tissue before closing the defect in the gastric wall.

All lacerations of the stomach should be closed with two layers of sutures. Small perforations are excised and converted into linear closures, so that the mucosal layer can be exposed and accurately sutured and bleeding vessels can be identified and ligated. A continuous inverting 2-0 chromic catgut or synthetic suture through the entire gastric wall is recommended for the first layer as it provides hemostasis in the very vascular submucosa of the stomach. Interrupted Lembert sutures of 3-0 or 2-0 silk are then used for the second layer of the closure. Pursestring sutures are not used because they are not as effective for controlling gastric wall bleeding.

Portions of the stomach should be resected, if necessary, for debridement of devitalized tissue, and occasionally partial gastrectomy is required for extensive injury. Spilled gastric contents are removed from the peritoneal cavity and the lesser sac, and subhepatic spaces are lavaged copiously to minimize the likelihood of later abscess formation. The need for draining the peritoneal cavity is a matter of judgment in individual cases and is influenced by the degree and quality of contamination. Postoperative gastric decompression is provided by leaving a nasogastric tube in place, attached to suction.

Administration of antibiotics, intraoperative lavage of the peritoneum, and drainage of potential sites cannot be depended upon to prevent abscess formation. Intra-abdominal sepsis is a common postoperative complication that is frequently fatal unless recognized and promptly treated; therefore, one should be alert for its occurrence in the postoperative period.

Intramural Hematomas of the Stomach

Intramural gastric hematomas may be caused by emesis or trauma, either local or remote. "They have also occurred spontaneously as a complication of many types of bleeding diathesis, including hemophilia, leukemia, idiopathic thrombocytopenic purpura, and anticoagulant therapy. The stomach has been involved much less often than the small bowel and colon. Mahoney (1974) reported a 22-year-old man, a known hemophiliac, who was admitted to the hospital with a history of sudden onset of severe, unrelenting epigastric pain associated with nausea and vomiting of eight hours' duration but no history of hematemesis, melena, or changes in bowel habits. Physical examination disclosed diffuse upper abdominal tenderness with a questionable epigastric mass. An upper gastrointestinal x-ray contrast film showed a 12 by 6 centimeter mass projecting into the lumen of the stomach from the greater curvature. The surface of the mass appeared slightly irregular. The patient was given supportive therapy and cryoprecipitated antihemophilic globulin. He was free of pain and eating normally on the third day after admission. A repeat gastrointestinal x-ray contrast study done 6 months later showed resolution of the mass with a completely normal stomach.

Mahoney advised that a careful history and appropriate testing for bleeding diathesis are essential to diagnosing any gastrointestinal lesion of rapid onset, because surgical intervention in such a case can be disastrous. Spontaneous regression occurs with control of the bleeding and conservative management.

The fact that both the Mallory-Weiss syndrome and intramural gastric hematomas have been reported in association with emesis suggested to Watts (1976) that in some cases these two emetogenic lesions might coexist and that intramural gastric hematomas may be a variant of the Mallory-Weiss syndrome. In order to determine whether or not there is a significant association of these two lesions, Watts reviewed 44 patients seen with demonstrated Mallory-Weiss lesions in San Francisco General Hospital. Small hematomas were seen in nine (20 per cent). Five of these hematomas straddled the cardioesophageal junction. The remainder were divided equally between the distal esophagus (2) and stomach (2). In eight patients, hemorrhage ceased spontaneously. One patient required surgical intervention because of continued bleeding from the tear. In summary, nine (20 per cent) of the 44 patients with Mallory-Weiss syndrome had endoscopic evidence of small submucosal hematomas lying in or adjacent to the region of the tear. Watts believes that these small hematomas occur most commonly as a variant of the Mallory-Weiss lesion.

GASTRIC INJURIES BY PENETRATING TRAUMA

Penetrating wounds, such as gunshot or stab wounds of the upper abdomen or lower thorax frequently injure the stomach, often penetrating through both its anterior and posterior walls and injuring adjacent structures. The stomach also may be injured by penetrating wounds through the back, perineum, or buttocks.

Missile Wounds of the Stomach

These wounds may be caused by bullets fired from high-velocity or low-velocity weapons or by high-explosive fragments of various types. Similar wounds may be made by stones, nails, and other sharp objects projected at high velocity, as by rotary lawn mowers.

Much has been learned about managing missile wounds of the stomach from reports by military surgeons (Wolf, 1955; Whelan, 1975), who described their extensive experiences with the management of these wounds in World War II and the Korean and Vietnam Wars. The principles learned on the battlefield are applicable for civilian practice.

Wolf (Surgery in World War II, 1955) reported that in the 3154 penetrating wounds of the abdomen treated by the 2nd Auxiliary Surgical Group during World War II, the stomach was wounded in 416 instances (13.2 per cent), an unexpectedly high incidence. Wounds of this organ were complicated by injuries to other viscera in 9 of every 10 cases. The case fatality rate in gastric injuries (40.6 per cent) was significantly higher than it was in injuries of the colon, small intestine, liver, spleen, or genitourinary tract. Of the 416 gastric injuries, 196 (47.1 per cent) were by missiles that traversed the diaphragm, resulting in 85 deaths (43.4 per cent). In the remaining 220 cases, the missiles entered or traversed only the abdominal cavity, resulting in 84 deaths (38.2 per cent). In the 416 cases with gastric injuries, the injury was univisceral in 42 (10.1 per cent), 12 of whom died (28.6 per cent). The injury involved more than one viscus in 374 cases (89.9 per cent), of whom 157 (42.0 per cent) died. The mortality rate increased in almost arithmetical progression with each additional viscus injured (Table 7–2).

Wounds of the stomach varied widely in type (Table 7–3), and the mortality rate was related to the type of the wound. The 258 perforating wounds were caused by small missiles, which perforated one or both walls of the stomach in a nearly perpendicular plane, and often caused little or no peritoneal contamination since the gastric mucosa tended to seal off the injury. Shock was not severe usually. Of the 117 lacerating wounds, 16 were simple tangential lacerations of the stomach wall without penetration into the lumen. In five cases, however, the stomach was completely transected. The remaining patients had extensive lacerations with profuse leakage and severe peritoneal contamination, resulting in the higher mortality rate (see Table 7–3).

Madding and Lawrence (Surgery in World War II, 1955) reported that "in 12 of the 3154 abdominal injuries observed by the 2nd Auxiliary Surgical Group during World War II, injuries of the abdominal viscera occurred without penetration of the abdominal wall by the wounding missile." In 10 of the 12 cases the missile caused a through-and-through wound of the abdominal parietes but did not injure the peritoneum. In the other 2 cases, the foreign body was retained within the abdominal wall. Apparently the energy associated with im-

Table 7–2. Influence of Multiplicity Factor on Case Fatality Rates in 416 Wounds of Stomach

Organs Injured	Cases	Deaths	Case Fatality Rate
Stomach only	42	12	28.6
Stomach and 1 viscus	174	47	27.0
Stomach and 2 viscera	112	44	39.3
Stomach and 3 viscera	50	29	58.0
Stomach and 4 viscera	23	23	100.0
Stomach, other viscera, and great vessels	15	14	93.3
Total	416	169	40.6

(From Wolf, L. H.: Wounds of the stomach. In Surgery in World War II. Vol. 2, General Surgery. Washington, D.C., Office of the Surgeon General, Department of the Army, 1955.)

Table 7–3. Case Fatality Rates in Relation to Type of Injury in 416 Wounds of Stomach

Type of Injury	Cases	Deaths	Case Fatality Rate
Perforating	258	91	35.3
Lacerating*	117	71	60.7
Not stated	41	7	17.1
Total	416	169	40.6

*Includes 5 complete transections. (From Wolf, L. H.: Wounds of the stomach. In Surgery in World War II. Vol. 2, General Surgery. Washington, D.C., Office of the Surgeon General, Department of the Army, 1955.)

pact of the missile was sufficient to produce an explosive effect in the abdominal wall, and this effect was imparted to the intra-abdominal structures. Hollow viscera containing gas and liquid were injured in 9 of the 12 cases, indicating that this type of viscus may be particularly prone to injury from indirect trauma because of transmission of the force of the missile by the visceral contents. The experience of these surgeons with injuries of the abdominal wall that did not involve the peritoneal layer convinced them that it would be an error to assume there is no intra-abdominal visceral injury merely because the missile did not enter the peritoneal cavity. Whenever there is clinical evidence of intraperitoneal involvement, exploration should be regarded as mandatory. The visceral injuries found in their experience proved the wisdom of that policy.

Madding and Lawrence also reported that the peritoneal cavity was penetrated in 41 of the 3154 abdominal wounds (13 per cent) without significant damage to any of the intraperitoneal viscera. However, a more important observation was that in not a single instance did a missile traverse a major diameter of the peritoneal cavity without causing visceral injury. Since every injury in which there was evidence or suspicion of peritoneal penetration in these 3154 cases was explored, perforating wounds of the peritoneal cavity in which there is no injury to the intraperitoneal structures must be extremely uncommon. "Although some wounds of the gastrointestinal tract seal over, and clinical recovery has occasionally ensued in such cases without surgery, and therefore without diagnosis, the risks involved in the nonsurgical management of this type of wound seem unjustified when good surgical service and facilities are available," the investigators concluded.

Missiles that penetrate through the skin may course straight through the body and escape through a wound of exit on the opposite side. Sometimes, however, the course within the body may be deflected so that the wound of exit is in a bizarre location. Two visible external wounds, one of entrance and the other of exit, suggest that the missile itself does not remain within the body, but a fragment may. The wound of exit is usually larger than the wound of entrance. If the missile lodges in the tissues, it remains as a foreign body and there is no wound of exit. This is an important observation. Penetrating wounds may contain foreign bodies of various types and sizes. A missile may have fragmented into widely separated parts. Furthermore, it may have carried into the tissues particles of infected clothing, dirt, gravel, or other contaminants. In addition, tissue in and adjacent to its course through the body is devitalized, and multiple viscera may be injured.

Wolff, Childs, and Gittings (Surgery in World War II, 1955) reported that in their series of 3052 abdominal wounds, the case fatality rate for bullet wounds was 24.7 per cent and for high-explosive fragments, 23.1 per cent. Three hundred forty-one wounds of entrance (13.2 per cent) were in the buttocks or the region of the hips, and 11 (0.4 per cent) were in the perineum. In practically every case in this series, the course of the missile within the body was a straight line. Bizarre or circuitous tracks were extremely uncommon. A seemingly erratic course could almost invariably be explained by an accurate reconstruction of the position of the soldier when he was struck. Changes of posture caused significant displacement of viscera and altered their customary relationships.

DIAGNOSIS

In penetrating injuries, the location of the wound of entrance and the absence or presence and location of a wound of exit are of diagnostic importance. In penetrating wounds of the chest and abdomen, the back, perineum, rectum, and vagina should be examined for wounds of entrance or exit. An imaginary line from a wound of entrance to a wound of exit suggests the course of the missile and the structures most likely to have been injured. When there is no wound of exit and the offending object has not been withdrawn through the wound of entrance, it remains as a retained foreign body somewhere within the patient. If the object is radiopaque, a plain x-ray film will show its location, size, and shape. An imaginary line from the entrance wound to the object may suggest the course within the body and the structures potentially injured.

Plain x-ray films of the chest and abdomen should be obtained in all patients with penetrating missile wounds that may have entered the peritoneal cavity. They provide valuable information by detecting injuries to bones, pneumothorax, hemothorax, pneumoperitoneum, and the absence or presence and location of radiopaque foreign bodies; they also influence the choice of operative incision.

Urinalysis should be obtained. If the patient is unable to void, insertion of a Foley catheter into the urinary bladder will provide an immediate specimen of urine, which is examined for blood. A positive test suggests injury to a kidney, the urinary tract, or both. A cystogram and intravenous pyelogram are indicated when hematuria is present in a patient with a penetrating wound that could have injured renal structures, because with preoperative knowledge that they are intact, their operative exposure may be avoided. Should a renal injury that might best be treated by nephrectomy be discovered, the preoperative status of the other kidney is critically important.

A nasogastric tube should be inserted. When the stomach has been injured, bloody aspirate can usually be obtained from the tube. Gastrografin injected through the tube into the stomach followed by an x-ray study will demonstrate whether or not this viscus is perforated.

Wolf (Surgery in World War II, 1955) reported that in his experience with 416 wounds of the stomach, the only two conclusive signs on physical examination in preoperative diagnosis were (1) emission of undigested food from the abdominal wound, and (2) observation of a perforation or laceration in an eviscerated stomach. Vomiting was no more frequent in gastric wounds than in wounds of other viscera. It was recorded in only 7 of the 416 cases and was neither a prominent nor a reliable sign of gastric injury. However, blood in the vomitus or in the aspirated gastric contents was both suggestive and reliable. It was noted in 41 of the 416 gastric wounds (4 times in vomitus) and was a valuable clue to the nature of the injury, when blood swallowed in wounds of the head, neck, or lungs could be ruled out. The absence of blood in the gastric contents was of no diagnostic value.

Preoperative passage of a Levin tube in suspected wounds of the stomach proved a useful diagnostic and therapeutic measure. Accumulations of gas and fluid were released, thus decreasing leakage of gastric contents and preventing more serious contamination. Leakage of gas from the damaged stomach was sometimes a valuable diagnostic sign, manifested by subcutaneous emphysema of varying degrees in the abdominal or chest walls. In some cases gas bubbled from the abdominal wound. If the gastric wound were thoracoabdominal, gas from the stomach might escape into the pleural cavity through the lacerated diaphragm and produce pneumothorax.

Pneumoperitoneum was recorded in only 6 of the 375 soldiers with gastric wounds who received radiologic studies preoperatively. In doubtful cases the absence of audible peristalsis was a useful diagnostic aid, but peristalsis might be present if soiling were localized to the retroperitoneal space or to the lesser peritoneal cavity.

MANAGEMENT OF MISSILE WOUNDS OF STOMACH

All patients with nonsurgical penetrating wounds should be protected against tetanus.

Treatment

There is general agreement that all patients with a perforating missile wound of the abdomen should be considered to be candidates for operation. When a patient with an abdominal wound is in shock, effort should be made to stabilize his or her condition preoperatively by use of lactated Ringer's solution and transfusion of whole blood. If prompt resuscitation does not result in improvement in the patient's condition, and no other obvious explanation is available, laparotomy should be performed. Further efforts at restoring blood volume will be futile until the hemorrhage is stopped. When bleeding is controlled, the patient's condition will improve and a definitive operation can be performed under less urgent circumstances.

"Surgical treatment should never be withheld until the signs and symptoms of oligemic shock appear, and should never be withheld because of indications of 'irreversible' shock" (Whelan, 1975).

Whelan also pointed out that it is important for the surgeon to know the wounding potential of the weapon, to assist in evaluating the extent of injury in order to treat it most effectively. This is true for both military and civilian surgeons.

The wounding potential of any missile is a summation of the following factors:

(1) The amount of energy transmitted to the body upon impact by a missile, which is determined in part by the mass and size of the missile, but chiefly by its velocity.

(2) The amount of energy expended is expressed by the formula:

$$KE = \frac{m(v_1^2 - v_2^2)}{2g}$$

where KE refers to kinetic energy in foot pounds, m refers to mass of the missile in pounds, v_1 stands for initial velocity in feet per second, v_2 stands for the final velocity in feet per second, and g is the acceleration due to gravity in feet per second^2.

(3) The behavior of the missile upon penetration is influenced by the density of the tissues injured and the elasticity of the skin and other tissues.

(4) The direction of the transmitted energy is determined by the shape of the missile, its motion in flight, and stability at the time of impact.

Velocity is the most important factor in wounding. The terms high velocity and low velocity are arbitrary; 2500 feet per second is chosen as the dividing line between them. Civilian injuries usually are inflicted with low-velocity weapons. For example, the .38-caliber pistol has a muzzle velocity of approximately 680 feet per second, compared with the high-velocity military rifle bullet (M-16) which has a muzzle velocity of approximately 3250 feet per second. "The energy expended is directly proportional to the mass and to the square of the effective velocity. Thus, doubling the velocity quadruples the kinetic energy of the missiles" (Whelan, 1975).

LOW-VELOCITY MISSILE WOUNDS. Low-velocity missiles injure only those tissues with which they come into contact. No significant energy is imparted to the nearby tissues so the damage is entirely localized—the missile simply creates local damage and pushes other tissues aside. Therefore, only minimal debridement is required. Spent high-velocity missiles produce wounds equivalent to those produced by low-velocity missiles.

HIGH-VELOCITY MISSILE WOUNDS. The high-velocity wound is a totally different entity. The kinetic energy of the missile upon impact is imparted to the adjacent tissues, which are suddenly hurled forward, laterally, and then backward, creating a large space or cavity that is approximately 30 to 40 times the size of the missile, in which pressures of 100 atmospheres (1500 p.s.i.) have been recorded. This effect is termed cavitation. The temporary cavity becomes a vacuum which draws in air from both the entrance and the exit sites. Its maximal size is attained within a few milliseconds, and it pulsates quickly to rest, forming the permanent cavity. This permanent wound tract is visible to the clinician, but the damage at a distance may not be immediately apparent. The effect of the cavity becomes more damaging when bone is fragmented and acts as a secondary missile. The high-velocity missile neatly shears the tissue, while the violence of the expansion of the missile tract as the cavity is created disrupts tissues, ruptures blood vessels and nerves, and may even fracture bones at a distance removed from the path of the missile. This force of cavitation simulates compression or crushing injuries similar to those sustained in blunt trauma.

The explosive nature of high-velocity wounds is such that a high-velocity rifle bullet passing near a blood vessel produces intimal lesions at a distance from the missile tract. Though externally appearing grossly normal, vessels may be thrombosed.

According to Whelan (1975), Kocher demonstrated in 1876 that tissues that contain large quantities of water were most severely damaged, and Daniel in 1944 correlated the severity of high-velocity wounds with the specific gravity of the tissue involved. Muscle is severely damaged because of its density. "In contrast, the lung sustains less extensive local destruction because of its low density, resulting in absorption of less energy and a smaller temporary cavity. Tissues of varying density, such as fascia or bone, may divert the direction of the missile, resulting in bizarre wound tracts."

Clinical Considerations. Because of their devastating local effects, high-velocity wounds must be debrided widely and completely. This includes removal of all devitalized tissue and foreign bodies. Tissues that do not bleed promptly when incised are considered to be devitalized. Structures distant to the missile tract are likely to be overlooked and remain as devitalized tissues. The risk of infection is increased in high-velocity wounds because the pulsation of their kinetic cavitation draws in foreign material and bacteria at both the entrance and the exit sites.

"It is fallacious to believe that bullets are sterile because of the heat generated in the firing process. Experiments have shown that bacterial infections were transmitted to animals shot with contaminated bullets. Thorsby, in 1967, demonstrated that heat-labile bacteria, inoculated on missiles fired at 1600 feet per second, uniformly grew along the bullet track. These facts should be appreciated when planning the extent of wound excision" (Whelan, 1975).

OPERATION

Preoperative Preparation

Aspiration of gastric contents is a serious hazard in trauma patients. Evacuation of the stomach by nasogastric tube is advisable before induction of anesthesia. Gastric lavage is contraindicated if the clinical findings suggest that perforation of the esophagus or stomach may have occurred. A cuffed endotracheal tube should be used during anesthesia.

Blood typing and cross-matching, hematocrit, and hemoglobin values are checked. Blood transfusion is given according to the indications in each case. Intravenous fluids are administered, and antibiotics are given preoperatively. If the patient is unable to void, catheterization is indicated; urinalysis is obtained.

Technic of Surgical Treatment

An upper right or left paramedian or upper or lower midline incision may be selected, depending upon whether the wound of entrance is in the upper, middle, or lower part of the abdomen. A generous midline incision provides the quickest and best access to the entire abdomen. In patients with known or suspected thoracoabdominal injury, exploration above and below the diaphragm is indicated. This may be done through a separate laparotomy and thoracotomy, or either one of these incisions can be extended across the costal arch to form a continuous thoracoabdominal incision that permits exploration both above and below the diaphragm. This approach makes the anterior and posterior surfaces of the gastric fundus accessible and greatly facilitates repair of injuries to the fundus and body of the stomach. The incision should be made generously, as free exposure is essential. Only in exceptional instances should the wound of entrance be included in the incision, because the penetrating tract may be heavily contaminated.

Finding abnormal odor, fluid, and/or gas upon opening the peritoneum indicates perforation of a hollow viscus. It is often difficult to determine whether the gas originated in the stomach, from the chest through a perforation of the diaphragm, or from some other hollow viscus. Careful exploration is necessary to determine its source. The presence of gas in the abdomen might also be due to an anaerobic infection. Crepitus and discoloration of tissue might be the result of leakage of gas and acid secretions from perforation of the stomach, but it might also be explained by an early infection.

If the fluid is bright red blood, active bleeding is probably still taking place. Free exposure is then particularly important, and one should not hesitate to enlarge the incision to obtain it. The blood is removed as rapidly as possible by suction and sponging with *dry* gauze packs, and the site of hemorrhage is sought. The mesenteric vessels, vena cava, aorta, portal vein, liver, and spleen are the most common sources of large intra-abdominal hemorrhage in penetrating wounds of the abdomen. As soon as the site of hemorrhage is identified it is dealt with appropriately. Any fluid remaining should be removed by aspiration. If blood loss threatens exsanguination, it may be necessary to cross-clamp the aorta to obtain control. Once the hemorrhage has been stopped, the patient's condition will improve, and the operation can proceed in a more leisurely fashion.

The anterior wall of the stomach is easily inspected; inspection of the posterior wall is more difficult. To accomplish this, it is advisable to divide part of the gastrocolic omentum and lift the stomach forward to visualize the posterior gastric wall and permit thorough examination. The entire surface of the stomach is examined, the site or sites of perforation are identified, and their extent is assessed. If the wound in the stomach is small, it may be difficult to find as it may be plugged by mucosa that permits little leakage to aid in identification. If a wound is found in one wall of the stomach, it is imperative to determine whether there is also another wound in the opposite wall.

Perforating wounds of the stomach should be treated by adequate debridement and a two-layer closure. Every effort should be made to approximate the gastric mucosa by suture in all wounds of the stomach. Although the simplest method for closing small, circular, smooth-edged perforations of the stomach appears to be by use of a pursestring seromuscular suture reinforced by a second such suture, military experience has demonstrated that the pursestring suture is unsatisfactory for this purpose. Wolf (Surgery in World War II, 1955) reported that "in six cases, all simple gastric perforations closed by the reinforced pursestring method, severe postoperative hemorrhage from the stomach occurred and was fatal in three. This was the largest number of postoperative hemorrhages encountered in the entire series of 3154 abdominal injuries.

"Since the pursestring suture does not include the gastric mucosa, the mucosal edges retract, thus exposing blood vessels which traverse the submucosa, and the resulting pathologic picture simulates that of acute peptic ulceration. Erosion of the previously sealed underlying vessels and subsequent hemorrhage are therefore possibilities when this method is used."

As a result of this report and others like it, the recommended policy for treating all gastric perforations is:

(1) Every effort should be made to approximate the gastric mucosa by suture in all wounds of the stomach.

(2) Small perforations may be enlarged transversely so that the mucosal layer can be exposed and accurately sutured.

(3) Pursestring suture should be avoided in managing wounds of the stomach.

When the gastric wound edges are jagged and contused, the devitalized parts should be excised and the resultant enlarged wound repaired in two layers. Occasionally the stomach will be so severely injured that a partial or, rarely, a total gastrectomy may be required. In suturing a wound near the pylorus or near the cardia, care must be taken not to constrict the lumen. After the wound in the stomach wall is closed, the remainder of the intestinal tract and the abdominal organs are carefully examined to see whether further wounds are present. If found, they are dealt with appropriately. The pylorus is also examined to make certain that the closure of the gastric wound did not encroach upon its lumen. If the pylorus has been obstructed, a gastroenterostomy or pyloroplasty must be performed in addition to the foregoing surgical procedures.

The need for peritoneal drainage differs in individual cases and depends upon the time elapsed between the injury and operation, the severity of the injury, the security of its closure, and the presence of contamination. If drainage is indicated, the drain is brought to the outside through a separate stab wound.

The incision and wounds in the abdominal wall should be closed in anatomic layers. A jagged and contused wound of the abdominal wall is treated separately from the abdominal incision. After it is excised and debrided, the muscle and fascia are closed immediately, but the skin and subcutaneous tissue are packed and left for delayed closure (Fig. 7–6). After 4 to 5 days of antibiotic therapy, and if the patient's condition permits, the pack is removed and the skin and subcutaneous tissue are closed

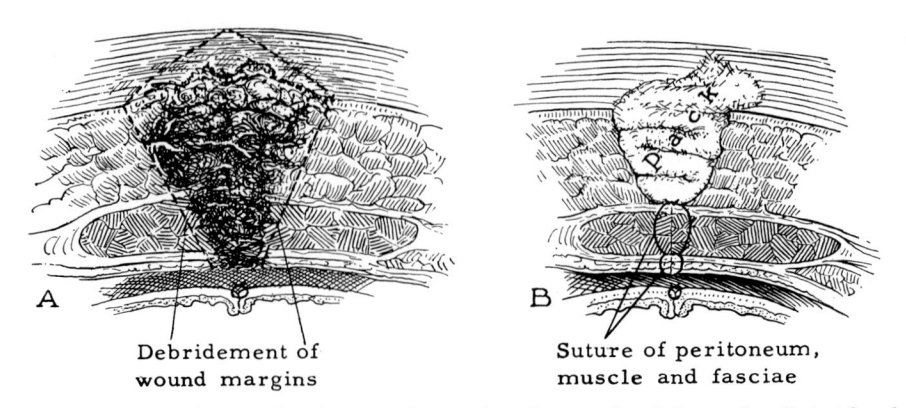

Figure 7–6. Treatment of a jagged and contused wound perforating the abdominal wall. *A*, After debridement, the peritoneum, muscle, and fasciae are closed, but the skin and subcutaneous tissue are packed and left open. *B*, Sectional views.

A, Debridement of wound margins
B, Suture of peritoneum, muscle and fasciae

secondarily by suture. This method of delayed primary closure of gunshot wounds was one of the valuable advances in surgery resulting from World War II and has been confirmed by subsequent experiences in both military and civilian surgery.

In any operation such as this, in which the gastrointestinal tract is opened, the abdominal wall incision is exposed to bacterial contamination. It is advisable, therefore, to close the muscle and fascia of the abdominal incision with No. 30 stainless steel wire or similar monofilament suture, which is nonabsorbable and is less likely to become infected than silk or other braided material. The peritoneal layer is usually sutured with catgut or a synthetic suture and the skin is subsequently closed with *interrupted* sutures of nylon.

If intraperitoneal drainage is unnecessary, the abdominal wall incision may be closed primarily. However, if the incision is grossly contaminated it is advisable to close the muscle and fascia but leave the skin and subcutaneous tissue open with a sterile dressing in place. A delayed primary closure of the skin can then be carried out in 4 to 5 days without undue risk of infection.

If the patient's condition is critical, and speed in closure of the abdomen is imperative, mass closure may be done by placing steel wire or heavy braided sutures of Prolene or silk through all the layers of the abdominal wall. This type of mass closure saves time and may be life-saving, but it does not provide an anatomic closure in layers and frequently results in later development of a postoperative hernia. Furthermore, great care must be taken in tightening these sutures to make sure that the intestine or omentum is not caught between the suture and anterior abdominal wall. Although mass closure has a place in the management of patients in precarious condition, it should only be used as an emergency measure.

Postoperative Care

Postoperatively, a nasogastric tube is left in the stomach and attached to suction. Fluids, electrolytes, and alimentation are given intravenously until after the patient is passing gas per rectum spontaneously, and normal peristalsis has returned. Then the tube is removed and oral feeding is commenced.

GASTRIC INJURIES BY STAB WOUNDS

Stab wounds may be caused by sharp objects, such as icepicks, knives, bayonets, glass, scissors, screwdrivers, and many other articles not intended for weapons but so used. The wound may be inadvertent, accidental, or self-inflicted.

The frequency with which penetrating wounds of the stomach occur in patients with stab wounds of the abdomen may be estimated by combining the incidences reported by investigators in three different localities (Perry, 1970; Nance and Cohn, 1969; Wilson and Sherman, 1960, 1961). The combined total of their patients was 602, of whom 77 had penetrating wounds of the stomach, an incidence of 12.7 per cent in the three series.

In contrast to the general agreement that all gunshot wounds that may have penetrated the abdominal cavity are best treated by routine laparotomy, controversy exists about the proper management of abdominal stab wounds. Some advocate routine, immediate laparotomy, and some advocate selective management of stabbed patients.

"In World War I, it was first shown that mortality could be lowered from 90 to 53 per cent by exploration of all penetrating wounds, including stab wounds, of the abdomen. This policy was confirmed by the experiences in World War II and in Korea when the mortality was respectively 25 per cent and 12 per cent" (Nance and Cohn, 1969). So the policy of routine laparotomy for all patients with wounds, including stab wounds, of the abdomen that *might* have entered the peritoneal cavity likewise became the policy for treating stab wounds of the abdomen in civilians. This policy permitted no exercise of surgical judgment in the management of patients with stab wounds of the abdomen and resulted in a 25 to 75 per cent incidence of negative laparotomies, which in turn were associated with a significant number of early and late postoperative complications.

If all patients with stab wounds undergo routine laparotomy, those with no penetration, or with trivial injury, are exposed to the risks of a major operation that offers them no benefit. However, some surgeons believe that it is so difficult to decide which patients have significant intra-abdominal injuries on the basis of history, physical examination, and the usual laboratory tests that anything short of exploration of the wound or laparotomy will result in missed visceral injuries and accompanying morbidity and mortality.

Selective management of penetrating abdominal stab wounds was popularized by Shaftan (1960), who adopted a policy of not performing laparotomy on patients with abdominal stab wounds unless clinical signs on admission or during a period of clinical observation, repeated hourly in the hospital, suggested intraperitoneal hemorrhage or visceral injury. He believed the risk of observing patients with abdominal stab wounds but without clinical signs of hemorrhage or peritoneal irritation was less than the risk of unnecessary laparotomy. He stressed, however, that for *some* patients with abdominal stab wounds, laparotomy is mandatory. The mandatory indications for immediate laparotomy include shock, signs of peritonitis (rebound tenderness, muscle guarding, absent bowel sounds), gastrointestinal bleeding, free air in the peritoneal cavity, evisceration, and massive hematuria.

Shaftan reported 535 patients with penetrating wounds of the abdomen, 90 per cent of whom had stab wounds. Only 28 per cent underwent laparotomy. The mortality of the operated group was 7.3 per cent and of the nonoperative group, 0.3 per cent; the overall mortality was 2.6 per cent. The morbidity of the operative group was 31 per cent and of the nonoperative group, 3.3 per cent. No deaths could be attributed to delay or failure to recognize the need for exploratory laparotomy.

Nance and Cohn (1969) reported that in their comparative study of "routine" laparotomy versus selective management in 600 patients with abdominal stab wounds, the overall complication rate had been reduced from 27 to 12 per cent. The average period of hospitalization was reduced from 7.9 to 5.4 days after the policy of routine laparotomy was superseded by the policy of selective management of patients with abdominal stab wounds. They also found that virtually all the deaths following stab wounds of the abdomen had been from hemorrhage, pulmonary complications, or other associated injuries. There were 14 deaths in their 1700 patients treated for abdominal stab wounds; none died of peritonitis. From the literature they collected 15 reports totalling 5005 patients with abdominal stab wounds, 72 (1.44 per cent) of whom died, but only 12 (0.24 per cent) died of peritonitis, indicating a remarkable rarity.

Several other surgeons have also documented reductions in overall morbidity and the same or improved mortality by the policy of selective management.

Although selective management of abdominal stab wounds appears to decrease morbidity and hospitalization time, it has some disadvantages. (1) It requires frequently repeated (usually hourly) examinations, preferably by the same examiner, so that changes for better or worse can be recognized; hence full-time physician coverage must be available for this purpose. For a surgeon in solo practice and without the support of a skilled house staff, routine exploratory laparotomy may serve the patient best. (2) It entails definite risks for those patients with serious abdominal injuries who initially do not display abdominal findings and for those who cannot be evaluated or observed properly because they are intoxicated, narcotic-addicted, psychotic, or comatose.

Zuidema and his associates (Cornell, Ebert, and Zuidema, 1965; Smithwick, Gertner, and Zuidema, 1968; Zuidema, 1969) emphasized the frequency of patients with abdominal stab wounds being intoxicated and unable to cooperate, so intra-abdominal injury is difficult to diagnose clinically. They described a simple radiographic procedure (sinography) for determining peritoneal penetration that could be used in patients who are unable to cooperate, thus sparing those with superficial wounds a needless laparotomy.

Technic of Sinography. Following sterile skin preparation, the wound edges are infiltrated with local anesthetic to permit placement of a pursestring suture. A small (14 F.) rubber catheter (polyethylene catheters are too rigid for this purpose) is placed in the ostium of the wound with its tip immediately underlying the dermis. The skin edges are tightly secured around the catheter with a 2-0 silk pursestring suture. Then 60 to 80 ml. of 50 per cent sodium diatrizoate (Hypaque), with 1 ml. of methylene blue added, are injected manually under moderate pressure from a syringe through the catheter. The catheter is clamped and recumbent. Lateral and oblique roentgenograms of the abdomen are promptly made. These demonstrate whether the wound has or has not penetrated the peritoneum. Failure to show contrast material within the peritoneal cavity is considered reliable evidence that the wound is superficial and the peritoneum has not been penetrated, so laparotomy is not performed, and the patient is observed in the hospital. Demonstration of contrast material within the peritoneal cavity is evidence that the peritoneum has been perforated, and laparotomy is indicated.

Indications for Sinography. "The use of sinography should be limited to patients who have abdominal stab wounds. It is not recommended in any way for patients with bullet wounds" (Zuidema, 1969).

Sinography may be used in any patient with a truncal stab wound that might have penetrated the peritoneal cavity, unless shock, peritonitis, protruding viscus, or other mandatory indication for immediate laparotomy is present; it is not used in patients who have a history of sensitivity to contrast media. It is particularly helpful in avoiding unnecessary exploration when multiple trauma or intoxication complicates clinical evaluation and adds to operative risk. The procedure does not require a cooperative patient or general anesthesia. It may be performed in the emergency room and provides a diagnostic decision shortly after the patient's arrival there, facilitating overall management.

Sinography must precede diagnostic peritoneal lavage, to avoid intra-abdominal dilution of contrast medium. Multiple stab wound tracts are injected individually and filmed, thus minimizing confusion in interpretation resulting from superimposition of contrast media. Although this procedure can reduce the number of negative explorations, it does not identify those patients with penetration of the peritoneum without serious injury.

Results of Sinography. Some surgeons have had good, and others poor, success with sinography. Zuidema (1969) reported one false-positive and three false-negative tests in 192 cases.

Steichen and colleagues (1967, 1969) reported only one false-negative test in sinographic studies of 95 patients but found that selective management by clinical signs alone resulted in a 7.3 per cent rate of unnecessary laparotomies, compared with 15.9 per cent by sinography.

Trimble (1969) reported on 50 patients in whom stab wound sinography had been used. In 12, the sinogram was positive and was confirmed by operation in 11, but one was a false-positive reading. In 38 patients, sinograms showed no peritoneal penetration. In 27 of these, there was no operation and early discharge. In 11, operation was performed on clinical grounds. Nonpenetration was confirmed in 5 of these, but, in 6, penetration has occurred (false-negatives).

Trimble concluded that sinographic evidence of nonpenetration must be confirmed by clinical observation in order to detect false-negative studies, and that exploration is indicated whenever there is clinical or sinographic evidence of peritoneal penetration. Attempts to eliminate unnecessary exploration by observation appear hazardous. The likelihood of significant injury and the dangers inherent in delayed operation greatly outweigh the risks associated with negative exploration.

Other methods for determining the presence or absence of peritoneal penetration include:

(1) Under local anesthesia, opening the stab wound sufficiently to visualize its complete course and depth. If the peritoneum has not been penetrated, the wound is closed by sutures and laparotomy is avoided. If the peritoneum has been penetrated or there is doubt, laparotomy is performed.

(2) Diagnostic peritoneal lavage and four-quadrant tap, which are described in the opening section on blunt abdominal trauma in this chapter, may also be used for patients with stab wounds.

(3) Netterville and Hardy (1967) recommended limited exploration through a small incision adjacent to the wound. If no penetration of the peritoneum has occurred, the procedure can be terminated and the incision closed. If penetration has occurred, laparotomy is performed.

A rigid policy for managing abdominal stab wounds can be impractical. Circumstances differ in each case and influence selection of the most appropriate diagnostic and therapeutic procedures.

If peritoneal penetration has not been demonstrated and the patient is alert and cooperative, frequently repeated examinations by the same clinician are necessary for good management. The presence of generalized abdominal pain, rebound tenderness, and rigidity usually indicate peritoneal irritation by blood or gastrointestinal contents from an injured intra-abdominal viscus, but may be due to injury of the abdominal wall or a rib. If these signs are equivocal or if the patient cannot be properly evaluated or observed, sinograms, local wound exploration, or peritoneal lavage can be used.

Mandatory indications for immediate laparotomy include shock, signs of peritonitis (rebound tenderness, muscle guarding, absent bowel sounds), gastrointestinal bleeding, free air in the peritoneal cavity, evisceration, and massive hematuria.

A useful policy for managing abdominal stab wounds has been described by Ballinger, Rutherford, and Zuidema (1979):

"1. Any patient with mandatory indications for laparotomy undergoes immediate operation.
2. Of the remaining patients:
   A. Those seen within 6 hours of stabbing have exploration of the wound under local anesthesia or a sinogram performed. If penetration into the peritoneal cavity is confirmed, laparotomy follows.
   B. Those seen after 6 hours of stabbing are observed. If questionable abdominal findings are present, wound exploration or sinography is done.
   C. Patients who cannot be properly evaluated or observed because of intoxication, narcotic addiction, psychosis, or coma are also subjected to sinography or local wound exploration.
   D. Patients with stab wounds through the lower rib cage, which have probably penetrated the diaphragm, are explored because of the risk of herniation through unrepaired diaphragmatic lacerations.
   E. Patients with multiple stab wounds seen within the first 12 hours require laparotomy.
   F. Abdominal paracentesis may be done under any of the circumstances dictating local wound exploration or sinography, but only positive taps are accorded any value."

The diagnostic procedures and indications for operation just described may determine whether or not the peritoneum has been penetrated and an intra-abdominal viscus injured, but do not identify which viscus or viscera. A specific diagnosis of gastric injury is suggested by hematemesis or aspiration of blood through a nasogastric tube inserted into the stomach. Whether or not the stomach has been perforated by the stab can be determined by injecting Gastrografin through the nasogastric tube, followed by radiographic study of the stomach and duodenum. If the stomach or some other intra-abdominal hollow viscus has been perforated, immediate laparotomy is indicated.

OPERATIVE TREATMENT

A stab wound is a low-velocity wound. No significant energy is imparted to the nearby tissues, and only the tissues with which the blade comes into contact are severed. The size, shape, and length of the wounding instrument are important for estimating the potential extent and severity of the injury. Damage to the skin and subcutaneous tissue is usually insignificant and requires no special treatment.

The technic of laparotomy for penetrating wounds of the abdomen is described on pages 210 to 212 and can be modified according to the circumstances in individual cases. Since stab wound injury to intra-abdominal viscera is confined to the immediate area of penetration, only limited debridement is required. However, if a wound is found in one wall of the stomach it is imperative to determine whether there is also another wound in the opposite wall and adjacent structures. As emphasized, all perforations or lacerations of the stomach should be closed with two layers of sutures.

Stab wounds that are superficial and have not penetrated the peritoneum may be treated by simple cleansing and primary closure after all contaminated foreign material has been removed.

To assess the indications and complications of laparotomy in patients with suspected abdominal injury, Petersen and Sheldon (1979) retrospectively reviewed reports of 757 patients who had undergone exploratory laparotomy at San Francisco General Hospital because of blunt or penetrating abdominal trauma. Intra-abdominal injuries had occurred in 597 patients (79 per cent). At operation, 160 of these (21 per cent) had no identifiable visceral injury. There were negative findings at laparotomy in 42 (18 per cent) of the 231 victims of blunt trauma. Of the 367 patients with stab wounds of the abdomen, 106 (29 per cent) had insignificant or absent intra-abdominal injury. Sixteen complications occurred in 94 patients (17 per cent) whose celiotomies for stab wounds were negative. Most of the complications were minor and did not prolong hospitalization. The morbidity attributable to a negative laparotomy for abdominal trauma was negligible. The overall complication rate was 4.9 per cent. No deaths were associated with negative findings at explorations for gunshot or stab wounds. Seven patients with blunt abdominal trauma died (16.7 per cent), but all deaths occurred in patients with multiple injuries and were not secondary to laparotomy.

In summary, the investigators found that gunshot wounds, as opposed to stab wounds, have a 99.3 per cent likelihood of causing serious intra-abdominal injury when peritoneal penetration had occurred. The high probability of visceral injury and the mortality rate associated with intra-abdominal gunshot wounds justify mandatory laparotomy for gunshot wounds of the abdomen. They concluded that although it is undesirable to perform an unneeded laparotomy in patients with abdominal trauma, it is more serious to delay exploration and incur morbidity or mortality. Because a negative finding at laparotomy has a low incidence of complications, early exploration is justified when intra-abdominal injury is suspected. Although peritoneal lavage for blunt trauma and selective exploration for some stab wounds may reduce the incidence of unnecessary laparotomies, the high incidence of major injury associated with gunshot wounds precludes use of selective exploration as a reasonable policy.

FOREIGN BODIES OF THE STOMACH

A review of case reports and stories of foreign bodies in the stomach can entertain and can challenge one's imagination. Any large metropolitan hospital has its interesting stories of unusual objects retrieved from the stomach. These foreign bodies range from accidentally swallowed items such as tacks, pins, paper clips, dentures, and fishbones, to unusual items such as utensils, can openers, coins, and nail clippers. Most of the larger and more unusual items are discovered in mental patients. Fortunately, 90 per cent of these ingested articles are passed spontaneously. Occasionally several ingested foreign bodies may aggregate to form a bezoar (Bitar and Holmes, 1975).

Most of these objects are radiopaque

and can be seen and followed by x-ray study. Nonradiopaque materials, such as Styrofoam, plastics, and wooden objects, may require dilute barium or Gastrografin to outline them (McCaffery and Lilly, 1975).

SYMPTOMS

In the nonpsychiatric patient, accidental ingestion is generally recognized by the patient, and medical evaluation is usually sought. In psychiatric patients, actual observation of ingestion of a foreign body or incidental discovery on x-ray film is the usual way these objects are recognized. On occasion a complication originated by the ingested object may be the presenting symptom. Complications from ingestion of foreign bodies ordinarily are rare. The symptoms and complications associated with an ingested foreign body include abdominal discomfort, hemorrhage, obstruction, and perforation. The three latter complications generally require operation.

TREATMENT

In most cases the ingested foreign body will be passed spontaneously without specific treatment. If the object is large, pointed at both ends, or has sharp serrations or hooks, spontaneous passage may not occur (Kassner and associates, 1975). If a foreign body does not pass out of the stomach within 72 hours, removal is generally indicated. Noncomplicated extraction can be performed using a flexible fiberoptic endoscope, employing various devices such as snares, biopsy forceps, alligator forceps, and polypectomy snares (Dunkerley and associates, 1975; Waye, 1976). If bleeding, obstruction, or perforation occurs, operation is required to remove the foreign body and treat the complication.

Patients who have a history of ingesting foreign bodies should be isolated to minimize their access to such objects.

CORROSIVE INJURIES OF THE STOMACH

Corrosive gastritis is generally defined as severe mucosal inflammation related to the ingestion of toxic agents. Lesions in the stomach may be associated with oral and esophageal injuries. Owing to various factors, sparing of the oral pharynx, esophagus, or stomach may occur, and assessment of injury to each of these areas should be made independently. Caustic injuries of the duodenum are rare, probably because of pyloric spasm when an irritating material enters the stomach.

TYPES OF INJURY

Injuries are classified usually on the basis of the type of chemical ingested — alkalis or acids (Allen and associates, 1970). Acids, such as sulfuric, hydrochloric, nitric, phenolic, and formaldehyde, result in coagulation necrosis of the mucosa. Alkalis, such as sodium hydroxide, potassium hydroxide, hypochlorite, and other types of lye compounds, produce a liquefaction necrosis. Another group of compounds is the systemic poisons, such as mercury bichloride. It is important to determine the compound that was ingested, since this will influence treatment and possibly determine the prognosis.

FACTORS DETERMINING SEVERITY OF INJURY

The severity of injury is determined by the type of agent ingested, the amount of material ingested, and the status of the stomach. Compounds containing sulfuric acid are notorious for producing perforation and gangrene of the stomach, and compounds containing alkali are more corrosive. If small amounts of the toxic substance are ingested, lesions may be oral and esophageal rather than gastric. If the stomach had contained a large amount of food, the ingested substance may be neutralized. Since alkalis are more corrosive than acids, they generally have a greater effect on the squamous esophageal mucosa.

DIAGNOSIS

The patient may seek medical help following accidental ingestion or deliberate ingestion of a toxic substance in a suicide attempt. Sometimes a family member discovers the suicide attempt and brings the patient for treatment. The variability in response of the oral pharynx, esophagus, and stomach makes prediction of the extent of injury difficult. Complications from the use of rigid endoscopes and Ewald tubes are very common; however, cautious use of a fiberoptic endoscope to assess damage is generally recomended (Chong, Beahrs, and Payne, 1974; Chung and DenBesten, 1975). If an area of necrosis is seen, endoscopy should be terminated. Reassessment of damage may be required in several days.

TREATMENT

General supportive measures should be instituted. These include intravenous fluids, transfusions (if bleeding occurs), antibiotics, and steroids. The use of the latter is controversial, and there is no convincing evidence that steroids prevent late complications. A nasogastric tube is gently passed and the stomach aspirated. Emesis should not be induced. Aspiration of the stomach is important, especially if a systemic poison such as mercury bichloride has been ingested. If the material ingested is known, specific neutralization should be done (Chong, Beahrs, and Payne, 1974). If the material is unknown, checking the nasogastric aspirate with pH paper may provide the necessary information. Acid should be neutralized with any of the common antacids, and alkali can be neutralized with dilute vinegar.

COMPLICATIONS

Early complications include bleeding, perforation, and gangrene. If hemorrhage occurs, it should be treated initially with transfusions; operation usually is not required. Perforation and gangrene require resection of the stomach and, rarely, total gastrectomy (Nicosia and associates, 1974). In assessing endoscopic damage, it is important to distinguish between a mucosal eschar produced by acid and a blackened gangrenous area. The latter requires operation and resection to prevent perforation (Nicosia and associates, 1974).

Late complications include strictures of the esophagus and pyloric areas, usually occurring years after the initial injury. Because of the increased incidence of squamous cell carcinoma associated with lye injuries of the esophagus, esophageal resection is usually recommended (Eaton and Tennekoon, 1972). Fibrosis of the antrum may occur years after the injury and may resemble an infiltrating gastric carcinoma. Obstruction of the pylorus may later require a vagotomy and gastroenterostomy.

Chapter 8

INJURIES OF THE DUODENUM

TYPES OF INJURIES

The location of the duodenum deep within the abdomen protects it from injury by superficial wounds. It is also protected from external trauma on all sides by surrounding soft tissues and abdominal musculature. By far the majority of duodenal injuries, therefore, occur by penetrating wounds (Table 8–1).

The duodenum is partly retroperitoneal and mobile at the pylorus and at its terminal end, but its other portions are fixed. The fixed position of the duodenum against the lumbar spine makes it vulnerable to a crushing force directed anteroposteriorly, or to a shearing force applied tangentially. Cocke and Myer (1964) postulated that the mechanism responsible for such an injury by force is blunt trauma occurring when the abdominal wall is relaxed and the duodenum is distended with gas and is a closed loop, due to a closed pylorus and an acutely flexed duodenojejunal angle secondary to the contracted fibromuscular ligament of Treitz. In such circumstances, even a relatively minor force may produce a blow-out type of perforation of the duodenal wall. The simultaneous presence of these anatomic factors producing a closed duodenal loop occurs infrequently, so this mechanism is not responsible for every duodenal rupture by blunt trauma. Many are caused by the crushing of the duodenum against the vertebral column.

A review of five large series (Cave, 1955; Burrus, Howell, and Jordan, 1961; Stone and Garoni, 1966; Morton and Jordan, 1968; Corley, Norcross, and Shoemaker, 1975) with a combined total of 503 patients treated for traumatic duodenal injuries revealed that duodenal injuries are relatively common in patients with either blunt or penetrating trauma of the abdomen (3 to 5 per cent), although the occurrence of injuries is relatively infrequent. Because of the relation of the duodenum to other intraabdominal viscera, it is seldom the only organ injured.

Duodenal injuries are of special significance because the viscus is partly retroperitoneal and because fistula formation from the duodenum is such a serious complication. The overall mortality rate in these five collected series ranged from 21 to 56.8 per cent.

Morton and Jordan (1968) reported 131 cases of traumatic duodenal injuries and divided them into four basic categories:

1. Tearing wounds resulting from sudden deceleration occurring where the organ changes from an intraperitoneal to a retroperitoneal location.
2. Crushing wounds when the third or fourth part of the duodenum is caught between the anterior abdominal wall and the vertebral column.
3. Blow-out injuries in which the fluid-filled duodenum is compressed, with its two ends effectively closed by the pylorus and the angulation of the ligament of Treitz.
4. Penetrating injuries.

Table 8-1. Mechanisms of Injury in 131 Patients with Duodenal Wounds

	No. of Patients	Per Cent
Penetrating	117	89
Knife	22	17
Bullet	87	66
Shotgun	8	6
Blunt	14	11
Total	131	100

(From Morton, J. R., and Jordan, G. L., Jr.: Traumatic duodenal injuries; Review of 131 cases. J. Trauma 8:127, 1968.)

BLUNT TRAUMA

The commonest cause of blunt injury to the duodenum is automobile accidents, usually when the lower chest, upper abdomen, or both crash against the steering wheel. Other causes are a blow to the upper abdomen resulting from a fall, a fight, a kick, a blast, an athletic contest, or impact against a fixed stationary object. The trivial nature of the trauma may be deceptive in relation to the severity of the injury to the duodenum.

Duodenal injuries caused by blunt trauma usually involve the second, third, or both portions of the duodenum and are of two types: (1) intramural hematoma, which may or may not involve the ampulla; and (2) rupture of the duodenal wall, which may be intraperitoneal or extraperitoneal. In one series (Burrus, Howell, and Jordan, 1961), 93 per cent of these ruptures were into the free peritoneal cavity, and 7 per cent were retroperitoneal.

Duodenal injuries caused by blunt trauma are more likely to be associated with severe injury than are penetrating injuries. In the series of Burrus, Howell, and Jordan (1961), 67 per cent of those injured by blunt trauma had severe injuries, while only 5.2 per cent of those injured by penetrating trauma had severe injuries.

In the study by Corley, Norcross, and Shoemaker (1975), 6 of 23 patients with duodenal injuries caused by blunt abdominal trauma suffered complete transection of the injured duodenum; in 7 others, over half of the duodenal wall circumference was injured. Eight additional patients with blunt injury had intramural hematomas of the duodenum; two of these had coexisting perforations.

PENETRATING WOUNDS

Of 98 patients with traumatic duodenal injuries, 75 were penetrating; of these, 51 resulted from small-caliber gunshot wounds, and 24 were stab wounds (Corley, Norcross, and Shoemaker, 1975). All but 2 of the 51 gunshot wounds were through-and-through wounds that penetrated the duodenal wall in two places. Many of the gunshot wounds produced large duodenal wall defects, but the duodenum was never completely transected by a missile in this series of cases. (This is in contrast to Cave's series of 112 casualties with duodenal wounds made by mainly high-velocity missiles, where the duodenum was transected in 20.) Seventeen of the 24 stab wounds were through-and-through injuries.

The second portion of the duodenum is the longest and is the part most frequently injured. In this series of 98 patients the second portion of the duodenum was injured in 49, the first portion in 5, the third portion in 16, and the fourth portion in 13. More than one portion was injured in 15

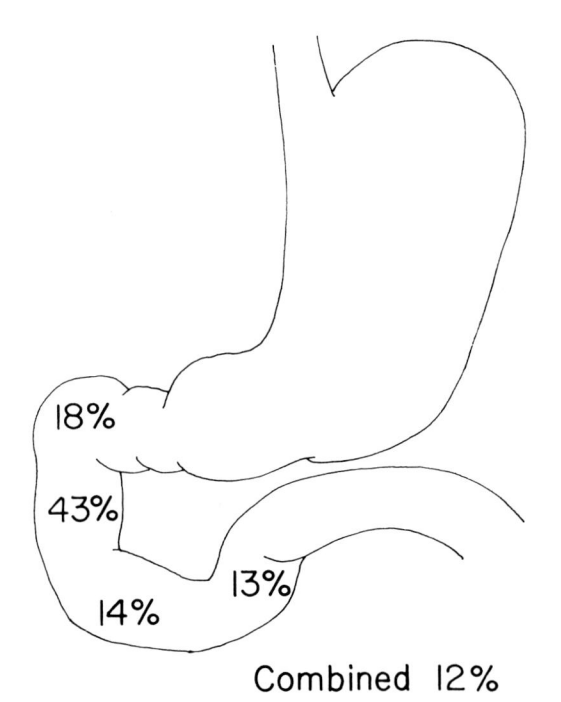

Figure 8-1. The incidence of wounds encountered in the four portions of the duodenum. Including those wounds involving more than one portion, the second portion was involved in almost 50 per cent of 131 patients. (From Morton, J. R., and Jordan, G. L., Jr.: Traumatic duodenal injuries; Review of 131 cases. J. Trauma 8:127, 1968.)

patients. The preponderance of the second portion of the duodenum as the site injured in traumatic duodenal injuries was documented in virtually all the reported series in which the sites of injury were recorded (Fig. 8–1).

In Cave's series (1955) of 118 casualties with duodenal injuries, 112 of the wounds were described in detail. The second portion of the duodenum was injured in 49.1 per cent, the first portion in 24.1 per cent, and the third portion in 13.4 per cent. In the remaining cases more than one portion was injured. Many injuries of the first portion were continuous with a wound of the pylorus, and some injuries of the third portion were continuous with wounds of the jejunum. Cave pointed out that the predominance of injuries of the second portion suggests that many patients with injuries of the first portion do not survive to reach a hospital because of associated lethal injuries to such adjacent structures as the vena cava, hepatic artery, and portal vein. Likewise, the paucity of injuries to the third portion suggests that associated fatal injuries to such adjacent structures as the aorta, vena cava, and mesenteric vessels preclude survival.

ASSOCIATED INJURIES

Because of the close association of the duodenum to major vessels and to other intra-abdominal viscera, it is seldom the only intra-abdominal organ injured. In Cave's series (1955), associated injuries to various other intra-abdominal viscera were present in 116 (98.3 per cent) of the 118 cases. The overall mortality rate was 56.8 per cent. Both patients with injury limited to the duodenum survived, but the mortality rate was 57.8 per cent in the 116 cases with multiple injuries. The visceral injuries in this series included 69 of the liver, 59 of the colon, and 37 of the right kidney.

In only 9 (7 per cent) of Morton's and Jordan's series (1968) of 131 patients treated for duodenal injury was the duodenum the only intra-abdominal organ injured. A major vascular injury occurred in 32 per cent of these patients, and most of the deaths occurred in this group. Pancreatic injury occurred in 28 per cent; many of these patients developed associated postoperative complications.

Some of the associated injuries to adjacent organs that commonly accompany and complicate duodenal injuries are shown in Table 8–2. Multiplicity greatly increases the lethality of wounds of the duodenum. In many, the associated intra-abdominal injuries present a much greater problem than the duodenal injury.

In the series of Burrus, Howell, and Jordan (1961), injuries of adjacent intra-abdominal viscera occurred in 81 of 86 patients with traumatic duodenal injuries; the duodenum was the only organ injured in just 5 patients. The liver was the adjacent organ most frequently injured, and there were 24 associated injuries of major vessels. Of particular importance were the associated injuries of the pancreas, which significantly complicated the postoperative course in a number of patients.

Extra-abdominal injuries may also accompany duodenal injury, especially in patients with multiple injuries by blunt trauma or by gunshot wounds. In one series, three of the patients with blunt trauma had concomitant chest injuries, including fractured ribs, hemothorax, and pneumothorax (Corley, Norcross, and Shoemaker, 1975). The major surgery required in multivisceral wounds plays an important part in the increase in mortality rates (Table 8–3). Cave (1955) reported that the mortality was 57 per cent in 21 cases which required nephrectomy, 75 per cent in 8 cases requiring cholecystectomy, 70 per cent in the 13 small

Table 8–2. Associated Intra-Abdominal Injuries in 88 Patients

Type of Injury: No. of Cases:	Gunshot 51	Stab 20	Blunt 17	Total 88
Organ Injured				
Pancreas	18	10	9	37
Liver	23	6	3	32
Colon	18	4	2	24
Stomach	18	2		20
Small bowel	15	3	1	19
Vena cava	14	4	1	19
Genitourinary	10	33	1	14
Extrahepatic	10	2	1	13
Major arterial	10	3		13
Retroperitoneum	1	2	2	5
Spleen	2	1	1	4
Diaphragm	1	2	1	4
Aorta	2			2
Total	142	42	22	206

(From Corley, R. D., Norcross, W. J., and Shoemaker, W. C.: Traumatic injuries to the duodenum; A report of 98 patients. Ann. Surg. 181:92, 1975.)

Table 8-3. Influence of Multiplicity Factor on Case Fatality Rates in 118 Wounds of Duodenum

Organs Wounded	Cases	Deaths	Case Fatality Rate
Duodenum only	2	0	0
Duodenum and 1 viscus[1]	28	16	57.1
Duodenum and 2 viscera	45	20	44.4
Duodenum and 3 viscera	21	14	66.7
Duodenum and 4 viscera	20	15	75.0
Duodenum and 5 viscera	2	2	100.0

[1]One fatality in this category was a univisceral wound, complicated by a wound of the portal vein, which was primarily responsible for the fatal outcome.
(From Cave, W. H.: Wounds of the duodenum (118 casualties). In Surgery in World War II. Vol. II. General Surgery. Washington, D.C., Office of the Surgeon General, Department of the Army, 1955, p. 240.)

bowel resections, 77.7 per cent in the 9 cases requiring colectomy, and 80 per cent in the 5 cases requiring splenectomy. Wounds of the major blood vessels played a particularly important part in the high case fatality rate of duodenal injuries. Eight of the nine patients with lacerations of the vena cava died; the only survivor was not in shock when first seen. Death also occurred in two injuries of the portal vein, the two injuries of pancreaticoduodenal artery, and the injuries of the hepatic and right spermatic arteries (one each).

Combined injuries of the pancreas and duodenum resulted in much higher mortality and morbidity rates than either injury alone, and the treatment was much more difficult. Pancreatic injuries were also highly fatal; eight of nine such cases died, though in only one was the head of the pancreas so badly damaged that the duct was severed.

In 15 of the 118 duodenal injuries, an associated chest injury was present, varying in severity from a simple perforation of the diaphragm to severe lacerations or contusions of the lung. Eleven of these 15 patients died.

CORROSIVE INJURIES AND FOREIGN BODIES OF THE DUODENUM

Foreign bodies of the duodenum and corrosive injuries of the duodenum are included in discussion of these topics in Chapter 7, Injuries of the Stomach.

DIAGNOSIS

A preoperative specific diagnosis of duodenal injury may be difficult and seldom is necessary. The diagnostic work-up is similar to that described for gastric injury (pp. 207–208). When an intra-abdominal injury is known or strongly suspected, the patient should be explored as soon as is feasible. Mandatory indications for immediate operation are similar to those listed for patients with gastric injuries. The specific diagnosis is made at exploratory operation.

RADIOLOGIC STUDIES

Plain scout films of the chest and abdomen should be obtained in all patients with blunt or penetrating injuries of the abdomen that may have caused intra-abdominal injury. They are not helpful in all cases but may provide valuable information by detecting injuries to bones, pneumothorax, hemothorax, the absence or presence and location of radiopaque foreign bodies, pneumoperitoneum, gas in the retroperitoneal area and along the upper pole of the right kidney, and the "more subtle, nonspecific findings of scoliosis and obliteration of the right psoas shadow which are often overlooked" (Lucas and Ledgerwood, 1975).

Corley and associates (1975) reported that 7 of their 17 patients with ruptures of the duodenum by nonpenetrating trauma had radiologic findings compatible with intraperitoneal organ injury; 3 had free intraperitoneal gas. In all 12 patients with penetrating trauma, free or retroperitoneal gas was demonstrated on scout films of the abdomen.

Donovan and Hager (1966) reported that free intraperitoneal air or retroperitoneal gas was noted on scout films of the abdomen in 7 of 10 patients with duodenal perforation by blunt trauma, but scout films revealed free intraperitoneal air in only 3 of 12 patients with duodenal perforation by penetrating trauma and were indeterminate in the other 9.

Stone and Garoni (1966) reported that in 2 of their 70 patients with duodenal injury, radiologic demonstration of extraluminal gas in the retroperitoneal area provided the first clue to the correct diagnosis.

It is inadvisable, and may be harmful, to routinely obtain emergency upper gastrointestinal tract radiologic studies with swallowed barium for contrast medium in an attempt to make, or rule out, a preoperative specific diagnosis of duodenal perforation in acutely injured patients. Many such patients are in shock and may be unable to withstand the additional manipulations required; others are unable to cooperate, and therefore may aspirate the barium. Also, the use of barium is contraindicated in patients suspected of having perforation of the bowel; if there is a duodenal perforation, the insoluble barium will escape into the peritoneal cavity or retroperitoneal tissues.

Better is the use of a water-soluble contrast medium, such as diatrizoate (Hypaque). This sometimes can be helpful in diagnosing a duodenal perforation, whether it be retroperitoneal or free intra-peritoneal. Hypaque can be administered orally or through the nasogastric tube, which is usually placed as an integral step in the diagnostic work-up. The latter route of administration seems preferable, as it lessens the risk of aspiration; since the nasogastric tube is already in place, active cooperation is not required.

Donovan and Hagen (1966) reported that Hypaque was administered orally in all four of their patients with retroperitoneal perforation of the duodenum by blunt trauma. In each instance, x-ray films showed spill of the contrast material outside the duodenum and also retroperitoneal gas outlining the right kidney. Their experience with the oral administration of Hypaque for radiologic examination of the stomach and duodenum convinced them that this valuable diagnostic study was reliable for the diagnosis of duodenal perforation. They recommended that such an examination be performed "in every patient with blunt trauma to the upper part of the abdomen in whom the serum amylase is elevated and in whom there are no clear indications for surgery." They thought that widespread use of this study would be a major factor in preventing delay in establishing the diagnosis of retroperitoneal perforation of the duodenum. A negative examination makes duodenal perforation less likely and may help to avoid operation on selected patients with multiple blunt injuries.

An upper gastrointestinal x-ray study with barium is indicated in a patient who initially is treated nonoperatively, but in whom duodenal obstruction later develops owing to the presence of an intramural duodenal hematoma. The typical radiologic findings show obstruction and the appearance of a coiled spring of barium in the first portion of the duodenum, and deviation of the duodenal lumen. These findings were noted by Roman, Silva, and Lucas (1971) in both of their patients who were operated upon 8 and 10 days after injury.

Corley and associates (1975) also made a correct preoperative diagnosis of intramural hematoma in four patients with blunt abdominal trauma by use of an upper gastrointestinal contrast x-ray study.

OTHER DIAGNOSTIC AIDS

Additional aids that may be used for diagnosing duodenal injuries are the same as those described for the diagnostic workup of gastric injuries (see pp. 198 to 204), but their value seems to differ. Donovan and Hagen (1966) reported that the level of amylase in the serum was determined preoperatively in 20 of their 29 patients with duodenal injuries, and that this test was of less assistance in establishing a correct diagnosis than anticipated. An elevated serum amylase arouses suspicion of pancreatic injury, and, because of the high incidence of combined duodenal and pancreatic injury, the possibility of duodenal perforation, particularly in blunt injury, should be considered. However, in their series, normal levels were observed in patients with gross pancreatic injury.

Conversely, elevated levels were observed in patients without pancreatic injury but with duodenal injury. Pancreatic injury was seen at operation in 2 of 11 patients with normal preoperative serum amylase levels. In four other patients, the preoperative level of amylase in the serum was above 250 Somogyi units (normal is 50 to 150). The pancreas was grossly normal in two of these four patients, and clinical pancreatitis developed postoperatively in only one of the four. (Compare this with the serum amylase determination in gastric injury on page 200.)

Stone and Garoni (1966) reported that, in their series of 70 patients with traumatic perforations of the duodenum, peritoneal aspiration with a needle and syringe was of no help in making an earlier diagnosis; in fact, it was often misleading. However, in two patients, radiologic demonstration of *extraluminal gas in the retroperitoneal area* gave the first clue to the patient's true condition. Although x-ray films, laboratory evaluation, and peritoneal aspirates may be unreliable, they are helpful when positive.

The most reliable sign influencing the decision for operation is that of *peritoneal irritation*, obtained by repeated physical examinations.

TREATMENT

Blunt Trauma

Rupture of the gastrointestinal tract by blunt abdominal trauma has been recognized for centuries. Aristotle noted that "a slight blow will cause rupture of the intestine without injury to the skin" (Poer and Woliver, 1942). Such injuries are relatively common, and the duodenum has been injured in approximately 10 per cent of the reported cases (Oglesby and associates, 1968).

Patients with nonpenetrating abdominal trauma are much more difficult to diagnose than are those with penetrating injuries because the clinical manifestations of blunt abdominal trauma may be unimpressive early in the postinjury period, until leakage into the peritoneal cavity or hemorrhage produces symptoms and signs that suggest intra-abdominal injury and indicate the need for laparotomy.

RETROPERITONEAL RUPTURE

Duodenal rupture may be into the free peritoneal cavity or it may be retroperitoneal. A retroperitoneal rupture may communicate with the peritoneal cavity, or it may be confined to the retroperitoneal space so signs of peritonitis are absent, as occurred in 25 per cent of the 32 patients with retroperitoneal rupture in one reported series (Matolo and associates, 1975).

In 1963, Cleveland and Waddell (1963) analyzed and tabulated the experiences with retroperitoneal rupture of the duodenum in the 39 cases that had been recorded in the literature since 1951, and included their own experience with 9 additional cases. Of particular interest are two of their patients — children in whom the injury resulted from blows to the abdomen during parental beating, the "battered child syndrome." A five-year old boy sustained a 10-cm. laceration of the fourth part of the duodenum at the ligament of Treitz and was treated successfully by duodenojejunostomy and drainage. A 1-year-old girl sustained complete transection of the third part of the duodenum and was treated successfully by duodenojejunostomy and drainage. The investigators noted that survival was possible even when therapy was delayed days, weeks, or, in one case, months. It is significant that all the fatalities occurred in patients in whom the interval between injury and operation was 24 hours or longer. However, among the survivors were six patients in whom retroperitoneal rupture of the duodenum went undiagnosed and more or less untreated for 2.5, 5, 6, 14, 18, and 210 days, which indicates the relative sterility of duodenal contents in many patients, the localization of contaminating duodenal content by intact peritoneum, and, perhaps, the tendency of surrounding tissues to seal intestinal defects.

When symptoms appear they usually consist of varying degrees of abdominal, flank, and/or back pain. The pain may be localized at any site from the right lower abdomen to the chest. Occasionally, pain referred to the testicle and shoulder has been reported (Butler and Carlson, 1931). "Testicular pain or priapism can occur due to soilage of the retroperitoneal space about the sympathetic nerves." Occasionally, also, "air can dissect retroperitoneally into the pelvis and can be palpated rectally and/or in the scrotum" (Oglesby and associates, 1968).

Nausea, vomiting that may be bilious, hematemesis, and shock are sometimes present. Most patients with rupture of the duodenum have upper abdominal tenderness and mild to moderate leukocytosis. Hematuria occurs occasionally, probably caused by injury of the right kidney. Plain abdominal roentgenograms without contrast media may aid in the diagnosis. Several radiologic abnormalities may suggest rupture of the duodenum (Jacobs, Culver, and Koenig, 1944; Jacobson and Carter, 1951): (1) Gas in the retroperitoneal space dissecting around the right kidney, about the right crus of the diaphragm, and along the psoas muscle. Gas may dissect upward into the mediastinum. Subcutaneous emphysema in the neck has been reported in at least one case (Adnopoz and Fortuna, 1961); (2) Obliteration of the right psoas muscle and kidney shadows due to extravasation of blood and fluid; and (3) "Scoliosis and obliteration of the right psoas muscle shadow are subtle, significant, nonspecific x-ray findings that suggest this injury but are often overlooked" (Lucas and Ledgerwood, 1975).

When injury is suspected early, it may be best to confirm it by an emergency x-ray study with swallowed water-soluble contrast media. When perforation or rupture is diagnosed or is strongly suspected, immediate laparotomy is indicated. However, in patients whose condition is not too critical, and particularly if hematuria is present, preoperative intravenous pyelography can be done to investigate possible associated renal or urinary tract injury, as described on page 208. These radiologic findings are not present in all patients with retroperitoneal rupture of the duodenum. In some cases they are present but either not recognized or, if recognized, their diagnostic significance is not appreciated.

More than 50 per cent of the 36 patients with duodenal injury by blunt abdominal trauma in one reported series (Lucas and Ledgerwood, 1975) had the diagnostic finding of retroperitoneal air along the upper pole of the right kidney, the right psoas muscle, and overlying the transverse mesocolon. Blurred psoas shadows and perirenal air were visualized in 17 of the 48 patients with retroperitoneal rupture of the duodenum reported in a collected series (Cocke and Meyer, 1964). As noted, these signs are not specific for duodenal rupture but suggest injury in that area and the urgent need for laparotomy.

INJURIES OF THE DUODENUM AND PANCREAS

Severe injuries of the duodenal wall other than the second portion of the duodenum, which contains the ampulla of Vater, may be treated by segmental resection of the damaged segment and primary anastomosis.

When the wound involves pancreas as well as duodenum, or if there is significant loss of duodenal substance, there may be no alternative but to proceed with a larger resection procedure.

Inactivated pancreatic enzymes do not digest living tissue. Therefore, when the pancreas alone has been injured, external drainage of the pancreatic area is adequate treatment in most of these cases, but fistula formation is common. When both the duodenum and pancreas have been injured, duodenal, biliary, and pancreatic secretions often combine, and pancreatic enzymes are activated. A suture line exposed to this mixture of activated enzymes is precarious. Reported mortality rates (Talbot and Shuck, 1975; Brawley, Cameron, and Zuidema, 1968) of combined pancreatic and duodenal injury have been as high as 73 per cent. In these cases extensive measures must be taken to prevent mixed duodenal and pancreatic contents from entering the peritoneal cavity.

Brawley, Cameron, and Zuidema (1968) have shown that for patients with complex wounds of the head of the pancreas and second and third parts of the duodenum, pancreaticoduodenectomy provides an effective means of removing all devitalized tissue and minimizing the leakage of combined digestive juices. They reported three such cases (Fig. 8–2).

They emphasized that, with previous methods of therapy, simultaneous injury to both the duodenum and the pancreas carries a considerably higher mortality than isolated wounds of either organ. Since pancreaticoduodenectomy removes traumatized and devitalized tissue, the occurrence of postoperative pancreatic complications decreases. They pointed out that pancreatic insufficiency rarely occurs if 20 per cent or more of the gland remains.

These investigators also mentioned that the only one of their three patients treated by pancreaticoduodenectomy in whom vagotomy was not also performed developed a marginal ulcer. They warned that when pancreaticoduodenectomy is performed for trauma, a vagotomy should be included routinely to protect the jejunum from marginal ulceration.

Although pancreaticoduodenectomy is being performed with an acceptable mortality, the consensus appears to be that it

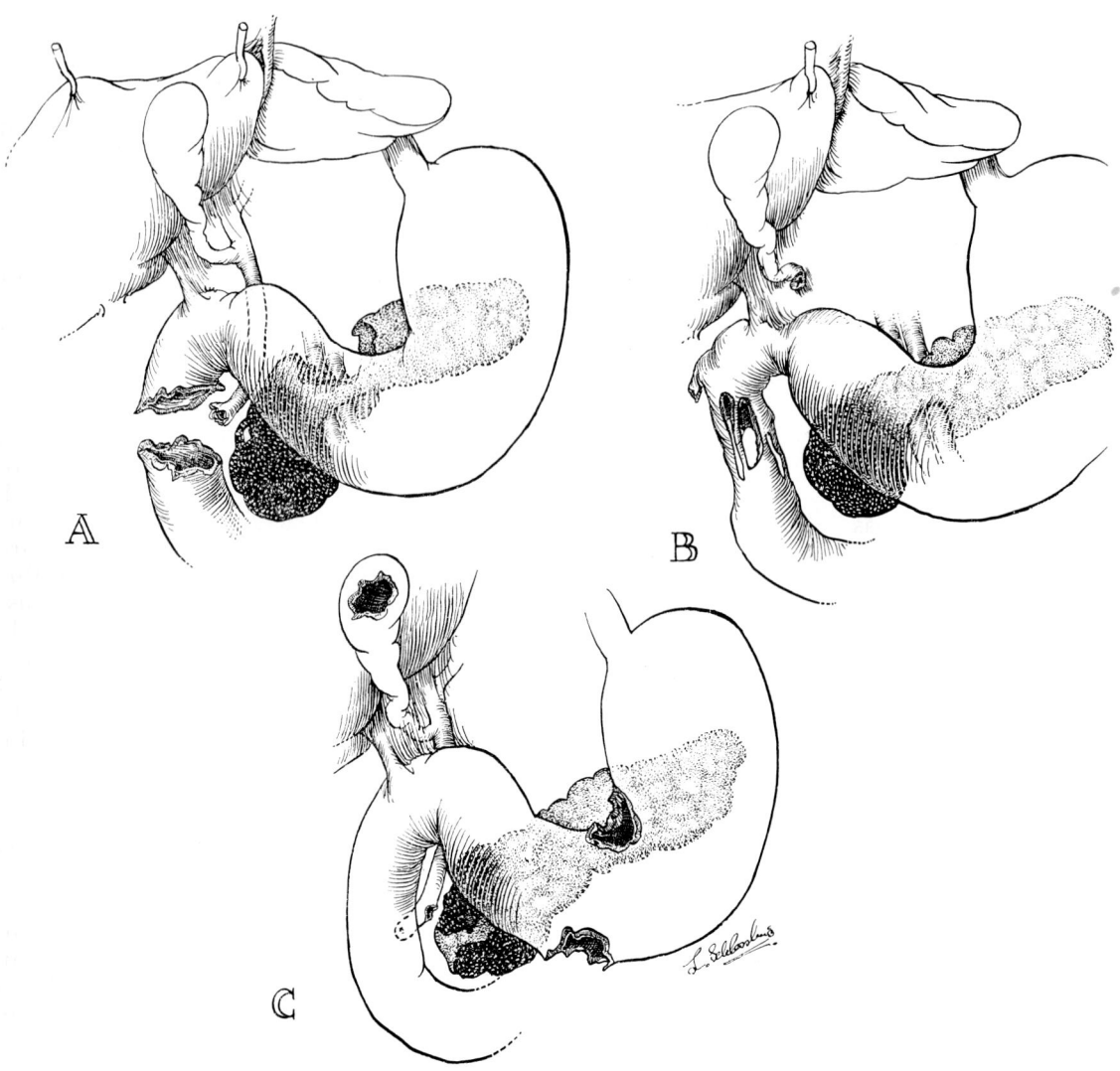

Figure 8–2. *A*, Drawing of the injury encountered in Patient 1. The second part of the duodenum was transected and the ampulla of Vater, with a cuff of duodenal mucosa, avulsed. The pancreas was partially transected in the area of the superior mesenteric vessels. *B*, Injury sustained by Patient 2. The proximal portion of the duodenum was virtually destroyed and the distal portion of the common bile duct divided. There was severe contusion of the pancreas. *C*, The drawing shows the severe upper abdominal injury found in Patient 3. There were lacerations of the spleen, stomach, small intestine, gallbladder, and common bile duct. The extent of the pancreatic injury was not appreciated at initial laparotomy.
(From Brawley, R. K., Cameron, J. L., and Zuidema, G. D.: Severe upper abdominal injuries treated by pancreaticoduodenectomy. Surg. Gynecol. Obstet. *126*:512, 1968.)

should be reserved for injuries in which the duodenum and the head of the pancreas are so severely damaged that no other form of therapy seems feasible.

RUPTURE OF DUODENUM WITH AVULSION OF THE AMPULLA OF VATER

This injury has been caused by blunt abdominal trauma in occasional cases. It creates two major problems for treatment: (1) The need for restoration of the integrity of the duodenum, and (2) re-establishment of patent entrances of the biliary and pancreatic ducts into the intestinal tract.

In 1965, Fish and Johnson reported such a case and at that time could find no other case recorded in the literature of avulsion of the papilla of Vater by blunt abdominal trauma. Their patient was a 23-year-old man who was injured in an automobile accident and admitted to the Martin Army Hospital an hour later with a laceration of the scalp and the complaint of right flank pain. His abdomen was soft, without muscle guarding or rebound tenderness. There was no external evidence of body injury. Routine laboratory tests and chest and abdominal x-ray films were negative. After 9 hours of observation, his abdominal pain suddenly became much worse, and he developed a rigid, quiet abdomen.

At operation, 200 ml. of bloody fluid were found in the peritoneal cavity. The omentum adjacent to the second portion of the duodenum was necrotic and surrounded by white plaques of fat necrosis. Elevation of the second and third portions of the duodenum revealed bile-stained intestinal fluid coming from a 2-cm. laceration in the posteromedial duodenal wall just below the inferior edge of the pancreas. The surrounding tissue was friable and partially digested by spilled duodenal contents. The surface of the head of the pancreas was similarly inflamed but not otherwise injured.

The duodenal rent was closed, and further exploration found a 1-cm. patch of mucosa on a stalk at the inferior edge of the pancreas. This proved to be the papilla of Vater avulsed from the duodenum. Since the duodenum was so friable, the ampulla was inserted into a Roux-en-Y limb of proximal jejunum. The anastomosis was performed by suturing the open end of jejunum to the capsule of the pancreas around the ampulla. Two drains were placed in the area of injury. The postoperative course was uneventful. T-tube cholangiograms at 10 and 27 days showed no ductal dilatation or stenosis. The T-tube was removed one month later. The surgeons suggested that the mechanism of this injury was a traction tear mediated through the hepatoduodenal ligament and common bile duct.

TRANSECTION OF DUODENUM WITH AVULSION OF THE COMMON DUCT

Lee, Zacher, and Vogel (1976) reported an 18-year-old boy whose car ran into a telephone pole. During observation in the emergency room, his abdomen became rigid, a peritoneal tap yielded blood, roentgenograms showed air around the right kidney extending upward toward the mediastinum, and his hematocrit dropped from 43 to 33 per cent. Emergency laparotomy was performed. Operation revealed almost complete transection of the second part of the duodenum at the ampulla of Vater, with avulsion of the common bile duct and main pancreatic duct. Intraoperative cholangiography through a tube in the gallbladder showed that the right and left hepatic ducts, the common hepatic duct, and the common bile duct were intact down to the level of injury. The pancreas was incompletely avulsed from the duodenum. The accessory pancreatic duct appeared intact. Further exploration showed no other injuries.

Instead of choosing a diverting or resectional procedure, which has greater risks, the surgeons performed a simple two-layer closure of the duodenum and primary repair of the ampulla, but leakage around the distal end of the common bile duct was seen. Retrograde cholangiography suggested that the main pancreatic duct was intact. A short distance below the transection of the duodenum, an opening was made through the duodenal wall, and the ampulla of Vater was pulled through this opening and anastomosed by sutures. It thus was transposed to this lower level in the duodenum. Through a 32 F. Pezzer catheter in the duodenum, an 18 F. Robinson catheter was placed through the pylorus and the duodenal anastomosis, producing both a gastrostomy and a transgastrojejunostomy. A long-arm T-tube was placed in the common duct and brought through the anastomosis of the ampulla to the duodenum. Secretin-Boots (1 u./kg) was injected intravenously, and a short time later watery fluid issued from the area of the transposed ampulla of Vater. A small opening had been made inside the long-arm T-tube near the ampulla of Vater to promote drainage. A sump drain was placed in the duodenal area. Intravenous hyperalimentation was begun on the fourth postoperative day, and skim milk by the jejunostomy tube on the seventh postoperative day. The transgastrojejunostomy tube was removed on the eleventh postoperative day, and the gastrostomy tube through which the previous tube had been inserted was removed, along with the sump drain, on the sixteenth postoperative day. The only postoperative problem was a mild pancreatitis, manifested by a peak serum amylase value of 1092 units/dl. on the fourth postoperative day, which returned to normal and remained so thereafter.

The patient remained completely asymptomatic after operation and regained his preoperative weight. The excellent result persisted more than two years later.

The investigators pointed out that the surgical approach for treating two similar patients recorded in the literature differed from theirs. In one, a pancreatoduodenal resection was done, while in the other only choledochoduodenostomy was performed. Since their result was excellent, they recommended that consideration be given to this operative approach in a similar anatomic situation: complete transection of first portion of duodenum at the *pyloroduodenal junction*.

It is unusual for blunt trauma to cause complete disruption at the pylorus, particularly without other significant associated injuries. Oglesby and associates (1968) reported the first such case recorded in the American literature.

The patient was a 45-year-old man whose car struck a tree head-on. At operation, complete transection of the duodenum immediately adjacent to the pylorus was found. The free ends were separated 2 to 3 cm. The duodenal end was mobile and relaxed and slowly oozed bile from the lumen and blood from the transected wall. The pyloric end was tightly contracted, bled very little, and spilled very little of the gastric contents, although the stomach contained a large amount of blood clots and ingested food. Complete abdominal and retroperitoneal exploration revealed only a mild contusion of the head of the pancreas and a small right retroperitoneal hematoma.

A 1-cm. portion of the duodenum and the gastric antrum was resected, and a two-layer gastroduodenal anastomosis was performed. Thorough peritoneal lavage was done, and the abdomen was closed with wire sutures. Large Penrose drains were placed in the lesser sac and Morison's pouch and brought out through a separate stab wound. Postoperative management included administration of antibiotics, continuous nasogastric suction, and fluid and electrolyte replacement. Urine and serum amylase values were slightly elevated initially but returned to normal by the third postoperative day. There was mild postoperative ileus, which resolved by the sixth postoperative day, and convalescence was uneventful.

TRAUMATIC PYELODUODENAL FISTULA

This is an uncommon but serious injury that is occasionally associated with injuries of the duodenum. McDougal and Persky (1972) reviewed the literature and tabulated the 46 cases of pyeloduodenal fistula recorded. Eight of the 46 cases were caused by trauma. Three of these followed blunt trauma (a fall in one and crush injuries in two), and five were caused by foreign body erosions or perforations. Specifically, these included swallowed bobby pins lodged in the second portion of the duodenum, which perforated the renal pelvis in three cases; two were due to iatrogenic perforation of the ureter during catheterization. The remaining 38 cases were spontaneous.

McDougal and Persky added a detailed report of their own case of traumatic pyeloduodenal fistula caused by a gunshot wound. Their patient was a 37-year-old man who had sustained a gunshot wound in the right flank. After initial resuscitation, laparotomy was performed. Operation revealed a tear in the spleen, which required splenectomy; a through-and-through wound of the stomach, which was debrided and closed; multiple wounds of the jejunum, which required resection of an 8-cm. segment with end-to-end anastomosis; a tangential wound of the transverse colon, which was treated by exteriorization; a laceration of the inferior vena cava, which was closed by suture; a through-and-through wound of the duodenum, which was closed in two layers by sutures, a lacerated right kidney, which was debrided and hemostasis achieved with a mattress suture; and a transected right ureteropelvic junction, which was debrided and anastomosed over a splinting catheter with a nephrostomy and slash pyelotomy. The wound was drained and closed.

Postoperatively, the patient's fever gradually subsided. Parenteral hyperalimentation was begun. The nephrostomy functioned well. An excretory urogram on the seventeenth postoperative day showed bilateral function. On the 24th postoperative day, fever and abdominal tenderness appeared. A nephrogram showed the ureter was patent, and three days later a lesser sac abscess was drained. On the 42nd postoperative day, the nephrostomy was removed, and the patient was discharged on the 53rd postoperative day. He was afebrile, fully ambulatory, and eating a regular diet.

He did well for 3 months but then developed right flank pain, fever, a tender mass in the right flank, and pyuria. Retrograde pyelography showed a perinephric abscess cavity with a fistulous communication between the pelvis of the right kidney and the duodenum. A No. 8 ureteral catheter was left in the right renal pelvis; it drained 200 ml. of purulent material, which cultured coliform bacteria. After 31 days of ureteral catheter drainage, a retrograde pyelogram showed persistence of the fistula, so a right subcapsular nephrectomy was performed through the flank. Much inflammatory and scar tissue was found, with distortion of the normal anatomy. The duodenum was bound in scar tissue. No attempt was made to close the fistulous portion of the duodenum. The area was drained. The pathologic specimen revealed acute and chronic nephritis. The patient made an uneventful recovery from this operation. Before discharge, an upper gastrointestinal tract x-ray contrast study showed no evidence of fistula, and 6-month follow-up was negative.

McDougal and Persky (1972) found that spontaneous and traumatic pyeloduodenal fistulas have a similar pathogenesis. The pathologic process uniformly begins in the kidney, progresses to involve the perinephric tissues, and culminates in the formation of a duodenal fistula. In the spontaneous type, pyelonephritis or tuberculosis occurs, resulting in perinephritis, abscess, or calculus formation. Subsequent rupture or erosion into the duodenum occurs, resulting in the fistula.

Of the nine traumatic cases, the three caused by blunt trauma resulted in extravasation of urine, followed by perinephritis, pyelonephritis, and abscess and drainage into the duodenum. The other five (plus the author's case), caused by foreign bodies, resulted in the same sequence of developments described above for those resulting from blunt trauma. A swallowed bobby pin that lodged in the second portion of the duodenum perforated the renal pelvis in three cases. Perinephritis and pyelonephritis occurred. However, the foreign body created the fistula. In all but one of the collected cases, the flow of contents was from pelvis to duodenum. This proved true in their case also, as duodenal contents were not detected in the urine, and a 24-hour collection of urine from the right kidney revealed a negligible instead of a high level of amylase.

Except for a history of trauma, the clinical presentations of both traumatic and spontaneous pyeloduodenal fistulas are identical. Flank or abdominal pain is the most common presenting symptom, occurring twice as frequently as urinary, gastrointestinal, or systemic symptoms. Pyuria and hematuria are the most frequent physical findings, closely followed by a flank or abdominal mass and fever. Less commonly, flank tenderness and elevated white blood count occur, and least often a draining sinus is noted. "All but one of the fistulas in this series involved the right kidney, and significant electrolyte abnormalities did not occur, not even a single instance of hyperchloremic acidosis"(McDougal and Persky, 1972).

The most valuable procedure for diagnosing pyeloduodenal fistula is retrograde pyelography. In this series, all the preoperative or premortem diagnoses were invariably made by retrograde pyelography. Intravenous pyelography usually fails to visualize the involved kidney. Upper gastrointestinal tract x-ray series with contrast media are usually not diagnostic, but they did demonstrate a fistula in two of the cases. In the case just described, intravenous pyelography revealed nonvisualization of the right kidney; upper gastrointestinal tract x-ray contrast studies showed duodenal distortion but no fistula; and retrograde pyelography was diagnostic.

The treatment of traumatic pyeloduodenal fistula is surgical. Seven of the eight patients with traumatic pyeloduodenal fistula in McDougal's and Persky's series were operated upon: one died, but six survived and had satisfactory results. The patient not operated upon died.

Two procedures, ureteral catheter drainage and subcapsular nephrectomy, were used for treating the surgeon's own patient. This illustrates several important points. Cystoscopic placement of a large ureteral catheter into the affected renal pelvis for drainage not only decompresses the abscess and reduces perinephric inflammation but also serves as a conduit through which antibiotic solutions may be introduced for lavage of the involved area. In this case, "Maintenance of ureteral catheter drainage was responsible for decompression and subsequent disappearance of the patient's flank mass and for cessation of the flank pain, fever, and elevated white blood count. Although continued ureteral catheter drainage did not result in closure of the fistula, it did make the operation less difficult with less risk, and minimized postoperative complications without violating the anticipated operative site" (McDougal and Persky, 1972).

Because a previous abdominal procedure had demonstrated dense fibrous adhesions with obliteration of identifiable land marks in the area of the duodenum, common bile duct, head of the pancreas, and right kidney, there would have been a high risk of injury to thse vital structures if an abdominal approach were used. Therefore, a subcapsular nephrectomy through the flank was performed. A subcapsular approach allows easy access to a plane of dissection without endangering the surrounding structures, in contrast to an extracapsular approach.

In their review of the literature, these surgeons found that nephrectomy is the procedure of choice for treating pyeloduodenal fistula. Nephrectomy had been performed in 18 cases; the postoperative course was satisfactory in 15, but complications ended in death in 1 patient and in fistulous drainage in 2 patients. In one of the latter, the tract closed spontaneously and in the other it persisted. Of the six patients in whom a nephrectomy was not performed, three died, one had a poor result in which flank pain necessitated repeated ureteral dilatations and irrigations, and only two had satisfactory results. In the surgeons' own patient, the fistulous tract was left open and the flank was drained. The fistula healed, and there was neither clinical nor radiologic evidence of persistence. McDougal and Persky stated "It is apparent that when the fistula is small and of the low output variety, and inflammation and scar tissue about the vital structures make dissection hazardous, a trial of spontaneous closure after the kidney has been removed and the area adequately drained is justifiable, since closure may be anticipated." If possible, however, the origin of the fistula in the duodenum should be closed primarily. Of the six operative cases in which the duodenal fistula was left open, there were two deaths, two persistent fistulas, and two satisfactory results.

In 17 cases the duodenum was primarily closed, resulting in 2 deaths, 1 fistula, and 14 satisfactory postoperative results.

McDougal and Persky pointed out that their approach to therapy by use of ureteral catheterization for drainage and the use of subcapsular nephrectomy lessens operative risk and reduces morbidity in patients with traumatic pyeloduodenal fistula.

INFLUENCE OF PREVIOUS GASTRECTOMY ON MAJOR BLUNT DUODENAL INJURY

Strauch (1972) reported a case of duodenal injury by blunt abdominal trauma, caused by an auto accident, in a patient who had undergone vagotomy and a Billroth II partial gastrectomy with an antecolic gastrojejunostomy for peptic ulcer disease 6 years previously.

The patient was brought to a hospital immediately after the accident; although he complained of some abdominal pain, serious intra-abdominal injury was not suspected, so he was released after repair of a minor lip laceration. Later the same evening he returned to the emergency room complaining of abdominal pain and stated that he had vomited blood, but again the examining physician advised the patient to return home. The following morning he returned to the hospital complaining of persistent abdominal pain and was hospitalized.

Examination revealed that he was in severe pain, his abdomen was rigid, and bowel sounds were absent. Laboratory studies included serum amylase that was over three times the normal value. Abdominal and chest roentgenograms and emergency intravenous urography were not helpful.

Exploratory laparotomy was performed because of presumptive evidence of severe injury to the pancreaticoduodenal region. The peritoneal cavity was seen to contain serosanguineous fluid. Exploration confirmed the patient's previous Billroth II partial gastrectomy with a normal-appearing antecolic gastrojejunostomy. Mobilizing the duodenum by the Kocher maneuver and dividing Treitz's ligament allowed evacuation of a large amount of bile and blood clot and exploration of the retroperitoneal duodenum, which revealed two longitudinal tears in its wall, one an 8-cm. anterior rent parallel to a 6-cm. tear in its posterior wall. The upper end of the latter was 2 cm. distal to the ampulla of Vater. The caudal margin of the head and body of the pancreas had been completely separated from the duodenum at the site of duodenal laceration. The head and body of the pancreas were grossly edematous and swollen, but the pancreatic capsule was intact (Fig. 8–3). It was apparent that a crushing type of trauma with associated shearing force had produced the injury. Fortunately, no vascular structure had been opened.

The duodenum at the site of injury was too damaged to be repaired, so it was segmentally resected. End-to-end anastomosis of the duodenum was precluded because of the short length of duodenojejunum between the transected end and the gastrojejunostomy; therefore, the distal duodenum was sutured closed in two layers. The efferent jejunal limb of the gastrojejunostomy was anastomosed side-to-end to the end of the duodenal stump in two layers, with care taken to avoid compromising the ampulla of Vater by the anastomotic suture lines. Cholecystostomy was performed, using a Foley catheter for drainage.

Stamm gastrostomy also was performed with use of a Foley catheter. The entire repair is shown in Figure 8–4. A sump drain was placed at the site of pancreatic contusion, and a Penrose drain was placed to the infrahepatic space. The postoperative course was uneventful except for a 3-day psychotic period, after which his postoperative course was uncomplicated. At 12 days, postoperative cholangiography through the cholecystostomy catheter visualized a normal biliary tree. A barium contrast x-ray study of the upper gastrointestinal tract showed the gastrojejunostomy to be functioning. The drains and gastrostomy catheter were removed and the patient was discharged 18 days after operation. During the next month he required two readmissions to the hospital because of gastrointestinal symptoms and abdominal signs highly suggestive of pancreatitis. Thereafter he remained well.

Strauch pointed out the problems in the diagnosis and management that the combination of circumstances in this case presented, which may be expected occasionally in other patients who have sustained duodenal injuries after having undergone gastrectomy.

The *diagnostic problem* in a patient who has previously undergone Billroth II gastrectomy may be magnified by periduodenal scarring and adhesions due to previous dissection, which may limit the spread of contamination and reduce the area exposed, thereby producing less impressive symptoms and misleading or delayed physical signs, compared with previously anatomically intact persons. Because the duodenal stump is bypassed by the gastrojejunostomy, there is no obstruction of the duodenum by a duodenal intramural hematoma, and neither air nor orally administered contrast material is likely to enter

Figure 8–3. Depiction of duodenal injury (segment of transverse colon omitted for clarity). (From Strauch, G.: Influence of gastrectomy on major blunt duodenal injury. Am. J. Surg. *124*:400, 1972.)

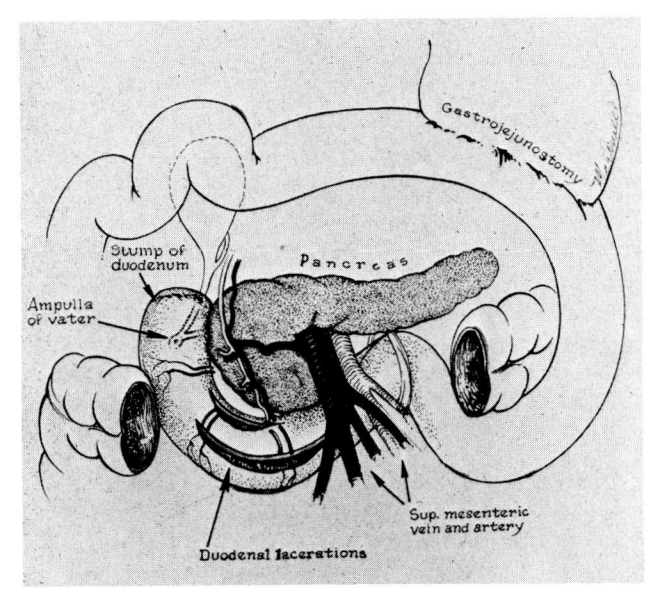

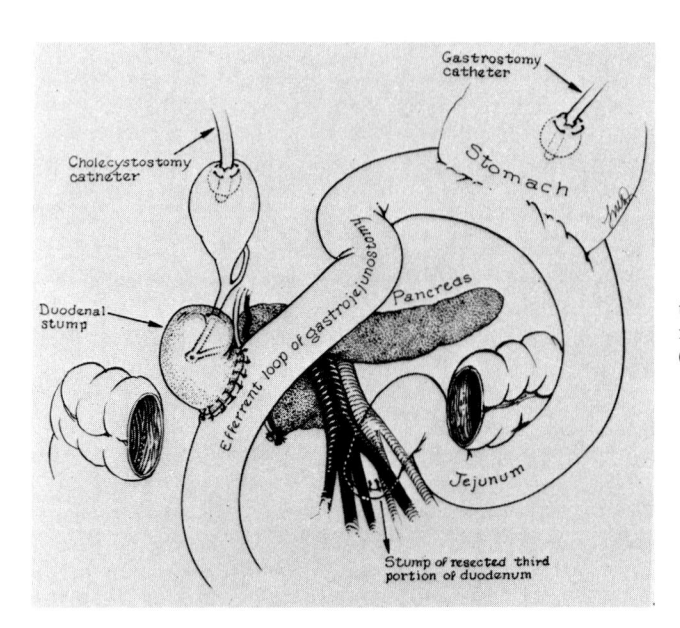

Figure 8–4. Completed reconstruction after resection of third portion of duodenum (segment of transverse colon omitted for clarity). (From Strauch, cited in previous figure.)

the injured segment. Consequently, plain films may fail to reveal periduodenal air, and contrast studies may fail to demonstrate either extravasation when there is duodenal rupture, or the coiled-spring pattern when there is an intramural hematoma, so the diagnosis may be missed altogether.

The nature of blunt traumatic duodenal injury may also be altered by previous gastrectomy. Strauch (1972) speculated that, after a Billroth I gastrectomy, absence of the pyloric musculature might decrease the potential for the closed-loop blow-out injury postulated by Cocke and Meyer (1964), and that a Billroth II gastrectomy might increase the potential for a blow-out injury because of the blind stump, but this potential is offset by the probability of there being less gas and fluid in the duodenum. He also pointed out that most duodenal ruptures occur as transverse duodenal tears involving more or less of the duodenal circumference. The extensive longitudinal tearing of the duodenum in this case is not commonly seen in blunt duodenal injury. "What role the prior gastrectomy played in this aspect of the injury can only be conjectured" (Strauch, 1972).

The operative management of a patient with traumatic duodenal rupture and a prior Billroth II gastrectomy presents two problems not otherwise encountered. First, the presence of a gastrojejunostomy limits the potential for end-to-end anastomosis if the magnitude of duodenal disruption requires duodenal resection. The retroperitoneal duodenum and gastrojejunostomy site being relatively fixed points, duodenal resection may preclude reanastomosis, as was the case in Strauch's patient.

Second, if major duodenal resection is required and end-to-end anastomosis is impossible, the most readily available provision for internal biliary and pancreatic drainage requires use of the jejunum distal to the gastrojejunostomy. However, this results in a modified ulcerogenic Mann-Williamson preparation (Mann and Williamson, 1923) so is not applicable in a patient such as Strauch's with a known ulcer diathesis, who is severely stressed because of serious injury and major operative intervention. In these circumstances, the simplest available course is to provide for entrance of bile and pancreatic secretions into the jejunum as near as possible to the gastrojejunal stoma, to encourage reflux of alkaline contents. Such a reconstruction was performed in the cases reported here (Fig. 8–4). Strauch commented that "because removal of pancreaticobiliary flow from the vicinity of the stomach in an ulcer-prone patient may result in peptic ulcer and its complications, jejunal interposition between the duodenum and gastrojejunostomy might be considered, but this seemed unwise in this patient whose chances for mere survival seemed limited."

Retroperitoneal Rupture of Duodenum by Blunt Trauma Complicated by Gas Gangrene in Patients with Previous Gastrectomy

Yeo and McNamara (1973) reported two patients with retroperitoneal rupture of the duodenum by blunt trauma due to an automobile accident. Both patients had undergone previous partial gastrectomy and vagotomy for duodenal ulcer, 5 years and 1 year, respectively, before the accident. Following the accident, both patients developed gas gangrene of the peritoneal and retroperitoneal areas.

The diagnosis and operation were delayed in both cases, and both died despite antitoxin, large doses of antibiotics, and as much debridement as could be done within limits compatible with life.

Yeo and McNamara pointed out that Turner (1964) and also Pyrtek and Bartus (1962) had shown that clostridia are known to exist in the diseased gallbladder in a saprophytic state, and Draser, Shiner, and McLeod (1969) have shown that bacterial growth occurs in gastric contents when achlorhydria is present as a result of either mucosal atrophy or gastric surgery. Since both of these patients had previous gastric surgery, the clostridial contamination may have come directly from the gastroduodenal contents. Standard treatment of gas gangrene, including extensive debridement, antibiotics, and clostridial antitoxin were used in both cases without effect.

INTRAMURAL HEMATOMA OF THE DUODENUM

This lesion is a collection of blood that has extravasated from a ruptured intramural blood vessel and has localized in the wall of the duodenum. Occasionally a perforation may be associated with the hematoma.

The hematoma in the bowel wall may be subserosal, submucosal, or within the muscular coat (Shannon, 1962–1963). The presumed mechanism of traumatic intramural hematoma is a shearing of the layers of the bowel wall, which tears the submucosal vascular bed. As the hematoma enlarges, it extends up and down the wall of the duodenum, partially or completely obstructing the duodenum and sometimes the common bile duct (Moore and Erlandson, 1963). In occasional cases the hematoma may rupture and spill its contents into the retroperitoneal space or peritoneal cavity, but intestinal contents are not present in the spillage since the mucosa usually remains intact.

The first report of intramural hematoma was by McLaughlan (1838), who described a false aneurysmal tumor that involved nearly the whole of the duodenum. The tumor was an organized hematoma between the mucous and muscular coats, which obstructed the duodenum with a fatal result. There was no apparent cause for it.

The etiology of intramural hematoma of the bowel remained obscure until 1855, when Thompson suggested that blunt abdominal trauma could cause an intramural hematoma in the bowel wall. Intramural hematomas have been described in almost every area of the gastrointestinal tract, ranging from the esophagus to the sigmoid colon. Hughes, Conn, and Sherman (1977) reviewed the 260 cases of intramural hematoma of the gastrointestinal tract reported in the world literature since 1838 and reported 17 cases of their own. The duodenum seemed to be the most susceptible portion; it was the site of 93.5 per cent of the traumatic intramural hematomas. This may be explained by the relatively fixed position of the duodenum anterior to the vertebral column, where it is vulnerable to a shearing force by blunt abdominal trauma.

Additional factors that have been cited to explain the higher incidence of duodenal involvement include the tangential insertion of the mesentery at the duodenum and proximal jejunum; the varying tensile strength of the three layers of the duodenal wall; the rich submucosal vascular plexus in the duodenum; and the lack of a completely circumferential, well-developed serosal layer in the retroperitoneal portion of the duodenum, resulting in decreased ability to tamponade active intramural hemorrhage.

The prevalence of intramural duodenal hematoma in children has been attributed to the high flared costal margin common in children and less well-developed abdominal musculature.

"Intramural hematoma of the duodenum is primarily a condition of males in children and young adults. The one case reported in a child less than 1 year old involved a newborn with a fatal bleeding diathesis. A history of trauma is present in nearly 80 per cent of cases. However, it is not unusual, particularly in the pediatric age group, in which minor blows to the abdomen occur frequently, for the trauma to pass unnoticed or be considered insignificant" (Margolis, Carnazzo, and Finn, 1976).

Incidence

Jones and associates (1971) analyzed the 125 cases of duodenal intramural hematoma recorded in the world literature and added one of their own. They found that no estimate of the incidence of intramural duodenal hematomas had been made. "Although it is being recognized with increasing frequency, it is a relatively rare surgical entity. About 50 per cent of intestinal hematomas are in the duodenum. This percentage is probably higher when trauma alone is the etiologic agent. Only 28 of 123 (22.8 per cent) of the patients were females."

The young are most frequently affected: 51.7 per cent (60 of 116) occurred in children less than 14 years age; 63.8 per cent (74 of 116) were in patients less than 20 years of age; and 75 per cent (87 of 116) were in patients less than 30 years of age. The youngest patient reported was a 7-day-old male infant, in whom the hematoma caused intestinal and biliary obstruction (Glass, 1937), and the oldest was a 76-year-old man.

Margolis, Carnazzo, and Finn (1976) reviewed 174 cases of intramural hematoma of the duodenum collected from the literature and an additional five of their own. Eight-two per cent occurred in patients less than 30 years old. The ratio of males to females was 3 to 1. There was a history of recent trauma in 79 per cent of patients, but in patients older than 30 years a history of recent trauma was absent in 55 per cent. In these, alcoholism, hyperamylasemia, anticoagulant therapy, pancreatitis, bleeding diathesis, and tumor were other factors that may have contributed to the development of an intramural hematoma of the duodenum.

Etiology

Blunt abdominal trauma is the most common cause of duodenal intramural hematoma. A history of previous blunt abdominal trauma was elicited in 89 of 120 cases (74.2 per cent) of duodenal intramural hematoma reviewed by Jones and associates (1971). The trauma may be major or minor and all but forgotten by the patient. Characteristically, the trauma occurs several hours or days before the onset of symptoms.

Other causes or contributing causes include underlying blood dyscrasias (Glass, 1937), hemophilia (Moore and Erlandson, 1963), Henoch-Schönlein purpura (Althausen, Deamer, and Kerr, 1937), use of anticoagulants (Wiot, Weinstein, and Felson, 1961), surgical trauma, peritoneal dialysis, vascular trauma, vascular malformation, peroral small bowel intubation biopsy (Toblin, Schlang, and James, 1966), pancreatic disease (Altemeier, 1963), alcoholism, severe hiccoughs (Felson and Levin, 1954), ruptured aortic aneurysm, epilepsy, mesenteric adenitis, and duodenal ulcer with hemorrhage.

Katsas, Sapountzis, and Leoutsakos (1970) reported an obstructing intramural hematoma of the duodenum that occurred in the immediate postoperative period after truncal vagotomy and Heineke-Mikulicz pyloroplasty had been performed for duodenal ulcer. Its apparent cause was mild manipulation in preparation for the pyloroplasty.

Laboratory Findings

"The white blood cell count is usually elevated (10,000 to 31,000 cells per cubic millimeter)" (Moore and Erlandson, 1963).

"Anemia was present in 20 of 86 cases (23 per cent), but hemoconcentration secondary to dehydration was the rule. [Studies] should be performed to rule out clotting defects. Increased serum bilirubin was present in 9 of 116 cases (7.8 per cent) due to a combination of hemolysis and ampullary obstruction by the hematoma. An elevated serum amylase was found in 19 of 116 cases (16.4 per cent) resulting from direct pancreatic trauma, ampullary obstruction by hematoma, or a combination of both. Serum electrolytes showed a typical hypochloremic metabolic alkalosis when the vomiting was protracted" (Jones and Associates, 1971).

Clinical Findings

The cases of blunt abdominal trauma that result in intramural hematoma of the duodenum without perforation usually involve the second portion of that viscus and follow relatively minor trauma. Frequently, the trauma is so insignificant that initially it is forgotten by the patient and the family.

"The trauma characteristically occurs several hours to days prior to the onset of symptoms. In 70 of 124 reported cases, this lag period from abdominal trauma to onset of symptoms averaged 53.6 hours" (Jones and associates, 1971). These patients frequently disclose minimal pain and vomiting 1 or 2 days after the injury.

Judd, Taybi, and King (1964) pointed out that duodenal hematoma appears clinically as two distinct syndromes: one as high bowel obstruction of insidious onset, and the other as an acute abdominal lesion with obstructive symptoms resembling acute appendicitis.

Intractable vomiting usually develops about 24 to 48 hours after the trauma. The vomiting could contain bile if the obstruction is below the papilla of Vater; otherwise it consists of gastric contents. Melena or hematemesis does not occur unless the patient has a clotting defect or the hematoma has evacuated its contents into the bowel.

Some abdominal pain, varying in degree and in time of appearance, is present in all patients with intramural hematoma of the duodenum. "The pain is in the right upper quadrant when the first, second, and third portions of the duodenum are involved, and in the left upper quadrant when the fourth portion of the duodenum is involved. Occasionally there may also be testicular and scrotal pain if a retroperitoneal hematoma is present, and shoulder pain if free intraperitoneal blood is present. The patient may complain of constipation, but passes flatus without difficulty" (Jones and associates, 1971).

Physical Examination

The findings on physical examination usually are of abdominal tenderness and guarding. A tender abdominal mass was palpable in 44 of 110 cases (40 per cent) reviewed by Jones. The mass may not be felt until after induction of general anesthesia. Abdominal distention is absent, and bowel sounds are usually normal unless there is free intraperitoneal blood. A gastric splash was heard over the region of the stomach in the three patients (2 children and 1 adult) with duodenal intramural hematoma reported by Shannon (1962–1963).

"The psoas sign is occasionally positive. On at least one occasion, the hematoma was palpable on rectal examination. The stool is usually Hematest-negative. Contusion of the abdominal wall is rare" (Jones and associates, 1971).

Jaundice was present in 7 of 116 cases (6 per cent) in Jones' collected series. "The diagnosis often has been confused with appendicitis, retroperitoneal hematoma, rectus hematoma, and pancreatitis" (Margolis, Carnazzo, and Finn, 1976).

Janson and Stockinger (1975) analyzed 56 cases of intramural duodenal hematoma reported in the English literature since 1966 and found that the presenting signs most frequently were those of upper gastrointestinal obstruction or abdominal pain. Forty-one of 54 patients (76 per cent) presented obstruction, 22 per cent with pain, and 2 per cent with hypotension secondary to an associated large retroperitoneal hematoma. In 80 per cent of the patients (44 of 56), the diagnosis was either made or suspected after an upper gastrointestinal x-ray contrast series or plain roentgenograms of the abdomen. Jansen and Stockinger noted that differentiation between types of duodenal hematomas can be made radiologically. "Barium contrast studies in traumatic hematomas show an acute duodenal mucosal angle of the proximal area of the hematoma, whereas spontaneous hematomas will have a more diffuse intramural spread and less angle."

Radiology

Characteristic radiologic signs may confirm the diagnosis. A plain supine x-ray film of the abdomen may show a large gas bubble and fluid level in the stomach and also, at times, in the first part of the duodenum, with no air in the remainder of the small bowel. It may also show obliteration of the psoas shadow or an abdominal mass.

Barium swallow x-ray studies of the stomach and duodenum are the most valuable for making a specific diagnosis of intramural hematoma of the duodenum. These may show obstruction, a dilated stomach and duodenum with an intraluminal filling defect in the duodenum, deviation of the duodenal lumen, and the diagnostic coiled-spring of barium in the involved portion of the duodenum, as was described by Felson and Levin (1954). These investigators, in 1954, described the characteristic barium meal x-ray findings of obstruction of the second part of the duodenum, with a rounded filling defect, a widening of the lumen near the duodenojejunal junction, and crowding of the edematous valvulae conniventes to give a pathognomonic coiled-spring appearance.

Since partial intussusception of the bowel mucosa distal to the hematoma has been reported in at least three cases, others (Devroede and associates, 1966) have postulated that the coiled-spring sign probably results from partial intussusception of bowel wall distal to the hematoma. "These characteristic x-ray signs were present in approximately half the cases in which upper gastrointestinal x-ray contrast studies were made in one large collected series" (Margolis, Carnazzo, and Finn, 1976).

METHODS OF TREATMENT

Both nonoperative and operative methods have been used successfully for the treatment of intramural hematoma of the duodenum. Each method has its proponents.

At first, intramural hematoma of the duodenum was considered to be a surgical condition, and most of the cases were treated operatively. In 1954, Schatzki emphasized the rapid resorption of duodenal hematomas and suggested that spontaneous regression should be expected. A number of investigators began trials of nonoperative treatment for selected patients and compared results with those obtained by operative treatment.

Nonoperative Treatment

Nonoperative treatment consists of restriction of oral intake, nasogastric suction, intravenous replacement of fluid and electrolytes, and observation for 7 to 10 days to allow the obstruction to resolve.

Experience has shown (Wiot, Weinstein, and Felson, 1961; Fullen and associates, 1974; Janson and Stockinger, 1975; Maull, Fallahzadeh, and Mays, 1978) that resolution of the hematoma sufficient to relieve the obstruction has required an average of 6 to 7 days (range, from 5 to 16 days) of nasogastric suction. Complications requiring surgical intervention have occurred during this period of observation in some cases (28 per cent in one series) (Wiot, Weinstein, and Felson, 1961). Also, there have been reports that even though the patient may survive the injury, the healing process will sometimes result in fibrosis and some degree of permanent duodenal obstruction by an organized hematoma.

Proponents of nonoperative treatment (Wiot, Weinstein, and Felson, 1961; Fullen and associates, 1974; Maull, Fallahzadeh, and Mays, 1978) believe that prolonged nasogastric decompression will resolve the hematoma and restore duodenal patency. They argue that conservative nonoperative treatment must be considered any time it can be done safely, with less mortality, less morbidity, and less cost, and they call attention to the high incidence of reoperation for persistent obstruction following operative treatment.

They recommend nonoperative treatment for intramural hematoma of the duodenum only after perforation of the duodenum and other associated intra-abdominal injuries requiring laparotomy have been excluded. Altemeier (1963) also pointed out that the operative treatment proponents' claim that surgical evacuation of the hematoma is a small operation often is not so. In some of his patients, the extravasation of blood had been largely into the wall of the duodenum, being not localized and not easily excised.

Izant and Drucker (1963) recommended nonevacuation of the hematoma, citing the difficulty in effectively releasing the clot, and they believed that incision and drainage encouraged late stricture.

Operative Treatment

On the other hand, numerous investigators endorse evacuation of the clot, citing the experience of Judd, Taybi, and King (1964), which showed that late stricture may result and enlargement of the hematoma may occur by the hyperosmotic effect of the liquefying hematoma.

Proponents of operative treatment believe that, without operation, even though the patient may survive the injury the healing process will frequently result in fibrosis of an organized hematoma, with some degree of permanent duodenal obstruction. "In these cases, some type of shunt, such as a juxtapyloric bypass, may be considered. However, gastroenterostomy also may not relieve symptoms of complete distal duodenal obstruction, since a competent pylorus will, to some degree, offset the benefits of the gastroenteric stoma" (Herrington, 1969).

Proponents advocate operation as the treatment of choice for the majority of patients with intramural hematoma of the duodenum because of the advantage of speedier recovery, less nutritional imbalance, and relative benignity of the postoperative course, and also the importance of determining the presence of any associated injuries to intra-abdominal viscera, particularly the duodenum, jejunum, pancreas, or liver.

Proponents of both methods of treatment generally agree that mandatory indications for prompt surgical intervention are associated perforation of the duodenum and/or other intra-abdominal viscera, ampullary obstruction by the hematoma causing obstructive pancreatitis, or pre-existing traumatic or alcoholic pancreatitis, biliary obstruction, and long-term cicatrization and stenosis of the duodenum secondary to organized intramural hematoma. The mortality is low when there are no complicating diseases.

Comparison of Nonoperative and Operative Treatment

Fullen and associates (1974) reported 14 patients in whom the diagnosis of intramural duodenal hematoma was made. Eleven of these patients were treated nonoperatively; all survived without complication. The remaining three patients were operated upon; there was one major complication, but all survived. On the basis of this experience, the surgeons recommended nonoperative treatment for intramural hematoma of the duodenum, "after perforation of the duodenum and other associated injuries requiring laparotomy have been satisfactorily excluded."

Jones and associates (1971) reviewd 125 cases of intramural duodenal hematoma reported in the literature, plus 1 of their own. Nonoperative treatment was used initially in 47 of 115 patients (40.9 per cent). Of these, 13, or 11.3 per cent, were successful, with four patients having clotting defects or taking anticoagulants. Twenty per cent (23 of 115) were treated nonoperatively and later required operation for obstructive symptoms, and 9.6 per cent (11 of 115) were treated without operation and died.

Operation took place in 80 per cent (96 of 120) of the patients, and 18 of these (18.8 per cent) required reoperation. Simple evacuation of the hematoma was done in 54.2 per cent (52 of 96) and was successful in 86.5 per cent (45 of 52).

The most frequent indication for reoperation after simple evacuation was continued obstructive symptoms, and the most frequent reoperation was gastrojejunostomy, with or without further evacuation of the hematoma. Hematoma evacuation and gastrojejunostomy were combined initially in 16.6 per cent of the cases (16 of 96) and was successful in 75 per cent. Four reoperations were done for malfunction of the gastrojejunostomy.

In 4 of 96 patients, no procedure was performed at operation and no further therapy was required. In 8.3 per cent (8 of 96), bowel resections were performed, and reoperation was required in 4 of these.

Biliary decompression with cholecystojejunostomy was required in three patients. Duodenal perforations were present in three and were closed. The data showed that exploratory laparotomy with simple evacuation of the hematoma with or without added gastrojejunostomy is statistically the most effective method of cure and decreasing morbidity. It also appeared from the data that conservative therapy with nasogastric suction and fluid and electrolyte replacement should be instituted initially when the hematoma is induced by clotting defects, or when obstructive symptoms and radiologic changes are minimal.

Jones and associates concluded that the best management for most patients with intramural duodenal hematoma is by surgical intervention and simple evacuation of the hematoma, but, in patients with hematomas induced by clotting defects and in those with only minimal duodenal obstruction, a trial of conservative management with nasogastric suction and fluid and electrolyte replacement may be given. If the patient fails to improve or worsens, surgical intervention may be necessary.

However, early operation is indicated if associated duodenal perforation, ampullary obstruction by hematoma causing obstructive pancreatitis, or pre-existing traumatic or alcoholic pancreatitis, biliary obstruction, or long-term cicatrization and stenosis of the duodenum secondary to organized intramural hematoma are present.

Wiot, Weinstein, and Felson (1961) reported a patient with intramural hematoma of the duodenum induced by anticoagulant therapy with coumarin. They stated that "although no long-term follow-ups have been reported, conservative therapy should be tried first, but numerous reports of obstruction and narrowing of the duodenum have caused a large majority of authors to recommend operation, and advise removing the blood and blood clot and draining the area when resection is not necessary. When gastroenterostomy has been performed to bypass the obstruction, healing is much more rapid if the hematoma is also evacuated."

In 1976, Margolis, Carnazzo, and Finn collected 174 cases of intramural duodenal hematoma from the literature and reported 5 additional cases of their own. They reviewed the clinical management of the 179 patients, of whom 44 were treated nonoperatively and 135 by operation.

In the nonoperative group, the average hospital stay was 14.6 days. There were 11 deaths (25 per cent) and 5 nonfatal complications. Five patients required readmission after discharge, and two were operated upon for persistent obstruction. Four of the 11 deaths occurred in patients without a history of trauma. Severe pancreatitis in association with intramural hematoma was found at autopsy in all four patients. Causes of death in the others include acute tubular necrosis, bronchopneumonia, and sequelae of high intestinal obstruction.

Of the 135 patients treated operatively, 2 were operated upon after previous hospitalization in which they were treated nonoperatively. At operation, the hematoma was most commonly found in the second and third portions of the duodenum and most frequently was subserosal. Associated injuries to viscera other than the duodenum were few. In several cases, partial intussusception of the bowel mucosa distal to the hematoma was noted.

The postoperative course was benign in 105 patients (77 per cent). Mortality for the entire operated group was 2.9 per cent (4 of 137). Sixteen patients required reoperation to treat persistent symptoms of obstruction.

Comparison of the results in the two groups showed that the average hospital stay was 50 per cent longer; the mortality rate was 22.1 per cent higher (25 per cent versus 2.9 per cent); and the incidence of complications was higher in the nonoperated group than in the operated group.

Because of the advantages of speedier recovery, less nutritional imbalance, and relative benignity of the postoperative course, Margolis and associates advocated operation as the treatment of choice for the majority of patients with intramural hematoma of the duodenum.

Margolis, Carnazzo, and Finn (1976) noted that the choice of operation affected not only the length of hospital stay but also the morbidity and mortality rates.

Laparotomy alone and resection of the duodenum were associated with the longest periods of postoperative recovery. The most common complication was persistent obstruction, which frequently required reoperation. Gastrojejunostomy with evacuation of the hematoma was associated with the largest number of patients with persistent obstruction.

They concluded that gastrojejunostomy is seldom indicated for primary treatment, and resection of the duodenum should be reserved for selected cases. They also pointed out that an intramural hematoma has a striking resemblance to gangrenous bowel at the operating table; however, in none of the cases reported thus far has necrosis of the bowel been confirmed on histologic examination.

Simple evacuation of the hematoma without a bypass procedure was associated with the lowest incidence of complications and the shortest hospital stay. Margolis and associates recommended "operative therapy with simple evacuation of the hematoma as the procedure of choice for treating intramural hematoma of the duodenum in most cases, and reservation of resection and bypass procedures for selected cases."

Maull, Fallahzadeh, and Mays (1978) reported 14 patients with obstructing intramural hematoma of the duodenum. They divided the patients into two clinical groups for treatment:

Group 1 includes patients who are seen in the immediate postinjury period because of symptoms directly referable to an obstructing injury of the duodenum, or because of associated injuries. In these, early exploration is performed. Selective treatment is recommended.

If complete involvement of the duodenum by the hematoma is found at exploration, a small transverse incision is made at its distal end, and the hematoma is milked empty. Small hematomas or those involving only portions of the duodenum are left alone. Because of the high incidence of stomal dysfunction and reoperation reported in the literature, gastroenterostomy is seldom justified as a primary procedure.

Group 2 includes the usual patient with an isolated post-traumatic intramural hematoma of the duodenum who is seen hours or days after an injury, during which time there has been a latent or asymptomatic period or, more commonly, the patient has noted increasing abdominal pain and vomiting and presents with persistence of these symptoms. In these cases plain x-ray films of the abdomen and water-soluble contrast studies of the stomach and duodenum safely provide information about the integrity of the upper gastrointestinal tract. After perforation has been excluded, barium swallow x-ray studies are added to more clearly visualize the hematoma.

Diagnostic peritoneal lavage and peritoneoscopy are useful to exclude associated intraperitoneal injury. Celiotomy is indicated when intraperitoneal or other serious injury is suspected. Maull and associates' data and the data of others strongly suggest that in the typical patient with increasing symptoms of bilious vomiting and pain in the upper abdomen, seen 48 hours after injury, celiotomy for evacuation of the intramural hematoma is not needed.

They concluded that for an isolated intramural duodenal hematoma found at laparotomy, or in the typical patient with an isolated intramural hematoma in whom no other indications for operation are identified, aggressive nonoperative therapy is the preferred treatment. This opinion is clearly debatable.

In 1975, Janson and Stockinger reviewed 56 cases of intramural duodenal hematoma reported in the English literature since 1966. In order to analyze the most recent treatment technics, they limited their review to only those cases that had not been reviewed previously. Thus the series was modern. Duodenal hematoma occurred most commonly in a male child with blunt abdominal trauma. The age range was 18 months to 56 years. Fifty-six per cent (28 of 50) were younger than 12 years of age, and 73 per cent (38 of 52) were younger than 25 years. Seventy-two per cent of the patients (36 of 50) were male. A history of trauma was present in 70 per cent (40 of 56). In addition to trauma, other suspected etiologic factors included acute alcoholism, hemorrhagic pancreatitis, intestinal biopsy with the Crosby capsule, anticoagulation therapy, and postoperative complication of Heineke-Mikulicz pyloroplasty.

The presenting signs and symptoms were most frequently those of upper gastrointestinal obstruction or abdominal pain: 76 per cent (41 of 54) had obstruction; 22 per cent, pain; and 2 per cent, hypotension secondary to an associated large retroperitoneal hematoma.

Janson and Stockinger (1975) found that the period between the causative trauma and onset of symptoms varied from 3 hours to 5 days, although most frequently patients became symptomatic after approximately 24 hours.

Physical findings in the patients varied from mild tenderness in the right upper quadrant to symptoms of complete obstruction with severe dehydration and electrolyte imbalance. An abdominal mass was frequently palpable. Some cases were diagnosed at surgery before diagnostic studies could be carried out, owing to an emergency situation. Laboratory findings generally revealed moderate leukocytosis and occasionally anemia. Two of the 56 cases had an increased bilirubin level, probably indicating obstruction of the common duct at the ampulla of Vater. Ten of the 56 (18 per cent) had an elevated serum amylase level. The two patients receiving coumadin had significantly low prothrombin time values, and the two alcoholic patients had abnormal liver function.

In 44 of the 56 cases (80 per cent) the diagnosis was either made or suspected after an upper gastrointestinal series or plain x-rays of the abdomen. Three basic characteristics are seen on the plain film: (1) gastric dilation, (2) an air-fluid level in the duodenum, and (3) absence of the right psoas shadow. Upper gastrointestinal barium contrast x-ray studies show the coiled-spring sign, described by Felson and Levin, in which elevated mucosal folds assume a helical pattern. It has been suggested that differentiation between origins of duodenal hematomas can be made radiologically. Barium contrast studies in traumatic hematomas show an acute duodenal mucosal angle at the proximal area of the hematoma, whereas spontaneous hematomas have a more diffuse intramural spread and less angle.

Of the 56 patients, 21 (38 per cent) were treated nonoperatively and 2 died, a mortality of 9.5 per cent in this subgroup. However, 19 of the 56 patients (34 per cent) had been treated successfully with nonoperative treatment. A mass was palpable in several cases. Resolution of the duodenal obstruction required 4 to 16 days with nasogastric suction in these cases.

Thirty-five (62 per cent) of the 56 patients were treated operatively, with no mortality. Six (11 per cent) underwent operation promptly after trauma because of findings of an acute abdomen, and 29 (51 per cent) were observed initially but subsequently underwent operation for persistent obstructive symptoms. Some surgical procedures were performed 24 hours after the trauma with prompt obstruction, but others were performed as late as 14 days after the onset of obstructive symptoms.

Examination of pathologic specimens demonstrated that the hematoma may dissect submucosally or in the intramuscular or subserosal layers. In most cases the mucosa remained intact. The hematoma may involve one or all portions of the duodenum.

Operative findings ranged from duodenal hematoma with no associated abnormality, treated only by simple evacuation and closure of the hematoma, to an acutely ill, hypotensive patient with 1500 ml. of blood in the retroperitoneal space and an intramural hematoma of the second and third portions of the duodenum. This patient was treated by drainage and evacuation of the hematoma and subsequently required reoperation for duodenal obstruction, which was relieved by gastrojejunostomy.

Janson and Stockinger concluded, "From the results reviewed, it appears that

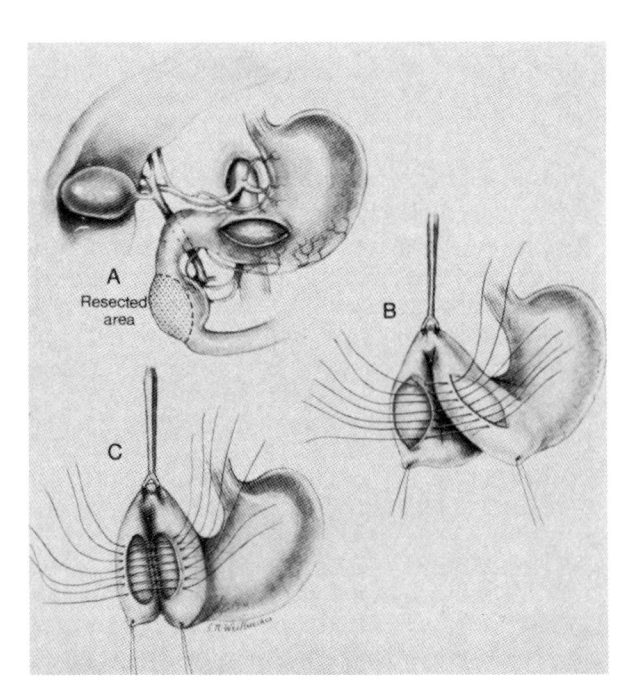

Figure 8–5. *A*, The area of the duodenum involved with intramural hematoma formation and the portion resected; *B* and *C*, The subsequent gastroduodenostomy. (From Janson, K. L., and Stockinger, F.: Duodenal hematoma; Critical analysis of recent treatment technics. Am. J. Surg. *129*:305, 1975.)

conservative management is indicated if the patient's clinical condition remains stable, and he seems able to tolerate a prolonged period of intravenous feeding and nasogastric suction; such management is especially indicated if the patient has any bleeding disorder.

"Patients with evidence of peritonitis, shock, or retroperitoneal air obviously require prompt exploration. Patients with a diagnosis of duodenal hematoma who do not have resolution of obstructive symptoms within a 10- to 14-day period of conservative treatment should be explored surgically."

In analyzing surgical patients, they found that 12 per cent (2 of 18) treated by simple evacuation of the hematoma required reoperation for obstruction. In patients treated by evacuation and gastrojejunostomy, 21 per cent (3 of 14) required subsequent reoperation for marginal ulceration. These results suggest the need for procedures with less risk of reoperation. In a patient they operated on, the lateral duodenal wall was resected because of its questionable viability (Fig. 8–5). Gastroduodenostomy (Jaboulay pyloroplasty technic) was used successfully for closure. They believed that "evacuation of the hematoma, combined with gastroduodenostomy, may lessen the risk of reoperation. This procedure would protect the patient from reobstruction even if the hematoma were to recur. In addition, marginal ulceration would be less likely since the duodenal mucosa is not as vulnerable to breakdown."

Summary

The information obtained from these reported experiences is helpful for selecting appropriate management of patients with intramural hematoma. The important findings can be summarized as follows:

1. Nonoperative treatment consists of restriction of oral intake, nasogastric suction, intravenous replacement of fluids and electrolytes, and observation for 6 to 7 days to allow time for the hematoma to resolve and relieve the duodenal obstruction.

Objections to this method of treatment are (1) resolution of the hematoma has required 4 to 16 days, and complications requiring surgical intervention have occurred during this period of observation in some cases (28 per cent in a series of Wiot, Weinstein and Felson [1961]); (2) in some cases the healing process has resulted in fibrosis and some degree of permanent obstruction, requiring operation.

2. Some controversy continues as to whether nonoperative or operative treatment is the method of choice for these patients. Comparison of the results obtained by these two methods of treatment in one large series of unselected patients (Margolis, Carnazzo, and Finn, 1976) showed that the average hospital stay was 50 per cent longer, the mortality rate was 22.1 per cent higher (25 per cent versus 2.9 per cent), and the incidence of complications was higher in the nonoperated than in the operated group.

In a modern series (Janson and Stockinger, 1975) 2 of the 21 cases treated nonoperatively died, a mortality rate of 9.5 per cent, but 35 cases were treated operatively without a death.

3. In regard to morbidity, in one series (Jones and associates, 1971), all 23 cases treated nonoperatively later required operation for obstructive symptoms. In another series, 5 of the 44 patients treated nonoperatively required readmission after discharge, and 2 were operated upon for persistent obstruction.

In the series of Jones and associates (1971), the data showed that when the hematoma is induced by clotting defects, or when obstructive symptoms and x-ray changes are minimal, a trial of nonoperative treatment should be instituted initially. If the patient fails to improve or worsens, surgical intervention is indicated.

It is now generally agreed that both nonoperative and operative therapy have a place in the treatment of intramural hematoma of the duodenum, and that each method has its specific indications. *Nonoperative treatment* is indicated for initial treatment when the hematoma is induced by clotting defects, or when obstructive symptoms and radiologic changes are minimal. If the patient fails to improve or becomes worse, surgical intervention is indicated. Nonoperative treatment should not be used until after the presence of intra-abdominal injury has been excluded.

There is mutual agreement by proponents of both methods of therapy that early *operative treatment* is mandatory if associated duodenal perforation, ampullary obstruction by the hematoma causing obstructive pancreatitis, or pre-existing traumatic or alcoholic pancreatitis, biliary obstruction, and long-term cicatrization and stenosis of the duodenum secondary to organized intramural hematoma are present. Surgical intervention has a low mortality when there are no complicating injuries or diseases. The operative procedure of choice varies with the condition of the patient and the findings at exploratory laparotomy.

Experience has shown that both methods of treatment have been associated with an undesirably high incidence of complications.

OPERATIVE TECHNICS

Simple Evacuation

In these patients, associated injuries to viscera other than duodenum are few. Direct pancreatic trauma is occasionally encountered. Active intra-abdominal or retroperitoneal hemorrhage is rare.

The patient is positioned supine on the operating table. The peritoneal cavity is entered through an upper midline or upper right paramedian abdominal incision. The duodenum and the site and extent of its hematoma are identified. After careful exploration for other intra-abdominal injury, the operative procedure that is most appropriate is elected. It varies with the abnormalities found at exploration.

A choice of methods is available for evacuating the hematoma. (1) If the hematoma is lengthy, it may be managed by making a short transverse incision through the serosa over the lower end of the hematoma and then finger-stripping the hematoma empty from top to bottom. (2) Another method is to make a longitudinal incision through the serosa over the full length of the hematoma, evacuating the hematoma by aspirating its semiliquid contents with a suction aspirator, and removing the clots with gauze swabs. When the hematoma is situated within the muscular layer, it may be difficult or even impossible to evacuate.

In Shannon's (1962-1963) experience when the hematoma was intramuscular, it could be removed by incising the serosa over the hematoma and evacuating its contents with a suction apparatus. The mucosal layer usually remains intact in these hematomas, and effort should be made to avoid violating its integrity during evacuation. However, in a few cases it has been necessary to make a short incision into the most proximal jejunum in order to reduce a small intussusception of the lower end of the hematoma. After reduction, the jejunotomy is closed in two layers.

It should be emphasized, that the duodenum should be widely mobilized by the Kocher maneuver so that its posterior surface and the full length of the hematoma can be exposed, to avoid overlooking a retroperitoneal hematoma or duodenal perforation and to permit an incision through the full length of the duodenal serosa over the hematoma. This permits the hematoma to be fully evacuated, which is particularly important when the distal portion of the duodenum is involved.

Failure to adequately evacuate the hematoma has been the leading cause of the high incidence of persisting obstruction requiring reoperation following simple evacuation. Simple evacuation of the hematoma was successful in 45 of the 52 patients, or 86.5 per cent, in which it had been used in one series (Jones and associates, 1971).

There is difference of opinion about how the operative area should be managed after the hematoma has been evacuated and before the abdominal incision is closed. Some surgeons believe that drainage of the area is unnecessary and advise that drains not be used because "drainage of the hematoma cavity with a rubber drain resulted in development of a duodenal valve with postoperative duodenal obstruction on one occasion" (Jones and associates, 1971). Some (Janson and Stockinger, 1975) prefer to close the duodenal serosal incision over the hematoma with interrupted 000 chromic catgut sutures, in order to tamponade any subsequent bleeding, and to close the abdominal incision without drainage.

At present most surgeons drain the area after the hematoma has been evacuated or use drainage selectively, according to the circumstances in each case.

Gastrojejunostomy

Although simple evacuation of the hematoma without a bypass procedure has been successful in about 85 per cent of the cases in which it has been used and has had the lowest incidence of postoperative complications, about 12 per cent of the patients have required reoperation. The most frequent indication for reoperation has been continued obstructive symptoms, and the most frequent reoperation has been gastrojejunostomy with or without further evacuation of the hematoma.

Gastrojejunostomy with evacuation of the hematoma is seldom indicated for primary treatment of intramural duodenal hematoma. This operation has been associated with the highest incidence of postoperative persistent obstruction that frequently required reoperation.

Nonviable Resection

Although most cases in which viability of the involved duodenum has been questionable have been treated by resection, its use should be reserved for selected cases, as it has some undesirable sequelae and alternative procedures are available. Resections of the duodenum have been associated with the longest periods of postoperative recovery. Almost half of them have been complicated by persistent postoperative obstruction, which frequently required reoperation — most often by performing a gastrojejunostomy — but the mortality has been surprisingly low. Two groups of 11 and 6 cases, respectively, with questionable viability of the involved duodenum were treated by resection without any mortality and with an average hospital stay of 17 days (Jones and associates, 1971; Margolis, Carnazzo, and Finn, 1976).

Alternative operative procedures in a questionably viable duodenum include (1) A diverting gastrojejunostomy. This was performed in two cases (Jones and associates, 1971). One patient was thought to have infarction of the duodenum and at a second operation was treated by gastrojejunostomy without resection.

(2) Janson and Stockinger (1975) reported a 54-year-old woman who, at operation for cholecystectomy, was found to have hydrops of the gallbladder, gallstones, and a submucosal hematoma in the duodenum. The vascular supply and viability of the lateral wall of the duodenum appeared questionable, so this area was excised and the resulting defect in the duodenal wall was closed by using it to form the stoma of a Jaboulay gastroduodenostomy in order to restore the size of the duodenal lumen and assure gastric outflow. Cholecystectomy was performed, and a liquefied intramural submucosal hematoma in the second portion of the duodenum was evacuated through an incision made in the anterior wall of the duodenal mass.

PEDIATRIC DUODENAL HEMATOMA

Intramural duodenal hematoma occurs most commonly in the pediatric population. It is usually the result of nonpenetrating abdominal trauma, often of mild or even trivial force. The injury may relate to the close relationship of the duodenum and the

Figure 8–6. Age distribution of 100 children reported with intramural duodenal hematoma.

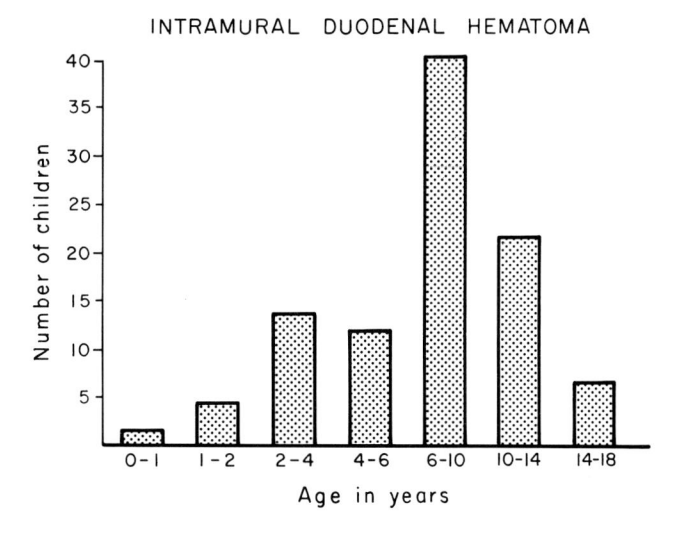

Table 8-4. Associated Injuries in Over 100 Cases of Pediatric Duodenal Hematoma

None	89
Closed head injury	1
Hiatus hernia	1
Skeletal trauma	4
Perforated bowel	1
Pancreatitis	2

Table 8-6. Treatment of 89 Pediatric Patients with Intramural Duodenal Hematoma

Nasogastric decompression until resolution	21
Evacuation of hematoma	43
Evacuation and bypass procedure	7
Bypass procedure	14
Exploration for diagnosis	3
Resection	1

vertebral column which presents an unyielding, fixed barrier to any force arising anteriorly. Such trauma may result in tearing of small blood vessels within the wall of the duodenum without actual disruption of the integrity of the bowel or pancreas.

In published reviews of over 100 pediatric cases of duodenal hematoma (Swaiman, Root, and Raile, 1958; Restel and associates, 1959; Davis and Thomas, 1961; Izant and Drucker, 1964; Freeark and associates, 1966; Darby, Johnson, and Till, 1968; Mahour and associates, 1971; Holgersen, 1977), there is a striking absence of significant associated injuries (Table 8-4). Furthermore, this injury is rarely seen as part of the multisystem, blunt trauma pattern seen most commonly with automobile-pedestrian or automobile-passenger trauma. The mechanism of injury is usually a moderate force pushing into the epigastrium of the unsuspecting child (Table 8-5). The age distribution of 100 children reported with duodenal hematoma was between 7 days and 18 years, with a peak incidence between the years of 6 and 10 (Fig. 8-6).

Duodenal hematoma usually presents with the gradual onset of gastric outlet obstruction over several days following the injury. Vomiting without anorexia several days after a blow to the abdomen was the most common complaint. Physical findings may include upper abdominal tenderness or a mass, which may increase in size over several days. A decrease in hemoglobin was reported in several cases, but patients rarely required transfusion. Chemical evaluation of traumatic injury to the pancreas rarely demonstrated elevation of serum amylase or lipase or urinary amylase. Radiographic examination of the suspected high gastrointestinal tract obstruction usually demonstrated varying degrees of duodenal obstruction by compression of the lumen by an intramural mass.

Once the diagnosis of intramural duodenal hematoma is made, the treatment must be individualized to each patient's state. If the patient exhibits clinical signs of injury to other organs, such as the pancreas, or has clinical peritonitis from a possible leak of small bowel contents, the appropriate course after hydration is laparotomy. If one feels that the intramural duodenal hematoma is an isolated injury, supportive therapy with intravenous fluids and nasogastric decompression of the stomach are an acceptable alternative.

Evacuation of the hematoma by longitudinal incision of the serosa muscularis was the most common therapy employed in the 89 pediatric patients reviewed. (See Table 8-6.) Supportive therapy until resolution of the hematoma was the second most

Table 8-5. Mechanism of Injury of Pediatric Duodenal Hematoma

Multisystem blunt trauma	4
Fall onto angled object	29
Human blow (fist)	13
Kicked in abdomen	6
Fell over/on bicycle handles	12
Child abuse (all under 4 years of age)	4
Thrown from horse	3
Struck by hockey stick	3
Struck by rake or shovel handle	3
Fell over monkey bar	2
Struck by swing	1
Struck by see-saw	1

Table 8-7. Result of Treatment of Pediatric Duodenal Hematoma

Death (1 hemophiliac)	3
Multiple operations	3
Cardiac arrest during surgery (recovered)	1
Complete resolution after conservative treatment	21/21
Complete resolution after surgical drainage	38/43

common therapeutic course, followed by gastroenterostomy for bypass of the hematoma.

The result of the different therapeutic modalities is seen in Table 8–7. Conservative treatment was associated with a longer hospitalization than simple evacuation of the hematoma, although 5 of 43 patients underwent laparotomy. Of the 64 reported pediatric cases, the follow-up revealed 3 deaths, one occurring in a hemophiliac patient.

In summary, intramural duodenal hematoma is an injury seen most commonly in the 6- to 14-year old who has sustained blunt trauma to the epigastrium. The signs of gastric outlet obstruction usually evolve over the following 2 to 4 days and result in progressive vomiting. Barium upper gastrointestinal tract radiographic study is usually diagnostic, and subsequent treatment must be individualized to conform to the presence or suspicion of associated visceral injury.

Chapter 9

TUMORS OF THE STOMACH AND DUODENUM

Tumors of the stomach and duodenum may be benign or malignant. A tumor's histologic components may not always be obvious, and areas of malignancy may occur among areas of benign change. Tumors of the stomach require a series of examinations to establish their nature. These examinations include endoscopy with biopsy and brushings, cytology, upper gastrointestinal series, and careful follow-up. With the skills acquired by most endoscopists, mucosal tumors of the stomach should be completely excised where possible or multiple incisional biopsies should be performed.

Most tumors of the stomach remain asymptomatic for long periods of time before clinical manifestations, including bleeding, pain, and obstruction, occur.

BENIGN GASTRIC TUMORS

Benign tumors are unusual and comprise only 5 to 10 per cent of all tumors of the stomach (Beard and associates, 1968). These gastric tumors may arise from the mucosa or underlying connective tissue. The mucosal lesions are generally adenomas (polyps), and the connective tissue lesions are generally intramural. Leiomyomas are the most common benign gastric tumor, and may be found in 46 per cent of the stomachs that are examined at autopsy (Meissner, 1944). Gastric polyps are relatively rare lesions, with an incidence of 0.5 per cent in most autopsy series.

LEIOMYOMA

Leiomyomas are the most common benign gastric tumor. They are submucosal and intramural and are usually found in the distal part of the stomach. Expansion of the tumor generally occurs toward the lumen but may penetrate the serosal surface. Generally these tumors are asymptomatic and come to attention because of their weight and bulk, which produce symptoms of abdominal discomfort. Hemorrhage is another presenting complaint and is the result of ulceration of the central part of the tumor, which generally has outgrown its blood supply. When discovered, these tumors should be widely excised to relieve symptoms and to rule out the possibility of malignant degeneration.

GASTRIC POLYPS

Most polyps of the stomach were once considered adenomas. Currently, adenomas comprise less than 10 per cent of all polyps of the stomach (Wilson and associates, 1975). The majority of polyps are hyperplastic, are randomly distributed, consist of normal mucosal components, and rarely become malignant. Adenomatous polyps are generally found in the antrum and are associated with gastritis. True adenomatous polyps have an association with carcinoma.

Most gastric polyps produce nondescript symptoms such as vague abdominal discomfort. Occasionally the patient presents weakness and anemia due to occult bleeding. Demonstration of polyps is usually by barium studies of the stomach, with good mucosal detail. Gastroscopy is more reliable than barium studies in detecting the smaller polypoid lesions and offers the opportunity of obtaining a cytologic diagnosis as well as being a therapeutic tool.

Pedunculated polyps can usually be removed endoscopically with a snare and electrocautery. Exfoliative cytology is a sensitive test to determine the malignancy of these lesions; however, the preparation of the sample and pathologic interpretation require expertise and experience.

Polyps 2 cm. or greater in diameter should be removed. This generally can be done using the endoscope for pedunculated polyps as large as 3 to 4 cm. in diameter. Larger or sessile lesions will usually require an exploratory laparotomy and wide excision of the lesion. Excision in all cases is preferred to multiple biopsies because of the risk of cancer.

Gastric polyps can be found in about one-fourth of patients with Peutz-Jeghers syndrome, as well as in patients with other familial polyposis syndromes.

MISCELLANEOUS BENIGN TUMORS OF THE STOMACH

Other tumors of the stomach are intramural lesions and are very unusual. They include, in decreasing order of frequency, fibromas, neurogenic tumors, aberrant pancreas, lipomas, vascular tumors, and cystic tumors.

FIBROMAS AND FIBROMYOMAS. Fibromas and fibromyomas are similar to the leiomyomas and contain either connective tissue (pure fibromas) or a mixture of connective tissue and smooth muscle (fibromyomas). They should be widely excised.

NEUROGENIC TUMORS. Most of the neurogenic tumors are neurilemmomas (70 per cent), and they usually occur in the distal stomach (Beard and associates, 1968). These arise from the nerve sheath (schwannomas). Approximately 25 per cent of the neurogenic tumors are neurofibromas and may be associated with generalized neurofibromatosis (von Recklinghausen's disease). The remaining 5 per cent of tumors arise from the sympathetic system and consist of neuroblastoma and periganglioneuroma. Ulceration and hemorrhage as well as abdominal pain are common symptoms of these tumors. Treatment consists of adequate excision.

ABERRANT PANCREAS. Most of the gastric pancreatic rests are located in the antrum, usually along the greater curvature, and are the most common form of gastric hamartoma (Beard and associates, 1968). These tumors are usually asymptomatic and discovered incidentally at the time of operation. Local excision is generally indicated.

LIPOMAS. Lipomas of the stomach are rare and may be submucosal or project into the lumen. Usually lipomas are sessile, but pedunculated lesions also occur. Larger lesions may ulcerate in the center. When discovered, wide excision is recommended.

VASCULAR TUMORS. These tumors include angiomas and endotheliomas of blood vessels and lymphatics (Beard and associates, 1968). Frequently these lesions ulcerate and result in severe hemorrhage. They also have a predilection to malignant change. Glomus tumors originating from capillary pericytes frequently ulcerate and require operative treatment.

BENIGN TUMORS OF THE DUODENUM

Benign tumors of the duodenum are extremely rare. They may produce hemorrhage, pain, or obstruction. In a review of 367 benign duodenal tumors, adenoma, leiomyoma, and lipoma were the most common, and each accounted for 20 per cent (Wilson and associates, 1975). The remaining benign tumors consisted of fibroma, angioma, and neurogenic tumors. Generally these lesions can be locally excised.

MALIGNANT TUMORS OF THE STOMACH

CARCINOMA

Ninety to 95 per cent of gastric tumors are malignant, and of these 95 per cent are carcinomas (Dupont and associates, 1978).

The remaining 5 per cent are sarcomas. The prognosis for gastric carcinoma is very poor, and 65 per cent of the patients who have gastric carcinoma are incurable. The gross characteristics of the tumor are generally good predictors of outcome. The polypoid and ulcerating but noninfiltrating tumors have the best prognosis, while the ulcerative infiltrating and the diffuse infiltrating, including linitis plastica, have a very poor prognosis. Superficial spreading tumors and carcinoma in situ have an excellent prognosis; however, they are rarely diagnosed at this stage in the United States. In Japan, where the incidence of carcinoma of the stomach is extremely high, a screening program was instituted for early detection. Routine use of endoscopy has revealed early lesions, resulting in very favorable 5-year survival figures.

Several predisposing factors have been implicated in gastric carcinoma. It is difficult to determine whether these factors are coincidental with carcinoma or have a significant role in the development of gastric carcinoma. These factors include gastric polyps (especially adenomatous polyps), achlorhydria, atrophic gastritis, and gastric ulcer.

Staging and Classification

The gross appearance of the tumor has served as a reliable guide for prognosis. To standardize the extent of disease, a staging classification has been proposed. This is based on the TNM system, where T refers to primary tumor; N, the regional lymph nodes; and M, distant metastases (Kennedy, 1970).

American Joint Committee for Cancer
Staging and End-Results (1978)

Stage	Finding
I	Tumor confined to mucosa and submucosa
II	Tumor penetrates through serosa without invasion of contiguous structures
III	Invasion of contiguous structures but resectable and/or nodal metastasis
IV	Not resectable and/or distant metastasis

Clinical Aspects, Symptoms, and Findings

Early stages of carcinoma of the stomach are usually asymptomatic, and this is perhaps the major factor that determines the dismal prognosis of this disease. Abdominal discomfort is one of the more common presenting symptoms. Pain, anorexia, weight loss, and hematemesis are other presenting symptoms and are usually associated with more advanced disease. Physical examination is usually unremarkable in the early stages; emaciation, abdominal mass, lymph nodes in the neck (Virchow's node), anterior mass on rectal examination (Blumer's shelf), ascites, or enlarged ovaries (Krukenberg's tumor) are findings associated with advanced disease.

Upper gastrointestinal barium studies may reveal a mucosal lesion or poor gastric contractions. The findings on barium studies may be suggestive of a malignancy, but cytologic confirmation is imperative. Exfoliative cytology and endoscopy with multiple biopsies and brushings are the most useful tests in establishing the diagnosis.

Other tests such as liver function tests, chest x-ray film, carcinoembryonic antigen, and computed axial tomography may be useful in assessing the extent of the disease. Palpable nodes and ascitic fluid should be biopsied and aspirated and analyzed for malignant cells.

Preoperative Treatment

While the patient's undergoing these various diagnostic and evaluative tests, the lesion should be presumed to be resectable for cure until distant metastases have been proved. Any electrolyte imbalance and anemia should be corrected early, and, if oral alimentation is poor, which it usually is, parenteral nutrition should be initiated. Adequate nutritional support will decrease the operative morbidity and mortality but has little effect on the overall prognosis.

Operative Treatment

If the patient has a complication of the tumor, such as bleeding, obstruction, or perforation, and emergency operation is required, the procedure should be designed to alleviate the complication and provide for reasonable palliation.

In the absence of distant metastases, a curative operation should be planned. At the time of operation, the surgeon should determine whether the tumor is resectable for cure. If there is evidence of distant metastases, such as widespread nodal involvement, a palliative procedure should be considered. Lymph nodes should be examined in the lesser and greater omentum, celiac axis, and portal area. Tissue confirmation of extension should be determined in all cases. Occasionally, adherence to a contiguous structure may not represent extension of the tumor through the serosa but an inflammatory response to the tumor.

The extent of the resection is determined by the location of the tumor and the lymph node drainage (Fig. 9–1). For distal gastric lesions, a generous subtotal gastrectomy, including en bloc removal of lymph nodes in the lesser and greater omentum, should be done. For lesions in the body of the stomach, a proximal gastrectomy and splenectomy are recommended. It is advisable to obtain frozen section examination of the proximal margin of the gastric resection. If tumor cells are seen, additional stomach should be resected. Favorable lesions near the cardia may require a total gastrectomy. Generally, a total gastrectomy is reserved for curative purposes. However, it may be required occasionally in a few selected patients to obtain adequate palliation. When total gastrectomy is performed as a palliative procedure, the operative mortality and morbidity must be acceptable. An antecolic Billroth II reconstruction is generally used when a gastric resection is performed for malignancy. A Roux-en-Y esophagojejunostomy or some modification of it is recommended following total gastrectomy.

In considering palliative resection, assessment must be made of the patient's symptoms and the location and nature of the tumor. In a relatively asymptomatic patient with an extensive tumor that presents a technically difficult problem, resection is not recommended. For obstructing and bleeding lesions, resection is preferred. A gastrojejunostomy may effectively palliate an obstructed patient and should be constructed in a manner to avoid reobstruction from the expanding tumor.

The overall 5-year survival rate for carcinoma of the stomach is 12 per cent. In a review of 1497 cases of adenocarcinoma of the stomach (Dupont and associates, 1978), 82 per cent of the patients were operable, and 48 per cent were resectable. The 5-year overall survival rate was 7.4 per cent and was as high as 30 per cent in those with localized disease. In this series, an extensive subtotal gastrectomy gave the best results; esophagogastrectomy and bypass procedures had a high mortality rate and a low survival rate. Adjuvant therapy did not significantly improve the survival figures. Most of these tumors are not sensitive to radiotherapy, and most chemotherapeutic regimens have not been successful.

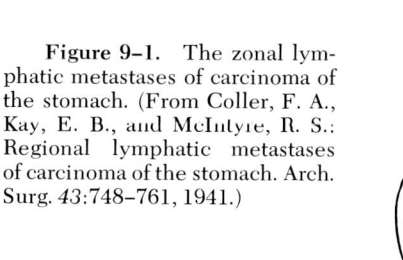

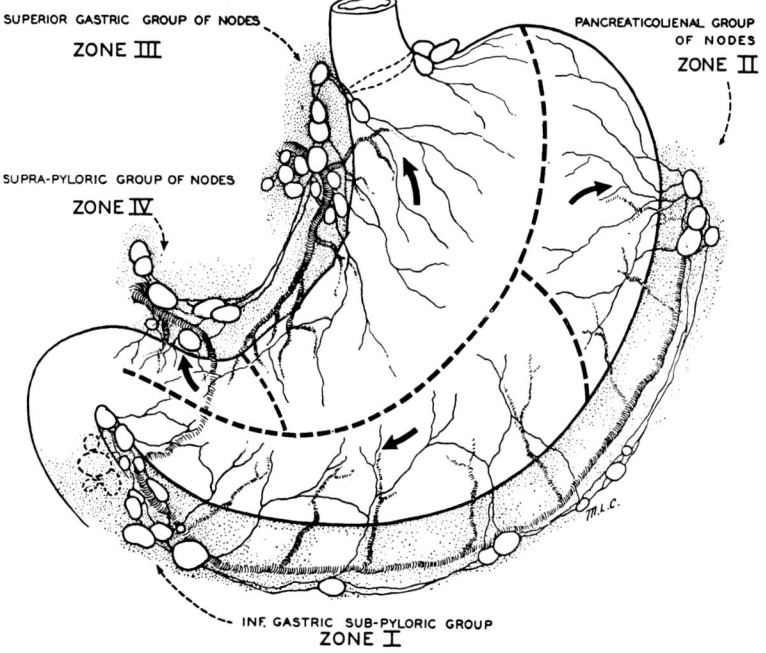

Figure 9–1. The zonal lymphatic metastases of carcinoma of the stomach. (From Coller, F. A., Kay, E. B., and McIntyre, R. S.: Regional lymphatic metastases of carcinoma of the stomach. Arch. Surg. 43:748–761, 1941.)

GASTRIC LYMPHOMA

Lymphomas comprise 2 to 5 per cent of all gastric malignancies (Hertzer and Hoerr, 1976). Most gastric lymphomas are secondary to disseminated disease; however, a primary lymphoma of the stomach can arise from the submucosal lymphoid tissue. The stomach is the most common site of primary gastrointestinal lymphoma. Primary lymphomas are usually large, bulky tumors, with central ulceration. These lesions are generally slow to metastasize, and with wide excision the 5-year survival rate approaches 50 per cent. It is important to distinguish these bulky tumors from extensive adenocarcinoma, since the lymphomas have a significantly better prognosis. These tumors are generally sensitive to radiotherapy, and this should be combined with surgical resection when the latter was not curative.

LEIOMYOSARCOMA

Leiomyosarcomas are generally bulky tumors; the large mass may be either intragastric or exogastric. The central area may ulcerate, and bleeding may be the presenting symptom. Leiomyosarcomas are usually well-localized tumors, and metastases and invasion generally occur late. These lesions are best treated by partial gastrectomy, since they are usually confined to the distal part of the stomach. If the proximal part of the stomach is involved, a total gastrectomy may be required. Other gastric sarcomas include fibrosarcoma, liposarcoma, angiosarcoma, and neurogenic sarcoma.

Other malignant lesions of the stomach are extremely rare and include gastric plasmacytoma, squamous cell carcinoma, chorioepithelioma, carcinosarcoma, and carcinoid tumors. All should be widely excised.

MALIGNANT TUMORS OF THE DUODENUM

Primary malignant tumors of the duodenum are extremely rare. In a review of 14 patients (Kerremans, Lerut, and Pennickx, 1979), 12 were patients with adenocarcinoma and 2 had lymphomas. In two-thirds of the patients with carcinoma the lesion was resectable (seven by pancreaticoduodenectomy and one by segmental resection). The 5-year survival was 14 per cent. Since the mean survival period for resection with lymph node invasion was 6 months and without lymph node invasion, 56.5 months, resection is not advised for those with positive regional lymph nodes except when hemorrhage is a complication.

Chapter 10

GASTRIC AND DUODENAL ULCERS

Gastric and duodenal ulcers are generally discussed under the common term *peptic ulcer disease*, although the natural history as well as the pathogenesis of these two diseases is quite different, and they do not have the same etiology. Pepsin is no longer thought the common denominator of duodenal and gastric ulcers. These two diseases are discussed separately in this chapter, except for the complications they have in common.

GASTRIC ULCERS

ETIOLOGY

Johnson (1965) divides gastric ulcers into three categories: Type I, Type II, and Type III. Type I gastric ulcers develop without a present or previous history of duodenal ulcer disease and occur generally along the lesser curvature, usually within a 2-cm. area between the parietal cells and the pyloric mucosa. They are generally associated with normal or low gastric acid output and an elevated serum gastrin level. Type II gastric ulcers are associated with a duodenal ulcer and gastric acid hypersecretion. Type III gastric ulcers are prepyloric ulcers associated with gastric acid hypersecretion. Types II and III resemble duodenal ulcer in their behavior and response to treatment.

Rhodes (1972) reviewed the multiple factors associated with gastric ulcers. Gastric ulcers can occur following chronic ingestion of salicylates or other irritating substances. In the absence of specific agents, reflux of bile into the stomach has been incriminated as a causative factor. Dysfunction of the pyloric sphincter may be the initiating factor in bile reflux gastric ulceration. Components of bile (bile acids and lysolecithin) can damage the gastric mucosa. Pancreatic enzymes alone are not an important intrinsic source of gastric mucosal damage. Although the precise pathogenesis of gastric ulcer has not been delineated, bile and pyloric dysfunction appear to be important factors. Other factors associated with gastric ulcer include tobacco smoking, alcohol ingestion, and anxiety.

PATHOLOGY

Atrophic gastritis is generally present in patients with gastric ulcer. The ulcers are generally 0.6 to 2 cm. in diameter, with the larger ulcers usually located more proximal from the pylorus. Ninety-five per cent of gastric ulcers are on the lesser curvature, with most located within 2 cm. of the pylorus. Gastric ulcers are multiple in 2.3 per cent of patients, and 42 per cent of patients with a gastric ulcer have an associated duodenal ulcer. In the Mayo Clinic series (Davis and coworkers), only 18 per cent of chronic gastric ulcers were associated with duodenal ulcer or duodenal scarring.

Three-fourths of gastric ulcers will heal completely within 12 weeks, on a good treatment program. There is a relationship between the size of the ulcer and the time required for complete healing. Seventy per cent of the ulcers less than 0.6 cm. in diameter will heal within 3 weeks, whereas only 18 per cent of those 2 cm. in diameter will be healed within 3 weeks. Despite this rapid healing rate, 42 per cent of patients will have one or more recurrences, generally within the first 6 months, and the recurrence is generally at the site of the original ulcer. Recurrence does not seem to be related to any specific factors or age. The complication rate for gastric ulcer include hemorrhage, 2.5 per cent; obstruction, 1.2 per cent; and perforation, 0.6 per cent.

CLINICAL FINDINGS

The highest incidence of gastric ulcer is generally in the 40 to 60-year-old age groups, which is slightly older than the age groups of duodenal ulcer. The pain is characteristically located in the epigastrium, usually between the xiphoid and umbilicus. The pain is often described as a gnawing or a burning sensation. In some cases it may be atypical in location and character. Although the pain may be relieved by food or antacids, it tends to appear earlier after eating than in duodenal ulcer disease. The symptoms are usually more severe than those of duodenal ulcer disease and may incapacitate patients, with loss of time from work. Duration of symptoms is as long as 4 weeks.

The relationship of symptoms to meals has been described by Edwards and Coghill (1968) — a triad consisting of food, comfort, pain. The period of comfort following a meal lasts from 0.5 to 1.5 hours. This is in contrast to the description of pain associated with duodenal ulcer, in which the neutralization of acid by food is important. In duodenal ulcer disease, the period of comfort following a meal usually lasts from 2 to 4 hours, and the pain that ensues is not relieved unless antacids or food is ingested to neutralize gastric acidity.

DIAGNOSTIC STUDIES

Four studies are important in a patient with gastric ulcer. These studies not only confirm the diagnosis and provide a therapeutic end-point but also rule out the possibility of a gastric cancer.

X-RAY STUDY. A barium study of the stomach will determine the presence of a gastric ulcer and possibly its malignant potential. The presence of a duodenal ulcer or a deformed pylorus favors a benign ulcer. The shape, size, and the completeness of healing are important characteristics in differentiating a benign from a malignant ulcer. A smooth appearance along the edge of the ulcer suggests a benign ulcer. A benign ulcer is also suggested if the base of the ulcer does not project beyond the estimated gastric wall. Ulcers less than 2 cm. in diameter are generally benign. Complete healing indicates a benign ulcer. Although these radiographic findings are helpful, they generally are not sufficient to rule out a malignancy. Occasionally an ulcer is missed because the crater becomes filled with food particles. Unlike the case with duodenal ulcer disease, it is important to follow these patients with barium studies to establish that complete healing has occurred. Air contrast barium swallows provide excellent detail of the mucosal surface and improve diagnostic accuracy.

GASTROSCOPY. Flexible fiberoptic gastroscopy has become an important diagnostic tool in the evaluation of gastric ulcers. Visual inspection of the ulcer can often determine the possibility of a malignancy. A gastric ulcer consists of an excavated area with whitish scar tissue surrounding the area of excavation. Around the edges of the ulcer, the mucosal pattern is intact and may show mild signs of inflammation. An ulcerated gastric carcinoma generally appears as an exophytic or fungating lesion with considerable heaping up and irregularity of the surrounding mucosa. The benign appearance of a gastric lesion does not rule out a neoplasm. Even though an ulcer appears benign, it should be biopsied in multiple areas and brushings should be taken. The biopsies preferable should be done at the edge of the lesion. Endoscopy is not mandatory as a follow-up once malignancy is ruled out; however, barium studies must be repeated until complete healing occurs.

GASTRIC WASHINGS AND CYTOLOGY. Gastric cytology can be a valuable aid in detecting gastric carcinoma. Expertise is needed not only in the methods of collecting gastric aspirate but also in preparing and reading the slides. With this expertise, gastric cytology can have an accuracy of 95 per cent.

GASTRIC ANALYSIS. A basal and stimulated gastric analysis (Histalog test) can be useful in evaluating a patient with a gastric ulcer. Patients with Type I gastric ulcer generally have a low or normal basal and stimulated acid secretion level. An elevated level of gastric acid secretion suggests that some obstruction is present or that the gastric ulcer is secondary to a pre-existing duodenal ulcer. Achlorhydria suggests that the ulcer is malignant.

Ulcer-Cancer Relationship. (Gastric carcinoma is discussed in more detail in Chapter 9). The relationship between a benign gastric ulcer and gastric carcinoma is more a diagnostic problem than an etiologic consideration. The incidence rate of carcinoma of the stomach is generally highest in the sixth decade. Approximately 25 per cent of carcinomas are ulcerating. Gastric carcinoma appears to be associated with a low fiber and a high carbohydrate intake. In most series that deal with the treatment of gastric ulcer, the incidence of a missed underlying carcinoma is approximately 0.8 to 4 per cent (Kraus, Mendeloff, and Condon, 1976; Grossman, 1971). With the combination of barium study, endoscopic examination with biopsy and brush biopsy, and cytology, a 95 per cent accuracy rate of diagnosis can be expected. As noted, the most important study in assessing malignancy is the follow-up barium study to insure that complete healing of the ulcer has occurred. Unless complete healing occurs in 6 to 12 weeks, carcinoma should be suspected and the patient referred for operative treatment.

Because of the high diagnostic accuracy rate that has been achieved, an initial trial of medical treatment for a gastric ulcer rather than immediate operation seems reasonable. However, failure to heal, recurrence, or another complication such as bleeding, perforation, or obstruction is an indication for operative treatment.

TREATMENT

Medical Treatment

Several factors have been associated with gastric ulcer — alcohol, tobacco smoking, spices, drugs that irritate the gastric mucosa or alter pyloric function, and stress. All should be eliminated. Treatment with carbenoxalone has been shown to be effective in the healing of gastric ulcer. Patients not responding to outpatient treatment or those with severe symptoms may require hospitalization. Bed rest and cessation of smoking are important therapeutic measures.

Although gastric hypersecretion is generally not a problem with gastric ulcer, antacid treatment has been used. Antacids are no better than placebo in gastric ulcer healing. The use of an H-2 receptor antagonist such as cimetidine is being evaluated. European studies have shown that cimetidine is of benefit in healing gastric ulcers. Studies from the United States showed no statistical difference in the percentage of ulcers healed at 2 or 6 weeks, comparing cimetidine with placebo or cimetidine plus antacid with placebo plus antacid (Fordtran and Grossman, 1978; Morgan and associates, 1978).

Surgical Treatment

Those patients with Types II and III gastric ulcers secondary to or associated with duodenal ulcer should have a standard duodenal ulcer operation. For patients with a Type I gastric ulcer, a partial gastrectomy is the recommended operation. The recurrence rate is low, and long-term results are good. Duthie and Kwong (1973) studied 50 patients treated with a Billroth I partial gastrectomy and 50 patients treated with vagotomy and pyloroplasty with biopsy of the ulcer. The functional results between the two groups were similar. Seven patients required reoperation after vagotomy: three for recurrent ulceration, three for gastric cancer, and one for bleeding. No patient who had a gastrectomy required reoperation. In a Mayo Clinic series (Davis, Verheyden, and Van Heerden, 1977), those patients with channel ulcers (gastric ulcers that behaved more like duodenal ulcers) had a lower recurrence rate if vagotomy accompanied partial gastrectomy. The recurrence rate for ulcers elsewhere in the stomach was the same whether or not vagotomy accompanied gastrectomy. Eighty-six per cent of 173 patients were treated by gastric resection without vagotomy. The recurrence rate was 1.3 per cent, compared with 16 per cent of 249 patients treated nonoperatively. The operative mortality ranged from 0 per cent in the series of Duthie and Kwong (1973) to 6 per cent in the series of Kraus, Mendeloff, and Condon (1976) for elective procedures. The mortality rate rises significantly when the patient requires emergency operation for perforation or bleeding and reached 34 per cent in the latter series.

With distal gastric resection, the ulcer is generally incorporated in the excised portion of the stomach. When the ulcer is in the more proximal part of the stomach, it is not necessary to do a more extensive gastrectomy in order to incorporate the gastric ulcer. The ulcer can be locally excised and oversewn, or biopsied and oversewn (Kelling-Madlener procedure). In poor-risk patients who cannot tolerate a distal gastrectomy, vagotomy and pyloroplasty can be useful to avoid the consequences of a technically difficult gastrectomy. Farris and Smith (1973) reported a 90 per cent rate of good results for vagotomy and pyloroplasty. This contrasts with a 38 per cent recurrence rate noted by Stemmer (1973) when vagotomy and pyloroplasty were performed. No recurrences were noted when gastric resections were done.

In a Scandinavian symposium on gastric ulcer (Fenger and coworkers, 1973; Nielsen and coworkers, 1973; Christiansen and coworkers, 1973) it was reported that 28 per cent of the patients treated also had a duodenal ulcer. Of those operated on, no recurrence was reported in 39 per cent. Good results were obtained with a Billroth I or II operation, but there was a 20 per cent recurrence rate if only a segmental resection was done. The mortality rate for elective operation was 2 per cent, which increased to 18 per cent for emergency operations.

These observations have been confirmed by the prospective randomized series done by Duthie and associates (1968, 1970, 1973) comparing vagotomy and pyloroplasty with resection, and proximal gastric vagotomy with resection.

DUODENAL ULCERS

ETIOLOGY

The cause or causes of duodenal ulcer are complex and involve genetic, psychologic, environmental, and local factors. The genetic factor is typified by the higher incidence of duodenal ulcer among monozygous than among dizygous male twins. Other genetic factors include the presence of blood group O and the absence of salivary blood group antigens, both of which are associated with a higher incidence of duodenal ulcers. Samloff (1975) showed that high levels of a specific serum pepsinogen are associated with patients who have a duodenal ulcer.

The incidence of duodenal ulcer over the last few decades is decreasing; it now averages 1.7 cases per 1000. This is attributed to the increase in the age of the population, and is also associated with the stabilization of urbanization in this country, with relatively fewer young people living in the cities.

Other factors include the use of coffee and other caffeine-containing beverages, cigarette smoking, and the chronic ingestion of aspirin, all of which are associated with an increase of ulcer incidence. It is surprising that alcohol has not been established as an important risk factor, although it is often implicated.

The pathogenesis of duodenal ulcer is better established than that of gastric ulcer (Ippoliti and Walsh, 1976). The two major mechanisms are (1) increased acid delivery into the duodenum, and (2) impaired neutralization of or impaired defense mechanisms for acid in the duodenum. The increased capacity for secreting acid is correlated with the parietal cell mass, and the number of parietal cells is significantly increased in patients with duodenal ulcer. Although the capacity of normal individuals and patients with duodenal ulcer to secrete a maximum amount of acid overlaps, duodenal ulcer patients generally are capable of secreting a larger total amount of acid. Associated with this ability is an increased serum pepsinogen I; this elevation of pepsinogen I is still under investigation.

Another factor in acid secretion is the sensitivity of the parietal cells to gastrin. The dose of gastrin needed to produce maximal secretion is significantly less in ulcer patients. Increased vagal tone and increased gastrin secretion also increase acid secretion. Establishing the vagus as a factor in the pathogenesis of duodenal ulcer is difficult since no tests are available to assess vagal tone. Serum gastrin, however, can be easily determined by most laboratories. The most common elevation in serum gastrin occurs in the Zollinger-Ellison syndrome, which is discussed later in this section. In some patients, such as those with pernicious anemia, hypergastrinemia is not associated with high levels of acid secretion. Hypergastrinemia is associated with hypersecretion in retained antrum, in which the antrum is incompletely resected and is excluded from the remaining stomach. This may occur with the Billroth II type of reconstruction. Hypergastrinemia occurs in G (gastrin) cell hyperplasia, in which the gastrin-producing cells are abnormally sensitive to amino acids and secrete large amounts of gastrin, which stimulate excess gastric acid.

Another factor postulated in the pathogenesis of duodenal ulcer is impaired inhibition of gastrin release. Normally, acid in the stomach (lowering of the pH) serves as an autoregulatory mechanism to shut off gastrin secretion. Impairment of this autoregulatory mechanism may be the cause of excessive acid secretion and ulceration in some patients. The defense mechanism — neutralization of acid by pancreatic and duodenal bicarbonate — has not been established as a causative factor. The single exception to this concept is the Zollinger-Ellison syndrome. In this disease, massive amounts of acid overwhelm the buffering capacity of the pancreas and duodenum and result in ulceration, as well as in inactivation of pancreatic enzymes and steatorrhea.

Although all of these factors are implicated in duodenal ulcer, acid is the most important. Duodenal ulcer patients secrete more acid than normal subjects. Medical and operative treatment that decreases acid secretion results in healing of the ulcer. Conditions that produce excess acid secretion result in ulcer formation. Inadequate neutralization of acid results in ulceration (e.g., marginal ulcer following gastrojejunostomy without vagotomy or gastric resection). Animal experiments in which excessive acid (chronic stimulation with histamine) or inadequate neutralization of acid (Mann-Williamson experiment) is produced result in ulceration similar to that occurring in humans.

PATHOLOGY

Duodenal ulcers are rarely malignant. They occur within the distal 1 to 2 cm. of the pyloric sphincter and are found with equal frequency on the anterior or posterior wall. Occasionally both walls may be affected. They may occur in the second portion of the duodenum or even more distally, but this is very unusual. The location of an ulcer in the distal part of the duodenum or in the jejunum should arouse suspicion that the patient may have Zollinger-Ellison syndrome or may have ulcerations secondary to ingestion of drugs like enteric-coated aspirin.

CLINICAL FINDINGS

Duodenal ulcers occur more frequently in males than in females and may occur at any age, with the middle of the third decade being most common. In neonates, ulcers are usually acute and multiple and cause either hemorrhage or perforation. In adults, a chronic ulcer is most common. In adults, acute ulcers generally indicate a drug-related cause, or they may occur in extremely stressful situations, as in burn and trauma patients.

The pain is generally similar to that of a gastric ulcer: a gnawing or burning sensation in the epigastrium. Unlike gastric ulcer pain, it generally occurs when the stomach is empty. The usual sequence is food, comfort, then pain, which is relieved by food or antacids. Seasonal recurrences or exacerbations are more common in duodenal ulcer patients generally occurring in the spring and fall, with remissions in the winter and summer.

Routine physical examination is generally unrevealing. During the acute stages, epigastric tenderness may be present.

DIAGNOSTIC STUDIES

The diagnostic studies that have been mentioned for gastric ulcer are also applicable for a duodenal ulcer. In patients with duodenal ulcer, concern about malignancy is negligible; therefore, biopsy, cytology, brushings, and repeat barium studies are unnecessary. For the patient with a typical duodenal ulcer history, it is generally sufficient to initiate treatment empirically and proceed to diagnostic studies only if the patient fails to respond. The usual studies for a patient with duodenal ulcer include upper gastrointestinal barium examination, endoscopy, gastric analysis, and examination of stool for blood. Barium studies and endoscopy are used to establish a diagnosis or document a recurrence.

GASTRIC ANALYSIS. Gastric analysis generally is not necessary unless the patient requires operation. Although gastric analysis does not significantly influence the type of operation that is performed, it is helpful as a baseline if problems develop following ulcer operation. With a successful vagotomy, maximal acid output can be expected to fall by 50 per cent. This occurs regardless of the type of vagotomy — whether truncal, selective, or proximal cell. With antrectomy, the maximal acid output can be expected to fall by 40 per cent. Combining vagotomy and antrectomy, maximal acid secretion is reduced by 90 per cent. Gastric analysis is also useful in diagnosing the Zollinger-Ellison syndrome. In patients with this syndrome, the ratio of basal acid output to maximal acid output is greater than 0.6. If low or negligible amounts of acid are secreted, this correlation no longer applies.

ENDOSCOPY. Routine endoscopy is generally not necessary in a patient with duodenal ulcer. Endoscopy is usually reserved for patients with duodenal ulcer symptoms whose barium x-ray study is normal. In such cases gastritis and duodenitis may be detected, which will help explain the cause of the patient's symptoms.

STOOL EXAMINATION FOR BLOOD. The stools of patients suspected of having an ulcer, whether duodenal or gastric, should be examined for occult blood. If the stool is black and gives a strongly positive reaction for blood, bleeding has occurred, presumably from the ulcer. The benzidine test is more sensitive than the guaiac test. If benzidine is used, the patient should be on a red meat–free diet for 3 days prior to the test. If bleeding is suspected, several stools should be examined to rule out intermittent bleeding. When occult blood is found, it is wise to perform a sigmoidoscopy and barium enema to rule out other causes of bleeding.

SERUM GASTRIN. A serum gastrin level is not routinely obtained in all patients who have duodenal ulcers. Serum gastrin determination is reserved for those individuals who fail to respond to conventional treatment and for patients with endocrine disorders. It is indicated in patients with elevated serum calcium levels, with recurrent complications of duodenal ulcers, and with continued ulcer symptoms following an ulcer operation. Serum gastrin levels greater than 600 picograms per milliliter strongly suggest the Zollinger-Ellison syndrome. Normal serum gastrin levels, in most laboratories, are less than 200 picograms per milliliter.

TREATMENT

Medical Treatment

The treatment of duodenal ulcer has four facets:

1. *Discontinue the use of agents* that have been closely associated with the formation of duodenal ulcers: tobacco smoking, aspirin (acetylsalicylic acid), coffee (and other xanthine-containing compounds), and secretagogues such as spices. Stress must be avoided. The use of sedatives should be discouraged, and, if significant emotional problems are present, psychiatric counseling can be very beneficial.

2. Although various types of *antacids* have been used in the treatment of duodenal ulcer, one must compromise between the palatability of various antacids for patients versus the buffering capacity of the antacids. Most important is to use one that the patient will accept and that has adequate buffering capacity. The side effects of antacids include diarrhea and constipation. Diarrhea is generally associated with the magnesium-containing antacids, and constipation with the calcium-containing type. Occasionally the use of both kinds may be required to minimize the side effects from either. Since calcium-containing antacids may result in an acid rebound, aluminum-containing antacids have become more popular compounds.

3. *Anticholinergics* used alone generally offer no significant benefit to patients with duodenal ulcer. To achieve therapeutic effect they usually have to be used in such high doses that the side effects are

extremely bothersome and incapacitating. If anticholinergics are used, they should be given in combination with antacids or cimetidine (Ivey, 1975).

4. An *H-2 receptor antagonist* (cimetidine) has been shown in several studies to be effective in the treatment of duodenal ulcer. Cimetidine works by blocking the H-2 receptor and inhibiting gastric acid secretion. This receptor is located on the parietal cell and is independent of vagal stimulation and gastrin concentration. Stimulation of the H-2 receptor results in acid secretion, whereas blockade, as is done by cimetidine, results in inhibition of acid secretion, regardless of other stimuli. Several clinical trials have shown that cimetidine was significantly different from placebo in healing duodenal ulcers after 4 to 6 weeks of treatment (Fordtran and Grossman, 1978).

Cimetidine is approved for the treatment of duodenal ulcer and hypersecretory states. Its long-term side effects are not completely known, and it is recommended for the patient who does not respond to antacids or cannot comply with antacid treatment. Cimetidine in a dose of 300 milligrams is given with meals and at bedtime.

Operative Treatment

Operative treatment for duodenal ulcer generally is recommended for a patient who remains symptomatic despite adequate medical treatment or in whom a complication has occurred. The indications for operation are obstruction, perforation, bleeding, and intractability. Because the long-term prognosis associated with the nonoperative treatment of obstruction or perforation is so unfavorable, operation is highly recommended. A patient experiencing minor hemorrhage from an untreated ulcer generally is given the initial benefit of medical treatment; however, if bleeding continues or recurs, operation is recommended. Intractability is defined as a persistence of symptoms (pain) despite good medical treatment. In such cases, it is important to document, by barium study or endoscopy, the presence of a duodenal ulcer.

Preoperative evaluation, therefore, consists of a barium study or endoscopy. Other worthwhile tests include a gastric analysis and a serum gastrin determination. Although gastric analysis is not a reliable indicator of predicting ulcer recurrence, there is evidence that the maximal acid output is higher in patients with recurrence. This has prompted Robbs and associates (1973) to recommend vagotomy and antrectomy if the maximal acid output exceeds 25 mEq. per hour.

Operations for duodenal ulcer are those that effectively reduce acid secretion. The two main components responsible for 90 per cent of acid secretion are vagal innervation and antral gastrin secretion. An effective vagotomy reduces stimulated acid secretion by approximately 50 per cent. Antrectomy, which removes the gastrin cells, reduces acid secretion by approximately 40 per cent. This physiologic observation is supported by the low recurrence rate achieved by combining vagotomy and antrectomy.

Four randomized prospective studies compare (1) subtotal gastrectomy, (2) vagotomy and resection (antrectomy), and (3) vagotomy with drainage (pyloroplasty or gastroenterostomy) (Goligher and coworkers, 1972; Jordan and Condon, 1970; Kennedy and coworkers, 1973; Price and coworkers, 1970, reviewed by Wise and Ballinger, 1974). The average mortality was less than 1 per cent in all groups. The recurrence rate was lowest for vagotomy and resection (average, 1 per cent), whereas with subtotal gastrectomy the recurrence rate averaged 4 per cent, and with vagotomy and drainage, 6 to 7 per cent. The average incidence of diarrhea as a complication in those with subtotal gastrectomy was 4 per cent; with vagotomy and resection, 12 per cent; and with vagotomy and drainage, 9 per cent. The incidence of dumping averaged 36 per cent for subtotal gastrectomy, 29 per cent for vagotomy and resection, and 25 per cent for vagotomy and drainage.

These studies show that these three types of operation are comparable when performed electively in good-risk patients under favorable operative conditions. If the intraoperative findings do not permit a resection, then vagotomy with drainage is a satisfactory option. No single operation is best for elective operative treatment of duodenal ulcer; when the preoperative and intraoperative findings are favorable, vagotomy and antrectomy are associated with the lowest recurrence rate.

Another operation, which has not yet stood the test of time, is the proximal gastric vagotomy, also termed parietal cell vagotomy, superselective vagotomy, and highly selective vagotomy. This operation consists of dividing the branches of the nerve of Latarjet; these branches innervate the parietal cells on the anterior and posterior aspects of the stomach along the lesser curvature. The technic consists of severing the branches to the stomach, along with the vascular bundle. The dissection includes skeletonizing the entire lesser curvature of the stomach from the cardioesophageal junction to a point 6 cm. proximal to the pylorus. In this area, a branch from the nerve of Latarjet spreads out in three prongs, resembling a crow's foot. The point of dissection is stopped at this distal landmark. Early results reported by Kronborg and Madsen (1975) had a recurrence rate of 22 per cent. Subsequent reports have a recurrence rate of 2 to 8 per cent (Johnson, 1975). The drop is probably accounted for by difference in technic, since there are vagal branches innervating the cardia and upper portion of the fundus that come directly from the main trunks off the esophagus. These have been termed the nerves of Grassi. In a proximal gastric vagotomy, it is important that the dissection continue up the esophagus for 4 to 5 cm., and that these nerves of Grassi fibers, which go directly to the cardia and superior part of the fundus, be interrupted.

Randomized prospective studies compare the proximal gastric vagotomy with other ulcer operations but have not been published yet. Kennedy and associates (1975), comparing proximal gastric vagotomy with selective vagotomy and gastroenterostomy, indicate that in a 2 to 4 year follow-up the recurrence rate was comparable in both groups, and the postoperative sequelae, such as dumping and diarrhea, were less with proximal gastric vagotomy. The recurrence rate from several nonrandomized studies is about 7 per cent (Hallenbeck and associates, 1976; Holt-Christensen and associates, 1977). Although the proximal gastric vagotomy is being enthusiastically accepted by most surgeons, technical expertise is required in performing this operation since it is important that the branches of the nerve of Latarjet be severed and that the nerves of Grassi be identified and interrupted.

This operation is most suitable for thin, young individuals, especially women, since women have a high incidence of sequelae following vagotomy and gastrectomy. The proximal gastric vagotomy has been advocated by some for complications of duodenal ulcer such as bleeding, perforation, and obstruction. This operation has not been shown to be of any special benefit under emergency conditions and because of its technical difficulties, a standard type of operation for these complications is recommended. Long-term follow-up is required to confirm the effectivenss of this operation under emergency conditions.

Giant Duodenal Ulcer

A giant duodenal ulcer is one that is greater than 2 cm. in diameter. Generally this is considered a subgroup of duodenal ulcer disease with ulceration in the duodenum ranging from 3 to 6 cm. The ulcer is generally posterior, with the pancreas forming its base. These ulcers have a higher mortality and morbidity than the typical duodenal ulcer (Klamer and Mahr, 1978; Lumsten, MacLarnon, and Dawson, 1970). The mortality rate in various series ranges from 8 to 40 per cent (Eisenberg, Margulis, and Ross, 1978; Klamer and Mahr, 1978). Medical treatment generally is not satisfactory, and, unless a close follow-up on these patients is possible, operative treatment is generally recommended before complications occur. Because of their size, operative treatment of these ulcers has a high mortality.

DIAGNOSIS

Patients usually complain of typical ulcer symptoms; in some patients weight loss and malnutrition may be present. On barium study of the gastrointestinal tract several features are important in making the diagnosis (Eisenberg, Margulis, and Moss, 1978).

Distinguishing features of this deformed area consist of a constancy in the size of the ulcer during the barium study, and abnormal mucosal pattern in this area, and possible granular protrusions at the base. The area does not have normal contractions. Giant ulcers have been described as appearing as an ulcer within an ulcer or as a large duodenal bulb. Endoscopy confirms the size of the ulcer and its posterior location.

TREATMENT

Patients with giant duodenal ulcers generally have a long history of ulcer disease, and treatment for the disease has usually been marginal. In the report by Eisenberg and associates, the diagnosis of giant duodenal ulcer was made early, and follow-up was included. Half the patients did well on medical management, and the mortality rate was 8 per cent. By most standards, these results would not be considered good for the treatment of typical duodenal ulcers; however, this represents a significant improvement compared with other reports in the literature. These results were attributed to early diagnosis. Most other reports in the literature do not support medical treatment in these patients and recommend early surgical intervention (Klamer and Mahr, 1978; Lumsten, MacLarnon, and Dawson, 1970).

Because of the large size of the ulcer and involvement of the pancreas, resection may not always be possible. When possible, vagotomy, antrectomy, and gastrojejunostomy should be performed. If the inflammatory mass surrounding the ulcer prevents safe dissection, vagotomy and gastrojejunostomy should be done.

Klamer and Mahr (1978) reviewed 16 patients with giant duodenal ulcer. In 8 of the patients, a truncal vagotomy, modified Bancroft resection, and gastrojejunostomy were performed. In 6 patients, a truncal vagotomy, antrectomy including resection of the duodenum distal to the ulcer, and gastrojejunostomy were done. In 2 patients, a truncal vagotomy and gastrojejunostomy without resection were performed. The latter operation was done because of the large size of the inflammatory ulcer. In assessing the feasibility of the resection, it is important to determine whether the duodenum is freed distal to the ulcer to allow safe closure of the stump. The base of the ulcer is left behind since this usually represents a full thickness penetration of the duodenum and represents the anterior surface of the pancreas. Good results were achieved in all 16 patients.

If emergency operation is required for bleeding, vagotomy, ligation of the bleeding site in the ulcer, and a drainage procedure are recommended.

COMPLICATIONS OF GASTRIC AND DUODENAL ULCER

The common complications of ulcer disease, both duodenal and gastric, are perforation, obstruction, and hemorrhage.

Perforation

Perforation generally occurs with an ulcer located on the anterior surface of the duodenum. If the ulcer is walled off or perforates into an adjacent structure, gastric juice and air do not escape into the abdominal cavity. The typical finding of free air under the diaphragm is therefore absent. The majority of perforated ulcers have free air in the peritoneal cavity, demonstrable radiographically in about 75 per cent of cases. Occasionally, the perforation can occur posteriorly and be localized in the lesser sac. A posterior perforation should be suspected when an irregular air fluid level is seen in the area of the lesser sac on the upright abdominal x-ray film. Although perforated duodenal ulcers are much more common than perforated gastric ulcers, the mortality and morbidity with a perforated gastric ulcer are considerably higher than in a duodenal ulcer. This is due in part to the older age of the group in whom gastric ulcers occur.

SYMPTOMS AND DIAGNOSIS

About three-fourths of patients with a perforated ulcer have antecedent symptoms of ulcer disease. The majority of patients have a history of sudden, abrupt onset of excruciating abdominal pain. The radiation of pain to the shoulder tip is common and is a result of diaphragmatic irritation. Gradually the pain improves and may localize to other parts of the abdomen, especially to the right lower quadrant where it may simulate appendicitis. Nausea and vomiting are accompanying symptoms. On physical examination the abdomen is rigid, and initially the temperature may be slightly below normal. The patient is apprehensive and appears shocky. These findings are attributed to the release of gastric contents and chemical peritonitis. Over the subsequent hours and days, the white blood count and the temperature become elevated, indicating progressive inflammation and bacterial infection.

TREATMENT

Because of the high mortality, *perforated gastric ulcers* should be treated operatively. Generally the treatment consists of a distal gastric resection which incorporates the ulcer. However, in poor-risk patients, oversewing the ulcer may be indicated. Multiple biopsies should be performed to rule out malignancy, if oversewing is elected for management.

A *perforated duodenal ulcer* can be treated by (1) nasogastric suction, (2) simple closure, or (3) definitive operation. *Nasogastric suction* has been recommended by Taylor and Warren (1956). They reported a series of patients who were successfully treated with nasogastric suction, antibiotics, and intravenous fluids. Most of the patients with acute ulcers did not subsequently require operation whereas those with a chronic ulcer required one. This treatment is reserved for poor-risk patients in whom operative treatment would carry undue risks. An important aspect of this form of treatment is continuous monitoring of the patient. Meticulous attention must be given to the nasogastric tube to insure its patency and function, since gastric decompression and thorough aspiration of the stomach are an essential part of treatment. Gastrografin studies must be obtained and repeated as indicated to confirm that the perforation remains sealed. If the perforation is open, either initially or on subsequent Gastrografin studies, operation is recommended. Abscess formation is a significant complication of this treatment. In general, this form of treatment is not recommended.

Simple closure of a duodenal ulcer is perhaps the standard form of treatment. In some series (Cohen, 1971; Steiger and Cooperman, 1976), a significant mortality is associated with simple closure, attributable to the types of patient in whom it is used. It is generally reserved for the most seriously ill patients. In this group, the existence of other concomitant diseases accounts for a mortality as high as 30 per cent. Simple closure consists of oversewing the ulcer with several silk sutures and then buttressing the closure line with a piece of omentum.

Definitive treatment is reserved for those patients who are good risks and who have minimal soilage of the peritoneal cavity. Several definitive types of operations have been advocated for treatment of patients with perforated ulcer. The best known series is that of Jordan and DeBakey (1961). They reported a mortality rate of 2.2 per cent of immediate subtotal gastrectomy, which was comparable to the mortality rate for simple closure. Since 30 to 40 per cent of the patients who have a perforated ulcer will require an ulcer operation in the future, definitive operation at the time of perforation is preferred since it decreases the days of hospitalization and the number of operative procedures. A definitive operation should only be done under favorable conditions, however, or if other complications such as hemorrhage or obstruction are also present. Jordan and associates (1976) and Sawyers and Herrington (1977) have advocated closure of a perforated ulcer combined with a proximal gastric vagotomy. This approach may be applicable in highly selected patients, but additional experience is needed before it can be recommended as standard treatment.

Obstruction

Obstruction due to a gastric ulcer is rare. When obstruction is seen in association with a gastric ulcer, the ulcer is probably malignant. Generally, prepyloric and duodenal ulcers can result in obstruction, but this is less common than perforation. Obstruction can result from edema during the acute phase of ulceration. Once the edema subsides, the obstruction is relieved, and the patient improves. Obstruction can also result from recurrent attacks of inflammation or a chronic ulcer causing permanent scarring of the pyloric canal, with gradual contraction and narrowing of the pyloric sphincter. In these cases, nonoperative treatment is not successful, and delays in operation can result in nutritional depletion of the patient. (See also Hourglass Stomach, p. 188).

SYMPTOMS AND DIAGNOSIS

Most patients with pyloric obstruction have a previous ulcer history. Crampy abdominal pain, nausea, and vomiting are the usual symptoms. Vomiting may be induced by the patient to relieve symptoms. Another common complaint is a sense of uncomfortable fullness after eating. At times, the patient may vomit food which is recognized as having been eaten 2 or 3 days previously. On physical examination, a succussion splash may be present. It is unusual to see gastric peristalsis or an outline of the stomach unless medical treatment is sought very late. Depending upon the amount of vomiting, the patient may be dehydrated and may have severe electrolyte imbalance with neuromuscular irritability. A barium study of the stomach may reveal a dilated stomach with considerable amounts of food and fluid. In patients who have chronic obstruction, the stomach may appear relatively normal in size; the emptying of barium will be significantly delayed, sometimes for as long as 12 or 24 hours.

A saline load test is also helpful in establishing a diagnosis of outlet obstruction. This is performed by emptying the stomach with a nasogastric tube and instilling 750 ml. of saline. The patient is placed in a sitting position, and 30 minutes later the nasogastric tube is aspirated. Normally, less than 400 ml. should remain in the stomach, and 90 per cent of subjects without gastric retention have a residue of less than 200 ml.

Additional details of the symptoms and findings of gastric outlet obstruction are discussed by Boyle and Goldstein (1968).

TREATMENT

If the patient is well nourished and the electrolyte imbalance is minimal or easily corrected, the stomach should be emptied completely with a large Ewald tube. The patient should be placed on nasogastric suction and receive total parenteral nutrition for 3 to 4 days. Generally, this is sufficient time for the stomach to regain adequate tone, as well as to supply adequate caloric needs to the patient. Operation can then be performed.

In patients who are malnourished or have severe electrolyte imbalance and neuromuscular irritability, the stomach likewise should be emptied completely, using an Ewald tube. The Ewald tube should then be replaced by a regular nasogastric tube and the stomach kept decompressed continuously. The electrolyte disturbances and anemia should be corrected. If the patient has lost significant amounts of weight, total parenteral nutrition for 2 to 3 weeks is recommended before an operation. The operations of choice consist of vagotomy and drainage or vagotomy and antrectomy (DeMatteis and Hermann, 1974; Hermann, 1976). Selection of either procedure should be determined by the severity of the ulcer disease, as well as by the degree of duodenal scarring. Delay in gastric emptying has occurred after both types of procedures. If gastric emptying is retarded and a mechanical cause is ruled out, treatment with metoclopramide, which has recently been released for use in this country, should be tried (Metzger and associates, 1976).

Hemorrhage

It is estimated that 15 to 20 per cent of patients with ulcer disease will have at least one hemorrhage (Chinn and Weckesser, 1951). Duodenal ulcers bleed with a slightly greater frequency than do gastric ulcers. Three-fourths of these patients will stop bleeding with medical treatment, and the remaining 25 per cent will require an operation. Massive hemorrhage is defined generally as blood loss that reduces the hematocrit to less than 30 per cent, with signs of clinical shock. Another definition includes the need for transfusions exceeding 1500 ml. of whole blood without restoration of normal vital signs. Chronic or repeated hemorrhage can also be an indication for operation when continued blood loss requires transfusions exceeding 4 to 6 units of blood or greater over 24 hours.

Other factors that influence the timing

of operative intervention is age and the existence of other diseases. Statistically, patients over age 60 do not tolerate blood loss as well as younger patients. Other preexisting diseases, especially pulmonary, cardiac, and renal disease, are associated with increased mortality from a bleeding ulcer. Patients older than 60, or with concomitant diseases, should have operative intervention at an earlier stage than those younger (Foster, Hall, and Dunphy, 1966).

In the evaluation of upper gastrointestinal hemorrhage, it is important that the site of bleeding be determined since this will influence the operative approach. Valuable aids for this are gastroscopy and arteriography. Barium studies are of limited value since they may detect a lesion that is not the source of bleeding and may hinder the later use of arteriography because of residual barium in the stomach or intestines.

If the bleeding site is from a gastric or duodenal ulcer, and bleeding is massive or persistent, early operative intervention is recommended. If the bleeding is from a Mallory-Weiss tear or diffuse gastritis, aggressive medical measures should be pursued (see Mallory-Weiss syndrome, pp. 81–87, in Vol. 1). Bleeding esophageal varices can often be controlled with intravenous pitressin or a Sengstaken tube. Diagnostic tests should be pursued early even in those patients who have a known previous history of gastrointestinal disease, for other sources often prove to be at fault (Himal, Perrault, and Mzabi, 1978).

SYMPTOMS AND DIAGNOSIS

A patient with massive hemorrhage may have symptoms of lightheadedness, hematemesis, or melena. In a patient with melena, a nasogastric tube should be placed to determine whether there is any bleeding from the upper intestinal tract. Physical examination generally reveals an anxious patient who usually shows signs of shock.

A useful sign in determining the severity of blood loss consists of measuring the patient's pulse rate and blood pressure in the reclining position and then in the upright position. An increase in the pulse rate of 30 or more beats per minute or a decrease in the systolic pressure of 20 mm. of mercury or more indicates a blood loss of 25 per cent or greater. Laboratory tests include a complete blood count and clotting studies to rule out any bleeding disorders. The hematocrit and hemoglobin levels may initially be normal, and only with hydration will they significantly decrease. The clotting studies are useful in determining the presence of any underlying diseases which may contribute to or may be a primary cause of the hemorrhage. At the time of drawing these blood studies, a specimen should be sent for typing and cross-matching.

TREATMENT

Resuscitation and diagnosis should proceed simultaneously. A large-bore intravenous line should be placed, and, if signs of significant blood loss are present, fluids should be infused rapidly through several intravenous sites. Monitoring the vital signs, central venous pressure, and urine output is essential. A large Ewald tube should be inserted into the stomach and blood clots evacuated. This is essential so that endoscopy can be performed and the rate of blood loss assessed. The stomach should be irrigated until clear fluid returns and endoscopy performed as soon as possible. The various nonoperative measures that have been used to control bleeding include irrigation with iced saline, intragastric instillation of Levophed (Douglass, 1974), intra-arterial perfusion with vasopressin (Johnson and Windrich, 1976), and intra-arterial embolization with various substances (Eisenberg and Steer, 1976). Most of these methods, when successful, will arrest hemorrhage for a limited time.

Other, more recent therapeutic approaches include the spraying of a bleeding lesion with acrylic resins and clotting factoors, via an endoscopic catheter. Endoscopic laser treatment has also been reported with an amazing success rate of 94 per cent (Kiefhaber, Nath, and Moritz, 1977). None of these techniques has been uniformly successful, and control trials may be necessary to determine their indications and outcome.

If the underlying cause is not corrected, bleeding generally resumes. If it continues despite treatment, operative intervention is necessary. Indications for operative treatment include the inability to maintain blood pressure despite rapid fluid infusion through large intravenous routes, inability to correct hypotension after more than 2000 ml. of blood, continued blood loss requiring greater than 500 ml. of blood every 8 hours, recurrent bleeding during hospitalization, age of 60 or greater, the existence of other significant concomitant diseases, and gastric ulcers. These factors have been associated with a high mortality rate if bleeding is allowed to continue (Halnagyi, 1970).

Operative Approaches to Hemorrhage

When emergency operation is required for massive bleeding, resuscitation must be continued in the operating room until shock is corrected. Controlling the bleeding is the first operative priority. The next consideration is to perform an operation that will prevent rebleeding. A controversy exists as to whether vagotomy and pyloroplasty with suture ligation of the ulcer are as effective as gastric resection in controlling bleeding. Comparison of the overall mortality rates favors vagotomy and pyloroplasty. Rebleeding occurs with about equal frequency with either operation. When the bleeding site is known, the approach should be directed to that area. If the site of bleeding is questionable or unknown and no lesions are palpated in the stomach, the first recommendation is to open the pylorus to inspect the duodenum. If an ulcer is found, it is transfixed with a nonabsorbable suture. If the bleeding cannot be controlled by this method, identification and ligation of the gastroduodenal artery behind the duodenum is recommended. The pyloroplasty can then be completed and a truncal vagotomy performed.

If the bleeding is not from the pyloric area, or if a gastric ulcer is known to be present, a gastrotomy should be made. Gastric ulcers are best treated by incorporating the ulcer in a distal gastric resection (Stafford and associates, 1967). When the ulcer is very high in the fundus, the recommended procedure consists of oversewing the ulcer, ligation of the left gastric artery, vagotomy, and pyloroplasty. When technically feasible, a local resection of a high gastric ulcer combined with vagotomy and pyloroplasty is another acceptable approach. Occasionally, a total gastrectomy may be required to control a bleeding ulcer; however, the mortality rate is significantly higher. Mallory-Weiss tears can generally be repaired with a running suture starting at the most distal aspect of the tear. Treatment of hemorrhagic gastritis and varices is discussed in their respective sections. Those patients who bleed at a slow rate or who bleed recurrently can be operated on in a more elective manner (Hallenbeck, 1970). Under these conditions, the patient may be able to tolerate a more extensive ulcer operation, such as truncal vagotomy and resection (Schiller, Truelove, and Williams, 1970). If this procedure is not technically feasible, then vagotomy with drainage is acceptable. However, the ulcer crater must be oversewn to prevent bleeding in the immediate postoperative course (McGregor and associates, 1976).

ZOLLINGER-ELLISON SYNDROME
(Gastrinoma)

The Zollinger-Ellison syndrome was first reported in 1955. Zollinger and Ellison cited two patients who had recurrent problems with ulcers despite previous gastric operation. They had persistent ulcers with gastric acid hypersecretion and non-β islet cell tumors of the pancreas. Many patients have since been reported in other series, and it has become well established that the Zollinger-Ellison syndrome is caused by a malignant or nonmalignant tumor of the pancreas, proximal duodenum, or periduodenal area that secretes excessive amounts of gastrin (gastrinoma). The gastrin produced by these tumors stimulates the parietal cells to secrete hydrochloric acid. Acidification of the antrum, which is a feedback pathway to decrease gastrin release, does not alter the continued production of gastrin by the tumor. As a result, acid is produced at a high and constant rate.

The incidence of gastrinoma is unknown but is estimated at less than 1 per cent of patients with ulcer disease. The sex distribution slightly favors males, and it has been reported in patients ranging in age from 7 to 90 years. The most common mean age distribution is between 40 and 60 years of age. The primary tumor (gastrinoma) usually occurs in multiple sites, and attempts to excise the tumors have not been successful. These tumors are slow growing, and most of the morbidity and mortality is a result of gastric acid hypersecretion. Since it is difficult to provide sufficient antacid to neutralize the enormous quantities of gastric acid, removal of the target organ has evolved as the most successful form of treatment. The H-2 receptor antagonists inhibit acid secretion even when the gastrin level is markedly elevated. Cimetidine has become a potent and successful agent in controlling gastric acid secretion and is being used in patients with a gastrinoma.

Ten to 40 per cent of these patients will have other nonpancreatic endocrine tumors (Ballard and associates, 1964). There are two recognized syndromes of multiple endocrine adenopathies (MEA). MEA type I involves abnormalities of the parathyroid glands, pancreas, and pituitary glands, although the adrenal and thyroid glands may also be involved (Craven and associates, 1972). MEA II is characterized by pheochromocytoma, hyperparathyroidism, and medullary carcinoma of the thyroid. Manifestations of these endocrine disorders may appear over a period of time in random order.

SYMPTOMS AND FINDINGS

The symptoms associated with the Zollinger-Ellison syndrome include: pain, 74 per cent; diarrhea, 36 per cent; vomiting, 26 per cent; melena, 22 per cent; and acute perforation, 18 per cent (Ellison and Wilson, 1964).

The diarrhea and steatorrhea in these patients are due to inactivation of pancreatic lipase and precipitation of bile salts by the enormous amounts of acid which overwhelm the buffering capacity of the duodenum. Physical examinaton may not be remarkable. There may be mild epigastric pain. Patients with severe diarrhea may show dehydration.

The most common x-ray finding is a duodenal ulcer. Other, less common findings which suggest gastric acid hypersecretion include prominence of the gastric folds with rapid dilution of barium and multiple ulcers of the stomach and jejunum. Angiography has not been particularly helpful in detecting or localizing tumors. Pancreatic scans lack the resolution to identify these tumors since most of them are small. Gastric acid secretion is helpful in establishing the diagnosis and is characteristically high. A 12-hour overnight secretion of greater than 100 mEq. of acid or a 1-hour basal value greater than 15 mEq. per hour suggests the diagnosis, although these levels of acid secretion can sometimes be found in patients with duodenal ulcer disease. A ratio of 0:6 or greater of basal acid secretion to maximal acid secretion is also suggestive of a gastrinoma, provided significant amounts of acid are produced.

Serum gastrin is generally elevated in patients with a gastrinoma. Values of 1000 picograms per ml. strongly suggest the presence of a gastrinoma in a patient with gastric acid hypersecretion and the absence of gastric retention. In a patient with virulent ulcer disease and gastric acid hypersecretion, gastrin values in the range of 200 to 800 picograms per ml. represent a diagnostic problem. Two provocative tests are used to detect an early gastrinoma when the serum gastrin is in the 200 to 800 range. The calcium infusion test consists of infusing 12 to 15 mg. per kg. of calcium over 3 hours. Patients without gastrinoma will have a modest increase in both serum gastrin and acid secretion. An increase of more than 500 picograms per ml. in the basal serum gastrin strongly suggests gastrinoma (Deveney and associates, 1977). A more discriminative test is the secretin infusion. A single infusion of 3 to 5 units per kg. of secretin is given; blood for serum gastrin determination is drawn before infusion, and then at 2, 5, 10, 15, and 30 minutes. Normally the serum gastrin level will be decreased when compared with the preinfusion value. This occurs in normal subjects as well as in patients with duodenal ulcer, pernicious anemia, and retained antrum. If the serum gastrin increases at least 100 picograms per ml. above the basal value, a gastrinoma is present (Deveney and associates, 1977).

TREATMENT

Medical

These patients respond poorly to the usual medical treatment of antacids and anticholinergic drugs; however, the hypersecretion can be reduced with cimetidine and other H-2 receptor antagonists. Cimetidine acts by inhibiting acid secretion and works directly on the parietal cells. It significantly reduces acid secretion without altering serum gastrin levels. It has become increasingly popular as a form of definitive treatment for patients with gastrinoma (McCarthy, 1978). The recommended regimen is 300 mg. every 6 hours plus 600 mg. at bedtime, in combination with antacids. The initial results of cimetidine treatment have been good, although long-term results are not yet available. It is also used preoperatively to reduce acid secretion and correct the electrolyte imbalance that results from gastric hypersecretion.

Operative Treatment

The standard operative treatment of a gastrinoma is total gastrectomy (Schrock and Way, 1978; Deveney, Deveney, and Way, 1978). The mortality from other, less extensive ulcer operations is signficantly higher. This is attributed to complications resulting from gastric acid hypersecretion in the immediate postoperative period. An interesting observation reported by Friesen (1967) is regression of metastatic tumor and a decrease in serum gastrin in certain patients following total gastrectomy. It is postulated that removal of the target organ may account for the regression of the primary tumor. Whether this represents one aspect of the natural history of these tumors or a relationship between the target organ and the spread of the tumor has not been resolved (Zollinger and associates, 1976). If the latter postulate is correct, total gastrectomy may remain the preferred treatment of choice in good-risk patients. Gastrinoma is usually a slow-growing tumor and does not commonly result in widespread metastasis. Following total gastrectomy, only 20 per cent of the patients will die as a result of malignancy. This figure needs to be compared with that obtained from patients who are being treated with cimetidine. At present, most patients with the Zollinger-Ellison syndrome are being treated with cimetidine and antacids. For those patients who fail to respond or are noncompliant, total gastrectomy is recommended.

The evaluation of patients with the Zollinger-Ellison syndrome should include periodic determination of serum calcium. If hypercalcemia develops and there is evidence of primary hyperparathyroidism, removal of the parathyroid adenoma is recommended. This may result in decreased acid secretion and serum gastrin levels.

POST-TRAUMATIC STRESS ULCERATION

Upper gastrointestinal hemorrhage occurring in patients already subjected to overwhelming physiologic stress further complicates a difficult clinical situation. Over the past 10 years, the knowledge and spectrum of this disease have changed. In 1971, Lucas and associates reported a marked increase in stress-related gastric bleeding in their critically ill, intensive care unit patients, which had surpassed both peptic ulcer and esophageal varices as the most common cause of upper gastrointestinal bleeding. Although it was not stated by the investigators, this report and others at that time described an increase in this type of bleeding that coincided with the development of modern supportive care which prolonged the life of critically injured or seriously ill patients.

Around this same time, numerous others were pointing to the continuing challenge of stress ulcers and bleeding. Eiseman and Heyman (1970) published an account of deliberations of the Conference of the Committee on Trauma of the National Research Council. Since then, however, the incidence of this type of bleeding has steadily decreased. The reason for this, as in many changing disease states, is not clear. Knowledge from both civilian and recent military experience has greatly aided our care of critically injured patients, the awareness of the potential for this type of postoperative complication has made early intervention more effective. In a 3-year period, the incidence of gastrointestinal ulcerations and bleeding in patients at the Brooke Army Hospital Burn Unit fell from 28 to 5 per cent (Lescher, Teegarden, and Pruitt, 1977). Although the incidence of bleeding sufficient to require a transfusion has decreased, if the disease is sought endoscopically it can be found in up to 80 per cent of patients with body burns greater than 35 per cent.

A similar picture is seen in general intensive care units: early reports show a 25 to 40 per cent incidence of gastrointestinal bleeding in patients. In a study conducted in 1979 using 100 ICU patients untreated for gastrointestinal bleeding prophylaxis but carefully observed, a 20 per cent incidence of either stress erosion or nontransfusable, upper gastrointestinal hemorrhage was found. The rate of transfusable bleeding in this patient population was 7 per cent. This study was carried out in a general-surgical intensive care unit caring for all types of critically ill patients (Zinner and associates, in press).

The incidence of upper gastrointestinal bleeding varies, depending upon the ongoing physiologic insult and the underlying illnesses of the patient. Certain clinical common denominators exist: uremia, usually as a consequence of acute tubular necrosis; respiratory insufficiency requiring assisted ventilation; hypotension as a result of cardiogenic, hypovolemic, or septic shock; and sepsis, often arising from intraperitoneal sources. Using an illness severity index score (ISIS) rating of 0 to 9, depending upon the number of systems impaired (Table 10–1), a patient with a score of 0 to 2 has an incidence of bleeding of 11 per cent. If the patient were moderately ill with an ISIS of 3 to 6, the incidence of bleeding is 34 per cent, and if the ISIS is 7 or more, the incidence of upper gastrointestinal bleeding is 50 per cent (Fig. 10–1).

Although the etiology of these lesions is not clear, most investigators would agree that gastric mucosal ischemia and intraluminal acid play key roles in the pathogenesis of this disease. Numerous studies on gastric blood flow in various primates have shown that the gastric mucosa is very sensitive to changes in systemic arterial pressure. In addition, once a hypotensive state has been achieved in the experimental animal and the animal resuscitated with fluids, gastric mucosal blood flow does not return to control values as does the mucosal blood flow for the rest of the gastrointestinal tract.

Similarly, the presence of intraluminal acid has proved necessary for the production of experimental stress ulceration. If intragastric contents are neutralized, no stress ulcerations will occur. If animals are pretreated with an H-2 receptor antagonist (cimetidine or metiamide), stress ulcerations can also be prevented. Clinically, superficial mucosal erosions occur almost exclusively in the portion of the stomach concerned with acid and pepsin production. Usually, patients developing this lesion are not gastric acid hypersecretors. This phenomenon may merely reflect an increased acid back-diffusion into the gastric mucosal cells in these critically ill patients.

Reports in the literature describe a link between damaged gastric mucosal barriers and intensive care unit patients (Skillman and associates, 1970). Although the experimental evidence is not as convincing, it is clear that normal amounts of acid will produce ulceration of gastric mucosa which has been subjected to ischemia and anoxia sufficient to interfere with protection against increased back-diffusion of H^+ ions. The most potent experimental model for the production of stress ulcerations or acute superficial erosions includes intraluminal acid, ischemia, and an agent used to break the gastric mucosal barrier, such as bile salts (Ritchie, 1975). Refluxed duodenal contents containing bile are known to increase the gastric mucosal permeability to acid, leading to greater back-diffusion and autodiges-

Table 10–1. Stress Ulcer Prevention Study; Risk Factors as Indices of Illness Severity

1. Cardiac	A. Evidence of moderate CHF or myocardial infarction
	B. Significant arrhythmias requiring drugs for control
2. Pulmonary	A. Required ventilator longer than 24 hours postop
	B. Pneumonia
3. Shock	A. Blood pressure less than 90 mm. Hg systolic
	B. Required use of pressors
4. Sepsis	A. Documented systemic infection
	B. Positive blood cultures
5. Renal	A. Acute renal failure
	B. Creatinine >3.0 mg. % (normal = 0.7 to 1.5 mg. %)
	C. Bun >50 mg % (normal 8 to 23 mg. %)
6. CNS	A. Obtunded mental status—coma
	B. Seizures from organic causes
7. Steroid use	A. Solucortef >250 mg./24 hours
8. Coagulopathy	A. Platelets <50,000 (normal = 150,000 to 300,000)
	B. Prothrombin time <30% control
9. Hepatic	A. Bilirubin >5.0 mg. % (normal = 0.1 to 1.1 mg. %)
	B. Cirrhosis

(From Zinner, M. J., et al.: Surg. Gynecol. Obstet., 1981 (in press).

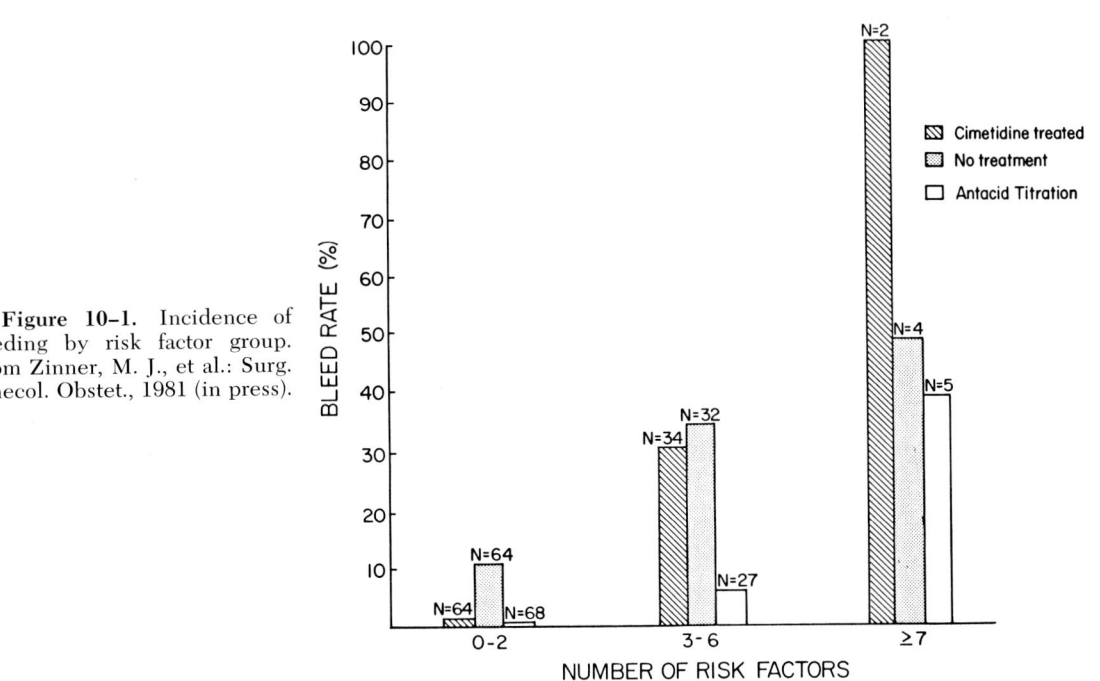

Figure 10-1. Incidence of bleeding by risk factor group. (From Zinner, M. J., et al.: Surg. Gynecol. Obstet., 1981 (in press).

tion and ulceration in the presence of ischemia.

TREATMENT

Once a diagnosis of acute superficial ulcerations has been made endoscopically, treatment should begin with nonoperative technics. These include iced saline or water irrigation and manipulation of intragastric pH with antacids. Although the trials were not randomized and controlled, Curtiss and associates (1973) reported the arrest of bleeding in patients with acute hemorrhagic gastritis by maintaining a gastric pH of 7.0 with vigorous instillation of magnesium and aluminum hydroxide antacids. LeVeen and coworkers (1972) attempted pharmacologic control of acute hemorrhagic gastritis by irrigating gastric contents with levarterenol solutions.

If these approaches fail, intra-arterial vasopressin has proved to be an effective technique for stopping bleeding from this type of lesion. Vasopressin is infused directly into the vessels under angiographic control, beginning at a rate of 0.2 unit per minute. If there is arteriographic evidence of constriction of the distal arterial bed, or cessation of bleeding, vasopressin is continued for an additional 24 hours at this rate. If hemorrhage remains stopped, the rate is decreased for 12 more hours. If bleeding continues, the rate of infusion of vasopressin is increased 0.1 unit per minute to a dose of 0.5 unit per minute. This form of therapy is effective in approximately 80 per cent of patients.

Nonoperative treatment for acute superficial ulcerations is successful in approximately 75 per cent of patients. If bleeding is not controlled by vigorous nonoperative measures, surgical intervention may be required. The choice of operative procedure remains controversial. Although truncal vagotomy and pyloroplasty can be done quickly with acceptable mortality rates, rebleeding can occur in 30 to 100 per cent of patients. Gastric resections and total gastrectomy have lower incidences of rebleeding but are more radical undertakings in desperately ill patients. Recently, Richardson and Aust (1977) recommended gastric devascularization as a useful salvage procedure for massive hemorrhagic gastritis. In a small group of patients, there were only a 9 per cent incidence of rebleeding, with no serious postoperative complications, and a mortality rate lower than that for gastric resections. Use of this surgical treatment deserves further investigation and consultation.

PREVENTION

Numerous clinical trials have been carried out showing the beneficial effects of vigorous antacid neutralization of gastric contents in the prevention of these lesions. In a randomized prospective clinical trial comparing antacids and cimetidine, antacids proved more effective and considerably less expensive than cimetidine (Priebe and associates, 1980). Whichever treatment is used, it is imperative that the gastric pH be regularly monitored and maintained at greater than 4.0.

The antacid titration regimen followed an every-two-hour dosing schedule (Fig. 10–2). It began by emptying the stomach and recording the pH, instilling 10 ml. of a concentrated antacid, clamping the tube for an hour, and then recording the pH. If the pH was greater than or equal to 4.0, the tube was put on straight drainage or intermittent suction for 1 hour, and then the cycle was repeated. If the pH was less than 4.0, the volume of antacid was doubled and the tube was clamped for an additional hour. At the end of that hour, if the pH was still less than 4.0 the amount of antacid was again doubled until the pH was greater than 4.0. Drainage for 1 hour was then allowed and the cycle repeated with the new dose of antacid. Cimetidine at a fixed dose was not effective in controlling intragastric pH in one-third of the patients in this study. With this treatment regimen, the incidence of acute superficial ulceration can be reduced to less than 5 per cent with a transfusable bleed rate of less than 1 per cent (Hastings and associates, 1978).

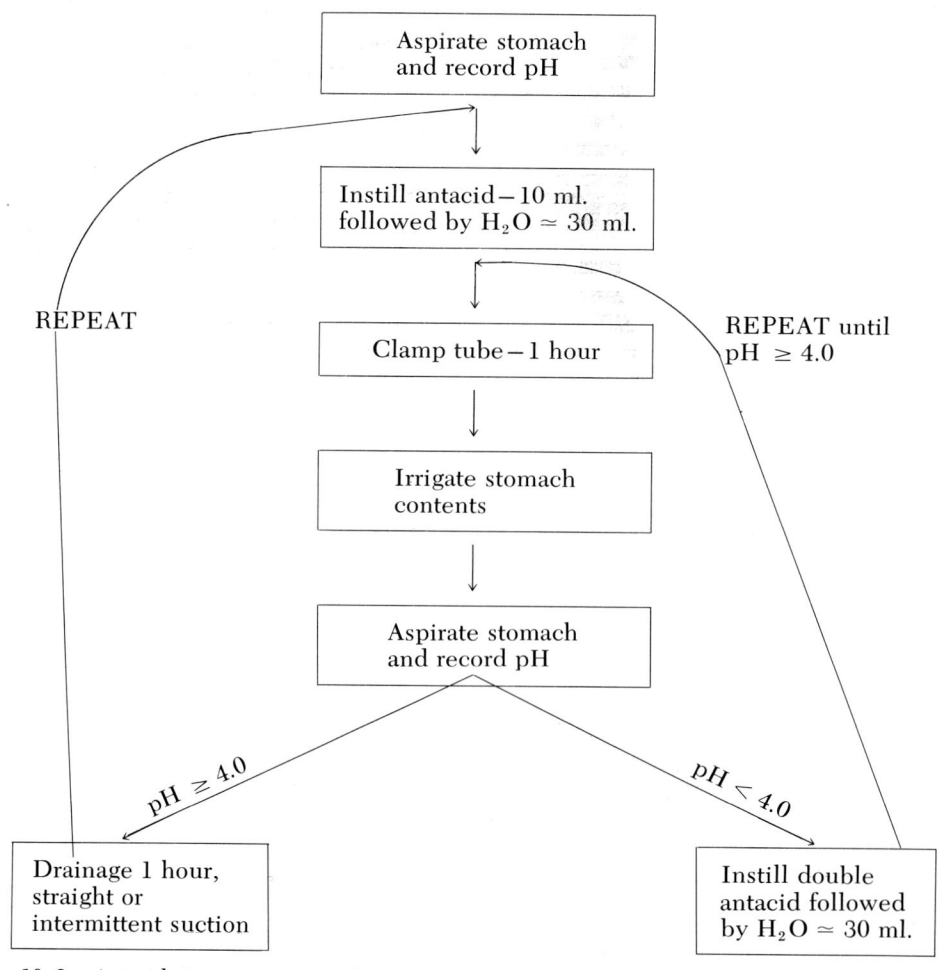

Figure 10–2. Antacid titration regimen. (From Zinner, M. J., et al.: Surg. Gynecol. Obstet., 1981 (in press).

SUMMARY OF OPERATIVE TREATMENT OF ULCER DISEASE

GASTRIC ULCERS

Chronic benign gastric ulcers are best treated with resection encompassing the ulcer. If the ulcer is associated with low acid secretion, a vagotomy generally is not required. Prepyloric gastric ulcer and all gastric ulcers associated with significant acid secretion are best treated with resection and vagotomy. Ulcers high on the greater curvature should be excised, using a sleeve resection. If technical difficulties exist with resection of the ulcer, a vagotomy and drainage procedure is then recommended.

Complications of Gastric Ulcer

Bleeding, perforation, and obstruction due to gastric ulcer disease require aggressive treatment, with resection of the ulcer. The high recurrence rate when lesser procedures are performed generally justifies the additional risks of the more extensive operation.

DUODENAL ULCER

The randomized prospective studies have shown that under favorable conditions the standard ulcer operations can produce good results. With recent experience the elective treatment of duodenal ulcer disease favors the use of proximal gastric vagotomy. This operation should be of special benefit in younger patients whose main indication for operation is intractability. Proximal gastric vagotomy offers all the advantages of an effective acid-reducing operation and has fewer disadvantages than the other standard ulcer operations. In good-risk patients, the proximal gastric vagotomy has the advantage of providing significant acid reduction without major sequelae, and, if the operation proves to be inadequate, vagotomy and antrectomy can be performed at a later time.

Complications of Duodenal Ulcer

The magnitude of the operation for such complications as hemorrhage, perforation, and obstruction is determined by the severity of the complication and the overall condition of the patient. If either are unfavorable, a conservative operation is recommended to alleviate the complication. It may be necessary at a later date to perform a more extensive operation to control the ulcer disease, or to treat the patient with cimetidine. Under favorable circumstances, a definitive ulcer operation such as a vagotomy and antrectomy can be performed.

Chapter 11

GASTRIC AND DUODENAL FISTULAS AND PERFORATIONS

A fistula is an abnormal communication between organs, segments of bowel, or an organ or a segment of a bowel and the exterior of the body. Fistulas may be created to gain access to the bowel, such as a gastrostomy, jejunostomy, or colostomy, in order to improve the patient's treatment. At other times fistulas result from pathologic causes and are detrimental to the patient's well-being.

CAUSES OF GASTRIC AND DUODENAL FISTULAS

Of the multiple causes of gastrointestinal fistula, most are related to a gastrointestinal anastomosis. Following operations such as gastrojejunostomy or gastric resection and gastroduodenostomy, a fistula may develop from the area of anastomosis. Five major factors contribute to the development of an anastomotic fistula. Healing may be impaired because of the poor *nutritional status* of the patient. The anastomosis may have been performed with *tension* on the suture line, resulting in disruption of part or all of the anastomosis. In preparing the bowel for anastomosis, the *blood supply* may have been compromised, and this results in necrosis and perforation at the anastomotic site. Soiling of the operative field may have occurred during the operative procedure, or a site of *infection* already may have been present, resulting in excessive contamination of the anastomosis. Another factor is the presence of a *foreign body* at the site of anastomosis. This includes the placement of drains over an anastomosis with frequent development of a fistula.

A gastric fistula followed parietal cell vagotomy (Hoile and Turner, 1975). This was attributed to ischemic necrosis of part of the lesser curvature. Another cause of gastric and duodenal fistulas is trauma to the stomach and duodenum, such as stab wounds, gunshot wounds, and blunt injuries. A perforated ulcer may fail to seal and fistulize to another organ or to the exterior. Other diseases, such as inflammatory bowel disease and diverticulitis, have been associated with intestinal fistulas. Erosion of a gallstone into the stomach or duodenum may result in a biliary tract–intestinal fistula, and this is usually complicated by intestinal obstruction (gallstone ileus).

TYPES OF FISTULA

Fistulas can be classified according to their location, such as gastrocutaneous, gastrojejunocolic, and duodenal cutaneous. Additional descriptions of fistula include not only its location but also the output of the fistula when it is to the exterior. Usually volumes of 1 liter or greater per day, generally from the upper intestinal tract, are regarded as high-output fistulas; whereas those with volumes less than 1 liter per day, usually located in the lower intestinal tract, are classified as low-output fistulas. The

TYPES OF FISTULA

classic description of fistula includes not only the segment of bowel from which the fistula originates but also the type of communication of the fistula. If the fistula communicates to the skin, it is an *external* fistula; if there is no external communication, it is an *internal* fistula.

Gastrojejunocolic Fistula

Following ulcer operation, a gastrojejunocolic fistula is rare and constitutes 1 to 2 per cent of the complications following ulcer disease (Lahey, 1936; Marshall and Knud-Hansen, 1957; Wychulis, Priestley, and Folk, 1966). If it is associated with recurrent ulcer disease, factors such as incomplete vagotomy, G-cell hyperplasia, and Zollinger-Ellison syndrome should be suspected. Once the cause of the fistula is determined and the patient has received adequate nutritional support and bowel preparation, a one-stage procedure can be successfully performed (Aguirre, Fisher, and Welch, 1974). This includes resection of the involved portions of stomach, jejunum, and colon, together with the fistulous

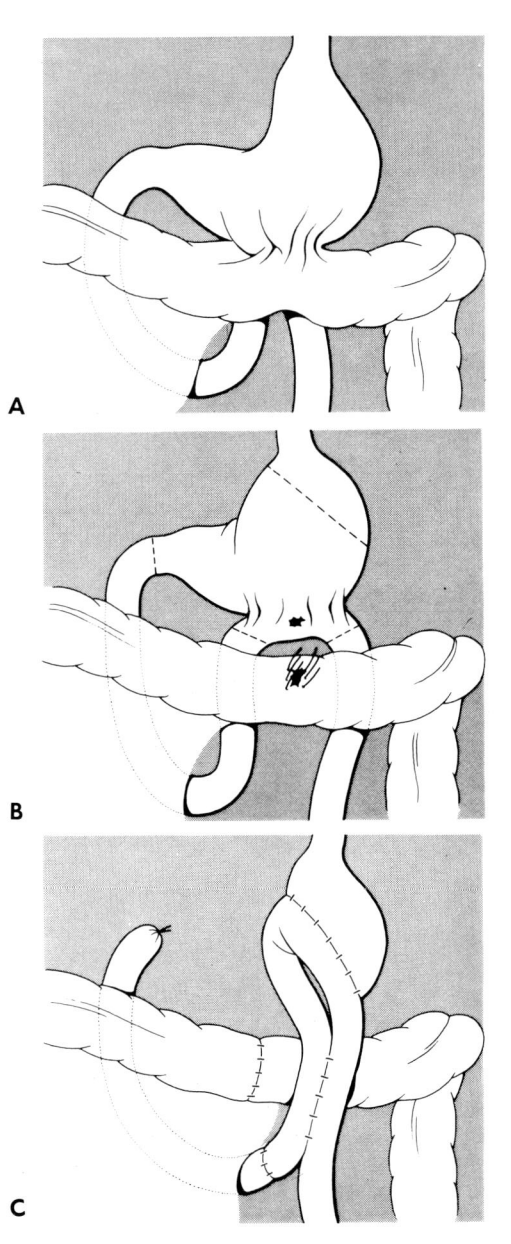

Figure 11–1. Gastrojejunocolic fistula following retrocolic gastroenterostomy. *A*, In the very complex operating area, the transverse colon is first identified and then, starting from a free segment, carefully isolated along the anterior gastric wall. The fistula is approached from both sides. The removal of the fistula-containing area follows only after circular mobilization has been completed. Careful draping of the abdomen is essential.

B, The colonic fistula is first dealt with. When a well-serosed portion of colon around the fistula is successfully prepared, the transverse fistula may be sewn across the longitudinal axis of the transverse colon using two rows of sutures. In the presence of large serosal defects or changes, resection of the altered colonic segment with subsequent end-to-end or side-to-side anastomosis is recommended. After freeing the gastroenterostomy from the mesocolon, the afferent and efferent jejunal limbs are transected close to the fistula. A typical two-thirds resection of the stomach is then performed.

C, The transected limbs of the jejunal loop are joined end-to-end. After suturing the duodenal stump and the mesocolic defect, a gastrojejunostomy is performed antecolically, followed by a Braun's anastomosis between the afferent and efferent limbs of the jejunal loop.

(From Grewe, H.-E., and Kremer, K.: Atlas of Surgery. Philadelphia, W. B. Saunders Company, 1980, pp. 131–132.)

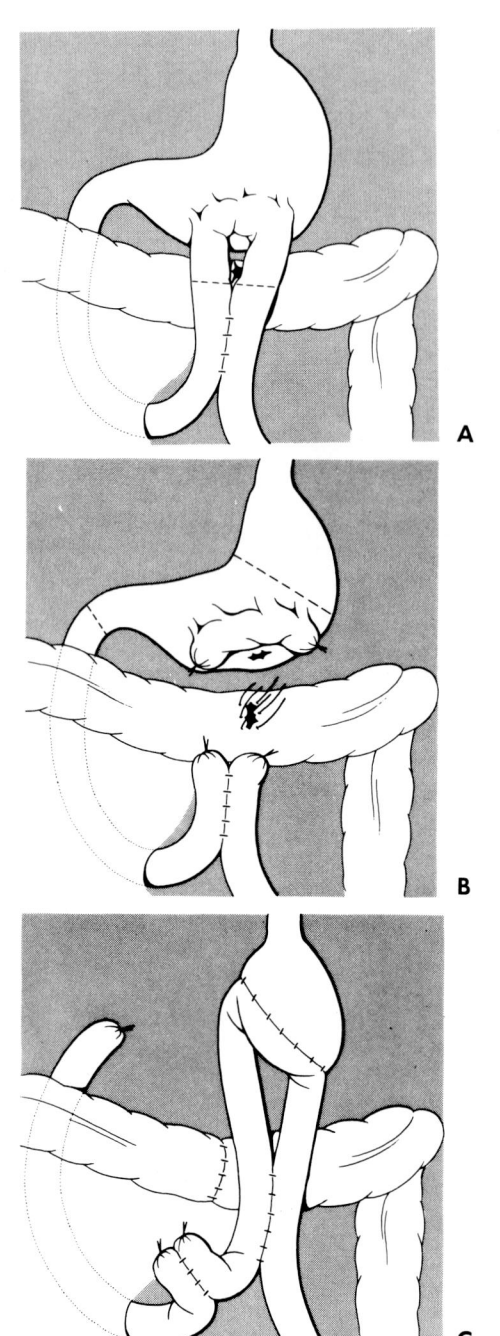

Figure 11–2. Gastrojejunocolic fistula following antecolic gastroenterostomy. *A,* After skeletonizing the stomach along the extent of the planned resection, the afferent and efferent limbs of the gastroenterostomy are identified. Both limbs are transected above the Braun's anastomosis, and the stumps are closed blindly. The Braun's anastomosis is left in place.

B, After incising the fistula, the stomach can be well prepared and clearly separated from the transverse colon. The colonic fistula is sewn using two rows of sutures. Subsequently, the stomach is skeletonized for a typical two-thirds resection.

C, After the gastrectomy has been performed, the anastomosis is carried antecolically to a lower jejunal loop.

(From Grewe, H.-E., and Kremer, K.: Atlas of Surgery. Philadelphia, W. B. Saunders Company, 1980, pp. 132–133.)

tract, and reconstruction by gastrojejunostomy, jejunojejunostomy, and colocolostomy. If free perforation occurred in a gastrojejunocolic fistula, a multistaged procedure may be necessary, consisting of a completely diverting transverse colostomy; interval resection of the fistula and associated stomach, jejunum, and colon; and a third-stage colocolostomy (Pfeiffer and Kent, 1939).

Operative treatment for gastrojejunocolic fistula following gastroenterostomy is illustrated in Figures 11–1 and 11–2.

Duodenal Fistula

A duodenal fistula following a Billroth II anastomosis occurs when there is severe scarring in the area of attempted duodenal closure. This complication can be avoided if the duodenal area is carefully inspected. If severe scarring is seen, a gastroenterostomy rather than a gastric resection should be performed. If the involvement of the duodenum is not recognized until after a gastric resection is performed, the duodenal closure can be protected with a tube duodenostomy by inserting a 16 French catheter through a stab wound in the lateral superior aspect of the duodenum (Pearsons, MacKenzie, and Ross, 1963; Welch and Rodkey, 1954). This tube is then exteriorized through a separate stab incision in the right upper quadrant. The tube is placed on gravity drainage and gently irrigated to insure its patency. This results in a controlled duodenal fistula. Once bowel motility returns and the drainage of the duodenostomy tube is negligible, the tube can be withdrawn. This is usually possible by the tenth to the fourteenth day.

If the duodenal fistula presents through the wound accompanying a wound dehiscence, a duodenostomy tube should be placed when the dehiscence is repaired. Direct attempts to repair the disrupted duodenal stump are generally unsuccessful. This complication may also result from a duodenal injury, as from a stab wound, gunshot wound, or blunt trauma (Smith and associates, 1970). Following repair of any duodenal injury, a duodenostomy tube should be placed to insure adequate drainage and decompression of the duodenum.

DIAGNOSIS

The clinical presentation of a patient with a fistula will depend upon the location of the fistula and type of communication. The common presenting symptoms are generally those of sepsis. The patient appears toxic, with pain, fever, weight loss, drainage from a wound, or severe diarrhea. Laboratory confirmation consists of an elevated white blood cell count, anemia, hypoalbuminemia, and electrolyte imbalance. Acidosis is present if there is considerable pancreatic and bile loss, such as from a fistula high in the small bowel. Alkalosis is present if the fistula is from the stomach, with loss of gastric secretion.

A patient with a fistula from an anastomosis may have a low-grade fever and wound dehiscence, and then intestinal fluid may appear at the incision.

TREATMENT

Priorities in the management of any intestinal fistula have been described by Sheldon and colleagues (1971). These priorities consist of resuscitating the patient with fluids, correcting the acid-base imbalance, restoring specific electrolyte losses, and correcting anemia. If there is evidence of an abscess, adequate drainage must be achieved and appropriate antibiotics administered. Drainage of the abscesses should not be delayed but made part of the resuscitative efforts. Control of the fistula must be achieved. If the fistula is external, careful insertion of a catheter to the source of the fistula may provide adequate control. At times operative treatment may be required with gastric and duodenal secretion controlled by a nasogastric tube. Occasionally a long tube may be necessary to decompress the bowel. Since most of these patients are nutritionally depleted, it is important to begin total parenteral nutrition as soon as possible (usually within 72 hours).

Delineation of the fistula becomes the next priority. This should be done at an early stage, after the patient's condition has stabilized. If there is no improvement in the clinical condition of the patient within 5 to 7 days, an undrained abscess should be suspected. Once the fistula is delineated and there is no evidence of distal obstruction, oral alimentation with elemental diets can be initiated (Kaminsky and Dietel, 1975). If the patient tolerates a low-volume, iso-osmotic oral diet without any significant increase in the fistula output, the oral alimentation can gradually be increased. Oral alimentation is usually possible if there is no distal obstruction. On this regimen most fistulas will close. If the fistula has not closed within 1 or 2 months, operation and resection of the fistula are usually necessary. Simple closure of the fistula is generally unsuccessful, and the area of fistula should be resected or excluded.

NEONATAL GASTRIC PERFORATIONS

A specific cause for perforation of the stomach in newborn infants continues to perplex neonatologists and pediatric surgeons. The condition may, in fact, be the result of a variety of factors which defy unification under a single etiology. To understand the difficulty in pinpointing an exact pathogenesis, one must analyze the setting in which gastric perforations occur.

Gastric perforation is most commonly seen in premature infants who have incurred a significant hypoxic insult at birth, often as a result of immature lungs. Endotracheal ventilation with maintenance of positive end-expiratory pressure is the generally accepted therapy for the respiratory distress syndrome. Such ventilatory management frequently results in a significant amount of air/oxygen mixture overflowing into the esophagus and stomach. The resultant gastric distention is generally treated by insertion of a small polyethylene nasogastric feeding tube. The end of this tube will usually be directed toward the greater curvature of the stomach. Documented instances of tube perforation of the stomach provide one unchallengeable etiology for acute gastric perforation. This should place an obligation upon the responsible physician to examine radiographically the position of such tubes, since longitudinal movement of the tube will occur frequently during the course of ventilatory management. Because of the small size of the catheter used (usually 5 French), the risk of occlusion of the small lumen increases the likelihood of perforations of the distended stomach by the catheter tip.

After 3 to 5 days, treatment is directed toward providing higher levels of caloric input. This is usually provided by intermittent gavage feedings through the small nasogastric feeding tube. Because of the small nasal passages in the premature infant and the obligatory nasal breathing typical of the neonate, these feedings are usually accomplished by introducing an oral gastric nasogastric tube, instilling the feeding, then withdrawing the tube. Tube introduction is checked for proper gastric position by auscultation of the left upper quadrant with a stethoscope while rapidly insufflating 0.5 to 1.0 ml. of air down the tube. This technique obviously will not distinguish tubes within the confines of the stomach from tubes passed through the stomach wall. Figure 11–3 is an abdominal radiograph showing a tube passed through the stomach depositing 10 ml. of Isomil into the retrogastric space. In spite of the dangers associated with such feeding procedures, adequate safeguard procedures are still lacking. Frequently such infants are fed as often as every 2 to 3 hours around the clock, so it is impractical to obtain radiographic documentation of proper tube placement with each feeding. Transillumination of the abdomen in the supine infant might afford some protection from perforations into the free peritoneal cavity (Hashimoto and associates, 1977).

Touloukian (1973) has espoused the theory that the *ischemic insult* following an initial hypoxic episode causes the subsequent gastric perforation. He found a significant perinatal complication leading to asphyxia in 69 per cent of infants who developed acute gastric perforations. Perfu-

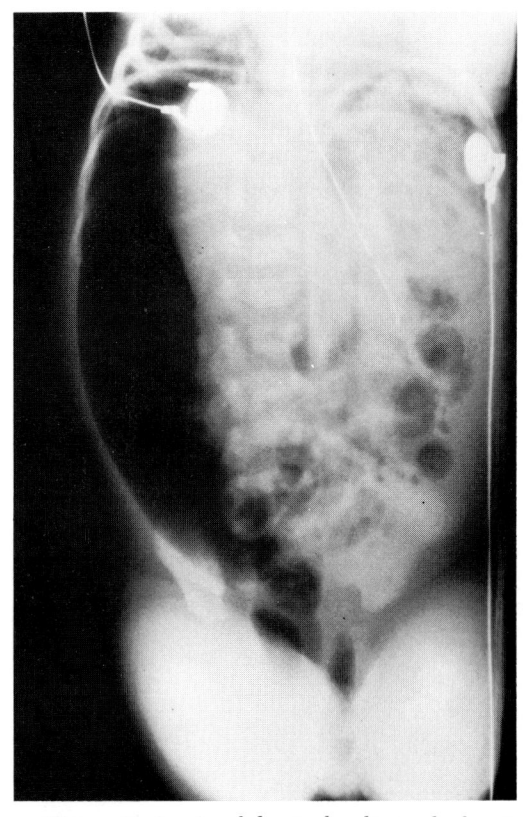

Figure 11–3. An abdominal radiograph showing a tube passed through the stomach depositing 10 ml. of Isomil into the retrogastric space.

sion studies in newborn piglets who were given asphyxic stress demonstrated marked reduction of blood flow to the mucosa of the stomach, distal ileum, and colon. This phenomenon of selective ischemia was originally described in the porpoise by Scholander (1963) as the "diving reflex." Such selective ischemia occurring in the premature infant with respiratory disease syndrome would be a significant prodromal event to perforations from subsequent aerophagic distention alone.

The potential role of *aerophagia* as a contributing cause of perforation has been evaluated by Shaker and associates (1973). They postulate that in our nurseries the standard management of infants in a supine position allows for pooling of formula and gastric secretions in the cardiac and pyloric regions, since these are the most dependent anatomic regions. This fore and aft pooling may act as a fluid trap valve. They collected the swallowed air in infants who had gastrostomy tubes and calculated a 6-hour average volume of 360 ml. Instillation of 20 ml. of barium in experimental animals in the supine position provided a fluid trap valve resulting in linear gastric tears with the addition of 90 to 300 ml. of air and with an increase of 40 to 300 ml. Hg in pressure.

The concept of *congenital deficiency* of the muscular wall of the stomach has been questioned in light of Shaw and associates' (1965) analysis of infants with gastric perforations and animal models. The histologic appearance in the infants was similar to that in their experimental model, in which normal young animal stomachs were perforated by gaseous distention. They felt that there are naturally occurring weak points in the muscular wall of the stomach at points where blood vessels perforate to supply the mucosal layer. With distention, these weak spots are enlarged and act as the lead point in a linear perforation. With the actual perforation, retraction of one or more of the three muscle layers resembles a congenital absence of that layer.

It is likely that one or all of the factors just cited may be involved in neonatal gastric perforation. Wilson's (1968) review of the literature contained 143 reports of neonatal gastric perforation to 1964, with only 39 survivors. The major survival factors were prompt recognition and surgical repair. Early signs and symptoms include sudden onset of lethargy, tachypnea, hypothermia, and abdominal distention. Radiographic examination of the abdomen, particularly a cross-table lateral with the infant in a supine position, may provide evidence of free abdominal air and fluid. The abdominal radiograph should be examined for evidence of subserosal air pockets (pneumatosis intestinales) indicative of necrotizing enterocolitis. This condition will most commonly be incurred by those patients at most risk of developing acute perforation. The proper treatment of either condition, once evidence of free intraperitoneal air has been radiographically documented, is immediate laparotomy. Occasionally both conditions will be encountered in the same infant.

Because of the poor condition of an infant with acute gastric perforation, the surgery should be carried out with careful attention to proper fluid resuscitation, acid-base balance, and maintenance of normothermia.

Abdominal exploration must be carried out through an incision that will allow examination of the entire intestinal tract — either a midline or a long, upper abdominal transverse incision. Evacuation of spilled gastric contents and copious irrigation with warm saline solution may aid in decreasing the extent of chemical peritonitis. Mobilization of the stomach to allow thorough examination of both the anterior and posterior surfaces, as well as proximally to the back of the esophagogastric junction, is essential for complete diagnosis and appropriate reconstruction. The majority of perforations will occur as longitudinal tears along the greater curvature of the stomach, usually close to the course of the gastroepiploic vessels. Closure of the gastric tear requires placing absorbable sutures back from the actual defect to assure approximation of all three muscle layers. While attempts to preserve the blood supply to the greater curvature are commendable, the principle of approximating all muscle layers should not be sacrificed.

A decompressing gastrostomy will protect against subsequent postoperative gastric distention during the healing process. This is preferable to nasogastric tube decompression because of the potential injury to the anastomosis by the end of the nasogastric tube. The gastric closure is best accomplished in two layers: the first a full thickness running suture, the second a seromuscular row.

Postoperative management must include antibiotic therapy and close monitoring of fluid and electrolyte replacement, since significant fluid shifts will occur secondary to the peritonitis. In those patients in whom early diagnosis and prompt surgical repair were accomplished, sepsis was the leading complication and ultimate cause of death.

Chapter 12

PYLORIC STENOSIS AND OTHER GASTRIC DISORDERS

CONGENITAL HYPERTROPHIC PYLORIC STENOSIS

Congenital hypertrophic pyloric stenosis (CHPS) is a genetic abnormality in which the pyloric sphincter hypertrophies and obstructs outflow from the stomach. This abnormality generally occurs in neonates and is usually diagnosed in the second to fourth week of life.

One of the first clinical reports of congenital hypertrophic pyloric stenosis (CHPS) was by an American physician, Hezekiah Beardsley, in 1788. Hirschsprung cited two further cases 100 years later and attributed the condition to a defect in the innervation of the pyloric muscle. The treatment for the condition was gastroenterostomy until 1907 when Fredet introduced the concept of the pyloromyotomy without incision of the pyloric mucosa. He concluded his surgical procedure by resuturing the muscle over the pyloromyotomy incision. In 1912, Ramstedt modified the procedure to simple pyloromyotomy without resuturing the pyloric muscle. This has remained the procedure of choice in the management of infants with congenital hypertrophic pyloric stenosis.

INCIDENCE AND ETIOLOGY

It is estimated that the incidence of congenital hypertrophic pyloric stenosis is between 1 and 2 patients per 1000 live births. The definite male preponderance is in the ratio of 3:1. Analysis of birth weight in infants with CHPS suggests that it is more common in infants weighing over 3500 to 4000 grams, although prolonged gestation has not been statistically related (Czeizel, 1972). Contrary to the widely held opinion that first-born infants are at highest risk, Huguenard and Sharples (1972) have shown that CHPS is randomly distributed with respect to birth rank.

Although a genetic basis for CHPS has been advocated, Dodge (1974) feels that environmental factors such as social class, season, and type of feeding have more influence on the incidence of the condition. Pentagastrin administered to pregnant dogs experimentally resulted in a condition in newborn puppies similar to human CHPS. Serum gastric analysis in infants with CHPS revealed significant elevations, but it is difficult to determine whether this represents a cause or an effect of the CHPS (Spitz and Zail, 1976).

Jaundice was initially reported in relation to CHPS by Martin and Siebenthal (1955). Woolley and associates (1974) reported an 8 per cent of incidence of infants with CHPS and jaundice and demonstrated a deficiency of hepatic glucuronyl transferase on liver biopsy of these infants.

Smith, Stone, and Swischuk (1971) described a distinct bundle of circular muscle in the pylorus as Torgersen's muscle, which extends from the pyloroduodenal juncture to the gastric antrum in a corkscrew pattern.

In CHPS, the coiled muscle contracts and hypertrophies, resulting in the luminal obstruction. Ramstedt's pyloromyotomy must include complete longitudinal division of the muscle bundle to decompress successfully the gastric outlet obstruction.

Ultrastructure examination of the pyloric muscle in CHPS suggests either reduction in the number of ganglion cells in the myenteric plexus or degenerative changes within the ganglion cells, although it is difficult to state whether this is a cause or effect of the muscular hypertrophy (Challa, Jona, and Markesberry, 1972).

CLINICAL SIGNS AND SYMPTOMS

While vomiting has been reported in the first week of life, the infant with CHPS is usually seen initially with nonbilious vomiting at 3 weeks of age. Children with central nervous system disorders may present the classic symptoms and findings of CHPS at a much older age. The vomiting usually begins insidiously, one or two times at first, progressing to encompass all the feedings over several days. The vomiting may be described initially as slight "spitting" with progression to "projectile" vomiting, indicating the progressive degree of gastric outlet obstruction. The character of the vomiting may change from clear, nonbilious to brownish. Brownish discoloration is usually related to the presence of blood from insult to the distal antral mucosa or, with repeated vomiting, mucosal injury of the esophagogastric juncture. Pellerin, Bertin, and Touar (1974) cite a 13 per cent incidence of functional or anatomic evidence of incompetent esophagogastric sphincters in infants with CHPS. When incompetent esophagogastric sphincters were present, hematemesis in association with CHPS was six times greater than in patients, with normal sphincters and CHPS.

Sanfilippo (1976) reported an increased incidence of CHPS during a single year which was temporally related to oral erythromycin estolate therapy. This experience represents an isolated report.

The association of CHPS with other gastrointestinal tract anomalies was reported to occur in 12 per cent of 1422 cases reviewed from the Los Angeles Children's Hospital (Pollock, Norris, and Gordon, 1977). There were 36 cases of esophageal atresia, followed by the development of CHPS.

Diagnosis

Important features in the diagnosis of congenital hypertrophic pyloric stenosis are the age of the patient, the history of vomiting, and examination of the abdomen. The infants to be considered at risk for CHPS usually are at the end of their first month of life or entering the second month. The vigorous, healthy infant begins spitting up portions of each feeding, with increasing frequency and volume. The condition is usually nonbilious and progresses to massive eruptions of the total intake with sufficient force to warrant the characteristic description of "projectile" vomiting. Of great significance in the history of these infants is the keen or avid interest in replenishing the lost feeding immediately after vomiting. This continuous desire to feed differentiates the vomiting of the mechanical obstruction caused by congenital hypertrophic stenosis from sepsis.

If allowed to continue over several days, the vomiting will cause weight loss and will frequently be associated with constipation secondary to dehydration. It is not uncommon eventually to have coffee-ground emesis from gastric irritation or small lacerations of the mucosa about the gastroesophageal junction (similar to the Mallory-Weiss lacerations described in the adult population).

Physical Examination

The history, coupled with the finding upon examination of the upper abdomen of a palpable pyloric "olive" (seen by most experienced examiners in over 80 per cent of all patients) makes a firm diagnosis of CHPS.

The means of carrying out a proper examination of the abdomen in an infant suspected of CHPS is of utmost importance. Of first importance is total evacuation of the air and fluid from the massively distended stomach. With gastric distention, the dilated antrum will frequently lie directly over the pylorus. This prevents ready identification of the firm, hypertrophic pylorus. Following insertion of a nasogastric tube for decompression of the stomach, the infant should be allowed to become quiet. The distressed, crying infant is a poor candidate for deep epigastric palpation. Once relaxed, the area to the right of the xiphoid process and extending to the umbilicus should be examined. The firm mass may lie as low as the umbilicus or may be found up under the edge of the right lobe of the liver, reflecting the tremendous mobility of the infant pylorus. Palpation of the mass is facilitated by compressing it over the lumbar vertebrae, which satisfies the examiner that it is indeed firm and mobile.

In some long-standing cases, when the distended stomach is not decompressed with a nasogastric tube, peristaltic waves from left to right in the upper abdomen may be seen.

Other signs of importance are the skin turgor, the amount of tearing, and the moistness of the oral mucous membranes, all of which provide some estimate of the degree of the severity of dehydration. Laboratory studies of extreme importance are serum electrolyte determinations; imbalances of these represent the major emergency of this diagnosis. The metabolic hypochloremic alkalosis resulting from repeated loss of gastric fluid must be promptly dealt with before there is any consideration of surgical intervention. This most frequent electrolyte abnormality is easily corrected by intravenous infusion of isotonic normal saline solution at a rate calculated to correct both the electrolyte abnormality and the total water deficit over 24 hours. Fluids of an infant weighing 6 kg. may be replaced at a volume of 100 ml. per kg per 24 hours of normal saline, requiring the addition of 20 mEq. per liter of potassium chloride at an hourly infusion rate of 25 ml. per hour. There is little need to consider preoperative hyperalimentation to correct the malnourished state, since the surgical correction will allow resumption of aggressive enteral alimentation within days, with subsequent correction of the caloric deficits.

If the vomiting has gone on for weeks, the electrolyte abnormality may be confused by the metabolic acidosis seen in severe malnutrition or starvation. Sequential correction of the electrolyte problem may require an additional day, with hypertonic glucose added to the preoperative therapy.

Initial radiographic examination of the abdomen prior to tube decompression usually will show a massively distended gastric bubble containing large air-fluid levels, with little gas beyond the stomach. A chest radiograph is advised to rule out aspiration in the face of chronic vomiting, and as a base line prior to the general anesthesia required for surgical correction. An upper gastrointestinal study with barium is to be done only when history or physical examinations are out of the normal pattern. It will usually demonstrate gastric outlet obstruction with a very thin pyloric channel classically referred to as the "string sign." It is important that as much as possible of the residual barium placed in the obstructed stomach be removed following the radiographic study, to prevent barium aspiration if vomiting should occur.

Surgical Procedure

When the states of electrolyte imbalance and dehydration have been corrected, the patient is scheduled for surgery. The anesthesia employed must be designed to minimize the chances of gastroesophageal regurgitation and aspiration. Endotracheal halothane anesthesia is the preferred method.

The surgical procedure as described by Fredet-Ramstedt over 50 years ago has been found to need little improvement or modification. The mobility of the infant pylorus allows its delivery through a variety of upper abdominal incisions. Whether a vertical midline or right upper transverse abdominal incision is used, the goal is to deliver the entire pylorus outside the abdominal cavity. With one finger at one end of the pylorus and the thumb on the other end, a shallow incision is made longitudinally at the upper margin of the pylorus. Once the serosal surface and superficial muscle fibers have been incised for 2 mm., a spreading instrument is inserted into the groove and the incision widened to the level of the glistening smooth submucosa.

The distal extent of the hypertrophic circular muscle fibers ends abruptly with slight superficial overhanging of the duodenal mucosa, so care must be taken to not overly stretch the distal end of the pyloromyotomy or the duodenal mucosa will be disrupted. If this happens, it is important to recognize the leak of bilious fluid and repair the *mucosal* tear with one or more sutures. Failure to correct the gastric outlet obstruction occurs most commonly for lack of proximal extension of the myotomy onto the gastric antrum, which may not be as thick as the main body of the pylorus but may extend a greater length. Bleeding at the operative site is insignificant and usually self-limiting. Some surgeons prefer instillation of air or saline through a nasal or oral gastric tube at the completion of the pyloromyotomy to assure an intact mucosa. Return of the pylorus to its proper location and closure of the abdominal incision are standard procedure.

Postoperative management is variable, with many pediatric surgeons electing to resume oral feedings of clear liquids once the general anesthesia has completely worn off. Others prefer to keep the stomach decompressed for a varying period of postoperative time to allow complete resolution of postoperative ileus. Invariably, enteral alimentation will be sucessfully resumed within 24 hours of the surgical decompression and the malnourished state rapidly resolved.

Little in the way of postoperative evaluation or study is warranted except to make sure that the goal of relief of gastric outlet obstruction has been achieved. Laparotomies for unassociated abdominal diseases, years after the pyloromyotomy, have shown little evidence of the early surgical procedure. The degree of satisfaction by parents and surgeons with the results is among the highest of any type of surgical therapy.

Because of the unique, narrow age range of patients and the similarity in presentation of each case of CHPS, the differential diagnosis is slim: intolerance of a change of diet, such as lactose intolerance, and infantile chalasia occurring rarely as a sequela to hiatal hernia, but most commonly caused by an immature, lower gastroesophageal sphincter mechanism.

CONGENITAL HYPERTROPHIC PYLORIC STENOSIS IN ADULTS

The discovery of congenital hypertrophic pyloric stenosis in adults is unusual and no data are available concerning its incidence. This abnormality must be differentiated from other causes of pyloric stenosis (Skoryna, Dolan, and Gley, 1959).

CAUSES

Hypertrophic pyloric stenosis in adults has the same histologic and anatomic appearances as in infants, and there is evidence supporting a genetic predisposition to this disease (Woo-Ming, 1961; Zavala and associates, 1969). Congenital hypertrophic pyloric stenosis must be differentiated from pyloric stenosis due to other causes, such as ulcer disease, cancer, and pancreatitis.

DIAGNOSIS

The symptoms of congenital hypertrophic pyloric stenosis in the adult are similar to the symptoms in infants (Wellman, Kagan, and Fang, 1964). Nausea, vomiting, anorexia, and weight loss are the most common. There may be a history of mild but similar episodes during childhood, and there is usually a family history of the disease. The diagnosis is made by ruling out other causes of pyloric stenosis; by taking a history of other diseases; by barium study of the upper gastrointestinal tract; and by endoscopy with brushings, cytology, and biopsy. Upper gastrointestinal series shows slow emptying of barium from the stomach and a narrow, elongated pylorus without evidence of ulceration or carcinoma. Endoscopy demonstrates a narrow pyloric area resembling the cervix, called the "pyloric cervix sign" (Schuster and Smith, 1970). There is no evidence of ulceration or tumor on visualization and biopsy.

TREATMENT

After electrolyte abnormalities and nutritional deficiencies have been corrected, definitive treatment consists of pyloromyotomy or distal gastric resection including the pyloric area (Wellman, Kagan, and Fang, 1964). The latter treatment is recommended if pyloric stenosis is due to other causes, especially if a localized malignancy is suspected.

GASTRIC DUPLICATION

A duplication of the gastrointestinal tract may be defined as a spherical or tubular structure which has a wall of smooth muscle, is lined by a mucous membrane similar to some part of the gastrointestinal tract, and is usually attached directly to or contained within the mesentery of the adjacent bowel. The mucosal lining of the duplication may not be identical to that of the attached normal portion of the gastrointestinal tract.

McLetchie, Purves, and Saunders (1954) have postulated that duplications arise from the development of an endoectodermal adhesion, resulting in local disorganization of vertebral precursors and a neurenteric band or connection between the spinal canal and a segment of the gastrointestinal tract. The band is responsible for the formation of a duplication as a traction-type diverticulum at one or both points of its attachment. The high incidence of vertebral anomalies seen in association with duplication of the esophagus and rectum supports such a mechanism.

A gastric duplication is identified by the presence of the normal three layers of the muscular wall. It usually shares a common wall and blood supply with the stomach. Reviews of gastric duplication (Kremer, Lepoff, and Izant, 1970; Bishop and Koop, 1964) show that most duplications involve the greater curvature and pyloric region. This location explains the common mode of clinical presentation, gastric outlet obstruction. Vomiting, hematemesis or melena, and weight loss are often encountered with gastric duplication. Most infants have a palpable upper abdominal mass (Bishop and Koop, 1964). Roentgenographic demonstration of a mass is common, with frequent displacement of the transverse colon.

Sixty-five per cent of gastrointestinal duplications are seen in the first year of life (Bishop and Koop, 1964). Gastric duplications are found predominantly in females, while the other gastrointestinal duplications are more commonly seen in males. Thirty-five per cent of gastric duplications are associated with other enteric duplications. Therefore, the latter should be ruled out radiographically or during the exploratory laparotomy.

SURGICAL MANAGEMENT

The two emergency complications of gastric duplication that require immediate surgical treatment are massive hemorrhage, arising from erosion through the common gastric wall, and perforation into the peritoneal cavity. Other indications for surgical intervention include gastric outlet obstruction, and suspicion of malignancy.

A midline or upper abdominal transverse incision will permit sufficient exposure of this gastric anomaly. Occasionally, the massive size of a duplication may interfere with safe resection. Resection may be facilitated by needle aspiration of the contents prior to removal. Excision of the mass by submucosal dissection of the common wall is the procedure of choice, provided this does not compromise the pyloric channel. Excision of the entire duplication, including the adjacent, shared gastric wall, may be done in those duplications involving only the greater curvature of the stomach. In complex anomalies, combined resection of a portion of the enteric cyst and mucosal stripping of the remaining part may be the procedure of choice (McLetchie, Purves, and Saunders, 1954).

SPONTANEOUS RUPTURE OF THE STOMACH IN ADULTS

This acute abdominal catastrophe occurs rarely in adults and is associated with a high mortality. It occurs in females more frequently than in males. According to Evans, who, in 1968, reported its occurrence in a 20-year-old woman with anorexia nervosa and reviewed the literature, the first recorded case of spontaneous rupture of the stomach was a 20-year-old woman reported by Thompson in 1842. The first survivor was the third patient operated upon, reported by Steinman in 1917. Evans reported that 49 patients with this condition, including his own case, had been recorded. Thirty-eight were female and 11 were male, a greater than 3:1 preponderance. The average age of the patients was 43 years with a range from 13 to 89 years; 24 of the 49 recorded cases occurred in patients under 40, and 25 in patients over 40 years of age.

ETIOLOGY

The exact etiology and mechanism of spontaneous gastric rupture are unknown, and in many cases no adequate explanation can be found.

The mechanism of rupture is apparently a closed-loop type of obstruction in the stomach associated with a sudden rise in intraluminal pressure caused either by attempts to vomit or by ingestion of sodium bicarbonate for relief of ulcer symptoms.

Most cases of spontaneous rupture have been associated with acute dilation of the stomach. The stomach is a very mobile muscular organ capable of enormous distention. "It can distend up to a volume of 7 liters without tearing" (Morris, Ivy, and Maddock, 1947). Revilliod (1952) demonstrated in cadavers that distention with 4 to 5 liters of fluid was required before rupture occurred.

The cardiac and pyloric sphincters act as safety valves. The stomach may be emptied by internal pressure in two directions: via the cardia and via the pylorus. Anything that prevents regurgitation or interferes with pyloric relaxation can lead to dangerous levels of gastric distention. Violent attempts to vomit or labored coughing aggravates the condition. Hence, as pointed out by Zer and associates (1970), at least two factors are necessary for the occurrence of spontaneous rupture of the stomach: (1) *"sudden distention* of the stomach which produces a more or less fixed shape, reduces mobility, and predisposes the thinned wall to rupture; and (2) *disturbance in the emptying mechanism* of the stomach." There is a close similarity between the etiology of this condition and that of spontaneous rupture of the esophagus (see pp. 67–79 in Vol. 1), in which the usual mechanism is distention of the viscus with obstruction at each extremity.

Etiologic Factors in Spontaneous Rupture of the Stomach

Distention of the stomach may occur after overeating or after drinking excessive amounts of alcohol or beer. Acute gastrointestinal bleeding can also cause sudden distention of the stomach with tears. Bolt and Hennessy (1955) reported two cases of gastric rupture caused by acute bleeding from a source other than the gastric tear itself.

The principal cause of sudden distention is the accumulation of gas within the stomach. Morris, Ivy, and Maddock (1947) showed that 7 liters of gas can accumulate in the stomach within minutes as a result of a "gastric-suction mechanism" when the patient has not even swallowed. They postulated that normally a valve-like mechanism prevents air entry and only in certain instances as in severely ill patients, does this mechanism fail to operate because of vagal inhibition, with the result that air is sucked into the stomach.

Spontaneous rupture of the stomach has been known to occur as a result of oxygen inhalation in pediatric patients (see Neonatal Gastric Perforation in Chapter 11). Walstad and Conklin (1961) described its occurrence in three adults to whom oxygen was given through a nasal tube at a rate of 4 liters/minute. "There was no reasonable explanation for gas accumulation in the stomach except the debilitated status of the patients," they wrote.

Jefferiss (1972) pointed out, "Some cases of gastric rupture, reported as spontaneous, resulted from administration of oxygen per nasal route to patients with a normal stomach, or have followed endotracheal intubation, and should be reported as traumatic, as would be a compression injury of the rectum. In these cases the site of rupture is commonly along the lesser curve or on the anterior wall. A mucosal tear is followed by dissection in the deeper layers of the stomach, and a longer tear in the serosa. The tears are usually described as being difficult to suture, and in cases in which organic outflow obstruction was present from peptic ulceration, vagotomy and gastrojejunostomy was usually successful."

Any surgical procedure should be done early, possibly preceded by abdominal paracentesis to relieve tension. In a case reported by Mirsky and Garlock (1965) there was a delay of 11 days before surgery, but the patient had an anterior perforation which sealed off spontaneously. This would seem to be unlikely with an extensive lesser curve rupture.

Another occasional cause of sudden accumulation of gas within the stomach resulting in spontaneous rupture of the stomach has been ingestion of sodium carbonate. In 1926, Murdfield performed experiments on fresh cadavers and proved that it was possible to create tears of the stomach by ingestion of sodium bicarbonate added to 2 to 3 liters of dilute hydrochloric acid solution.

In 1970, Zer and colleagues reported the case of a 47-year-old man with a duodenal ulcer who took 1 teaspoonful of sodium bicarbonate powder without dissolving it and followed this by drinking water. Immediately after drinking the water he felt a sharp pain in the epigastrum which he described as an explosion; this was followed by large quantities of bloody vomitus. He was admitted to the hospital as an emergency and in critical condition, in shock, and with a tender abdomen. X-ray films of the abdomen showed free air in the peritoneal cavity. Perforated peptic ulcer was diagnosed and immediate operation was performed. At operation a tear was found in the posterior wall, near the lesser curvature of the stomach, also massive bleeding into the stomach, and a large hematoma of the gastric wall. No ulcer was visible. A partial gastrectomy was performed. The postoperatives course was uneventful. Histologic examination of the specimen revealed no pathologic lesion in the wall of the stomach nor in the margins of the tear, except for the bleeding that had infiltrated between the layers of the stomach. Zer and colleagues found only three other reported cases of spontaneous rupture of the stomach following ingestion of sodium bicarbonate (Murdfield, 1926; Lemmon and Paschall, 1941; Kregel, 1955), despite the wide use throughout the world of an antacid powder containing sodium bicarbonate. In two of the cases, an additional factor of excessive eating or drinking prior to ingestion of sodium bicarbonate was present.

Impairment of gastric emptying is also an important factor. Any obstruction at the cardia or pylorus, as may be caused by tumors or by scarring secondary to peptic ulceration or esophagitis, may impair decompression of the stomach, thus leading to rupture. The most common cause of distal obstruction in the stomach is pyloric stenosis due to peptic ulcer. Jefferiss (1972) reported such a case and found three others in nine patients with spontaneous rupture of the stomach recorded in the literature.

Spontaneous rupture of the stomach has occurred as a rare complication of an inguinal hernia. Gue (1970) reported its occurrence in a 64-year-old man whose stomach was included in the sac of a long-standing, incarcerated, left inguinal hernia. The distal stomach became obstructed in the sac of the hernia and the stomach became distended with air, gastric juice, and beer, leading to distention of the fundus, obstruction of the cardia, and rupture of the stomach along the lesser curve. Gue reported that since 1802 45 patients with stomach in an inguinal hernia have been reported, but spontaneous rupture of the stomach occurred in none. Also, 43 cases of spontaneous rupture of the stomach have been found in the world literature by Albo, DeLorimier, and Silen (1963), but only one of these was associated with an inguinal hernia, and in this case rupture was due to a perforated peptic ulcer, making Gue's case unique.

The 20-year-old woman with spontaneous rupture of the stomach reported by Evans (1968) had symptoms of weight loss, amenorrhea, and anorexia of 16 months' duration. Her weight had dropped from 54 to 39 kg. A clinical diagnosis of anorexia nervosa was made, and she was admitted to the hospital. Chlorpromazine and insulin therapy were begun, and her appetite returned to normal. Five days later, she developed constant abdominal pain and started to vomit. After 4 hours the vomitus became blood-stained; 2 hours later, examination by a surgeon revealed that she was in shock and the abdomen was distended and hyperresonant to percussion. Bowel sounds were absent, and there were signs of peritonitis. Plain x-rays of the abdomen revealed a grossly dilated viscus. Laparatomy was performed 9.5 hours after the onset of symptoms. When the peritoneum was opened, the grossly enlarged stomach ruptured and released a vast quantity of gastric contents into the peritoneal cavity. The rupture was on the anterior surface of the greater curvature. The stomach was viable for 2.5 cm. distal to the cardia and then was infarcted down to the incisura. The cardia, pylorus, duodenum, and remaining intestinal tract were normal. Segmental gastrectomy was performed, the gastric remnants anastomosed, and pyloroplasty performed. The patient recovered uneventfully and was discharged on the nineteenth postoperative day.

Pathologic examination of the specimen demonstrated bluish-black discoloration, several perforations, congested vessels, and venous thrombosis. The pattern was one of venous infarction of the stomach.

Evans stated that no case of spontaneous rupture of the stomach in anorexia nervosa had been reported previously, but that in 1966 Russell reported a case of acute gastric dilatation in a girl suffering from anorexia nervosa. She responded to conservative treatment, and Russel felt that although the existing malnutrition and attempts at refeeding might have been partly responsible for the gastric dilatation, it was difficult to exclude emotional distress as an etiologic factor. Evans pointed out that Markowski (1947) had recorded four cases of acute dilatation in prisoners of war who had suffered starvation. Commencement of feeding precipitated the condition.

We (Shackelford, 1976) had a similar experience with over 200 emaciated prisoners of war returned to Hungary after long imprisonment in Russia in World War II. These patients could not tolerate unrestricted or forced feeding, which caused regurgitation though spontaneous rupture of the stomach did not occur in any to my knowledge. As suggested by Evans, "It appears that a stomach deprived of food for a long time may undergo contraction and muscular atrophy; stress of a large meal in these circumstances might lead to gastric atony and precipitate acute dilatation." Hence, forcibly feeding a starvation patient is dangerous.

Brea, Albites, and Otenasek (1963) reported spontaneous rupture of the stomach and duodenum in an 11-year-old boy with a spongioblastic pinealoma and commented that the alimentary tract lesions, malacia, and ischemia present in this patient coincide with other reports.

CLINICAL CHARACTERISTICS

Spontaneous rupture of the stomach occurs so rarely in adults that its presence often has not been thought of. In 1965, Mirsky and Garlock reviewed the 44 cases then recorded in the literature and reported that the diagnosis had never been made prior to operation or autopsy.

The diagnosis of spontaneous rupture of the stomach is suggested when sudden severe abdominal symptoms and shock develop in a patient with a distended abdomen. Very few cases have been associated with vomiting. A combination of abdominal distention, shock, and subcutaneous emphysema should lead to consideration of gastric rupture as a possible diagnosis.

The characteristic clinical manifestation of gastric rupture is the sudden onset of severe epigastric pain, which some patients may describe as an explosive sensation. Respiratory distress is usually present. There is distention of the abdomen and exquisite tenderness and peritoneal irritation in the epigastric region, but "no rigid board-like abdomen, in contradistinction to that in peptic ulcer perforation." (Zer and associates, 1970). Peristaltic sounds are absent. The patient soon becomes critically ill and is in shock. Often there is vomiting and sometimes hematemesis. "Subcutaneous emphysema appears in 18 per cent, occurring when the tear is near the cardioesophageal junction. The site of the tear is on the lesser curvature in 73 per cent of the cases" (Mirsky and Garlock, 1915).

According to Millar, Bruce, and Paterson (1957), "The diagnostic criteria for rupture of the stomach are severe abdominal pain, tympanitic distention with rigidity, subcutaneous emphysema, and shock," but many of the cases lack subcutaneous emphysema, particularly when diagnosis and laparotomy have been early.

Plain radiographs of the upper abdomen may show free air in the peritoneal cavity and/or dissecting the tissues along the lesser curvature and the subcutaneous tissues of the upper abdomen, chest, or neck.

The prognosis of spontaneous rupture is very grave. Its course is much more fulminating than cases of perforated ulcer. Within a few hours the patient is in severe shock and unless operated upon dies within

24 to 36 hours (Baglio and Fattal, 1962). The reason for this rapid mortality is unclear. The bleeding is usually not massive. A possible explanation is the liberation of large quantities of gases and digestive secretions into the abdominal cavity (Zer and associates, 1970). Air embolism has been suggested (Millar, Bruce, and Paterson, 1957), but neither of these theories has been substantiated.

TREATMENT

Immediate explorotory celiotomy is indicated. Lemmon and Paschal (1941) reported a case in which the patient died because surgical intervention was delayed for 14 hours in order to improve the patient's general condition prior to surgery. In retrospect they regretted this delay because "it is obvious that the general condition of a patient with a ruptured viscus cannot improve unless surgery is performed as rapidly as is possible." If the abdomen is greatly distended by a tension pneumoperitoneum, the tension can be rapidly relieved by needle paracentesis of the abdomen prior to operation, if desired.

Celiotomy may be performed through an upper midline or right or left paramedian incision. When the peritoneal cavity is opened, usually air, gas, and free fluid escape in a rush. The stomach is collapsed but greatly enlarged and cyanotic.

In most cases the tear is along the lesser curvature or on the anterior wall. A mucosal tear is followed by dissection in the deeper layers of the stomach and a longer tear in the serosa. Often the tear may be difficult to suture because the tissues are friable. The friable margins should be debrided back to normal tissue and the tear repaired in two layers, with an inner row of continuous absorbable 2–0 chromic catgut or its equivalent and an outer seromuscular row of interrupted nonabsorbable sutures of silk or its equivalent. After completing closure of the tear, the periotoneal cavity is thoroughly lavaged. One drain is placed down to the region of the rupture and another down into the pelvis. Jefferiss (1972) reported that when organic overflow obstruction was present from peptic ulceration, vagotomy with anterior gastrojejunostomy was also performed and had usually been successful.

In the majority of cases in the literature no organic obstructive abnormality was found at operation. Zer and colleagues (1970) postulated that the cause of rupture was a functional spasm simulating pylorospasm or cardiospasm which prevented gastric emptying. It has been reported (Walstad and Conklin, 1961; Albo, De Lorimier, and Silen, 1963) that such muscular spasm may result from forceful coughing, sudden vomiting, exertion, parturition, epileptic seizures, and so on. Severe vomiting may produce mucosal lacerations in the region of the cardioesophageal junction and result in massive bleeding into the stomach or intramural hematoma similar to the Mallory-Weiss syndrome or both.

In Zer and associates' (1970) case of spontaneous rupture due to ingestion of sodium bicarbonate, at operation a tear was found in the posterior wall, near the lesser curve of the stomach; there was also massive bleeding into the stomach and a large hematoma of the gastric wall. A partial gastrectomy was performed, which was followed by an uneventful recovery.

In Evan's (1968) case of spontaneous gastric rupture in a patient with anorexia nervosa, the rupture was on the anterior surface of the greater curvature, and the stomach was viable for 2.5 cm. distal to the cardia, but was infarcted down to the incisura. The cardia, pylorus, duodenum, and remaining intestinal tract were normal. Sleeve resection of the infarcted segment, anastomosis of the remaining gastric remnants, and pyloroplasty were performed. The patient recovered uneventfully.

The mortality rate has been significantly lower in patients who have been operated upon early. Postoperative management includes antibiotic therapy and some form of gastric decompression.

GASTRITIS

Gastritis refers to an inflammatory process of the stomach and in general is not a specific disease requiring surgical or operative intervention. It is generally asymptomatic but may present with abdominal pain and tenderness, blood loss, iron deficiency anemia, or vitamin B_{12} deficiency. Gastritis is generally classified as acute or chronic (Whitehead, Truelove, and Gear, 1972; Wood and Taft, 1958). Acute gastritis generally refers to those conditions discussed previously under gastroduodenal mucosal erosions. Chronic gastritis is divided into several subcategories, depending upon the degree of mucosal change and the depth of infiltration with chronic inflammatory cells. When there is complete loss of the gastric glands with thinning of the mucosa, gastric atrophy is present.

Specific types of gastritis, such as granulomatous gastritis, occur in patients with tuberculosis, regional enteritis, and sarcoidosis. Eosinophilic gastritis is diagnosed by biopsy and an eosophilinic infiltration of the entire stomach is present. Hypertrophic gastritis involves hyperplasia of the surface epithelial cells. Chronic atrophic gastritis may occur as a result of ingestion of various drugs, such as aspirin and alcohol, or as a result of duodenal reflux into the stomach.

Following ulcer operations, the reflux of bile into the stomach has been incriminated as a cause of gastritis, then frequently called postoperative reflux alkaline gastritis. The components in bile which have been implicated in injuring the mucosa include bile acids and lysolecithin. The syndrome is generally characterized by epigastric pain unrelieved by food or antacids, evidence of gastritis on endoscopy and biopsy, and bile present in the gastric remnant. Some patients may have anemia and weight loss. Bile vomiting may be a prominent feature in some patients. Other, more common causes of epigastric pain must be eliminated, such as marginal ulcer, gallbladder disease, and chronic pancreatitis.

Treatment with antacids and cholestyramine generally has not been successful in these patients, and those who are incapacitated by pain or have blood loss or weight loss should be considered for operation. The operative approaches in the past have consisted of converting a Billroth I to a Billroth II or vice versa. These types of interconversions have generally been unsuccessful. Procedure that divert bile away from the stomach are successful if the diagnosis is correct. Before contemplating such a procedure, however, it is important to establish that gastric acid hypersecretion is not occurring. This can be performed by fluoroscopic placement of a nasogastric tube and performance of a gastric analysis. Intragastric pH should also be treated. If there is a significant amount of acid or if the pH is low, the diagnosis of alkaline reflux gastritis should be questioned, since the patient's symptoms more likely represent gastric irritation due to hypersecretion. If gastric acid hypersecretion is not present and the pH is alkaline, the two most successful operations are interposition of a 40-cm. segment of jejunum or construction of a Roux-en-Y. This has been reported with good success by Van Heerden and associates (1975).

The specific factor producing gastritis has not been definitely identified. However, Gadacz and Zuidema (1978) in a small group of patients, have shown alteration in the composition of bile, in which deoxycholic acid was elevated.

Chapter 13

GASTRIC RESECTION AND RECONSTRUCTION

GASTRECTOMY

Gastrectomy refers to removal of any portion of the stomach. There are four types. (1) A hemigastrectomy or antrectomy consists of removing the distal 30 to 40 per cent of the stomach. (2) A partial gastrectomy consists of removing the distal 40 to 70 per cent of the stomach. (3) A subtotal gastrectomy consists of removing the distal 70 to 90 per cent of the stomach. (4) A total gastrectomy consists of removing the entire stomach, from the esophagus to the duodenum; this subject is discussed later in this chapter.

The first three types of gastrectomy usually include most of the lesser curvature and varying portions along the greater curvature. All include removal of the pylorus and the proximal 1 to 2 cm. of duodenum. Subtotal gastrectomy is usually performed for malignancies of the stomach or when a more conservative gastric resection is not sufficient to control ulcer disease. At one time subtotal gastrectomy without vagotomy was a popular operation for duodenal ulcer disease. It is seldom used for benign diseases, except for gastric ulcers that are high on the greater curvature. Partial gastrectomy is generally performed for the treatment of duodenal and gastric ulcer disease and for malignant lesions in the antrum. Antrectomy or hemigastrectomy is also performed for ulcer disease but seldom for malignant lesions of the distal stomach.

For benign disease, the greater omentum and gastrohepatic ligament and lymph node drainage usually are not included in the resection. For malignant disease in the antrum, the omentum and gastrohepatic ligament usually are included in the resection; and for malignancies in the body of the stomach, the spleen and its lymphatic drainage also are sacrificed.

Following gastric resection, several types of reconstruction have been described. The two standard types of reconstruction are gastroduodenostomy (Billroth I) and gastrojejunostomy (Billroth II). Segments of the stomach have also been removed (sleeve resection), generally for benign gastric ulcer.

HISTORY (Figure 13–1)

The history of the various gastroduodenal operations has been reviewed by Frederick and Osborne (1965). The first successful partial gastrectomy was reported by Billroth in a letter to Wittelshofer dated February 4, 1881. Péan had previously reported a similar operation, which was unsuccessful. The procedure, now known as a Billroth I operation, consisted of a pylorectomy and anastomosis of the distal stomach and proximal duodenum. The lesser curvature of the stomach was approximated. Von Haberer modified the Billroth I operation by performing an end-to-end anastomosis of

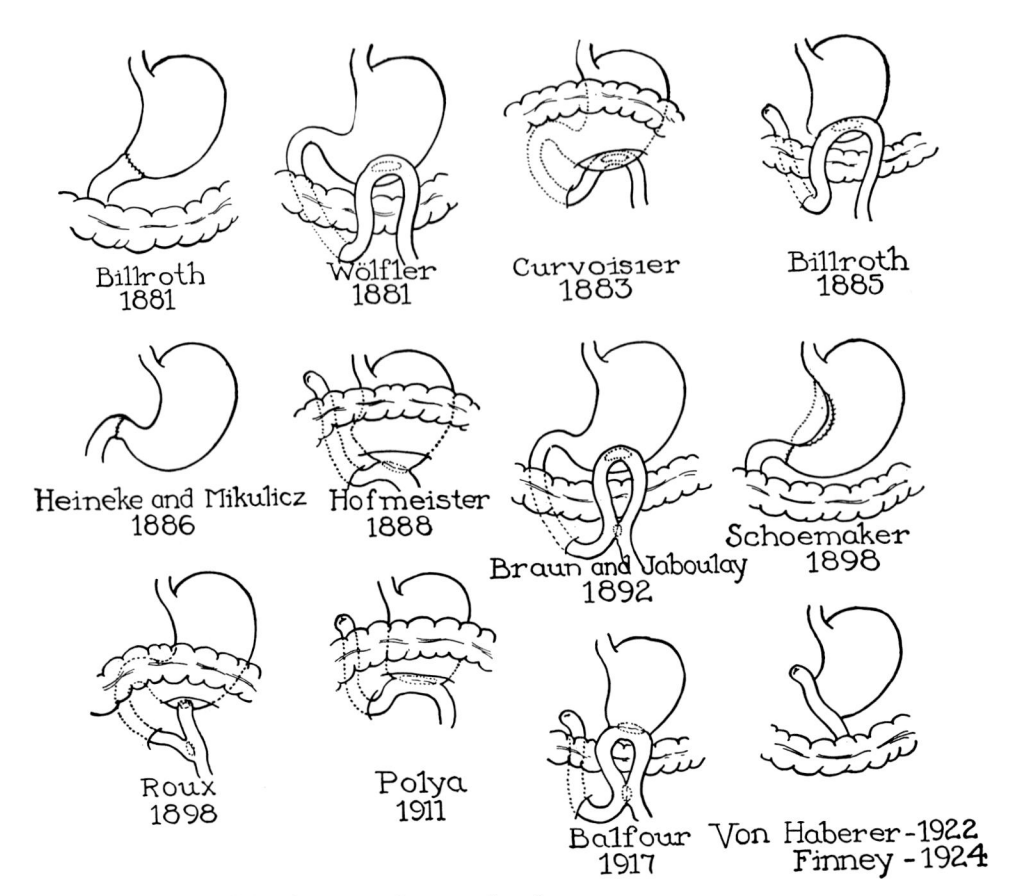

Figure 13–1. Historical development of surgery for ulcer.

Billroth I Operation: Gastric resection utilizing cut ends of stomach and duodenum as end-to-end anastomosis. *Wölfler:* Anterior gastroenterostomy executed in such a manner that it was antiperistaltic, and the frequent occurrence of regurgitant vomiting was thought to be due to this. *Curvoisier:* Posterior gastroenterostomy. *Billroth II:* Cut ends of stomach and duodenum are closed after resection; the jejunum is anastomosed to the most dependent portion of the stomach, as in antecolic long-loop gastroenterostomy.

Heineke and Mikulicz: Pyloroplasty for benign stricture of pylorus. *Hofmeister:* Modification of Billroth II, closing the upper portion of the cut end of the stomach, using only the lower portion in establishing continuity with the jejunum following partial gastrectomy. *Braun and Jaboulay:* Anastomosis between the afferent and efferent loops of jejunum in order to drain the dependent portion of the proximal loop and thus avoid regurgitation. Particularly useful where the proximal loop is unusually long, as in the antecolic type of anastomosis. (Objection: draining alkaline duodenal juices away from anastomosis, thus predisposing to marginal and jejunal ulcer.) *Schoemaker:* Modification of Billroth I by means of a special clamp with two wide-angled blades manipulated so as to remove a large portion of the lesser curvature and a smaller portion of the greater curvature. The upper arm of the angle was closed and the smaller opening, which was left between the lower angles, was then united directly to the cut end of the duodenum.

Roux: Y-shaped gastroenterostomy — the jejunum is divided, the distal end implanted into the stomach and the proximal end into the side of the distal end. (Same objection as to the Braun and Jaboulay operation.) *Polya:* Partial gastrectomy — the cut end of the duodenum was closed and a loop of jejunum brought up through the mesocolon as an end-to-side anastomosis with the cut end of the stomach. *Balfour:* Principle of Polya and making a long-loop anterior anastomosis and an enteroanastomosis at the dependent part of the afferent loop if the acidity was low. *Von Haberer-Finney:* Partial resection closing the cut end of the duodenum and making an end-to-side anastomosis between the stomach and the second portion of the duodenum.

the entire distal stomach to the proximal duodenum.

In 1885, Billroth published a description of his second operation, which consisted of removal of the distal portion of the stomach, closure of the distal stomach and duodenal stump, and anastomosis of another opening made into the gastric remnant to the side of a loop of jejunum. This procedure is now known as the Billroth II operation or gastrojejunostomy.

In 1888 von Eiselsberg first performed the modification of the Billroth II operation reported by Hofmeister in 1889 and now commonly known as the Hofmeister-Finsterer operation. In this procedure the upper portion of the cut end of the stomach is closed and the opened lower portion is anastomosed to the side of the jejunum.

In 1892 Braun and Jaboulay first performed and reported an anastomosis between the afferent and efferent loops of jejunum to provide better drainage of the dependent portion of the proximal loop as an additional step to a Hofmeister-Finsterer operation.

In 1893 Kocher reported his modification of the Billroth I operation. He closed the distal end of the remaining stomach and implanted the cut end of the duodenum into a new gastric incision.

In 1911, Polya popularized the modification of the Billroth II operation that bears his name, which consists of anastomosing the entire open end of the distal stomach to the side of the jejunum. This procedure was suggested by von Hacker in 1885, first performed by Krönlein in 1887, and later by Reichel in 1908, but Polya's reports popularized it and associated his name with the operation. In 1917 Balfour added enteroenterostomy to the Polya operation, but the procedure had been previously performed by Hofmeister. It is now referred to as the Balfour-Polya operation.

In 1922 Von Haberer and in 1923 Finney reported independently their modification of the Billroth I operation in which the cut end of the duodenum is closed and the open end of the remainder of the stomach is anastomosed to the side of the first portion of the duodenal stump.

Schoemaker, in 1911, was among the first surgeons to perform gastric resections for benign lesions of the stomach.

EXTENT OF GASTRECTOMY IN RELATION TO DISEASE

For a benign disease, such as duodenal or gastric ulcer, antrectomy or hemigastrectomy is usually performed. For gastric ulcer disease, the resection should be high enough to encompass the ulcer. In duodenal ulcer disease, antrectomy is performed to eliminate the gastrin-producing cells of the antrum. This procedure reduces stimulated acid output approximately 40 per cent. A more extensive gastric resection removes some of the acid-producing cells as well as the gastrin-producing cells. Patients with recurrent ulcer disease who have had a previous vagotomy and drainage or resection may require an extensive gastric resection to effectively decrease acid secretion. Before such an operation is planned, it is necessary to determine the completeness of the vagotomy.

For malignant disease, a margin of at least 4 to 5 cm. proximal and distal to the tumor should be obtained. It is often helpful to check the proximal margin by frozen section examination for intramural tumor cells. Gastric resection for malignancy requires extensive resection, including the greater omentum, gastrohepatic ligament, spleen, and celiac nodes, depending upon the location of the tumor (Sunderland and associates, 1953) (Fig. 13–2).

RECONSTRUCTION

Following antrectomy, a gastroduodenostomy (Billroth I) can be performed provided the stomach and duodenum are adequately mobilized and there is no tension on the anastomosis. For more extensive gastric resections, or if it is not possible to mobilize the duodenum, a gastrojejunostomy (Billroth II) should be done.

Technic

An upper midline incision is generally made for partial gastrectomy. Depending upon the body habitus, the incision may have to be extended below the umbilicus and upward to the left of the xiphoid proc-

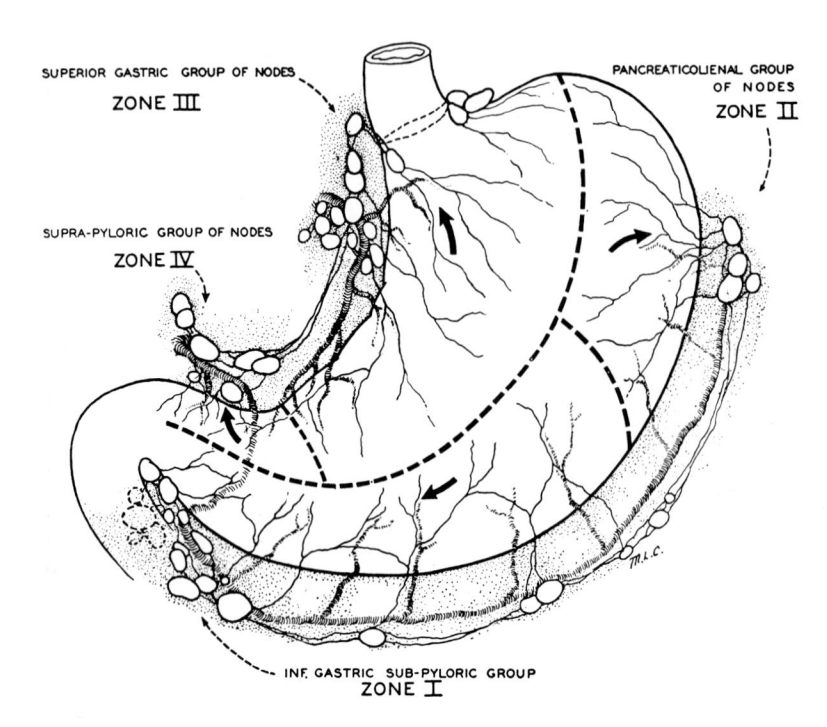

Figure 13–2. The zonal lymphatic metastases of carcinoma of the stomach. (From Coller, F. A., Kay, E. B., and McIntyre, R. S.: Regional lymphatic metastases of carcinoma of the stomach. Arch. Surg. *43*:748, 1941.)

ess. A paramedian incision may be used, but it may not provide sufficient exposure if a high gastric resection is undertaken. Exposure through a paramedian incision can be improved by extending the upper end transversely to the left for 5 cm. and cutting through the ninth costal cartilage without entering the pleural cavity.

Once the patient's abdomen has been explored and operability assessed, the first step should be to make a small incision through an avascular portion of the gastrocolic omentum and enter the lesser sac. This step is important since it enables the surgeon to establish the proper plane for dissection and permits accurate identification of subsequent structures, such as the middle colic artery (Fig. 13–3). The lesser sac should be entered in an area along the greater curvature between the body and antrum. If an attempt is made to enter the lesser sac from a more dependent part along the greater curvature near the pylorus, it may not be possible to establish a good plane, and the middle colic artery may be inadvertently injured. After the lesser sac is entered, the branches of the left gastroepiploic vessel are divided close to the stomach. For malignant disease of the antrum the greater omentum should be dissected free of the colon and included in the speci-

men. For lesions in the fundus and along the lesser curvature, the gastrohepatic ligament should be dissected free from the liver and included in the resection, and the spleen should also be removed. These modifications should be made to the following description.

The dissection is generally carried cephalad along the greater curvature, depending upon the extent of the resection. The area between the branches of the left gastroepiploic vessel and the short gastric vessels will usually result in a 40 to 50 per cent gastric resection. Once the proximal margin of the greater curvature is cleared, the greater curvature is then freed distally toward the pylorus. The stomach along the greater curvature is retracted anteriorly and cephalad, and the posterior wall of the stomach is separated from the transverse mesocolon in an avascular plane. Gentle retraction on the transverse mesocolon aids in establishing and identifying this plane. Mobilization of the greater curvature is continued distally to a point 2 cm. distal to the pylorus. Care is taken not to injure the pancreas or the small branches from the gastroduodenal and pancreaticoduodenal arteries.

If an extensive gastric resection is to be performed, the vasa brevia are not divided,

GASTRECTOMY

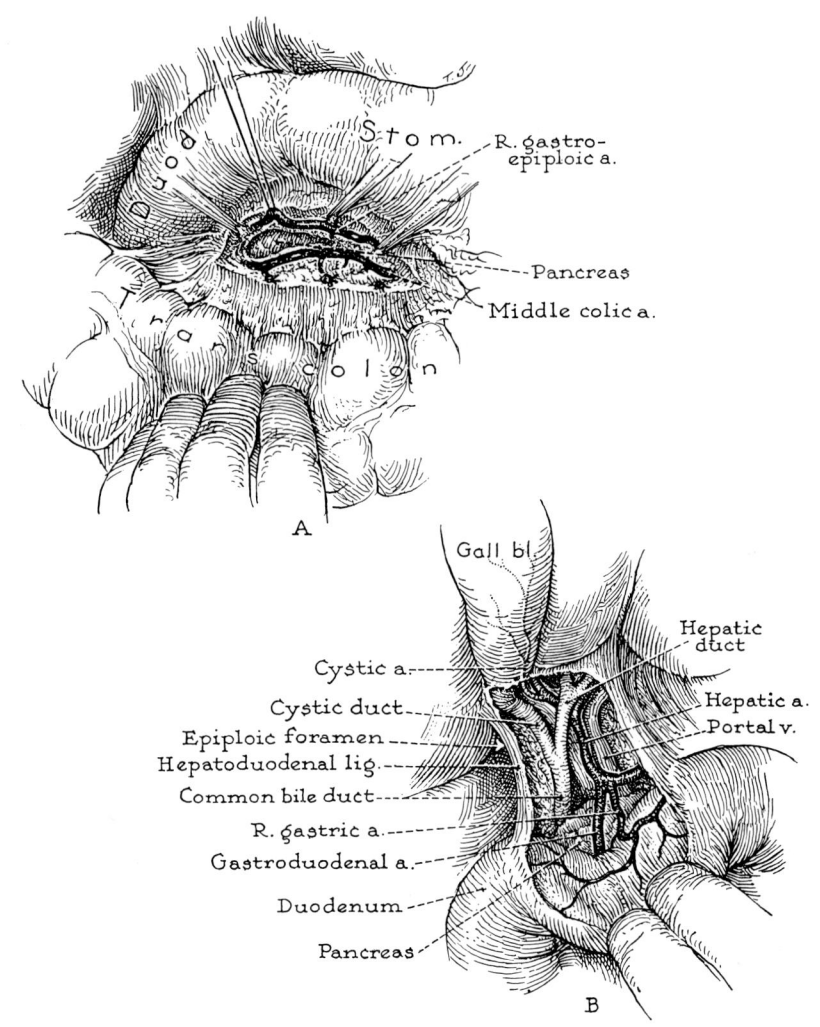

Figure 13–3. *A*, This drawing shows the close relationship of the gastroepiploic to the middle colic artery. It is very important to realize the close proximity of these two arteries when performing a gastrectomy or allied operations. *B*, The relationship of the biliary ducts and blood vessels as seen upon dissection of the hepatoduodenal ligament. The duodenum has been rotated downward.

but the splenic artery is transected at the upper margin of the pancreas so that the spleen can be removed with the stomach. If the spleen is not to be removed, division of all the vasa brevia permits a high transection of the stomach.

The dissection along the lesser curvature is performed by making an opening in an avascular area in the gastrohepatic omentum. Gentle downward traction is placed on the stomach, and the right gastric vessels are identified and divided. Prior to ligation and division of the right gastric artery, the hilar structures must be identified and safeguarded. For benign disease, the gastrohepatic ligament is divided near the lesser curvature. For malignant disease, the gastrohepatic ligament is divided near the liver. The dissection distally along the lesser curvature is continued until the gastroduodenal artery is identified and divided. The smaller supraduodenal branches are divided close to the superior margin of the duodenum. If the gastroduodenal artery is difficult to locate, this can be facilitated by incising the peritoneal layer over the superior margin of the duodenum and sweeping the peritoneum and the fat away, exposing the vessel. The gastroduodenal artery can also be identified by following the right gastroepiploic artery back to the duodenum, which has been freed circumferentially 1 to 2 cm. distal to the pylorus.

The dissection around the duodenum must be meticulous to avoid injury to the pancreas, portal triad structures, and pancreaticoduodenal vessels. The short, small branches from the pancreaticoduodenal artery must be clamped and ligated (Fig. 13–4). At this point or later when the dissection along the lesser curvature is completed, the duodenum can be transected between two clamps (Stone, Kocher, or small Payr clamps can be used). If the duodenal stump is not to be used in the anastomosis, it is generally closed with a double layer of absorbable sutures. The first layer is a horizontal mattress placed distal to the clamp. The clamp is then removed, the crushed tissue excised, and the absorbable suture continued back to its origin in a simple running over-and-over manner. A layer of nonabsorbable Lembert sutures is placed in the seromuscular layer. The various methods of obtaining a secure closure of a scarred duodenum are illustrated in Figures 13–5 through 13–11. If a gastroduodenostomy is to be performed, the clamped and transected margin of the duodenum is covered with a laparotomy pad.

The proximal portion of the lesser curvature is freed by continuing dissection through the avascular portion of the gastrohepatic ligament. At a point 2 to 3 cm. distal to the cardioesophageal junction, the lesser curvature is cleared and the left gastric artery identified, ligated, and divided. The stomach is freed posteriorly from the avascular tissue connecting it with the retroperitoneal area. The extent of the resection is determined, and clamps are placed along the site of transection. Two clamps are placed from the greater curvature to the midportion of the stomach, encompassing a suitable distance to perform the anastomosis either to the duodenum or the jejunum.

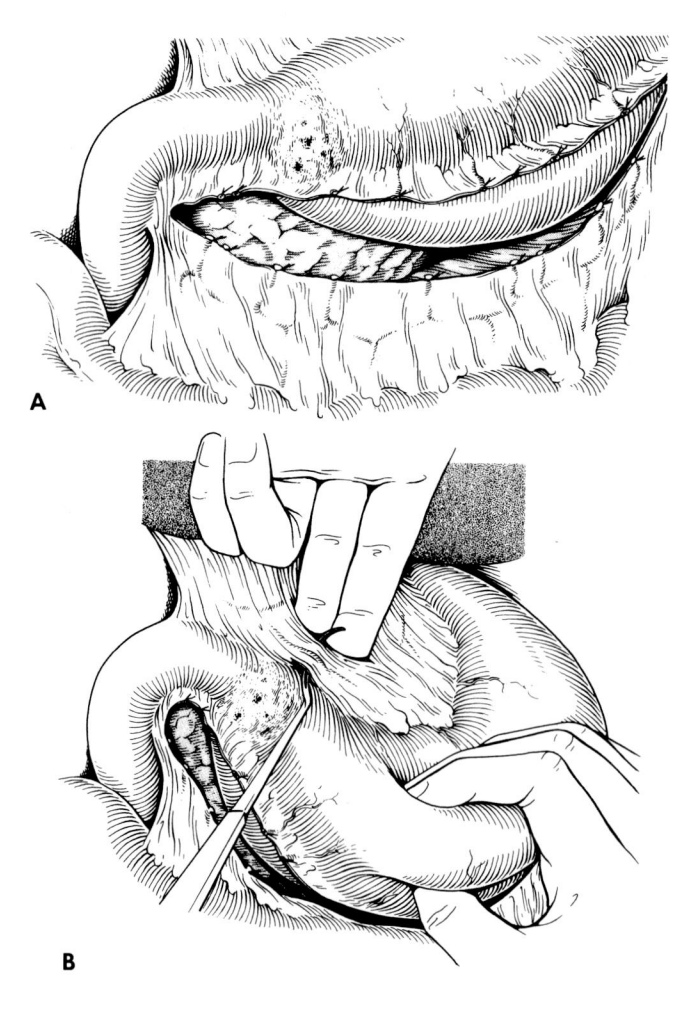

Figure 13–4. Skeletonization of the stomach. *A*, This starts at the greater curvature with the opening of the lesser sac. The middle portion of the vascular arcade of the gastroepiploic artery is initially preserved. The upper extent of the skeletonizing process ceases with the division of the branches of the left gastroepiploic artery. When skeletonizing in the duodenal direction, the anatomic relations must be kept in mind. It is advisable to proceed step-by-step close to the duodenal wall. If there is a penetrating ulcer crater at the posterior wall, it is advisable to first mobilize the lesser curvature.

B, The stomach is raised and a hole is dissected bluntly within the pars flaccida. A rubber tube is inserted around the stomach through the hole. By pulling at the ends of the tube, the stomach is stretched and the lesser curvature is, therefore, more easily prepared. The duodenum is approached from the mid-portion. The right gastric artery is ligated, whereas the gastroduodenal artery should be spared. The hepatoduodenal ligament requires special attention. When marked adhesions are present, the course of the common bile duct should be determined precisely. The dissection close to the duodenal wall must be performed very cautiously, taking only small amounts of tissue at one time.

Illustration continued on opposite page

GASTRECTOMY

Figure 13–4 *Continued. C,* The fingers of the left hand are introduced behind the lesser omentum up to the site chosen for the resection. The left gastric artery is now grasped at this site between the fingers and the thumb. The borderline between the stomach and the lesser omentum is easily palpable, and possible gastric injuries due to blind, sharp dissection are avoided. The artery is ligated proximally, using a double ligature.

D, Following adequate skeletonization at both curvatures, the stomach and the duodenum are re-examined and any adhesions at the posterior wall are detached.

(From Grewe, H.-E., and Kremer, K.: Atlas of Surgery. Philadelphia, W. B. Saunders Company, 1980, pp. 97–98.)

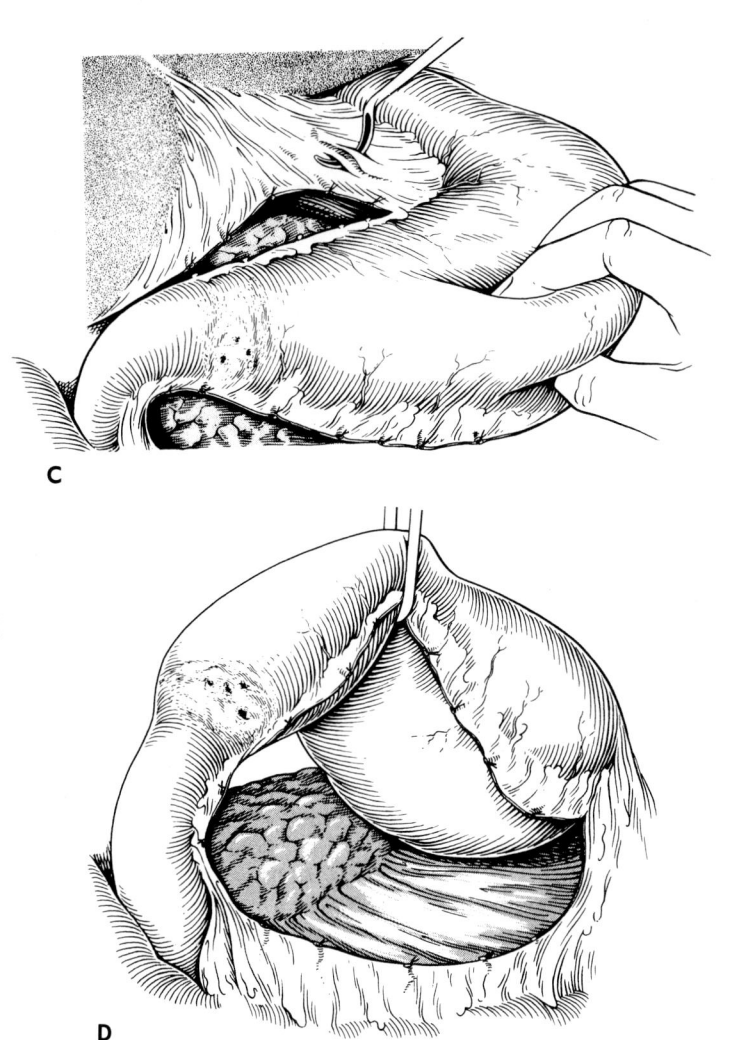

The line of transection from the tips of these clamps to the desired point on the lesser curvature is marked by two other clamps. These may be placed from the lesser curvature or beyond the first pair of clamps. The stomach is then divided between the clamps, using either the scalpel or electrocautery.

If a Polya type of reconstruction is to be performed, the entire cut margin of the stomach is anastomosed to the jejunum. If a Hofmeister reconstruction of either a gastroduodenostomy or gastrojejunostomy is to be performed, the portion of the stomach along the lesser curvature is closed with a running absorbable suture. The clamp along the lesser curvature is removed, the crushed tissue excised, and the absorbable suture is then returned to the point of origin at the lesser curvature by a simple over-and-over stitch. The serosa is approximated using interrupted seromuscular Lembert sutures.

If a gastrojejunostomy is to be performed, a site on the jejunum is selected. This should be as proximal as possible, while avoiding tension. A posterior layer of interrupted nonabsorbable sutures is placed between the stomach and small bowel. Once this layer is secured and tied, the clamps are removed from the stomach and the small bowel. An inner row of absorbable sutures is then placed on the posterior and anterior aspects. The anastomosis is then completed with an outer row of interrupted nonabsorbable sutures on the anterior surface.

If a gastroduodenostomy is to be per-

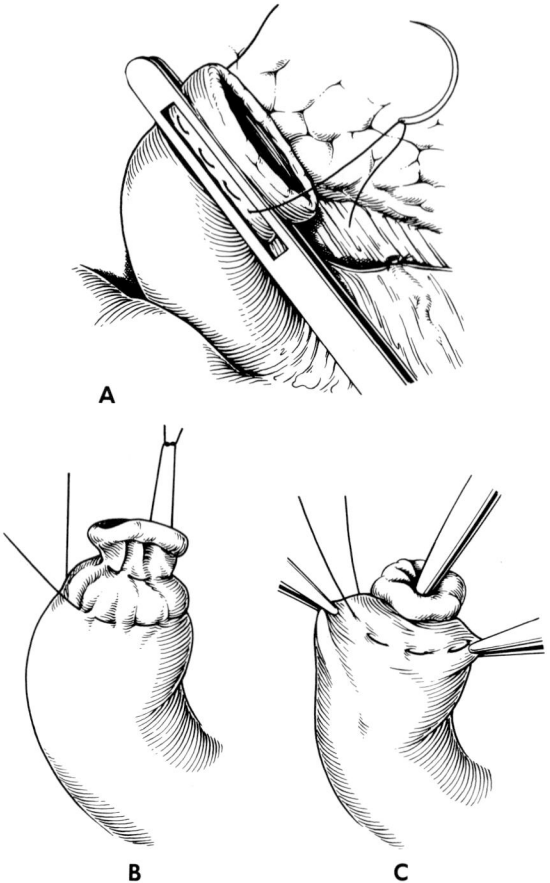

Figure 13–5. Pursestring suture according to Doyen. *A,* The duodenum is grasped within a Graser clamp and sutured using a continuous mattress catgut suture. A straight or round needle may be used. *B,* Before removing the atraumatic clamp, a silk pursestring suture is applied below the clamp. After removing the clamp, the catgut suture is knotted. *C,* The opposing duodenal walls are pulled upward and outward, using two anatomic forceps, and the stump is buried with the help of a third forceps. The pursestring suture is then tied. A second similar suture makes duodenal closure even safer.

(From Grewe and Kremer, p. 102, cited in previous figure.)

Figure 13–6. Duodenal closure using the so-called three-corner stitch according to Gohrbandt and Guleke. *A,* The duodenum is ligated, previous crushing being optional. When a short stump results after transection, slipping of the ligature can be avoided by placing a securing suture. *B,* The stump is inverted using a three-corner suture (simplified pursestring suture). The first and the third stitch are placed as far as possible at the anterior wall parallel to the axis of the duodenum; the second stitch is located at the posterior wall close to the pancreaticoduodenal junction. *C,* By tensing the duodenum with the help of two forceps and by pulling apart the threads of the suture, the duodenal stump can be easily buried. The threads are now crossed over and tied. The stump is then completely covered with serosa. A second similar suture makes the closure safer.

(From Grewe and Kremer, p. 103, cited in Figure 13–4.)

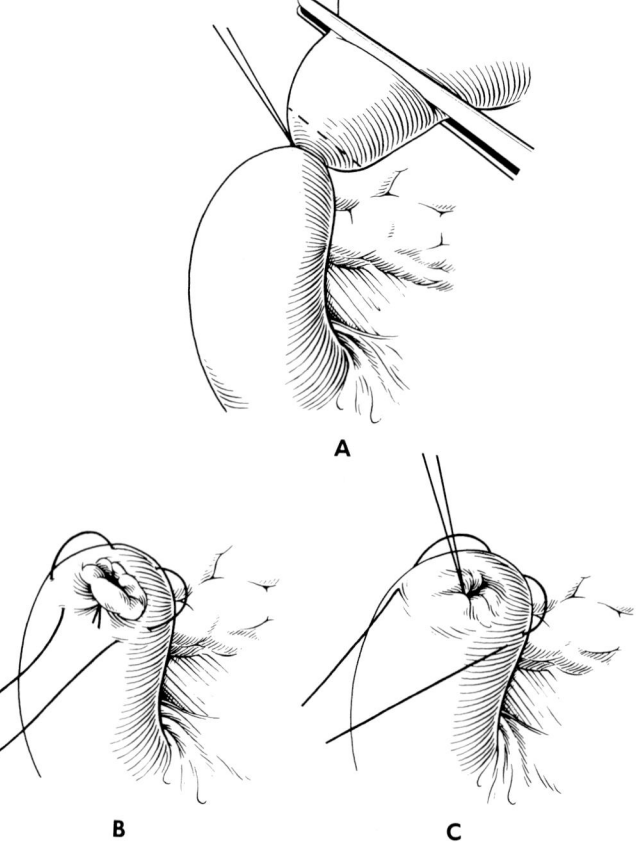

GASTRECTOMY

Figure 13–7. Closure of a short duodenal stump. *A*, The pursestring suture is applied close to the margin of the open duodenal stump and then tied. As a result, the stump is only partially covered by serosa. *B*, By applying a second pursestring suture at a lower level, the stump is given a full serosal coat. If the duodenum allows, it is advisable to perform a third suture at an even lower level.
(From Grewe and Kremer, p. 103, cited in Figure 13–4.)

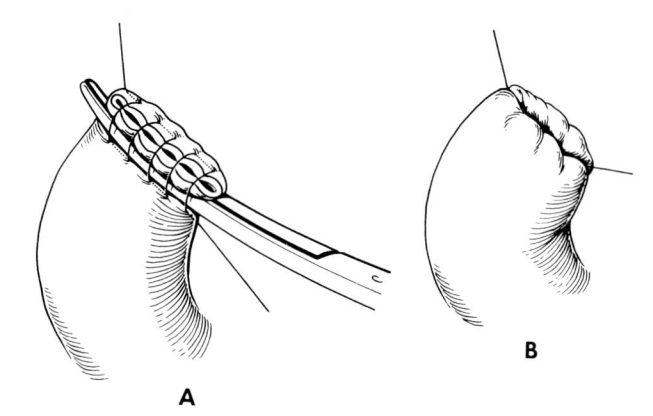

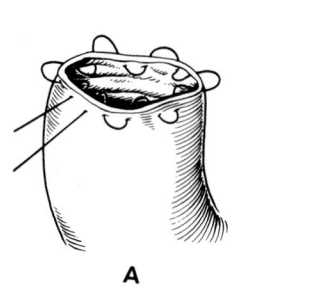

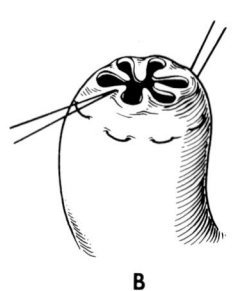

Figure 13–8. Duodenal closure according to Moynihan. *A*, The duodenal stump is grasped within a noncrushing clamp. The anterior and posterior walls of the duodenal stump are approximated loosely over the clamp with a continuous mattress suture (seroserous). *B*, After completion of the suture and removal of the clamp, the mucosa is invaginated and given a serosal coat by pulling at the threads. The serosal surfaces are now sutured in a retrograde direction using the medial-lying thread. The threads are then knotted; this provides a safe closure of the duodenal stump.
(From Grewe and Kremer, p. 104, cited in Figure 14–4.)

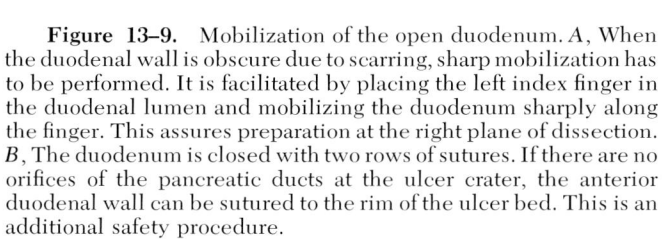

Figure 13–9. Mobilization of the open duodenum. *A*, When the duodenal wall is obscure due to scarring, sharp mobilization has to be performed. It is facilitated by placing the left index finger in the duodenal lumen and mobilizing the duodenum sharply along the finger. This assures preparation at the right plane of dissection. *B*, The duodenum is closed with two rows of sutures. If there are no orifices of the pancreatic ducts at the ulcer crater, the anterior duodenal wall can be sutured to the rim of the ulcer bed. This is an additional safety procedure.
(From Grewe and Kremer, p. 104, cited in Figure 13–4.)

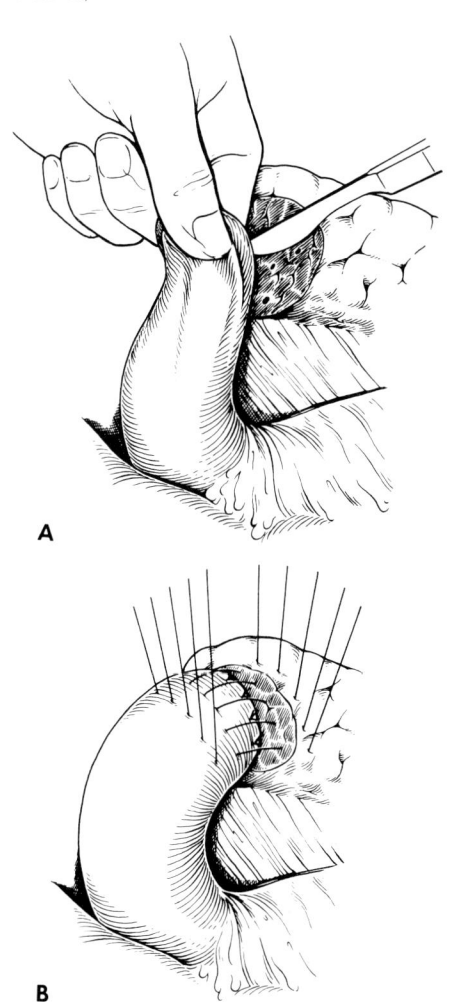

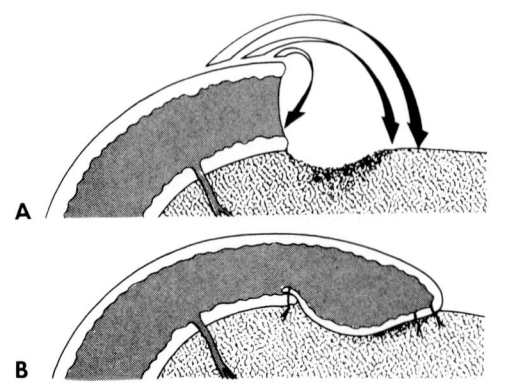

Figure 13-10. Duodenal stump closure using the mobilized anterior wall according to Gohrbandt and Nissen. *A*, The principle of this procedure is that when the posterior duodenal wall fails, closure of the stump can be achieved by mobilizing the anterior wall and including the scarred ulcer crater within the sutures. This method can be recommended only when no secretory pancreatic ductule is found at the ulcer crater. The sutures are made as shown in the figure. The first row of sutures provides a provisional closure of the duodenum. *B*, The second row of sutures buries the duodenal stump and at the same time covers the ulcer crater. The diagram is a cross section showing the position of the suture rows. The third row of sutures approximates the serosa of the anterior duodenal wall to the pancreatic capsule.

(From Grewe and Kremer, p. 105, cited in Figure 13-14.)

formed, the greater curvature portion of the gastric remnant is anastomosed to the duodenum, end to end.

The details and modifications of these two basic techniques of reconstruction are included in the sections that follow.

BILLROTH I OPERATION (Fig. 13-12)

After removal of the desired amount of stomach, the duodenal stump is approximated to the remaining gastric remnant to determine whether an anastomosis can be performed without undue tension. If this cannot be accomplished without tension, then the duodenum should be closed and a Billroth II reconstruction performed. Resection for carcinoma of the stomach generally is extensive, and a Billroth II reconstruction commonly is required. If the duodenum and stomach can be approximated without tension, a Billroth I (gastroduodenostomy) can be performed.

The diameters of the duodenum and stomach should be equal. The clamps should be placed on the greater curvature of the stomach at a distance that would approximate the diameter of the duodenum, to avoid any discrepancies in size between the opening of the stomach and the diameter of the duodenum.

Kocher's maneuver is generally performed, and the stomach is freed posteriorly to avoid tension. Stay sutures are placed from the lesser curvature to the superior aspect of the proximal duodenum. A posterior row of interrupted seromuscular Lembert nonabsorbable sutures is placed on the posterior wall, approximating the serosal surfaces of the stomach and duodenum. The clamps are removed from the stomach and duodenum after this posterior row of sutures is tied. The crushed margin of the tissue is excised, and bleeding points on the stomach and duodenum are controlled with fine sutures or ligatures or with electrocautery. A hemostatic inner posterior row of absorbable sutures is placed. In this stitch, it is advantageous to use two separate running sutures, starting each at the midportion of the posterior row, where each is tied to itself and then to each other. These sutures run as a continuous full-thickness suture in opposite directions until each reaches its corresponding angle. At this point the angle is turned in, and the stitches are continued toward each other as either a simple over-and-over stitch or as Connell stitches, to form the anterior wall of the anastomosis until they meet. This method places the the bulky knots in the mid-

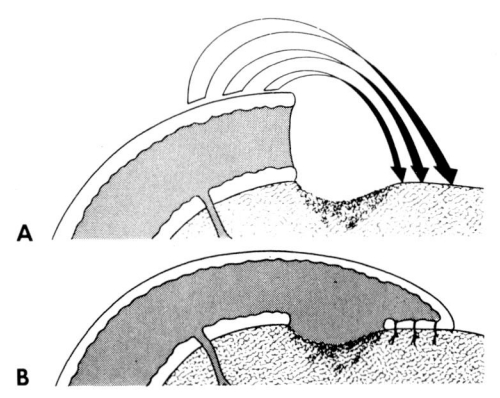

Figure 13-11. Duodenal stump closure using the mobilized anterior wall according to Bsteh. *A*, The secretory pancreatic ductules at the ulcer bed are drained into the duodenal lumen. The duodenal stump closure begins with suturing of the anterior duodenal wall to the margin of the ulcer crater. *B*, Two further rows of sutures are applied between the pancreatic capsule and the seromuscular layer of the anterior duodenal wall. This concludes the pancreas-draining procedure.

(From Grewe and Kremer, p. 105, cited in Figure 13-4.)

GASTRECTOMY

Figure 13-12. The extent of gastric resection. The lesser curvature is closed proximal to the curved clamp, and the crushed margin is excised and inverted. The duodenum and stoma at the greater curvature are approximated with a posterior row of interrupted, nonabsorbable sutures. The clamps are removed and the crushed portions are excised. After hemostasis is obtained, a hemostatic inner row of continuous absorbable sutures is placed. The anastomosis is completed with an anterior row of interrupted, nonabsorbable sutures.

Once the extent of the resection is determined, atraumatic intestinal clamps are placed on the proximal stomach and distal duodenum. This eliminates the need to excise additional tissue under a crushing clamp.

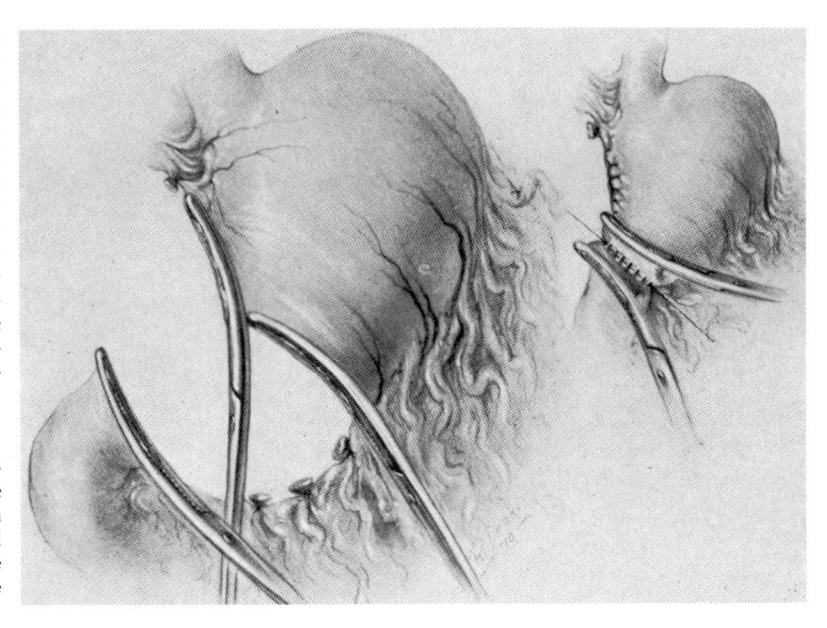

portion of the suture lines and not at the less secure angles. An outer anterior layer of nonabsorbable sutures is placed, generally using Lembert stitches.

Both angles are reinforced by seromuscular stitches of nonabsorbable material, including the anterior and posterior walls of both the stomach and duodenum, further inverting these danger areas. Particular care should be taken at the superior angle where the anastomosis is joined into a Y-shaped fashion by the stomach, to be sure that all points of the suture line are inverted. This completes the anastomosis.

A nasogastric tube is positioned in the stomach proximal to the anastomosis, and the abdominal incision is closed in layers.

Comments

If an ulcer is located in the region of the pylorus and has inflammatory adhesions fixing it to the pancreas and other surrounding structures, it may be advantageous to begin the operation by incising the gastrocolic and lesser omentum at the level of the midportion of the stomach. The fingers of the left hand can then be inserted behind the ulcer to assess the feasibility of doing a safe resection.

In the early days of the Billroth I operation, fears were expressed that closure of the lesser curvature of the stomach would form a cul-de-sac or diverticulum in which food would collect and stagnate. For this reason oblique transection of the stomach was advocated, severing the lesser curvature at a higher level than that of the greater curvature. The closed lesser curvature portion of the open end of the stomach would then form a funnel to guide food to the gastroduodenal stoma. For this purpose the Schoemaker clamp was devised. Although moderately popular, it is not essential. To prevent possible diverticulum formation in the stump of the stomach, Mayo devised and described a method of removing more of the lesser curvature than of the greater curvature of the stomach. Both the Schoemaker and Mayo procedures are minor modifications of the Billroth I operation. Today it is important to extend the resection high on the lesser curvature to encompass as many of the gastrin-producing cells as possible for reduction of acid secretion. Several modifications of the Billroth I operation have been described (Fig. 13-13).

VON HABERER MODIFICATION

In this procedure, the open end of the stomach is reefed by sutures until its lumen approximates the size of the lumen of the duodenum, after which an end-to-end anastomosis of the stomach and duodenum is performed. The posterior outer row of nonabsorbable sutures is placed. An incision is made in the seromuscular layer of the stomach down to the mucosa, and interrupted

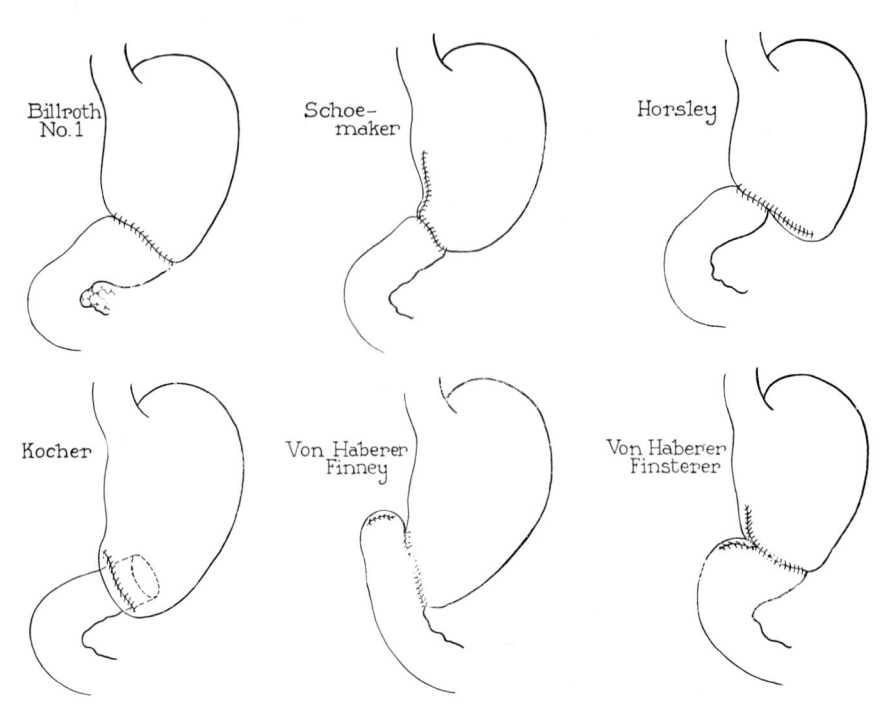

Figure 13–13. Billroth I type of operation, and some of its modifications. (From Eusterman, G. B., and Balfour, D. C.: The Stomach and Duodenum. Philadelphia, W. B. Saunders Company, 1935.)

nonabsorbable sutures are used to reef the gastric mucosa, decreasing its circumference (Fig. 13–14). Traction sutures are placed at the superior and inferior margins of the anastomosis, enabling one to stretch the duodenum so that the diameter nearly conforms to that of the stomach. An incision is made through the mucosa of the anterior wall of the stomach, and interrupted transverse sutures are placed. These serve both

Figure 13–14. Billroth I–Von Haberer technic. The first continuous row of silk sutures approximating the peritoneal coat of the posterior wall of the duodenum and stomach has been applied. Incision has been made in the peritoneal and muscular coats of the stomach down to the mucous membrane, and interrupted sutures of silk have been used to reef the gastric mucosa, decreasing its circumference. Sutures have been placed in the superior and inferior margins of the anastomosis, enabling one to stretch the duodenum so that its diameter nearly conforms to that of the stomach. (From Walters, W., Gray, H. K., Priestley, J. T., et al.: Carcinoma and Other Malignant Lesions of the Stomach. Philadelphia, W. B. Saunders Company, 1942.)

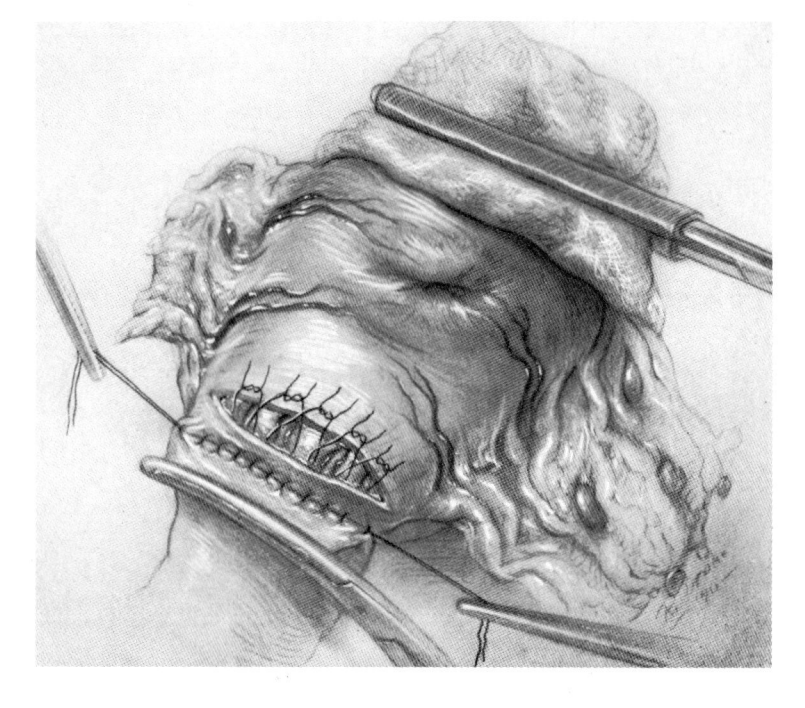

GASTRECTOMY

Figure 13-15. Billroth I–Von Haberer technic *(continued)*. The posterior sutures have been inserted. An incision has been made through the mucous membrane and muscularis mucosae of the anterior wall of the stomach, enabling one to ligate the branches of the gastric vessels of the submucosa and anterior wall of the stomach and also reefing the mucous membrane, thus decreasing the size of the gastric lumen of the anastomosis. (From Walters, Gray, Priestley, et al., cited in previous figure.)

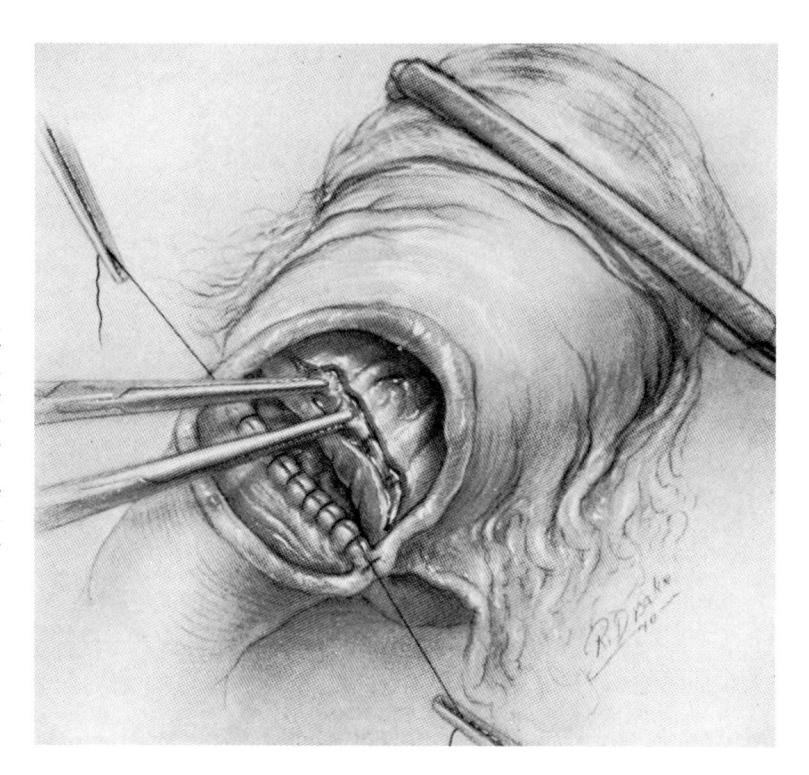

to ligate the blood vessels and to reef the circumference of the stomach. A continuous over-and-over suture of absorbable material is then placed to unite the entire thickness of the posterior walls of the cut edges of the stomach and duodenum. This is tied at each angle, and the ends are left uncut for further traction (Fig. 13–15). The anterior wall of the stomach is now completely severed. A point is chosen in the mid-portion of the edge of the anterior wall of the stomach, and this is approximated to a corresponding point of the duodenum with an absorbable suture. The diameter of the duodenum is stretched by the traction sutures previously placed on opposite margins of the duode-

Figure 13-16. Billroth I–Von Haberer technic *(continued)*. Posterior anastomosis completed and blood vessels of submucosa and anterior wall of stomach ligated. Interrupted sutures shown, the first suture being placed in the center in order to approximate as nearly as possible the mucous membrane of the stomach to that of the duodenum. (From Walters, Gray, Priestley, et al., cited in Figure 13–14.)

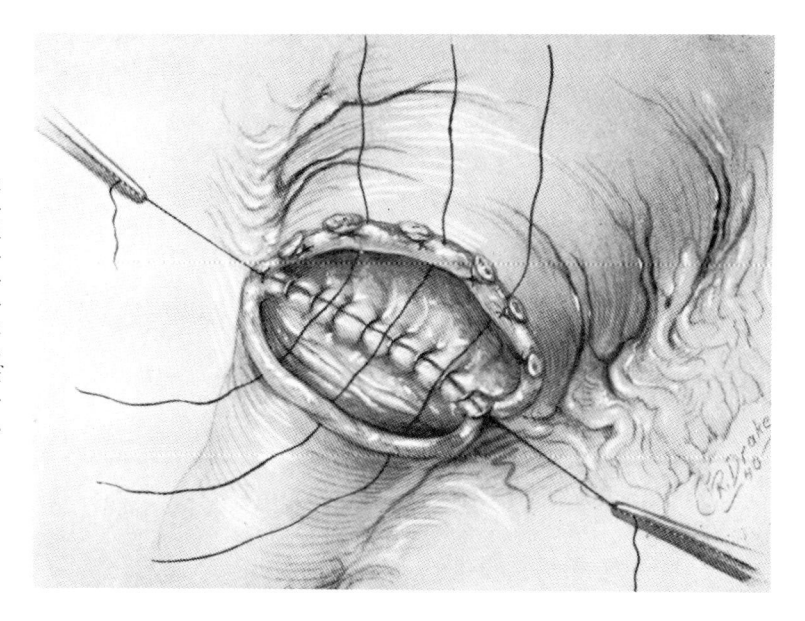

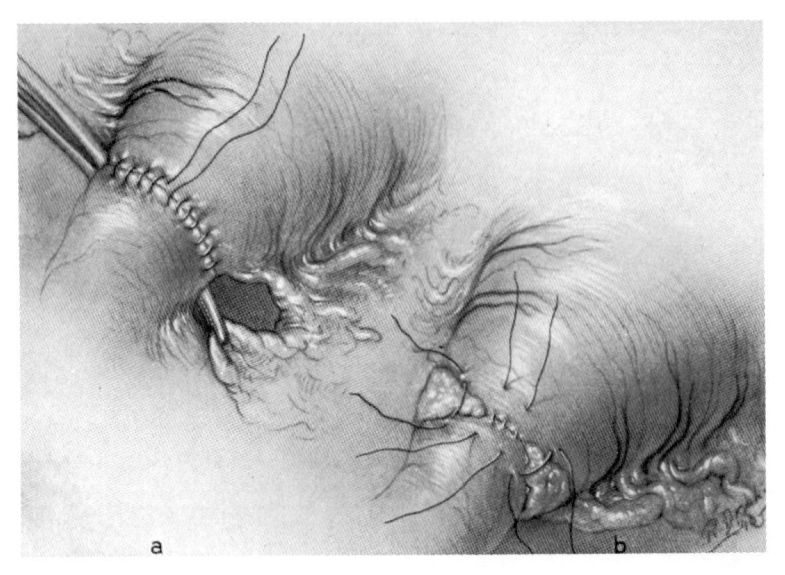

Figure 13–17. Billroth I–Von Haberer technic *(continued)*. *a*, Second row of sutures approximating the peritoneal coat of the duodenum nearly completed, separate sutures being started from the opposite sides and meeting in the center. Omentum brought posterior to the anastomosis and up over the upper angle to protect it. *b*, Interrupted sutures approximating peritoneal coats of stomach and duodenum in the anterior part of the anastomosis. Note the omentum protecting the upper and lower parts of the anastomosis. (From Walters, Gray, Priestley, et al., cited in Figure 13–14.)

num. If the diameter of the duodenal opening is smaller than that of the reefed stomach, it can be enlarged by making a small incision down the anterior wall of the duodenum at right angles to the circumference (Horsley's method, next paragraph). The stomach and duodenum are then approximated with additional interrupted sutures, inverting the mucosa. A second row of nonabsorbable sutures approximates the anterior walls of the stomach and duodenum and completes the outer anterior layer (Figs. 13–16 and 13–17).

HORSLEY MODIFICATION (Fig. 13–18)

Horsley modified the Billroth I operation by suturing the open end of the duodenum to the lesser rather than the greater curvature of the stomach. The greater curvature is not included in the anastomosis but

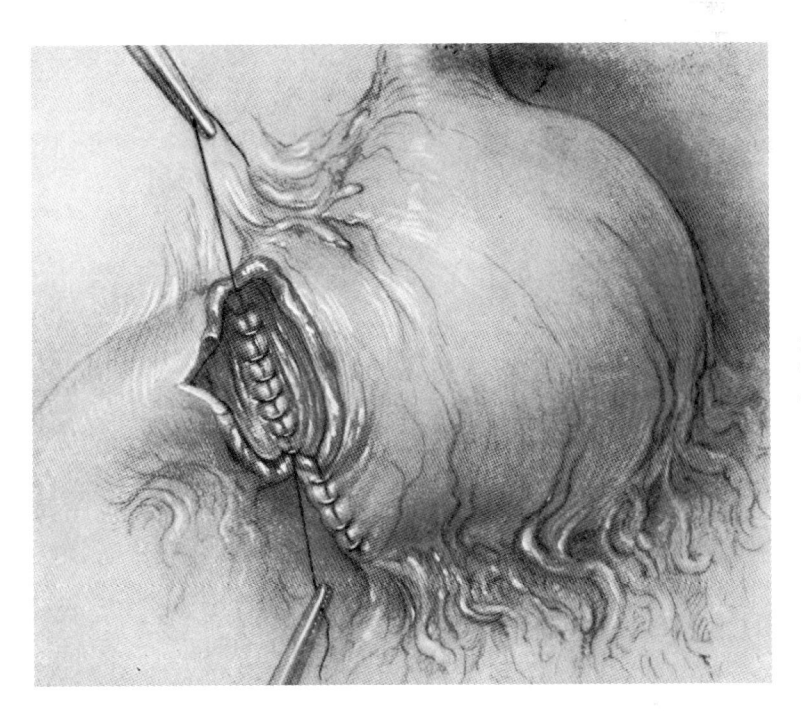

Figure 13–18. Horsley's modification of the Billroth I method. (Horsley and Bigger: Operative Surgery, 5th ed. Courtesy of the C. V. Mosby Company.)

is closed with nonabsorbable sutures. The method of enlarging the duodenal lumen is the main contribution of this procedure.

KOCHER MODIFICATION
(See Fig. 13-13)

Because of the difficulty encountered in matching the size of the lumen of the duodenum and stomach for an end-to-end anastomosis in the Billroth I operation, Kocher presented his modification in 1893. In this procedure, the entire cut end of the remaining stomach is closed by suture, and the end of the duodenum is anastomosed to a new incision made in the remaining stomach. This method requires an additional opening and suture line, with a corresponding increase in complications and longer operating time. Therefore the operation now is seldom employed.

VON HABERER–FINNEY MODIFICATION (Fig. 13-19)

In this procedure, the stomach is resected in the usual fashion. The open end of the duodenum is closed. The open end of the gastric remnant is anastomosed to a new opening in the side of the duodenal stump, as an end-to-side gastroduodenostomy (Fig. 13-19).

BILLROTH II OPERATION

Following gastric resection, intestinal continuity can also be re-established with a gastrojejunostomy (Billroth II). In the original Billroth II operation (a type that was also reported by von Hacker in 1885, the same year of Billroth's report), the distal part of the stomach and proximal part of the duodenum were removed and the cut ends of each closed by suture. A loop of jejunum was brought into antecolic position and anastomosed to a newly made opening in the remaining segment of stomach. This manner of performing the gastrojejunostomy has had minor modifications. The operation has advantages over a Billroth I type in that the freely mobile loop of jejunum can be brought up to a very short gastric remnant without tension, and the size of the anastomotic stoma in the jejunum can be made large enough to encompass the entire area of the transected stomach. This reconstruction has the potential disadvantage of development of a marginal ulcer if the resection is not extensive enough or if the vagotomy is incomplete. There is also an increased incidence of afferent loop syndrome, especially if there is a long segment between the closed stump of the duodenum and the gastrojejunostomy. Weight loss and fat malabsorption can also occur with a long afferent loop. This is attributed to poor mixing of food as it quickly enters the jejunum, while bile and pancreatic juice are delayed through the long afferent limb.

The Billroth II reconstruction is used when the gastric resection is extensive, or when there is considerable scarring of the duodenum and a Billroth I anastomosis cannot be safely performed. The anastomosis can be performed in several ways, depending upon the relationship of the jejunum to the colon and the segment of jejunum that is anastomosed to the lesser or greater curvature. The *antecolic* Billroth II anastomosis is performed by orienting the loop of jejunum anterior to the colon. This type of anastomosis is popular and is usually used if the gastric resection is very extensive, or if it is done for malignancy. Malignant lesion metastases may recur along the base of the transverse mesocolon and the middle colic artery. As a result, if the anastomosis is retrocolic, obstruction of the lumen or loops of jejunum may occur. A *retrocolic* anastomosis is performed by passing the loop of jejunum through an opening in an avascular portion of the transverse mesocolon. After the anastomosis is completed, the stomach is generally retracted downward through the opening in the transverse mesocolon, so that the limbs of the jejunum are located below the mesocolon. It is important to secure the edges of the transverse mesocolon to the stomach in order to prevent the transverse mesocolon from slipping down around the jejunum and possibly obstructing the jejunal segments. The stomach is more resistant to such compression since it is more muscular. Failure to secure the edges of the mesocolon to the stomach may also result in an internal hernia, with loops of small bowel entering the lesser sac and producing high intestinal obstruction.

The limb of jejunum leading from the oversewn duodenal stump is referred to as

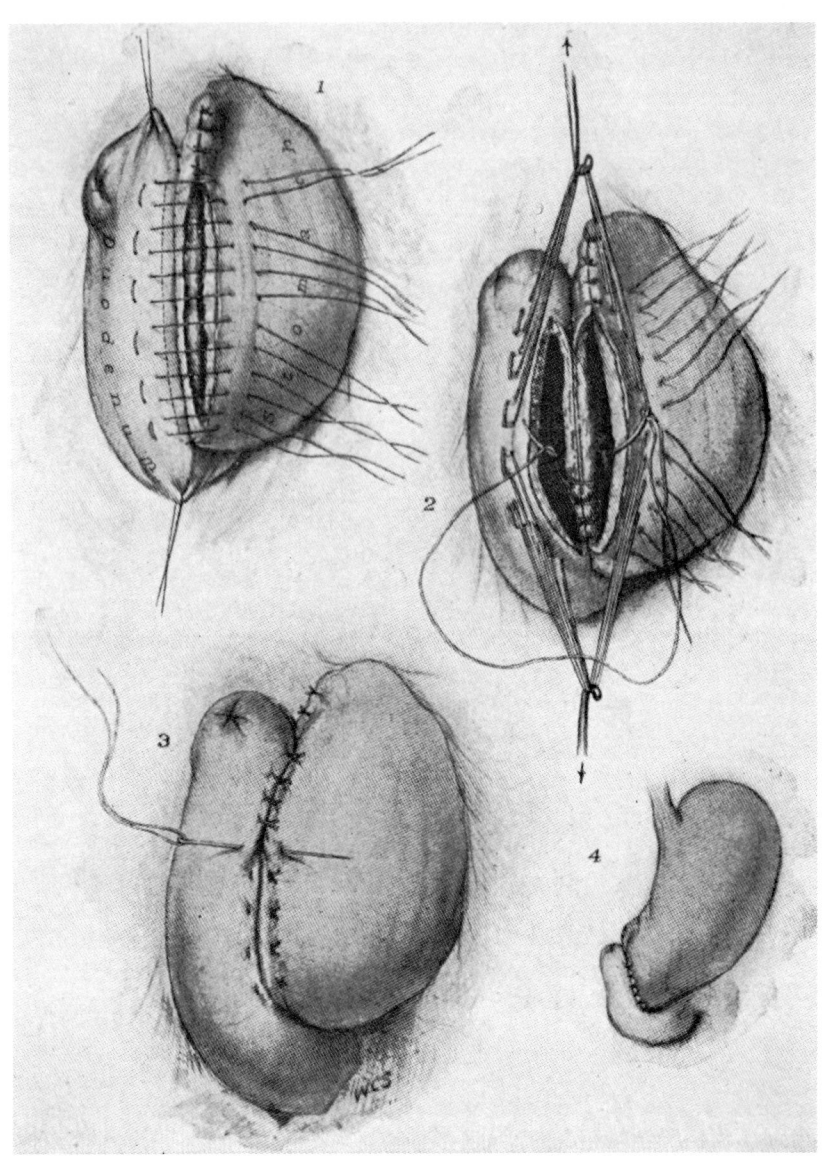

Figure 13–19. Terminolateral gastroduodenostomy (Von Haberer-Finney). *1*, The duodenum has been sutured to the posterior border of the stomach orifice. The anterior mattress sutures have been placed and are ready to be drawn aside for the incision in the duodenum. The line of this incision is indicated. *2*, The catgut suture of the mucosa, the anterior mattress sutures having been drawn aside. *3*, The anterior closure is made by releasing and tying the mattress sutures and is reinforced with Lembert sutures. *4*, The completed anastomosis. In this illustration, only the lower part of the stomach orifice has been used for the anastomosis. In many cases, the whole orifice may be used, and, if necessary, narrowed by appropriate placing of sutures (slightly wider bites on the stomach side).

the *afferent* segment. The remaining jejunum leading from the gastrojejunostomy to the rest of the small bowel is referred to as the *efferent* loop. If the afferent loop is near the lesser curvature and the efferent limb on the greater curvature, the anastomosis is antiperistaltic. If the afferent limb is on the greater curvature and the efferent limb near the lesser curvature, the anastomosis is said to be isoperistaltic.

Except for the instances just mentioned, construction of the Billroth II anastomosis in any of these fashions functions well. The differences are of little importance as long as the afferent loop is as short as possible and without tension. In choos-

GASTRECTOMY

ing between these alternatives it is best to select the procedure that results in an anastomosis which lies comfortably, without tension, and without any sharp kinks or bends in the small bowel.

The operative technique for the gastric resection is the same as that previously described. The Hofmeister reconstruction includes closing a part of the stomach along the lesser curvature. The Polya operation is performed in a similar manner, except that the entire cut edge of the stomach is used for the gastrojejunostomy. The Hofmeister method is most commonly used and is the technique that will be described (Fig. 13–20).

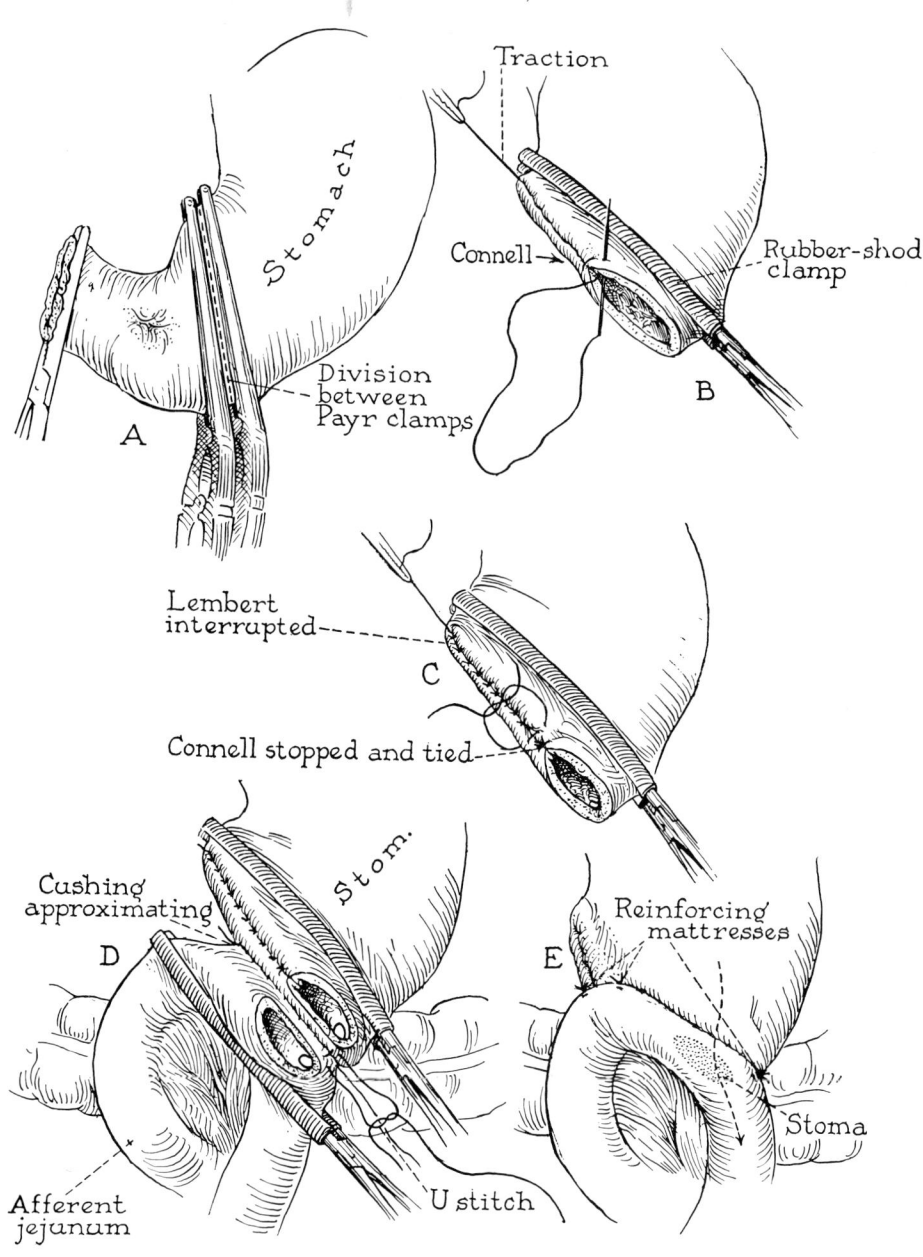

Figure 13–20. Hofmeister modification of Billroth II operation. Anterior gastrojejunostomy. *A*, Division of the stomach between Payr clamps. *B*, Rubber-shod clamp applied to stomach and remaining crushing clamp removed; placing of Connell inverting suture. *C*, Reinforcing of Connell with interrupted Lembert sutures. *D*, Initial suture line (Cushing) approximating posterior serous walls of stomach and jejunum; U-stitch placed as a beginning to through-and-through lock suture. *E*, Completed anastomosis. The jejunum, as shown, is brought above the line of stomach closure.

The duodenum is closed securely, as is a portion of the stomach along the lesser curvature. Approximately 6 cm. of the transected edge of stomach on the greater curvature are required for the anastomosis. If a retrocolic anastomosis is decided upon, the transverse colon is held forward and upward, and an opening is made in an avascular portion of the transverse mesocolon, generally to the left of the middle colic vessels. A loop of jejunum near the ligament of Treitz is selected and brought through the opening in the transverse mesocolon. When necessary, part of the ligament of Treitz can be incised to further decrease the length of the afferent limb. Noncrushing linen-shod clamps are placed on the small bowel proximal and distal to the area of planned anastomosis to prevent small bowel fluid from contaminating the field. Stay sutures are then placed between the jejunum and posterior wall of the stomach,

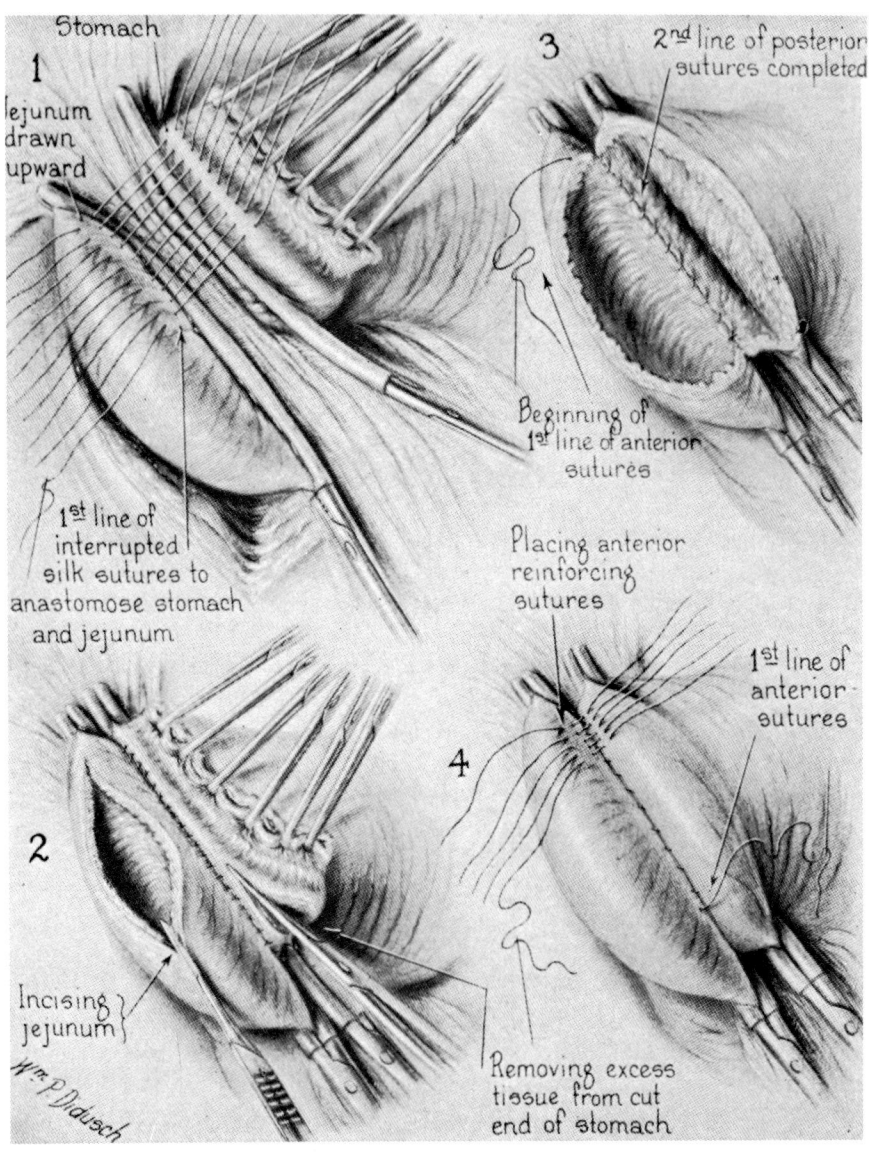

Figure 13–21. Polya technic of Billroth II operation. Method of re-establishment of continuity of gastrointestinal tract by antecolic gastrojejunostomy. Crushed tissue is removed from the stump of the resected stomach. (From Rienhoff, W. F., Jr.: An analysis of the results of the surgical treatment of 260 consecutive cases of chronic peptic ulcer of the duodenum. Ann. Surg. *121*:583, 1945.)

GASTRECTOMY

followed by a row of nonabsorbable seromuscular sutures. This posterior row extends for the entire 6 to 7 cm of the anastomosis. The crushing clamp is removed from the cut end of the stomach and the devitalized tissue removed.

An opening is then made in the small bowel the same length as that of the gastric opening. An inner row of absorbable sutures is placed in a manner similar to that described for a Billroth I operation. These are running hemostatic sutures extended as inner anterior sutures as well. The anastomosis is then completed with an outer anterior row of interrupted, nonabsorbable, Lembert seromuscular stitches. One or two sutures are then placed from the jejunum to the lesser curvature to secure that angle, and one or two sutures at the greater curvature angle as well. The noncrushing clamps are removed from the small bowel, and the anastomosis palpated for patency. The transverse mesocolon is then lifted upward, and slight traction is placed on the stomach to allow the jejunal loops to lie below the mesocolon. The transverse mesocolon is then fixed to the stomach circumferentially with 7 or 8 nonabsorbable sutures, 3 to 5 cm. proximal to the gastrojejunostomy.

The antecolic anastomosis is performed in a similar manner, except that the loop of jejunum is brought anterior to the trans-

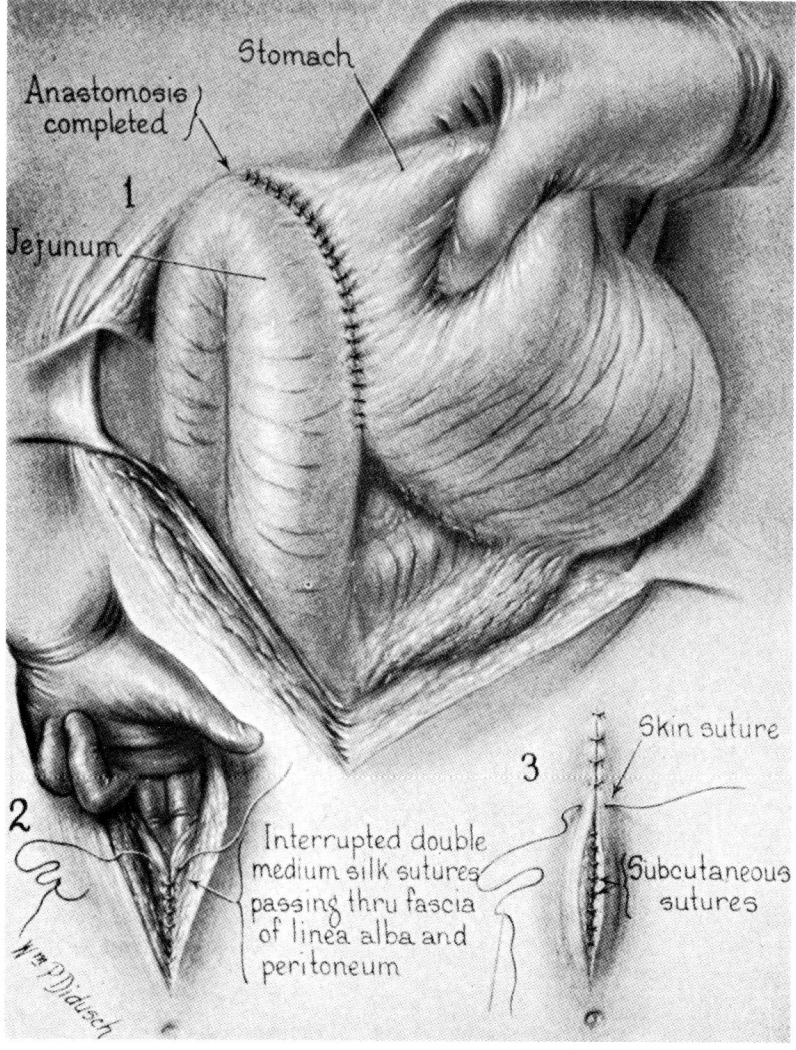

Figure 13–22. Polya technic of Billroth II operation *(continued)*. The antecolic gastrojejunostomy is completed. (From Rienhoff, cited in previous figure.)

verse colon instead of through the transverse mesocolon.

The Polya modification consists of using the entire length of the cut end of the stomach in constructing the anastomosis (Figs. 13–21 and 13–22).

POLYA-BALFOUR MODIFICATION

This operation differs from the Polya procedure only in the construction of an enteroenterostomy between the afferent and efferent loops of the jejunum (Fig. 13–23). It was first described by Balfour in 1917 but previously had been used by Hofmeister. It was devised in the anticipation that stagnation would occur in the long afferent jejunal limb. Experience has shown this to be not as important as was once thought. Furthermore, attempts are now made to make the afferent loop as short as possible. This operation is occasionally performed to allow bile and pancreatic juice to enter the efferent limb of the small bowel, preventing the duodenal juices from entering the stomach. To successfully accomplish this, the enteroenterostomy must be at least 6 cm. in length and sufficiently distant to the gastrojejunostomy (30 to 35 cm.).

DEVINE EXCLUSION

The Devine exclusion, usually performed as a two-stage partial gastrectomy, consists of transecting the stomach proximal to the lesion as the first stage. The open end of the gastric remnant is anastomosed to the side of the jejunum as in an anterior Polya operation, while the distal end of the stomach containing the lesion is sutured closed. In the second stage, the distal stomach is removed and the duodenal stump closed (Figs. 13–24, 13–25, and 13–26). This operation is rarely performed and is of historic interest.

FINSTERER PARTIAL GASTRECTOMY WITH ANTRAL EXCLUSION

The Finsterer exclusion operation consists of transecting the distal portion of the stomach at the junction of the body and antrum and stripping off and excising all the mucosal lining of the antrum. The cut end of the denuded antral stump is closed, and a large segment of the body of the stomach is resected. Alimentary continuity is restored by constructing a Hofmeister antecolic gastrojejunostomy. This type of operation is

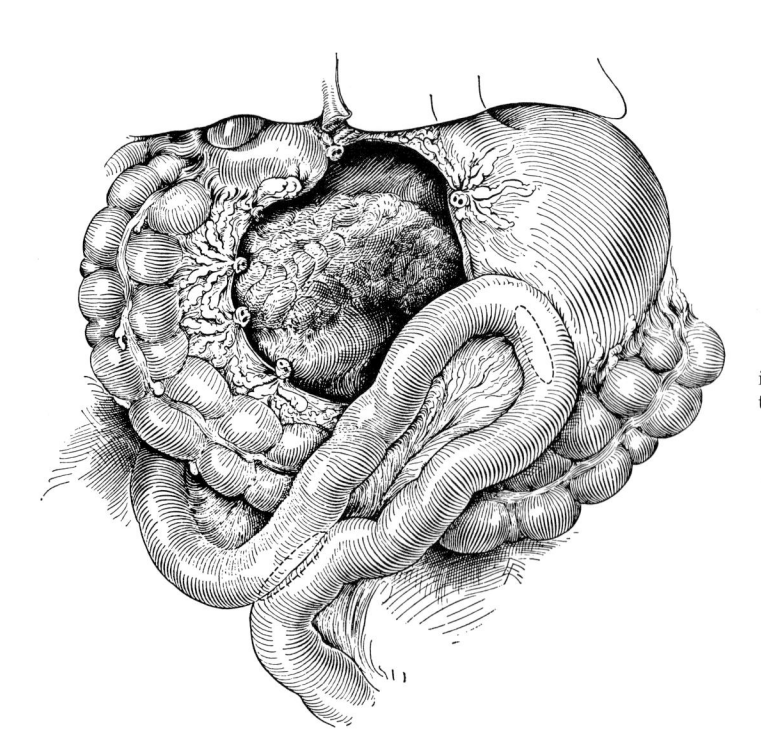

Figure 13–23. Polya-Balfour modification of Billroth II operation. Gastroenterostomy and enteroanastomosis.

GASTRECTOMY

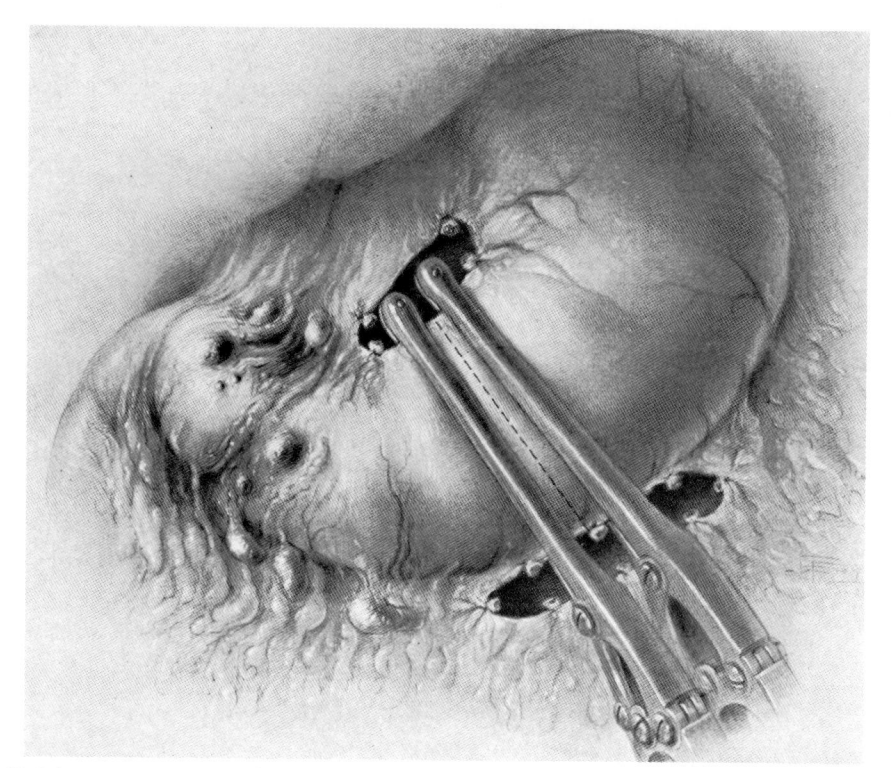

Figure 13–24. Two-stage partial gastrectomy for carcinoma or ulcer with end-to-loop transmesocolic gastrojejunostomy (Devine principle). First-stage procedure. The stomach is freed at its greater and lesser curvatures, proximal to the growth. Two Payr clamps are placed on the stomach at the proposed level of transection. (From Eusterman, G. B., and Balfour, D. C.: The Stomach and Duodenum. Philadelphia, W. B. Saunders Company, 1935.)

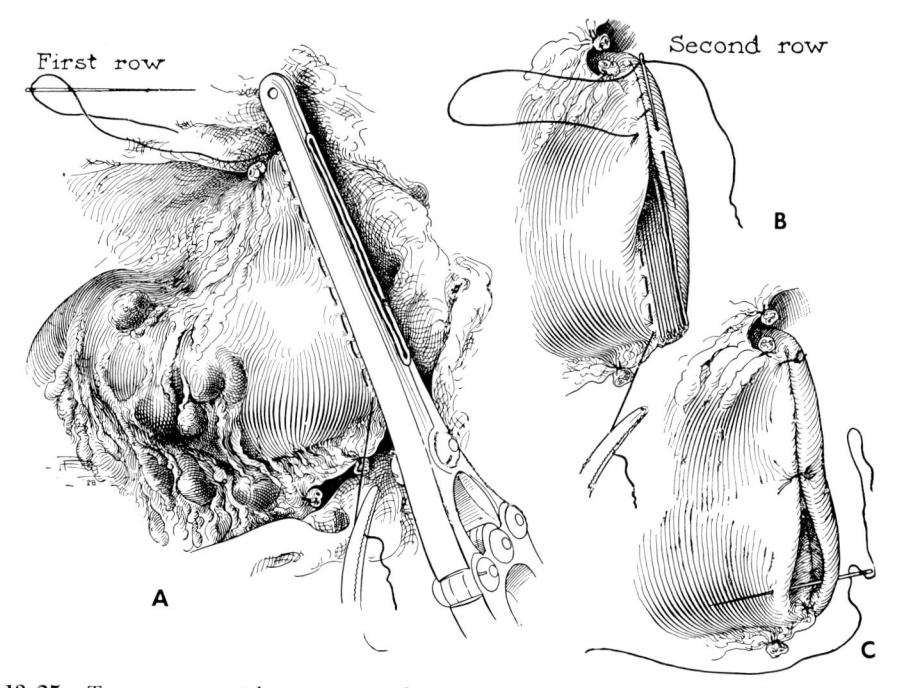

Figure 13–25. Two-stage partial gastrectomy for carcinoma or ulcer with end-to-loop transmesocolic gastrojejunostomy (Devine principle). First-stage procedure *(continued)*. *A*, The lower segment of the stomach is closed distal to its clamp by continuous through-and-through absorbable sutures. *B*, The through-and-through suture is continued as an invaginating seromuscular continuous suture of the Cushing type. *C*, A few seromuscular reinforcing nonabsorbable sutures are placed. (From Eusterman and Balfour, cited in previous figure.)

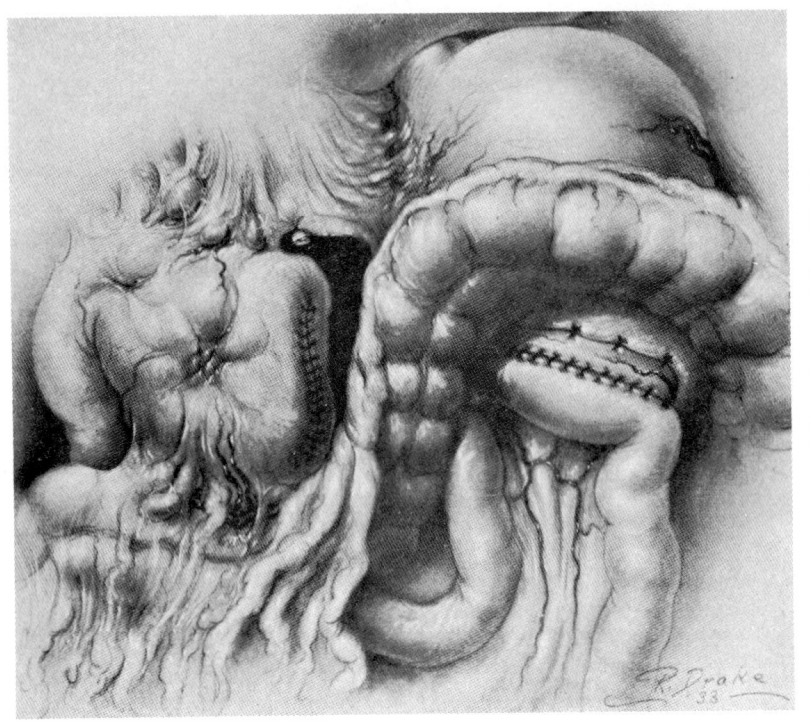

Figure 13-26. Two-stage partial gastrectomy for carcinoma or ulcer with end-to-loop transmesocolic gastrojejunostomy (Devine principle). First-stage procedure *(continued)*. The first stage is concluded when the antrum has been excluded, and the proximal segment of the stomach has been sutured end-to-side to the first jejunal loop. The anastomosis is retrocolic and is performed according to the posterior Polya modification of Billroth II operation described on pages 305–306. (From Eusterman and Balfour, cited in Figure 13-24.)

rarely performed, although occasionally it may be indicated in a patient with an antral carcinoma which technically cannot be removed with a standard gastric resection. If duodenal or pyloric obstruction is suspected, this type of operation should not be performed since the antral closure may disrupt.

ROUX-EN-Y MODIFICATION

In this procedure, the distal stomach and first portion of duodenum are resected, and the stump of the duodenum is closed. The jejunum is transected 6 to 10 cm. distal to the ligament of Treitz, and the open end of the distal segment is anastomosed end-to-end to the remaining segment of stomach. (As a further modification, the distal end also can be closed and the stomach can be anastomosed to the antimesenteric border of the jejunum in an end-to-side fashion.) The open end of the proximal jejunum is then anastomosed to a site on the distal jejunum, generally 35 to 45 cm. distal to the gastrojejunostomy (Fig. 13-27). This operation is generally not employed as a primary operation; however, Billroth I and Billroth II procedures can later be converted to a Roux-en-Y reconstruction if there is evidence of reflux alkaline gastritis. This operation has the advantage of preventing reflux of alkaline juice into the stomach, but

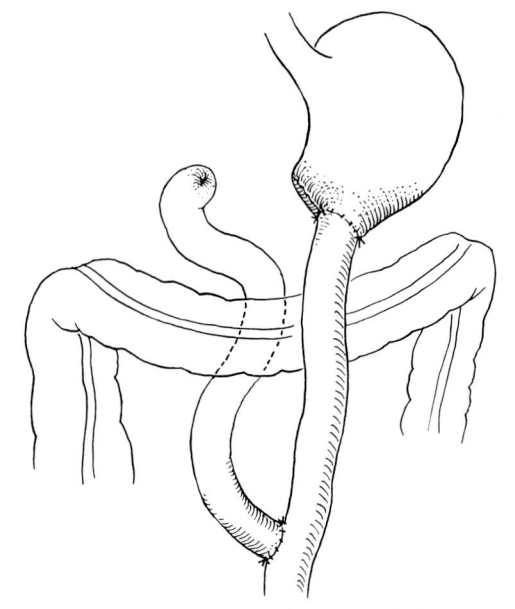

Figure 13-27. Antecolic gastrojejunostomy. Roux-en-Y modification of Billroth II operation.

a disadvantage is that alkaline material is not provided to the segment of jejunum that is in continuity with the stomach. If the ulcer operation is incomplete and there is significant acid secretion, a marginal ulcer may develop. Since the risks arising from marginal ulcer are considerably higher than the risks of bile gastritis, the Roux-en-Y reconstruction is not recommended as an initial procedure.

SLEEVE RESECTION

Sleeve resection refers to a type of partial gastrectomy with resection of the mid-portion of the stomach. It generally is indicated for a benign gastric ulcer located in the body of the stomach. The free edges of the remaining portions are anastomosed end-to-end. This operation is rarely performed.

TOTAL GASTRECTOMY AND RECONSTRUCTION

Total gastrectomy consists of the removal of the entire stomach, from the pylorus to the cardioesophageal junction. Total gastrectomy for a gastric tumor should include the stomach from the cardioesophageal junction to a cuff of the first portion of the duodenum, the greater and lesser omenta, the spleen, and the gastrohepatic ligament. All lymph nodes in these areas are included in the dissection. Total gastrectomy may also be required for benign conditions such as diffuse adenomatosis, for a gastric ulcer located at the cardia, or for hypersecretory states, such as gastrinoma. Generally for these benign conditions the omenta and spleen need not be removed.

For malignant lesions, total gastrectomy generally should be attempted as a curative procedure. Occasionally it may be a beneficial palliative operation, particularly if metastases are not widespread and the lesion is producing such symptoms as bleeding, obstruction, or perforation.

Conner in this country is credited with the first attempt at total gastrectomy. His operation, performed in 1883, was unsuccessful. Schlatter, in 1897, reported the first successful total gastrectomy. Since that time increasing numbers of these operations have been reported, with decreasing mortality rates.

Technic

Total gastrectomy is usually performed through an abdominal incision or a thoracoabdominal approach entering either the fourth or sixth intercostal space (Fig. 13–28). A transthoracic approach is rarely used. Following total gastrectomy several methods of reconstruction have been described: (1) esophagojejunostomy, (2) esophagoduodenostomy, and (3) esophagocolostomy (using colon to create a pouch).

Reconstruction by esophagojejunostomy is the most common type of reconstruction following total gastrectomy. Occasionally, esophagoduodenostomy as described by Madden (1951) is possible. Both the right colon and transverse colon have been described as a substitute gastric reservoir; however, this type of procedure is rarely performed. The jejunum or colon is not commonly used to form a gastric reservoir since these require multiple anastomoses and suture lines, and no nutritional benefit has been demonstrated by constructing a

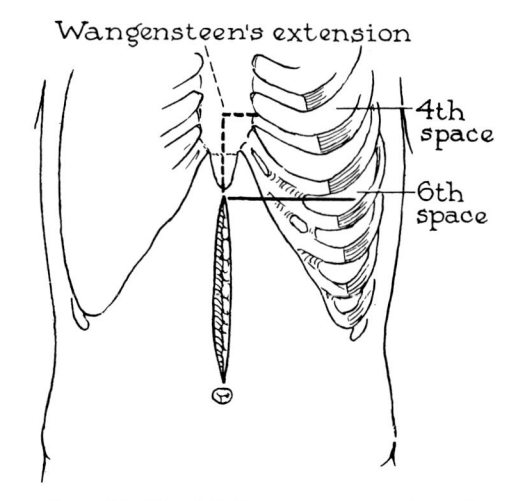

Figure 13–28. Midline incision which may be extended by splitting the sternum upward as high as the fourth intercostal space (Wangensteen) or by extending incision laterally through the sixth intercostal space.

reservoir. The most common type of reconstruction performed is a Roux-en-Y esophagojejunostomy or an end-to-side esophagojejunostomy to a proximal loop of jejunum with a large enteroenterostomy between the afferent and efferent limbs of the jejunum.

LONGMIRE METHOD
(Longmire, 1952)

A Levin tube is passed through the nose into the stomach. The stomach is lavaged and the tube is left in the stomach.

The abdomen is entered through the abdominal incision selected. It is explored to determine the operability of the lesion, taking particular care to determine that sufficient esophagus can be freed to form an anastomosis.

The great omentum is held up by an assistant, and it is severed from all attachments (see Fig. 13–34, p. 315) to the transverse colon by cutting those attachments at their juncture. While carrying out this step, great care must be taken *not* to include the transverse mesocolon with the omentum and to avoid injury to the middle (see Fig. 13–35, p. 316) and left colic arteries. The gastrocolic omentum is severed from its attachments to the transverse colon and is left attached to the stomach to be removed in one piece with that organ.

The right gastric and gastroepiploic arteries are identified (see Fig. 13–36, p. 316) in the pyloric region and divided as close to their origins as possible. The duodenum is freed down to the head of the pancreas where it is cut across between two small clamps.

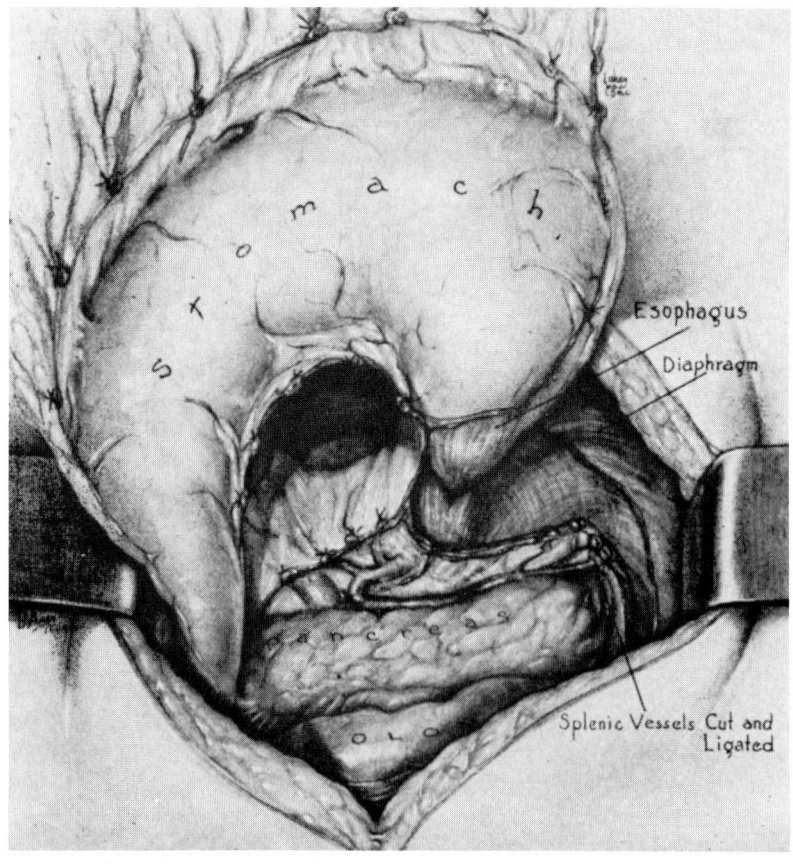

Figure 13–29. Total gastrectomy. In this illustration the spleen has been removed and the ample exposure of the esophagus following splenectomy is demonstrated. One can likewise see the peritoneum of the diaphragm as it extends over the esophagus, from which will be cut the apron of peritoneum with which to suspend the jejunum anastomosed to the esophagus. (From Lahey, F. H., and Marshall, S. F.: Combining splenectomy with total gastrectomy. Surg. Gynecol. Obstet. 73:341, 1941.)

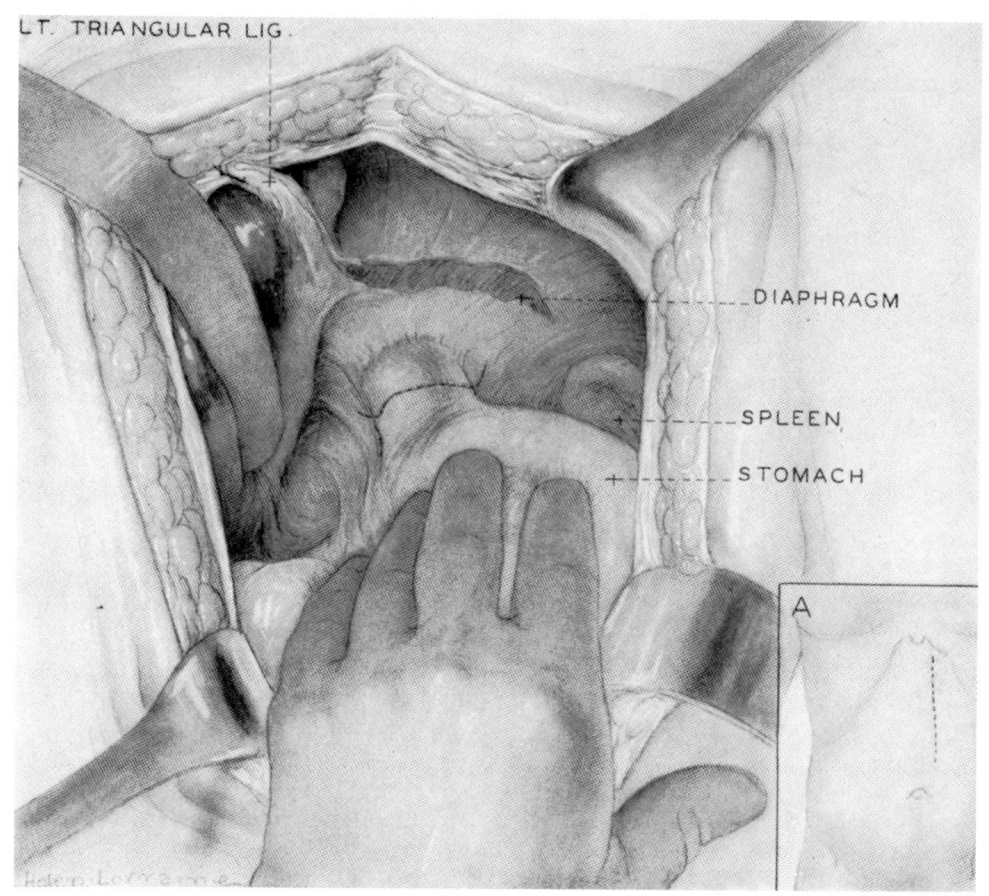

Figure 13-30. Total gastrectomy *(continued).* The left triangular ligament of the liver has been severed and sutured to the right abdominal wall to retract the left lobe of the liver. The broken line denotes the site of incision in the peritoneum for exposure of the esophagus. *A,* Line of abdominal incision. (From Orr, T. G.: Operations of General Surgery, 2nd ed. Philadelphia, W. B. Saunders Company, 1949.)

The distal stump of the duodenum is closed in two layers. The cut end of the stomach is covered with gauze to prevent contamination and held forward while that organ is freed posteriorly toward the cardia. If extension of the tumor or peritoneal implants make necessary the removal of the peritoneum of the posterior wall of the lesser peritoneal sac, it is resected. The greater curvature of the stomach is freed by severing and ligating the vasa brevia if the spleen is to be left in place. Usually in total gastrectomy it is desirable to remove the spleen with the stomach, in which case the splenic artery and vein are clamped, cut and ligated at the tail of the pancreas just prior to their formation of the splenic pedicle (Fig. 13–29). The spleen is mobilized by freeing its lateral peritoneal attachments, but it is left attached to the stomach with which it is later removed.

With the greater curvature and the spleen mobilized, the stomach is reflected upward and to the left. This maneuver exposes the left gastric vessels. The left gastric vein is traced down to its junction with the splenic vein, at which point it is divided and ligated.

The left gastric artery is traced to the celiac axis, where it is divided and ligated. All lymph nodes in these areas are dissected away with the stomach. The stomach is now free everywhere except at its attachment to the esophagus.

The left triangular ligament of the liver is incised (Fig. 13–30) and either retracted to the right or sutured to the right abdominal wall so as to retract the left lobe of the

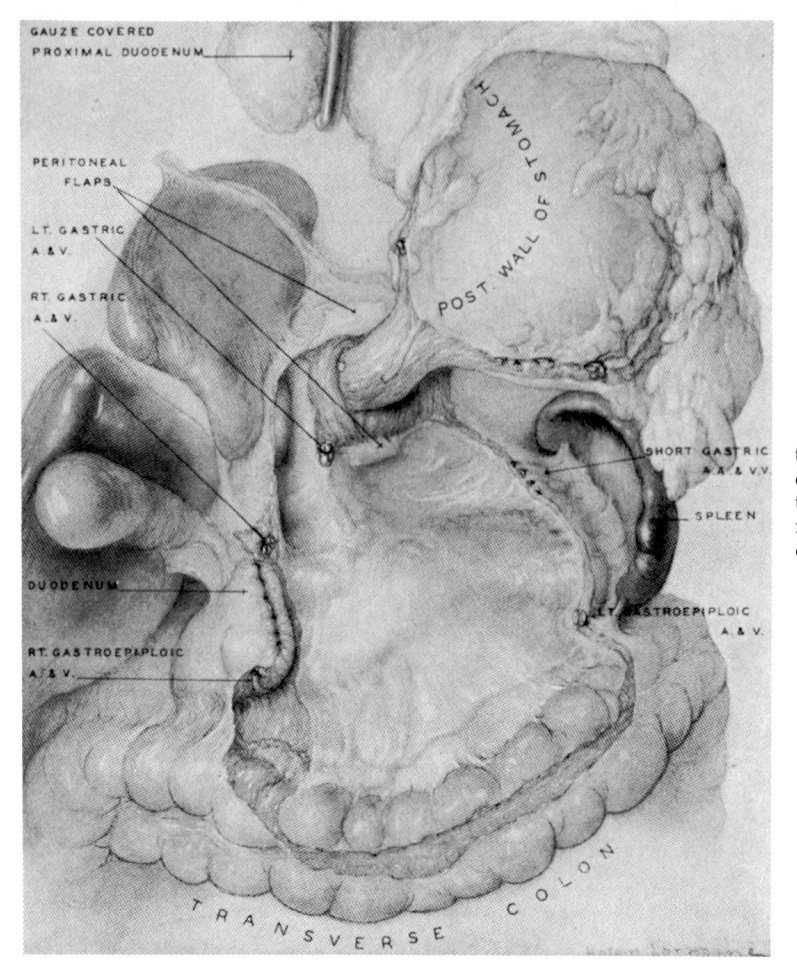

Figure 13-31. Total gastrectomy *(continued)*. The stomach and omentum have been freed and retracted. The esophagus is exposed, ready for anastomosis. (From Orr, cited in previous figure.)

liver to the right of the operative field. (The remaining part of the operation is much more easily done if the thoracicoabdominal incision recommended is used.)

A peritoneal flap is raised, which starts from the gastrohepatic omentum and extends across the anterior wall of the esophagogastric junction to the left side of the diaphragm (Fig. 13-30). This flap is continued around the posterior wall of the esophagus until that structure is circumcised through the peritoneal layer.

The anterior flap of peritoneum is elevated, and the vagus nerve on each side of the esophagus is exposed and cut. This procedure permits the esophagus to be pulled several centimeters farther into the abdomen (Fig. 13-31). A segment of jejunum is now identified by tracing it back to its origin at the ligament of Treitz. The decision is made whether to bring this loop of jejunum up to the esophagus in front of or behind the transverse colon. Longmire recommends a retrocolic type, as at times he has found the jejunal mesentery to be too short to permit the longer antecolic route. Even with the retrocolic method, on several occasions he has found it necessary to divide one of the primary mesenteric arteries to the jejunal loop to afford sufficient length for the anastomosis. Other surgeons prefer the antecolic route and have found it satisfactory.

When the decision has been made for a retrocolic anastomosis, an opening is made in the transverse mesocolon. The loop of jejunum is brought through this opening and approximated to the posterior wall of the esophagus while the stomach, serving as a retractor, is held upward and to the left, out of the operative field. A posterior row of interrupted Lembert sutures of silk is placed so as to unite the posterior wall of the esophagus to the jejunum (Fig. 13-32).

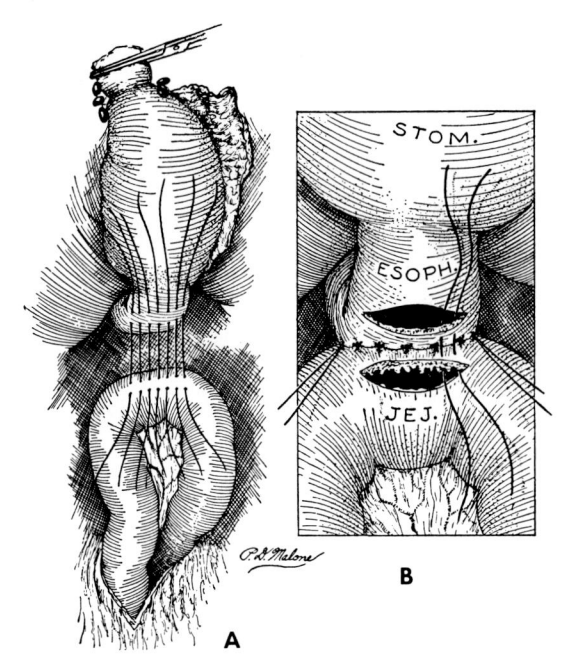

Figure 13–32. Total gastrectomy (continued). *A*, Stomach freed and retracted over upper angle of incision. Posterior row of interrupted silk sutures placed between jejunal loop and posterior wall of esophagus. *B*, Opening made into lumen of esophagus and jejunum. Second posterior row consists of interrupted catgut sutures which pass through the entire thickness of the wall of esophagus and jejunum. (From Longmire, W. P.: Total gastrectomy for carcinoma of the stomach. Surg. Gynecol. Obstet. *84*:21, 1947.)

These sutures are all placed before any are tied. After tying, the long ends of the first and last sutures placed are left uncut to serve as tractors. The long ends of the other sutures are cut (Fig. 13–32*B*). An opening is then made into the lumen of both the esophagus and jejunum (Fig. 13–32*B*). These openings should equal the diameter of the lumen of the esophagus. A second posterior row of interrupted 2–0 chromic catgut or silk sutures (some surgeons prefer a continuous lock-stitch suture here) swaged on an atraumatic intestinal needle is placed so as to pass through the entire thickness of the wall of the esophagus and jejunum and carefully approximate the mucosal edges.

The anterior wall of the esophagus is divided, and the specimen consisting of the stomach, spleen, omentum, and lymph glands is removed from the operating table. That part of the nasogastric tube that was in the stomach and now projects beyond the cut end of the esophagus is placed through the jejunal opening into the efferent loop of the jejunum.

The anterior suture line, consisting of a row of interrupted catgut or silk sutures, is reinforced by a second row of interrupted silk sutures as was previously done with the posterior suture line. Each angle is reinforced by a mattress suture of silk.

The peritoneal flap previously formed is now sutured over the anastomosis to the jejunum (Fig. 13–33). This step helps to support the jejunal loop as well as to reinforce the suture line.

The cut edges of the opening in the transverse mesocolon are sutured obliquely across the jejunal limbs to secure any opening against internal hernia later. The obliquity is to prevent later constriction of the jejunum by cicatrical contraction of the transverse mesocolon.

Longmire does not consider jejunojejunostomy between the afferent and efferent loops necessary in either antecolic or retrocolic esophagojejunostomy.

If a thoracicoabdominal incision was used (Longmire used an upper midline abdominal incision), a stab wound is placed in the ninth intercostal space in the midaxillary line through which a 14 F. catheter is left within the left thoracic cavity for drainage. Its outer end is attached to rubber tubing, the open end of which is placed under a water trap. This tube can usually be removed 48 hours postoperatively.

The diaphragm is sutured with interrupted stitches of heavy silk.

The thoracic part of the incision is closed by reapproximating the separated eighth and ninth ribs with a rib approximator or two temporarily placed perichondrial sutures of heavy silk, while the intercostal muscles are approximated with interrupted sutures of chromic catgut or silk. It is not necessary to suture the divided ninth and tenth cartilages as they will fall into place. In some instances, for greater exposure it is helpful to excise a 6- to 8-cm. segment of these cartilages. When this has been done, it is not necessary to replace those segments of cartilage.

The fascial layer is closed with interrupted sutures of stainless steel wire or silk. The subcutaneous layer is approximated with interrupted sutures of catgut or silk and the skin is closed with interrupted sutures.

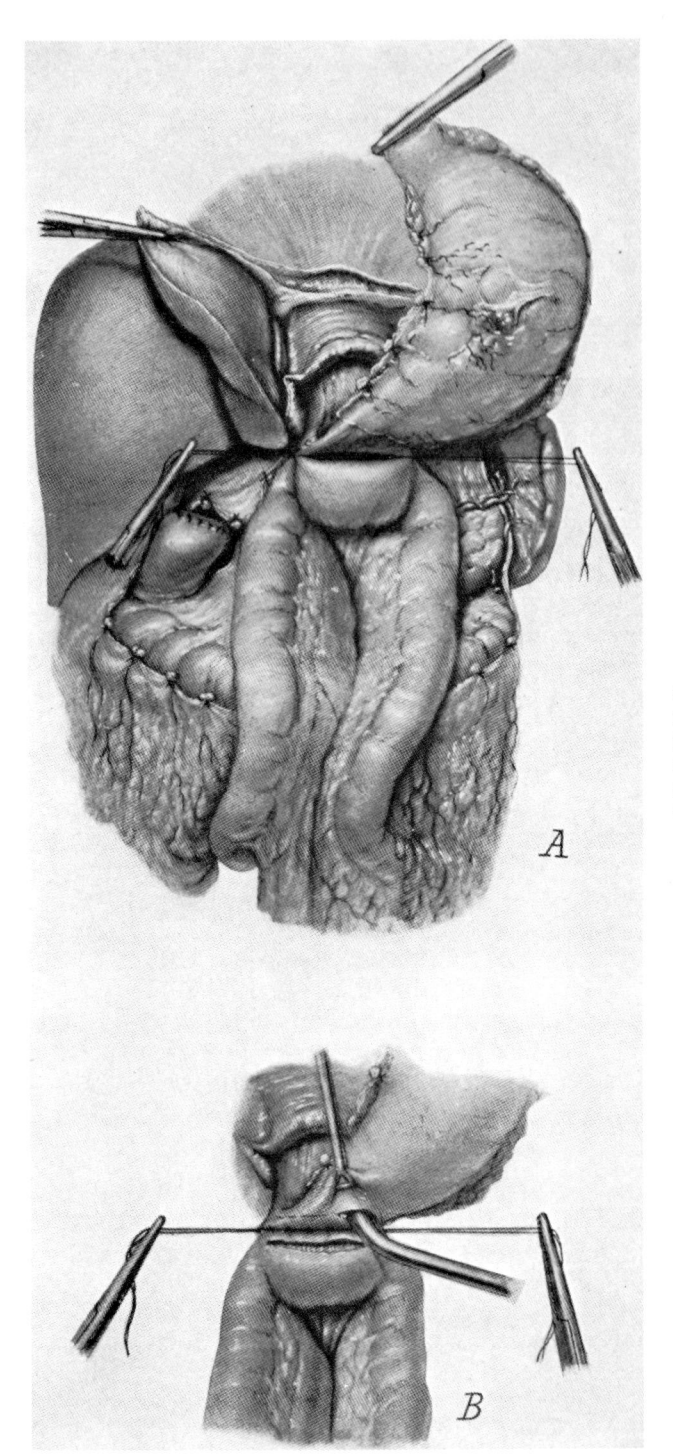

Figure 13-33. Total gastrectomy (continued). A, Stomach and lower end of esophagus mobilized. Stomach left attached for traction. Jejunum attached to esophagus with two traction sutures. B, First row of interrupted silk sutures completed. Esophagus opened and gastric contents aspirated.

Pre- and Postoperative Care

The patient is given a short course of antibiotic therapy.

Opinion is divided as to whether the nasogastric tube should be left through the anastomosis into the jejunum. It is a comforting safety valve should postoperative distention develop. Some surgeons claim that it may interfere with the healing of the anastomosis. However, if it is removed, difficulty in reinserting it through the anastomosis, should this be desirable, might be met. We leave it in place for the first 3 or 4 postoperative days, after which it is removed.

The patient is permitted nothing by mouth for the first 3 days. Then small amounts of liquid are permitted at frequent intervals, gradually increasing the volume as tolerated. A soft diet is not permitted until after the tenth day, and solids only after the twelfth day. Feedings are better tolerated if administered six times a day in half the normal portions rather than three times a day in full portions.

Intravenous feedings and frequently hyperalimentation are used until the daily oral intake becomes adequate for the patient's needs.

LAHEY METHOD

The operation is carried out exactly as is the Longmire technic, except that the loop of jejunum is brought anterior to the transverse colon for its anastomosis with the esophagus. In addition, a jejunojejunostomy is employed.

A long left upper rectus incision is used. The steps of the operation are well illustrated in Figure 13–34 through 13–43.

ORR METHOD

The mobilizing steps in this operation are the same as those detailed in the Longmire technic. The great omentum is dissected off the transverse colon. The duodenum is mobilized and cut across below the pylorus and its distal segment closed. The right gastric, gastroduodenal, right gastroepiploic, splenic, and left gastric arteries are cut and tied, and the stomach and spleen are mobilized upward as described under the Longmire method.

The Orr method (Orr, 1949) differs from those of Longmire and Lahey in that the esophagojejunostomy is performed in the manner of a Roux-en-Y anastomosis instead of as an end-to-side esophagojejunostomy (Fig. 13–44). This is accomplished in the following manner. After the stomach, spleen, and omentum have been mobilized up to the esophagus, the jejunum is identified and divided between clamps about 15

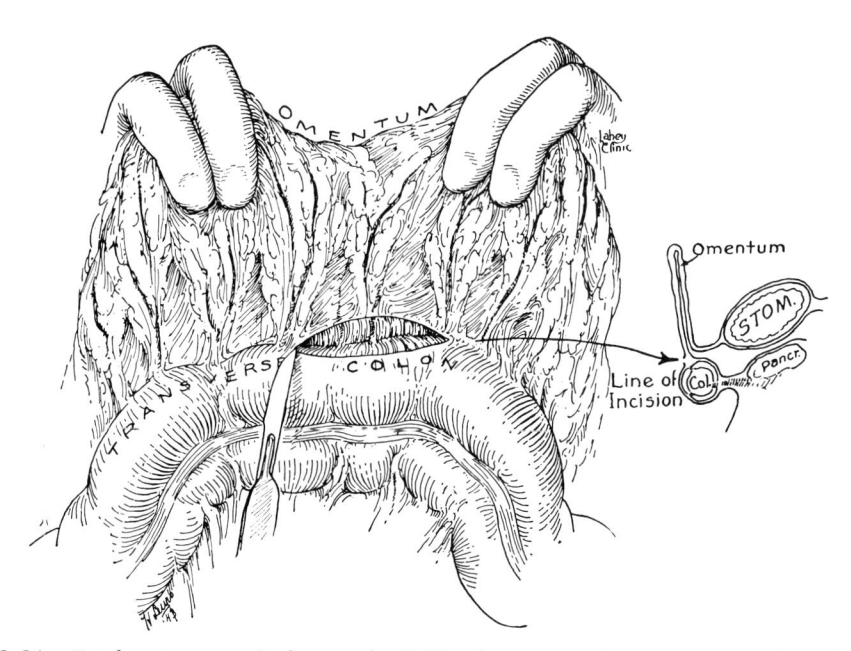

Figure 13–34. Total gastrectomy (Lahey method). The first step in the separation is sharp dissection of the omentum from the transverse colon. Note the avascular line of cleavage. Note the developmental line of cleavage and the line of incision in the avascular area (insert). (From Lahey, F. H., and Marshall, S. F.: Indications for, and experiences with, total gastrectomy based upon 73 cases of total gastrectomy. Ann. Surg. 119:300, 1944.)

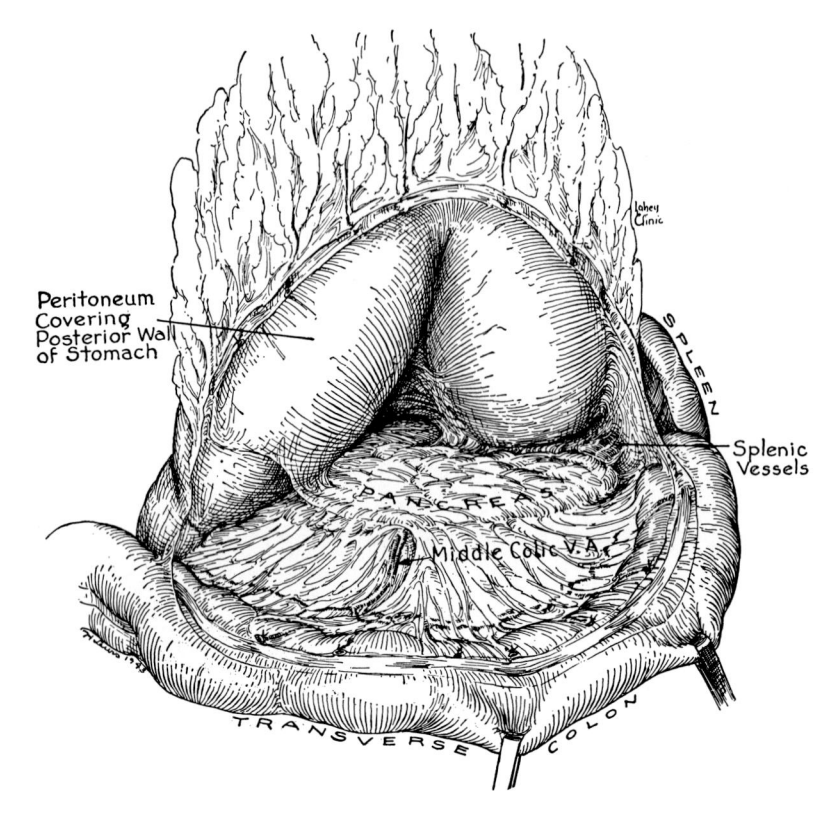

Figure 13-35. Total gastrectomy (Lahey method) *(continued)*. The omentum is completely separated from the transverse colon and is still attached to the greater curvature. The pancreas is visualized, and the stomach is turned up. Note the splenic vessels beyond the tip of the pancreas. (From Lahey and Marshall, cited in the previous figure.)

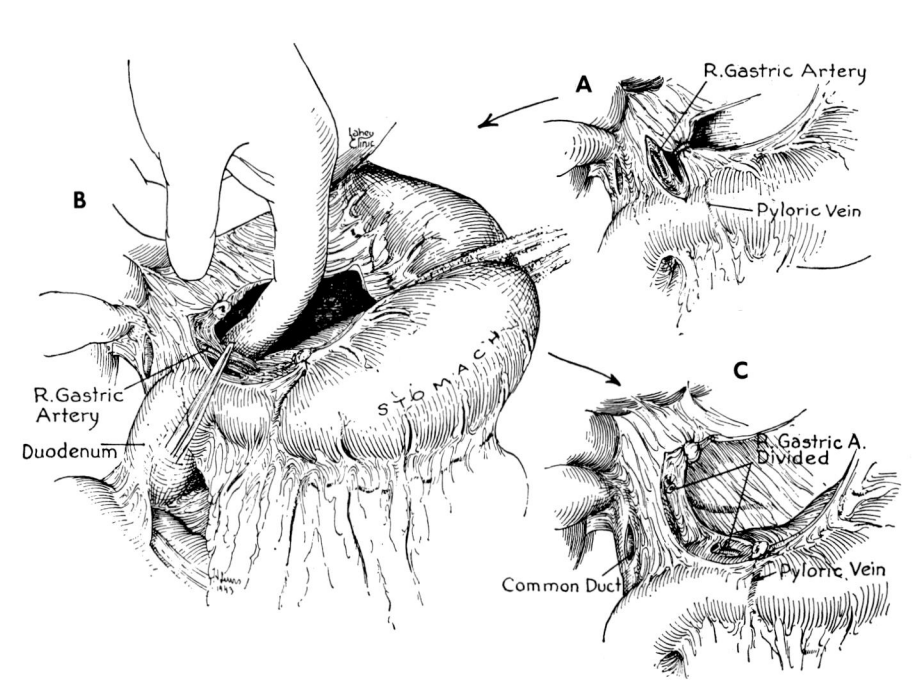

Figure 13-36. Total gastrectomy (Lahey method) *(continued)*. *A*, The lesser peritoneal cavity is opened through the gastrohepatic omentum. *B*, The right gastric artery and vein are clamped close to the pylorus. *C*, Vessels of the gastrohepatic omentum have been ligated, and the lesser curvature is cleared. (From Lahey and Marshall, cited in Figure 13-34.)

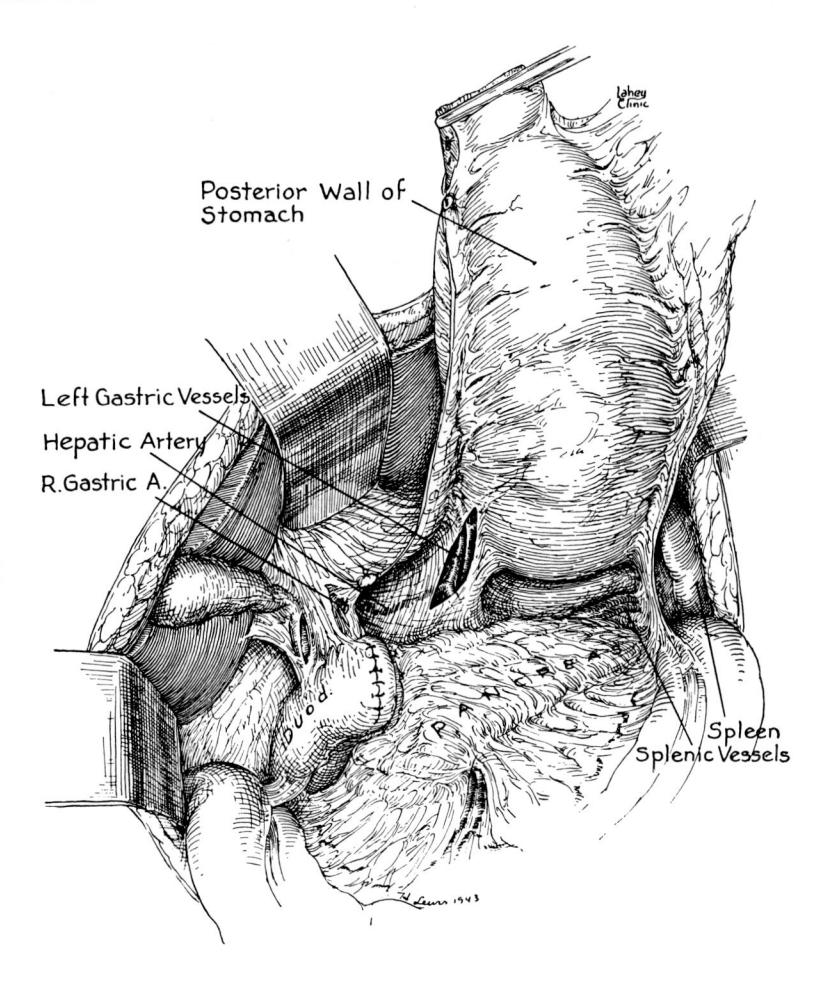

Figure 13-37. Total gastrectomy (Lahey method) *(continued)*. The duodenum has been cut across and inverted, and the stomach has been lifted higher. Note the exposure of the left gastric vessels ready for ligation (From Lahey and Marshall, cited in Figure 13-34.)

to 20 cm. below the ligament of Treitz. The proximal end is covered with gauze and held for later anastomosis. The distal end of the cut jejunum is closed in two layers.

An opening is made in the transverse mesocolon, and the distal jejunal segment is drawn through it and anastomosed to the esophagus 5 to 6 cm. distal to its closed end. The anastomosis is performed in the same manner as in the Longmire and Lahey technics. (The jejunal segment may be brought anterior to the colon instead of posteriorly through the transverse mesocolon if desired). Orr uses a continuous lock-stitch to unite the mucosal surfaces of the esophagus and jejunum instead of the interrupted sutures described in the Longmire technic; however, the outer serosal layer of sutures consists of interrupted silk sutures. This anastomosis line is covered with the peritoneal flap, as detailed in the Longmire technic.

Intestinal continuity is re-established by an end-to-side anastomosis between the proximal end of the severed jejunum and the side of the distal segment of the jejunum below the mesocolon. If the esophagojejunostomy is retrocolic, the opening in the transverse mesocolon is sutured about the jejunum and its mesentery. The jejunojejunostomy is performed 40 cm. from the esophagojejunostomy to prevent reflux of bile. The operation is illustrated in Figure 13-27 (p. 308).

The incision is closed as described in Longmire's technic. Orr's technic has the disadvantage of requiring an additional bowel closure. If later trouble develops, an antecolic type of esophagojejunostomy should be easier to reoperate upon.

Text continued on page 323

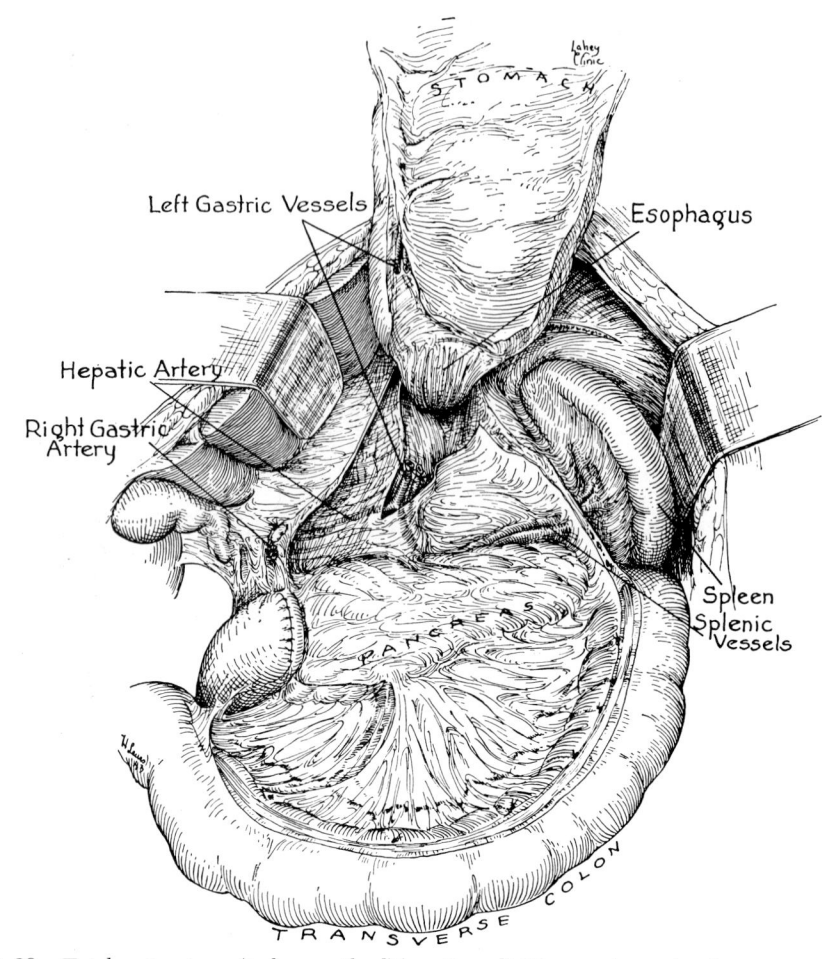

Figure 13-38. Total gastrectomy (Lahey method)*(continued)*. The esophagus has been exposed and freed, the stomach has been turned up, and the pedicle of the spleen has been visualized. The left gastric vessels have been ligated. The spleen is ready to be removed with the stomach. (From Lahey and Marshall, cited in Figure 13-34.)

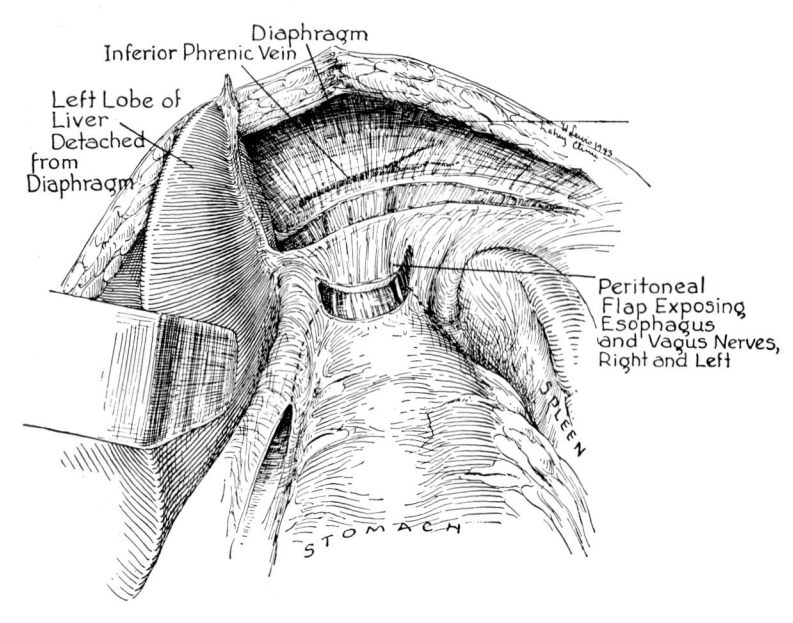

Figure 13-39. Total gastrectomy (Lahey method)*(continued)*. The left lobe of the liver is mobilized to the right, and the anterior flap of the peritoneum is reflected up over the esophagus. This is used later to suspend the jejunum in order to remove traction from the anastomotic line. (From Lahey and Marshall, cited in Figure 13-34.)

TOTAL GASTRECTOMY AND RECONSTRUCTION

Figure 13–40. Total gastrectomy (Lahey method) *(continued)*. *A*, The preliminary introduction of a posterior row of untied silk sutures before opening the jejunum. Note the ease with which the jejunum may be opened and trimmed to fit the esophagus. *B*, When the sutures are put in and tied before the jejunum is opened, satisfactory management as to size and fit of the jejunal opening is difficult with the jejunum pulled high up under the stomach. (From Lahey and Marshall, cited in Figure 13–34.)

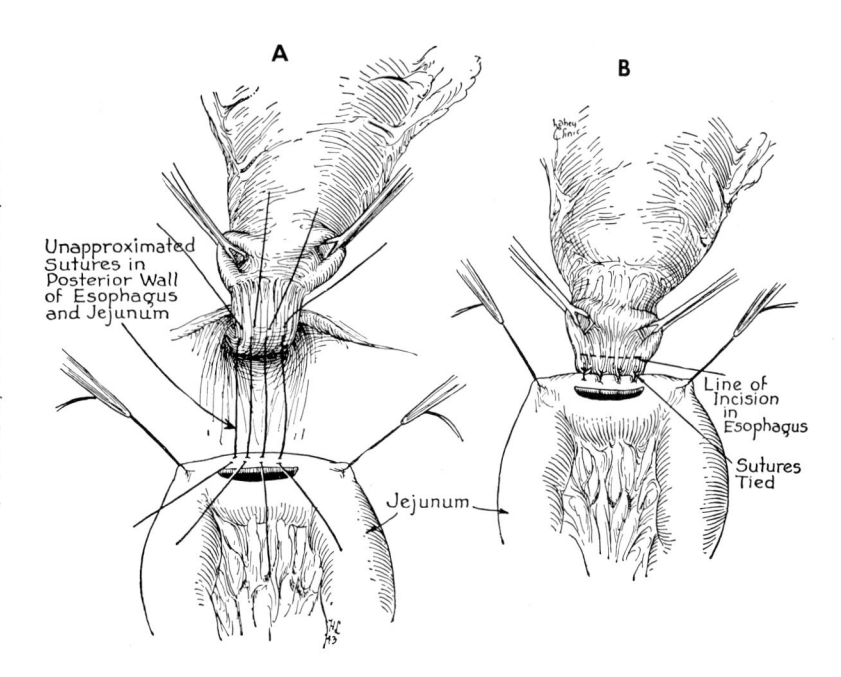

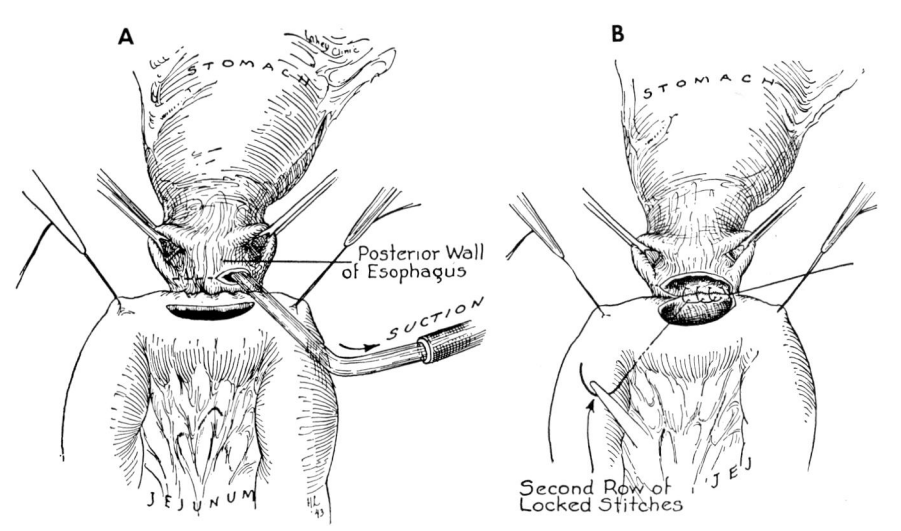

Figure 13–41. Total gastrectomy (Lahey method) *(continued)*. *A*, The traction stitches to hold the anastomotic opening are spread apart. The first row of silk stitches already has been tied. Note the small opening in the esophagus. *B*, Note the locked stitches employed a step at a time as the opening gradually is increased in size until the entire posterior second row of stitches has been inserted. (From Lahey and Marshall, cited in Figure 13–34.)

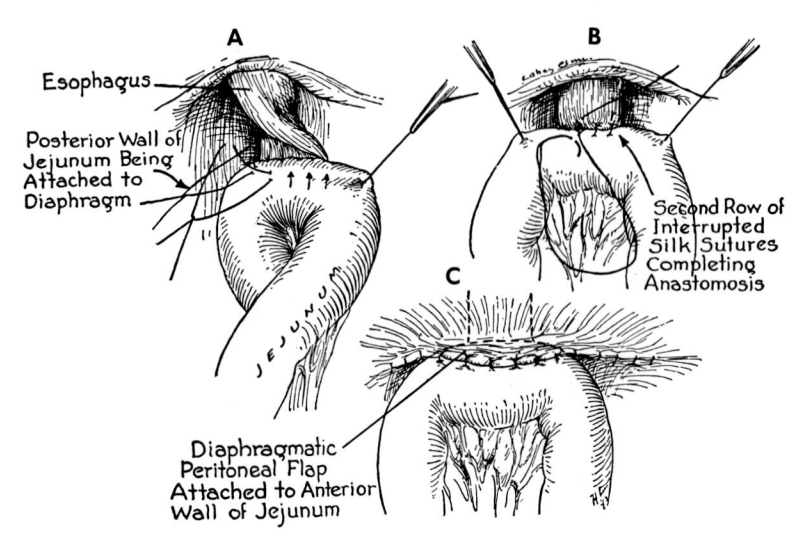

Figure 13-42. Total gastrectomy (Lahey method) *(continued)*. *A*, The method of twisting the esophagojejunal anastomosis in order to inspect the posterior row of sutures, and the insertion of suspensory jejunal sutures posteriorly to take the strain off the posterior row of the anastomotic suture line. *B*, The application of the anterior second row of silk approximation sutures. *C*, The previously fashioned flap of diaphragmatic peritoneum sutured to the jejunum over the anastomosis to reinforce it, to suspend the jejunum, and to relieve traction on the anastomotic line. (From Lahey and Marshall, cited in Figure 13-34.)

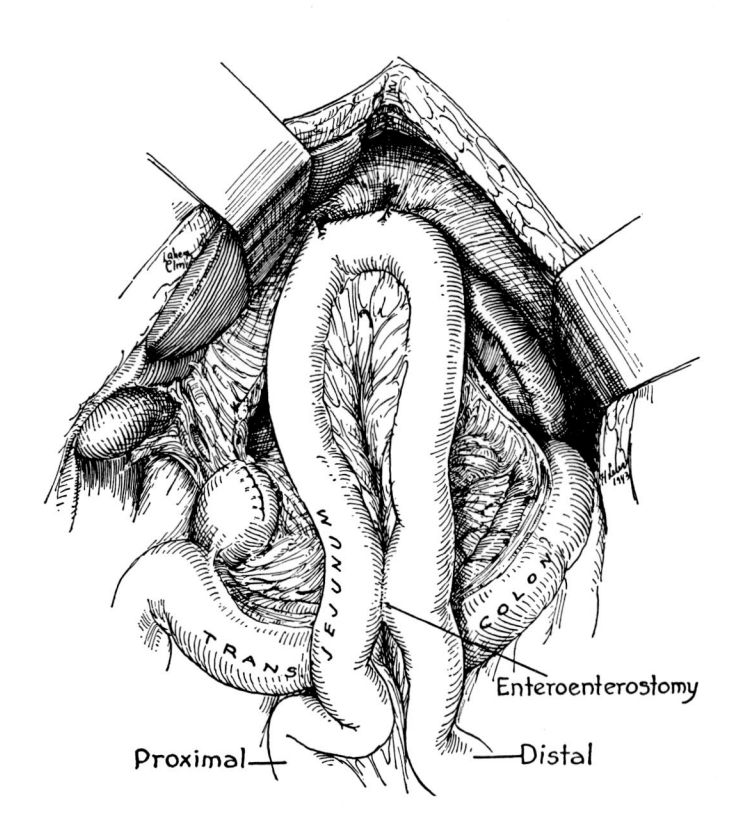

Figure 13-43. Total gastrectomy (Lahey method) *(continued)*. The antecolic esophagojejunal anastomosis with additional suspension sutures to the diaphragm. Note the enteroenterostomy. (From Lahey and Marshall, cited in Figure 13-34.)

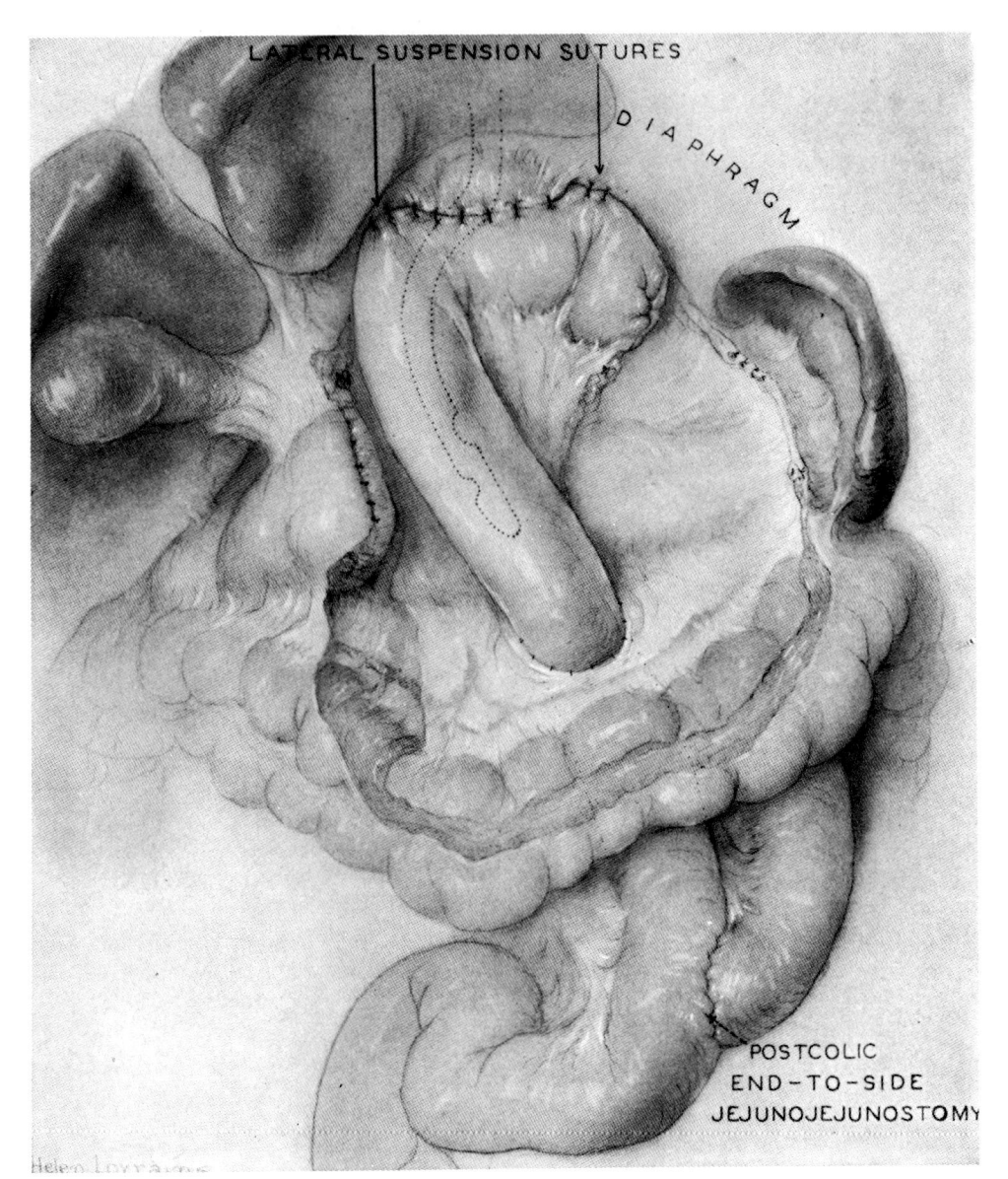

Figure 13-44. Total gastrectomy (Orr method). Anastomosis of esophagus to jejunum and end-to-side jejunojejunostomy completed. A tube is shown passed through the esophagojejunostomy. (From Orr, T. G.: Operations of General Surgery, 2nd ed. Philadelphia, W. B. Saunders Company, 1949.)

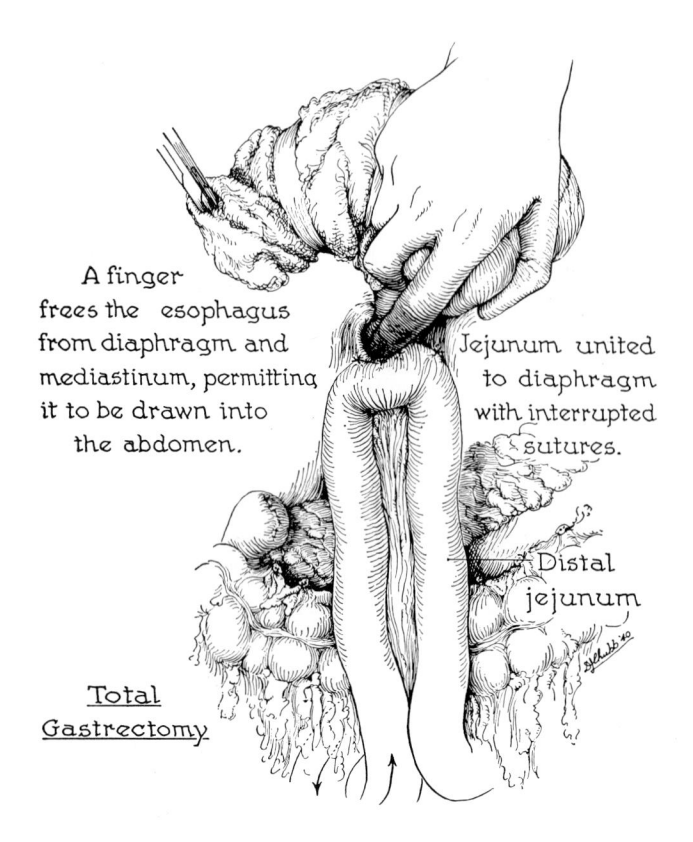

Figure 13-45. First stage of Graham's method of anastomosing the esophagus to the jejunum in performance of total gastrectomy. (From Graham, R. R.: A technic for total gastrectomy. Surgery 8:257, 1940.)

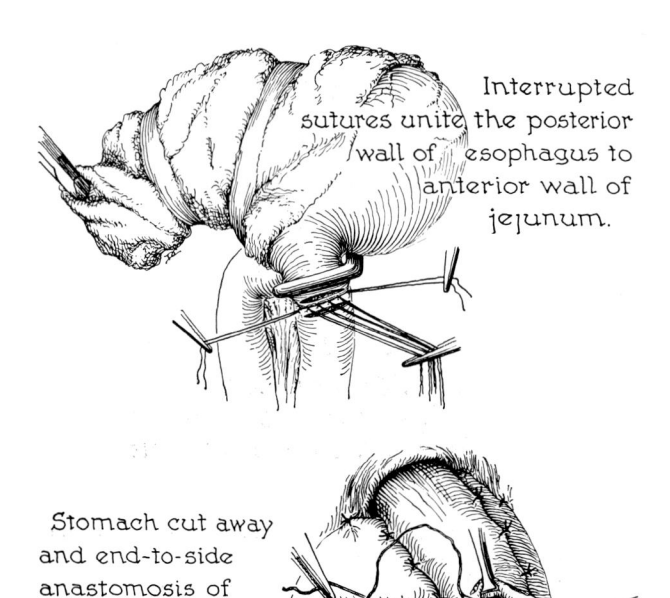

Figure 13-46. Third and fourth stages of Graham's method of total gastrectomy. (From Graham, cited in previous figure.)

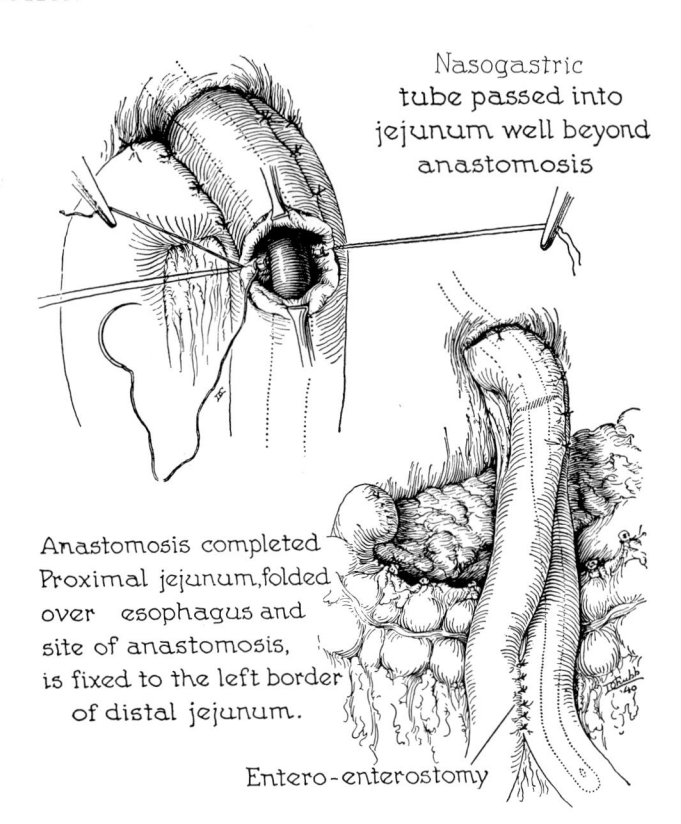

Figure 13-47. Fifth and sixth stages of Graham's method of total gastrectomy. (From Graham, cited in Figure 13-45.)

GRAHAM METHOD

This procedure (Graham, 1940) differs from the Longmire technic only in its method of esophagojejunal anastomosis and the fact that with it the *employment of a jejunojejunostomy is essential.*

The stomach is mobilized as described in the Longmire technic. The loop of jejunum is brought up in front of the colon and united to the diaphragm with interrupted silk suture (Fig. 13-45). The posterior wall of the esophagus is again united to the anterior wall of the jejunum by a layer of interrupted silk sutures, which will form the posterior layer of the esophagojejunostomy. A transverse incision is made in the posterior wall of the esophagus, and a matching transverse incision is made in the anterior wall of the jejunum. The posterior edges of these incisions are united by a 2-0 chromic catgut or silk continuous lock-stitch through all the layers (Fig. 13-46). Severance of the esophagus is completed, and the specimen is removed. The nasogastric tube is passed into the distal jejunum well beyond the anastomosis (Fig. 13-47). The anterior cut edges are approximated by a continuous inverting 2-0 chromic catgut or silk suture, which is reinforced by a second row of interrupted Lembert sutures of silk. Each angle is secured by a silk U-stitch (see p. 303).

After the anastomosis is completed, the proximal jejunum is folded over the esophagus and site of esophagojejunal anastomosis and is sutured to the left border of the distal jejunum (Fig. 13-47) with interrupted silk sutures. Thus the proximal jejunum becomes a patch over the anastomosis. This procedure *obstructs* the proximal jejunal loop, so it is essential that a *jejunojejunostomy* be performed (Fig. 13-47).

A side-to-side jejunojejunostomy is performed with an inner row of catgut sutures and an outer row of silk sutures at a level about 12 cm. below the esophagojejunostomy.

This method is more time consuming and not as widely used as some of the other methods described.

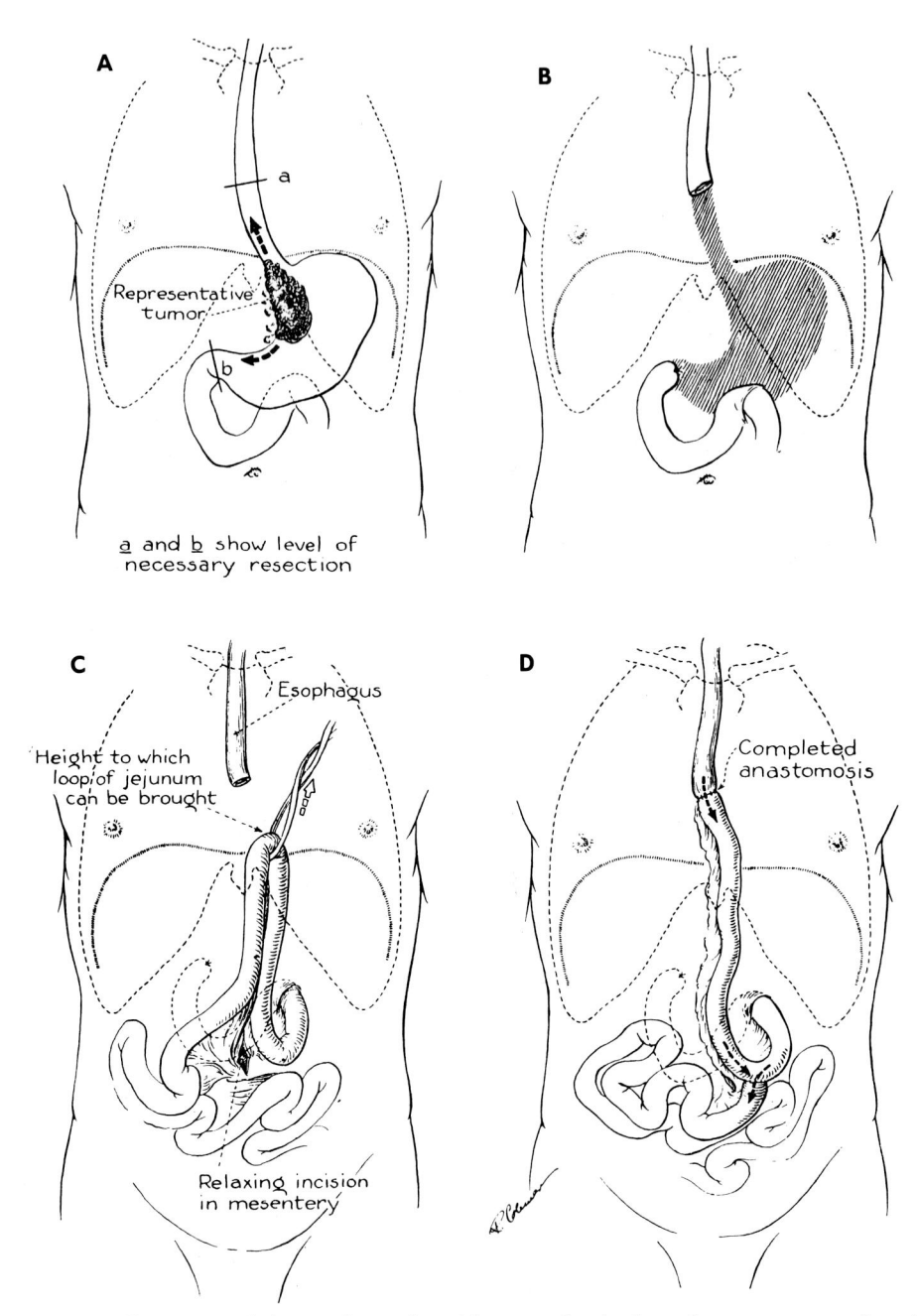

Figure 13–48. Illustration of the mechanical problem involved when the entire stomach and the lower esophagus must be removed. *A*, A representative tumor, the arrows indicating the direction of metastases; *B* emphasizes the extent of the defect after such a resection; *C* shows the difficulty (at times insurmountable) of bringing a loop of jejunum high enough to accomplish anastomosis; *D* illustrates the ease with which a Roux-en-Y loop will meet the esophagus. The importance of blood supply to this loop is more thoroughly emphasized in Figures 13–49 and 13–51. (From Reynolds, J. T., and Young, J. P.: Use of Roux Y in extending operability of carcinoma of stomach and of lower end of esophagus. Surgery 24:246, 1948. Correction, 24:731, 1948.)

TOTAL GASTRECTOMY AND RECONSTRUCTION

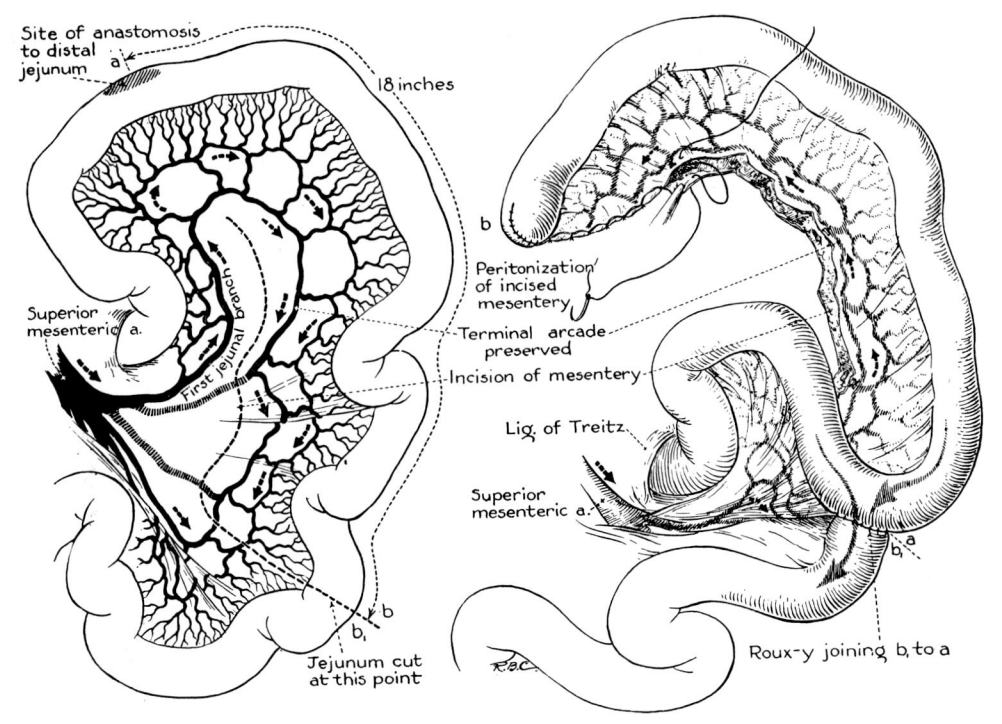

Figure 13–49. Roux-en-Y total gastrectomy as recommended by Rienhoff. Note the meticulous preservation of the first jejunal branch of the superior mesenteric artery; also note that the Roux Y so constructed provides the loop with peristalsis against intended direction. This does not seem to influence the course of food from the anastomosis with the esophagus on its course to the rest of the intestinal tract. Shaded arrows indicate the course taken by food and by bile and pancreatic juices. (From Reynolds and Young, cited in previous figure.)

ROUX-EN-Y TOTAL GASTRECTOMY

Antiperistaltic Segment

In some instances carcinoma of the cardiac end of the stomach extends up into the esophagus (Fig. 13–48A). To extirpate the tumor it may be necessary to resect a considerable length of esophagus (Fig. 13–48B). Transection of the esophagus at such a high level may make it difficult or impossible to bring a loop of jejunum to its proximal end (Fig. 13–48C) for anastomosis because the jejunal mesentery is not long enough to reach that high. In such instances the length of jejunum obtainable may be increased by transecting the distal portion of the loop (Fig. 13–49), severing its mesenteric vessels so as to preserve the arterial arch (see dotted line of Fig. 13–49) but meticulously preserving the first jejunal arterial branch (Fig. 13–49) and anastomosing this elongated segment to the esophagus (Fig. 13–48D). The cut end of the proximal segment of jejunum is anastomosed to the side of the elongated distal segment (Figs. 13–48D and 13–49) to complete a Roux-en-Y esophagojejunostomy. The fact that the loop of elongated jejunum is antiperistaltic apparently has no deleterious effect on the passage of food down it, but whenever possible an isoperistaltic segment is preferred.

The elongated loop of jejunum is brought through the transverse mesocolon behind the transverse colon, as this is the shortest route.

INDICATIONS. This method of total gastrectomy is used in treatment of carcinoma of the stomach or lower esophagus in which a jejunal loop is too short to be approximated to the cut end of the esophagus by an end-of-esophagus-to-side-of-jejunum anastomosis. Its principle can be applied in a palliative end-of-jejunum-to-side-of-esophagus esophagojejunostomy for inoperable carcinoma of the lower esophagus or cardiac end of the stomach (Fig. 13–50).

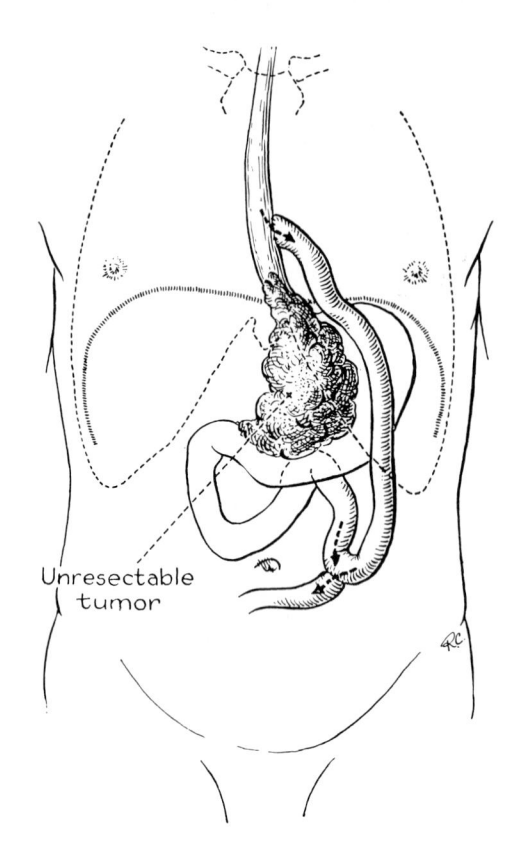

Figure 13–50. The use of a Roux-en-Y loop to circumvent obstruction due to unremovable tumor in the region of the cardia of the stomach. The procedure is also applicable for circumventing a tumor that is confined strictly to the stomach. (From Reynolds and Young, cited in Figure 13–48.)

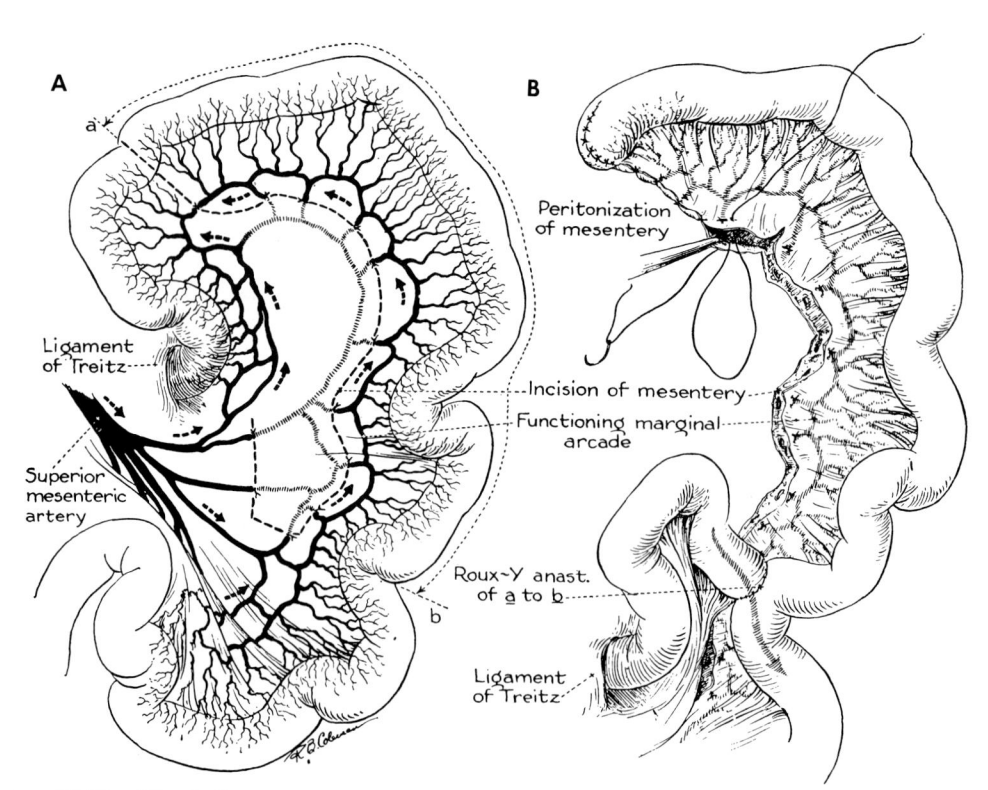

Figure 13–51. Classic Roux-en-Y anastomosis. *A*, The first portion of jejunum with blood supply from the superior mesenteric artery. Dotted line a to b indicates segment of bowel to be utilized in the anastomosis. Note that blood supply to this sector must come from short vessels supplied by small jejunal branches. *B*, Roux-en-Y anastomosis practically completed. (From Reynolds and Young, cited in Figure 13–48.)

TOTAL GASTRECTOMY AND RECONSTRUCTION

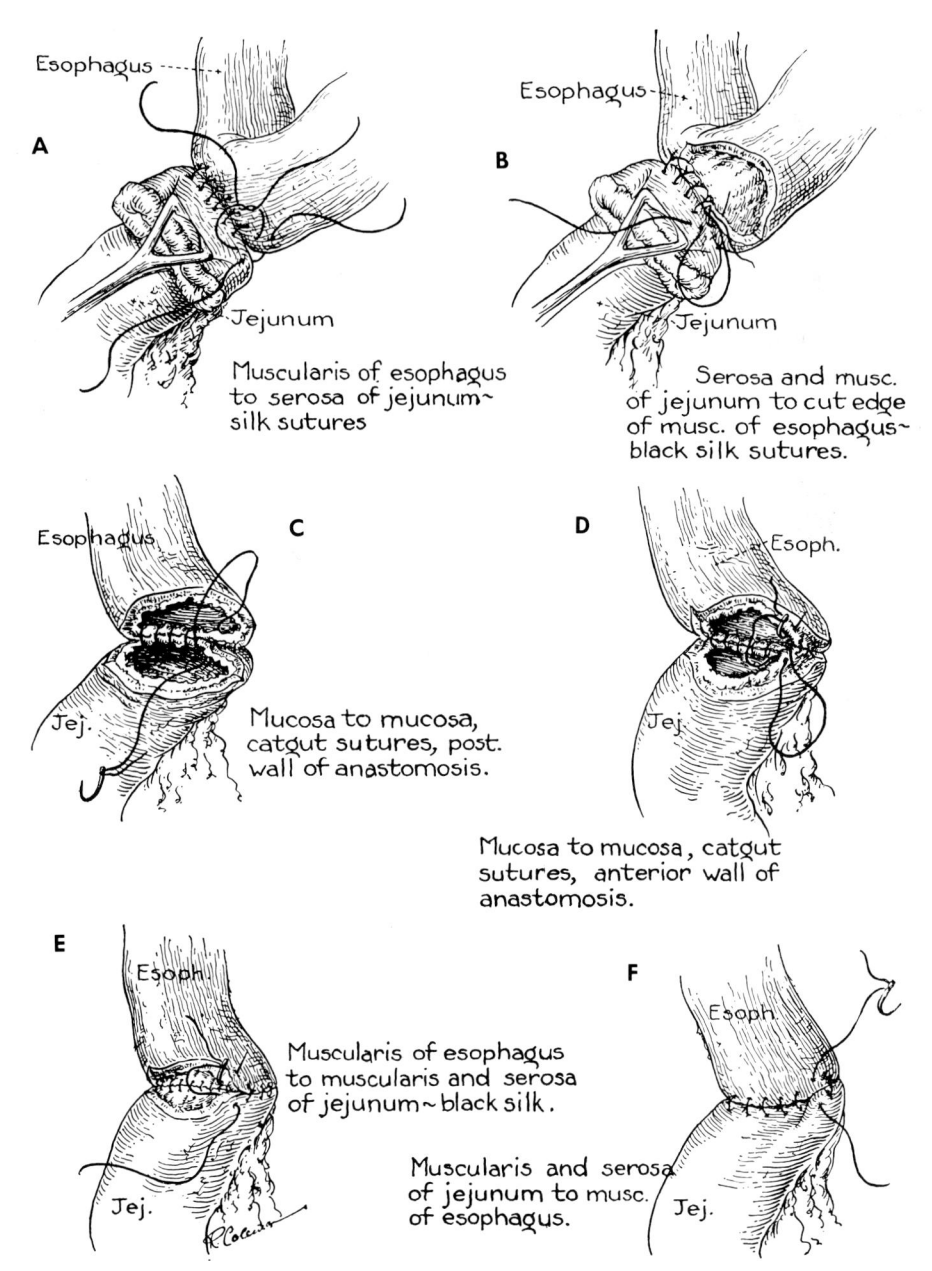

Figure 13–52. Roux-en-Y total gastrectomy. Technical details of anastomosis. *A*, Already placed interrupted sutures are shown being tied. *B*, The incision into esophageal muscularis shown should be at least 0.6 to 1 cm. distal to the first row of outer sutures. This is to allow for the muscular contraction that always follows. *C* and *D*, The use of continuous, very fine catgut in the mucosal stitch. *E*, The middle row of interrupted sutures. Black silk is used so it can be seen and excluded by the last layer, illustrated in *F*. (From Reynolds and Young, cited in Figure 13–48.)

Isoperistaltic Segment

The classic Roux-en-Y reconstruction consists of transecting the jejunum just distal to the ligament of Treitz and basing the distal cut end on the second and third jejunal vessels. The proximal end is oversewn and an end-to-side esophagojejunostomy is performed. Intestinal continuity is re-established by anastomosing the proximal end of the jejunum to the side of the jejunum 40 cm. distal to the esophagojejunostomy. This is represented in Figure 13–51, and also Figures 13–41 and 13–42. Occasionally an end-to-end anastomosis can be performed (Fig. 13–52). This method of re-

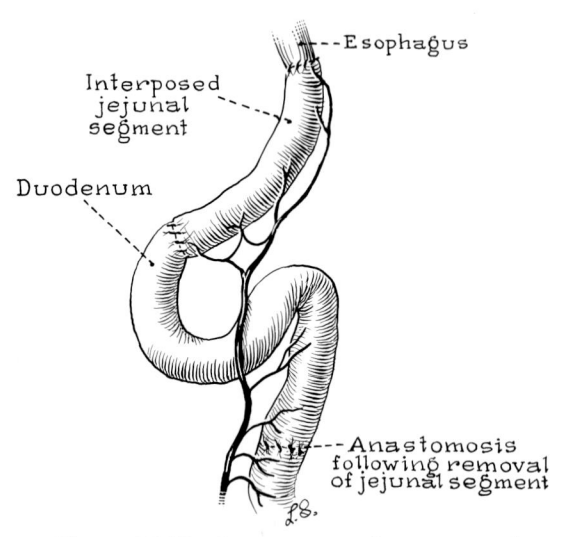

Figure 13–53. Interposition of a segment of jejunum between the esophagus and duodenum (Henle loop).

construction provides an isoperistaltic segment of jejunum from the esophagus.

The classic Roux-en-Y principle of transecting the jejunum near the ligament of Treitz, next anastomosing isoperistaltically the cut end of the distal segment end-to-side with the esophagus, and then anastomosing the cut end of the proximal segment of the jejunum to the side of the distal jejunal segment at a point at least 40 cm. below the esophagojejunostomy can also be used to bypass an unresectable esophageal or gastric tumor (Fig. 13–50).

JEJUNAL INTERPOSITION

Another method of reconstruction, described by Henley, consists of isolating a free segment of proximal jejunum on a vascular pedicle and interposing this segment by end-to-end anastomosis between the esophagus above and the duodenum below. When using this method of reconstruction, the duodenum is transected during the gastrectomy so that an end-to-end anastomosis with the jejunal segment is possible (Fig. 13–53).

RECONSTRUCTION WITH A RESERVOIR OR POUCH

Construction of a pouch or reservoir usually requires increased operative time as well as an increase in the number of anastomoses or suture lines. A simple pouch consists of a long enteroenterostomy either at or shortly below the esophagojejunostomy. Several types of reconstructions and pouches are shown in Figure 13–54.

TOTAL GASTRECTOMY WITH ESOPHAGODUODENOSTOMY

In some cases the duodenum can be mobilized sufficiently to be approximated end-to-end to the esophagus without tension after the entire stomach has been removed. When this is possible an esophagoduodenostomy is probably the most satisfactory method of restoring alimentary continuity because the duodenum seems to be less subject to irritation after an anastomosis than does the jejunum. The decision concerning performing an esophagoduodenostomy will depend upon the length of the duodenal and esophageal stumps that can be preserved, the amount that the duodenal stump can be mobilized, *the adequacy of the blood supply to the cut ends of both the esophageal and duodenal stumps, and the ability to approximate the esophagus and duodenum without the slightest tension.* If the latter criteria (given in italics) are not fulfilled, or there is doubt concerning them, the procedure should be abandoned and some type of esophagojejunostomy performed.

Technic

The entire stomach is mobilized as described in the Longmire technic for total gastrectomy, but as long a duodenal stump as is compatible with a safe margin below the lesion is preserved, and the duodenum is cut across immediately distal to a crushing clamp placed on the pyloric sphincter. No crushing clamp is placed on the duodenal side of the transection. The pyloric sphincter should be removed with the stomach as it is not satisfactory for use in the anastomosis. A rubber-shod occluding but *not crushing* clamp is placed across the duodenum below its cut edge to prevent

TOTAL GASTRECTOMY WITH ESOPHAGODUODENOSTOMY

SIMPLE RECONSTRUCTIONS

Esophago-jejunostomy

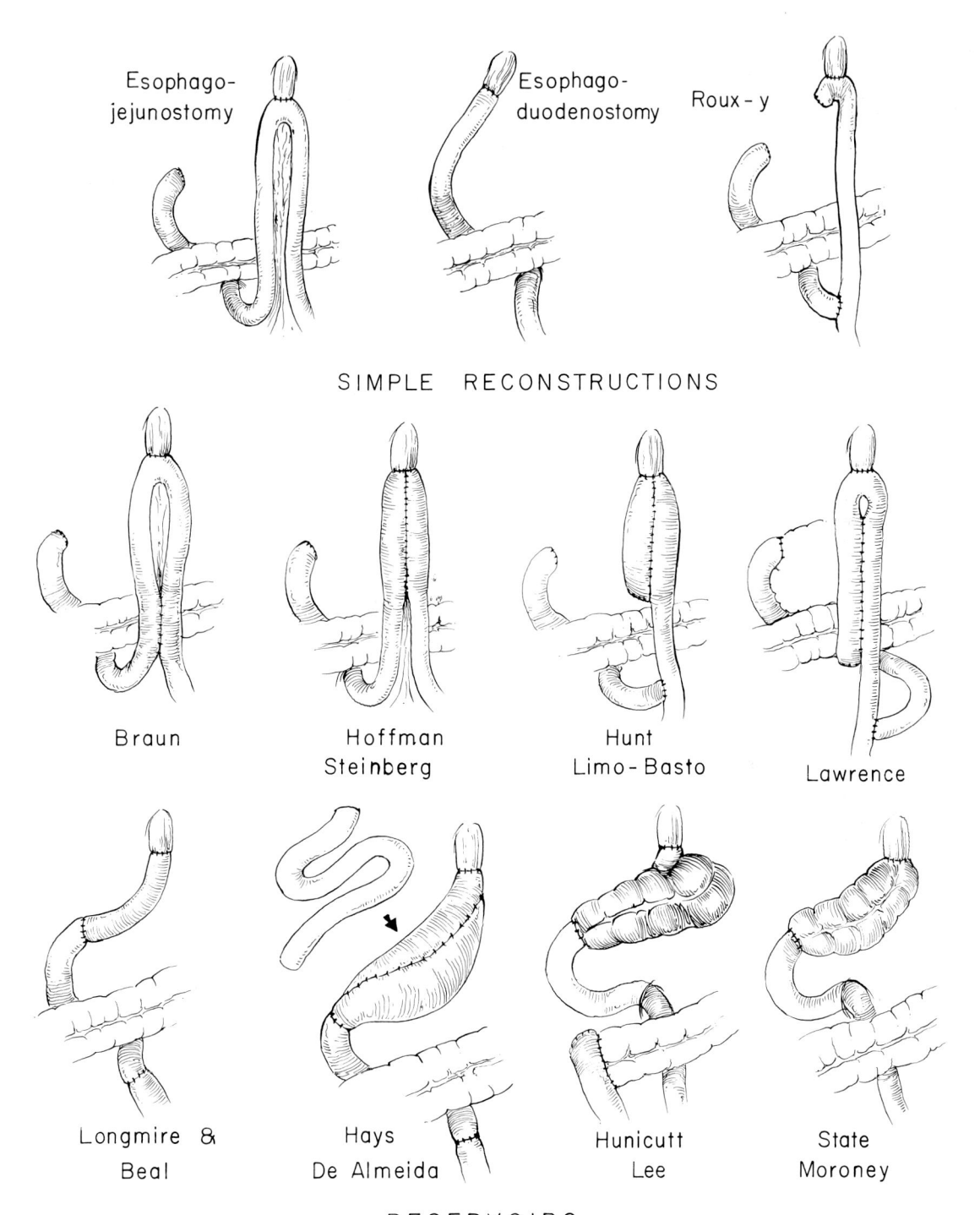

Esophago-duodenostomy

Roux-y

Braun

Hoffman Steinberg

Hunt Limo-Basto

Lawrence

Longmire & Beal

Hays De Almeida

Hunicutt Lee

State Moroney

RESERVOIRS

Figure 13–54. Variations of reconstruction following total gastrectomy. (From Nora, P. F. (ed.): Operative Surgery, 2nd ed. Philadelphia, Lea and Febiger, 1972, p. 437.)

spillage during the subsequent manipulations.

The esophagus is not transected until after the posterior suture lines of the anastomosis are completed, so that the attached stomach can serve for traction and thus the use of any clamps on the esophagus is avoided. After the duodenum is transected, however, an occluding clamp is placed across the upper portion of the stomach is held forward and upward during the placement of the posterior anastomotic suture line.

The duodenum is now mobilized by incising its lateral peritoneal reflection (see Fig. 2–3) along the descending portion. The superior margin (lesser curvature) of the duodenum is mobilized by dividing the supraduodenal branches of the gastroduodenal artery close to the duodenal wall, but if possible the main stem of the gastroduodenal artery is preserved so as to furnish a better blood supply through its superior pancreaticoduodenal branch (see Fig. 1–1) to the duodenal stump. In order to obtain adequate mobilization, it may be necessary to divide the main gastroduodenal artery, but if this is done the cut edge of the duodenal stump should be observed closely for duskiness, which may indicate an inadequate blood supply for it to be safely used in the anastomosis.

After the supraduodenal vessels have been divided, *the common duct, hepatic artery, and portal vein are identified and protected from injury* while the anterior peritoneal layer only of the hepatoduodenal ligament is divided. This permits the duodenal stump to be drawn as far medially and upward as the attachment of the common bile duct will permit. The common duct should not be purposely divided and reimplanted to provide greater mobility, as an esophagojejunostomy is preferable to this added step.

A centimeter or two of additional upward mobility can be obtained by dividing some of the small vessels on the inferior (greater curvature) margin of the duodenal stump, between it and the pancreas, but it is safer not to sacrifice too many of these because the pancreaticoduodenal vessels lie in that sulcus and may now be the chief source of blood supply to the duodenal stump.

The open end of the duodenal stump is now approximated to the esophagus at the level the latter is to be transected. If there is tension or if the cut ends have a dusky color indicating an inadequate blood supply, then esophagoduodenostomy should be abandoned and some type of esophagojejunostomy performed.

If, however, the duodenum and esophagus can be approximated without tension and the blood supply to their cut ends appears adequate, then esophagoduodenostomy is the procedure of choice, and this anastomosis is performed.

The posterior walls of the esophagus and duodenum are united with a row of interrupted mattress sutures of 2–0 silk, all sutures being placed before any are tied. After these sutures are tied, the long ends of the two end sutures are left uncut for traction while the long ends of the intervening sutures are cut. The posterior wall of the esophagus is now incised. The mucosal layers of the esophagus and duodenum are united by a row of interrupted or continuous sutures of 2–0 chromic catgut which first form a posterior row, after which the nasogastric tube is pushed down the esophagus and passed through the anastomotic stoma well down into the duodenum, in which position it is left. The anterior wall of the esophagus is divided and the specimen removed. The posterior row of catgut sutures is now continued around each angle and then as an anterior row to unite the mucosal layers of the anterior walls of the esophagus and duodenum, to complete the inner suture line of the anastomosis. This inner row of sutures penetrates all the layers of both the esophageal and duodenal walls. The anterior suture line is now reinforced by a row of interrupted mattress sutures of 2–0 silk which, like the posterior row of silk sutures, penetrates only the seromuscular coat of the duodenum and the muscular coat of the esophagus but does not enter into the lumen of either viscus. Each angle is reinforced by a 2–0 silk mattress suture which includes a bite in both the anterior and posterior walls of the esophagus and the duodenum. The peritoneal flap previously reflected off the diaphragm during the circumcision of the esophagus is now sutured over the anastomosis to the duodenum to support the duodenum and relieve tension of the anastomotic suture line, as well as to provide an additional seal.

This completes the operation. The incision is closed in layers.

TRANSPOSITION OF TERMINAL ILEUM AND ASCENDING COLON FOR SUBSTITUTE GASTRIC RESERVOIR (LEE)

Lee (1951) formed a substitute gastric reservoir by isolating the terminal ileum, cecum, and ascending colon with their blood supply preserved. After the entire stomach had been removed, this isolated segment of the right colon was rotated upward, and the stump of ileum was anastomosed end-to-end with the cut end of the esophagus. The transected hepatic flexure end of the ascending colon was anastomosed to the pyloric end of the duodenum. Continuity of the lower bowel was restored by a side-to-side ileotransversecolostomy (Fig. 13-55). Lee's case was successful; the cecum and ascending colon served satisfactorily as a substitute gastric reservoir.

Longmire and Beal (1952) employed this procedure in two patients, but in one of these gangrene of the ileocolic segment developed following the transposition and necessitated a later esophagojejunostomy. In the other a left subphrenic abscess occurred postoperatively, requiring drainage. They concluded that because of the hazards of a precarious blood supply in the transposed bowel and the large numbers of bacteria present in the colon, the dangers may outweigh the advantages of this type of substitute gastric reservoir.

TRANSPOSITION OF TRANSVERSE COLON FOR SUBSTITUTE GASTRIC RESERVOIR

In this procedure, after the entire stomach has been removed, a segment of the transverse colon is isolated, with its blood supply preserved. One end of this colonic segment is anastomosed to the cut end of the esophagus, and the other end of the colonic segment is anastomosed to the pyloric end of the duodenum. Colonic conti-

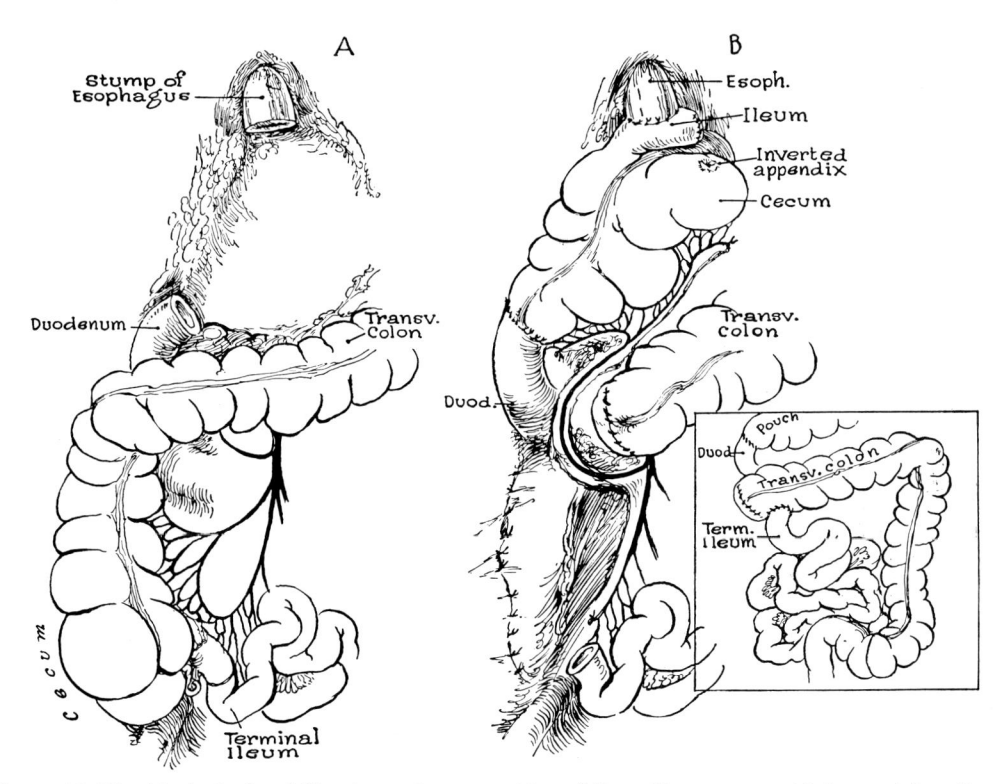

Figure 13-55. Method of mobilization and transposition of ileocolic segment with intact right colic vessels. (From Longmire, W. P., and Beal, J. M.: Construction of a substitute gastric reservoir following total gastrectomy. Ann. Surg. *135*:637, 1952.)

nuity is restored by mobilizing the hepatic and splenic flexures so that the right and left sides of the colon can be anastomosed to each other.

Successful use of this technic has been reported a few times, but the method appears to have the same hazards as those pointed out for employment of the right colon.

Comment

These rather extensive procedures for forming a substitute gastric pouch are not widely used as they add appreciably to the magnitude of an already complex operation and apparently are not essential for the patient's welfare. If it is desirable to form a substitute gastric pouch, the technic of the long jejunojejunostomy is probably the safest and most satisfactory for the average surgeon.

GASTROSTOMY

According to Gibbon, Nealon, and Greco (1956), Egeberg, a Norwegian Army Surgeon, in 1837 was the first to suggest the operation of gastrostomy. In 1844, Dr. Watson of New York was the first American to suggest the procedure. In 1849, the first gastrostomy on a human patient was performed by Sedillot (1853) of Strasbourg. The patient died 10 days later from peritonitis. In 1869, Dr. Maury of Philadelphia was the first American surgeon to perform a gastrostomy. The patient died.

The first successful gastrostomy was performed by Sydney Jones in 1875. This patient lived for 40 days following the operation. The gastrostomy was used for feeding during this period, but there was marked excoriation of the skin from leakage of gastric juice.

Definition

A gastrostomy is a fistula created between the lumen of the stomach and the anterior abdominal wall. This fistula permits access to the gastric lumen from the exterior. Fistulous tracts between the stomach and the skin have either a mucosal or a serous lining. Those with a mucosal lining are usually permanent gastrostomies; part of the wall of the stomach is so contructed to form a tubular channel between the lumen of the stomach and the exterior. The serous gastrostomy is usually temporary, and a tube generally is used to establish communication between the gastric lumen and the exterior. The fistulous tract that forms around the tube is serosa-lined (Farris and Smith, 1956).

The chief advantages of a serosa-lined gastrostomy are that it does not leak gastric juice, is simpler to perform than many of the elaborate modifications of a mucosa-lined gastrostomy, and will close spontaneously when the catheter is withdrawn from the stomach.

The disadvantage of the serosa-lined fistula is that the catheter must remain constantly in the stomach. If the catheter is removed, the fistula is rapidly obliterated by adhesion of serosal surfaces. Also, catheters occasionally slip out of the fistula or are pulled out by the patient. When this occurs, it may be difficult to replace the catheter or a false passage may be made. In three reported cases (Gibbon, Nealon, and Greco, 1956), a gastrostomy feeding entered the peritoneal cavity through a replaced catheter.

The advantages of a mucosa-lined gastrostomy are that the catheter need be inserted only at the time of the gastrostomy feeding and can be withdrawn without danger of obliteration of the tract. There is no risk of creating a false passage when reinserting the catheter.

A mucosa-lined gastrostomy, which will not leak gastric juice and can be simply and easily performed without opening the stomach during the operation, has certain advantages over the serosa-lined type.

Indications

A gastrostomy is performed either to feed a patient or to decompress and drain the stomach. Gastrostomy is used to provide nutritional support for patients with tumors of the larynx, pharynx, esophagus, and proximal stomach when the patient is unable to ingest sufficient calories to maintain adequate nutrition. Gastrostomy is also used for benign conditions, such as esophageal strictures and extrinsic compression of the esophagus from mediastinal masses. Gastrostomy in most of these patients is of limited benefit since the disease process also generally makes it difficult for the patient to handle saliva. Since most palliative or curative operations to bypass the obstruction require the use of the stomach, a previous gastrostomy may jeopardize this method of relief. Because of improved parenteral nutrition and low-residue liquid formulas, intravenous hyperalimentation and jejunal feeding tubes are usually preferable to feeding gastrostomies. One possible exception is the patient with a cerebral vascular accident who is unable to swallow. Another is the patient for whom expectations for recovery are high — a feeding gastrostomy may be preferable to a nasogastric feeding tube.

In selected patients, following trauma or extensive abdominal operations, a decompression gastrostomy may be helpful to avoid the use of a nasogastric tube. In such cases a simple tube gastrostomy is usually preferable to the more complex gastric mucosa-lined gastrostomy.

Types of Gastrostomy

The three classic types of gastrostomy are (1) the Stamm gastrostomy: a tube is inserted into the lumen of the stomach and its entrance into the stomach is secured with a pursestring suture. The tube exits to the exterior through a stab incision (Stamm, 1894); (2) the Witzel gastrostomy: a tube is inserted into the lumen of the stomach and secured with a pursestring suture. In addition, a 5- to 7-cm. segment of the tube is covered with the stomach before its exit through the abdominal wall to the exterior (Witzel, 1891); and (3) permanent mucosa-lined gastrostomies: a gastric tube is formed which is approximated to the abdominal wall (Janeway, 1913; Beck and Carrel, 1905; Glassman, 1939).

STAMM GASTROSTOMY
(Fig. 13–56)

In most patients this operation can be performed under local anesthesia. Access to the stomach can be gained by either an upper midline incision or a left rectus muscle–splittling incision. The stomach generally can be identified by its color and arrangement of vessels along the lesser and

Figure 13–56. Stamm method of gastrostomy superimposing pursestring invagination. A, A tube is shown inserted through the anterior stomach wall, and pursestring sutures are placed about it. B, The cone of stomach has been invaginated, and the stomach wall is being sutured to the posterior layer of the rectus sheath, transversalis fascia, and peritoneum. Sutures to close the outer layers of abdominal wall are indicated. C, Sectional view of the gastrostomy.

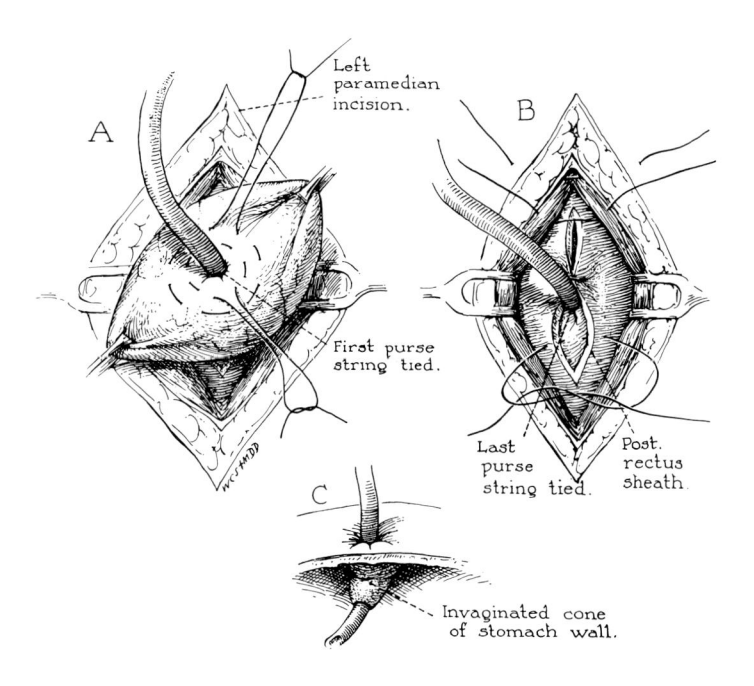

greater curvature. The greater omentum is of use in confirming the identification of the stomach. It is important to identify the transverse colon, which is usually recognized by the presence of a tenia.

A site on the anterior wall of the stomach is usually selected in the proximal antrum. It is important to avoid being too close to the pyloric area or the tube itself may obstruct the gastric outlet. Generally, the mid-portion of the anterior wall is chosen, to avoid the larger vessels on the greater and lesser curvatures. A point of entry for the tube is selected, and this may be grasped with an Allis clamp. Although the gastrostomy tube can be brought out through the main abdominal incision, it is usually preferable to use a separate stab incision for the gastrostomy tube. In planning the incision in the stomach as well as the site of the tube tract through the abdominal wall, it is important to coordinate the location of these two sites to insure as short a distance as possible between stomach and abdominal wall, to prevent tension between them. The location of the entrance site on the stomach should correspond to the site on the abdominal wall, so that the contact between the anterior wall of the stomach and the abdominal wall permits straight entrance of the tube into the stomach.

Once the sites on the stomach and abdominal wall have been selected, a stab incision is made through the abdominal wall, and the tube is passed from the abdominal cavity to the skin. A pursestring suture, generally of nonabsorbable material, is placed into the seromuscular layer of the stomach surrounding the planned site of entry. Once this suture is placed, an incision is made through the serosa and tunica muscularis. Generally the bleeding in the two layers is easily controlled with electrocautery; however, if any major vessels are incised a transfixion suture may be required. The mucosa is opened and a catheter inserted for a distance of 5 cm. The pursestring suture should be secured tightly enough to prevent the catheter from slipping out of the stomach. A second pursestring is generally placed about 1 cm. from the first, to invaginate the first pursestring. The anterior wall of the stomach is generally secured to the abdominal wall with 2 or 3 sutures to insure good contact between the stomach and abdominal wall and prevent any leakage into the peritoneal cavity.

Various tubes have been used for the gastrostomy. A French or Robinson catheter is a common choice, while some prefer a mushroom, de Pezzer, or Foley catheter. If the tube is to be used for decompression, it should be at least an 18 or 20 French. The tube is secured to the skin, and the abdominal incision is closed in layers.

WITZEL GASTROSTOMY (Fig. 13-57)

The Witzel gastrostomy is similar to the Stamm gastrostomy except that a segment of the tube is covered by the anterior wall of the stomach. After sites in the stomach and anterior abdominal wall have been selected, a pursestring suture is placed around the entrance site on the stomach. The tube is then brought through the anterior abdominal wall, and an incision is made into the stomach to insert the tube for a distance of approximately 5 cm. The pursestring suture is secured. Additional sutures are placed in the anterior gastric wall, imbricating the tube for a distance of 5 to 7.5 cm. Seromuscular Lembert-type stitches are usually used to form this serosal tunnel around the tube. The stomach is then secured to the anterior abdominal wall.

PERMANENT GASTROSTOMIES

Janeway Gastrostomy
(Figs. 13-58, 13-59)

This mucosa-lined gastrostomy tube is seldom used. It provides a permanent fistula, which generally requires reoperation for closure. A rectangular flap of stomach 5 to 6 cm. in width is made, with the base being at the greater curvature; the abdominal cavity is walled off against spillage of gastric contents. The free margin and sides of the flap are deepened through the mucosa, and any large vessels in the gastric wall are ligated. Two Allis clamps are placed on the edges of the free portion of the flap. After the stomach is opened, the gastric contents are removed by suction.

The flap is retracted gently toward the greater omentum, and a gastric tube is created by approximating the edges of the in-

GASTROSTOMY

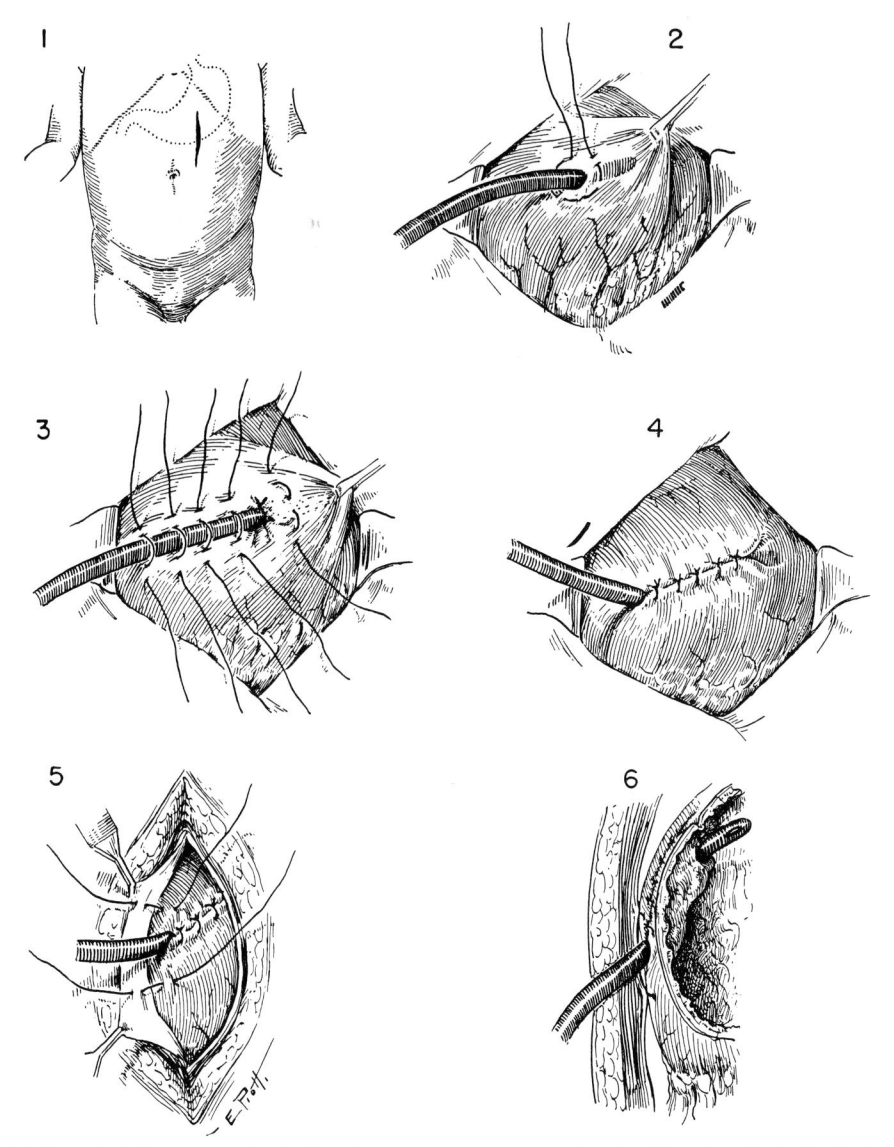

Figure 13–57. Satisfactory method of performing a gastrostomy by the Witzel technic. 1, Position of the left rectus muscle–splitting incision. 2, Stomach exposed and held up with an Allis clamp. Catheter thrust in through gastric wall and the opening is being closed with a pursestring suture. 3, Pursestring suture tied. Additional sutures of silk placed in gastric wall to form an oblique channel for the catheter. 4, Channel sutures tied, with the catheter imbedded in the gastric wall. 5, Stomach being anchored to the peritoneum so that it will not pull away from the abdominal wall. 6, Parasagittal view of completed operation, showing the oblique implantation of the catheter in the stomach and abdominal walls. (From Ladd, W. E., and Gross, R. E.: Philadelphia, W. B. Saunders Company, 1941.)

cised stomach, beginning at the lesser curvature. Usually an inverting layer of continuous 00 chromic catgut and another seromuscular layer of silk are used to create the tube. A 16 or 18 F. catheter is inserted into the stomach and may be directed through the pylorus into the duodenum. The neck of the gastric tube is then completed, and the appearance of the tube is checked to determine whether the blood supply is adequate. The tube is then brought through a stab wound in the abdominal wall, and the mucosa is sutured to the abdominal skin. The catheter is secured to both the gastric mucosa and skin. The abdominal incision is closed in layers.

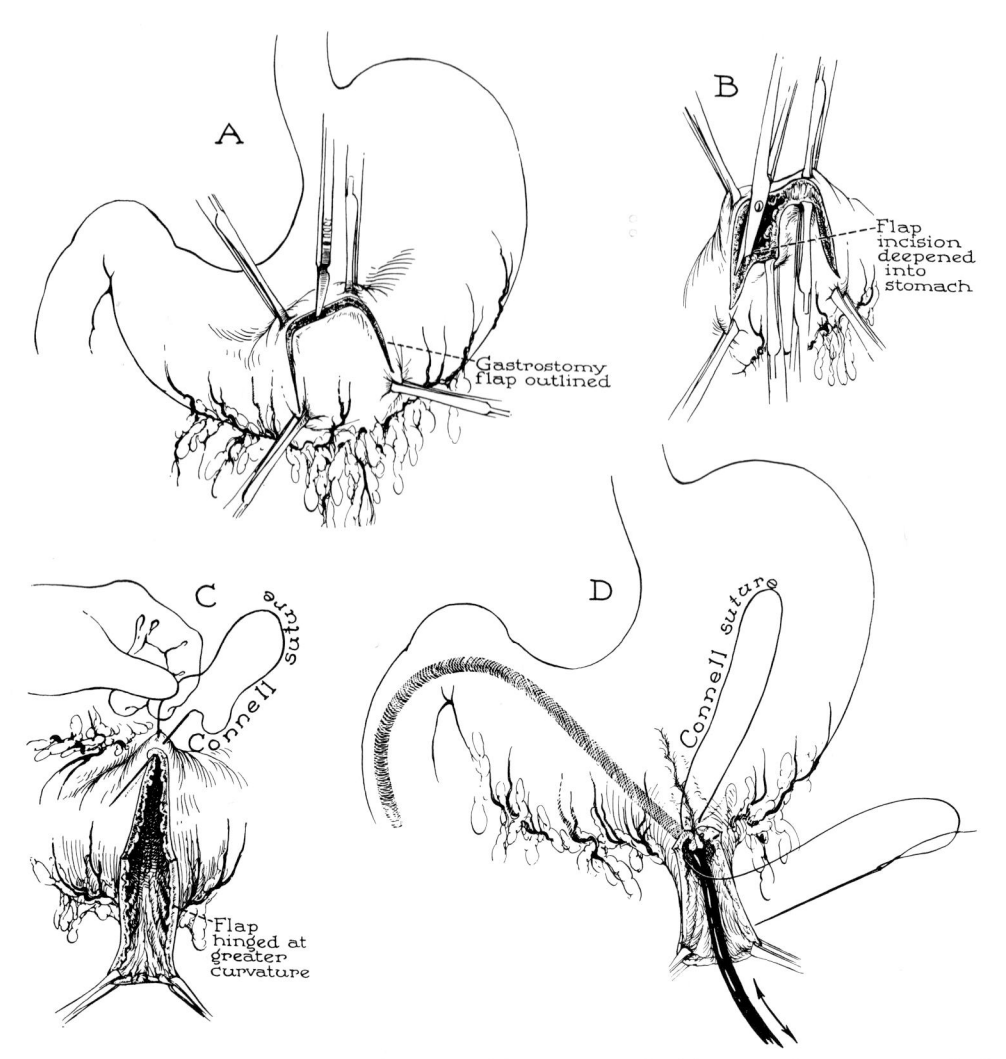

Figure 13–58. Janeway gastrostomy. *A*, The flap of the anterior wall of the stomach is outlined with a knife. *B*, The incision is deepened with scissors through all coats. *C* and *D*, Approximating the incised margins of stomach and stomach flap with a Connell suture. A rubber tube is shown inserted into the duodenum before the "gooseneck" of stomach is closed.

If the stomach is contracted, the gastrostomy flap may not be long enough to extend to the outside. A modification described by Thorek (1945) can be used in which the stomach is opened over its posterior as well as anterior surfaces. Access to the lesser sac and posterior surface of the stomach is obtained by dividing the gastrocolic ligament. The major complication of a Janeway type of gastrostomy is impairment of the blood supply to the distal part of the tube. This may interfere with a good anastomosis between the gastric mucosa and the skin, resulting in stenosis. A more extensive loss of the tube results in a peritoneal leak and is usually fatal.

Beck-Jianu Gastrostomy

Another type of permanent mucosa-lined gastrostomy is the Beck-Jianu (Fig. 13–60). This is a long gastric tube fashioned from the greater curvature of the stomach and based on the left gastroepiploic artery. This tube also has been lengthened and used to establish continuity following distal esophageal resection. The gastrocolic ligament and gastrosplenic omentum are divided about 2.5 cm. distal to the greater curvature, preserving the left gastroepiploic artery. It is important that an adequate margin of gastrocolic and gastrosplenic omentum be left on the stomach, or else the

GASTROSTOMY

Figure 13-59. Janeway gastrostomy *(continued)*. *A*, The stomach tube has been completed; the rubber tube is being stitched to it. *B* and *C*, The tube of stomach, brought to the skin surface through a left rectus stab wound, is sutured to the skin margins of the wound.

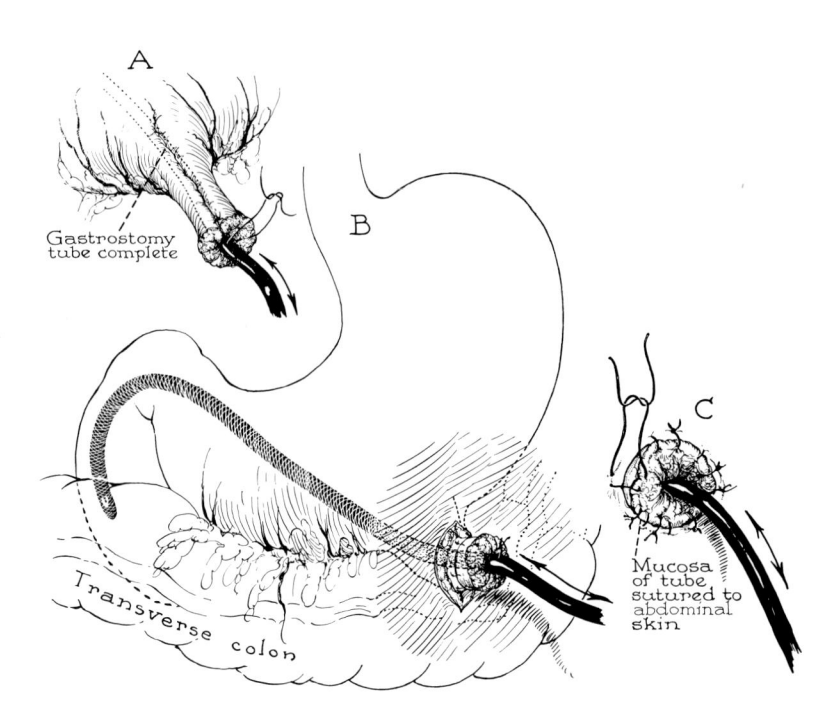

vascular supply of the tube is compromised. The right gastroepiploic vessels are ligated and divided proximal to the pyloric area. The stomach is grasped longitudinally between the antrum and the fundus at the junction of its middle and lower thirds by a pair of atraumatic clamps. The stomach is divided longitudinally between the clamps, and each of the clamp margins of the stomach is closed with an inner layer of running chromic suture and an outer layer of interrupted silk.

If the gastrostomy tube thus formed is to be used only for purposes of feeding, the gastrocolic ligament attached to the transverse colon reinforces the suture line on the stomach. This suspends the transverse colon and protects the gastric suture line. If the stoma of the gastrostomy tube is to be placed high on the chest wall or if the tube is to be used for anastomosis to the esophagus, the ligament is not sutured to the stomach since this exerts undue tension on it.

The gastrostomy tube is exteriorized onto the abdominal wall, and the mucosa is secured to the skin. A 12 or 16 F. catheter is inserted through the fistulous tract to decompress the stomach.

A similar type of gastrostomy can be constructed easily with use of the gastrointestinal stapling device.

Glassman's Gastrostomy

In 1939, Glassman described a mucosa-lined gastrostomy in which leakage of gastric juice is prevented by creating two areas of constriction in a cone-shaped diverticulum formed of the anterior wall of the stomach. The operation can be easily performed with local anesthesia, which is also the anesthesia of choice in a very sick patient. If abdominal exploration is desired, or if the patient is psychiatric and uncooperative, general inhalation anesthesia is preferable.

The stomach is exposed through a vertical high left upper paramedian or a high left upper rectus muscle–splitting incision. The upper end of the incision should extend to the junction of the xiphoid and costal cartilages. When the operation is performed on patients with esophageal obstruction, the stomach is usually small and empty and lies cephalad in the abdominal cavity. If the incision is properly placed, its length need not exceed 8 to 10 cm.

The anterior wall of the stomach is grasped with a Babcock clamp in its central and most mobile portion and is pulled up into a cone-shaped diverticulum (Fig. 13-61).

The portion of the anterior gastric wall

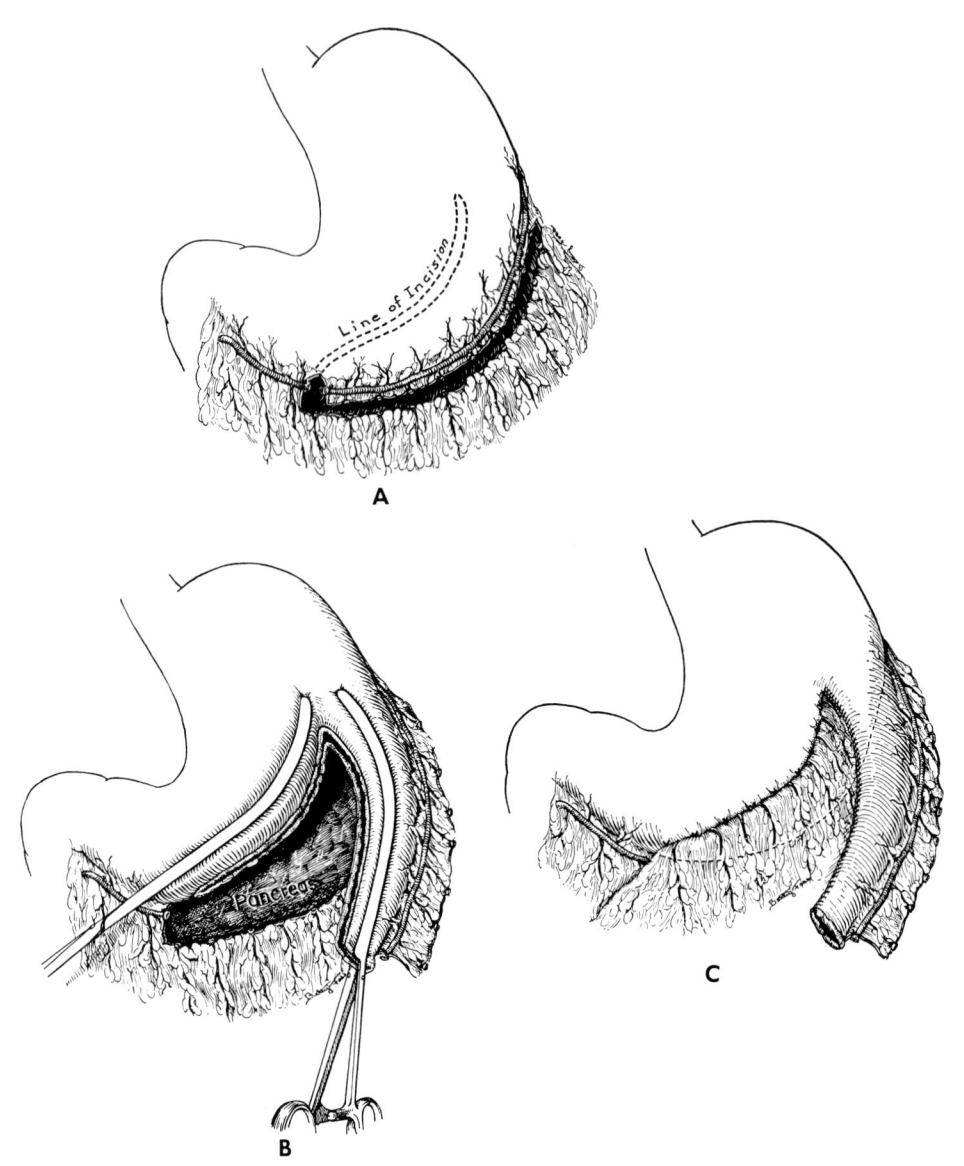

Figure 13–60. Beck-Jianu gastrostomy. *A*, Division of the gastrocolic omentum; ligation of the right gastroepiploic vessels. Dotted line shows direction and optimal length of incision through the stomach walls. *B*, Stomach divided and ready for suture. Note the preservation of the left gastroepiploic vessels on the gastric tube. Clamps shown in place as actually used during the operation. *C*, Suture of the body of the stomach and gastric tube completed. Gastrocolic ligament resutured to the stomach. Gastric tube lies free and ready to be brought out over the costal margin. (Courtesy of Dr. Sweet and Surgery, Gynecology & Obstetrics.)

that can be drawn up to the level of the skin without tension is selected for the site of the gastrostomy. In this portion of the anterior wall, at a point equidistant from the greater and lesser curvature of the stomach, a traction suture is placed through the serosal and muscular coats of the stomach (Fig. 13–62). Traction on this suture produces a conelike elevation of the anterior wall of the stomach.

A heavy silk pursestring suture is now placed about the base of the cone and is tied tight enough to pucker the wall of the cone and constrict, but not occlude, its lumen. A second pursestring suture is placed 1 cm. above the first. When tied, the second suture creates a broader area of approximation of the gastric mucosa at the base of the pouch and provides added protection against leakage of gastric juice from the main body of the stomach.

A third pursestring suture is placed 1

GASTROSTOMY

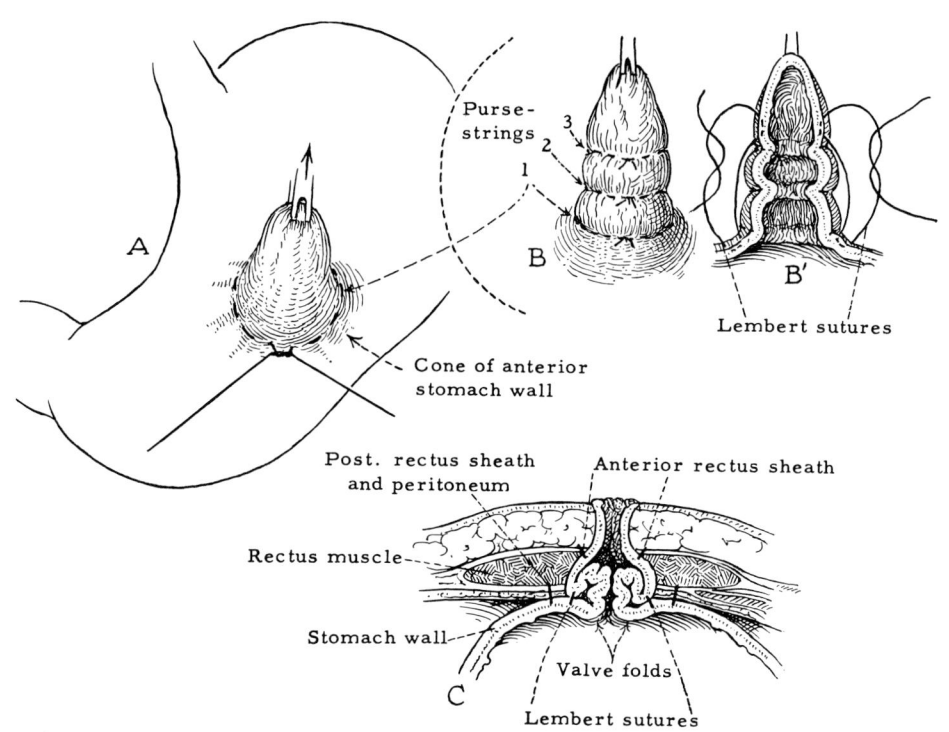

Figure 13–61. Glassman's gastrostomy. *A,* Anterior wall of stomach pulled into a cone-shaped diverticulum; pursestring suture placed at base of cone. *B,* Second and third pursestring sutures placed and tied. *B′,* Sectional view of *B,* with circular row of reefing Lembert sutures indicated. *C,* Lembert sutures tied and scheme of abdominal wall closure about stomach tube. Shown in section.

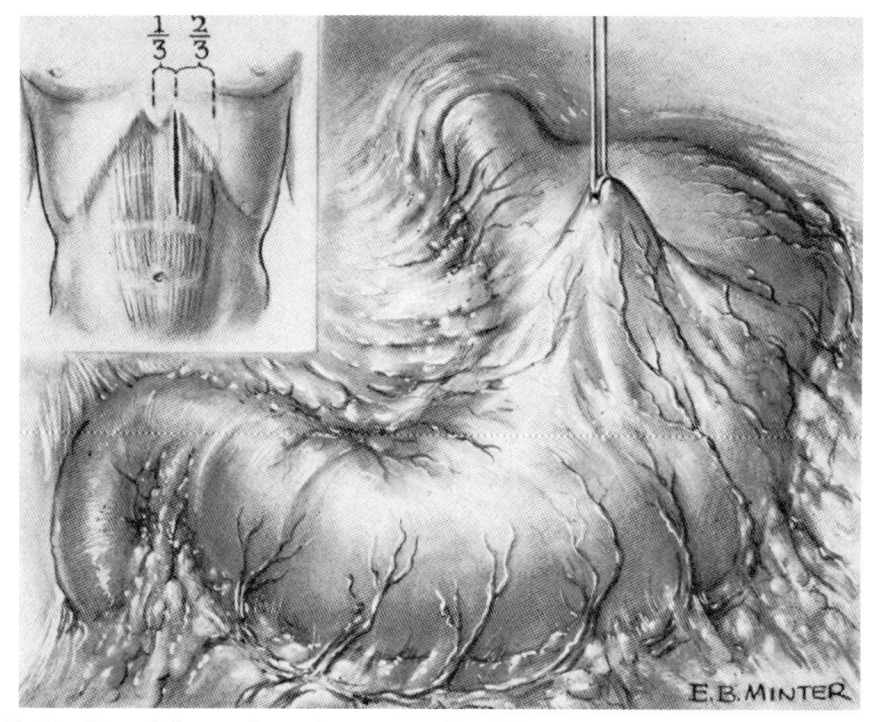

Figure 13–62. Upper left inset shows the position of the abdominal wound. The drawing shows the placement of a traction suture in the anterior wall of the stomach. (From Gibbon, J. H., Jr., Nealon, T. F., Jr., and Greco, V. F.: A modification of Glassman's gastrostomy with results in 18 patients. Ann. Surg. *143*:838, 1956.)

cm. above the second (Fig. 13–61B). Moderately heavy, nonabsorbable suture material should be used for these pursestring sutures.

Gibbon, Nealon, and Greco (1956) modified Glassman's original description of this procedure by pointing out and emphasizing that "in placing these pursestring sutures it is of utmost importance to pass the needle beneath all visible arteries and veins supplying the raised cone of the anterior gastric wall" (Fig. 13–63).

If this precaution is observed there will be no interference with the arterial supply or the venous drainage of the stomach pouch that is formed when the suture is tied. Neglect of this precaution results in a violaceous and edematous pouch which may slough.

It is also important to avoid traumatizing the gastric pouch or producing an extravasation of blood by injury to a blood vessel when placing a suture.

After completing the pursestring sutures, interrupted Lembert sutures of silk are placed in the stomach wall below the three pursestring sutures and inserted into the wall of the newly formed diverticulum above the three pursestring sutures (Fig. 13–61B'). When the Lembert sutures are tied, a circular valve is formed at the base of the diverticulum.

The anterior wall of the stomach around the base of the diverticulum is sutured with silk to the peritoneal edges of the abdominal wound after the diverticulum has been pulled through it to the outside of the abdomen.

The anterior sheath of the rectus muscle is also sutured to the cone about its circumference at the fascial level. The skin edges are sutured to the cone about its tip. The tip of the cone can be opened by a stab wound made with scissors or knife immediately, but, when conditions permit, asepsis is more certain if it is not opened until 48 or more hours postoperatively. Figure 13–61C shows the arrangement at the completion of the operation.

After opening the tip of the cone, a tube should be inserted through the pouch into the main body of the stomach and left there for 4 or 5 days until the margins of the small incised wound in the gastric pouch have healed. After this the tube need only be inserted for gastrostomy feedings. A properly constructed gastrostomy of this type will

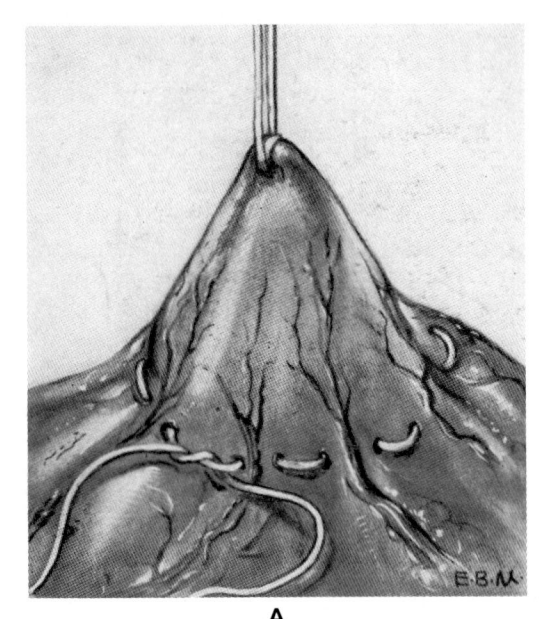

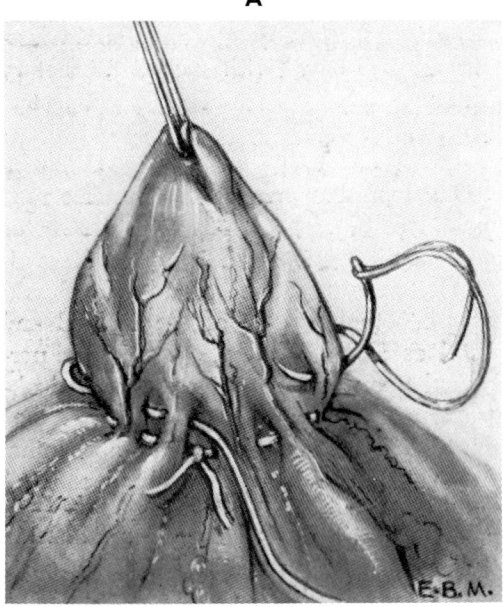

Figure 13–63. *A*, The first pursestring suture has been placed around the base of the cone formed by traction on the anterior wall of the stomach. The suture has been so placed as to pass beneath the arteries and veins supplying the wall of the stomach in the elevated cone. *B*, Placement of the second pursestring suture 3 or 4 mm. above the first suture. Care is again taken to pass the suture beneath the vessels supplying the gastric wall. (From Gibbon, Nealon, and Greco, cited in previous figure.)

not leak gastric juice on the skin surface, and there is no danger of creating a false passage when inserting the catheter for feeding. The appearance of the wound scar and the open gastrostomy 6 days after operation is shown in Figure 13–64.

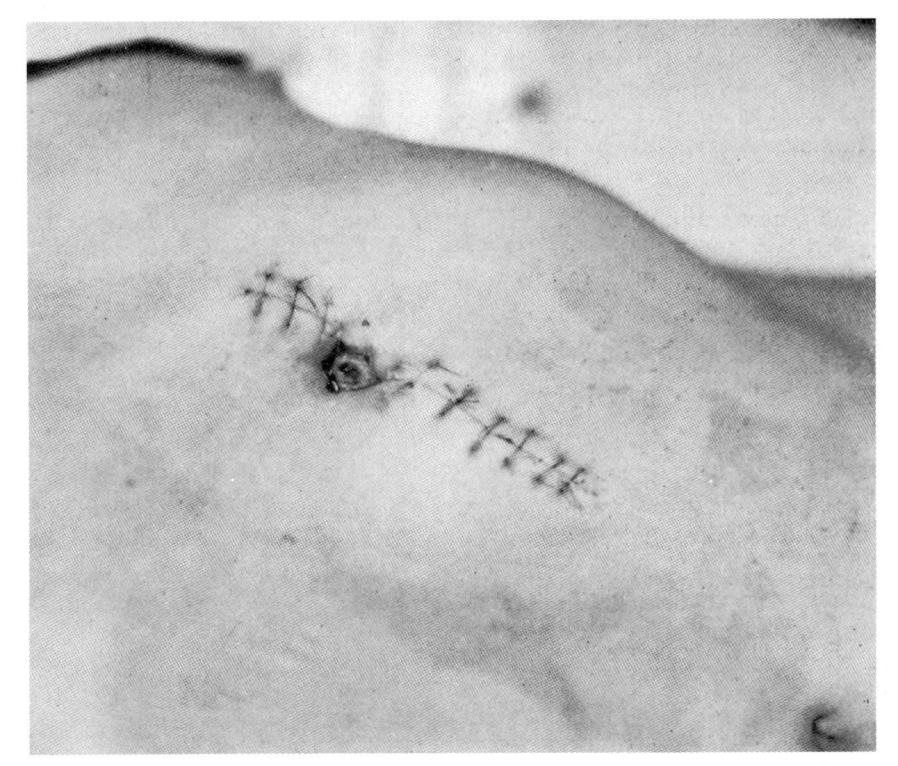

Figure 13–64. Photograph of the gastrostomy opening and abdominal wound on the sixth postoperative day. Note the position of the vertical wound overlying the left upper rectus muscle just beneath the chondral margin. (From Gibbon, Nealon, and Greco, cited in Figure 13–62.)

Gibbon, Nealon, and Greco (1956) reported 18 consecutive gastrostomies with this technic. Sixteen were opened and used; 14 of the 16 functioned excellently. There was slight leakage and skin irritation in one patient, and one complete failure from marked leak of gastric juice.

Our house staff has frequently used Glassman's gastrostomy for making a permanent mucosa-lined feeding gastrostomy in patients who either cannot or will not swallow and have a life expectancy that is indefinite and may be long. The operation has been easy to perform without opening the stomach during the operation, leakage of gastric juice does not occur, the tube can be removed and reinserted at will without danger of creating a false passage, and the patient can live at home without special care.

PEDIATRIC GASTROSTOMY

The Stamm gastrostomy is an excellent means of gastric decompression following major abdominal and gastrointestinal reconstruction, as well as an efficient means of feeding patients unable to accept oral alimentation. Its use in pediatric surgery, particularly in neonates and infants, has been strongly advocated by many experienced surgeons (Martin and Pultz, 1959; Holder and Gross, 1960; Meeker and Snyder, 1962; Berg, Schuster, and Colodny, 1964; Cox and Gillesby, 1967).

The only alternative way to accomplish these goals is by nasogastric tube, but the gastrostomy tube has these advantages:

1. It is more efficient, since a much larger gastrostomy than nasogastric tube can be used in the infant.

2. It is the only means possible in infants with esophageal atresia or large cervical cystic hygromas.

3. It does not interfere with respiration in the neonate who is an obligate nose breather.

4. Overall nursing care of the patient is enhanced since mobility is increased, with less chance of accidental displacement.

Since an operative procedure is required for the placement of the gastrostomy tube, its routine use must be weighed against its associated morbidity and mortality rates, especially in premature infants (Haws, Sieber, and Kiesewetter, 1968; Raffensperger and associates, 1968). Concern over these reports led to a series of technical modifications, which resulted in a significant decrease in both morbidity and mortality in patients of all ages. One of the most significant contributions toward improved results with the gastrostomy tube was by Holder, Leape, and Ashcroft (1972).

They presented their experience over a 7-year period, which included performing Stamm gastrostomies in 280 pediatric patients, half of whom were under 2 weeks of age, and one-quarter of whom weighed less than 2500 gm. One death was related to a gastrostomy tube, making a mortality rate of 0.4 per cent, and 7 major and 12 minor complications, making a morbidity rate of 6.8 per cent. The surgeons determined ten points of technic and management of importance in minimizing complications of the use of gastrostomy tubes in infants.

1. The operation must be performed under sterile conditions in the operating room.
2. The catheter used must be self-retaining.
3. The tube must be placed in the body of the stomach near the greater curvature.
4. Two pursestring sutures must be used to invert the collar of the gastric wall around the tube as it enters the stomach.
5. One must employ meticulous hemostasis.
6. One must provide suture fixation of the stomach to the anterior abdominal wall.
7. A proper dressing of the junction of the tube and the skin of the anterior abdominal wall is essential.
8. Simple gravity drainage is better than either constant or intermittent suction.
9. Frequent irrigation of the catheter is essential to allow continuous function.
10. The gastrostomy tube must be brought through a separate stab wound in the abdominal wall.

By adherence to these principles, morbidity and mortality rates in recent reports are similarly low (Thomas and Croom, 1970; Parrish and Cohen, 1972; Gallagher, Tyson, and Ashcroft, 1973; Campbell and Sasake, 1974).

The Pediatric Surgical Service at The Johns Hopkins Hospital has employed this protocol for gastrostomy tube placement in over 200 neonates between 1974 and 1978 without a major complication or death. The procedure has been facilitated by using a specially designed pediatric gastrostomy tube, constructed of Silastic with a steel coil support incorporated into the shaft. This prevents occlusion and minimizes rotational movement as the tube passes out through the stab wound in the abdominal wall.

The Silastic de Pezzer–type end of the tube is placed in the gastric lumen in the manner described, with double pursestrings of chromic catgut. At a distance of 0.5 cm. proximal to the de Pezzer end is an inflatable Silastic balloon, which is positioned on the surface of the anterior abdominal wall. After the double pursestrings in the seromuscular wall of the stomach are secured around the tube, inflation of the balloon fixes the catheter firmly in place, with the stomach wall and anterior abdominal wall compressed together between the de Pezzer end and the balloon. This prevents inward migration of the catheter. The balloon may be released after 3 days, by which time there is a fine seal of the gastric serosa to the parietal peritoneum. The Silastic construction obviates the need for dressings, and inflation of the balloon prevents any leak of gastric contents onto the skin.

When need for the gastrostomy is over, it is simply pulled out, and a pressure dressing is placed over the gastrocutaneous fistula, which invariably closes within 3 days.

Comments on Gastrostomy

The basic procedures all have various modifications, such as Brunschwig's gastrostomy in which a 26 F. de Pezzer catheter is used instead of an ordinary straight catheter. The procedure otherwise is identical to a Stamm gastrostomy. The Kader gastrostomy is a combination of the Stamm and Witzel, in which the catheter is invaginated into the stomach by means of a tier of Lembert interrupted sutures. This technic invaginates the tube by creating adjacent folds of stomach wall. In the Ssabanejew-Frank gastrostomy, a cone of stomach is pulled through an incision through the left rectus muscle and sutured to the skin. This is possible only with a large or relaxed stomach. Various modifications of this technic likewise depend upon a large and relaxed stomach. Other modifications include creation of a valve with the mucosa-lined gastrostomies. Interposing a 25-cm. segment of jejunum between the stomach and skin also provides a valvular effect, preventing reflux from the stomach to the exterior (Nyhus and associates, 1961).

Various types of tubes have been used for the serosa-lined gastrostomies. Nonreactive tubes like Silastic should be avoided since a good fibrous tract generally does not develop. If a de Pezzer or Foley catheter is used, gentle traction may be placed on the tube to push the stomach against the abdominal wall. The management of a gastrostomy in the immediate postoperative period generally consists of placing the catheter on gravity drainage to avoid gastric distention and promote adherence between the gastrostomy site and the anterior abdominal wall. Occasionally, gentle irrigation of the gastrostomy tube may be necessary to insure its patency. When used in trauma or in nutritionally depleted patients, it is best to allow 7 to 10 days for healing before infusion tube feedings. Initially the stomach should be aspirated every 6 to 8 hours to insure that adequate gastric emptying is occurring.

The gastrostomy tube is generally brought through a separate stab incision in the abdominal wall to minimize the problems of wound healing. Our preference is to insert the tube through the abdominal wall before placing it into the stomach to avoid pulling a potentially contaminated tube through the abdominal wall once it has been inserted into the stomach.

Significant complications can occur following simple tube gastrostomy, and, in severely depleted patients, these complications may be fatal (Connar and Sealy, 1956; Stenter, 1960). The most common complication is leakage around the tube, resulting in peritonitis or excoriation of the skin. Wound problems can be minimized if a separate stab wound is used for the tube exit. We prefer closing the main abdominal incision with wire.

The Stamm gastrostomy is most commonly used because it is simple to perform and does not have any long suture lines. With the advancements made in intravenous parenteral nutrition and jejunal feedings using a small polyethylene tube, gastrostomies are not frequently used.

GASTROENTEROSTOMY

Gastroenterostomy is an anastomosis between the stomach and small intestine. It is usually classified by naming the part of the small bowel used for the anastomosis, such as *gastroduodenostomy* or *gastrojejunostomy*. A gastroileostomy is never intentionally performed since an anastomosis between the stomach and distal small bowel results in diarrhea and malnutrition.

HISTORY

Gastrojejunostomy was first described by Wölfler in 1881 (see Fig. 13–71). For approximately 20 years the anastomosis consisted of a long afferent loop of jejunum anastomosed to the anterior part of the stomach in an antiperistaltic manner. The principal modification over a 20-year period consisted of moving the anastomosis to the posterior aspect of the stomach. This operation was performed primarily for pyloric or antral obstruction. Its major disadvantage was the regurgitant vomiting due to the long afferent limb.

This major problem of gastrojejunostomy was alleviated somewhat by creating an enteroenterostomy between the afferent and efferent limbs of jejunum. Roux introduced an en-Y anastomosis in 1897 which eliminated regurgitant vomiting; however, it was abandoned because of the high incidence of stomal ulcers. These operations were not accompanied by vagotomy.

Petersen in 1900 described the type of gastrojejunostomy that is currently used. This consists of a posterior short-loop gastrojejunostomy. This modification eliminated the long afferent loop and avoided the problem of regurgitant vomiting. The ideal gastrojejunostomy should be situated on the stomach so as to provide adequate drainage, and the afferent limb should be short enough that regurgitant vomiting and other afferent loop symptoms will be avoided (Stammers, 1961; Tanner, 1966).

INDICATIONS

Gastroenterostomy without vagotomy is indicated only in highly selected cases. If gastric acid secretion is normal or elevated, gastroenterostomy without an acid-reducing operation such as vagotomy will result in a marginal ulcer; gastroenterostomy alone can be safely performed if there is little or no acid secretion from the stomach. Gastroenterostomy is generally performed in combination with vagotomy for duodenal ulcer disease and is the procedure of choice when there is considerable scarring of the duodenum that makes gastric resection and closure of the duodenal stump or a pyloroplasty unsafe. In chronic obstructing duodenal ulcer disease with low acid secretion, gastrojejunostomy alone may be performed.

Other indications for gastrojejunostomy without vagotomy include palliative drainage of an obstructed stomach associated with carcinoma of the pancreas, a distal antral carcinoma, or metastatic disease obstructing the antral or pyloric area. When a gastrojejunostomy for malignant disease is done, it is important to select a site on the stomach that will provide adequate drainage and to locate the anastomosis anterior to the colon to avoid nodal metastases along the transverse mesocolon, which would eventually obstruct the jejunal limbs.

A gastroduodenostomy (Jaboulay pyloroplasty) is preferred by some surgeons as a drainage procedure accompanying vagotomy for the treatment of duodenal ulcer (Farris and DeLaria, 1976).

Technics

GASTRODUODENOSTOMY

Gastroduodenostomy consists of anastomosis between the antrum of the stomach and the duodenum. The pylorus is not interrupted. Although this operation is sometimes referred to as a Jaboulay pyloroplasty, this is incorrect since the pylorus is not incised. This operation provides a large opening between the distal stomach and duodenum and avoids the inflammatory process in the pyloric area (Fig. 13–65). It has the disadvantage of requiring a complicated reconstruction should it be necessary to take down the anastomosis.

The lateral aspect of the duodenum is mobilized (Kocher maneuver). The antrum of the stomach and the duodenum are lined up by placing a traction suture just proximal to the pylorus near the greater curvature of the stomach. The duodenum just distal to the scarred pylorus is selected and approximated to the stomach. A second traction suture is placed between a more proximal portion of the stomach along the greater curvature to a more distal portion of the duodenum. The distance between the first and second traction sutures should be 7 to 9 cm. A posterior row of interrupted nonabsorbable sutures is placed, approximating the serosal surfaces of the stomach and duodenum. An opening is made then in the stomach and duodenum. Hemostasis is secured, and an inner row of absorbable sutures is placed posteriorly and carried anteriorly. The anastomosis is completed with an anterior row of nonabsorbable sutures, using a Lembert stitch.

A popular modification of the gastroduodenostomy, described by Rienhoff, consists of performing the anastomosis between a more proximal part of the stomach and the transverse duodenum (Figs. 13–66, 13–67, and 13–68). The stomach is anastomosed in the most dependent part of the antrum, the duodenum is freed inferiorly, and the anastomosis is made distal to the ampulla of Vater. The basic technic is similar, and the size of stoma is 7 to 9 cm. Good results have been described by Farris and DeLaria (1976).

GASTROJEJUNOSTOMY

Gastrojejunostomy consists of an anastomosis between the stomach and the proximal jejunum. The loop of jejunum may be brought anterior to the colon (antecolic gastrojejunostomy) or through the transverse mesocolon and under the transverse colon (retrocolic gastrojejunostomy) (Fig. 13–69). If the afferent limb (limb leading from the duodenum) is at the more distal part of the

Text continued on page 349

GASTROENTEROSTOMY

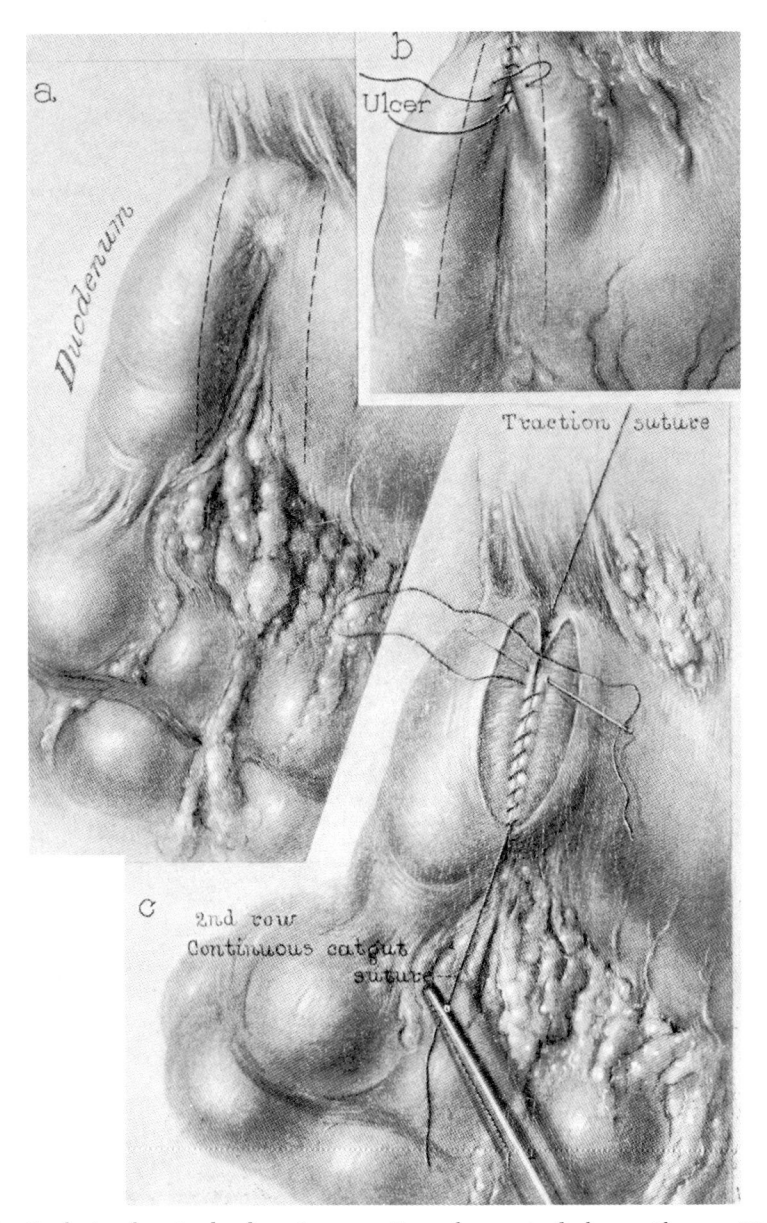

Figure 13-65. Technic of gastroduodenostomy. *a*, Serosal aspect of ulcer with apposition of stomach and duodenum; *b*, covering of the ulcer; *c*, beginning of gastroduodenostomy. (From Eusterman, G. B., and Balfour, D. C.: The Stomach and Duodenum. Philadelphia, W. B. Saunders Company, 1935.)

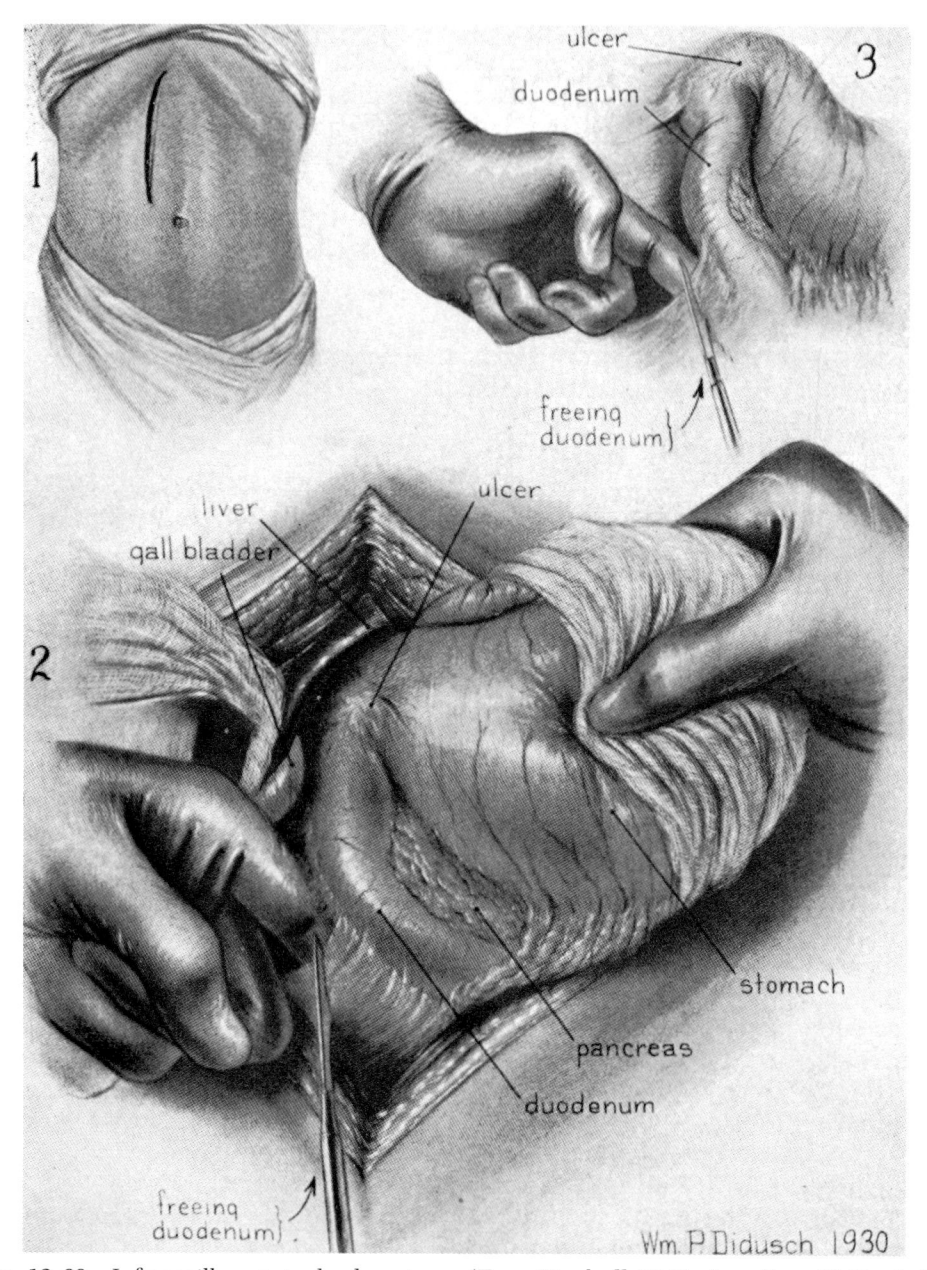

Figure 13–66. Infrapapillary gastroduodenostomy. (From Rienhoff, W. F.: Ann. Surg. 95:No. 1, 1932.)

GASTROENTEROSTOMY 347

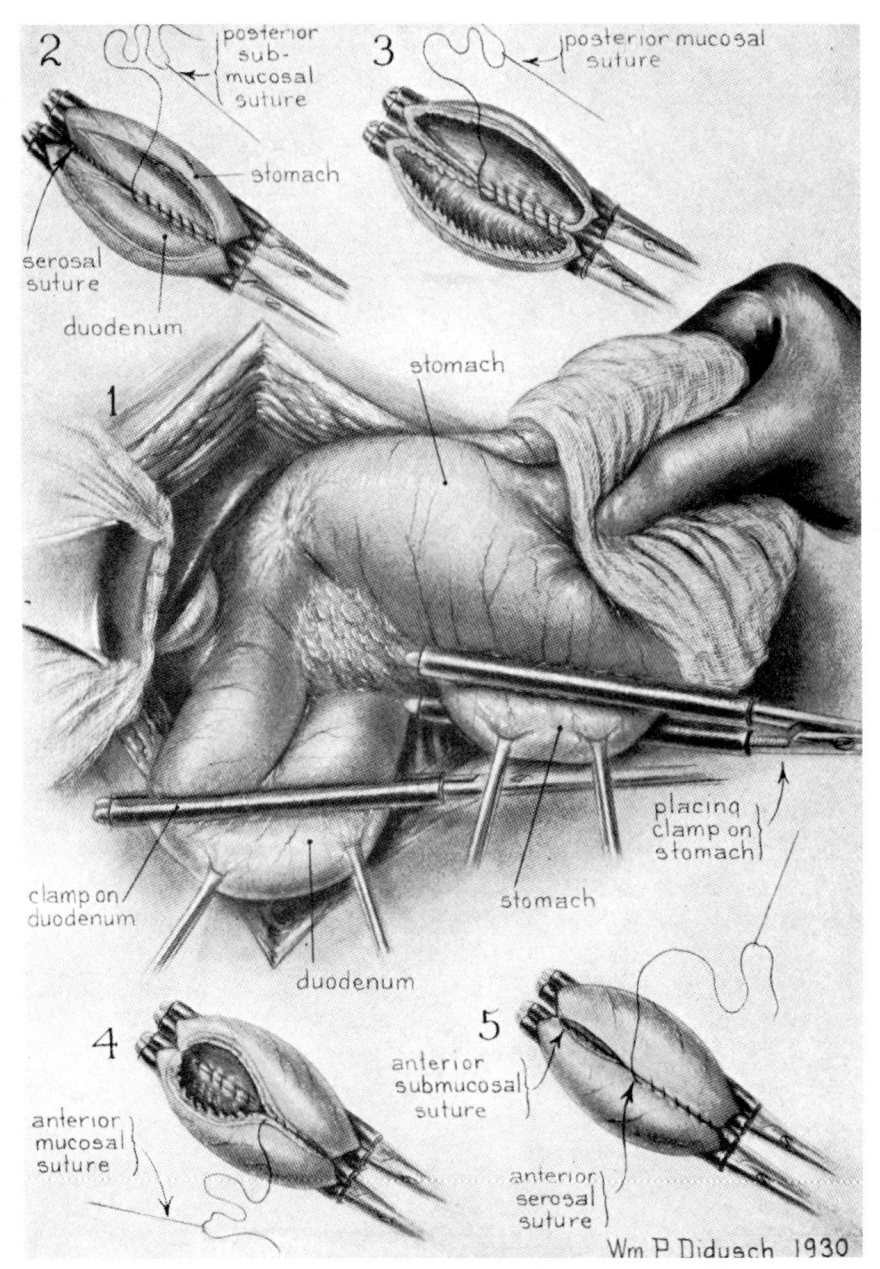

Figure 13–67. Infrapapillary gastroduodenostomy *(continued)*. (From Rienhoff, cited in previous figure.)

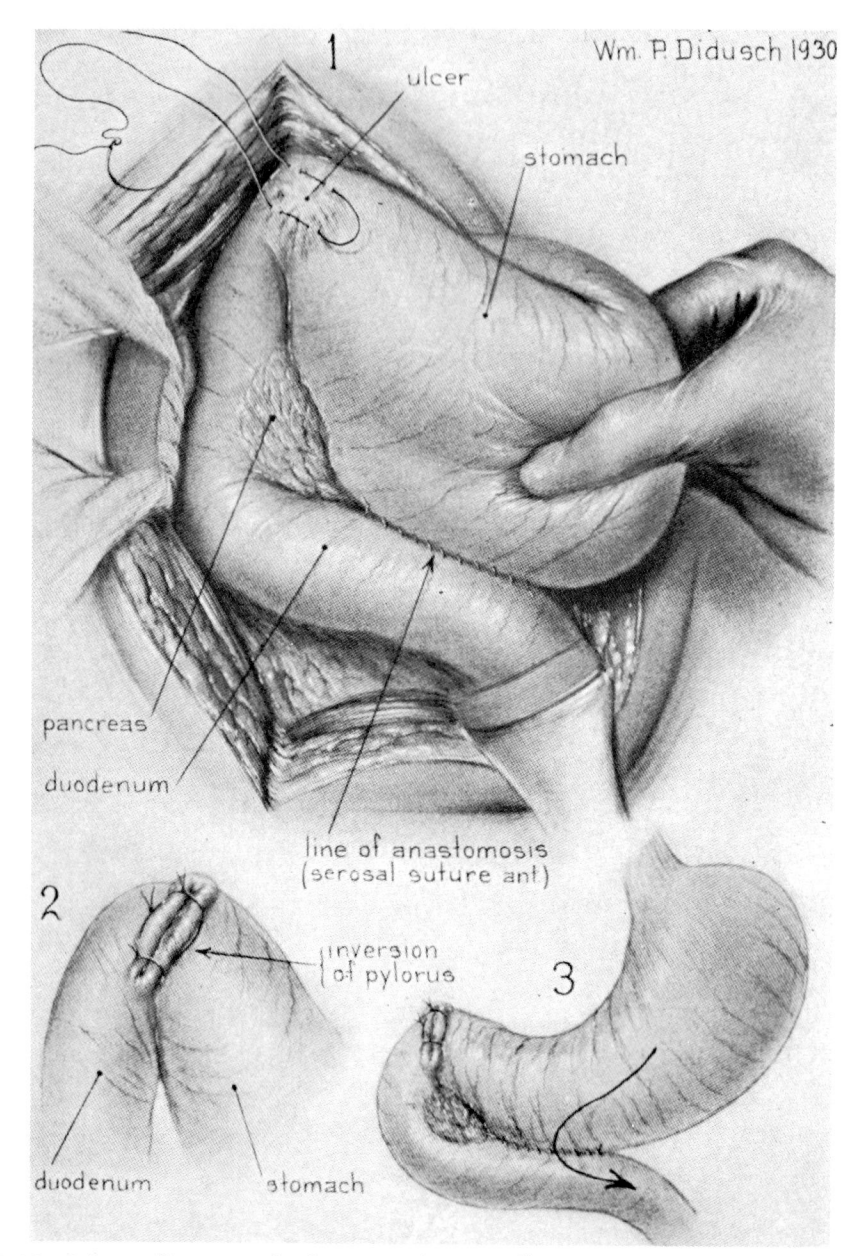

Figure 13–68. Infrapapillary gastroduodenostomy *(continued)*. (From Rienhoff, cited in Figure 13–66.)

GASTROENTEROSTOMY

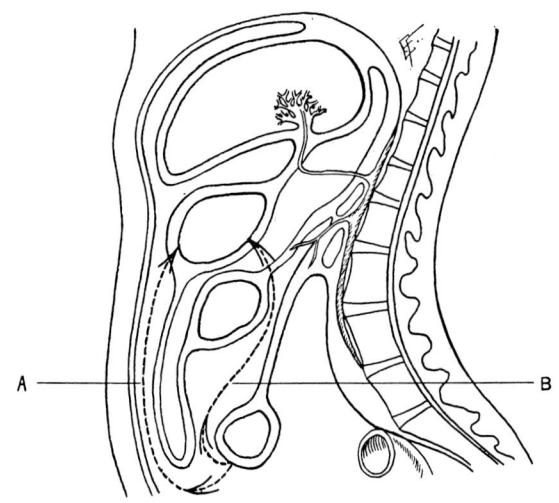

Figure 13–69. *A*, Antecolic gastroenterostomy—the jejunum is anterior to the transverse colon and omentum. *B*, Retrocolic gastroenterostomy—the jejunum is brought through the transverse mesocolon and is behind the transverse colon.

stomach, the gastrojejunostomy is antiperistaltic. If the afferent limb is at the more proximal part of the stomach, the gastrojejunostomy is isoperistaltic (Fig. 13–70). The afferent loop can be shortened by incising the ligament of Treitz and mobilizing the distal part of the duodenum and proximal jejunum. Care must be exercised in performing this maneuver to avoid hemorrhage from small vascular branches near the uncinate process of the pancreas and transverse mesocolon. For malignant disease, an antecolic anastomosis is usually preferred.

In selecting a site on the stomach for the anastomosis, the stomach and omentum should be retracted downward and the most dependent portion of the stomach selected for the anastomosis. In an obstructed and distended stomach, what appears to be the more dependent portion will actually be quite high on the greater curvature after the obstruction is relieved. In such cases it is preferable to select a more distal site on the antrum near the pylorus for the anastomosis. It is usually desirable to free a portion of stomach from the omentum along the greater curvature to allow the anastomosis to be performed in as dependent a portion of the stomach as possible.

Anterior Gastrojejunostomy

A site along the greater curvature of the stomach is selected for the anastomosis and freed from the gastrocolic ligament and omentum (Fig. 13–71). If the operation being performed is a palliative decompression of the stomach and the anastomosis is situated higher on the stomach, it is not necessary to free the stomach from the colon. The ligament of Treitz (Fig. 13–72) is identified and the jejunum is freed to allow as short a loop as possible between the duodenum and gastrojejunostomy. The transverse colon and omentum are gently retracted to the left to minimize the amount of tissue under the loop of jejunum. The omentum may also be separated from the distal greater curvature and reflected to the

Figure 13–70. The antiperistaltic and isoperistaltic methods of gastrojejunal anastomosis. The afferent loop in this illustration is excessively long. Antiperistaltic—the *a*fferent limb is at the distal aspect of the anastomosis. Isoperistaltic—the *e*fferent limb is at the distal aspect of the anastomosis.

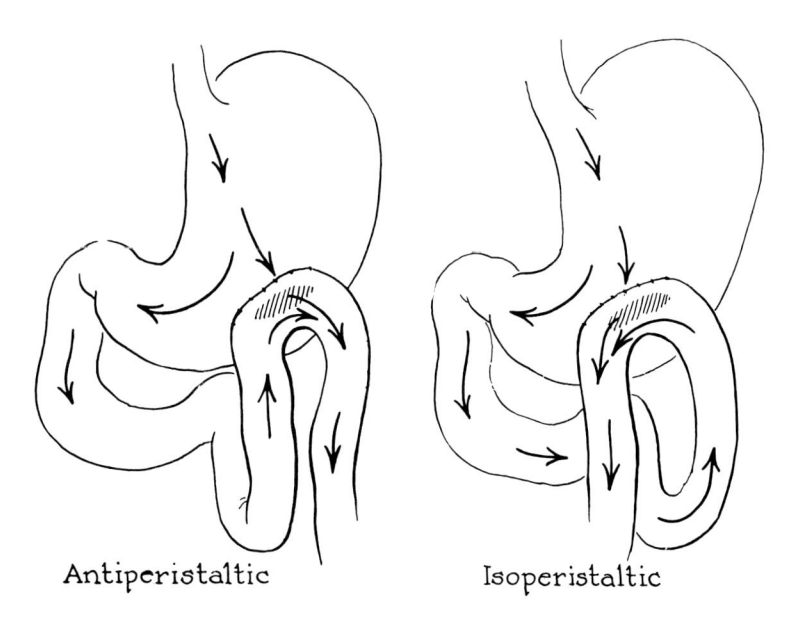

Antiperistaltic   Isoperistaltic

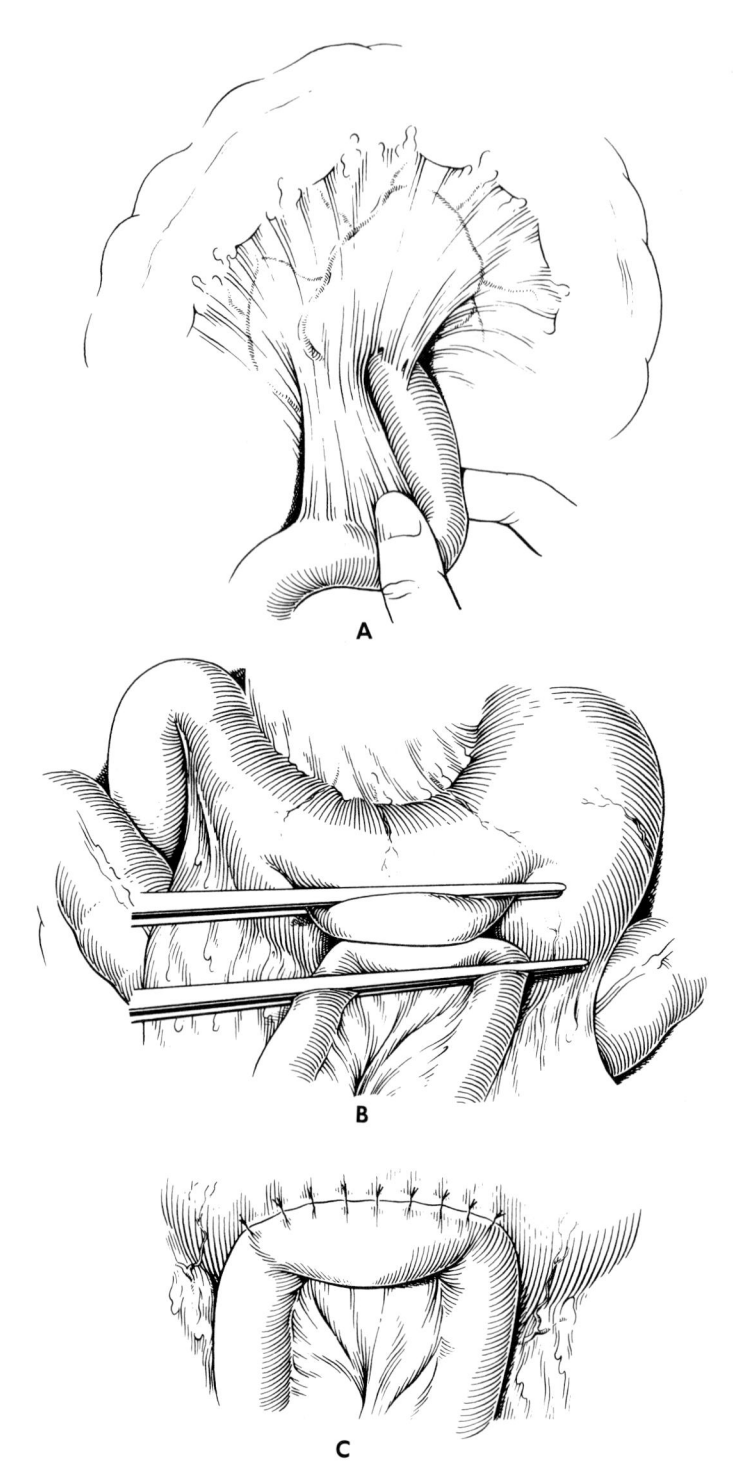

Figure 13–71. Wölfler's technique of anterior antecolic gastrojejunostomy. *A*, First, duodenojejunal flexure is exposed. With the left hand, the transverse colon is drawn upward while the right hand slightly stretches the uppermost jejunal loop. An intestinal clamp is applied approximately 50 cm. away from the flexure along the extent of the desired anastomosis (8 to 10 cm.).

B, The jejunal loop, fixed in the clamp, is brought to the stomach wall in front of the transverse colon, and its tension-free position is checked. The anterior stomach wall is caught with a rubber-covered clamp to the same extent, and both clamps are placed side by side. An isoperistaltic position (in the figure: to the right, the afferent jejunal loop; to the left, the efferent jejunal loop) is preferred by most surgeons.

C, The anastomosis can have one, two, or three rows of sutures. The clamps are removed after the anastomosis is completed.

(From Grewe, H.-E., and Kremer, K.: Atlas of Surgery, Philadelphia, W. B. Saunders Company, 1980, p. 93.)

left (Fig. 13–73). A site on the jejunum is selected so there will be a short loop of jejunum between the ligament of Treitz and the anastomosis, yet tension on the suture line is avoided. The anastomosis between the stomach and jejunum is performed with a posterior interrupted row of nonabsorbable sutures, using a Lembert stitch. Generally the loop between the ligament of Treitz and the anastomosis is about 10 cm. in length. The loop should lie comfortably over the transverse colon and be oriented so as to avoid kinking and torsion.

An isoperistaltic anastomosis is per-

Figure 13–72. Method of locating the first loop of jejunum. (From Partipilo, A. V.: Surgical Technique and Principles of Operative Surgery. Philadelphia, Lea and Febiger, 1949.)

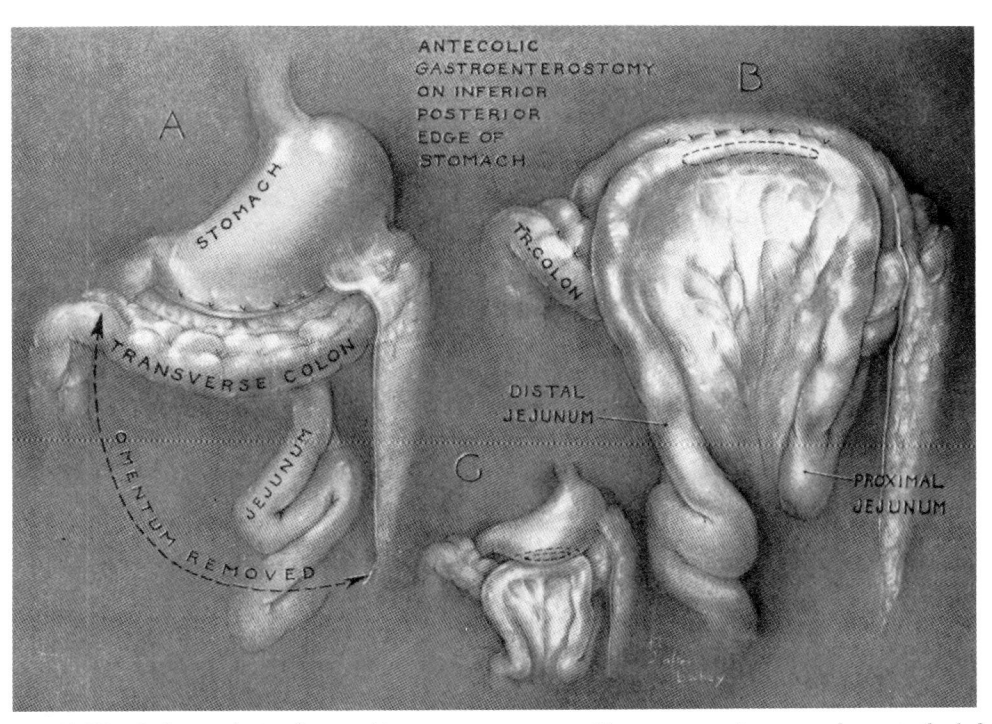

Figure 13–73. Lahey technic of antecolic gastroenterostomy. The omentum is removed over to the left side of the greater curvature. The greater curvature of the stomach is completely freed, and the gastrojejunostomy is made just behind the greater curvature edge.

351

formed in which the afferent limb is attached to the more proximal portion of the stomach, and the efferent limb of the jejunum is at the more distal portion of the stomach. The stoma should be at least 5 cm. long. A two-layer anastomosis is performed, with an outer posterior row of interrupted nonabsorbable Lembert sutures and an inner row of continuous absorbable sutures. The anastomosis is completed with an outer anterior row of nonabsorbable sutures, again using a Lembert stitch. Atraumatic clamps may be used on the stomach and jejunum to minimize any contamination from gastric or small bowel fluid. Generally one or two additional stitches are placed at either end of the anastomosis to alleviate any tension on the corner sutures.

Posterior Gastrojejunostomy

The posterior gastrojejunostomy is performed like the anterior gastrojejunostomy except for its relationship to the transverse colon. The site selected on the stomach for the anastomosis is freed from the colon, and the transverse colon is retracted upward to visualize the middle colic artery and its

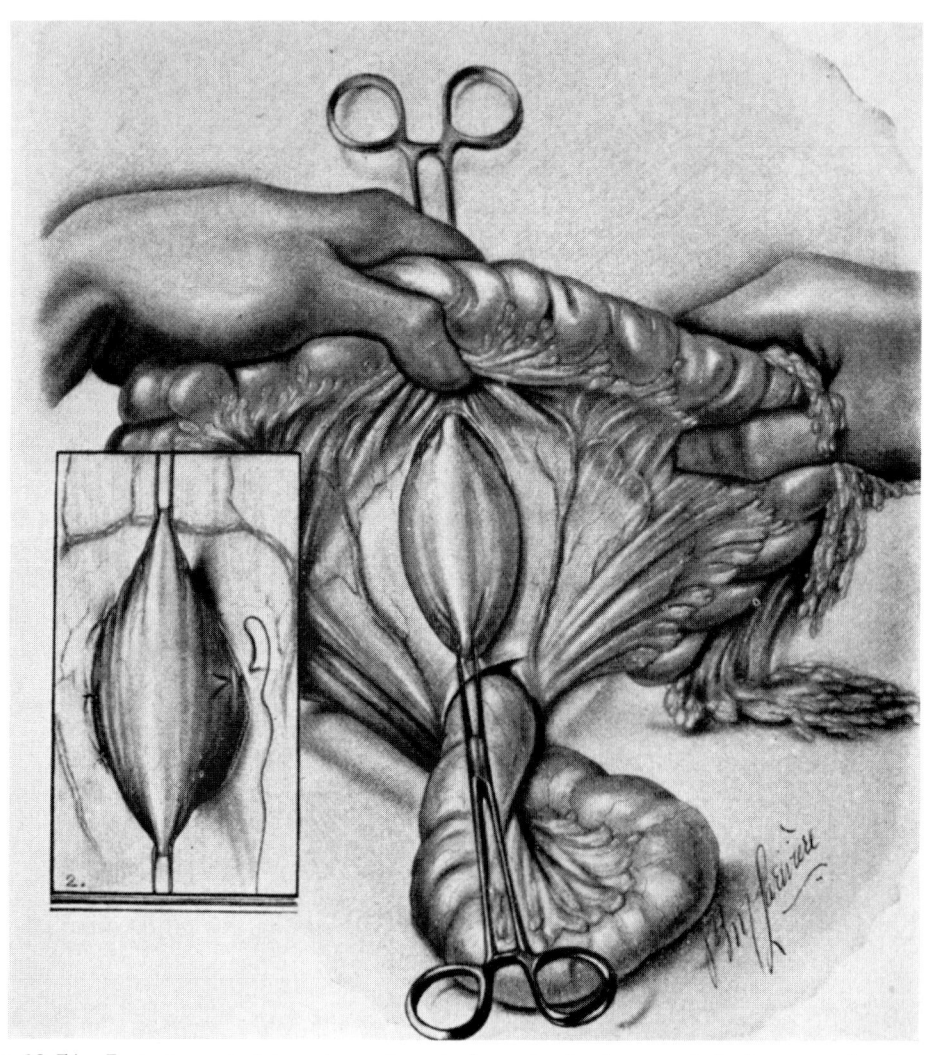

Figure 13–74. Posterior gastrojejunostomy. A vertical opening has been made in the mesocolon through one of the wide arches of the middle colic artery. The duodenojejunal flexure and the first loop of jejunum have been withdrawn from the abdomen. A vertical pouch of the posterior wall of the stomach has been drawn through the opening of the mesocolon. Inset shows the edge of the mesocolon being sutured to the posterior wall of the stomach. (From Maingot, R.: Abdominal Operations, 2nd ed. New York, Appleton-Century-Crofts, 1948, p. 327.)

GASTROENTEROSTOMY

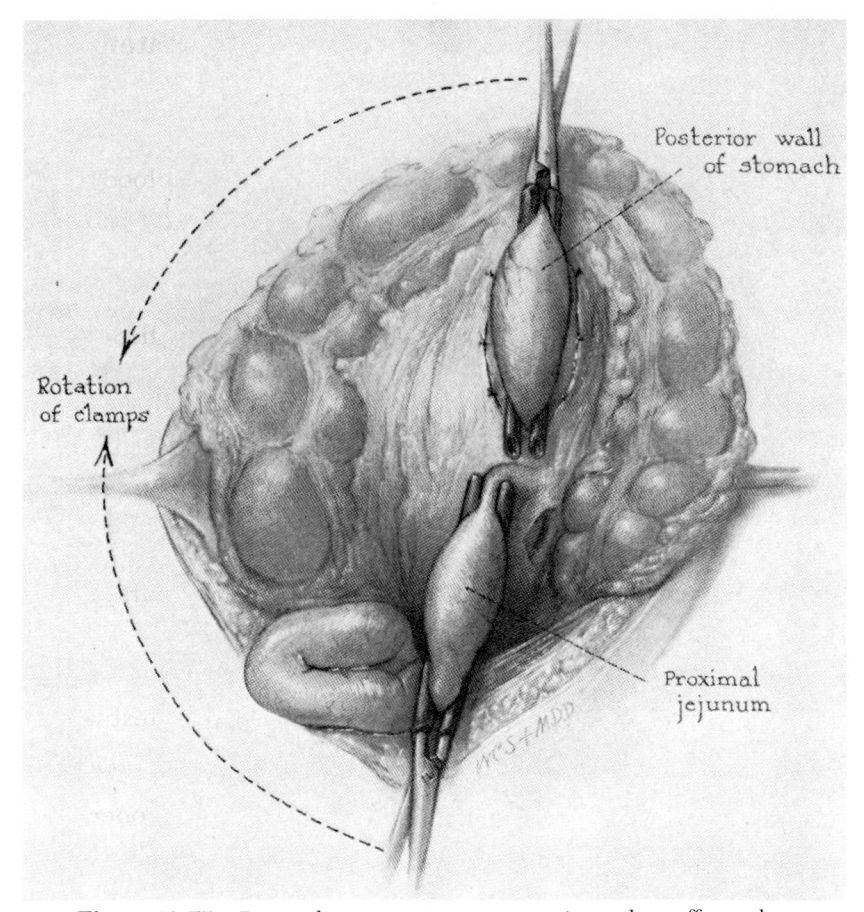

Figure 13–75. Retrocolic gastrojejunostomy, using a short afferent loop.

arching branches. An avascular area in the transverse mesocolon is selected, and an opening is made in the mesocolon at least 7 to 9 cm. in length (Fig. 13–74). If the mesocolon is excessively fat, short, or contracted because of previous adhesions, selecting an opening may be extremely difficult and injury to the vascular supply of the colon may result. In such cases it is preferable to perform an antecolic gastrojejunostomy.

The ligament of Treitz is identified and the jejunum is freed from the ligament, as described (Fig. 13–75). The site on the stomach selected for the anastomosis is gently drawn through the opening in the mesocolon with Babcock clamps. The anastomosis between the jejunum and stomach is performed as described. After completing the anastomosis, it is essential to secure the edges of the mesocolon to the posterior wall of the stomach. This prevents the transverse mesocolon from slipping over the jejunum and obstructing the jejunal limbs. The stoma should admit two fingers comfortably. The corners of the anastomosis should be palpated to insure that there has been no compromise of the lumen of the small bowel.

COMMENTS ON GASTROJEJUNOSTOMY

The essential feature of the technic of gastrojejunostomy is to select a dependent portion of the stomach to permit good emptying. The jejunal loop to the stomach should be as short as possible. This is easier to accomplish with a retrocolic anastomosis than an antecolic anastomosis, although no significant differences have been demonstrated when the two types of anastomoses were compared (ReMine and colleagues, 1978). An isoperistaltic anastomosis is preferred; however, there are no data to substantiate the efficacy of isoperistaltic over antiperistaltic anastomoses.

COMPLICATIONS AFTER GASTROINTESTINAL ANASTOMOSIS

Complications may occur after gastric resections and various types of gastrointestinal anastomoses. Their rate of occurrence has varied in the reports from different sources. Hardy (1964) reviewed 604 patients who had a gastric resection; the deaths and types of complications are listed in Table 13–1.

Complications that usually occur at a longer interval after gastric operations are malnutrition, marginal ulcer at the site of the gastrointestinal anastomosis, gastrojejunocolic fistula, obstruction of the gastrointestinal stoma from scar retraction, and reactivation of an ulcer that was not removed or occurrence of a new peptic ulcer.

Intussusception of the jejunum through a gastrojejunal stoma is rare but may occur early or late following a gastrojejunal anastomosis and is generally included with afferent loop syndromes.

The incidence of some of these complications can be minimized by careful attention to details at the time of the operation.

Table 13–1. Postoperative Deaths and Complications Following Gastric Surgery in 604 Patients

Death or Complication	Incidence (%)
Deaths	6
Wound problems	12
Pulmonary problems	9
Hemorrhage	5
Dumping and diarrhea	5
Malnutrition	5
Duodenal stump dehiscence	3
Jaundice	3
Gastric retention	2
Marginal ulcer	2
Intraperitoneal abscess	2
Fistulas (nonduodenal)	2
Proximal loop syndrome	1
Anastomotic leak	1
Common bile duct injury	0.3

(Modified from Hardy, J. D.: Problems associated with gastric surgery: A review of 604 consecutive patients with annotation. Am. J. Surg. 108:699, 1964.)

When complications do occur, in some instances surgical treatment will be required, and these procedures are discussed in the following sections.

Hematemesis

In the usual patient who has had an uncomplicated gastric resection, varying quantities of old blood pass through the indwelling nasogastric tube for the first postoperative day, then blood in the gastric contents gradually decreases in amount without evidence of fresh bleeding and usually is absent by the third day. If there is a large or protracted hemorrhage, fresh blood will siphon out of the nasogastric tube or be vomited around it. This is often accompanied by general signs of hemorrhage, such as an increase in pulse rate and fall in both the blood pressure and hematocrit.

Experience has shown that postoperative hemorrhage occurs far less frequently if the original gastroenterostomy was performed by the open technic, with ligation of the individual bleeders of the cut edges of the stomach and intestine, than when the closed method of anastomosis is used. For this reason the open technic is preferred.

Rarely, a postoperative intragastric hemorrhage may occur for the first time on the sixth to tenth postoperative day. This is presumably caused by sloughing of the anastomotic suture line. Such a hemorrhage is seldom severe and is usually self-limiting.

Intraperitoneal hemorrhage most commonly occurs within the first postoperative 24 hours when it is usually due to a bleeding vessel that was unnoticed at the time of the operation. Intraperitoneal hemorrhage that occurs on the second or third postoperative day may be from a ligature that has slipped off one of the larger arteries, particularly the left gastric. To minimize this occurrence, the larger arteries should be doubly ligated at the time of their division.

METHODS OF TREATMENT

When general signs of severe or prolonged hemorrhage occur, blood transfusions should be administered, and serious consideration must be given to reoperating upon the patient in order to find and ligate the bleeding point, which is nearly always at the anastomotic suture line. One should not procrastinate long enough for the patient to be depleted by a hemorrhage that is severe, persistent, or recurrent and is causing the patient to lose ground despite transfusions. Instillations of blood-clotting substances into the stomach are unreliable and usually ineffectual.

An intragastric hemorrhage occurring on or after the sixth postoperative day seldom requires surgical treatment, though a rare case may prove to the contrary.

Endoscopy may be performed to determine the site of hemorrhage since on rare occasions hemorrhagic gastritis may be the cause of postoperative hemorrhage. Under such circumstances endoscopy should be performed by an experienced endoscopist since excessive insufflation of air or manipulation may disrupt the anastomosis.

When intraperitoneal hemorrhage is diagnosed, a blood transfusion should be initiated, the patient promptly reoperated upon, and the bleeding point searched for and secured. Procrastination in this condition is futile and is often dangerous as the amount of blood lost is often underestimated. This type of bleeding rarely ceases spontaneously.

TECHNIC FOR LIGATION OF BLEEDING POINT

If reoperation is decided upon, when the abdomen has been opened the anastomotic suture line is identified, and several sutures in its anterior wall are removed so the operator can view the interior of the stoma. It is usually not necessary to take apart the entire anastomosis. (Reoperation is much easier if the gastroenterostomy is an antecolic rather than a retrocolic one.) As soon as the interior of the stoma can be viewed the bleeding point can usually be seen. Most frequently it is the cut edge of the stomach wall. The bleeding point is clamped and ligated. The small opening made in the anterior wall of the anastomosis is now closed with several interrupted sutures that approximate the mucosal layers. This is reinforced with several interrupted Lembert sutures which approximate the seromuscular layers. The abdominal incision is closed in layers.

Postoperative Gastric Retention

This is the most perplexing complication. It occurs in about 2 per cent of patients subjected to gastrectomy. The condition usually is manifest 1 to 14 days postoperatively but infrequently may first appear as late as 30 days or even years after the operation. It is more common after a retrocolic than an antecolic anastomosis.

The causes of obstruction in posterior gastrojejunostomy are listed by Hoag and Saunders (1939) as follows: (1) an improperly placed stoma; (2) a stoma which is too small or which because of its narrow attachment to the stomach produces an acute angulation of the jejunum (more trouble is caused by a small stoma than by a large one); (3) a loop too long or too short for the changing position of the stomach; (4) a mesocolon which fails to stretch when the stomach fills and its walls straighten out; (5) inadequate fixation by suture of the stomach to the cut edges of the transverse mesocolon; (6) adhesions about the stoma due to leakage or trauma (these usually cause obstruction, which appears late in the period of convalescence); (7) pressure on the two loops of jejunum by the middle colic artery; (8) marginal or jejunal ulcers at or near the stomach; and (9) adhesion distal to the anastomosis.

After an anterior gastrojejunostomy the same causes for obstruction may occur, with the exception of constriction by the mesocolon. However, as a substitute for this exception, in anterior gastrojejunostomy without a jejunojejunostomy, stagnation may occur in the long afferent loop and cause obstructive symptoms. This complication can be corrected by performing a subsequent jejunojejunostomy.

Hoag and Saunders state that patients in whom obstruction occurs may be divided into four groups: (1) Those in whom gastric retention occurs immediately following operation but in whom relief eventually is obtained by continued gastric lavage. The obstruction in these patients is due to edema and swelling. (2) Those in whom obstruction still persists after from 7 to 14 days of conservative treatment. The obstruction in these patients is of mechanical nature. (3) Those in whom food ingestion has been satisfactory during the early days of the postoperative period, but signs of obstruction subsequently appeared. The obstruction in these patients is usually mechanical and caused by adhesions, but occasionally it may be adynamic in nature. (4) Those in whom either complete or incomplete obstruction is manifest weeks or years following operation. The obstruction in these patients is due to a marginal ulcer or its complications.

DIAGNOSIS AND METHODS OF TREATMENT

Gastric retention manifest immediately or soon after operation should be treated conservatively at first by the use of a nasogastric tube indwelling in the gastric remnant for continuous drainage of gastric contents. During this time the patient is permitted nothing by mouth while fluids, nutrition, and electrolytes are supplied intravenously. If under this regimen the obstructive symptoms persist for more than 3 to 5 days, the patient should be given barium through the nasogastric tube or by swallow, and its passage through the gastroenterostomy stoma observed under the fluoroscope. Normally the stomach will empty itself rapidly through the stoma, and the barium will pass down the efferent loop of the small intestine. If this occurs, one can assume that the obstructive symptoms are functional. Most of these patients will recover spontaneously if conservative treatment is persisted in. Some of these patients have gastric atony, which usually responds to metoclopramide. Nutritional needs during this period must be adequate, and intravenous hyperalimentation is recommended.

In some cases the barium will be seen to stop abruptly at the stoma and only slowly trickle into the intestine or even appear to be completely held back by an obstruction. When this occurs, the prospect of escaping reoperation is less favorable. If the x-ray study has been made within the first 10 postoperative days, one should continue conservative therapy and close observation for a few more days and then restudy the patient under the fluoroscope. The stomal obstruction conceivably may be caused by edema of the suture line from the operative trauma, or it may be due to edema caused by a stitch abscess at the suture line. Either of these conditions may subside spontaneously, and the obstruction will be relieved within a few days. A localized peritonitis with abscess formation, or a hematoma in the lesser peritoneal sac, may cause the same obstructive signs and symptoms and should be searched for by careful physical examination and roentgenograms taken to determine whether the diaphragm is elevated.

If the obstruction persists and there is no other apparent cause for its presence, it must be assumed that the stoma is mechanically imperfect, and reoperation will be required. The time interval that one can wait before making this decision requires surgical judgment. There is no need to rush in precipitously, as such a patient can be maintained satisfactorily for a number of days by intravenous hyperalimentation. On the other hand, one should not procrastinate so long that the patient becomes depleted and a poorer operative risk. At reoperation the commoner causes of this obstruction are found to be an anastomotic stoma that is too small, an intestinal loop badly angulated at the site of the gastroenterostomy so as to obstruct the stoma, a hematoma or abscess in the anastomotic suture line, or a constricting narrowing of the opening in the transverse mesocolon causing compression if the gastrojejunostomy has been a retrocolic one. It will be necessary to take down and reform the gastroenterostomy stoma or carry out an appropriate procedure, such as a jejunoplasty, partial gastrectomy, or jejunojejunostomy, to correct the situation. *A simple jejunojejunostomy will be of no benefit if the obstruction is at the stoma.*

If at fluoroscopic study the barium is seen to pass freely through the stoma into the efferent loop where it becomes partially obstructed at a lower level with only small amounts of the opaque material passing farther down the intestine, the obstruction may be functional. Golden (1952) believes that this may be due to spasm which is a self-limited physiologic disorder that disappears spontaneously "provided the blood protein and electrolytes are maintained at normal levels by appropriate methods and the distention of the stomach pouch is relieved by suction evacuation." If the condition persists, one should suspect a mechanical intestinal obstruction and reoperate.

In a small number of postgastrectomy patients who develop persistent postoperative vomiting, a fluoroscopic study after a barium swallow will demonstrate that the barium passes easily from the stomach through the stoma into the afferent loop of the gastrojejunostomy with only small amounts passing into the efferent loop. If observed longer under the fluoroscope, the barium in the afferent loop will be seen to regurgitate back and forth into the stomach and afferent loop in which segment it is retained. These patients are usually not greatly disturbed by this condition as their only symptom is vomiting, which occurs only once or twice a day and which they prefer to put up with rather than undergo a second operation. As a result they may carry on for weeks or months with these symptoms and constantly lose weight before appearing for reoperation. The vomitus usually contains undigested food consumed some hours previously. When operated upon, the anastomotic stoma is found to be unobstructed and of satisfactory size, while the afferent loop of jejunum is somewhat but not greatly dilated. An opening should be made in both the afferent and efferent jejunal loops and simultaneously a finger passed up through the lumen of each to meet at the anastomotic stoma and satisfy the operator that the stoma is of adequate size and unobstructed. The cause of the difficulty may be found to be a high spur formed by a too sharp angulation of the two limbs of the jejunal loop as they fall away from the stomach. The spur guides the stream of gastric contents into the afferent loop and partially covers over the opening into the efferent loop. The condition can be easily and satisfactorily corrected by performing a jejunojejunostomy between the afferent and efferent loops or a Hoag jejunoplasty.

Obstruction at an anastomotic stoma that appears months or years after a previous gastric resection is usually caused by cicatricial contracture or marginal ulcer and requires appropriate surgical relief. If the previous gastric resection was for cancer, a recurrence of the malignant lesion should be the cause most suspected.

PREVENTION

Some cases of postoperative gastric retention can be prevented at the time of operation by careful attention to such details as providing a stoma of adequate size, approximating the intestinal loop to the open end of the stomach in such a way that it will not be too sharply angulated, and, in retrocolic anastomoses, by suturing the opening in the transverse mesocolon around the less compressible stomach rather than the jejunal walls. However, even the most careful technic will not always prevent this complication which at present must be accepted as a hazard, even though a small one, of gastric resections.

JEJUNOPLASTY

Hoag and Saunders (1939) published a report of a method of jejunoplasty based on the principle of the Finney pyloroplasty, in which the jejunal loops are utilized for the repair to be made contiguous to the stoma.

It is used for the treatment of obstruction at the gastrojejunostomy stoma or obstruction in a long-loop anterior gastrojejunostomy. If necessary, the procedure also permits simultaneous enlarging of the opening into the stomach and removal of a marginal ulcer. It may also be used for closure of the gastrojejunostomy stoma, thus restoring the original continuity of the alimentary canal in patients with an open pylorus and recurring marginal ulcers in whom local treatment of the lesions or subtotal gastrectomy is contraindicated. It affords an approach that permits complete closure of the stoma from inside and does not require the jejunum to be detached from the stomach or to be resected and anastomosed.

Technic

Hoag and Saunders' description of the procedure will be closely followed.

RELIEF OF OBSTRUCTION WITH OR WITHOUT REMOVAL OF MARGINAL ULCER. After the abdomen has been opened and the anastomosis identified, inspection is made for possible obstructive adhesions at a distance from the anastomosis. The apposed serosal coats of the jejunum are sutured together for about 2 to 4 cm. after the loops have been drawn downward from the attachment to the stomach (Fig. 13-76). The central point chosen for starting the suture line is determined by whether or not it is desirable to shorten the proximal

358　GASTRIC RESECTION AND RECONSTRUCTION

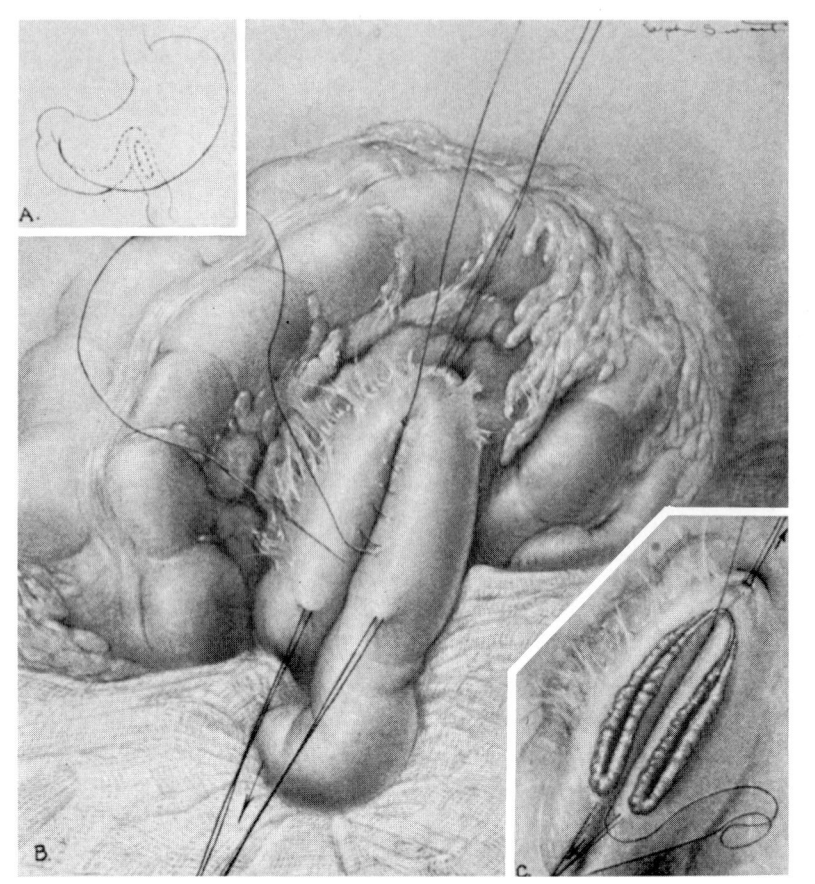

Figure 13-76. Jejunoplasty. *A*, Stomach and posterior gastrojejunostomy. *B*, Center point selected and the jejunum on either side of the anastomosis drawn parallel and united by running peritoneal sutures, forming the outer suture line. *C*, Horseshoe-shaped incision following the lumen of the gut and encircling the suture line. (From Hoag, C. L., and Saunders, J. B.: Jejunoplasty. Surg. Gynecol. Obstet. 68:703, 1939.)

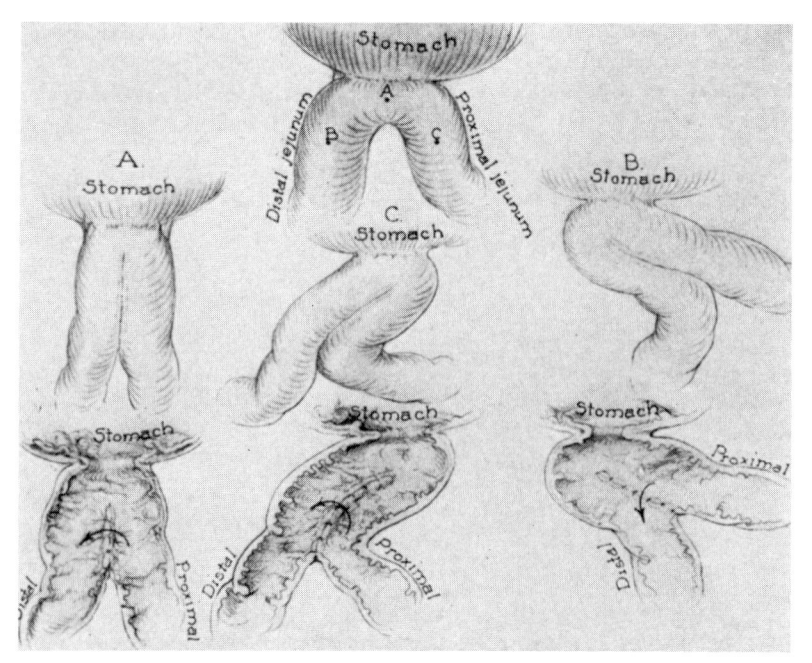

Figure 13-77. Jejunoplasty *(continued)*. Sketch showing how the selection of a central point for starting the jejunoplasty will permit changing the length of the short loop and the resulting change in the lumen of the gut. *A*, Central point using equal length of both proximal and distal jejunum, both shortened an equal amount. *B*, Length of short loop not changed by reflecting the distal jejunum against it. *C*, Maximum shortening of proximal loop by using it entirely for the jejunoplasty. (From Hoag and Saunders, cited in previous figure.)

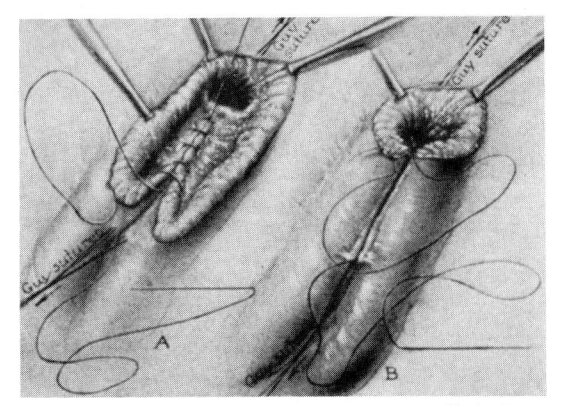

COMPLICATIONS AFTER GASTROINTESTINAL ANASTOMOSIS

Figure 13-78. Jejunoplasty *(continued)*. *A*, Outer edge of the incision retracted showing the stoma; inner catgut interlocking suture line completing the posterior wall. *B*, Inner catgut suture line carried to the anterior wall, completing the closure by use of the Connell stitch. (From Hoag and Saunders, cited in Figure 13-76.)

loop (Fig. 13-77). The point may be directly opposite the stoma or at either end. The viscera are carefully packed off and an inverted U-shaped incision is made around the suture line that approximates the jejunal loops, thereby opening both branches of the bowel (Fig. 13-76C). The edges of this incision are drawn apart so that the stoma in the stomach can be directly inspected and palpated (Fig. 13-78). If the stoma is adequate and no ulcer or faulty mechanics are present, the opening in the jejunum is closed as shown in Figures 13-78 and 13-79. The anterior suture line is reinforced with omentum. If a marginal ulcer is present, it may be excised or cauterized from within the jejunal lumen (Fig. 13-80) and its opening repaired without disturbing the anastomosis, prior to determining whether or not enlargement of the stoma is required.

Ulceration without obstruction may be treated by this method; by vagotomy; by partial gastrectomy with a new gastrojejunal anastomosis; or, if a gastroenterostomy only has been performed and the pylorus is still in continuity and patent, by closing the gastrojejunostomy stoma and returning the passage of food to its original and normal route.

ENLARGEMENT OF STOMA. When the stoma is too small, due to not having been made large enough originally, or has contracted because a marginal ulcer is present, or is narrowed following the excision of an ulcer, it can be enlarged as a final step in completion of the jejunoplasty.

For enlargement of the stoma a vertical incision is made to extend from the superior margin of the original inverted U-shaped incision across the stoma and as far into the stomach as is required for increasing the diameter of the opening (Fig. 13-81). The entire incision is then closed, after selecting a new center, by separating its ends with interposed gastric or duodenal tissues (Figs. 13-82 and 13-83), including more tissue in each stitch on the longer than on the shorter side.

CLOSURE OF STOMA. When closure of the stoma is desired, after completion of the

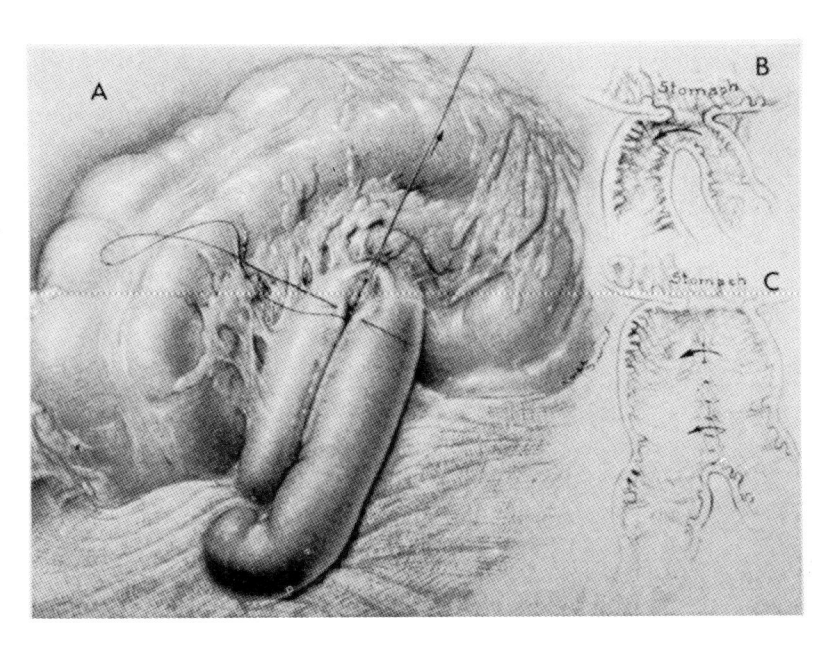

Figure 13-79. Jejunoplasty *(continued)*. *A*, Completion of outer peritoneal suture line by continuing it from the posterior wall. *B*, Sagittal section of stomach, stoma, and jejunum before jejunoplasty. *C*, After jejunoplasty. (From Hoag and Saunders, cited in Figure 13-76.)

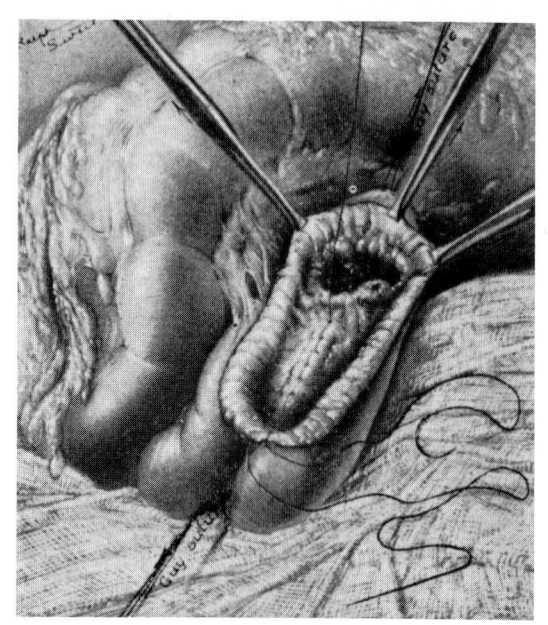

Figure 13-80. Jejunoplasty *(continued)*. First part of operation complete as an approach for the removal of a marginal ulcer. (From Hoag and Saunders, cited in Figure 13-76.)

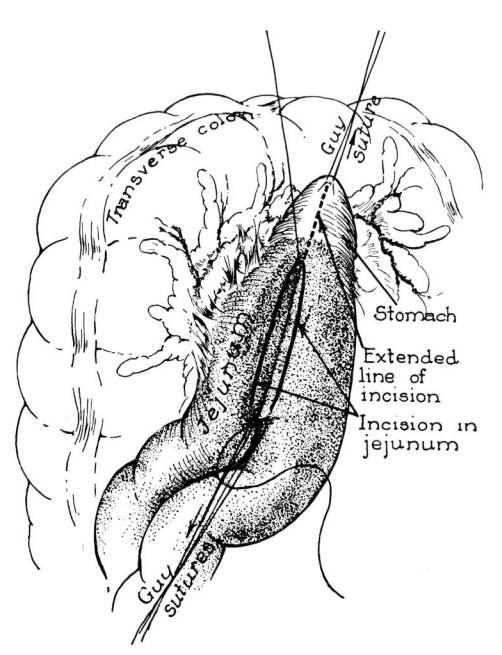

Figure 13-81. Jejunoplasty *(continued)*. Enlargement of the stoma. Line of incision from U-incision across stoma into stomach. (From Hoag and Saunders, cited in Figure 13-76.)

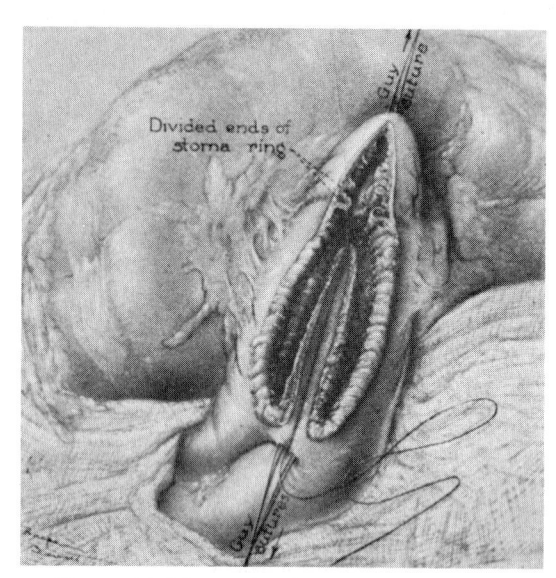

Figure 13-82. Jejunoplasty to enlarge the stoma *(continued)*. Incision is carried across the stoma into the stomach. (From Hoag and Saunders, cited in Figure 13-76.)

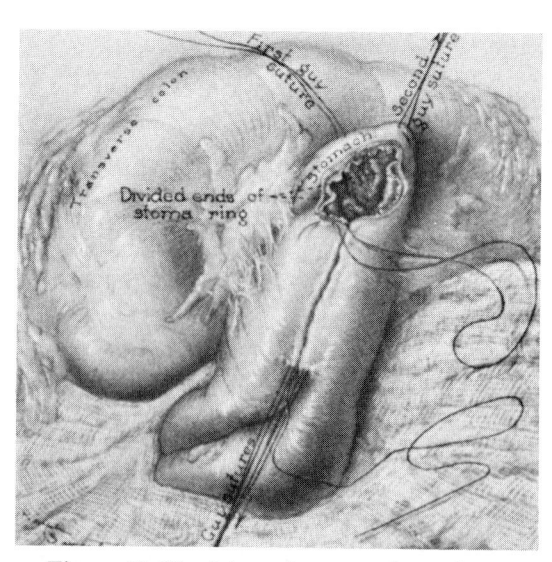

Figure 13-83. Jejunoplasty to enlarge the stoma *(continued)*. Closure of the anterior wall of the jejunum and stomach by staggering the suture line and interposing gastric wall between the ends of the divided stoma to increase its size. (Wider stitches on long side.) (From Hoag and Saunders, cited in Figure 13-76.)

first steps of the jejunoplasty for relief of obstruction, an assistant pushes the stoma forward well up into the operative field by placing a hand either behind the stomach or even in the lesser peritoneal cavity, should this be required, to permit the execution of this step with minimum traction and trauma. The surgeon excises the mucous membrane surrounding the rim of the stoma with curved scissors and then detaches the free edge of the muscularis mucosa around the circumference of the opening and places a double row of Connell sutures of fine gastroenterostomy catgut to evert it into the stomach. Interrupted sutures of silk are used to close the muscle layer of the ring, placing them in the same direction used when the stoma was originally made. These sutures penetrate the entire muscle layer and approach without penetrating the jejunal mucous membrane. A third row of sutures may or may not be required for approximation of the jejunal mucosa (Fig. 13–84). When used, catgut stitches are employed for this layer. The operation is completed by closing the opening in the jejunum (Figs. 13–78 and 13–79).

Comments

In the steps just described for jejunoplasty, except for the procedure involving closure of the stoma, the anastomosis of the jejunal loops should be as short as correction of the mechanical faults permits (usually 2 to 4 cm.) in order to minimize the hazard of marginal ulceration by permitting the alkaline duodenal secretions to continue to bathe the stoma. Since neutralization of acid is not a factor when the stoma is to be closed, a longer jejunal anastomosis is not only permissible but is necessary for the prevention of the encroachment of the swollen tissues about the closed stoma upon the jejunoplasty lumen.

By jejunoplasty, performed by the method described for relief of obstruction, by a minimum of surgery the stoma may be inspected, the opening into the small bowel increased in size, and the septum between the limbs of the jejunal loop cut down materially. Furthermore, the alkaline duodenal secretions are not shunted from the site of the anastomosis. A small secondary stomach with three openings having wider separation from each other than those resulting from the initial gastrojejunostomy has been formed. This cavity is similar to that frequently effected by the gradual dilatation and hypertrophy of the jejunum in patients with long-standing gastroenterostomy or subtotal gastrectomy. Continuity has been restored, permitting the jejunal contents to pass directly downward, to bathe the gastric stoma, or to pass into the stomach. If the jejunal loops had been twisted or compressed, the procedure brings about correction of this fault. If adhesions form over the new suture line they are not likely to cause obstruction.

Jejunoplasty performed by this method has several advantages. It is less time-consuming and is attended with less trauma than is the breaking up of adhesions to expose the anastomosis from without. While the jejunum is being split by the inverted U-shaped incision, the adhesions are divided and the stoma exposed. It is more quickly completed and is attended with no more shock than in an ordinary enteroanastomosis and, in addition, permits direct inspection of the stoma and the adjacent mucosa. It should be a more valuable procedure than the usual enteroanastomosis and should carry no greater operative risk.

Figure 13–84. Jejunoplasty for complete closure of the gastric stoma from within the gut. (Approach and closure as in Figs. 13–76, 13–78, and 13–79.) A, Mucous membrane covering the rim of the stoma excised, exposing a wall made up of muscularis mucosa of the stomach, combined muscle of the stomach and jejunum, and mucous membrane of the jejunum. B, Muscularis mucosa detached from around the stoma and everted into the stomach by the Connell stitch of catgut. C, Muscular layer closed with interrupted silk in the direction in which the stoma was originally made. These stitches approximate but do not penetrate the firmly attached jejunal mucosa, which falls together as the muscle is approximated, and usually does not require a separate suture. (From Hoag and Saunders, cited in Figure 13–76.)

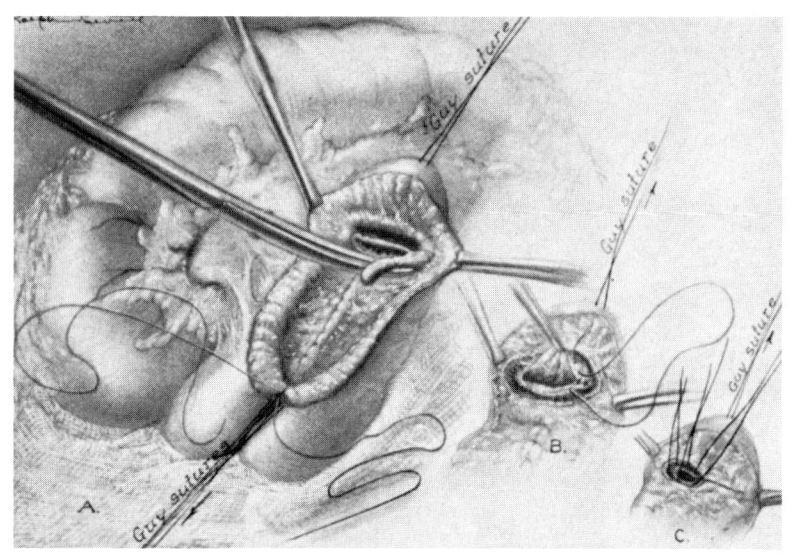

Leakage from Duodenal Stump

This serious complication occurs most frequently in patients having a Billroth II type of gastrectomy in which the duodenal stump is closed under tension or insecurely, or in which the cut end of the duodenum has been so denuded of its vascular supply that it is nonviable. This complication is probably the most common cause of death attending this type of operation.

Great care should be taken to prevent its occurrence. This can be done by mobilizing enough duodenal stump, without devascularizing its seromuscular coat, to invert its cut end with two rows of sutures that are free of tension. If there is any doubt about the security of the closure, a drain should be placed down to that area to convert any possible subsequent leak into a duodenal fistula.

While performing a partial gastrectomy for a duodenal ulcer, if it is apparent that resection of the ulcer will jeopardize the secure closure of the duodenal stump it is safer and wiser to abandon the standard gastrectomy and perform a vagotomy and gastrojejunostomy.

Postoperative leakage from a duodenal stump or gastrointestinal anastomosis, when it occurs, usually manifests itself on the third to seventh postoperative day. The symptoms and signs consist of a rather sudden change for the worse in a patient convalescing normally up to that time, an increase in pulse rate, increased upper abdominal pain and tenderness, and often vomiting. As soon as the diagnosis is made the patient should be reoperated upon and a drain placed down to the leak. At this time no effort should be made to close the leaking viscus as the tissues will be too inflamed to hold sutures satisfactorily. Later, appropriate steps as outlined for a duodenal fistula can be taken.

Rupture of Abdominal Incision

This complication may occur after gastric resections, particularly those that are performed for carcinoma, or those associated with postoperative coughing, hiccuping, distention, persistent vomiting, wound infection, or wound hematoma formation.

The complication usually occurs about the sixth to ninth postoperative day and is forewarned by drainage of a small amount of serosanguineous fluid from the wound. The wound may be partially or completely disrupted, accompanied by eventration of the intestine of a varying degree.

Whenever an abdominal wound disrupts and the intestine can be seen, even though only in the depth of the wound, no time should be lost by trying futile tamponades. The disrupted wound should be covered by a sterile towel which is held in place by suitable adhesive strips to prevent further eventration of the intestine. The patient is taken immediately to the operating room where under anesthesia the bowel is replaced in the abdominal cavity. The wound is closed with sutures of nylon or wire on large, curved, cutting-edge needles which are passed through all the layers (skin, fascia, muscle, and peritoneum) of the wound to reapproximate its separated edges. Care must be taken to avoid injuring the bowel with these sutures. The long ends of the wire are twisted together over a roll of gauze placed on the approximated edges to prevent their cutting through the tissues. In this condition, layer-by-layer closure of the wound is difficult or impossible owing to the friability and edema produced by the recent original operation. Postoperative cough and distention must be controlled by suitable measures.

The frequency of this complication has been reduced by using nonabsorbable instead of absorbable sutures for closing the abdominal incision, and by the use of stay sutures.

Prompt repair of an abdominal eventration carries a surprisingly low mortality, but in a number of subjects in whom repair has been successful an incisional hernia has developed later.

Jejunal Ulcer

Following gastrojejunostomy or partial gastrectomy with gastrojejunostomy for gastric or duodenal ulcer, an ulcer sometimes develops in the jejunum. Most of these postoperative ulcers begin in the jejunum just distal to the anastomosis and are designated as "marginal jejunal ulcers." They occasionally attain sufficient size to encroach on the anastomosis or extend to the gastric side of the stoma. Endoscopy is the most reliable diagnostic procedure for the detection of a marginal ulcer.

Jejunal ulcer can develop after any anastomosis of which the jejunum is part, regardless of whether none or all of the stomach has been resected.

Chronic, subacute, or acute perforation complicates some jejunal ulcers. Jejunal ulcers perforate into the transverse mesocolon, transverse colon, and abdominal wall, in this order of frequency. Perforation into the transverse colon is a grave complication of marginal ulcer which results in *gastrojejunocolic fistula*. That a fistula of this kind can occur is the greatest justification for operating early on intractable jejunal ulcer.

Surgical cure of jejunal ulcer is more certain than that of gastric or duodenal ulcer because it almost always is effected by disconnecting the stomach from the jejunum, and the ulcer does not recur if the jejunum is not used in restoring gastrointestinal continuity. Disconnecting the gastrojejunal stoma is not an unusually difficult operation unless perforation or a jejunocolic fistula has developed. It is easier to perform if the original anastomosis was made antecolic instead of retrocolic.

At operation the patient with jejunal ulcer is treated not only for the secondary or complicating jejunal lesion, but also for the primary duodenal or gastric ulcer for which the gastrojejunostomy was performed. The benefit from any procedure directed toward alleviation of the jejunal ulcer depends upon what can be done for the primary ulcer. For that reason the cause of the jejunal ulcer must be investigated thoroughly.

Identification of a penetrating or perforating jejunal ulcer at surgical exploration ordinarily is possible because signs of penetration and perforation usually are seen when the colon is mobilized, the mesocolon is exposed, and the area of anastomosis is examined from without. A nonpenetrating or nonperforating ulcer usually can be located by careful dissection after opening the anastomosis. There rarely is more than one jejunal ulcer.

A bleeding jejunal ulcer may be extremely difficult to recognize and may be missed even after the gastrojejunal stoma is taken down. An ulcer in the posterior part of the anastomosis also can be overlooked unless the anastomosis is taken down very carefully. Unless one searches through an incision in the jejunum, it is good practice to cut across the stomach 2.5 cm. proximal to the anastomosis and look for the ulcer in the jejunum through the stoma.

Marginal Ulcer

The evaluation, causes and treatment of recurrent ulcer have been reviewed by Stabile and Passaro (1976). When a recurrent ulcer is discovered, the factors leading to its development should be investigated. These factors can be divided into six major categories: (1) inadequate vagotomy, (2) inadequate drainage, (3) inadequate gastric resection, (4) inadequate alkaline neutralization, (5) G-cell hyperplasia or Zollinger-Ellison syndrome, and (6) drugs.

Incomplete vagotomy is probably the most common cause of recurrent ulcer. Acid secretion remains at a high level because vagal innervation is intact. Following a vagotomy, the maximal acid secretion should be reduced by at least 50 per cent. If preoperative acid studies are available for the patient, a postoperative test can provide valuable information about the status of the vagotomy. Completion of the vagotomy is recommended in a patient with recurrent ulcer disease following partial gastrectomy.

Inadequate gastric emptying resulting in stasis is the usual cause of the gastric ulcer following a previous ulcer operation. This is due to technical factors in which the stoma is narrowed or to subsequent scarring which impedes drainage of the stomach. Delayed emptying is usually evident on barium studies of the stomach and gastroscopy. On occasion the stoma can be gently dilated with the endoscope but usually reoperation is required to enlarge the gastroenterostomy.

When gastric resection is not combined with vagotomy, a generous gastrectomy (75 per cent) is necessary to prevent recurrent ulcer disease. Antrectomy and hemigastrectomy may not be adequate to sufficiently reduce acid secretion. Gastric analysis in these patients generally reveals significant amounts of stimulated acid. Vagotomy is recommended for these patients. Patients who have had a vagotomy and antrectomy and develop a marginal ulcer should be investigated for retained antrum or Zollinger-Ellison syndrome. In both groups of patients, the basal gastrin will be elevated; however, in the patient with retained antrum the gastrin level will be decreased by the secretin test.

Inadequate neutralization of acid produced by the stomach is another cause for marginal ulcer. This is generally seen in the patient with a Billroth II with a long afferent limb. Pancreatic and bile secretions may have lost their effectiveness by the time they reach the gastroenterostomy if the afferent limb is excessively long. Another factor in the long afferent limb is the delay between acid secretion coming in contact with the jejunum at the stoma and the arrival of biliary and pancreatic secretions. Gastroenterostomy without vagotomy is another cause of marginal ulcer due to inadequate neutralization of acid secretion. In both these circumstances, an acid-reducing procedure is recommended, and shortening of the afferent limb may be necessary.

Excessive amounts of gastrin, whether due to G-cell hyperplasia or to the Zollinger-Ellison syndrome, are hormonal causes of marginal ulcer. G-cell hyperplasia is characterized by an increase in serum gastrin following a protein meal and suppression of resting gastrin by the secretin test. The Zollinger-Ellison syndrome is diagnosed by gastric acid hypersecretion and markedly elevated serum gastrin levels or an increase in basal gastrin following intravenous injection of secretin. G-cell hyperplasia is successfully treated by antrectomy, and the Zollinger-Ellison syndrome can be treated by total gastrectomy, or, more recently, with the use of cimetidine.

Drugs such as salicylates, steroids, and anti-inflammatory agents have been implicated in causing ulcers. The ulcers may occur not only in the gastric remnant but also in the jejunum.

Other causes have been implicated in recurrent ulcers, such as hyperparathyroidism, pituitary adenomas, Cushing's syndrome, and stress.

DISCONNECTION OF GASTROJEJUNOSTOMY

Indications

This procedure is indicated for the treatment of gastrojejunal ulcer if the original peptic ulcer has healed and the pylorus is both patent and not obstructed. In such instances the gastrojejunal ulcer will promptly heal.

If the original peptic ulcer is still active, disconnection should be combined with partial gastrectomy accompanied by gastroduodenostomy or a new gastrojejunostomy.

Vagotomy alone has been very successful in treating gastrojejunal ulceration occurring after partial gastrectomy, but has been less successful than gastrectomy with removal of the gastrojejunal ulcer and gastroenteric stoma for gastrojejunal ulcer occurring after a simple gastroenterostomy.

Technic

Disconnection of an anterior gastrojejunostomy is easier to perform than that of a posterior gastroenterostomy, as the latter is adherent to the transverse mesocolon and is deeper within the abdominal wound. Disconnection of a posterior gastrojejunostomy will be described.

The site of the gastrojejunostomy and gastrojejunal ulcer is usually found densely adherent to the transverse colon.

The first step is to identify and mobilize the stomach by freeing it of adhesions to the anterior abdominal wall and liver, until the pylorus and duodenum are exposed. It should then be carefully inspected to discover whether the original ulcer is healed, whether other ulcers are present, and whether the pylorus is patent or obstructed. The duodenum is inspected to determine whether its second portion can be mobilized sufficiently to form a gastroduodenostomy if desired.

The transverse colon is then mobilized, and the gastrojejunostomy anastomosis is exposed so it can be inspected for signs of ulceration or inflammation. Usually the lesion is on the jejunal side of the anastomosis in either the proximal or distal jejunal loop. The mesocolon is usually adherent to the inflammatory mass.

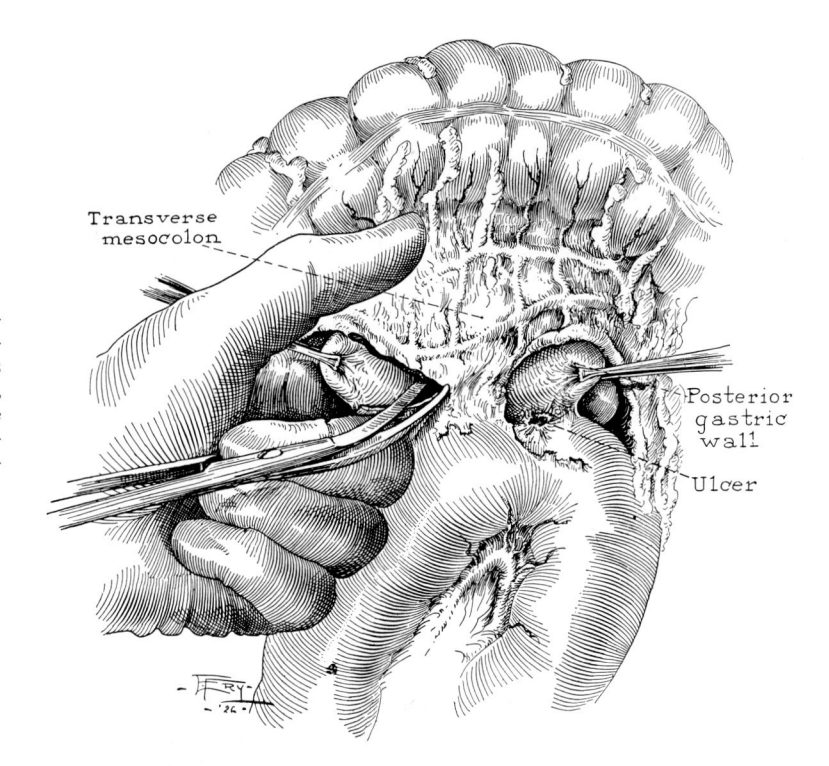

Figure 13-85. Disconnection of gastrojejunostomy. Freeing the mesocolon from its attachments. (From Eusterman, G. B., and Balfour, D. C.: The Stomach and Duodenum. Philadelphia, W. B. Saunders Company, 1935.)

The anastomosis is freed from its adhesions by exposing the posterior wall of the stomach through an opening made in the transverse mesocolon to one side of the gastrojejunal anastomosis, and then inserting a finger through this opening and dissecting the posterior wall of the stomach away from the mesocolon (Fig. 13–85). The anterior wall of the stomach is freed from the colon and mesocolon in the same way, and the anastomosis is mobilized intact.

Any perforation or defect in the wall of the colon is closed over at this time.

After mobilization of the anastomosis is complete, the stomach is brought down through the opening in the transverse mesocolon, and a rubber-shod clamp is placed across it 4 to 5 cm. proximal to the anastomosis (Fig. 13–86). Another rubber-shod clamp is placed across the two limbs of the jejunum, forming the anastomosis. The stomach is divided just distal to the clamp occluding

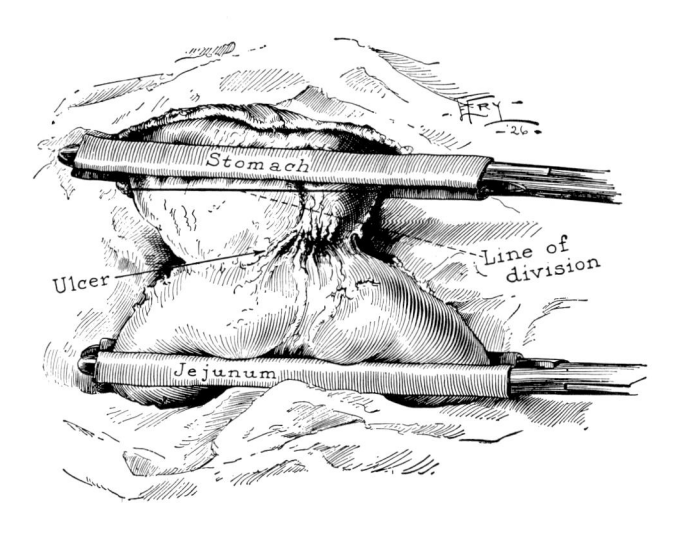

Figure 13-86. Disconnection of gastrojejunostomy *(continued)*. Application of clamps to stomach and jejunum on each side of the anastomotic ulcer. (Balfour, D. C.: Ann. Surg., Vol. 84. J. B. Lippincott Company.)

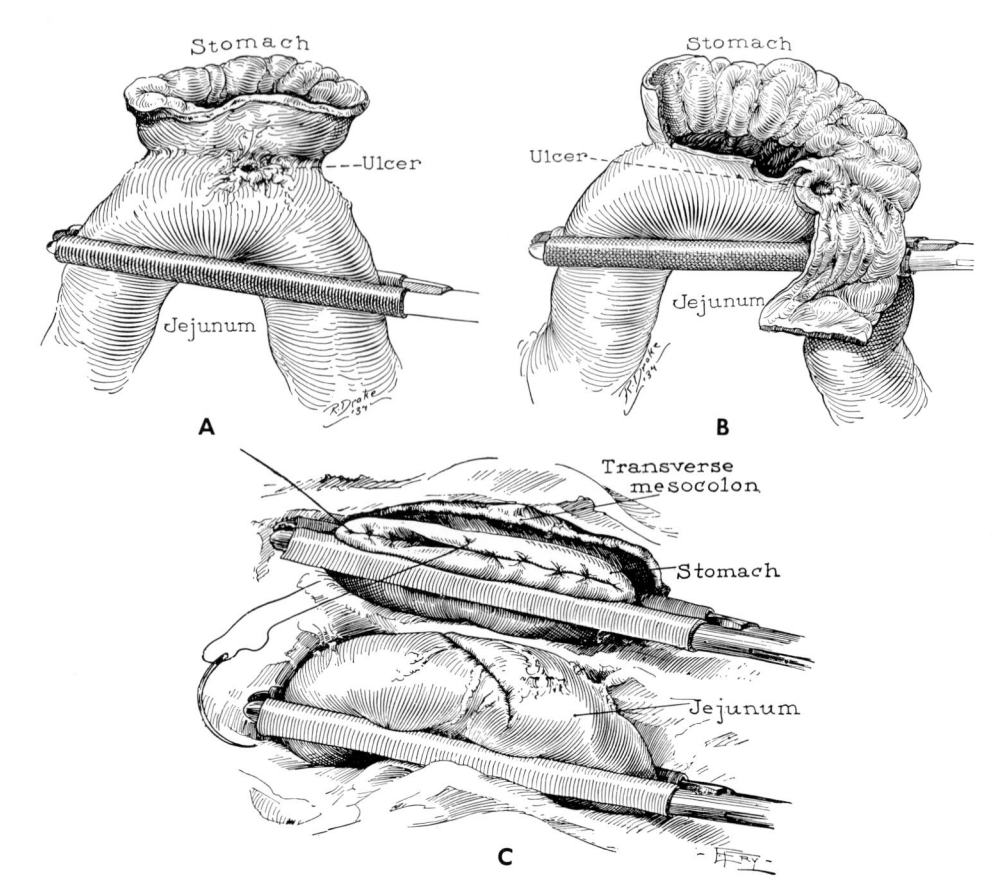

Figure 13–87. Disconnection of gastrojejunostomy *(continued)*. *A*, Jejunum mobilized by division of the stomach. *B*, Excision of gastric cuff, including ulcer in the jejunum. *C*, Closure of the site of gastroenterostomy in the stomach and jejunum preparatory to resection. (From Eusterman, D. B., and Balfour, D. C.: The Stomach and Duodenum. Philadelphia, W. B. Saunders Company, 1935.)

it (Fig. 13–87A), and the mucosal surface of the anastomosis inspected before it is damaged (Fig. 13–87B). If the ulcer is in the anastomotic line, the anastomosis with the cuff of stomach attached can be excised (Fig. 13–87B). If the ulcer is in the jejunum at some distance from the anastomosis it is not necessary to excise it, since healing will promptly occur if the jejunum is closed, if a gastroduodenostomy is performed, or if a new gastrojejunostomy is formed *distal* to the ulcer.

The opening in the jejunum is closed transversely with a row of continuous Connell sutures of chromic catgut reinforced by a row of interrupted Lembert sutures of silk.

If there is any possibility that the jejunum will be constricted by such a closure, the jejunal segment should be resected, and an end-to-end anastomosis performed.

If the primary peptic ulcer is healed and the pylorus is in continuity and fully patent, it may be desirable to restore the normal pathway for the passage of food, in which case the opening in the stomach is closed (Fig. 13–87C), the stomach is withdrawn above the transverse mesocolon, the opening in the mesocolon is closed, and normal anatomic relations are restored, completing the operation.

If partial gastrectomy is indicated, the desired amount of stomach is resected, and a gastroduodenostomy or new gastrojejunostomy is performed. If the latter, the anastomosis should be made to a new opening in the jejunum at least 6 cm. distal to the site of the original gastrojejunostomy. An antecolic anastomosis may be preferable for this, but a retrocolic one is often used.

The abdomen is closed without drainage.

Repair of Gastroileostomy

The formation of an anastomosis between the stomach and the ileum is a surgical error that occurs infrequently but may have serious consequences. If the error was made in attempting a simple gastroenterostomy, leaving intact a patent pylorus, the consequences may not be so severe, as sufficient food may pass through the pylorus into the small intestine to nourish the patient. If, however, all food passes through the gastroileostomy stomach — which it must if a partial gastrectomy was previously performed — marked malnutrition ensues.

In 2 of the 7 patients having gastroileostomy reported by Rivers and Wilbur (1932), an ileal ulcer developed just distal to the anastomosis.

The symptoms and signs of gastroileostomy usually begin in the immediate postoperative period and resemble those found in gastrojejunocolic fistula, except that in the latter there is a prolonged interval between operation and the onset of symptoms. They include diarrhea and marked loss of weight despite an adequate intake of food. Fecal belching and vomiting may or may not occur.

The diagnosis can usually be made by x-ray study made after the patient has had a barium meal.

The treatment is surgical. These patients are often in such a depleted condition when first seen that they will obviously not withstand a major surgical procedure. A vigorous attempt should be made to improve their condition by correcting anemia with blood transfusions; restoring serum protein with intravenous plasma; and correcting electrolyte, fluid and nutritional deficiency by intravenous hyperalimentation. If these efforts are unsuccessful, a preliminary nutritional jejunostomy may be performed.

When the general condition is restored satisfactorily, the gastroileostomy should be corrected by operation. The operation consists of taking down the gastroileostomy, closing the opening into the ileum (if closure constricts the ileum, the involved segment of ileum should be resected and a side-to-side ileoileostomy performed), and forming a proper gastrojejunostomy.

The technic is the same as that described for disconnecting a gastrojejunostomy.

Chapter 14

VAGOTOMY, PYLOROPLASTY, AND GASTRIC BYPASS

VAGOTOMY

Vagotomy consists of interrupting the vagus nerves by transection. The effects of vagotomy on gastric acid secretion are to ablate the cephalic phase of gastric acid secretion and to desensitize the parietal cells to gastrin. Following vagotomy, maximal acid secretion will be reduced 30 to 40 per cent. This degree of reduction of gastric acid secretion occurs regardless of the type of vagotomy performed and depends upon complete denervation of the acid-secreting cells. This reduction can be useful in determining the completeness of the vagotomy in the postoperative period if a recurrent ulcer develops. A reduction of less than 30 to 40 per cent of the maximal acid output is strong evidence that the vagotomy is incomplete.

The vagus also is an important determinant of gastric motility. It has two major influences: (1) on the emptying of liquids; and (2) on the emptying of solids. When liquids are received into the stomach, the stomach accommodates for the increase in volume without any significant increase in pressure. This mechanism is mainly under the control of the fundic area of the stomach and is termed *receptive relaxation*. When vagal innervation to the fundus is interrupted, as happens in all types of vagotomy, this mechanism also is interrupted, and, with an increase in volume, an increase in pressure occurs. This results in the rapid emptying of liquids. The emptying of solids is coordinated through the peristaltic action of the antrum and the relaxation of the pylorus. If disruption of vagal innervation to the antrum and pylorus occurs, then these coordinated movements are abolished, and emptying of solids is delayed.

Truncal vagotomy and selective vagotomy result in reduced acid secretion, increased emptying of liquids, and decreased emptying of solids. The latter is the result of denervation of the gastric antrum and generally results in gastric stasis. A drainage procedure is therefore required for a truncal vagotomy or selective vagotomy. Proximal gastric vagotomy results in reduced acid secretion, increased emptying of liquids, and no change in the emptying rate of solids. The increased emptying rates of liquids are the result of denervation of the fundus and loss of receptive relaxation. The normal emptying of solids is maintained because the antrum is not denervated. As a result, a drainage procedure is not required for a proximal gastric vagotomy.

Anatomy of the Vagus Nerves

The vagus nerves arise, one on each side, from the medulla oblongata. The great majority of the fibers of which they consist belong to the parasympathetic division of the autonomic nervous system. Branches of the vagus nerves are widely distributed, passing to the esophagus, heart, bronchi, lungs, stomach, small intestine, and other abdominal viscera (Fig. 14–1). Only the distribution to the stomach will be considered

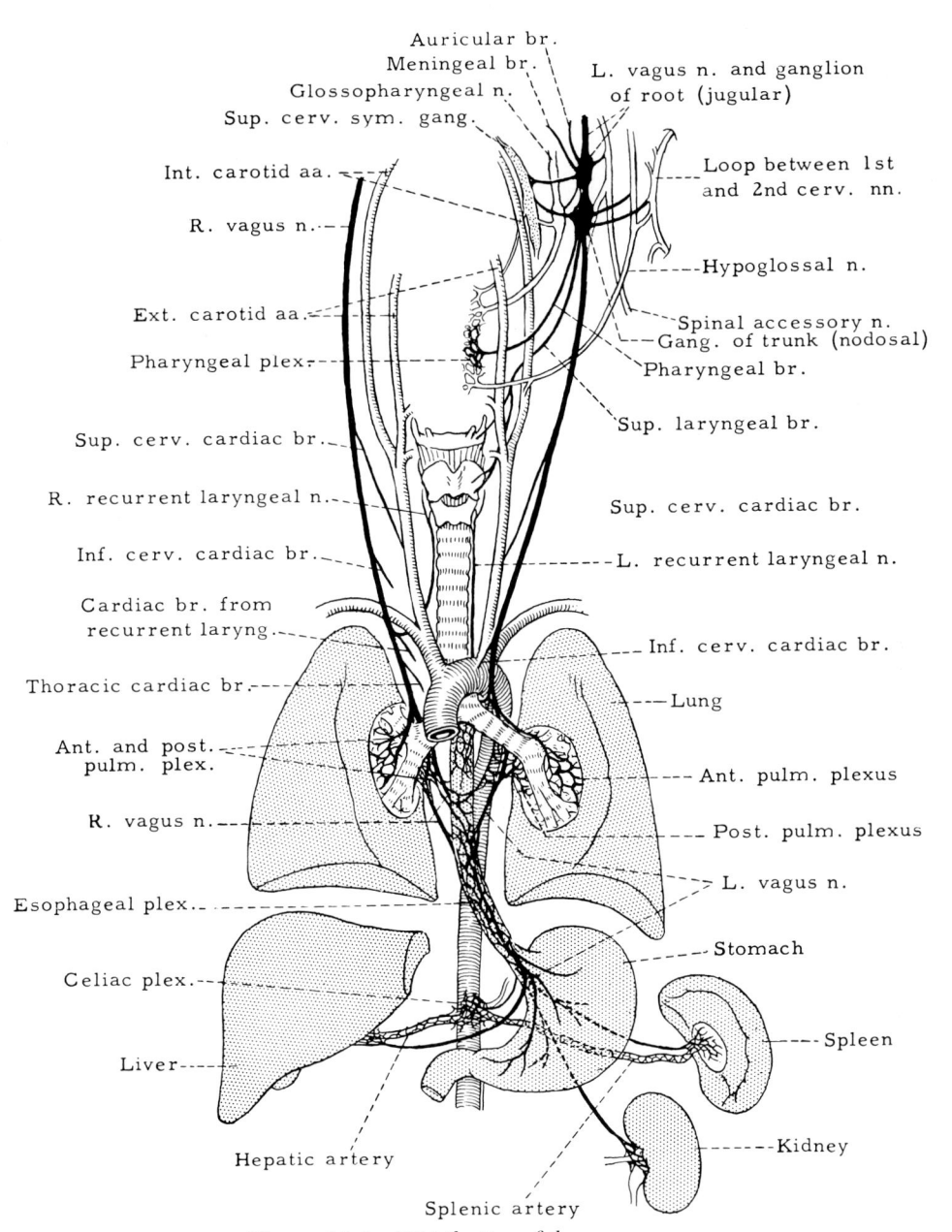

Figure 14-1. Distribution of the vagus nerves.

here, for in performing vagotomy for peptic ulcer the vagi are sectioned below the points of departure of their branches to the heart and lungs, none of which occur below the level of the hilus of the lung.

After forming a plexus about the hilus of the lung the vagus fibers on each side reunite to form a single nerve on each side. They continue along the corresponding wall of the esophagus to the diaphragm. (There is considerable variation in this anatomic arrangement (Fig. 14–2) as the nerves may continue as multiple instead of single trunks and in a variety of patterns, but the single-trunk pattern is the one most commonly found.) As they traverse the esophageal hiatus of the diaphragm, the left vagus nerve changes from a left lateral position to an anterior one, and below the diaphragm its trunk divides into many fibers which fan out over the anterior wall of the stomach.

Simultaneously, the right vagus

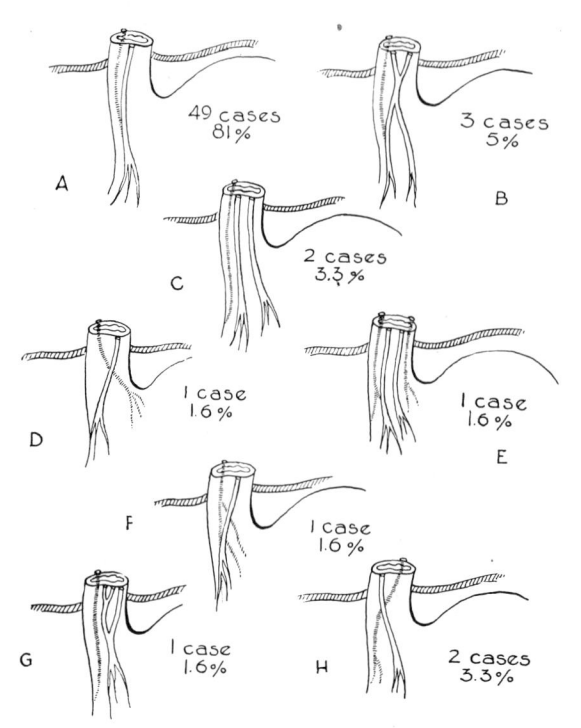

Figure 14-2. Sketches showing the distribution of the vagus nerves along the lower portion of the esophagus and upper stomach in 60 human dissection specimens. Note that in 81 per cent of the cases the distribution is as illustrated in A. (From Partipilo, A. V.: Surgical Technique and Principles of Operative Surgery. Philadelphia, Lea & Febiger, 1949.)

changes from its previous right lateral position to a posterior one, and below the diaphragm its fibers fan out over the posterior wall of the stomach. This is due to the left-to-right embryologic rotation of that part of the gut that forms the stomach.

Generally speaking, the fibers are concentrated into single trunks immediately above and immediately below the diaphragm. These are the points at which there will be the least chance of missing some of the fibers in sectioning the nerves.

Physiology of the Vagus Nerves

All the functions of the vagus nerves are not understood. In general they are inhibitors of the heart action and stimulators of gastric secretions and of the motility of the esophagus, stomach, and intestines.

For the treatment of peptic ulcer, they should be sectioned only below the points of departure of the branches to the heart and lungs, to avoid undesired effects upon those structures. Only the known effects upon the stomach of severance of the vagus nerves will be considered here. Bilateral complete vagotomy alters gastric secretion and intestinal motility. These alterations are discussed in greater detail under the types of vagotomy.

Types of Vagotomy

Four types of vagotomy are used in the treatment of peptic ulcer disease: truncal, selective, proximal gastric, and transthoracic.

TRUNCAL VAGOTOMY

Truncal vagotomy consists of severing the main vagal trunks as they emerge through the esophageal hiatus. A truncal vagotomy not only denervates the entire stomach but deprives the entire abdomen of parasympathetic innervation derived from the vagus. Another descriptive term for truncal vagotomy is total abdominal vagotomy. Often a segment of the vagal trunk is removed; this procedure more properly is termed vagectomy.

TECHNIC. The peritoneum overlying the esophagus is incised, and the esophagus is encircled with a Penrose drain. Care is taken to encircle the entire esophagus, avoiding perforation. With gentle traction, the anterior and posterior vagal trunks can be identified either visually or by palpation. The anterior or left vagal trunk is generally on the anterior surface of the esophagus and is easily identified visually. A segment of the trunk is freed from the esophagus and a segment excised. The ends of the trunk are either clipped with hemoclips or ligated. The posterior or right vagal trunk lies on the posterior part of the esophagus and is generally identified by palpation. A slight amount of downward tension on the Penrose drain encircling the esophagus usually results in the trunk being felt as a taut band. By deflecting the main trunk to either the right or left, the trunk is secured with a nerve hook or clamp and a segment removed similarly to the method used with the anterior trunk. Small vagal fibers are then sought to insure the completeness of a vagotomy. In general, excessive tension and dissection around the esophagus are to be avoided (Skandalakis, Rowe, and Gray, 1974).

SELECTIVE VAGOTOMY

Attempts have been made to minimize such troublesome postvagotomy problems as diarrhea and gallstones. The selective vagotomy denervates the entire stomach but preserves the innervation to the liver and biliary tree and to the celiac ganglia. This is accomplished by dividing the main vagal trunks after the hepatic branch is given off the anterior trunk and the celiac branch off the posterior trunk. The selective vagotomy requires meticulous isolation of the vagal trunks and identification of the fibers to the stomach and other visceral organs. The low recurrence rate following this type of vagotomy reported by Herrington and Sawyers (1978) is probably the result of the care required to perform this type of vagotomy to insure its completeness.

TECHNIC. The anterior trunk of the vagus is identified on the anterior surface of the esophagus and is traced to the lesser omentum after it gives off the hepatic branch. The trunk is divided at this point. The posterior vagus is identified as in a truncal vagotomy and is divided along its course adjacent to the left gastric artery. Usually the left gastric artery is ligated along with the posterior nerve. The remaining vagal fibers are best ablated by dividing the tissue along the lesser curvature of the stomach. The pyloric fibers which are a branch of the hepatic trunk innervate the antrum and are interrupted along the course of the right gastric artery. The right gastric artery is usually sacrificed along with the pyloric branch.

PROXIMAL GASTRIC VAGOTOMY

Truncal vagotomy and selective vagotomy denervate the entire stomach, and, as a consequence, antral stasis occurs in 10 to 20 per cent of the patients. To avoid the complications of antral stasis, some sort of drainage procedure is generally performed with either a truncal or selective vagotomy. The proximal gastric vagotomy is an alternative that provides a significant reduction in acid secretion without the necessity for a drainage procedure. The proximal gastric vagotomy also has been termed parietal cell vagotomy, highly selective vagotomy, and superselective vagotomy. The recurrence rates following proximal gastric vagotomy range from 5 to as high as 20 per cent. The high recurrence rates are generally associated with technical problems that result in an incomplete vagotomy. This generally is the result of a failure to interrupt the nerve of Grassi.

TECHNIC. As the main vagal trunks send off the hepatic and celiac branches, they continue along the anterior and posterior aspects of the lesser curvature. These two major trunks are then termed the nerves of Latarjet. From these two major trunks, branches are given to the stomach along the lesser curvature. These branches extend from the cardia to the pylorus. Approximately 6 cm. proximal to the pylorus, one of the branches further subdivides to resemble a crow's foot. It is approximately at this area that the parietal cell mass ends. Measurement of 6 cm. from the pylorus or identification of the crow's foot pattern marks the distal extent of the vagotomy.

A proximal gastric vagotomy consists of interrupting the branches of the nerves of Latarjet to the anterior and posterior aspects of the lesser curvature. These nerves are accompanied by vessels in the lesser omentum. The dissection may commence at the main trunks; however, it is generally easier to begin at the crow's foot and work proximally. The lesser omentum is placed on a slight stretch, and the anterior leaf of the lesser omentum is incised at the most distal branch, which is ligated and divided near the stomach. Care must be taken not to encroach on the stomach or to sacrifice the main trunk. Once the dissection is begun the individual neurovascular bundles are then ligated and divided. This is continued proximally until the entire anterior leaf of the lesser omentum is freed from the lesser curvature. The anterior nerve of Latarjet can generally be seen and palpated in the leaf.

The dissection is continued approximately 4 to 5 cm. up the esophagus and any branches from the main vagal trunk to the cardia of the stomach must be interrupted. The branches of the posterior nerve of Latarjet are ligated and divided in a similar fashion for a distance of 4 cm. up the esophagus. It is important to interrupt any fibers that are contained in the posterior peritoneal reflection to the stomach as well as any branches from the main posterior vagal trunk to the cardia and fundus of the stomach. The posterior fiber passing obliquely across the back of the lower esophagus is the nerve of Grassi, also referred to as the "criminal nerve." To complete this posterior division of nerves it is necessary to enter the lesser sac and elevate the stomach away from the celiac plexus. Attachments between the esophagus and angle of His should be divided to insure that these transverse fibers from the posterior vagus are interrupted.

The results from proximal gastric vagotomy are encouraging, and success depends upon meticulous technique. If the long-term recurrence rate remains low, proximal gastric vagotomy will probably become the operation of choice for the operative treatment of duodenal ulcer disease (Wise and Ballinger, 1974). This operation should be especially gratifying in asthenic women who have a significant incidence of postvagotomy and postgastrectomy sequelae (Herrington and Sawyers, 1978).

TRANSTHORACIC (SUPRADIAPHRAGMATIC) VAGOTOMY

Some surgeons believe that a more complete division of the vagus nerves can be accomplished through a transthoracic approach, which permits greater visualization of those nerves. This approach is usually reserved for reoperation because of a previous incomplete vagotomy.

TECHNIC. The patient is placed on his or her right side, with the left arm carried forward, and a long incision is made over the left seventh rib (Fig. 14–3A). The seventh rib is widely resected subperiosteally (Fig. 14–3B), and the seventh intercostal nerve is divided at the posterior margin of the incision. The left pleural cavity is then opened throughout the extent of this incision.

The left lower lobe of the lung is retracted, exposing the inferior pulmonary ligament (Fig. 14–4), which is divided between ligatures, and the left lung is retracted upward out of the operative field. The pleura over the lower 7.5 cm. of the esophagus is incised longitudinally and the esophagus identified by palpating the nasogastric tube previously inserted into the stomach. The esophagus is mobilized by finger dissection until the finger can be passed beneath it (Fig. 14–5). The vagus nerves will then be seen and palpated on each side of the esophageal wall. (Because of the patient's rotated position on the table, the left vagus will be found on the upper surface and the right vagus beneath the esophagus.)

The vagi are freed from the esophagus by finger dissection. At this level the vagi are usually formed as a single trunk, but each may consist of two or more fibers, so, to be certain of dividing all the fibers, it is well to clean off all adventitia of the esophagus around its entire circumference for a length of 5 cm. The vagi are isolated and divided between silk ligatures just above the diaphragm (Fig. 14–6A). A segment of nerve need not be removed. The proximal tied ends of the resected vagi are transplanted into the left pleural cavity (Fig. 15–6B), and the incision in the esophageal pleura is closed about them.

The lung is inflated, the pleura and intercostal muscles are closed with interrupted sutures of heavy silk, and the skin is

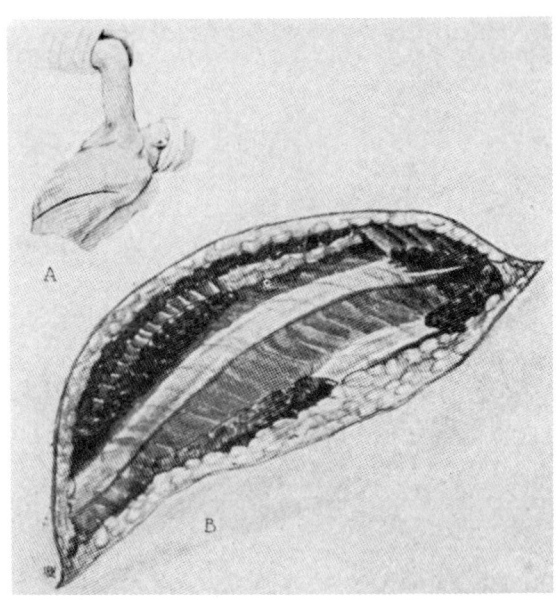

Figure 14–3. Incision (A) and exposure (B) of the seventh rib for transthoracic vagotomy. (From Dragstedt, L. R.: Vagotomy for gastroduodenal ulcer. Ann. Surg. *122*:973, 1945.)

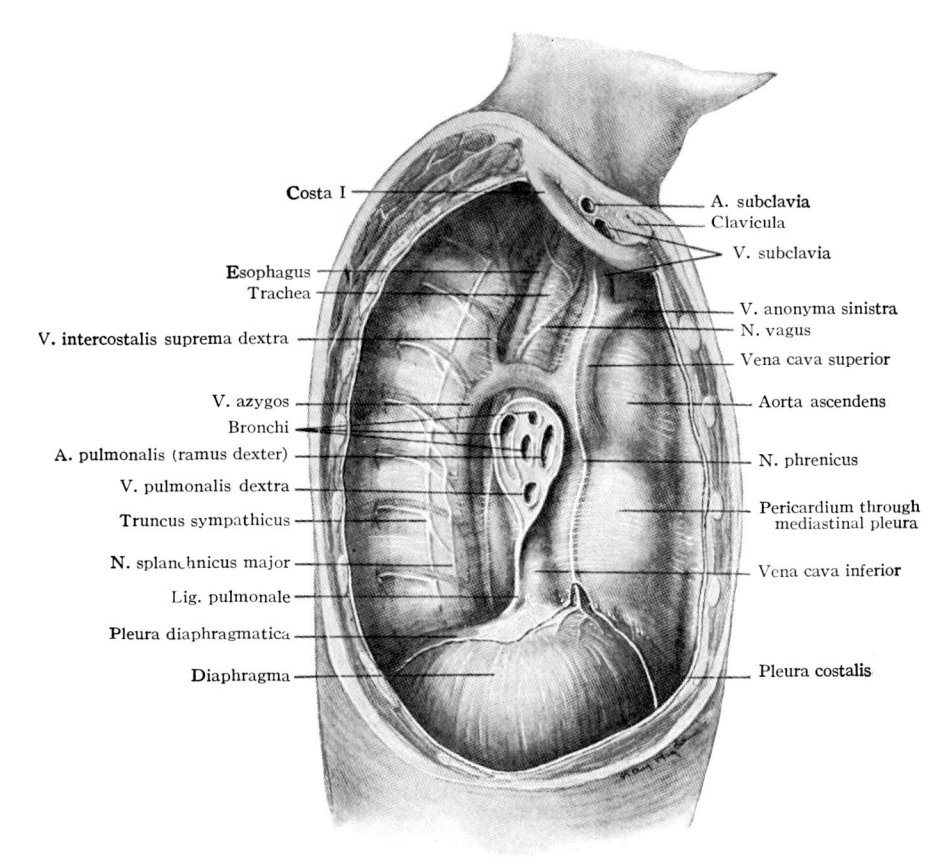

Figure 14-4. Structures on the right surface of the mediastinum.

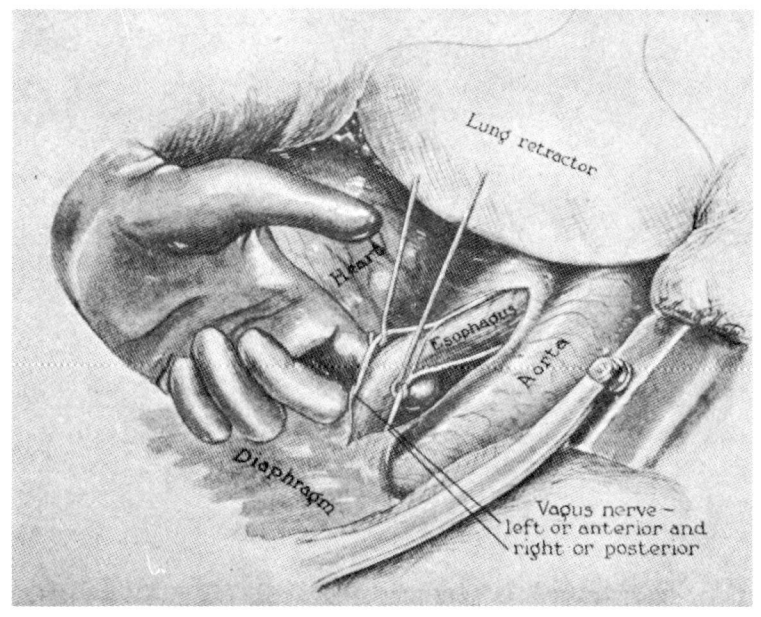

Figure 14-5. Mobilization of the esophagus and isolation of vagus nerves, showing the communication between the anterior and posterior trunks. (From Dragstedt, L. R.: Vagotomy for gastroduodenal ulcer. Ann. Surg. 122:973, 1945.)

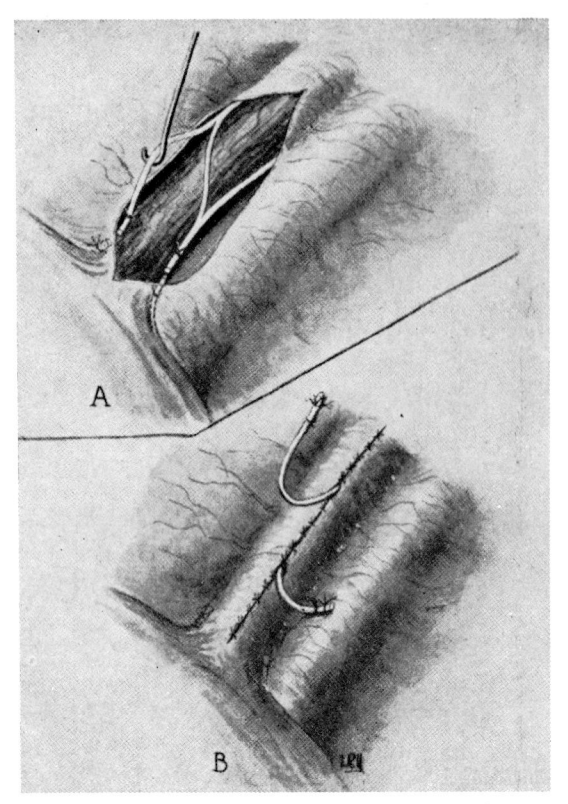

Figure 14-6. *A*, Ligature and division of vagus nerves just above diaphragm. *B*, Transplantation of proximal ends of cut vagi into the pleural cavity. (From Dragstedt, cited in previous figure.)

closed with continuous sutures of fine black silk, without drainage.

Postoperative Complications of Vagotomy

Most transthoracic vagotomies are complicated by postoperative pleural effusion. In about 10 per cent of patients the effusion is sufficiently great to require aspiration (Dragstedt, 1945). No empyema occurred in Dragstedt's series.

Pain in the region of the intercostal incision has been the most troublesome complication in transthoracic vagotomies. It has usually subsided within a week but in some older patients it has persisted for 3 to 4 months. It may be alleviated by procaine injections of the intercostal nerves near the vertebral border.

Gastric dilatation is common postoperatively owing to the atony of the stomach and its prolonged emptying time. This is prevented or treated by the postoperative use of continuous gastric suction through a nasogastric tube for 48 hours. In some instances, this condition has persisted and required a later gastroenterostomy for its relief.

Troublesome diarrhea has occurred in some patients but has usually been transient. Some vagotomized patients have lost weight and have been unable to regain their normal poundage.

Comments

Dragstedt (1945) reported the initial results for vagotomy without a drainage procedure for the treatment of peptic ulcer disease. With an experience based on 490 patients with varying types of peptic ulcer, including bleeding ulcers, he concluded that a benign peptic ulcer regularly may be expected to heal following this operation alone. All investigators agree, however, that if a gastric ulcer is questionably malignant then gastric resection should be carried out in preference to vagotomy. Dragstedt stated that if a gastric ulcer does not heal within 6 weeks after vagotomy, then it may be malignant and gastrectomy should be performed. In his series of patients followed for 6 years, only two ulcers recurred in those upon whom a complete vagotomy was performed.

Dragstedt and associates (1949) reported the performance of section of the vagus nerve supply in the stomach in 521 patients. In only 20 patients was the operation done for gastric ulcer, and in 5 of these vagotomy failed to bring the relief and healing usually resulting following this operation performed for duodenal and gastrojejunal lesions. In 197 patients with duodenal ulcers treated by vagotomy alone, gastric ulcers subsequently developed in 2. In 262 patients with duodenal ulcers treated by vagotomy and gastroenterostomy, no gastric ulcers developed. These workers found that in patients with duodenal ulcers and in those with coexisting duodenal and gastric ulcers the production of hydrochloric acid in the nocturnal secretion is from three to four times greater than the amounts in normal persons, whereas in patients with gastric ulcers the output of hydrochloric acid in the nocturnal secretion is the same as or less than that in normal persons. The absent hypersecretion in gastric ulcers suggests that these lesions are not due to an increase in the corrosive properties of the gastric contents. He concluded that vagotomy is not indicated in the treatment of gastric ulcers, except in those patients in whom a high ulcer is situated adjacent to the cardia. In these a vagotomy and gastroenterostomy may give as good a result as some type of resection, with less risk.

Grimson and coworkers (1950) followed nearly 100 vagotomized patients for 4 years. They found that vagotomy alone gave good results in about 50 per cent of the peptic ulcer patients, but some of the ulcers recurred and frequently there was persistence of abdominal distention, eructation of gas, and regurgitation of food.

Recent randomized prospective studies that compared various types of ulcer operations in good-risk patients showed little difference in mortality, morbidity, and postoperative sequelae among various operations (Cox and Williams, 1969). A vagotomy and drainage procedure was generally associated with a 5 per cent recurrence rate, whereas a vagotomy and gastric resection had a recurrence rate of 1 per cent or less. Since vagotomy is generally combined with other types of operative procedures for the treatment of ulcer disease, it is difficult to separate postoperative sequelae due to vagotomy alone.

Some of the sequelae following vagotomy include recurrent ulcer, generally due to an incomplete vagotomy, diarrhea, and postoperative gastric retention. Complaints such as epigastric fullness have also been associated with vagotomy and alterations in the patient's gastric tone. The higher incidence of cholelithiasis following ulcer operations has generally been attributed to a truncal vagotomy.

The postoperative abnormalities following proximal gastric vagotomy consist of an increase in the emptying time of liquids, which occasionally produces mild dumping-type symptoms and early satiety and in general is attributed to a loss of receptive relaxation. The incidence of nausea, reflux alkaline gastritis, and bile vomiting has remained very low. Avoidance of these postoperative sequelae has been attributed to the presence of an intact pyloric sphincter.

At present, a proximal gastric vagotomy is generally recommended for the elective treatment of duodenal ulcer disease, especially in women who have a high likelihood of postoperative sequelae of nausea, bile vomiting, and epigastric fullness. Long-term follow-up is needed for this operation to determine whether the recurrence rate is acceptably low. Surgeons wishing to perform this operation should become completely familiar with the technical details to insure completeness of the vagotomy.

PYLOROPLASTY

Pyloroplasty is an operation which consists of incising the pyloric muscle and reconstructing the pyloric channel so as to facilitate gastric emptying. The distal antrum and pylorus are responsible for the regulation of gastric emptying, and they also prevent reflux of duodenal fluids into the stomach. When Dragstedt introduced vagotomy in 1943, gastric acidity was effectively controlled in patients with duodenal ulcer, but, as a consequence of vagotomy, gastric tone and muscular activity were altered, resulting in gastric stasis (Thomas, 1957). Pyloroplasty alleviates this side effect of vagotomy and effectively facilitates gastric emptying.

Following truncal and selective vagotomy, gastric tone is impaired and a gastric drainage procedure is required. In parietal or proximal gastric vagotomy, now more frequently performed, vagal innervation to the distal antrum and pylorus is not destroyed, and an emptying procedure is unnecessary. Studies confirm normal emptying of solids following proximal gastric vagotomy.

Indications

Pyloroplasty generally is performed following truncal or selective vagotomy in the treatment of duodenal ulcer disease. It is also important to incise the pyloric area when operating for a bleeding duodenal ulcer, to get exposure of the ulcer and trans-fix the bleeding site with a suture. However, a pyloroplasty or any other procedure that involves the pyloric area is avoided if the pyloric area is severely distorted or inflamed as a result of the ulcer disease. In these patients some other form of drainage procedure, such as gastroenterostomy, is performed.

To perform a pyloroplasty, the anterior surface of the pylorus should be minimally involved and the duodenum sufficiently mobile to make the operation technically feasible. Occasionally, a pyloroplasty can be performed in the presence of an anterior ulcer if the tissue surrounding the ulcer is minimally involved. Technical modifications have been described which involve excision of the ulcer and pyloroplasty.

Types of Pyloroplasty

The two basic types of pyloroplasty are the Heineke-Mikulicz and the Finney procedures. The Jaboulay (1892) pyloroplasty is a gastroduodenostomy; the incision does not extend through the pylorus.

HEINEKE-MIKULICZ PYLOROPLASTY

This pyloroplasty was described independently by Heineke in 1886 and Mikulicz in 1888. It consists of a longitudinal incision through the pylorus, extending from the distal antrum to the proximal duodenum. The incision is then closed transversely, which results in ablating the continuity of the pyloric sphincter and increasing the diameter of the outlet of the pylorus (Fig. 14-7).

The pylorus is identified and the duodenum given Kocher's maneuver. If mobilization is adequate and scarring on the anterior surface of the pylorus is minimal, the pyloroplasty is technically feasible. Two traction sutures are placed about 1 cm. apart on the anterior surface of the pylorus. A longitudinal incision is made between the two traction sutures, extending proximally 2.5 to 3.5 cm. onto the antrum and a similar

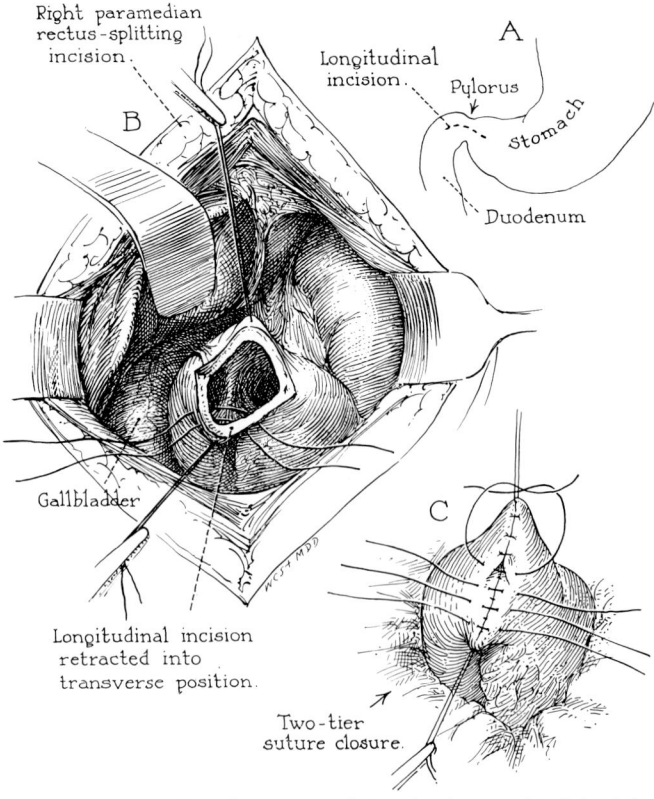

Figure 14-7. Heineke-Mikulicz pyloroplasty. *A* and *B*, The longitudinal incision is converted into one running transversely by traction on the marginal traction sutures. *C*, Two-tier closure is shown. Most surgeons prefer a single-layer closure, as described by Weinberg (1956).

distance distally on the duodenum. Bleeding, if it occurs, is controlled with fine silk ties or coagulation. The duodenum and proximal stomach are inspected for obstruction and ulceration. If there is any bleeding from the base of the ulcer, a nonabsorbable transfixion suture may be necessary.

Although a two-layer closure has been described for closing the incision transversely, the infolding of additional tissue that occurs detracts from the advantage of increasing the opening in this area. Weinberg and associates (1956) advocate a single-layer closure with interrupted nonabsorbable sutures. Various techniques have been described to accomplish this closure with slight inversion and good approximation of the serosa. Whatever method is used, it is important that the suture pass through all layers with good approximation of the serosa and inversion of the mucosa.

One of the popular methods for closing the Heineke-Mikulicz pyloroplasty is with the use of a Gambee stitch (Gambee, 1951). The suture is started from the serosa of the stomach through all layers including the mucosa. The suture is then passed through the mucosa to the junction of the submucosa and muscularis on the gastric wall. Mucosal approximation between the stomach and duodenum is insured by next passing the suture on the duodenal side from the junction of the submucosa and muscularis to the mucosa of the duodenum and then full thickness from the duodenal mucosa to the serosa of the duodenum. The suture is then tied. This helps invert the mucosa and gives good approximation to the serosal surfaces. A simple full-thickness stitch incorporating more of the serosal surface than the mucosa is also a very effective technic for closing the pyloroplasty.

To insure adequate closure and a good outlet, care must be taken in making the longitudinal incision. Some surgeons extend the incision slightly more on the gastric side than on the duodenal side, which may provide better alignment when the incision is closed transversely. If there is difficulty in determining the location of the pylorus, it is best to make a small incision in the area of the pylorus; once entrance into the stomach or duodenum is achieved, palpation from the inside can usually determine the exact location of the pyloric ring. The total length of the incision should be at least 5 cm., to insure an adequate outlet when it is closed transversely. Generally, it should not be more than 7 cm. or difficulty in closing the incision transversely without excessive tension may be encountered.

Horsley (1926) modified the Heineke-Mikulicz pyloroplasty by excising the ulcer. This has some advantage if the ulcer is limited to a small area on the anterior surface of the duodenum and the tissue in the area of the ulcer has produced a thinning-out of the duodenal wall. If the involvement of the ulcer on the anterior surface is more extensive and the tissue not suitable for a pyloroplasty, a gastroenterostomy should be performed (Figs. 14–8, 14–9).

FINNEY PYLOROPLASTY (Fig. 14–10)

A Finney pyloroplasty (Finney, 1902) consists of incision of the pyloric area with extension onto the stomach and first portion of the duodenum. The duodenal and gastric walls are approximated anteriorly and posteriorly. This results in a larger outlet and depends upon sufficient mobilization of the duodenum. Detachments of the gastric-hepatic ligament must be mobilized and the duodenum given Kocher's maneuver. A traction suture is placed in the superior margin of the pyloric ring and a second one on the greater curvature of the stomach, 10 cm. proximal to the pylorus. A third traction suture is placed on the duodenal wall, 10 cm. distal to the pyloric ring. Upward traction is placed on the suture at the pyloric ring and downward traction on the gastric and duodenal sutures. This opposes the anterior wall of the stomach and duodenum.

The opposed walls of duodenum and stomach are sutured with interrupted 000 silk. A U-shaped incision is then made into the lumen of the stomach and duodenum through the pylorus. Submucosal bleeding is controlled with fine ligatures or electrocoagulation. The posterior septum between the posterior walls of the stomach and duodenum is secured with a continuous 0000 chromic catgut suture. This is generally a through-and-through suture insuring hemostasis, and is begun at the pyloric end of the posterior wall. After the posterior suture is completed, it is then extended anteriorly, securing the anterior walls of the stomach and duodenum. An outer row of 000 inter-

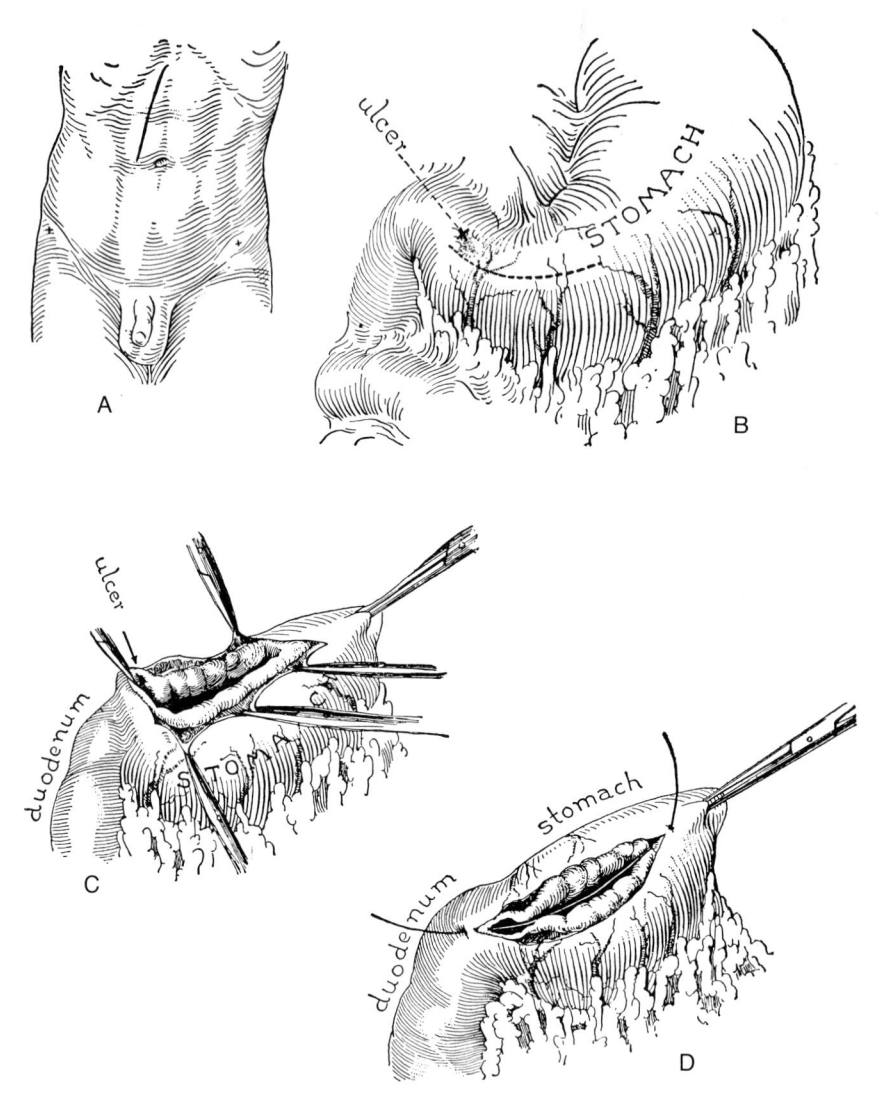

Figure 14-8. Horsley modification of Heineke-Mikulicz pyloroplasty. *A*, Abdominal incision for exposure of duodenum. *B*, Dotted line shows proposed incision for physiologic pyloroplasty. The gastric portion of the incision is at least twice as long as the duodenal portion. *C*, The incision is first made in the stomach side and the duodenal ulcer exposed to view. *D*, The ulcer has been excised and a traction suture is placed from the extremity of the incision in the stomach to the extremity of the incision in the duodenum. It penetrates only the peritoneal and muscular coats of the stomach but includes all of the duodenal wall.

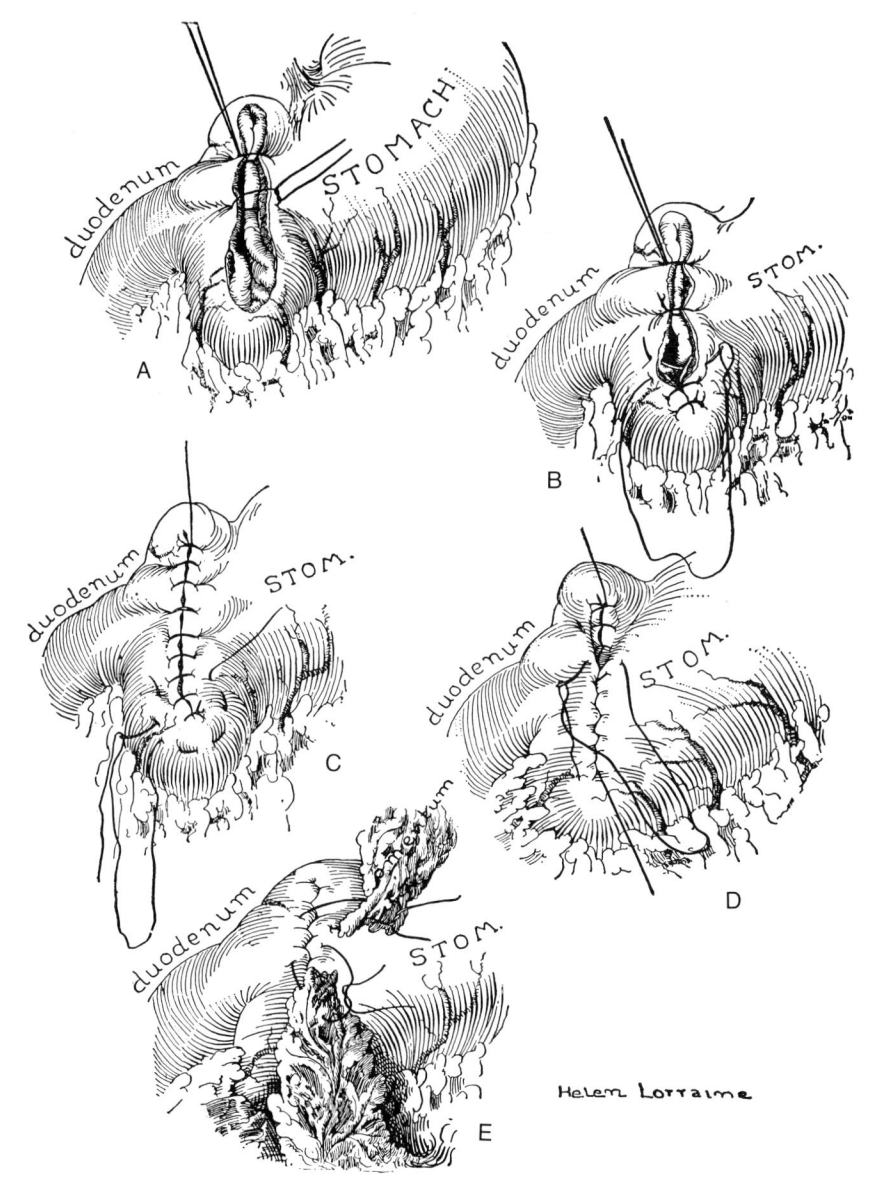

Figure 14-9. Horsley modification of Heineke-Mikulicz pyloroplasty *(continued)*. *A*, Another traction suture is placed in a similar manner about 1.25 cm. above the first. These sutures are tied and the ends left long. *B*, A continuous suture of absorbable suture material is applied, catching not only the peritoneal and muscular coats of the stomach but also the entire duodenal wall. *C*, The second row of sutures is begun at the lower end of the wound as a pursestring suture, invaginating the lower teat. *D*, This suture is continued upward as a right-angle suture with occasional backstitches until the upper teat is reached. It is then converted into a pursestring suture in order to bury the teat. *E*, Tags of gastrocolic and gastrohepatic omentum are brought over the suture line and fastened with a few interrupted sutures.

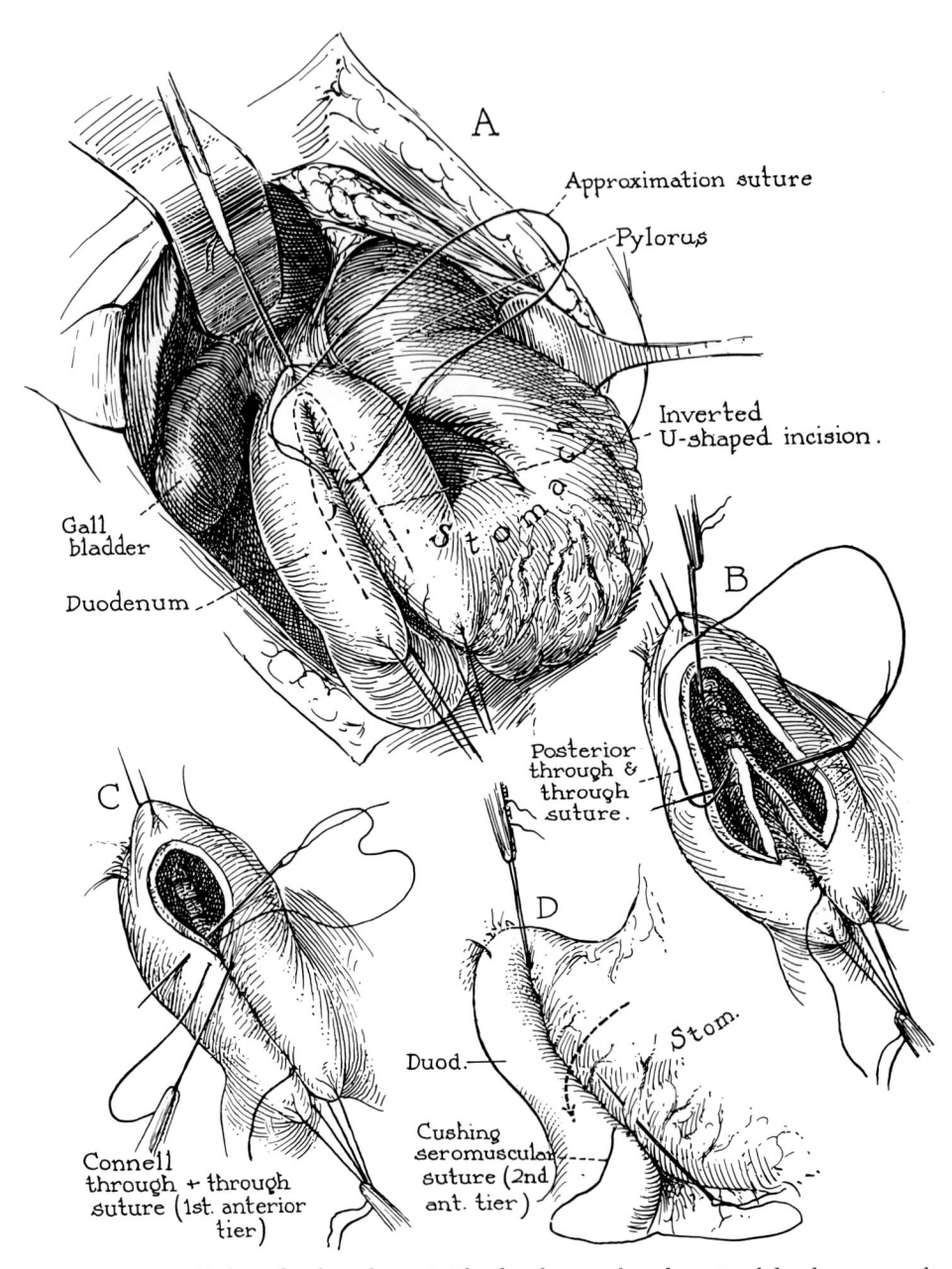

Figure 14-10. Finney U-shaped pyloroplasty. *A*, The distal stomach and proximal duodenum are aligned with traction strands and their adjacent walls approximated with a Cushing suture; the inverted U-shaped incision into the lumens of the stomach and duodenum is indicated. *B*, Suture of the posterior septum of stomach and duodenum. *C*, The first anterior tier of sutures (Connell) is placed. *D*, The operation is completed with a reinforcing tier of Cushing sutures.

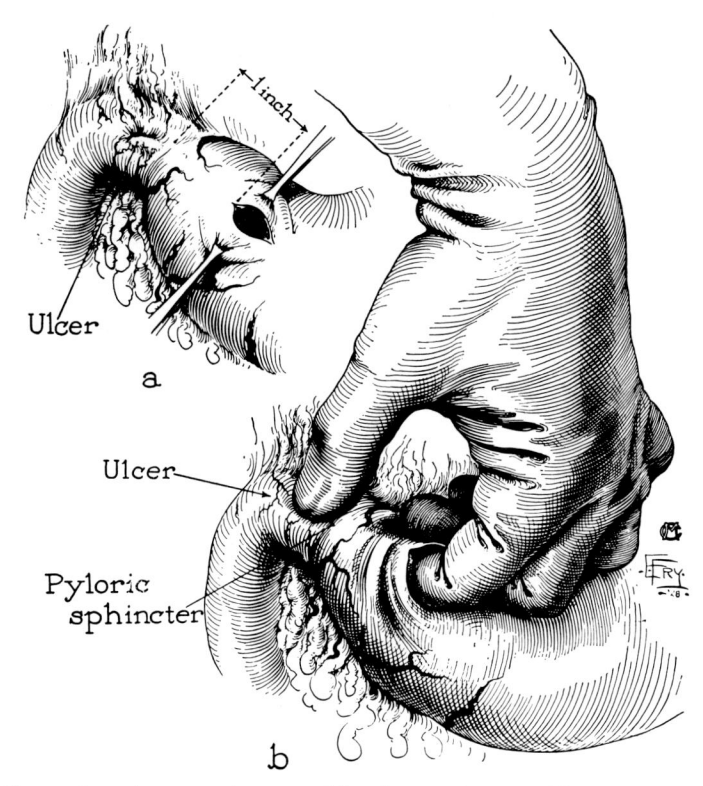

Figure 14-11. Balfour pyloroplasty. Exploration of duodenum. (From Balfour, D. C.: Surg. Gynecol. Obstet., Vol. 49.)

rupted silk Lembert seromuscular stitches approximates the anterior walls of the stomach and duodenum. The incision on the stomach and duodenum generally extends for a distance of 6 to 9 cm. on either side of the pylorus.

Balfour introduced a modification of the Finney pyloroplasty in which the ulcer on the anterior wall of the stomach or duodenum is excised. Although there are some descriptions of excising a posterior ulcer, generally this is not necessary and poses the hazard of bleeding, injury to the common duct, and injury to the pancreas (Figs. 14–11, 14–12).

JUDD PYLOROPLASTY (Figs. 14–13, 14–14)

Judd's pyloroplasty (Judd and Nagel, 1927) consists of excision of the anterior ulcer with removal of the anterior two-thirds of the pyloric sphincter. Because of the large amount of tissue removed and the failure to perform a vagotomy, recurrent ulceration and stenosis occurred. This and other modifications of the two standard pyloroplasties are generally of historic interest since our present understanding of duodenal ulcer disease does not support the need for excision of the ulcer bed.

MOSCHEL PYLOROPLASTY

The Moschel pyloroplasty consists of a Y-shaped incision, with the base of the Y extending through the pylorus onto the proximal duodenum and the arms of the Y onto the antrum. The Y must produce a short and broad flap on the antrum, otherwise the tip of the flap will not have an adequate blood supply. The flap of the antrum is then sutured to the duodenum, generally using a one-layer closure.

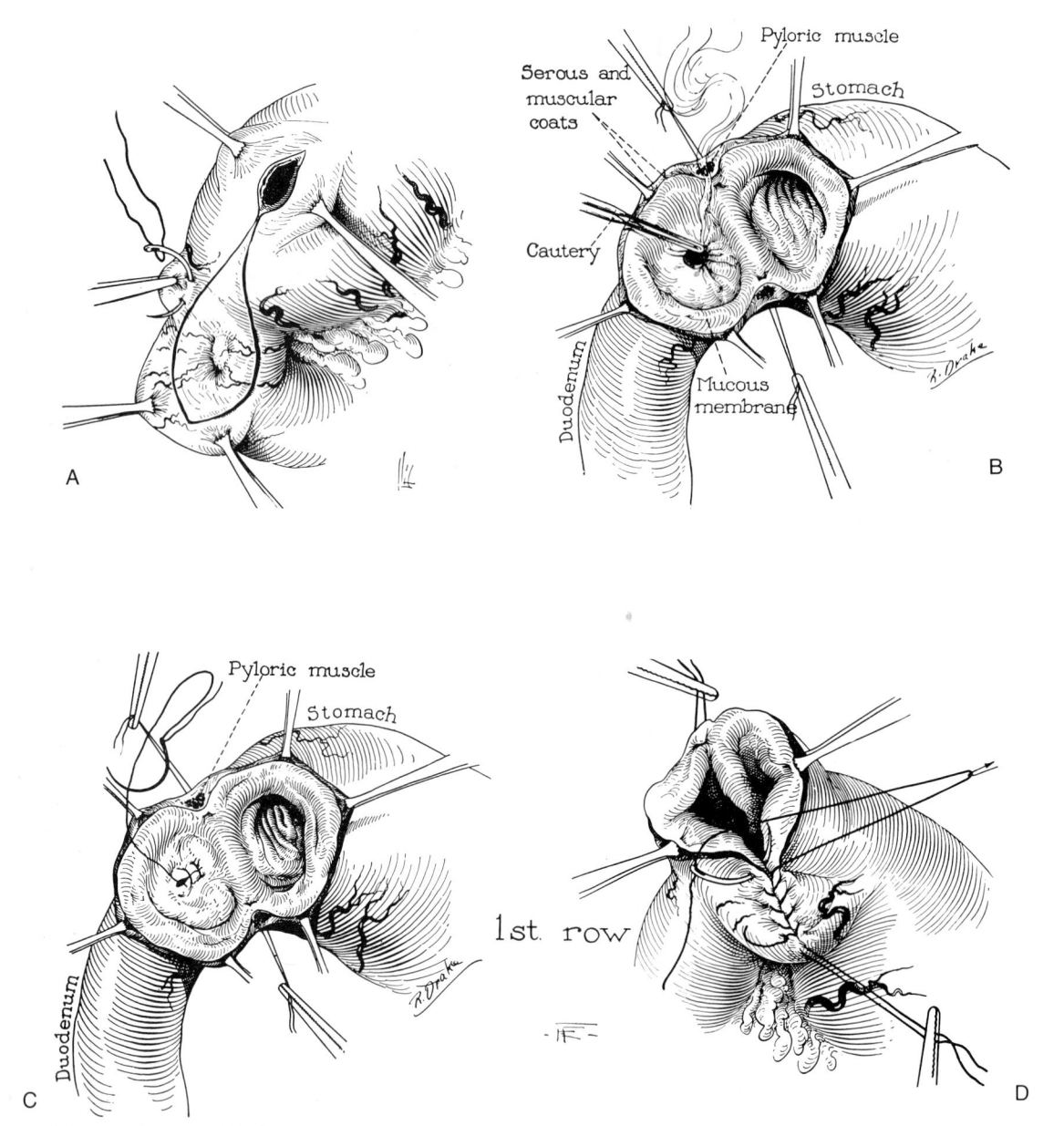

Figure 14-12. Balfour pyloroplasty *(continued).* A, Excision of ulcer on anterior wall of duodenum. B, Cautery excision of a posterior ulcer. C, Closure with chromic catgut of defect following cautery excision of ulcer. D, Reconstruction after excision of ulcer of the duodenum. (From Balfour, cited in previous figure.)

Figure 14-13. Judd gastroduodenostomy near the pylorus, with or without excision or cauterization of the ulcer. *A,* The area at each side of the pylorus is flattened to show the duodenal ulcer. *B,* The stomach and duodenum are mobilized to permit their approximation. (From Eusterman, G. B., and Balfour, D. C.: The Stomach and Duodenum. Philadelphia, W. B. Saunders Company, 1935.)

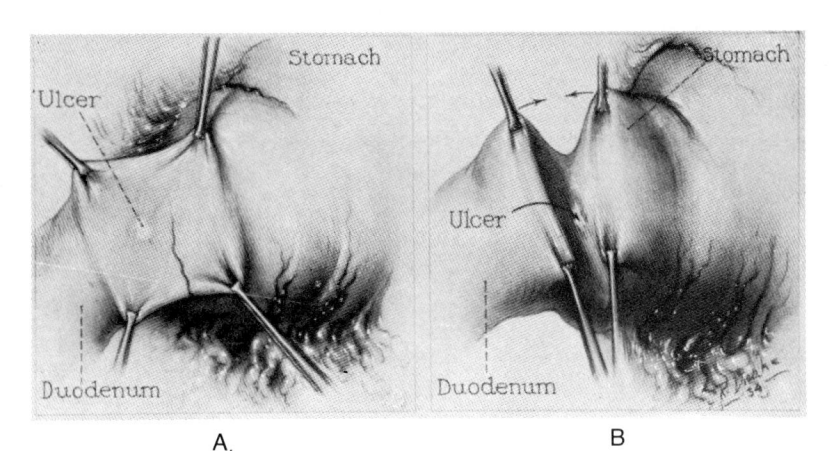

Comments on Pyloroplasty

Pyloroplasty is usually a safe and technically easy operation, provided the duodenal area is not severely scarred or inflamed. Although it has the advantage of facilitating gastric emptying (Davies and associates, 1974), it also has some disadvantages. Because of the rapid emptying of liquids and solids (Gustafson, 1967), symptoms such as dumping and diarrhea may occur following destruction of the pyloric sphincter. Likewise, reflux of duodenal fluid into the stomach can result in reflux alkaline gastritis.

From the randomized prospective studies which have been reported, there are no significant differences between pyloroplasty and gastroenterostomy in the incidence of recurrent ulceration and postoperative sequelae. The single exception to this is the study by Goligher and associates (1972), who reported a lower ulcer recurrence rate with gastroenterostomy compared with pyloroplasty.

There is some evidence that a Finney pyloroplasty provides better emptying than other types of pyloroplasties (Hayden and Reed, 1968). Lynch and associates (1965) have shown that the high recurrence rate after Heineke-Mikulicz pyloroplasty is due to impaired gastric emptying. Although the Weinberg modification using a single-layer closure has the theoretic advantage of providing a larger opening in the pyloric area, this has never been confirmed with any clinical studies.

Figure 14-14. Judd gastroduodenostomy *(continued).* *A,* The posterior seromuscular suture of the anastomosis is laid. *B,* Incision is made into the stomach and duodenum. (From Eusterman and Balfour, cited in previous figure.)

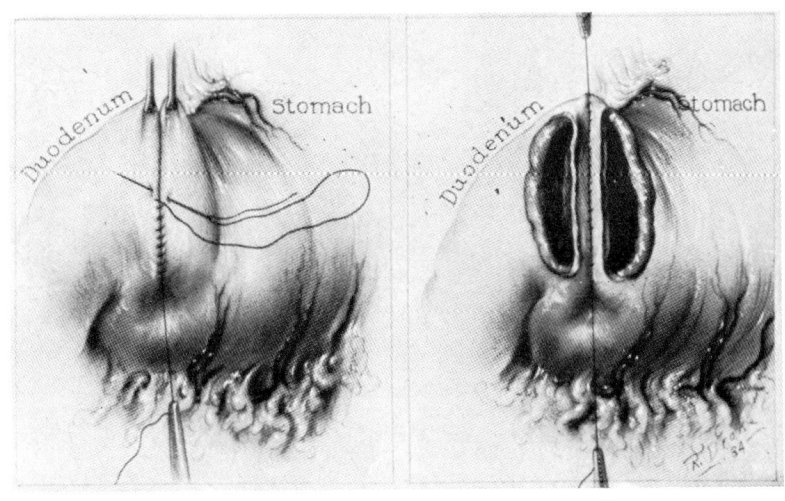

GASTRIC PROCEDURES FOR MORBID OBESITY

Gastric Bypass

In 1969, Mason and Ito introduced gastric bypass as a new procedure for the treatment of morbid obesity. The observation that subtotal gastric resection with gastrojejunostomy often resulted in weight loss triggered interest in gastric procedures for control of obesity. The gastric bypass is designed to limit the intake of food severely, both by creating a small gastric reservoir and by delaying gastric emptying. It is, in essence, a 90 per cent exclusion of the distal stomach combined with a gastrojejunostomy to the proximal pouch. The gastroenterostomy stoma must be small, no larger than 1.5 cm., to retard gastric emptying. Following gastric bypass, patients experience early satiety even after ingesting a very small meal. If they are tempted to eat more than the proximal gastric reservoir will allow, they will either vomit or experience epigastric pain secondary to acute dilatation of the proximal pouch. Occasionally, patients will experience dumping symptoms, particularly following ingestion of carbohydrate-rich fluids; further restriction of intake may result from a desire to avoid such symptoms (Mason and Ito, 1969).

Technic of Gastric Bypass

Mason and Ito (1969) recommend that gastric bypass be performed either through a long mid-line upper abdominal incision or a bilateral subcostal incision (Fig. 14-15). The suspensory ligament of the liver is divided so as to retract the left lobe to the right. The stomach will ultimately be transected to divide it into a proximal 10 per cent and distal 90 per cent pouch. To per-

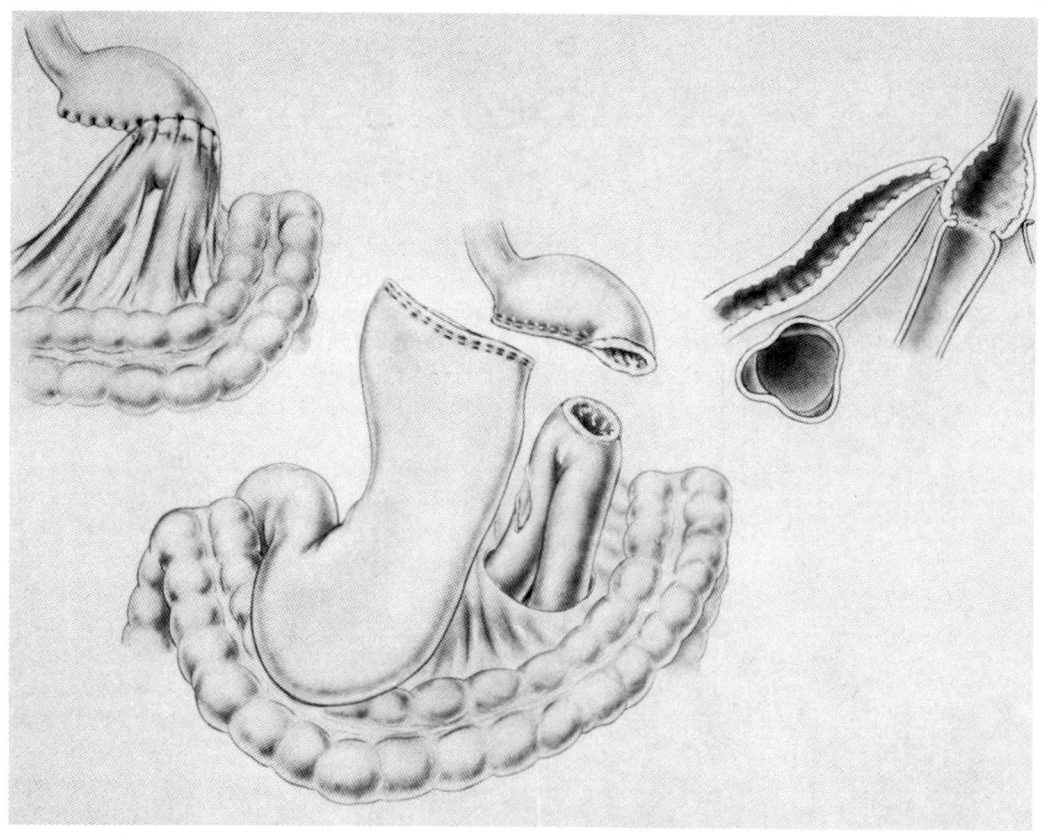

Figure 14-15. The potentially reversible 90 per cent gastric bypass operation with a short-loop retrocolic gastroenterostomy. The ligament of Treitz is divided. The mesocolon is secured to the 10 per cent stomach pouch, and the closed distal 90 per cent of excluded stomach is attached to the anterior wall of the fundic segment. These steps are important in preventing antral stasis. (From Mason, E. E., and Ito, C.: Gastric bypass. Ann. Surg. *170*:329, 1969.)

form the division, vessels are cleared along the lesser curvature for a length of 5 cm., beginning at the gastroesophageal junction. Five centimeters are also cleared on the greater curvature, beginning 10 to 12 cm. from the gastroesophageal junction.

The stomach is divided with the GIA stapler (see Chapter 23) so that two rows of staples are left on either side; the staples are then inverted with 3-0 silk Lembert sutures. In this way the distal stomach is closed completely and a Hofmeister-type closure of the upper pouch is carried out. Approximately 2 cm. of stomach on the greater curvature side of the pouch are amputated and used for the gastrojejunostomy. The ligament of Treitz is divided, and a short-loop retrocolic gastroenterostomy is performed. The division of the ligament of Treitz allows for the creation of a relatively short loop.

An opening is made in the mesocolon and the edges are sutured to the proximal pouch above the anastomosis. A 2-layer anastomosis is performed between stomach and jejunum. The colon is then retracted cephalad; the anterior edges of the mesocolon are sutured to the gastroenterostomy loop. It must be emphasized that the gastroenterostomy must be small, no greater than 1.5 cm. The excluded distal stomach is then sutured to the anterior surface of the proximal pouch in such a way as to prevent twisting or intussusception and antral stasis. Mason and Ito (1969) consider this a most important part of the procedure, as antral stasis might predispose to jejunal marginal ulceration.

Alden (1977) has described a modification of the gastric bypass introduced by Mason. In his modification (Fig. 14-16), the stomach is not transected and the gastrojejunal anastomosis is antecolic. The abdominal esophagus is encircled with a Penrose drain. The upper one-half of the greater curvature is mobilized up to the gastroesophageal junction. All the short gastric arteries are divided. A small opening is made in the lesser omentum to allow introduction of the 90 mm. thoracoabdominal stapler (TA-90). An antecolic loop of proximal jejunum is tacked to the proposed proximal gastric pouch, and an anastomosis is made with the gastrointestinal stapler set at 2 cm. The stab wound used for introduction of the GIA stapler is closed with 3-0 silk Lembert sutures. A nasogastric tube is passed through the gastroenterostomy and the stomach is partitioned transversely using the TA-90 with 4.8 mm. staples. The partitioning is done so as to create a small proximal 10 per cent pouch. The efferent limb of the jejunum is sutured to the anterior wall of the greater curvature of the stomach for about 8 cm. to prevent torsion of the jejunum (Fig. 14-16).

Buckwalter (1978) advocates the use of double lines of 4.8 mm. staples to partition the stomach as the staple lines of some patients have dehisced, permitting food to pass from the proximal to the distal pouch with resultant minimal weight loss. To minimize this possibility, patients are cautioned to eat small amounts of well-chewed food and to stop eating promptly when they feel full, uncomfortable, or nauseated.

Physiologic Consequences

A major objection of some to the use of gastric bypass in the treatment of morbid obesity is the possibility of it being an ulcerogenic procedure. Antral exclusion procedures are notorious for producing jejunal ulceration, with an incidence as high as 20 per cent. However, the incidence of stomal ulceration following gastric bypass is apparently low. In explanation, gastric bypass is postulated to exclude sufficient acid-secreting mucosa with the antrum that, after the stomach is stimulated to secrete acid, the antrum and first portion of the duodenum are bathed with acidified gastric juice unbuffered by food. This, in turn, inhibits release of gastrin, thereby tending to regulate gastric secretion at a relatively low-normal level.

The effects of gastric bypass on gastric secretion were reported in 1976: Mason and associates studied 393 morbidly obese individuals who had undergone gastric bypass to limit food intake severely. Stomal ulceration occurred in 1.8 per cent of these patients. In a much smaller number of patients, Mason and associates found that gastric bypass reduces acid production in the fundic pouch after Histalog stimulation, but that basal acid production is usually unchanged. Studies of aspirates from the distal pouch usually show a decrease in gastric acid secretion in comparison with collections from the entire stomach ob-

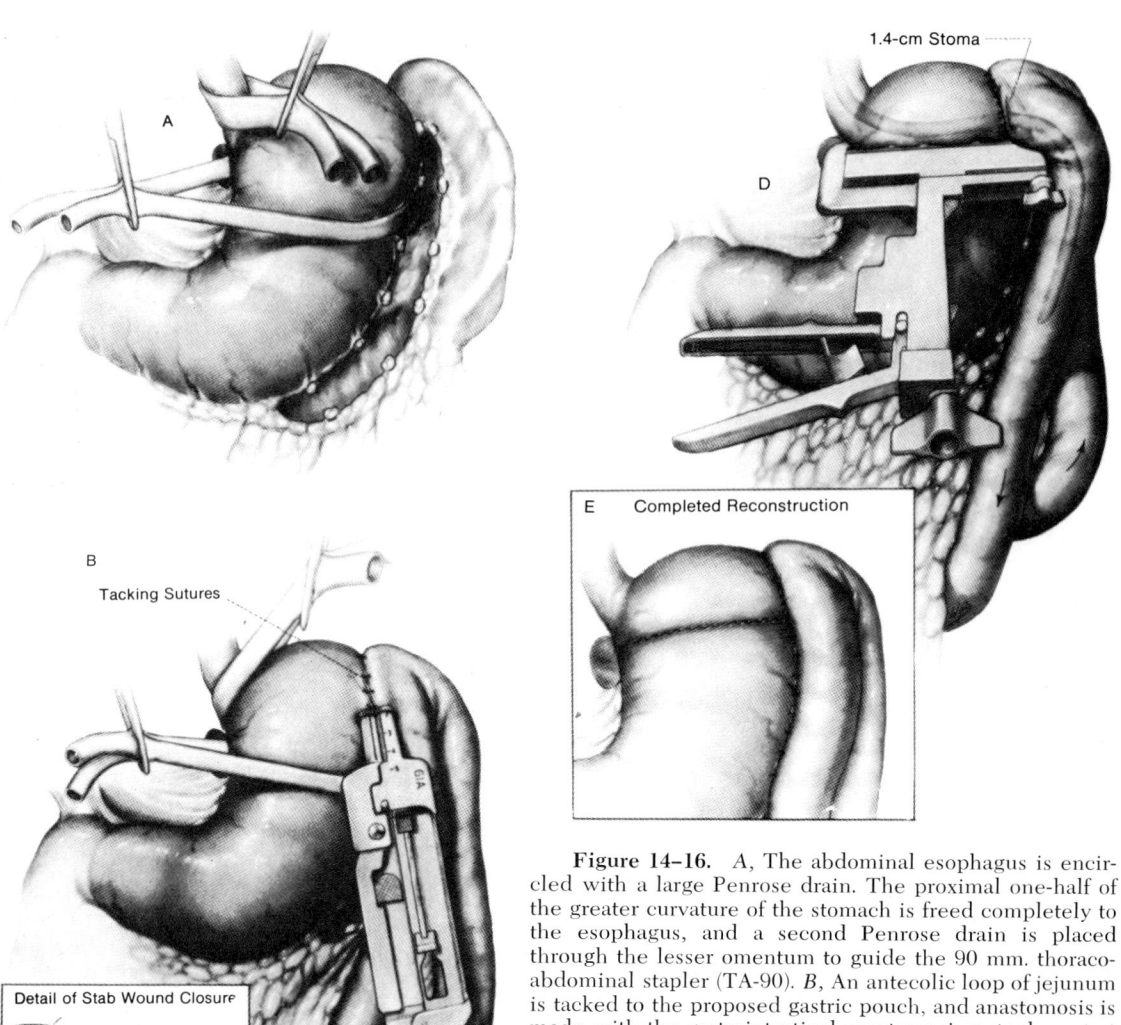

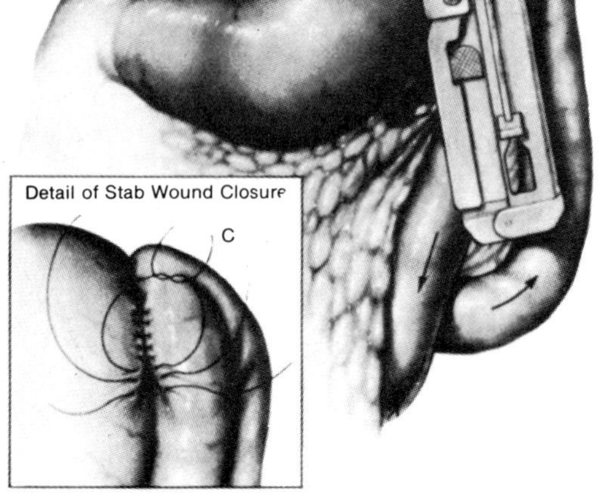

Figure 14–16. *A*, The abdominal esophagus is encircled with a large Penrose drain. The proximal one-half of the greater curvature of the stomach is freed completely to the esophagus, and a second Penrose drain is placed through the lesser omentum to guide the 90 mm. thoracoabdominal stapler (TA-90). *B*, An antecolic loop of jejunum is tacked to the proposed gastric pouch, and anastomosis is made with the gastrointestinal anastomosing stapler set at 2 cm. *C*, The remaining defect in the stomach and jejunum is approximated with 3-0 silk Lembert sutures. *D*, A gastric tube is placed in the efferent limb of the jejunum, and the stomach is transversely closed, using the TA-90 with 4.8 mm. staples. *E*, The efferent limb of the jejunum is sutured to the anterior wall of the greater curve of the stomach for about 8 cm. to prevent twisting of the jejunum. (From Alden, J. F.: Gastric and jejunoileal bypass. Arch. Surg. *112*:799, 1977.)

tained preoperatively; however, the pH almost always remains within the acid range. Some of the decrease in proximal pouch acid secretion is thought to be due to the smaller parietal cell mass present since not all of the stomach has been excluded. Following gastric bypass, postprandial gastrin secretion is almost invariably lowered. In patients known to have acid peptic disease, acid secretion from the fundic pouch is almost never lowered. However, in patients who do develop stomal ulceration after gastric bypass, a consistent pattern of acid secretion has not been demonstrated (Mason and associates, 1976).

Printen (1978) has studied the physiologic activity of the excluded stomach. To determine whether this segment retained vagal innervation, 25 patients underwent preoperative Hollander tests of their intact stomachs. The test was repeated after operation following resumption of oral intake. Postoperative specimens were collected from a gastrostomy placed in the excluded stomach. The percentage changes in volume and total acid production for both the pouches were the same. suggesting that normal gastric physiology is maintained after gastric bypass. This is not surprising, so long as great care is taken to preserve neurovascular structures in the lesser curvature when mobilizing the stomach for gastric bypass.

Results

In 1975, Mason and associates reported on 434 patients who underwent gastric bypass for morbid obesity. The overall mortality was 3 per cent, with an operative mortality of 2.6 per cent. The hospital deaths were due to pulmonary embolism (4 patients) and peritonitis (9 patients). Of the latter, one had primary peritonitis while the remainder had anastomotic problems of various types. Wound problems occurred in about 8 per cent of patients; the majority of these were subcutaneous infections, which responded to open drainage and dressing changes. Stomal ulceration was diagnosed in 1.8 per cent of patients, which was calculated to be one ulcer per 140 patient years of exposure. This complication was usually heralded by signs and symptoms of blood loss rather than by abdominal pain.

No metabolic or nutritional deficiencies were observed in long-term follow-up of gastric bypass. Specifically, decreased serum albumin, elevation of liver enzymes, and electrolyte abnormalities were not seen. The postoperative bowel habits tended toward constipation rather than diarrhea, although the majority of patients had normal bowel habits. Vomiting was an early postoperative complication and, occasionally, was a serious problem. Usually, patients vomit only when they overeat or eat too rapidly, losing only the food that has been recently ingested. Therefore, despite frequent vomiting episodes, hypochloremic alkalosis and dehydration usually do not occur. It is, of course, possible for obstruction to develop either at the gastroenterostomy stoma or distally, so that patients who are vomiting must be evaluated to rule out other causes. Initially, patients are encouraged to eat small meals to minimize the risk of suture line dehiscence, which might occur secondary to distention of the proximal pouch.

The average weight loss observed in Mason and associates' series was about 36 kilograms; however, great variation was seen. Preoperative weight and age, to a lesser degree, tended to correlate with weight loss. The best results were seen in the heaviest patients and in young adults. At three years, weight loss was 50 kilograms or more in one-third of patients, between 25 and 50 kilograms in one-third, and less than 25 kilograms in the remainder. Mason feels that the effectiveness of gastric bypass depends upon the bypass of the distal stomach and duodenum, the creation of a small gastroenterostomy measuring 1.5 cm., and the formation of a small reservoir between the esophagus and the stoma.

The creation of a small proximal pouch seems to be of particular importance in achieving adequate weight loss. Mason and associates now recommend that all the short gastric arteries be divided up to the esophagus to facilitate mobilization of the upper stomach into the wound, where it can be transected easily either with the GIA or TA–90 stapler or between Kocher clamps (Mason and associates, 1975) (Fig. 14–17). Alder and Terry (1977) recommend mandatory intraoperative standardization to assure reproducible pouch and stomal size. They suggest that the site of gastric transection can be accurately determined by inserting a nasogastric tube that has been marked from the tip with archbar rubber bands at 5 and 12 cm., respectively (Fig. 14–18). The surgeon guides the tube, which is palpated through the stomach wall, precisely along the lesser and greater curvatures. The lesser curvature is then cleared at a site 5 cm. from the gastroesophageal junction. The greater curvature transection site should be at 12 cm. from the gastroesophageal junction, as determined by palpation of the second marker. Alder and Terry (1977) also have suggested that the volume of the proximal pouch be determined before transection takes place. The amount of saline required to begin distention of the pouch is considered the pouch volume. The pouch volume should not exceed 50 ml. of saline in order to achieve satisfactory weight loss. In dividing the stomach, preservation of the proximal left gastric artery, which supplies the upper gastric pouch, is important, particularly when all the short gastric arteries have been divided to facilitate mobilization (Fig. 14–19) (Maini and associates, 1977).

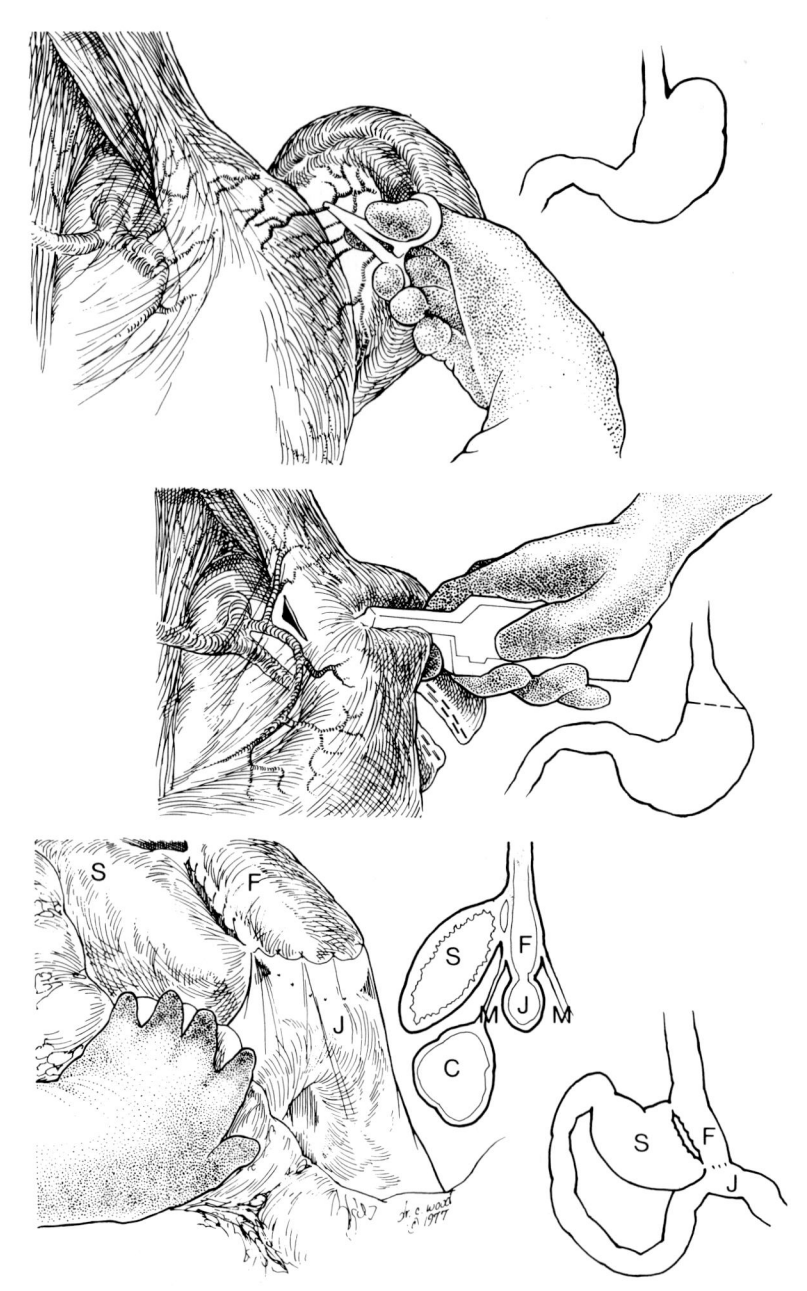

Figure 14–17. Technic of gastric bypass. The short gastric vessels are taken down. The stomach is transected with a GIA stapler, preserving the branches of the left gastric and ascending esophageal arteries. A 1 cm, retrocolic, short afferent loop anastomosis is created. The transected, closed stomach is sutured to the closed fundus. (From Knecht, B. H.: Experience with gastric bypass for massive obesity. Am. Surg. 48:496, 1978.)

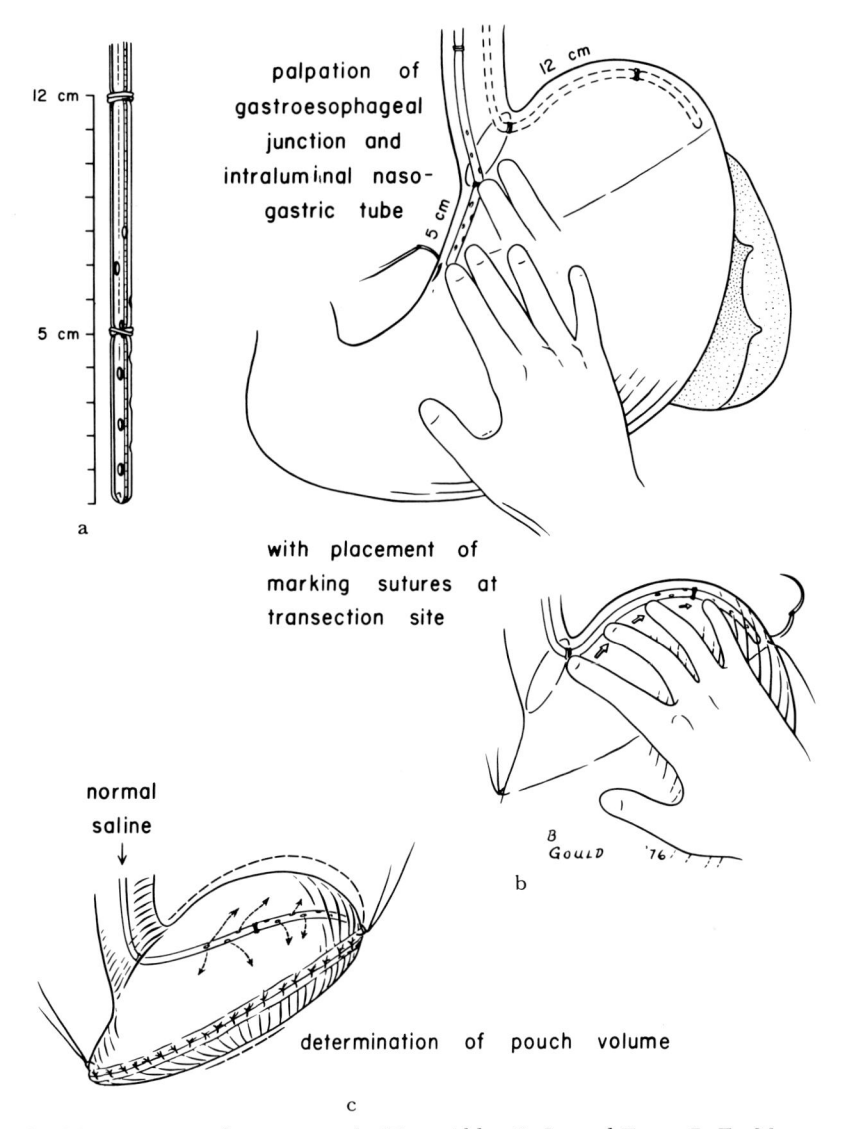

Figure 14-18. Measurement of gastric pouch. (From Alder, R. L., and Terry, B. E.: Measurement and standardization of the gastric pouch in gastric bypass. Surg. Gynecol. Obstet. *144*:762, 1977.)

Other investigators have now had considerable experience with the gastric bypass for morbid obesity. Hermreck and colleagues (1976) performed the procedure in 75 patients who averaged 31.4 years of age and had an average weight of 121.4 kilograms. No postoperative deaths occurred. Wound infections developed in 13 per cent of the patients and subsequently three of these developed incisional hernias. Postoperative stomal obstruction was noted in two patients, both of whom required reoperation. Four patients developed functional gastric outlet obstruction; all responded to extended nasogastric suction. Splenectomy is a possible complication of this operation, particularly when the gastric fundus is mobilized by taking down the short gastric arteries. This occurred in four patients in Hermreck's series. Fifteen of the 75 patients developed varying chronic gastrointestinal complaints, with vomiting being the most common. Prolonged vomiting is usually due to overeating and can be controlled by limiting the volume of meals. A certain number of patients, despite counseling, continued to overeat and complained bitterly of the experience. Hermreck and col-

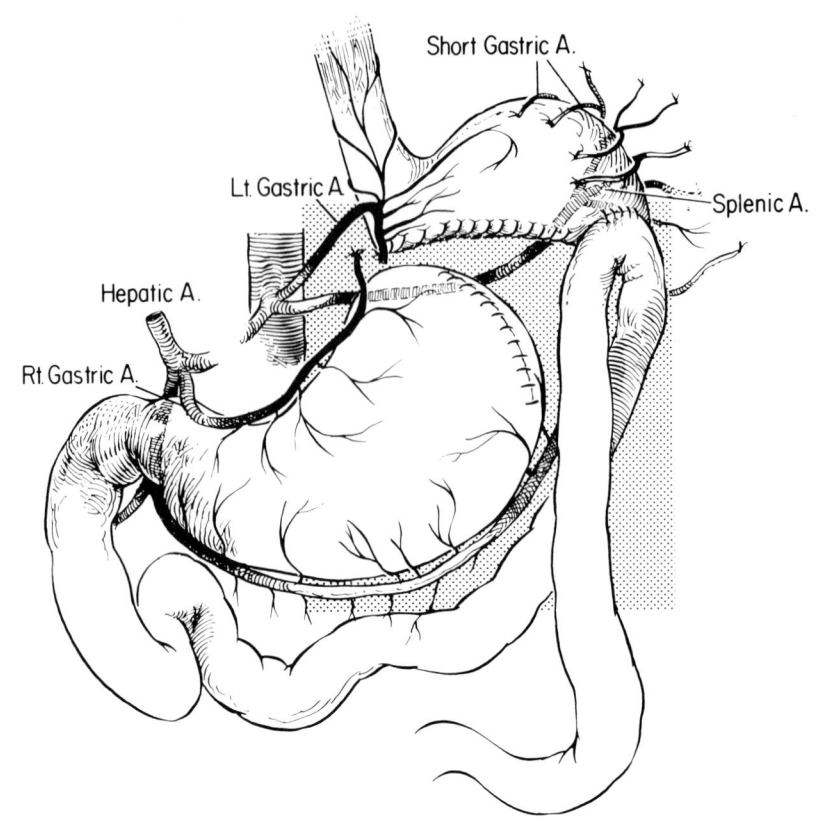

Figure 14-19. Gastric bypass. Viability of the fundic pouch is ensured by ligating the left gastric artery distal to the origin of the ascending esophageal artery and the upper gastric branches. (From Maini, B. S., Blackburn, G. L., and McDermott, W. V.: Technical considerations in a gastric bypass operation for morbid obesity. Surg. Gynecol. Obstet. *145*:907, 1977.)

leagues (1976) feel that this may represent a failure in adjustment on the part of the patient and perhaps a failure in judgment on the part of the surgeon in selecting candidates for the procedure. Severe dysphagia, gastroesophageal reflux, esophagitis, and diarrhea were occasional chronic problems. Vitamin deficiencies, especially of the B vitamins, can develop in patients who are in a starvation state following gastric bypass. Continuous vitamin administration is recommended during the period of weight loss to prevent polyneuritis and ataxia.

In Hermreck's series, about 80 per cent of the patients had excellent or good results. At 6 months, there was a 24.5 per cent average weight decrease, which progressed to 35.8 per cent by 12 months. In a comparison of weight loss with that of a series of patients undergoing small bowel bypass, no statistical difference was noted. Seven of 54 patients had inadequate weight loss; this was due either to stomal enlargement or to a pattern of continuous eating despite a small upper pouch and stoma.

The results of gastric bypass for obesity in three series are summarized in Table 14-1.

Table 14-1. Results of Gastric Bypass for Obesity

	Knecht[*]	*Hermreck*[†]	*Hornberger*[‡]
Number of patients	50	75	31
Average weight loss (1 year)	49 kg	—	50 kg
Hospital morbidity	10%	18%	50%
Wound problems	4%	13%	21%
Obstruction of stoma	2%	2.6%	0
Intra-abdominal abscess	4%	0	3%
Anastomotic leak	4%	0	0
Stomal ulceration	0	0	6%
Failure to lose significant weight	25%	9.3%	10%
Mortality	2%	0	6%

[*]Knecht, B. H.: Experience with gastric bypass for massive obesity. Am. Surg. 48:496, 1978.
[†]Hermreck, A. S., Jewell, W. R., and Hardin, C. A.: Gastric bypass for morbid obesity: Results and complications. Surgery 80:498, 1976.
[‡]Hornberger, H. R.: Gastric bypass. Am. J. Surg. 131: 415, 1976.

Complications

Mason and colleagues (1979), reporting on the complications associated with gastric operations for obesity, found that the procedure was associated with a significant risk of gastric perforation (40 in 863 operations, or 4.6 per cent). Perforation was noted to occur only in the early postoperative period and was associated with an overall mortality rate of 15/40 (37.5 per cent). These investigators emphasize the need for early recognition and reoperation after perforation has been identified. Perforation is generally associated with severe pain, in contrast to the usual uncomplicated course. Perforations were found to be equally common in the upper stomach, at the gastrojejunal anastomosis, or in the excluded pouch. Diagnosis of perforation in the distal stomach is difficult since ingested contrast material usually does not reach this segment. In this series, 17 of 30 upper gastrointestinal studies were negative despite the presence of perforation. At times, exploration must be undertaken on the basis of clinical signs and symptoms rather than on radiologic criteria alone.

Perforation following gastric bypass has many causes. Some are probably related to malposition and function of the nasogastric tube used to decompress the proximal pouch and jejunum. The nasogastric tube may fail to decompress the proximal stomach because the tube opening is beyond the gastroenterostomy stoma, located in the efferent limb of the jejunum (Fig. 14–20). As a result, the upper stomach, the efferent limb, the duodenum, and the excluded stomach may become markedly distended, with resultant perforation. Pressure of the nasogastric tube against the wall of the upper pouch also has produced necrosis and perforation (Fig. 14–21). Mason and associates suggested that the small size and boot shape of the

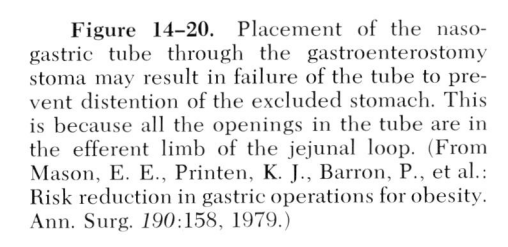

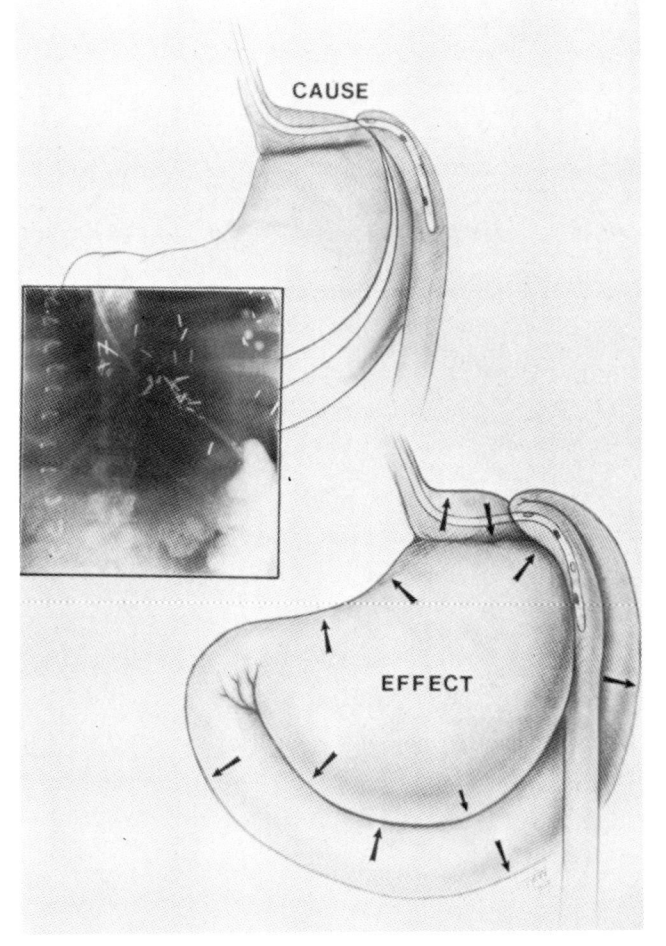

Figure 14–20. Placement of the nasogastric tube through the gastroenterostomy stoma may result in failure of the tube to prevent distention of the excluded stomach. This is because all the openings in the tube are in the efferent limb of the jejunal loop. (From Mason, E. E., Printen, K. J., Barron, P., et al.: Risk reduction in gastric operations for obesity. Ann. Surg. *190*:158, 1979.)

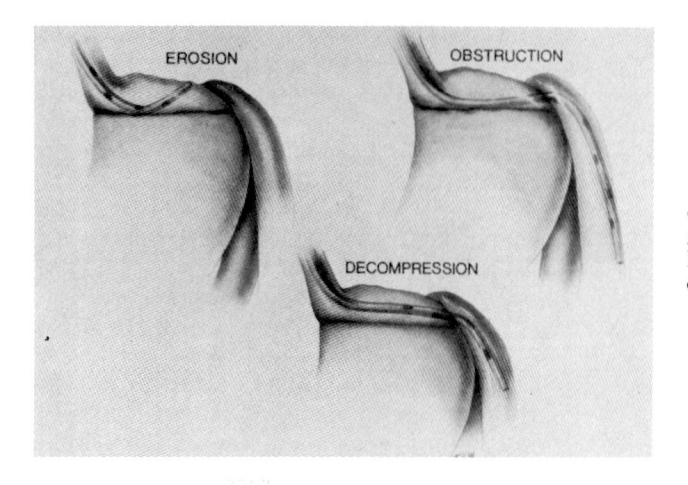

Figure 14–21. Too shallow, too deep, and correct placement of the nasogastric tube in gastric bypass. Both erosion and obstruction have caused perforation. (From Mason, et al., cited in previous figure.)

upper stomach contribute to the problem of perforation by the nasogastric tube. The tube must make two nearly right angle turns at the cardia and again at the gastroenterostomy stoma. The tube should be placed a few centimeters through the stoma, with holes on both sides of the anastomosis. In this way, decompression will be complete.

Early ventilation with a mask after extubation may lead to the introduction of air into the stomach, producing marked dilatation and possible perforation. Gomez (1980) has suggested that some perforations in the upper stomach are secondary to stress ulceration and recommends the routine administration of cimetidine or antacids. Some feel that many perforations, particularly at the anastomosis, are due to relative ischemia. Care must be taken to preserve the lesser curvature vasculature, particularly the ascending branches of the left gastric artery. Dissection in that area should be minimized and sufficient only for the toe of the stapler to be passed around the stomach. Blood supply can be compromised by staples or sutures used in partition or transection of the stomach. If, for example, two rows of staples are used to partition the stomach, the second row should be incomplete to preserve blood supply at the gastroenterostomy site (Fig. 14–22). In summary, these problems can be secondary to poor exposure and technical error, impaired blood supply, pressure necrosis from the nasogastric tube, inadequate decompression of one or the other portion of the anastomosis, or afferent loop obstruction.

Buckwalter and Herbst (1980) and Peltier and associates (1979) have emphasized the complications seen following gastric bypass procedures for obesity. Peltier and colleagues (1979) reported an experience with 400 consecutive patients undergoing gastric bypass at the University of Kansas. In half of these, the standard gastric division of Mason and Printen was used, while in the remainder the gastric stapling technique of Alder was employed. The mean weight loss

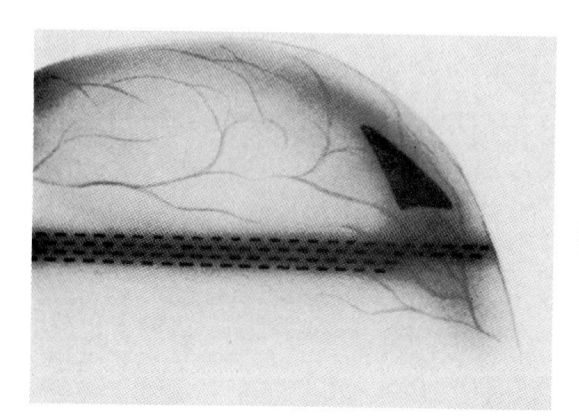

Figure 14–22. Staple line at greater curvature. The second set of staples is left incomplete to enhance the blood supply. (From Mason, et al., cited in Figure 14–20.)

was 31.5 per cent at 24 months. Twenty-three per cent of patients had a poor result because of inadequate weight loss or complications. A mortality rate of 2.5 per cent (10 patients) was reported, with the early deaths being secondary to anastomotic leaks (4), pulmonary embolism (2), and respiratory failure (1). Anastomotic leakage, in 2.5 per cent of the patients, required operative intervention in all but one patient. In addition to anastomotic leaks, nine patients developed an intra-abdominal abscess, usually subphrenic, requiring operative drainage. Anastomotic or marginal ulceration was seen in seven patients and gastric outlet obstruction in six patients. Seventeen wound infections and 17 wound hernias were seen. A few patients developed vitamin B complex deficiency states manifested by severe peripheral neuropathy. Peltier and coworkers conclude that gastric bypass results in a weight reduction equal to that of small bowel bypass, and that chronic complications are few. However, acute operative complications can be substantial and are usually technical in origin.

Comparison of Gastric and Jejunoileal Bypass in the Treatment of Morbid Obesity

A few prospective comparisons of gastric and jejunoileal bypass in the treatment of morbid obesity have been reported. Griffen and coworkers (1977), at the University of Kentucky, made a randomized prospective study of 49 patients (22 jejunoileal bypass patients and 27 gastric bypass patients). The patients were strictly comparable in age, preoperative weight, and incidence of concomitant diseases. For the jejunoileal bypass, an end-to-end anastomosis was created between 30 cm. of proximal jejunum and 25 cm. of terminal ileum; the bypassed segment of small bowel was decompressed by an end-to-side anastomosis to the transverse colon. The first seven gastric bypasses were done according to the method of Mason: the stomach was transected and a retrocolic end-to-side gastrojejunostomy was created. The remainder of the gastric bypass group underwent identical transection of the stomach. However, rather than use of a loop of small bowel for anastomosis, the jejunum was transected and the distal limb brought retrocolic for anastomosis to the stomach (Fig. 14-23). The proximal limb of the jejunum was then anastomosed to the jejunum 30 cm distal to the gastrojejunostomy in an end-to-side fashion. This Roux-en-Y technique was introduced because the greatest technical difficulty encountered was in bringing the stomach into such a position that the gastrojejunostomy resided below the opening in the transverse mesocolon. In addition, some loop patients had considerable difficulty with bilious vomiting.

In this series, there were no early deaths, and one patient in each group required takedown of the bypass. Two late deaths occurred, one in each group. In the jejunoileal bypass group, the late death was due to intractable weight loss and severe liver disease with hepatorenal syndrome. The gastric bypass patient was admitted to hospital for observation and died of what was suspected to be a pulmonary embolus. Ten patients in the small bowel bypass group required rehospitalization for severe electrolyte imbalance or for further surgical procedures, such as cholecystectomy or ventral hernia repair. Only four gastric by-

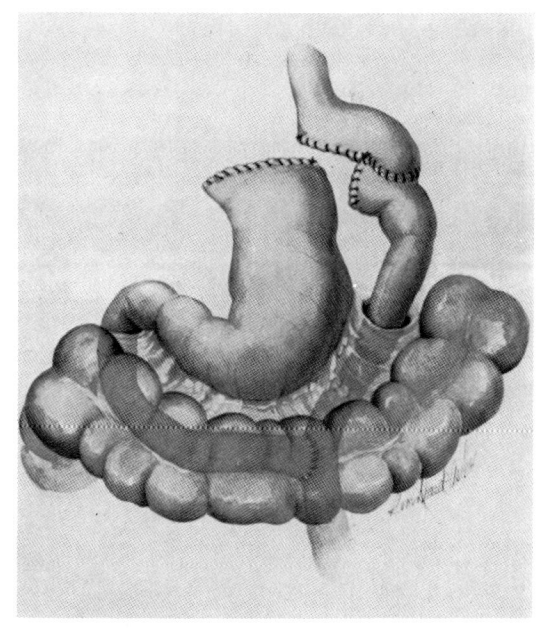

Figure 14-23. Technique of retrocolic Roux-en-Y anastomosis. (From Griffen, W. O., Young, V. L., and Stevenson, C. C.: A prospective comparison of gastric and jejunoileal bypass procedures for morbid obesity. Ann. Surg. *186*:500, 1977.)

pass patients required rehospitalization — one for a fistula after an anastomotic leak and the others for ventral hernia repair. The incidence of early surgical complications was greater in the gastric bypass group. The wound complication rate was similar in both groups, but the gastric bypass procedure was associated with three incidental splenectomies. When splenic injury is eliminated from consideration, the early complication rate is almost identical in the two groups.

The late complications in the two groups were somewhat different. Nausea and vomiting was a prominent symptom in patients after gastric bypass and was clearly the most troublesome postoperative complaint. In contrast, the small bowel bypass group displayed a high incidence of diarrhea, requiring antidiarrheal medications and electrolyte supplementation. Kidney stones developed only in those with small bowel bypass (four patients). The incidence of liver disease was strikingly different in the two groups. No patient undergoing gastric bypass demonstrated significant liver disease while two patients in the small bowel bypass group developed severe liver disease postoperatively. One of the latter patients died of this complication, and the other required takedown of the bypass. Liver biopsies done 1 year postoperatively in the two groups revealed entirely different patterns. All the patients who underwent gastric bypass showed either no change or improvement in the liver biopsy specimens. In the small bowel bypass group, 12 of 15 patients showed worsening of the liver pattern histologically, while only 3 were stable.

There was no difference in weight loss pattern or statistics between the two groups. Patients in both groups generally showed a weight loss of 20 to 30 kilograms in the first 2 to 3 months. Thereafter, they stabilized at a weight loss of 4 to 6 kilograms per month. At 1 year postoperatively, the mean weight loss was 51 kilograms in the gastric group and 57 kilograms in the small bowel bypass group. The results were not statistically different.

Several conclusions are suggested by this study and a smaller series reported by Buckwalter and Herbst (1980). Both the jejunoileal and gastric bypass procedures can be performed relatively safely in the morbidly obese individual. Anastomotic breakdown is uncommon, and the incidence of other complications, like wound infection, pulmonary embolus, and respiratory complications, is acceptable. The gastric bypass procedure is more demanding technically, and strict attention to details, particularly the size of the gastric pouch and the diameter of the gastrojejunostomy, are critical to success. Liver disease is a distinct threat following small bowel bypass, and it is often preceded by excessive weight loss. However, liver disease is exceedingly uncommon following gastric bypass. Complications such as renal calculi, post-bypass arthritis, colonic pseudo-obstruction, bypass enteritis, and electrolyte abnormalities do not occur following the gastric bypass. Several investigators have now concluded that gastric bypass is superior to small bowel bypass in incidence of long-term complications and is of equal efficacy for weight loss.

Gastric Partitioning for Morbid Obesity

In view of the technical difficulties encountered by some in the performance of gastric bypass, other gastric procedures for obesity have been proposed. Pace and colleagues (1979) have developed a technic of gastric partitioning as an alternative to standard or modified gastric bypass. They recommend that the procedure be done through an upper mid-line incision. The left lobe of the liver is retracted superiorly without dividing the triangular ligament. None of the short gastric arteries is divided (Fig. 14–24). By blunt dissection, the index finger of the surgeon is passed about the stomach from the greater to the lesser curvature, taking care to reflect the posterior vagus nerve. The thumb is then passed around the lesser curvature of the stomach to meet the index finger. The thumb is passed between the anterior vagus nerve and the anterior wall of the stomach. The left index finger is then passed through this opening in the lesser omentum, going from the lesser to the greater curvature of the stomach, and is used to guide the lower jaw of the TA-55 or TA-90 stapler about the stomach. The 4.8 mm. cartridges are used. Three staples are

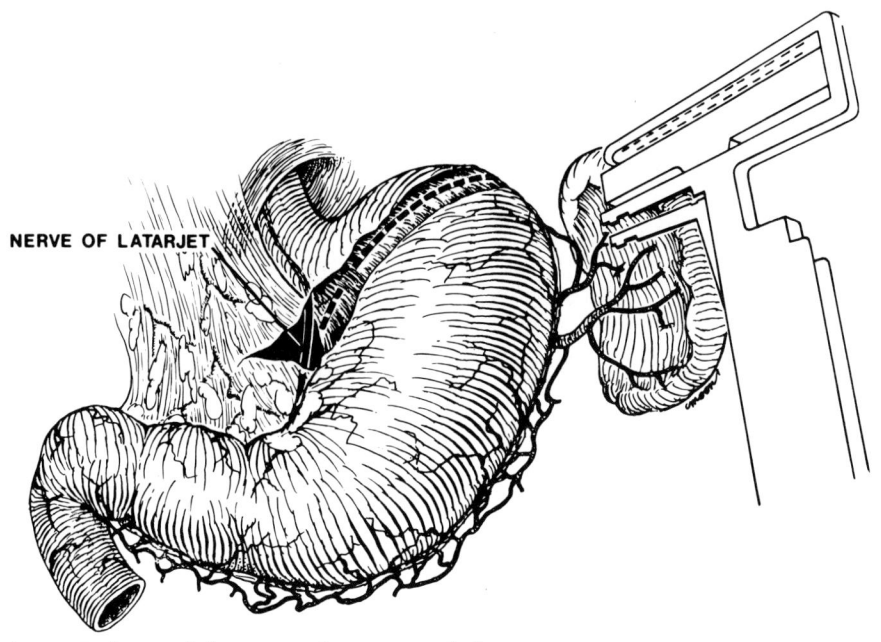

Figure 14-24. Isolation of the nerve of Latarjet and placement of the TA-90 above the vasa brevia. (From Pace, W. G., Martin, E. W., Tetirick, T., et al.: Gastric partitioning for morbid obesity. Ann. Surg., *190*:392,, 1979.)

removed from the mid-portion of the cartridge so as to create a channel between the upper and lower gastric pouches (Fig. 14-25). The nasogastric tube is withdrawn so that it lies completely within the esophagus. The stapling device is then tightened, with extreme care being taken to avoid bunching of the stomach as the staples will not fix properly under these circumstances. If the stomach fills the entire jaw area of the stapling device, the device is loosened and repositioned nearer the gastroesophageal junction. The staples are then discharged. When the device is removed, the nasogastric tube is passed through the defect into the lower stomach (Fig. 14-26). Utilizing the TA-90 stapler, the proximal gastric pouch should accommodate no more than 30 to 60 ml. of saline when calibration is performed.

The technical aspects of gastric partitioning are felt to be relatively straightforward. However, postoperative management is exceedingly important and occasionally difficult. Vigorous attention is paid to bronchopulmonary toilet. Nothing is given by mouth until ileus has resolved. When water is started following resolution of ileus, no more than 30 ml. at a time are given. Patients are warned that one 30 ml. cup represents the size of the gastric pouch and that no more than that quantity of fluid may be taken at any given time. It is imperative that the patient be instructed not to challenge the staple suture line with large quantities of fluid or with solid foods until after the eighth postoperative week. Tensometer studies performed in animal models have demonstrated that weakness of the staple suture lines persists for approximately 2

Figure 14-25. Removal of three staples from the TA-90 cartridge. (From Pace, et al., cited in previous figure.)

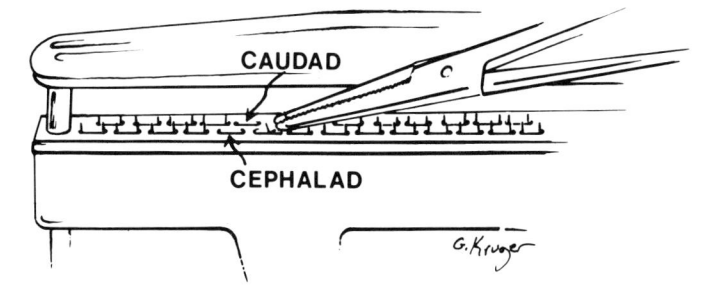

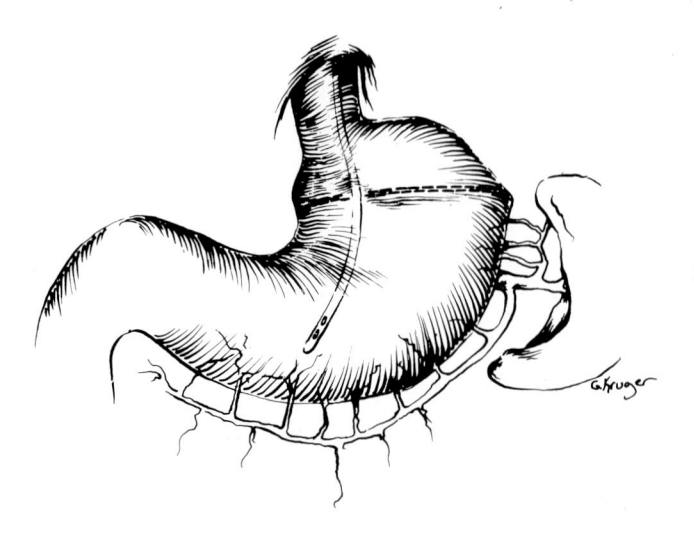

Figure 14-26. Completed TA-90 staple partition. (From Pace, et al., cited in Figure 14-24.)

weeks, after which strength increases to a maximum at about 8 weeks. It is essential to instruct patients concerning the thorough mastication of food. Failure to follow restrictions absolutely may result in dehiscence of the suture line and failure of the procedure.

Pace and coworkers (1979) have reported on 220 patients who have undergone gastric staple partitioning. The average preoperative weight was 290 pounds. There was a single death, resulting from a pulmonary embolus. Postoperative complications, which prolonged hospital stay, occurred in 5 per cent. These complications included stomal obstruction (2), pulmonary embolus (1), fistulas (2), and partial staple line necrosis with leakage (1). Four severe wound infections and two wound dehiscences were noted. Associated major technical problems included splenectomy (2) and posterior lacerations of the stomach (2). There was one misplaced staple line. Of the 220 patients, 82 per cent were considered to have successful results, while 18 per cent were considered to be failures. All patients in the failure group had disruption of the partition, usually secondary to ingestion of large amounts of solid food or large quantities of liquid shortly after the procedure. The average weight loss was approximately 5 pounds per month, with weight loss ongoing for 12 to 18 months. While the procedure seems to be safe and relatively simple, a successful outcome depends upon proper selection of patients and absolute cooperation of patients in the postoperative period to permit healing of the staple partitioning.

The long-term results following this procedure are yet to be determined.

Freeman and Burchett (1980) proposed some technical modifications of gastroplasty aimed at preventing dilatation of the gastrogastrostomy. They recommend mobilization of the greater curvature up to the esophagus, including division of the short gastric arteries (Fig. 14-27). A small opening is then created in the gastrohepatic omentum, taking care to avoid ligation of the branches of the left gastric artery or of the vagus nerve. The contemplated pouch is calibrated so as to create a 30 to 40 ml. proximal pouch manometrically (Fig. 14-28). A No. 14 nasogastric tube is then introduced and positioned along the greater curvature of the stomach. The TA-90 stapler, utilizing 4.8 mm. staples, is then aligned so that it lies close to the medial surface of the nasogastric tube (Fig. 14-29). It is introduced from the lesser to the greater curvature. The instrument is fired, reloaded, and fired again so that four rows of staples partition the stomach. To prevent dilatation of the gastrogastrostomy, mattress sutures are placed through and through in pairs around the nasogastric tube for a distance of 4 cm. This creates a longer gastrogastrostomy, and it is hoped that dilatation will be less likely (Fig. 14-30).

In comparing gastroplasty to gastric bypass, Freeman and Burchett (1980) have shown that weight loss is approximately the same over the initial 6 months. However, utilizing a double gastric staple line and vertical mattress sutures in performance of the gastroplasty, a mortality rate of 1 to 4 per

GASTRIC PROCEDURES FOR MORBID OBESITY

Figure 14–27. Mobilization of the greater curve from its mid-point to the angle of His. (From Freeman, J. B., and Burchett, H. J.: A comparison of gastric bypass and gastroplasty for morbid obesity. Surgery 88:433, 1980.)

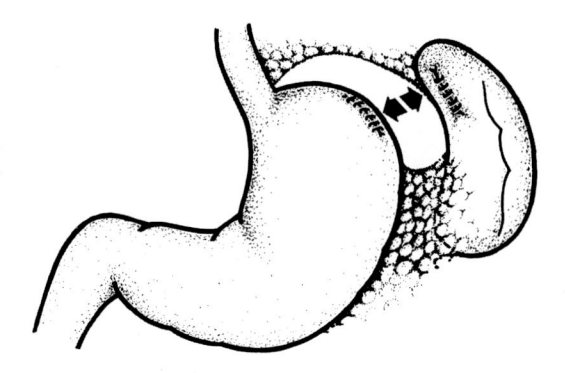

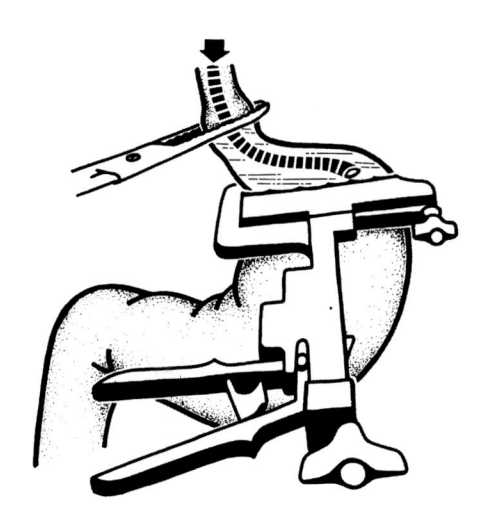

Figure 14–28. The TA-90 or 55 stapler is passed through a small opening in the gastrohepatic omentum and tightened, but not fired. Pouch size is measured manometrically by occluding the esophagus. (From Freeman and Burchett, cited in previous figure.)

Figure 14–29. Stapler moved from patient's left to right so the No. 14 nasogastric tube passes down the greater curve. (From Freeman and Burchett, cited in Figure 14–27.)

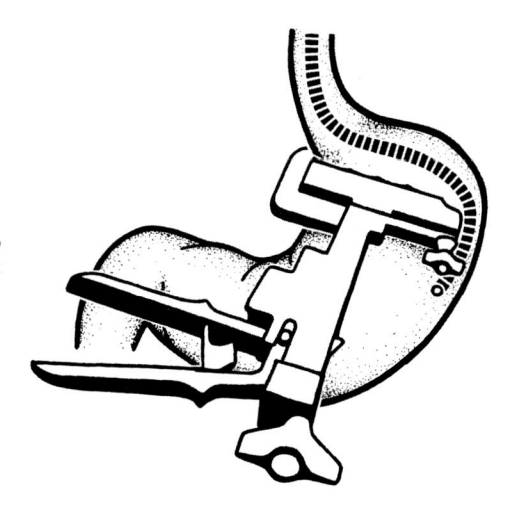

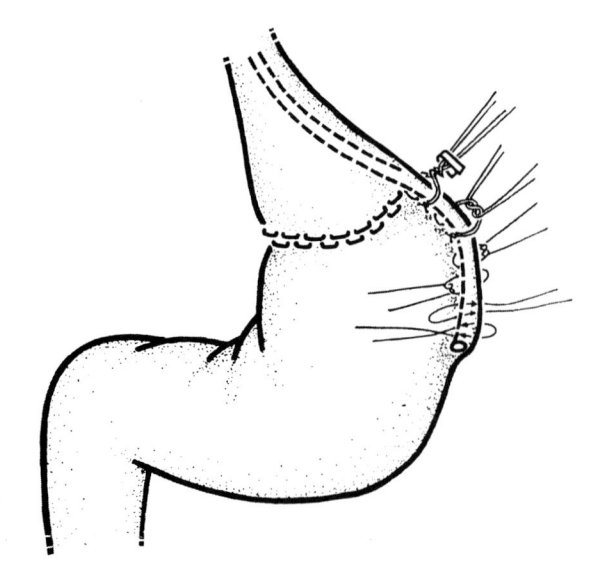

Figure 14-30. A double staple line is made, and interrupted vertical mattress sutures are tied around the tube. (From Freeman and Burchett, cited in Figure 14-27.)

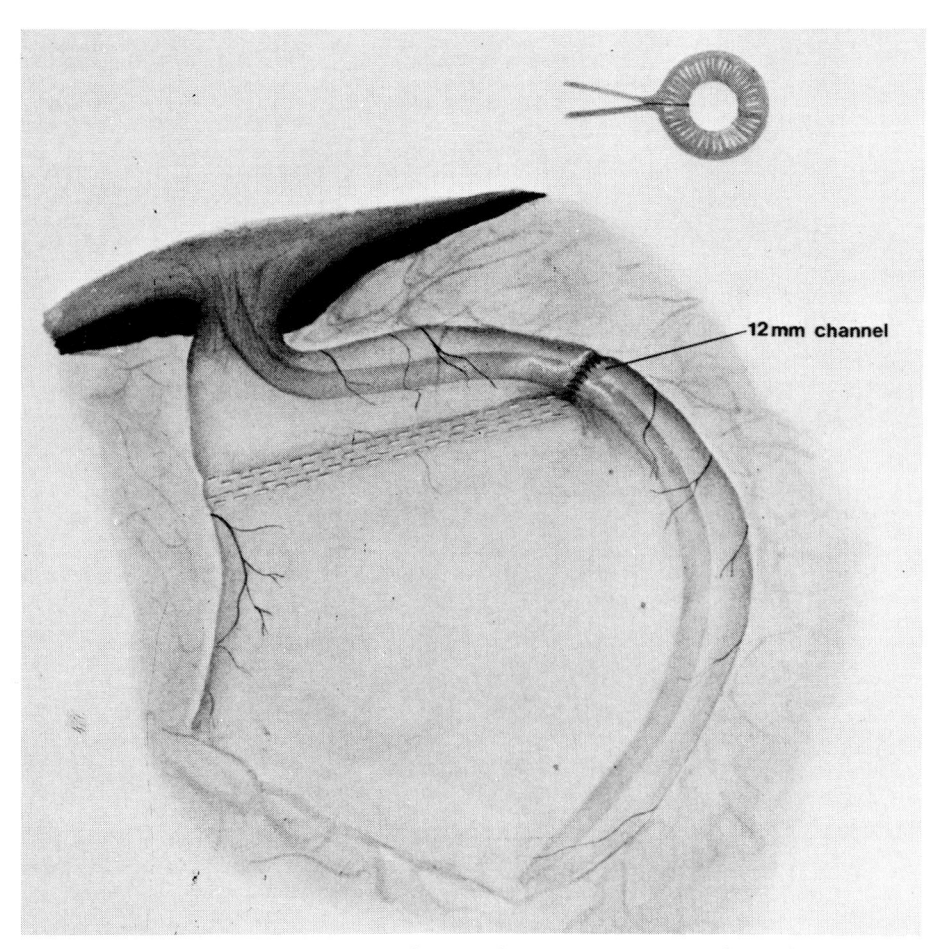

Figure 14-31. Operative technic. Completed gastroplasty with 12 mm. Maloney bougie through channel. (From Gomez, C. A.: Gastroplasty in the surgical treatment of morbid obesity. Am. J. Clin. Nutr. 33:406, 1980.)

GASTRIC PROCEDURES FOR MORBID OBESITY

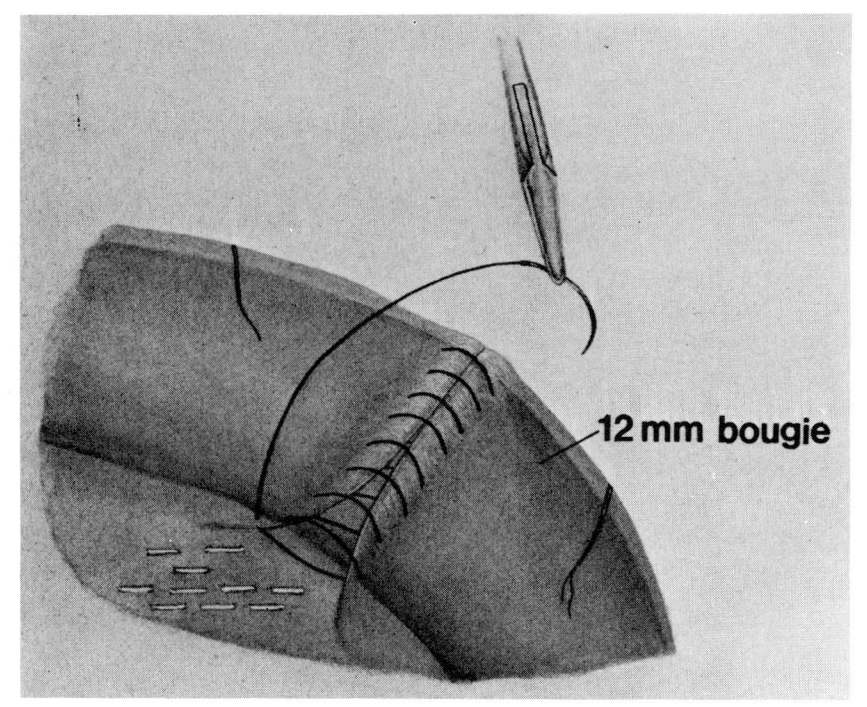

Figure 14–32. Operative technic. Seromuscular suture ring of 3-0 Prolene. (From Gomez, cited in previous figure.)

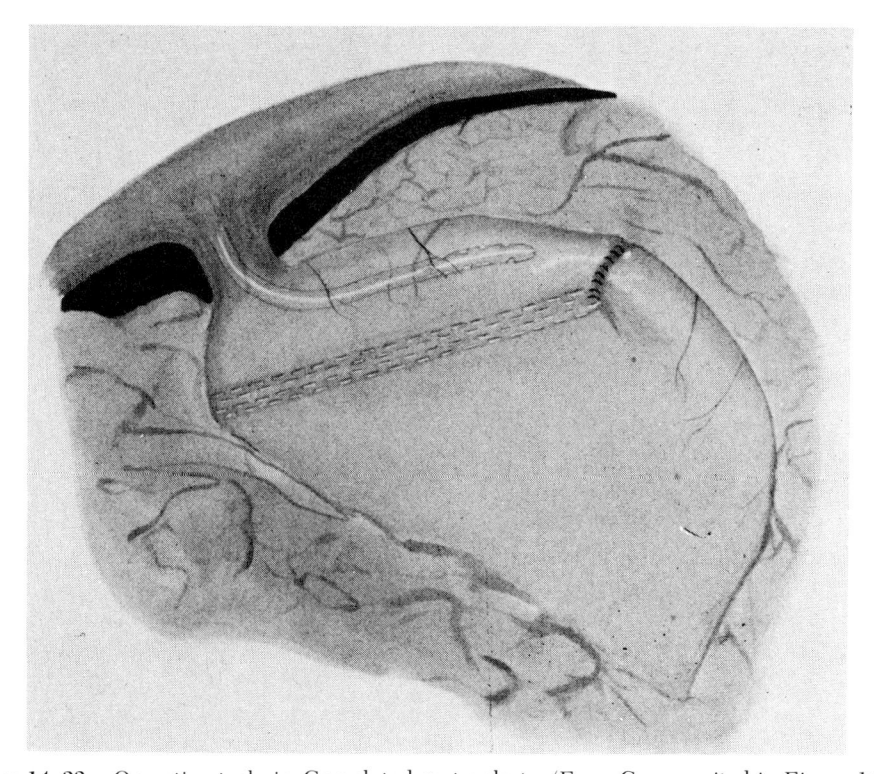

Figure 14–33. Operative technic. Completed gastroplasty. (From Gomez, cited in Figure 14–31.)

cent can be expected, with a leakage rate of 8 per cent. However, in the absence of a double staple line and stomal reinforcement, the failure rate as measured by weight loss may be as high as 30 per cent. A balance must ultimately be achieved between an unacceptably high incidence of disruption and the development of such significant complications as leakage due to ischemia. Gomez (1980) recommends that a seromuscular suture ring using 3–0 Prolene be employed to further narrow the stoma about an indwelling 12 mm. Maloney bougie. The last three to four staples are transfixed and the Prolene suture carried from the posterior to anterior gastric wall as an imbricating suture around the channel and against the bougie. Utilizing this technique in a small number of patients, no staple line disruption or stomal enlargements have been seen. Longer follow-up is needed for further evaluation of this modification (Figs. 14–31, 14–32, and 14–33).

Part 3

INCISIONS

INTRODUCTION

The ease of an operative procedure on the alimentary tract depends upon the selection, execution, and closure of the incision. The proper selection of an incision and the subsequent success of the operative procedure depend upon several variables:

1. The incision should provide the most direct and, if possible, the shortest approach to the organ upon which the operation is being performed.

2. The incision should be of sufficient length to permit ample retraction and adequate exposure of the operative field.

3. The incision must avoid injury to vital structures.

4. When possible, the incision should divide only tissues that are capable of strong repair.

5. When possible, the incision should be placed so as to heal with the best possible cosmetic result.

6. The incision will not heal without adequate nutrition.

A good cosmetic result may not be possible and should be of low priority. Nevertheless, the final appearance of the scar can be very important to the patient. There are few excuses for not making an attempt to obtain the finest-line scar possible under the circumstances at the time of wound closure. Tissue necrosis should be kept to a minimum. Atraumatic technic should always be practiced. The surgeon must use sharp cutting instruments. Hemostats, forceps, and electrocautery should be used meticulously and cause only minimal tissue damage. It is important to select the proper needle and the correct size and type of suture.

Despite years of experimentation, surgeons have yet to find the perfect suture material. The ideal suture would possess adequate tensile strength, tie with ease, be easy to sterilize, create no foreign body reaction, and undergo complete tissue absorption.

Chapter 15

EXPOSURE OF THE CERVICAL ALIMENTARY TRACT

The cervical esophagus is situated deep in the neck, where it lies in the *visceral space*, the space located between the pretracheal and prevertebral fascial layers of the neck (Fig. 15–1). Exposure of the esophagus in this area requires some knowledge of the anatomy of the neck.

Anatomy

The anatomy of the esophagus has been described in Volume 1 (pp. 6–23).

The neck is the portion of the body that lies between the head and trunk. Its superior boundary is the line of the inferior margin of the body of the mandible continued from the angle of the jaw through the mastoid process from the anterior to the posterior midline on both sides. Its inferior border anteriorly is delineated by the suprasternal notch and the superior margin of the clavicle, while posteriorly it is a line drawn from the acromioclavicular joint to the spinous process of the seventh cervical vertebra. This spinous process is the most prominent one of the cervical vertebrae and is easily recognized. Other recognizable surface landmarks of the neck are:

1. The sternocleidomastoid muscles, (Fig. 15–2), one on each side, form a prominence that runs from the mastoid process obliquely downward and medially (anteriorly) across the lateral surface of the neck to the medial portion of the clavicle and its junction with the sternum at the episternal notch. Each sternocleidomastoid muscle divides its side of the neck into an anterior and a posterior triangle.

2. The thyroid cartilage (Adam's apple), which is more prominent in men than in women. This is easily visible and palpable as it protrudes in the anterior midline (Fig. 15–2). It moves up and down when a person swallows.

3. The hyoid bone, which lies about 2.5 cm. above the thyroid cartilage. It moves on swallowing and cannot be seen, but, when steadied with fingers placed on both sides, it can be palpated. The greater horn of the hyoid bone lies about midway between the mastoid process and the thyroid prominence.

4. The arch of the cricoid cartilage, which can be felt (but not seen) in the anterior midline just inferior to the thyroid cartilage. It moves up and down on swallowing. Immediately below it the butterfly-shaped thyroid gland can be palpated (see Fig. 15–2). This gland cannot be seen as a surface landmark unless it is enlarged. The cricoid cartilage is at the level of the palpable anterior tuberosity (carotid tubercle of Chassaignac) of the sixth cervical vertebra. This tubercle can be identified by applying pressure at the anterior border of the sternocleidomastoid muscle at this level, and serves as a landmark in ligation of the common carotid artery. It also marks the level at

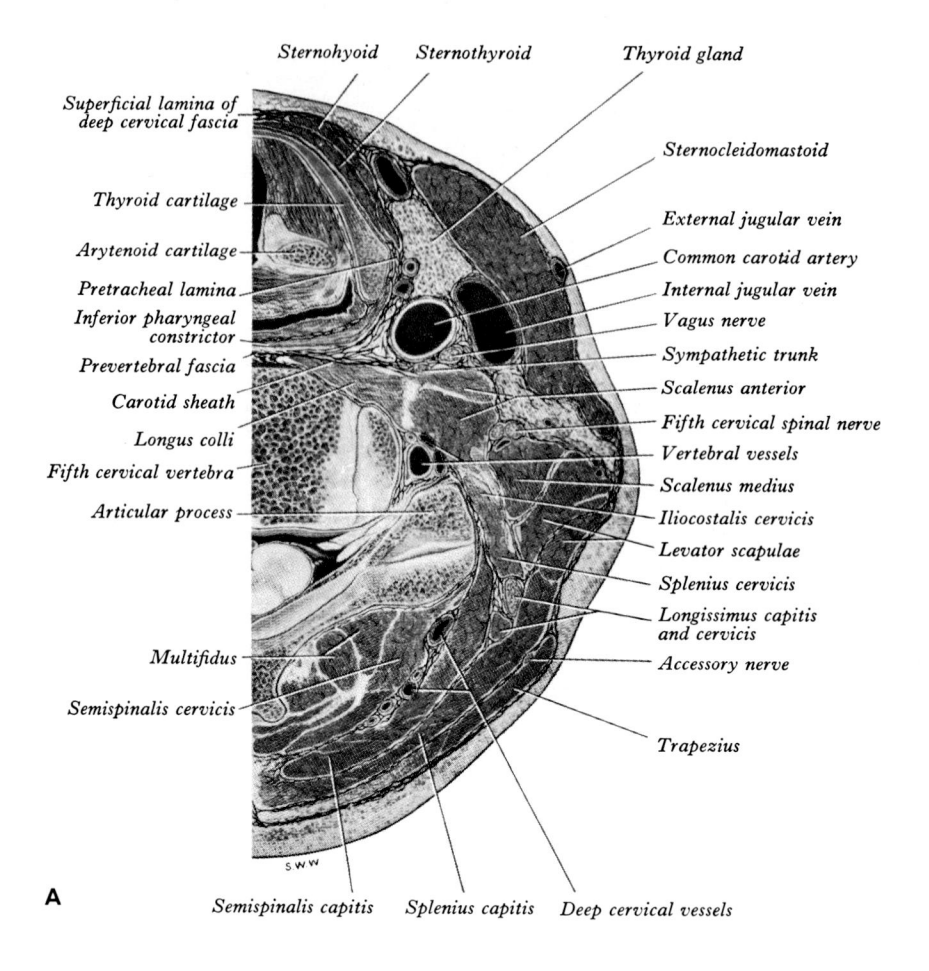

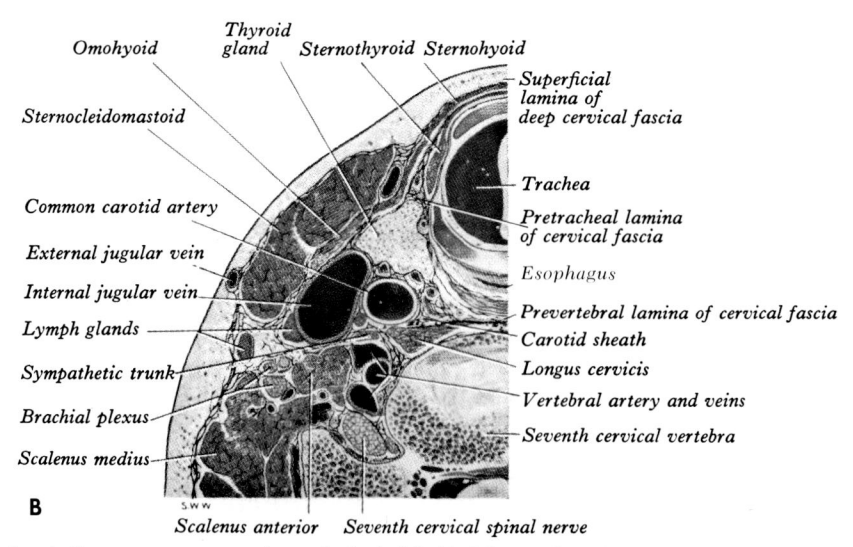

Figure 15–1. *A*, Transverse section through the left half of the neck to show arrangement of the deep cervical fascia. *B*, Part of a transverse section through the lower part of the neck at the level of the seventh cervical vertebra to show the arrangement of the deep cervical fascia. (Specimen provided by Prof. R. E. M. Bowden.) (From Warwick, R., and Williams, P. L. (eds.): Gray's Anatomy, 35th Br. ed. Philadelphia, W. B. Saunders Company, 1973.)

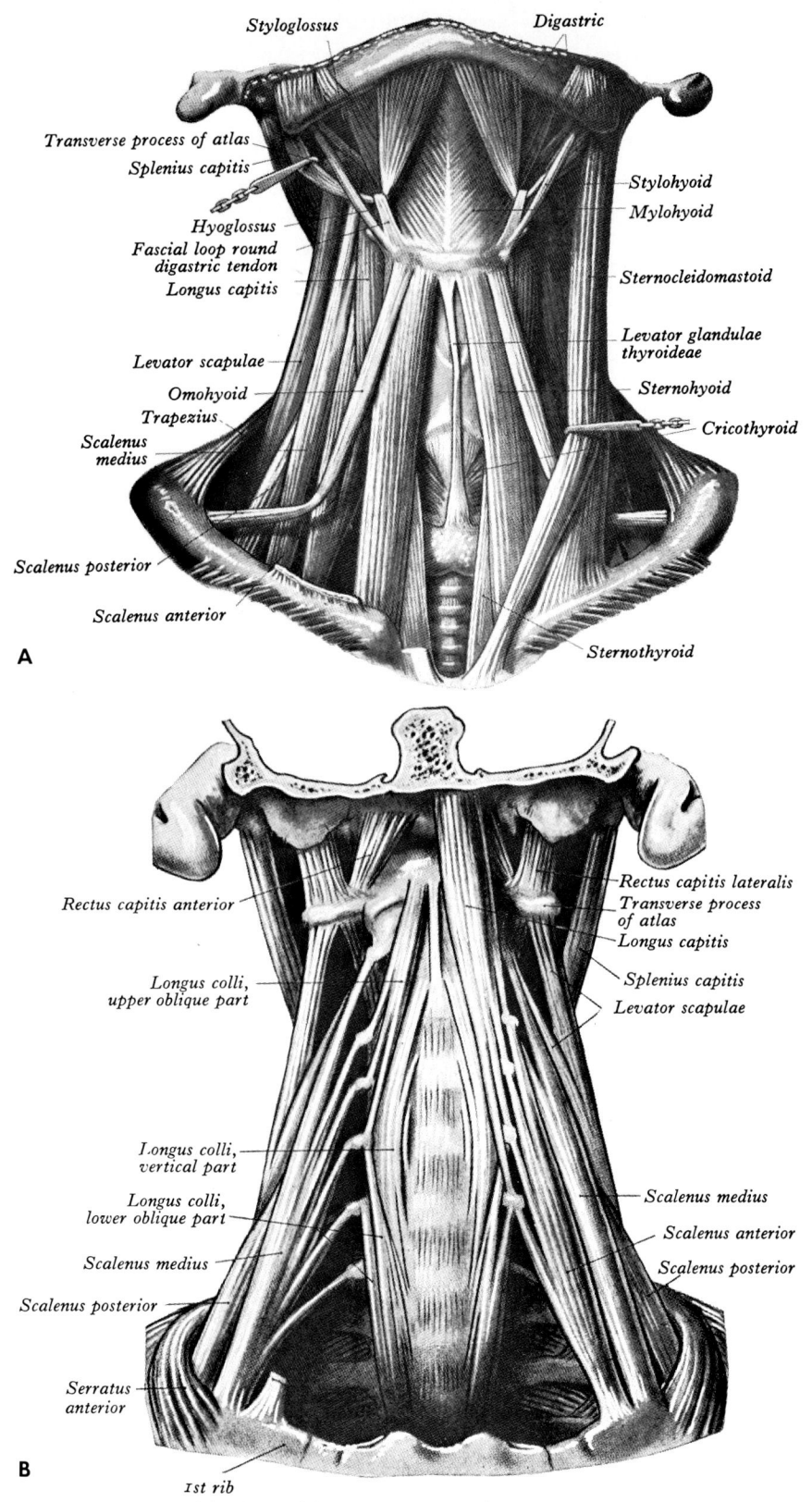

Figure 15–2. *A*, Muscles of the front of the neck. On the right side the sternocleidomastoid has been removed. In this subject, the origin of the scalenus medius extended up to the transverse process of the atlas. *B*, The anterior and lateral vertebral muscles. On the right side the scalenus anterior and the longus capitis have been removed. (From Warwick and Williams, cited in previous figure.)

405

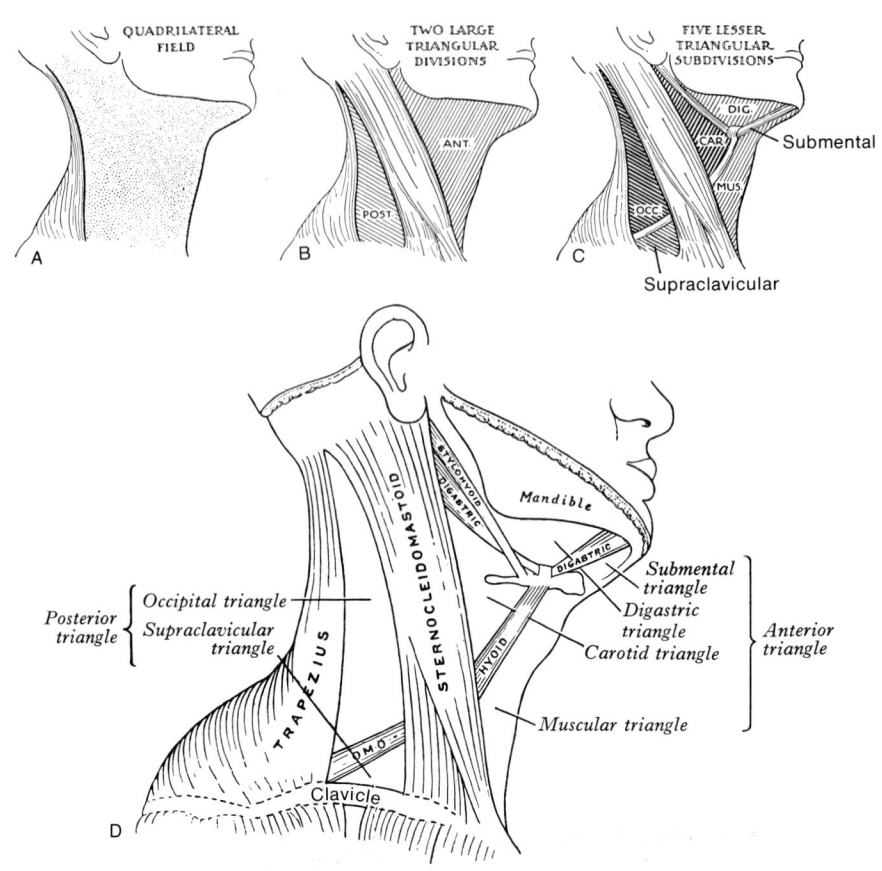

Figure 15-3. Subdivision of the anterolateral portion of the neck into triangular areas. A, Quadrilateral field bounded by the trapezius muscle (behind), mandible and occipital bone (above), midline of the neck (front), and clavicle (below). B, Subdivision into two triangular areas by the obliquely coursing sternocleidomastoid muscle. C, Further subdivision of the posterior triangle into occipital and supraclavicular triangles by the omohyoid muscle; comparable subdivision of the anterior triangle into submental digastric, carotid, and muscular triangles by the omohyoid and digastric muscles. D, the triangles of the right side of the neck. (D modified from Warwick and Williams, cited in Figure 15-1.)

which the pharynx merges into the cervical esophagus to form the beginning of that structure.

5. The anterior edge of the trapezius muscle, which can be palpated and sometimes seen as a ridge that forms the posterior boundary of the posterior triangle of the neck (Fig. 15-3).

Encasing the neck are two main fascial layers called the superficial and the deep cervical fascial.

The *superficial cervical fascia*, barely demonstrable as a separate layer, lies immediately beneath the skin around the entire circumference of the neck. It contains the superficial vessels, nerves (see Fig. 15-1), and adipose tissue. It is separated from the investing lamella of the deep cervical fascia by the platysma muscle extending over the anterolateral portion of the neck (Fig. 15-4). The platysma muscle arises from the deep fascia of the pectoral region and from the clavicle to pass upward to the inferior border of the mandible, beyond which it blends with some of the muscles of the face. In closing incisions made in the neck, it is important to approximate the cut edges of the platysma, including the superficial fascia, in order to minimize the unsightliness of the subsequent scar.

The *deep cervical fascia* consists of three layers, which invest and support the muscles, pharynx, trachea, esophagus, lymph glands, large vessels, and nerves (see Fig. 15-1). The *superficial (investing) layer of the deep cervical fascia* forms a complete

EXPOSURE OF THE CERVICAL ALIMENTARY TRACT

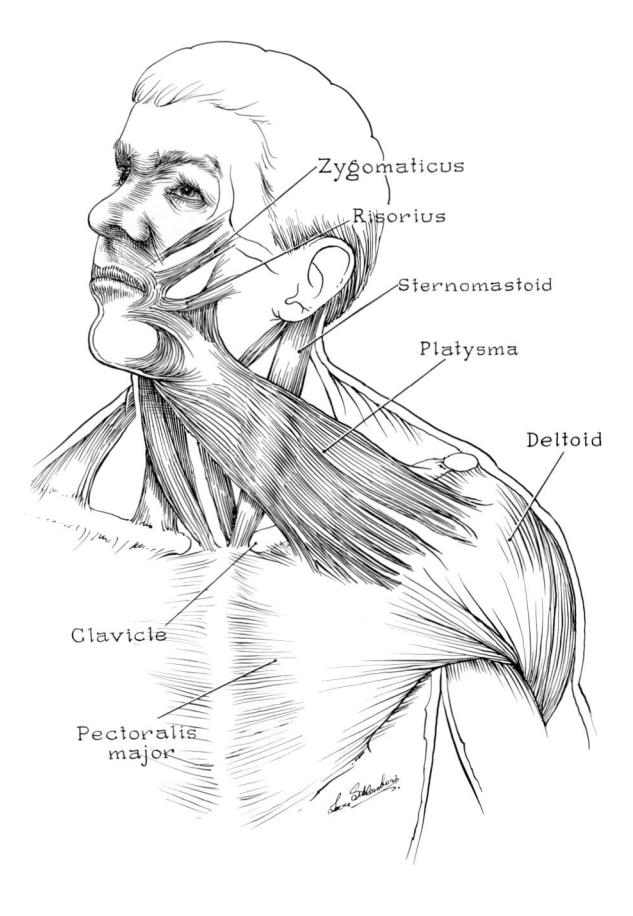

Figure 15-4. Platysma muscle and related muscles of facial expression. The platysma, like the corresponding muscles of the face and scalp, is situated in the superficial fascia. This layer of tissue has been dissected away to expose the platysma muscle, the related triangularis, and other facial muscles in the subcutaneous stratum.

envelope for all the cervical structures except the platysma and the superficial vessels and nerves. It is attached above to the inferior margin of the mandible; posterior to the angle of the jaw it continues upward to enclose the parotid gland and attaches to the zygomatic arch, mastoid process, occipital protuberance, and superior medial line. It splits and reunites at appropriate points to ensheathe the trapezius and sternocleidomastoid muscles. These lamellae are fused again to form a single layer anterior to the sternocleidomastoid muscle, and this layer fuses in the midline with its counterpart from the other side. This layer is attached to the hyoid bone, below which level the fascia splits to form a superficial and a deep layer. The former is attached to the anterosuperior border of the sternum and the latter to the posterosuperior border of the sternum. In the space (suprasternal space of Burns) between the two layers of the investing layer of deep cervical fascia lie the sternal heads of the sternocleidomastoid muscles. Through this space the anterior jugular veins and their transverse anastomosis (jugular arch) pass to join the external jugular veins (Fig. 15-5). The investing layer of the deep cervical fascia fuses with the fascial covering of both the anterior and posterior bellies of the digastric muscle, thus shutting off the submandibular and submental areas from free communication with each other or with other regions of the neck.

The *pretracheal (middle) layer of the deep cervical fascia* arises from the investing layer deep to the sternocleidomastoid muscle (see Fig. 15-1). It passes in front of the laryngotracheal tube and the infrahyoid muscles and descends deep to the investing layer into the lower neck and mediastinum to fuse with the covering of the aorta and the pericardium. Laterally it splits to form the carotid sheath. Its anterior lamella ensheathes the omohyoid and sternohyoid muscles, while its posterior lamella ensheathes the sternothyroid muscle.

The *prevertebral (posterior) layer of the deep cervical fascia* also originates from

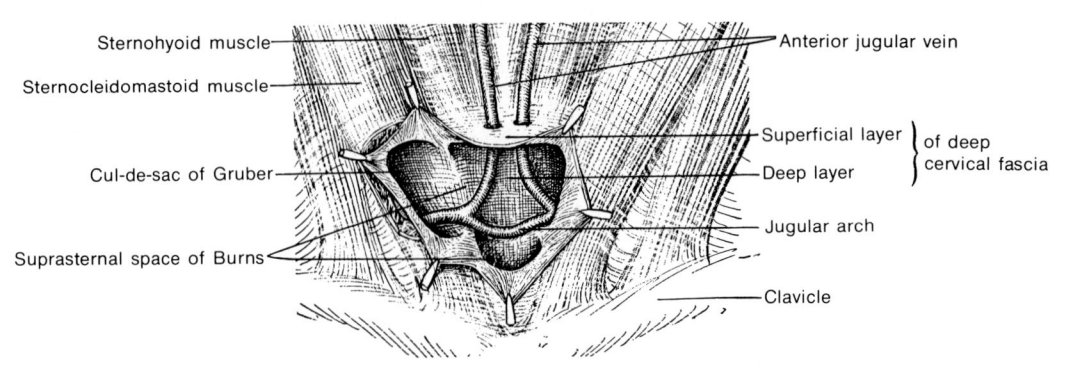

Figure 15-5. Vascular and fascial relation in the suprasternal space.

the investing layer (see Fig. 15–1). It passes across the neck over the prevertebral musculature and behind the pharyngoesophageal tube. It lies behind the great vessels of the neck and covers the muscles on which they lie. The prevertebral layer of the deep cervical fascia forms the floor of the supraclavicular triangle, where it overlies the cervical and the subclavian vessels. As these vessels leave the supraclavicular area they invaginate the prevertebral fascia to form the fascial axillary sheath which surrounds them. Hence pus that has collected beneath the prevertebral fascia may extend down the axillary sheath to present in the axilla or anywhere along the course of the brachial artery in the arm.

The superficial branches of the cervical plexus penetrate through the prevertebral fascia, but the phrenic nerve remains deep to it.

Various spaces are formed by the three layers of the deep cervical fascia. They are:

1. The *suprahyoid space* which lies between the investing (anterior) layer and the fascial layer covering the mylohyoid muscles. The submaxillary and submental divisions of this space may communicate with the visceral space.

2. The *visceral space* which lies between the pretracheal and prevertebral layers of the deep cervical fascia. This space contains the laryngotracheal tube, the pharyngoesophageal tube, the thyroid gland, and the great vessels of the neck. These structures are surrounded by loose areolar connective tissue which offers little resistance to the progress of accumulations of fluid or air. A collection of fluid, pus, or air in the visceral space may spread behind the clavicle into the mediastinum, or may pass along the subclavian vessels into the axilla, or may progress laterally into the posterior cervical triangles, or upward through the submaxillary area into the retromandibular spaces.

Topographically the anterolateral portion of the neck can be considered as a quadrilateral field bounded by the trapezius muscle (behind), the mandible and occipital bone (above), the midline of the neck (front), and the clavicle (below) (see Fig. 15–3). This quadrilateral field is subdivided into an *anterior* and *posterior triangular* area by the obliquely coursing sternocleidomastoid muscle.

The posterior triangle is subdivided into an *occipital* and a *supraclavicular triangle* by the omohyoid muscle; likewise, the anterior triangle is subdivided into a *submental, a digastric, a carotid,* and *a muscular triangle* by the omohyoid and digastric muscles.

The contents of the occipital and supraclavicular triangles are chiefly nerves (cervical plexus, brachial plexus, and spinal accessory nerve), of the carotid and digastric triangles are vascular and glandular structures (carotid arteries, jugular and its tributary veins, parotid and submaxillary glands) and of the muscular triangle are mainly visceral structures (larynx, trachea, esophagus, and thyroid gland).

In making an incision for operations on the cervical esophagus it is helpful to be familiar with the locations of the important veins, arteries, and nerves.

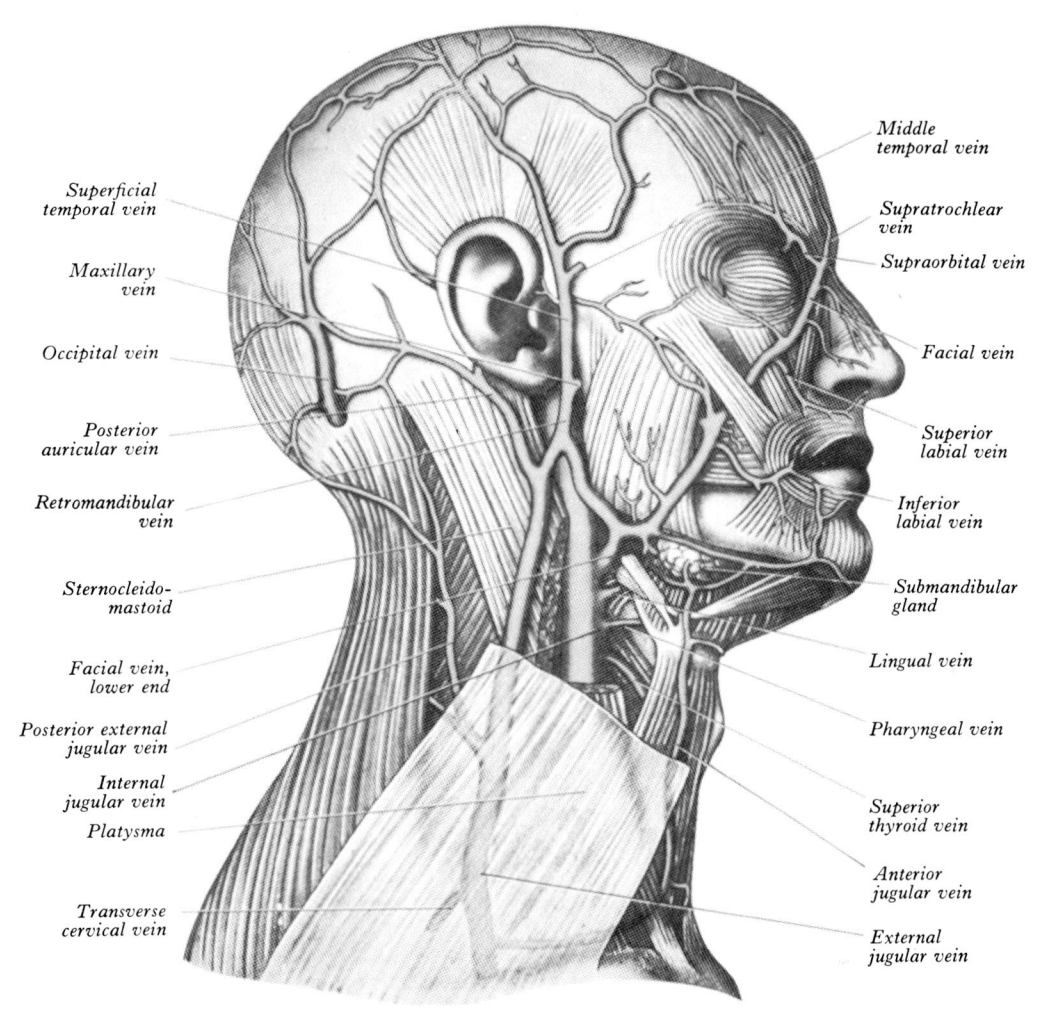

Figure 15-6. The veins of the right side of the head and neck. Parts of the right sternocleidomastoid and platysma have been excised to expose the trunk of the internal jugular vein. The external jugular vein is visible through the lower part of the platysma. (From Williams, P. L., and Warwick, R (eds.): Gray's Anatomy, 36th Br. ed. Philadelphia, W. B. Saunders Company, 1980.)

VEINS

Deep to the superficial fascia but superficial to the pretracheal layer of the deep cervical fascia are the anterior and external jugular veins, one of each on each side of the neck (Fig. 15-6).

The external jugular vein arises at the angle of the mandible, crosses the sternocleidomastoid muscle from its medial to its lateral border at the midportion of that muscle to pierce the pretracheal fascia either above or below the posterior belly of the omohyoid muscle to open into the subclavian vein near its junction with the internal jugular. Its course is along a line drawn from the angle of the mandible to the center of the clavicle. Just below the mandible it gives off a large branch which passes forward and downward to communicate with the facial vein. The external jugular vein can often be retracted laterally out of harm's way when approaching the esophagus, but when it is in the way it can be clamped, cut, and ligated with impunity.

The *anterior jugular vein* (Fig. 15-7) arises beneath the chin, upon the mylohyoid muscle by branches from the integument and superficial muscles of that area and by submental branches from the facial vein. It passes almost vertically down the neck, lying on the sternohyoid muscle a few

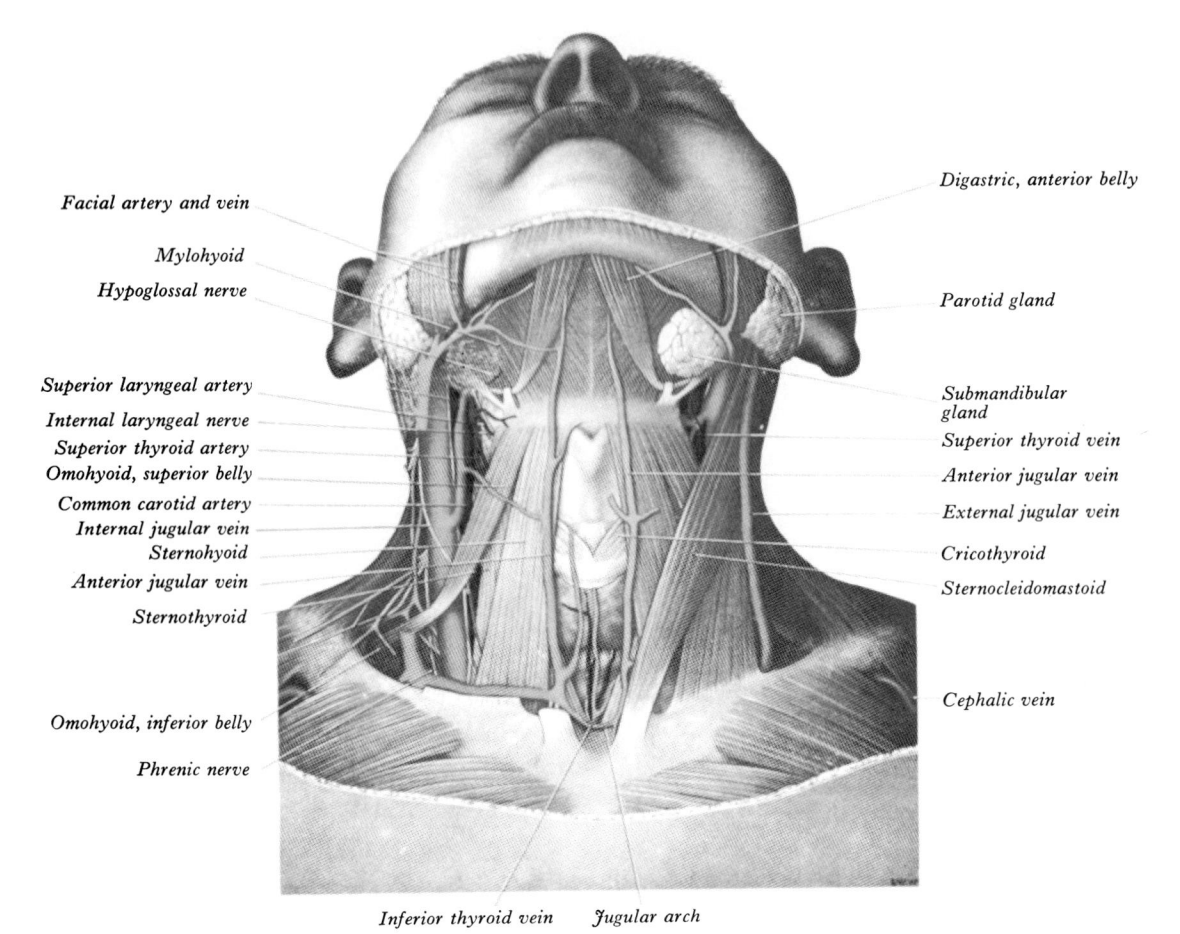

Figure 15-7. Anterior view of the veins of the neck. (From Williams and Warwick, cited in previous figure.)

centimeters lateral to the midline until it meets the anterior (medial) border of the sternocleidomastoid muscle near its sternal attachment. At this point it turns abruptly outward to pierce the pretracheal fascia and to run almost transversely beneath this muscle to open into the external jugular vein immediately above its termination. The right and left anterior jugular veins anastomose across the suprasternal space of Burns.

The anterior jugular vein usually must be divided in making a surgical approach to the cervical esophagus.

The *posterior external jugular vein* (see Fig. 15-6) runs obliquely downward along the posterior margin of the sternocleidomastoid muscle to empty into the external jugular at the lateral margin of that muscle. It is not encountered in operations upon the cervical esophagus.

The *internal jugular vein* is the princi-pal venous trunk of the neck. It arises at the jugular foramen and descends the neck in company with the internal and common carotid arteries and the vagus nerve, surrounded by the carotid sheath. Within the carotid sheath the internal jugular vein lies lateral to the carotid artery while the vagus nerve lies behind and between the two vessels. It joins the subclavian vein to empty into the brachiocephalic vein. During its course down the neck the internal jugular vein lies beneath the sternocleidomastoid muscle, rests upon the inner border of the scalenus anterior muscle, and receives some tributaries. The most important of these are the common facial vein and the superior, middle, and inferior thyroid veins. Some of these tributaries require division in order to procure an adequate exposure of the cervical esophagus, but the internal jugular vein itself is usually retracted out of harm's way. If it is inadvertently and irrep-

EXPOSURE OF THE CERVICAL ALIMENTARY TRACT

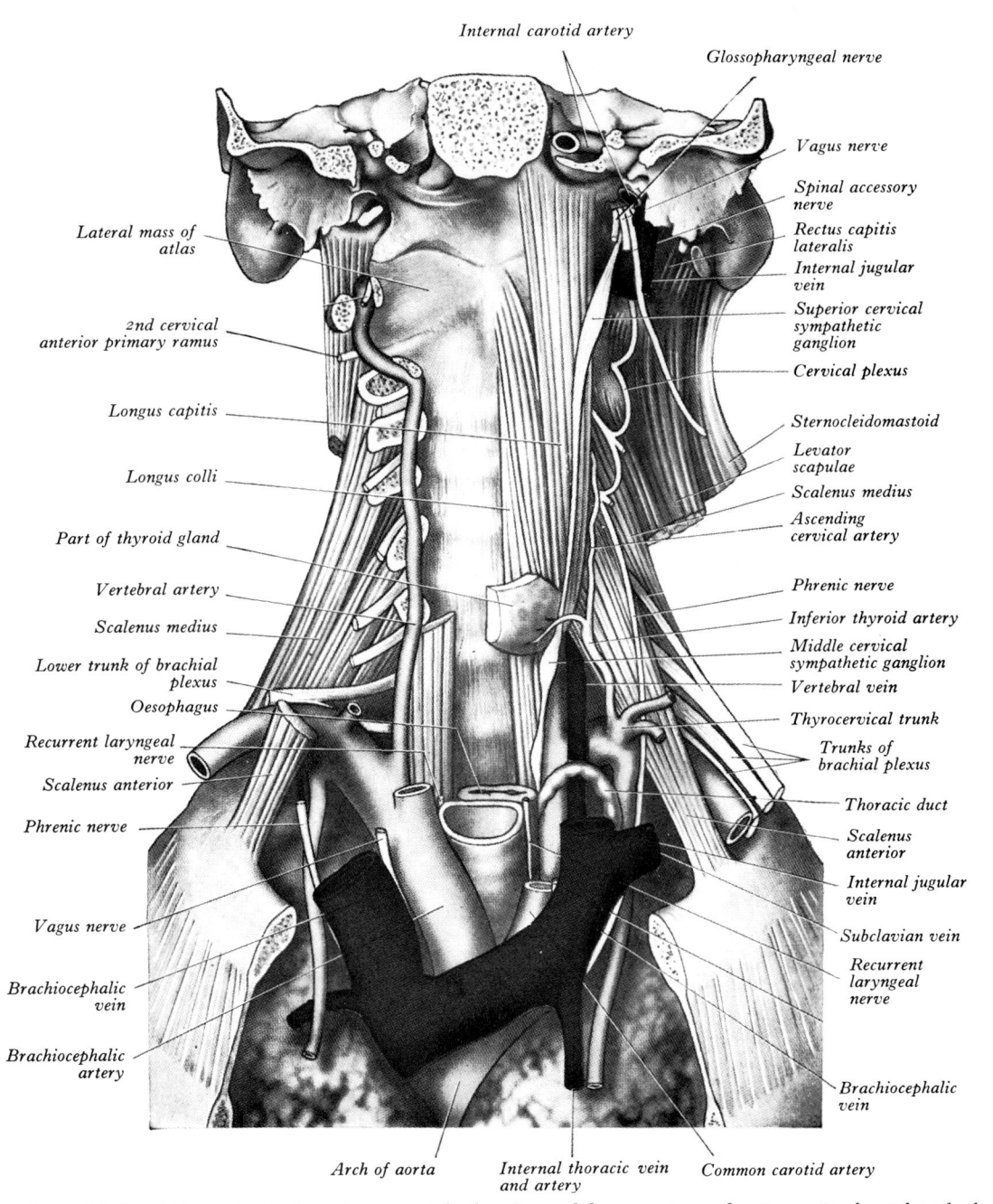

Figure 15–8. A dissection to show the prevertebral region and the superior mediastinum. On the right side the costal elements of the upper six cervical vertebrae have been removed to expose the cervical part of the vertebral artery. On the left most of the deep relations of the common carotid artery and the internal jugular vein are exposed. (From Williams and Warwick, cited in Fig. 15–6.)

arably injured it can be ligated without ill effects, but when doing so care should be taken to preserve the accompanying vagus nerve.

The terminal portion of the internal jugular vein passes just behind the space between the sternal and clavicular heads of the sternocleidomastoid muscle before joining the subclavian vein.

The *vertebral vein* (one on each side)

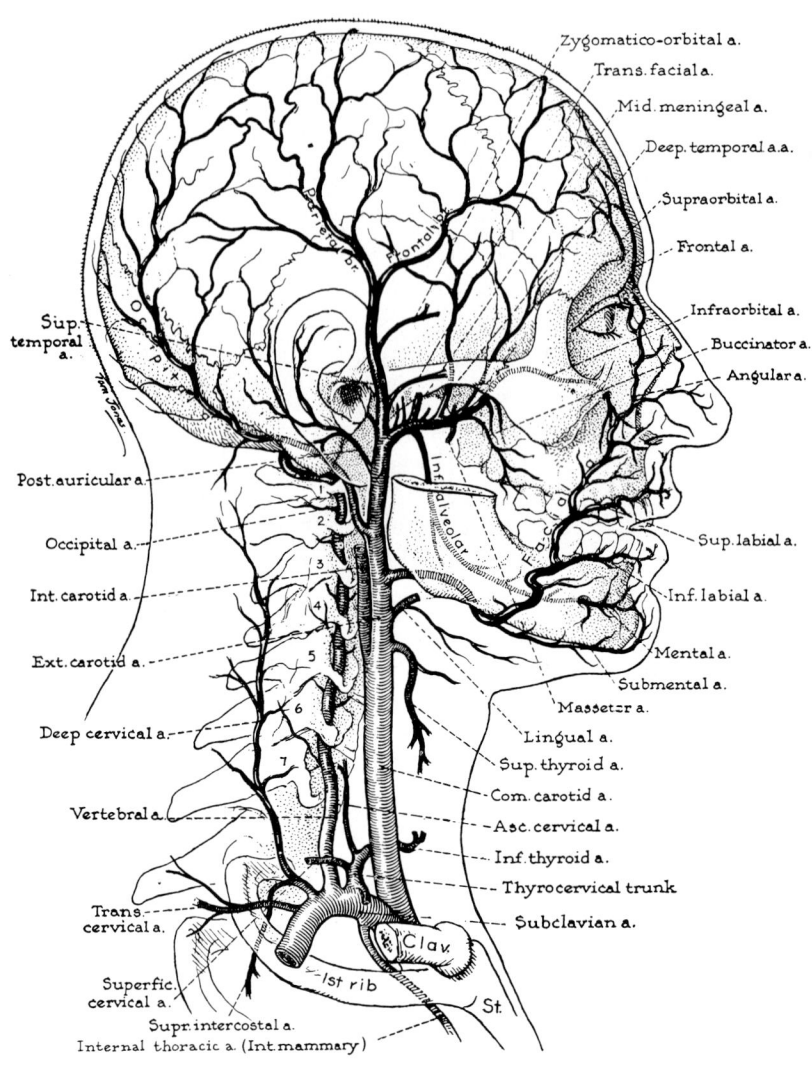

Figure 15–9. Arteries of the head and neck shown in relation to skeleton and body outline. (From Jones, T., and Shepard, W. C.: A Manual of Surgical Anatomy. Philadelphia, W. B. Saunders Company, 1945, p. 155.)

(Fig. 15–8) accompanies the vertebral artery as it passes downward through the foramina in the transverse processes of the upper five or six cervical vertebrae and is not encountered at this level. Below its exit from the foramen of the sixth cervical vertebra the vertebral vein passes obliquely forward and downward behind the inferior thyroid artery and internal jugular vein to pass in front of (occasionally behind) the subclavian artery and open into the brachiocephalic vein near its origin. In the lower portion of its course the vertebral vein may be injured during exposure of the cervical esophagus and require ligation.

ARTERIES

The carotids are the main arteries in the neck. The right *common carotid artery* arises from the brachiocephalic artery (Fig. 15–9) and the left one arises from the arch of the aorta. They both emerge from behind the ipsilateral sternoclavicular joint and ascend obliquely in the direction of the angle of the mandible, to terminate opposite the upper border of the thyroid cartilage by dividing into the external and internal carotid arteries. Throughout its course neither common carotid artery gives off any branches.

The *internal carotid artery* begins at the level of the superior margin of the thyroid cartilage and is a continuation of the common carotid that passes almost vertically upward, resting on the prevertebral fascia, to enter the carotid canal of the skull. The common and internal carotid arteries are enclosed, along with the internal jugular vein and vagus nerve, in the carotid sheath which is derived from the deep cervical fascia. At its origin the internal carotid lies a little posterolateral to the external carotid, but as it ascends it passes to the mesial side of the external carotid toward the pharynx. When it reaches the pharynx it runs vertically into the maxillopharyngeal space and carotid canal. The cervical portion of the internal carotid artery gives off no branches.

The *external carotid artery* arises from the common carotid artery at the same level but somewhat mesial and anterior to the internal carotid artery. It immediately leaves the carotid sheath to pass upward and backward to the angle of the mandible, where it changes direction and rises vertically to pass deep to the posterior belly of the digastric and the stylohyoid muscles to pierce the posteromesial surface of the parotid gland. It continues upward through the gland just behind the neck of the mandible, where it terminates by dividing into the maxillary and superficial temporal arteries. In its course the external carotid artery passes very close to the great horn of the hyoid bone, which serves as an excellent landmark for locating this artery and is the point of election for its ligation.

The external carotid artery gives off eight branches. From its anterior surface in order from below upward are given off (1) the superior thyroid, (2) the lingual, (3) the facial, and (4) the maxillary artery. From its posterior surface, and also in order from below upward are given off (5) the ascending pharyngeal, (6) the occipital, (7) the posterior auricular and (8) the superficial temporal, which is one of its terminations.

One or more of these branches may require division to obtain adequate exposure of the cervical esophagus, but the common internal and external carotid arteries are left intact and retracted out of harm's way in most operations on this area. When necessary or desired to reduce bleeding, the external carotid can be ligated with impunity. Ligation of the internal or common carotids should be avoided because of the danger of subsequent damage to the brain even though the collateral anastomotic channels are said to be adequate to maintain circulation.

The *vertebral artery* is the first and largest branch of the subclavian artery. It runs upward to enter the vertebral foramen of the sixth cervical vertebra. Since it lies deep to the prevertebral fascia it seldom presents a problem in exposing the cervical esophagus.

The *inferior thyroid artery* is one of the three terminal branches of the short thyrocervical trunk that arises from the subclavian artery. The other two are the transverse cervical and transverse scapular arteries, which are not encountered in exposing the cervical esophagus.

The inferior thyroid artery ascends along the mesial margin of the anterior scalenus muscle as far as the level of the cricoid cartilage, at which point it turns abruptly to run mesially in a transverse direction and then downward to divide into branches at the lower pole of the lateral thyroid lobe. In its course it passes deep to the carotid sheath.

The inferior thyroid artery and vein frequently require division in order to obtain an adequate exposure of the cervical esophagus.

The *thoracic duct* is applied closely to the left side of the esophagus as it leaves the thorax to ascend in the neck about 4 cm. above the clavicle, at which point it turns laterally behind the carotid sheath and in front of the inferior thyroid and vertebral arteries. When it reaches the medial margin of the scalenus anterior muscle it runs inferiorly to enter the angle of union of the internal jugular and subclavian veins. In operations upon the lower portion of the cervical esophagus, care must be taken to avoid injury to the thoracic duct, or else to identify and ligate it, which causes no untoward aftereffects.

NERVES

The *vagus* is the tenth cranial nerve. It passes from the skull down the neck in the carotid sheath where it lies posterior and between the carotid artery and internal jug-

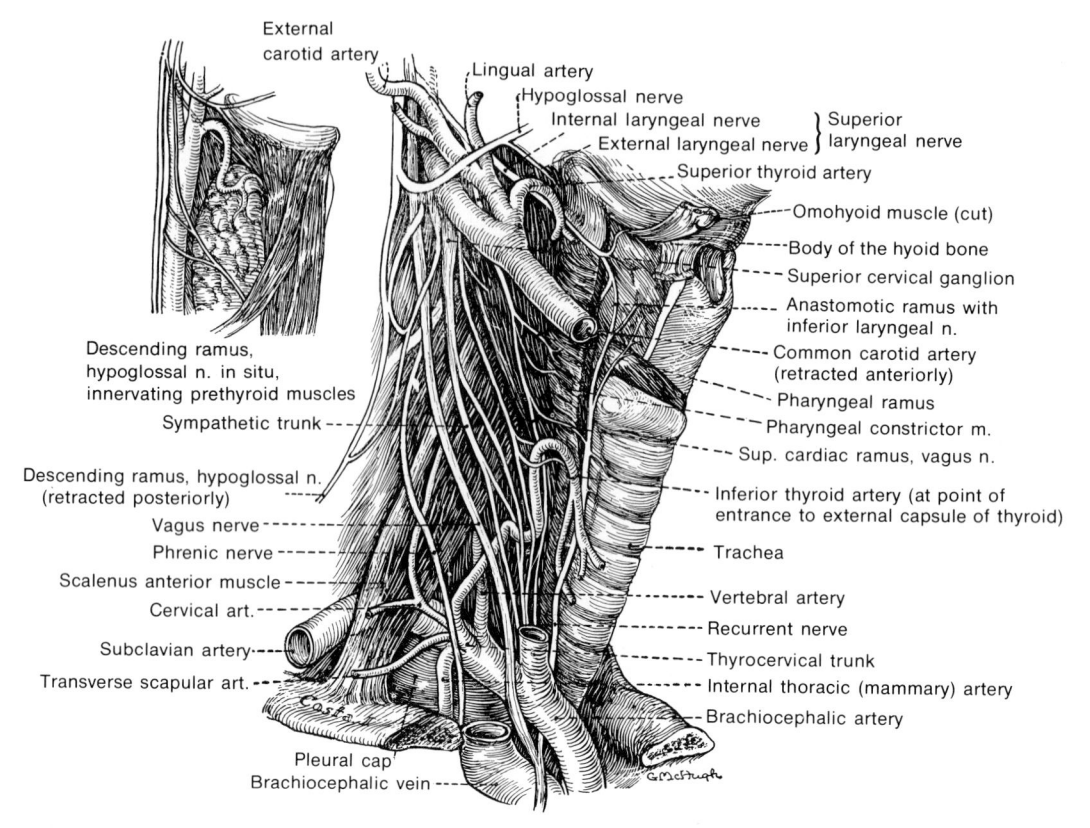

Figure 15-10. Dissection of the right side of the neck to show relations of the superior and inferior laryngeal nerves. (Nordland: Surg. Gynecol. Obstet. Vol. 51.)

ular vein. When ligating or exposing either of these vessels care must be taken to avoid injury to the vagus nerve, for its injury in the neck produces serious consequences.

In its course down the neck the vagus gives off its *superior laryngeal branch* which passes behind the carotid artery to penetrate the thyrohyoid membrane with the superior laryngeal vessels (Fig. 15-10).

The vagus nerve passes anterior to the subclavian artery on the right and to the arch of the aorta on the left to enter the thorax. At the inferior margin of these vessels the vagus gives off the inferior (recurrent) laryngeal nerve which loops around the arch of the aorta on the left or the subclavian artery on the right to ascend in a groove between the esophagus and trachea to reach the larynx (Fig. 15-11). At the thyrocricoid articulation it divides into branches that supply the main motor muscles of the larynx (Fig. 15-12). At the lower pole of the thyroid the recurrent laryngeal nerve may lie 1 to 2 cm. lateral to the trachea and is in close relation with the branches of the inferior thyroid artery. Its most intimate relations to the thyroid gland are on the posterolateral surface of the junction of the middle and upper thirds of the gland, which is also the level at which the main branches of the inferior thyroid artery enter the gland.

Injury to the superior laryngeal nerves produces a loss of sensation in the laryngeal mucous membrane and a paralysis or relaxation of the cricothyroid muscles.

Injury to the inferior (recurrent) laryngeal nerves paralyzes the vocal cords.

Injury to either of these nerves should be avoided. The inferior laryngeal nerve is in particular danger when the cervical esophagus is exposed.

The *phrenic nerve* is a branch of the cervical plexus (C3, C4, C5) (Figs. 15-13 and 15-14), which descends the neck on the anterior surface of the anterior scalenus muscle, crossing that structure obliquely downward from its lateral to its medial border. It courses lateral to the carotid sheath and enters the thorax between the subclavian artery and vein. Its injury paralyzes the ipsilateral leaf of the diaphragm and should be avoided.

The *hypoglossal* is the twelfth cranial nerve. It passes downward from the skull to course between the internal carotid artery and internal jugular vein to enter the submaxillary space betwen the hypoglossal muscle and posterior belly of the digastric muscle (Fig. 15–13), descending to the inferior margin of the latter muscle where it hooks around the occipital artery and runs through the greater portion of the suprahyoid space before entering the sublingual compartment through the cleft between the hyoglossal and mylohyoid muscles. At about the point at which the hypoglossal nerve hooks around the occipital artery, it gives off a descending branch (the *descendens hypoglossi or the upper root of the ansa cervicalis*) which runs downward and inward in front of or within the carotid sheath. At about the middle of the neck it is joined by the *lower root of the ansa cervicalis* cervical plexus to form a loop called the *ansa cervicalis*, branches of which innervate the sternohyoid, sternothyroid, and posterior belly of the omohyoid muscles.

In exposing the uppermost portion of the esophagus and pharynx, only the main hypoglossal nerve is encountered, but the descending branches and ansa cervicalis may be seen when exposing lower parts of

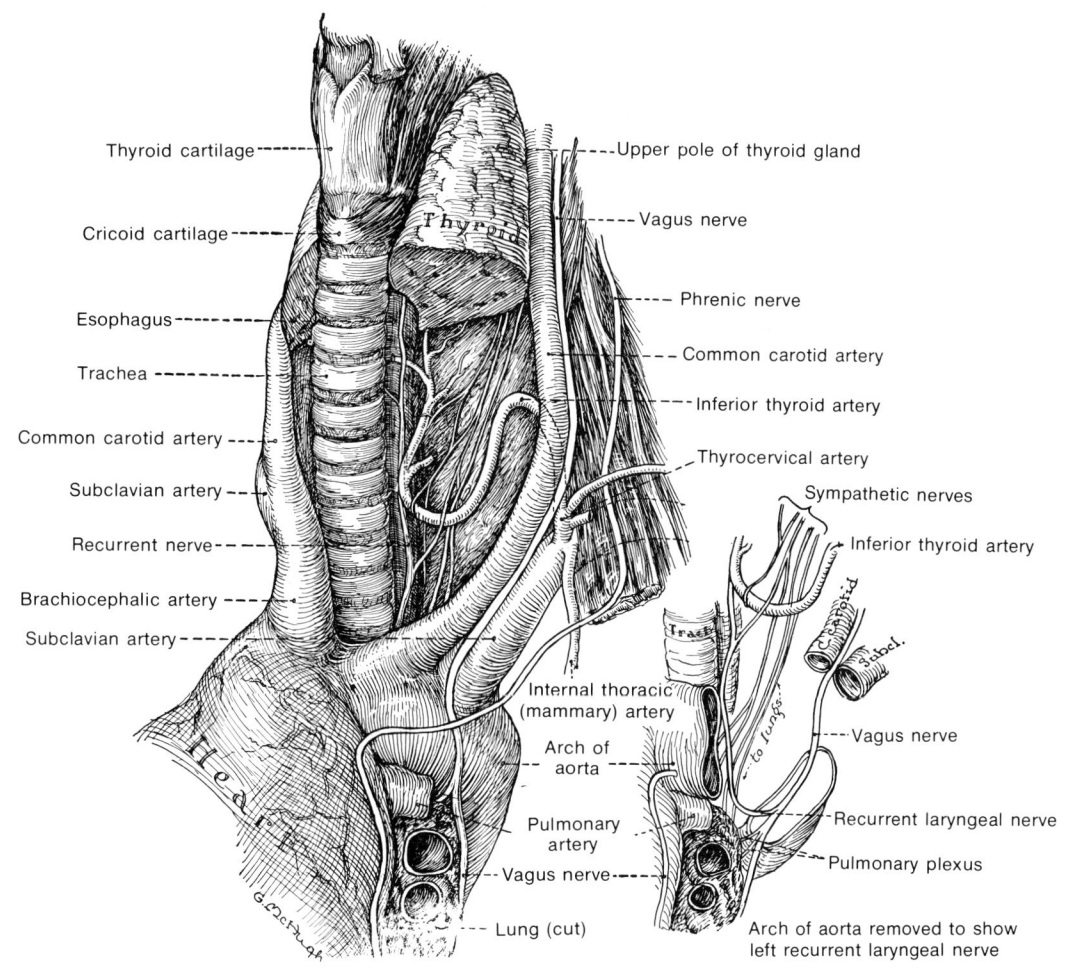

Figure 15–11. Dissection of the left side of the neck to show relations of the recurrent laryngeal nerve. (Nordland, cited in previous figure.)

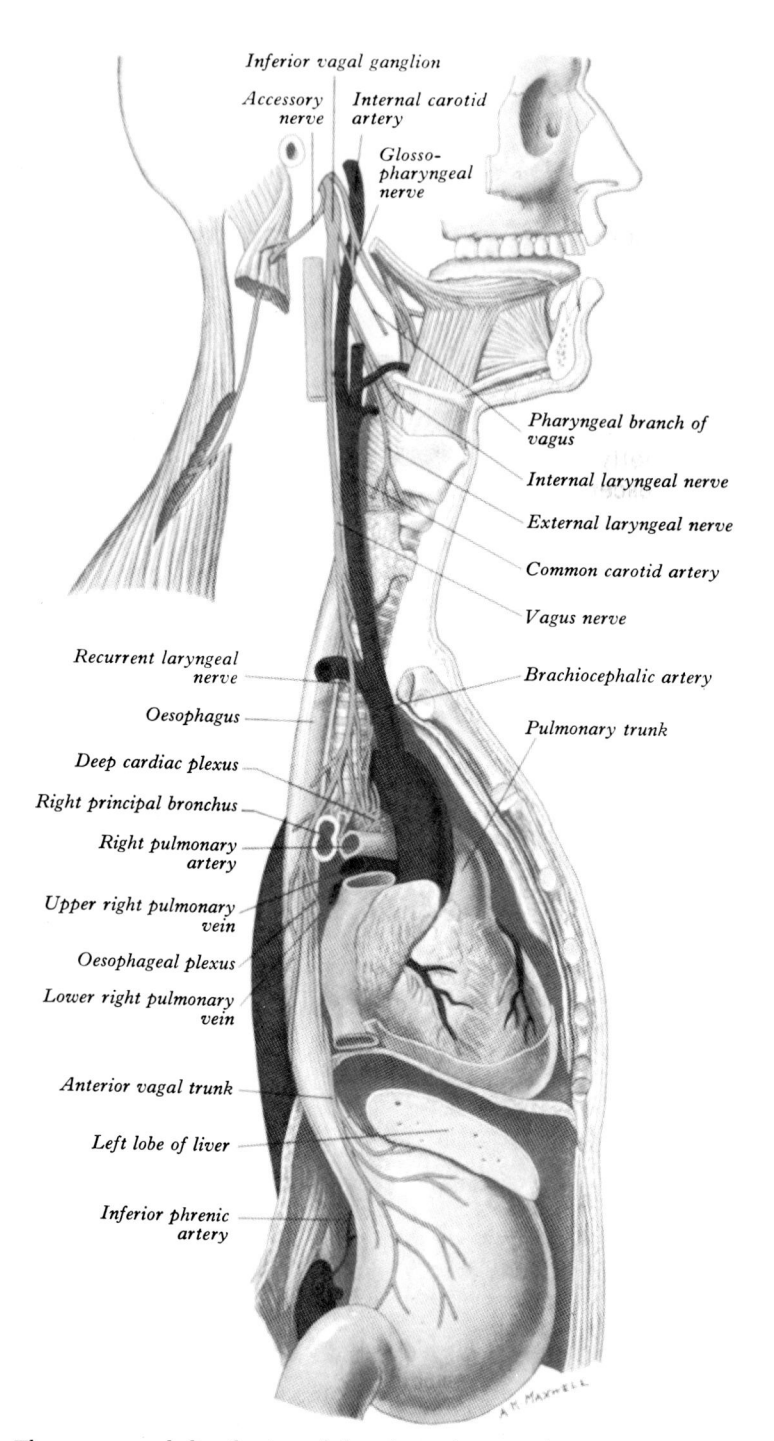

Figure 15–12. The course and distribution of the glossopharyngeal, vagus, and accessory nerves. (From Williams, P. L., and Warwick, R. (eds.): Gray's Anatomy, 36th Br. ed. Philadelphia, W. B. Saunders Company, 1980.)

EXPOSURE OF THE CERVICAL ALIMENTARY TRACT

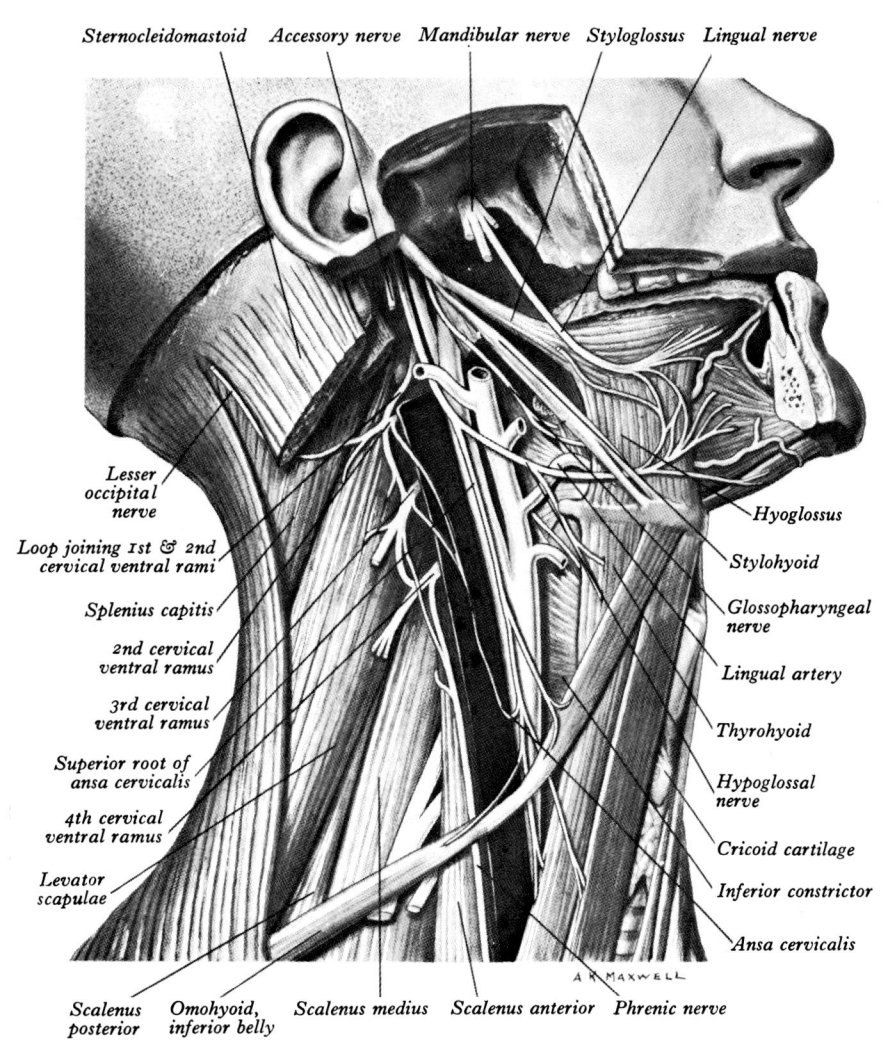

Figure 15–13. A dissection to show the general distribution of the right hypoglossal and lingual nerves, and the position, constitution, and some of the cervical plexus of the right side. (From Williams and Warwick, cited in previous figure.)

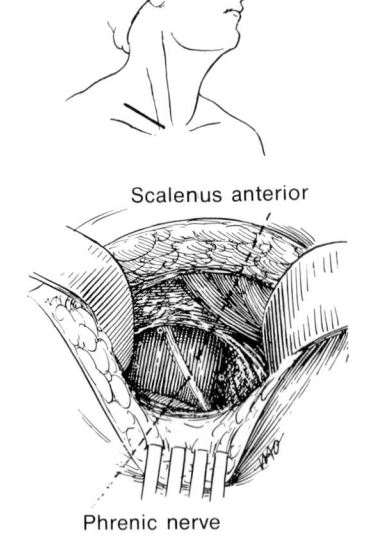

Figure 15-14. Surgical approach to the phrenic nerve through a supraclavicular incision.

the cervical esophagus. They should be preserved when possible, but the ansa cervicalis frequently must be divided to increase the exposure. Its division apparently causes no serious harm.

The *spinal accessory* is the eleventh cranial nerve. It emerges from the skull and descends between the internal carotid artery and the internal jugular vein to about the angle of the mandible where it passes backward, either anterior or posterior to the jugular vein, to enter the deep surface of the sternocleidomastoid muscle. It enters the substance of this muscle near the junction of the middle and upper thirds of the muscle, which is about 4 cm. inferior to the tip of the mastoid. It crosses obliquely downward, laterally and posteriorly through this muscle, emerging near the middle of its posterior border, to continue its course across the posterior triangle to the trapezius muscle (see Fig. 15-18). The deep guides to the nerve are the posterior belly of the digastric muscle and the internal jugular vein, both of which the nerve crosses obliquely downward, laterally and backward.

The spinal accessory nerve is seldom encountered in exposures of the esophagus but might be injured if the sternocleidomastoid muscle is transected at a high level. Its injury should be avoided.

The *cervical sympathetic ganglion chain* lies on the prevertebral fascia, just mesial to the tuberosities of the cervical transverse processes, and is held in place by fibers from the underlying fascia. It lies beneath the carotid sheath and is not disturbed while exposing the cervical esophagus.

The plexus of *cervical nerves* passes laterally from the vertebral column deep to the scalenus anterior muscle. This protects the cervical nerves from injury during operations on the cervical esophagus (Fig. 15-15).

APPROACHES TO THE CERVICAL ESOPHAGUS

The cervical esophagus may be approached by one of three different routes:

1. An anterior approach, splitting the neck muscles in the anterior midline, retracting the sternothyroid and other muscles laterally while slipping a finger down along the side of the trachea to the esophagus (Fig. 15-16). This route does not afford a good exposure and endangers the recurrent laryngeal nerve. The skin incision can be a transverse collar type or the oblique incision used for the other routes.

2. An anterolateral approach by retracting the sternocleidomastoid and omohyoid muscles and the carotid sheath laterally while the sternothyroid muscle and thyroid gland are displaced medially. This route provides a good exposure, can be followed with relative safety and is the one of choice for approaching this portion of the esophagus (Fig. 15-16).

3. A retrosternocleidomastoid approach by retracting the sternocleidomastoid muscle and carotid sheath forward so as to pass behind them to the esophagus. This route is longer than the anterolateral one but can provide a good exposure. When this route is contemplated, the oblique incision should be made along the middle or posterior margin of the sternocleidomastoid muscle instead of along its anterior margin (Fig. 15-16).

The cervical esophagus is usually and most easily approached from the left side unless the lesion presents on the right side, in which case the incision which is to be described is made on the right by an identical technic.

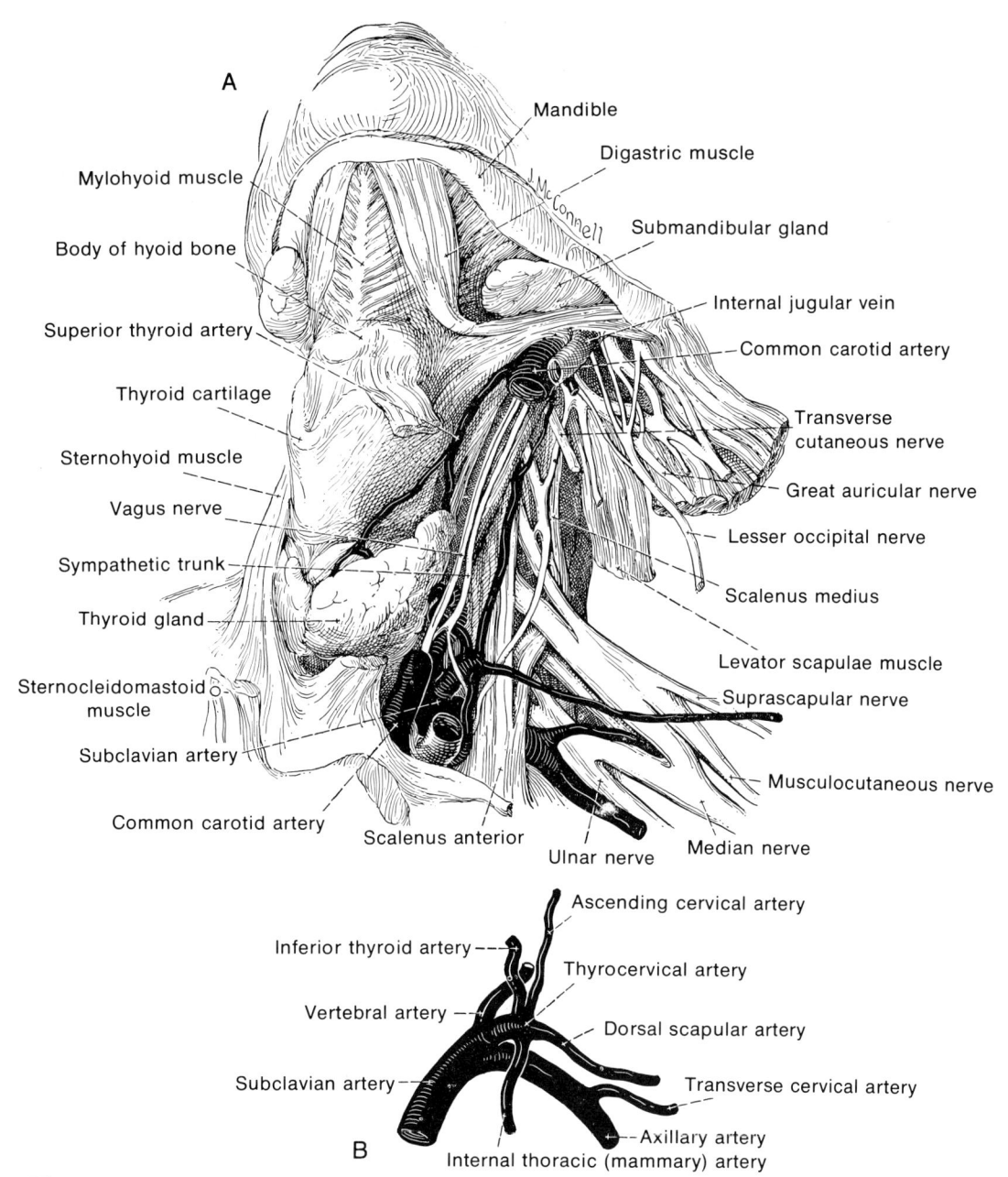

Figure 15–15. *A*, Structures in the deep portion of the neck; anterolateral view. The sternocleidomastoid and the infrahyoid muscles have been partially removed, together with the clavicle and the subclavius muscle; the carotid artery and jugular vein remain as proximal and distal segments. The following structures are exposed: branches of the common carotid artery and subclavian artery; the constituents of the cervical and brachial plexuses of nerves; the middle and anterior scalenus muscles; the vagus nerve and spinal accessory nerve; the thyroid gland and its arteries of supply. In this specimen the cervical rami contributory to the trunks of the brachial plexus passed through a cleft in the scalenus anterior muscle, not between the latter and the middle scalenus. *B*, The left subclavian artery and its branches.

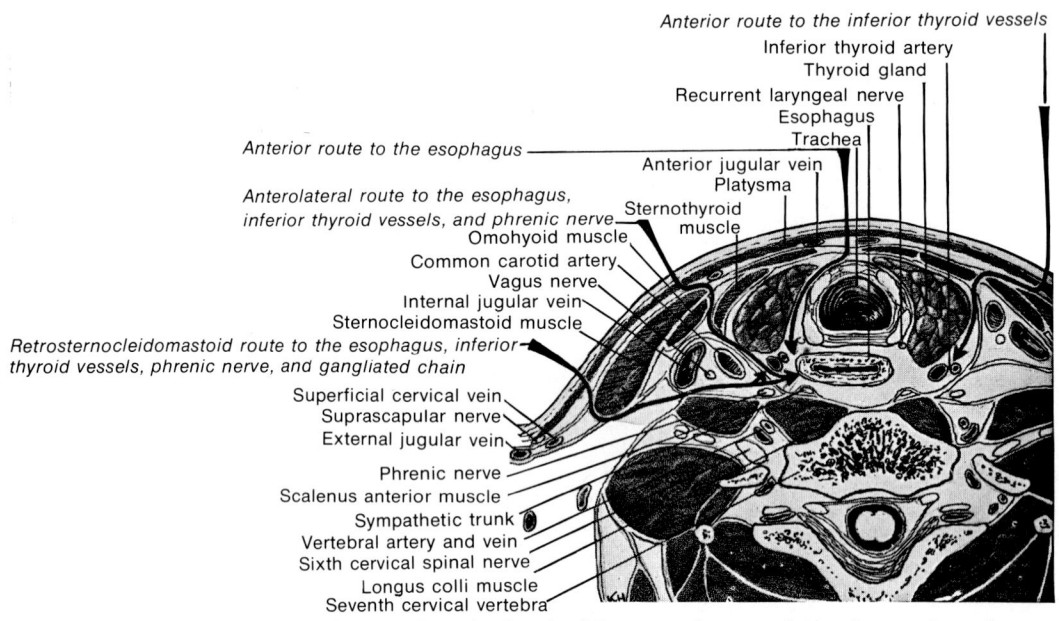

Figure 15–16. Cross section of the neck at the level of the seventh cervical vertebra to show the cervical approaches to the esophagus, inferior thyroid artery, phrenic nerve, and sympathetic gangliated chain.

TECHNIC OF ANTEROLATERAL APPROACH (LEFT SIDE)

The patient is placed supine on the operating table with the head turned away from the side to be incised. The anterior margin of the left sternocleidomastoid muscle can be seen as a surface landmark passing obliquely down the neck. An incision is made over the anterior margin of the sternocleidomastoid muscle from the level of the angle of the mandible obliquely down-

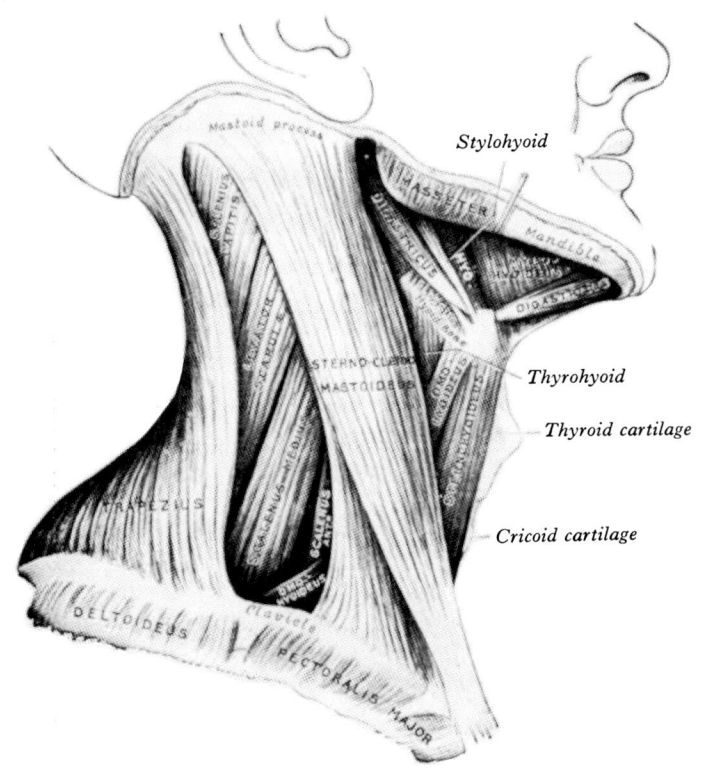

Figure 15–17. Muscles of the neck. Right lateral aspect. (From Warwick, R., and Williams, P. L. (eds.): Gray's Anatomy, 36th Br. ed. Philadelphia, W. B. Saunders Company, 1980.)

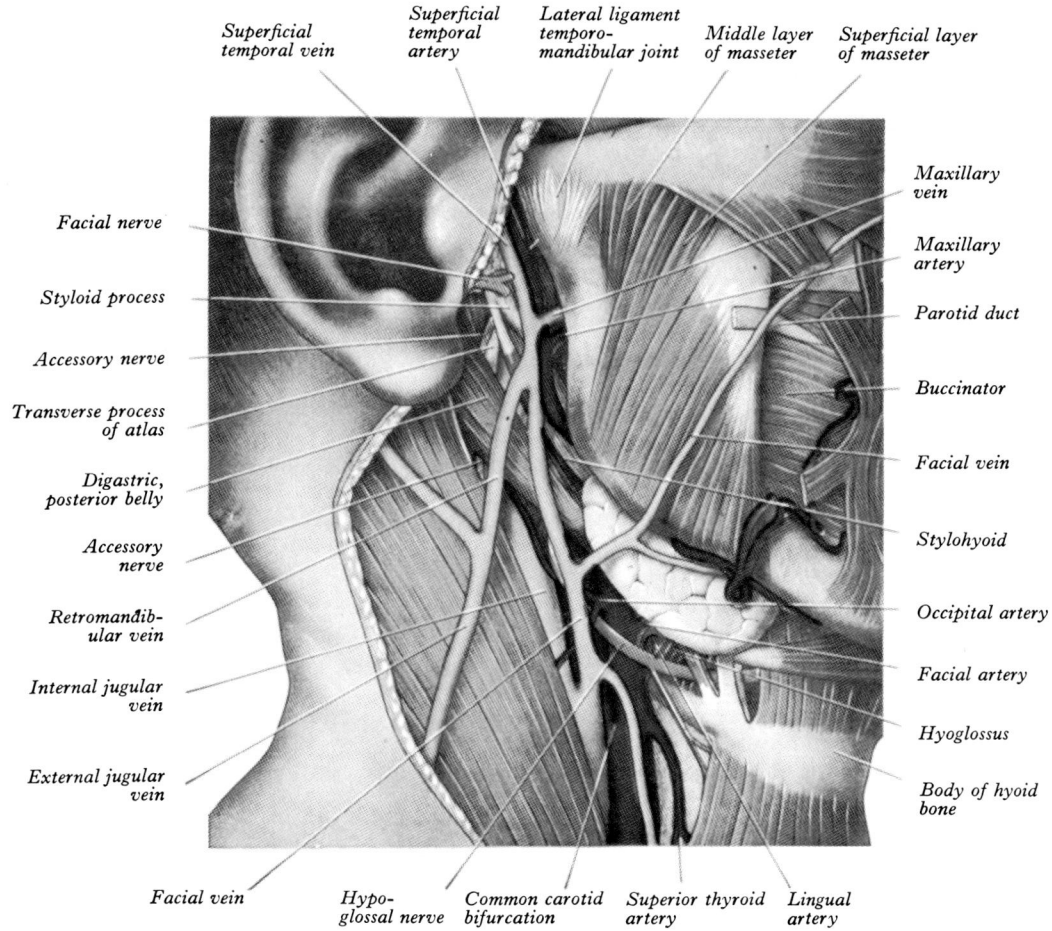

Figure 15–18. Relations of the posterior belly of the digastric, exposed by the removal of skin, fasciae, parotid gland, and cutaneous branches of the cervical plexus. (From Williams and Warwick, cited in previous figure.)

ward and medially to the sternal notch (Fig. 15–17). This incision is deepened through the skin, fat, and platysma muscle, the edges of which are retracted to expose the anterior margin of the sternocleidomastoid muscle. The investing layer of the deep cervical fascia is opened along the anterior margin of this muscle (see Fig. 15–1) and the muscle is retracted posterolaterally, exposing the sternohyoid and sternothyroid muscles overlying the lobe of the thyroid gland. The superior belly of the omohyoid muscle, the superior thyroid vessels, the carotid sheath, and the ansa cervicalis are also seen (see Figs. 15–2, 15–13, and 15–18). The omohyoid muscle can usually be retracted downward and medially a sufficient amount without division, but if its integrity limits the exposure it can be divided without subsequent ill effects. Likewise, the superior thyroid vessels can be divided and the ansa cervicalis can be cut at the apex of its loop if additional exposure is desired.

The carotid sheath is freed, and the lateral margin of the left lobe of the thyroid gland is exposed by dividing the sternothyroid musculofascial layer. This permits the carotid sheath and its contents to be retracted laterally with the sternocleidomastoid muscle while the left lobe of the thyroid, the larynx, and trachea with their overlying muscles and fascia are retracted medially.

The loose areolar tissue between the thyroid and carotid sheath is then opened by blunt dissection, exposing the left inferior thyroid vessels. These may be divided if they interfere with a satisfactory expo-

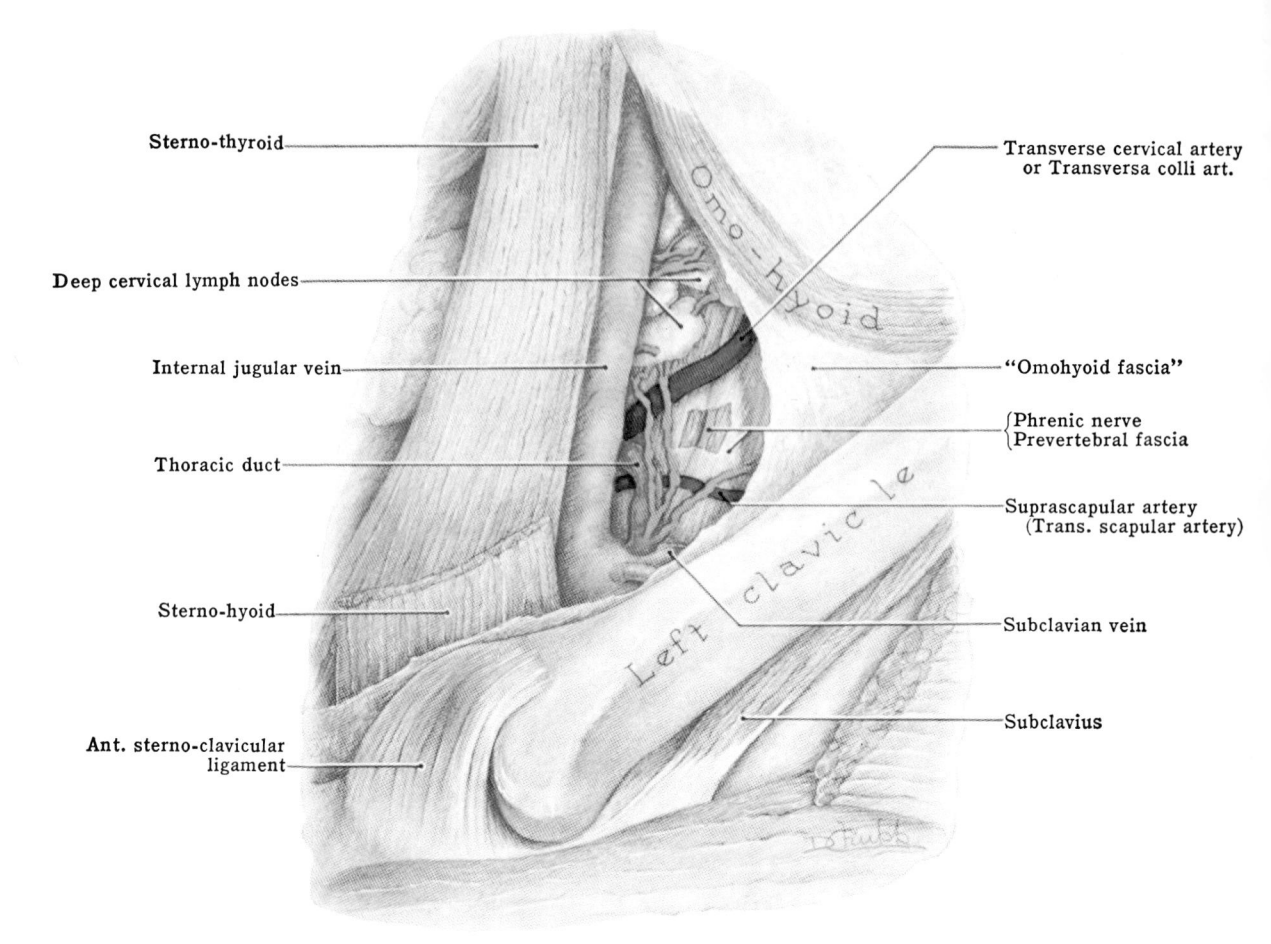

Figure 15-19. Left side of neck. (From Boileau Grant, J. C.: An Atlas of Anatomy. 5th ed. Baltimore, Williams & Wilkins, 1962.)

sure, care being taken while doing so to avoid injury to the recurrent laryngeal nerve.

The anterolateral wall of the esophagus can now be seen, and by blunt dissection the retropharyngeal space (Fig. 15-19) can be entered to mobilize the esophagus to a limited extent.

After the operation has been completed, the retractors are removed and the retracted structures are allowed to fall back into their normal position. If the esophagus has been opened during the operation, a drain is placed down to that area. The cervical fascia is approximated loosely with a few interrupted sutures. The cut edges of the platysma are approximated with interrupted sutures.

The skin incision is closed with interrupted sutures of 4-0 silk, nylon, or stainless steel staples.

COMMENTS. This incision is employed for removing diverticula, benign tumors, and foreign bodies in the cervical esophagus. It is also used for cervical esophagostomy or esophagotomy, and for draining periesophageal abscesses in this area. It is not used for resections of this portion of the esophagus for malignant lesions as such procedures require special incisions which are described with the specific operative procedures.

Chapter 16

EXPOSURE OF THE THORACIC ALIMENTARY TRACT

The esophagus continues downward from the neck to enter the posterior mediastinum of the thoracic cavity wherein it is called the thoracic portion of the esophagus. It is the only portion of the alimentary tract that is normally situated within the thorax. The anatomy of the esophagus is described in Volume 1 (pp. 6–22), but it is necessary to have some understanding of the anatomy of the thorax when discussing the incisions used for an approach to this part of the alimentary tract.

Anatomy

The *thorax* is that portion of the body that lies between the neck and the abdomen. It consists of a bony cage which is covered by important muscles beneath an integument. It contains the principal organs of respiration and circulation, nerves, blood vessels, and the thoracic portion of the esophagus. The entire interior of the thorax is accessible to some route of surgical approach.

The bony cage of the thorax is formed by the sternum, ribs, and vertebrae.

The thorax is shaped like a truncated cone, with its smaller base (superior) at the inlet and its larger (inferior) at the diaphragm (Figs. 16–1 and 16–2).

For convenience of description the surface of the thorax is arbitrarily marked by longitudinal lines which parallel the long axis of the body. The *midsternal line* is the anterior midline of the thorax and bisects the sternum. The *midclavicular (mammary) line* (one on each side) runs vertically downward from the midpoint of the clavicle. It usually passes somewhat mesial to the nipple. The *parasternal line* (a right and a left) parallels and lies midway between the midclavicular and midsternal lines.

The *anterior, posterior and midaxillary lines* (right and left) run vertically downward from the anterior and posterior axillary folds and from the middle of the axillary space.

The surface area of the thorax is also arbitrarily divided into regions, which are named according to their relation to its various components (Figs. 16–1 and 16–2).

THORACIC WALLS

The *sternal region* occupies the median anterior portion of the thoracic wall and consists of the sternum with its three segments and its clavicular and chondral attachments (Fig. 16–1). The three segments of the sternum are, from above downward, the manubrium, the body (gladiolus), and the xiphoid (ensiform) process. The sternal region is bounded superiorly by the suprasternal notch, inferiorly by the tip of the xiphoid, and laterally by the sternoclavicular and sternocostal joints. The superior margin of the sternum lies in the same

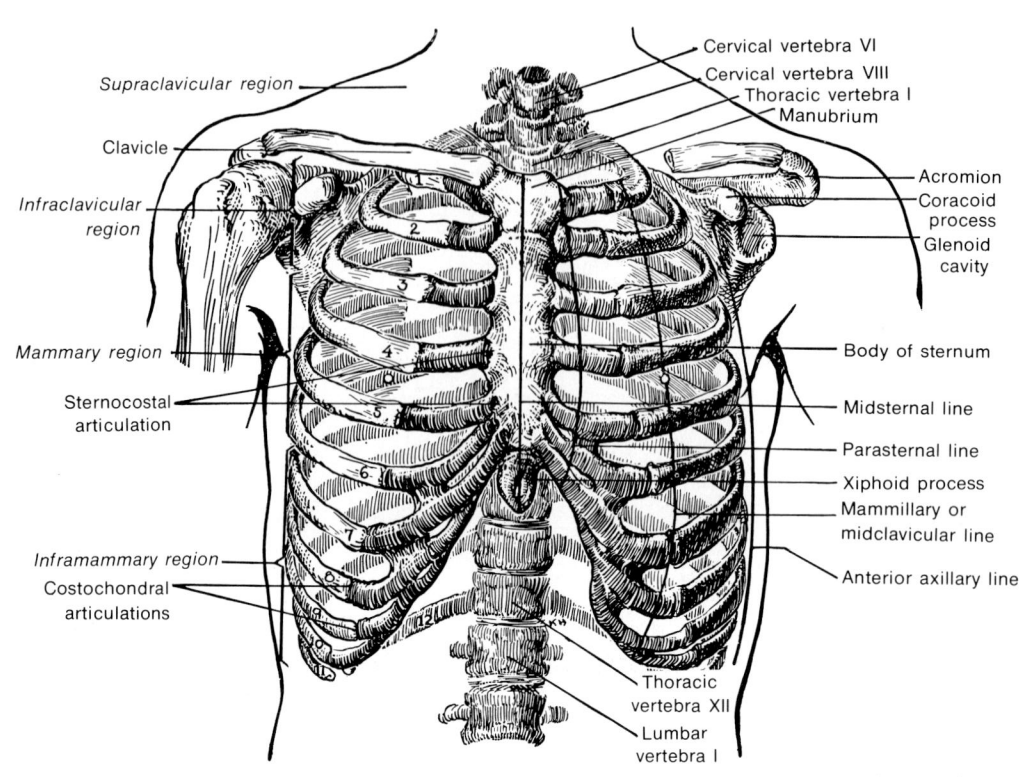

Figure 16–1. Anterior view of the bony thorax to show regions, landmarks, and surface markings.

horizontal plane as the inferior border of the body of the second thoracic vertebra; the distance between them is about 5 cm. This distance is the anteroposterior diameter of the inlet of the thorax.

At the junction of the manubrium and body of the sternum there is an anterior prominence which can usually be seen and palpated. It is named the sternal angle or the angle of Ludwig or the angle of Louis and serves as a helpful surface landmark. It lies in the same horizontal plane as the body of the fifth thoracic vertebra and also marks the junction of the sternum and the second ribs. The xiphisternal junction lies in the same horizontal plane as the cartilage between the ninth and tenth thoracic vertebrae.

The sternum articulates laterally on each side with the clavicle and with the superior seven costal cartilages at the sternoclavicular and sternocostal joints, which are reinforced by ligaments. These joints permit free movement of the clavicles on the sternum and more restricted motion between the ribs and the sternum.

The sternum is superficially situated, being covered only by the skin, subcutaneous tissue, and a thin musculotendinous layer derived from the origins of both major pectoral muscles superiorly, and of both rectus abdominis muscles inferiorly.

The *costal region* of the chest wall is that part which lies between the sternum and the vertebral column and extends in depth to the parietal pleura. This area contains the ribs and a portion of the shoulder girdle, with their attached muscles, as well as the breast.

The *ribs* are paired and are twelve in number. The upper seven ribs are *true* or *sternal* ribs in that they articulate directly with the sternum. The lower five ribs are *false*, having no direct attachment to the sternum. The upper three false ribs (eighth, ninth, and tenth) are connected with the sternum through the intermedium of the cartilage of the seventh rib. The eleventh and twelfth ribs have neither a direct nor indirect attachment to the sternum and are called *floating ribs.*

The body of the first rib (occasionally the second rib also) is shaped so that its superior and inferior surfaces are flat. In the

EXPOSURE OF THE THORACIC ALIMENTARY TRACT

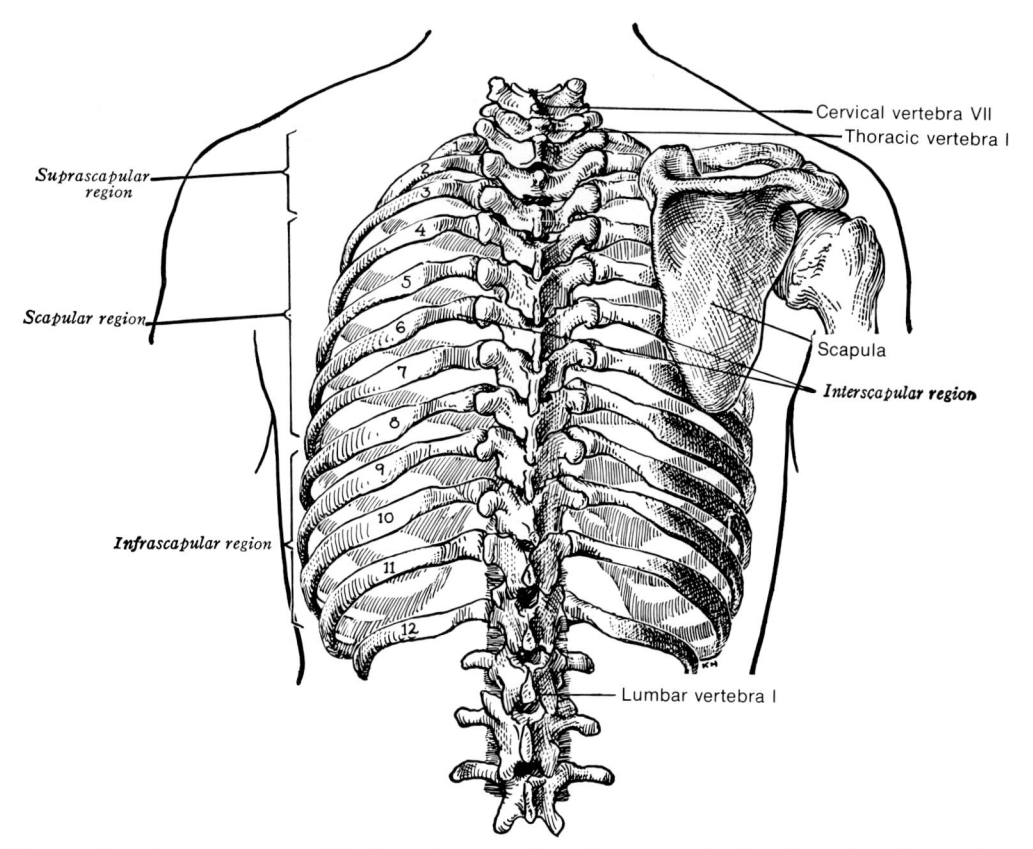

Figure 16-2. Posterior view of the bony thorax to show the regions, landmarks, and surface markings.

middle portion of the superior surface are two transverse grooves — a posterior groove through which the subclavian artery runs, and another groove just anterior to it through which the subclavian vein runs. Between these two grooves lies the scalene tubercle to which the scalenus anterior muscle is attached. The remaining ribs are shaped so that their flat surfaces present laterally, with their narrow edges presenting superiorly and inferiorly.

Identification of the ribs prior to or during an operation is important for the accurate placing of an incision. This is done by counting the ribs from some known point. Before the skin incision is made it can be accomplished posterolaterally by counting upward from the palpable lower edge of the twelfth rib, or if the arm is not abducted, by identifying the seventh rib which usually lies beneath the tip of the scapula (inferior angle) (Fig. 16-3). However, the latter method is unreliable because the scapula changes position with movements of the shoulder girdle.

Anterolaterally the ribs can be identified by counting down from the second rib which lies at the level of the angle of Louis (Fig. 16-4).

After an incision has been made and the latissimus dorsi muscle has been severed, the ribs can be identified by thrusting a hand beneath the scapula to palpate the first rib and counting down. The attachment of the scalenus anterior muscle to the first rib will prevent the finger from hooking over the superior surface of this rib and make its identification less certain than desired. When in doubt or if identification is important, a metal clip can be placed on a rib and a roentgenogram made with a portable x-ray machine, following which it and the other ribs can be enumerated.

When within the thoracic cavity the unique shape of the first rib can be easily identified by palpation and then the other ribs enumerated downward therefrom.

Each rib has an enlargement at its posterior end called the *head*, which contains facets that articulate with the body of the

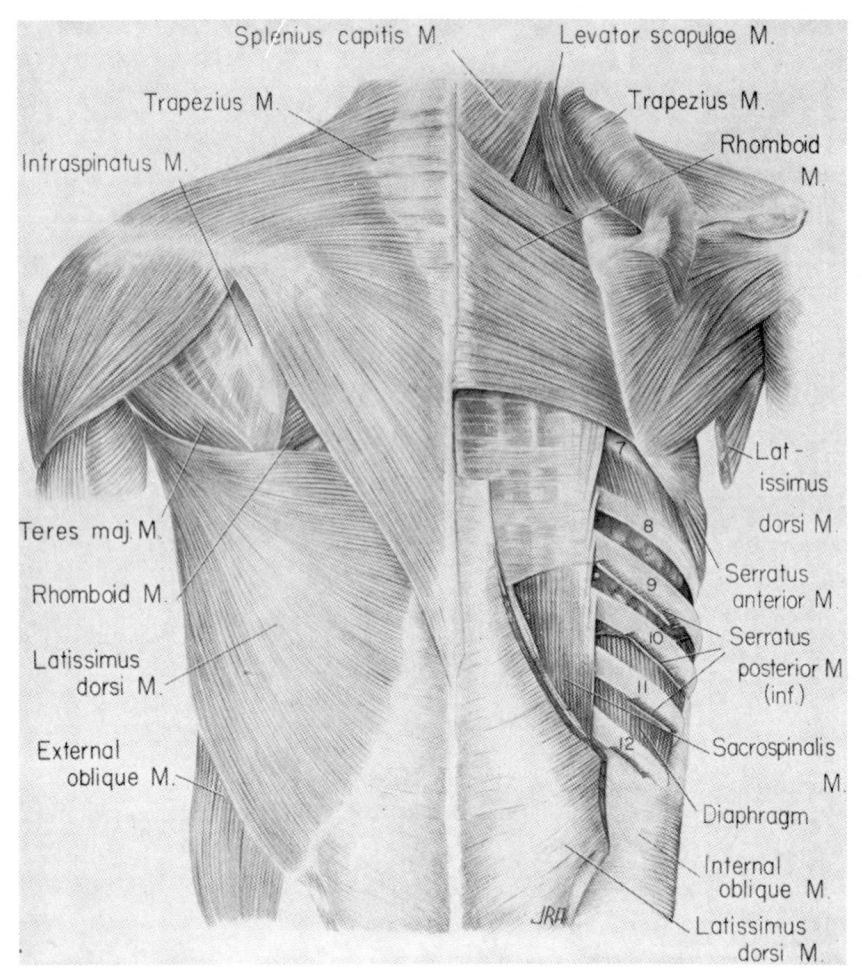

Figure 16-3. Posterior view of the thorax and contiguous portions of the neck and abdominal wall. The left half illustrates the superficial muscles. The right half illustrates the deeper muscles and topographic relations of the lung and diaphragm. (From Sweet, R. H.: Thoracic Surgery, ed. 2. Philadelphia, W. B. Saunders Company, 1954, p. 71.)

vertebra. Just anterior to the head is the short *rib neck*, and just anterior to it is a *tubercle* on the posterior surface of the rib containing a facet that faces backward and downward to rest on the transverse process of the vertebra. Thus it can be seen that there are two articulations between the rib and the vertebrae. From the tubercle the *shaft (body)* of the rib continues laterally to its *angle* (the first rib has no angle) where it changes direction to run obliquely downward and forward. Before terminating anteriorly the bony shaft of the rib is continued by a costal cartilage to articulate with the sternum in the case of the upper seven ribs, or with the seventh costal cartilage in the case of the eighth, ninth, and tenth ribs or to terminate as a free end in the case of the eleventh and twelfth ribs. The costal cartilages grow progressively longer from the first to the seventh, while the eleventh and twelfth are short and pointed.

Costal cartilages are more flexible than the bony parts of the rib and are of soft enough consistency to be easily cut through with an ordinary scalpel. These two characteristics have surgical significance. Since the costal cartilage is more flexible than the bony posterior portion of the rib, greater exposure can be obtained with less risk of fracturing a rib by transecting with a bone-cutter the posterior portion of the ribs just above and just below a thoracotomy incision. The ribs can then be spread more widely apart. Also, when desired to extend a thoracic incision into the abdomen or vice versa, the costal arch can be cut across without the necessity of special bone-cutting instruments.

The bony part of the rib is tightly en-

EXPOSURE OF THE THORACIC ALIMENTARY TRACT

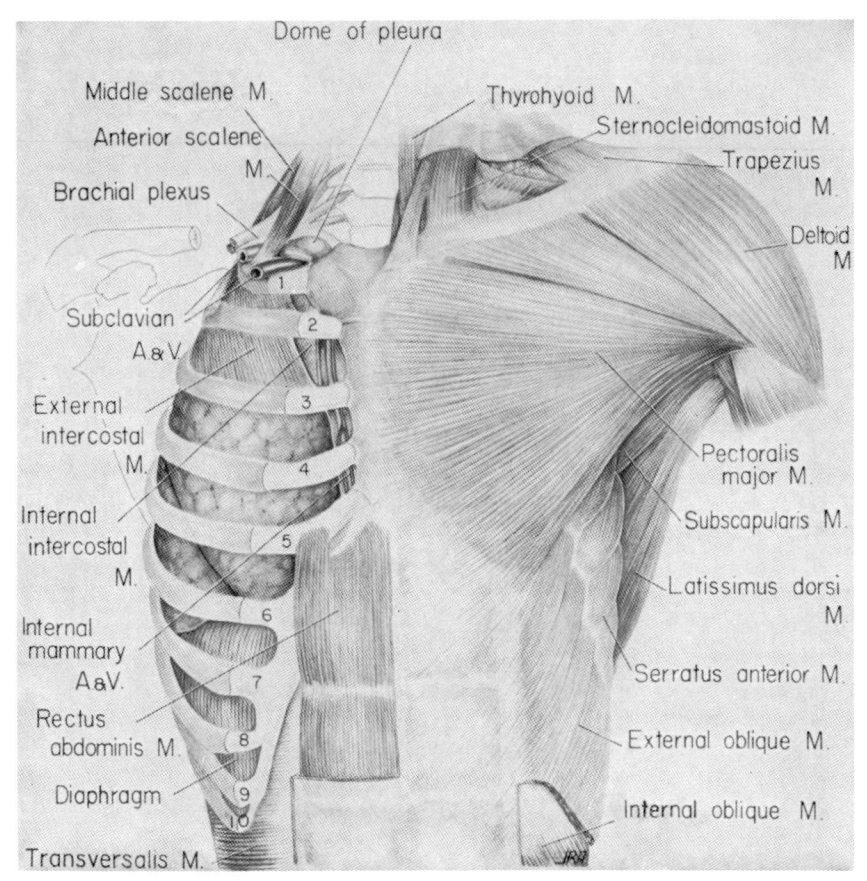

Figure 16-4. Anterior view of the thorax and contiguous portions of the base of the neck and the anterior abdominal wall. The left half illustrates the superficial layer of muscles and fascia. The right half illustrates the relations of the deep muscles of the neck and abdomen to the rib cage; the intercostal muscles; the diaphragm; the internal mammary vessels; the relations of the muscles, nerves and vessels with the first rib; and the anterior relations of the lung. (From Sweet, cited in previous figure.)

cased in a fibrous *sheath* called the periosteum, which is continuous with the fibrous sheath that envelops the costal cartilage, known as the perichondrium. It is from this sheath that new cartilage and new bone are derived to replace a rib that has been removed or to repair one that has been fractured. The periosteum and perichondrium can be incised and easily stripped off the rib to be left in place when a part or all of the rib is removed (subperiosteal rib resection) or its posterior surface can be separated from the underlying parietal pleura so that it can be removed with the rib. In the former case, a new rib will be formed by the remaining periosteum. In the latter, a new rib will not be formed.

Ribs lose their elasticity and strength with age. Therefore, although intercostal thoracotomies are often satisfactory in young adults and preferable in children, they are less satisfactory than a rib resection type of thoracotomy in older patients.

The *intercostal spaces* between the ribs average about 2 cm. in width. They are wider anteriorly than posteriorly and are broader between the upper ribs than between the lower ones. Their width is modified in movements of flexion and extension. They are occupied by two layers of intercostal muscle with their fascial investments, and the intercostal nerve, artery, and vein (Fig. 16-5).

BLOOD VESSELS AND NERVES

The thoracic wall contains no arteries of major size. The principal ones are the intercostal and internal thoracic (mammary) arteries.

The first two or three pairs of *intercos-*

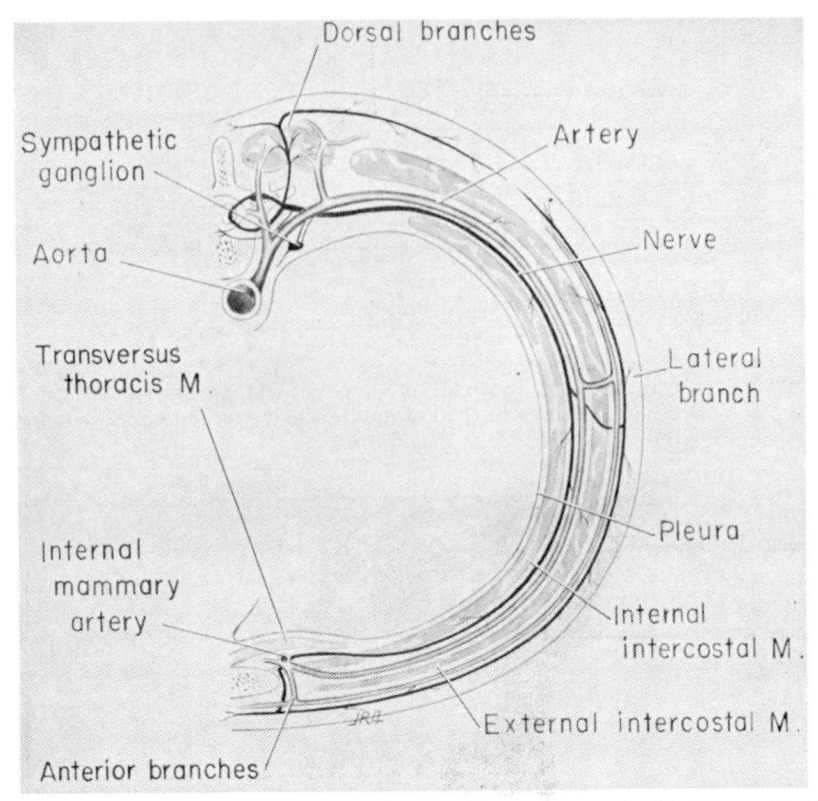

Figure 16–5. Diagram of an intercostal space. (From Sweet, cited in Figure 16–3.)

tal arteries arise from the superior intercostal branch of the costocervical trunk from the ipsilateral subclavian artery; the inferior nine pairs arise directly from the aorta. The intercostal arteries course from their origin through the corresponding intercostal space, passing along the subcostal groove (along with the intercostal vein and nerve), which runs along the entire length of the inner surface of the inferior margin of its corresponding rib, except posterior to the rib angle where the nerve, artery, and vein traverse the middle of the intercostal space (Fig. 16–6). Anteriorly they anastomose directly with the internal thoracic (mammary) artery. Small anastomotic branches cross the intercostal spaces to connect intercostal arteries with the one immediately above and below (Fig. 16–7). From their origin at the aorta the intercostal arteries pass between the pleura and the external intercostal muscle as far as the angle of the ribs where they continue between the internal and external intercostal muscles to the parasternal line. Here they penetrate the internal intercostal muscle to communicate with the internal thoracic artery. The intercostal veins accompany the arteries to empty into the azygos and hemiazygos veins posteriorly and the internal thoracic vein anteriorly.

The intercostal vessels are capable of serious and persistent hemorrhage. When injured or transected, both cut ends should be securely ligated. They are most frequently injured in the course of freeing the inferior margin of a rib, or when a rib is fractured. The location of these vessels along the inferior margin of a rib explains the desirability of proceeding along the superior margin of a rib in aspiration of pleural exudates and in performing an intercostal type of thoracotomy.

The *internal thoracic artery* (one on each side) arises from the inferior surface of the ipsilateral subclavian artery opposite the origin of the thyrocervical trunk. It passes inferiorly, anteriorly and mesially on the parietal pleura. It lies behind the sternal end of the clavicle and descends into the chest deep to the lateral margin of the sternum, parallel to and about 1.25 cm. from it. At the level of the sixth intercostal space the internal thoracic (mammary) artery divides into a lateral branch, the muscu-

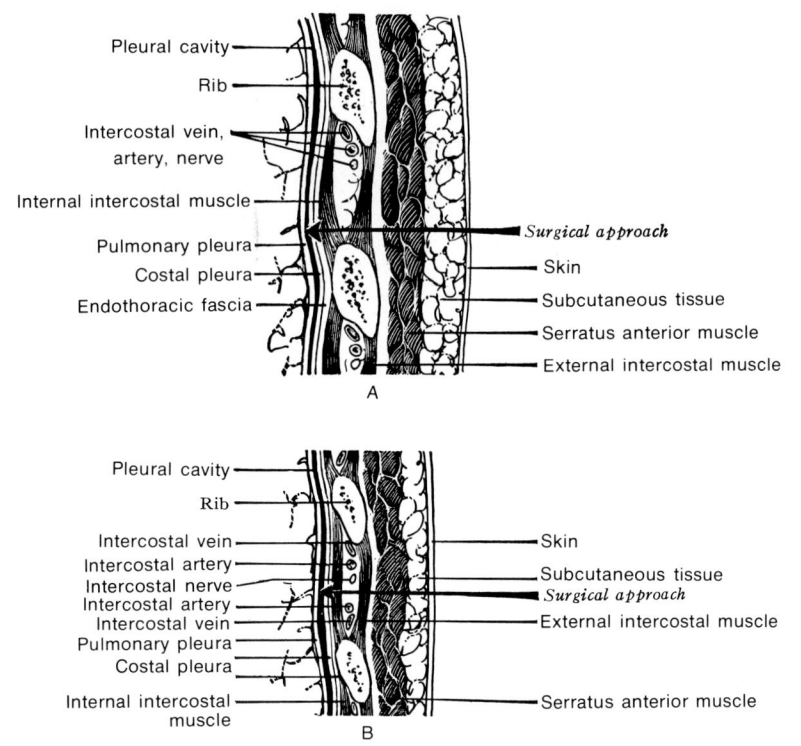

Figure 16-6. Vertical sections through the ribs and intercostal spaces. *A*, Posterior to axilla; *B*, anterior to axilla. To show the differences in the location of the intercostal vessels and nerves and the importance of these relations in intercostal thoracotomy.

lophrenic, which passes to the diaphragm, and a medial terminal branch, which continues downward on the abdomen where it is called the superior epigastric artery. The *internal thoracic (mammary) vein*, which empties into the ipsilateral brachiocephalic (innominate) vein, accompanies its artery.

The internal thoracic (mammary) vessels are capable of severe hemorrhage when injured, in which case both cut ends should be ligated. This can be done fairly easily in the relatively wide upper three intercostal spaces but is more difficult to accomplish in the narrower fourth or fifth intercostal space. Their injury should be avoided while making the anterior portion of a long thoracotomy incision.

The *intercostal nerves* provide the

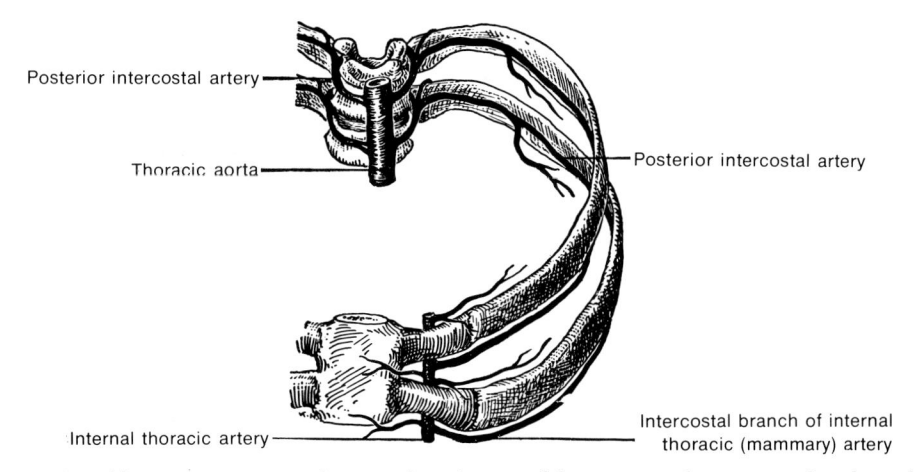

Figure 16-7. Oblique cross section showing the relations of the intercostal arteries to the ribs and intercostal spaces. Posterior to the axilla, the arteries are protected; anterior to the axilla, they are more exposed.

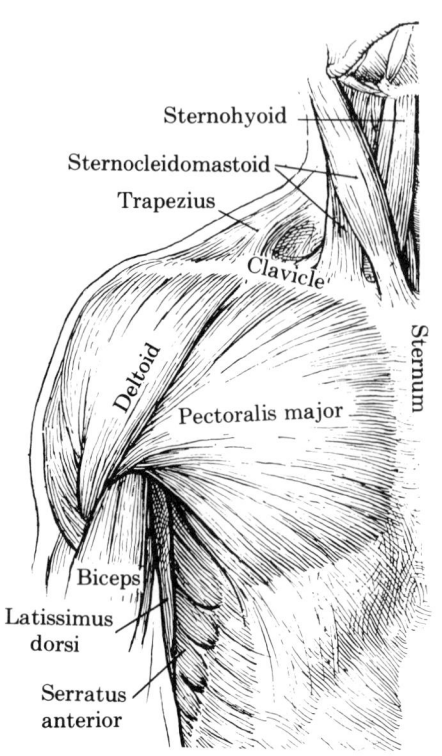

Figure 16–8. Muscles of the trunk, anterior view. (From Dorland's Illustrated Medical Dictionary. Philadelphia, W. B. Saunders Company, 1974. Jones and Shepard.)

The *pectoralis major* is a fan-shaped muscle which arises from the inner half of the anterior border of the clavicle, from the anterior surface of the sternum and the upper six costal cartilages, and from the upper part of the anterior sheath of the rectus abdominis (Fig. 16–8). Its fibers run transversely, converging toward the proximal extremity of the arm where they insert into the lateral lip of the intertubercular sulcus of the humerus. Its inferior border is free. This muscle forms the anterior wall and fold of the axilla. The pectoralis major muscle is encountered and partly severed when a long thoracotomy incision is made at or above the level of the fifth rib; the higher the incision, the more of its fibers must be divided. The amount of this muscle requiring division can be minimized by using a curved submammary incision and retracting the pectoralis major upward and medially.

The *pectoralis minor* is a thin triangular muscle at the superior portion of the

main innervation to the muscles of the chest and abdominal walls. These nerves arise from the spinal cord and enter the intercostal spaces to accompany the intercostal vessels between the external and deep intercostal muscles.

In their course the nerves lie inferior to the vessels and at a greater distance from the rib next above. The lower intercostal nerves pass beneath the costal arch to the abdomen where they innervate the musculature of the abdominal wall. They anastomose with each other frequently both in the intercostal space and on the abdominal wall. When deliberating the severance of an intercostal nerve, one should consider its effect on the abdominal musculature. The severance of one or two intercostal nerves will have no deleterious effect, but division of three or more will produce some degree of paralysis of the muscles they innervate.

MUSCLES AND MAMMARY GLAND

The costal region of the thoracic wall is covered by a considerable *extrinsic musculature*.

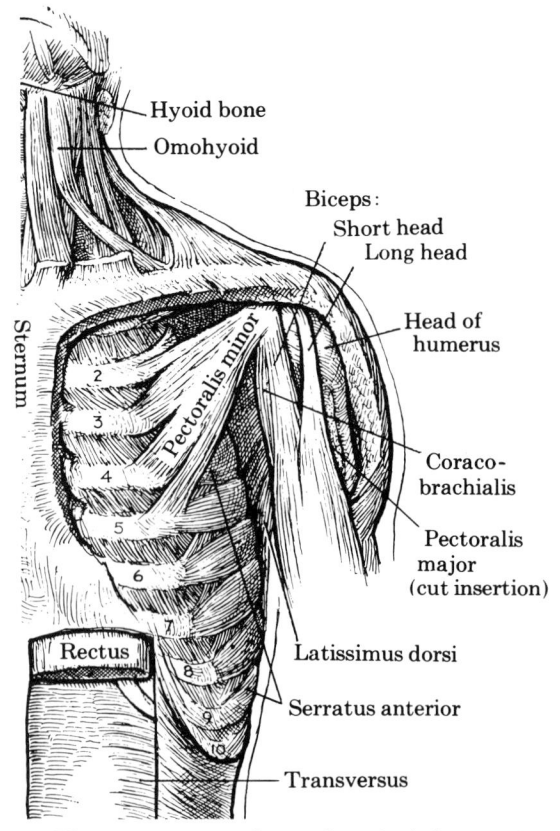

Figure 16–9. Trunk muscles. The left sternocleidomastoid, pectoralis major, external oblique, and a portion of the deltoid have been removed to show underlying muscles. (From Dorland's, cited in previous figure.)

EXPOSURE OF THE THORACIC ALIMENTARY TRACT

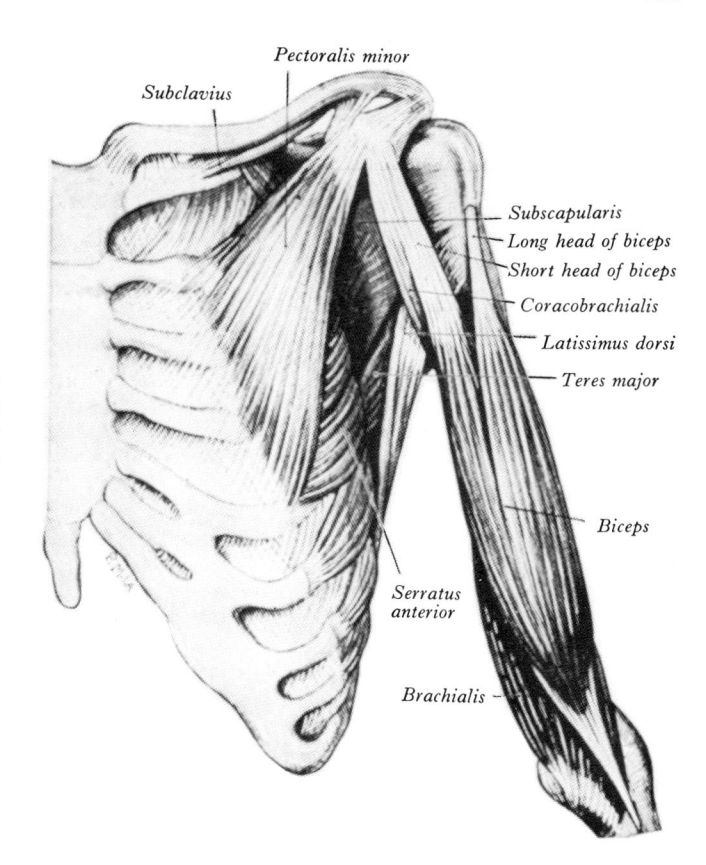

Figure 16–10. The deep muscles of the front of the chest and arm. Left side. (From Warwick, R., and Williams, P. L.: Gray's Anatomy, 35th Br. ed. Philadelphia, W. B. Saunders Company, 1973.)

thorax immediately deep to the pectoralis major. It arises from the third, fourth, and fifth ribs near their costal cartilages and from their intercostal aponeuroses. Its fibers run obliquely upward and laterally to insert into the coracoid process of the scapula (Figs. 16–9 and 16–10). It is not disturbed in the usual thoracotomy incision.

The pectoralis major and minor are both innervated by anterior thoracic nerves (C5, C6, C7, C8, and T1).

The *serratus anterior* muscle occupies the side of the chest and medial wall of the axilla (Fig. 16–10). It arises by nine or ten fleshy digitations from the outer surfaces of the eight or nine upper ribs, the second rib giving attachment to two slips. Its fibers run laterally beneath the scapula to insert into the entire length of the vertebral border of the scapula and function by pulling the scapula forward on the chest. The serratus anterior is innervated by the long thoracic nerve (C5, C6, C7) of Bell which appears from behind the axillary vessels and runs vertically downward to enter the muscle on its superficial aspect.

A considerable portion of the serratus anterior muscle is divided when carrying out the anterior part of most thoracotomy incisions (Fig. 16–11).

The *external intercostal muscles* are 11 (on each side) in number, stretching across all the intercostal spaces from the lower border of one rib to the upper border of the next inferior rib. Its fibers, which are largely interspersed with strands of connective tissue, are directed obliquely downward and forward, and form in each intercostal space a muscular sheet which extends in the upper spaces from the tubercle of the rib to the junction of the rib with its costal cartilage, and, in the lower spaces, it is continued upon the cartilages. The interval between the medial borders of the upper muscles and the lateral border of the sternum is occupied by a sheet of connective tissue called the *external intercostal fascia* or *anterior intercostal aponeurosis* (Fig. 16–12).

The muscles are innervated by the corresponding intercostal nerves.

Because of the direction of their fibers these muscles are stripped most easily from the superior margin of the ribs by passing

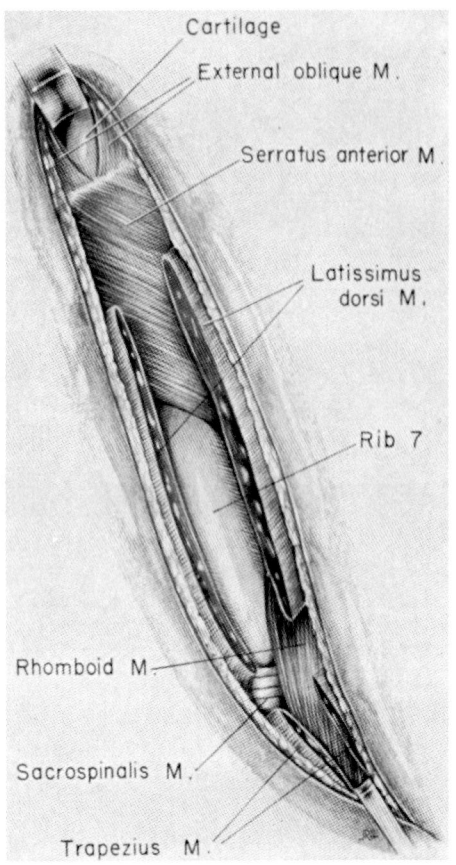

Figure 16-11. Standard thoracotomy incision. View of the incision after division of the latissimus dorsi muscle and partial division of the lower portion of the trapezius muscle; rib partially exposed. (From Sweet, R. H.: Thoracic Surgery, ed. 2. Philadelphia, W. B. Saunders Company, 1954.)

the periosteal elevator from a posterior to anterior direction, while they are most easily freed from the lower rib margins by passing the elevator in a reverse (anterior to posterior) direction.

The *internal intercostal muscles* lie immediately deep to the external, and, like these, extend across each of the intercostal spaces. The fibers are directed obliquely downward and backward (Fig. 16–12) (nearly at right angles to those of the external intercostals) from the lower border of one rib and its costal cartilage to the upper border of the next inferior one. The muscle sheets so formed extend from the medial extremity of each intercostal space as far back as the angles of the ribs, becoming there continuous with an internal intercostal fascia *(posterior intercostal aponeurosis)* which continues backward to the tubercles of the ribs.

The internal intercostal muscles are innervated by their corresponding intercostal nerves. These muscle fibers are most easily stripped from the superior and inferior margins of the ribs by passing the periosteal elevator in reverse directions from those recommended for freeing the external intercostals.

The *mammary gland (breast)* consists of a group of highly specialized cutaneous glands. In the male it is usually so small that it can almost be ignored in planning an appropriate incision. In the female, howev-

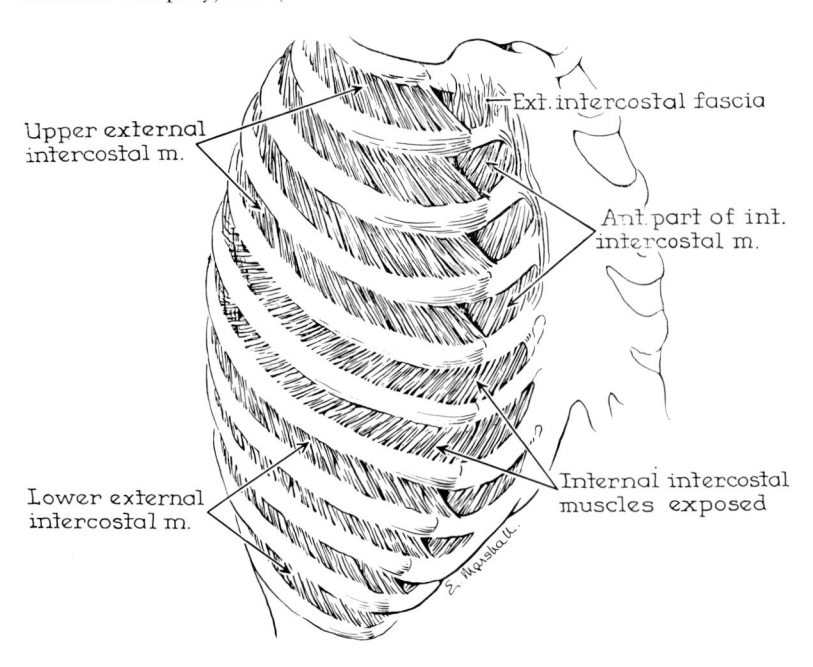

Figure 16-12. Diagram showing the direction taken by the fibers of the external and internal intercostal muscles, which extend across the intercostal spaces.

er, thoracotomy incisions should be planned so as to spare the breast, to avoid going through its tough substance, and to be closed with the least cosmetic disturbance of the breast contours. For these purposes an incision placed along the inferior margin of the breast, reflecting that organ upward, is usually the most satisfactory.

The female mammary gland with its fibrous and fatty tissue lies deep to the skin and superficial to the pectoralis major muscle from which its deep surface can easily be separated by an easily developed line of cleavage. The gland occupies an area bounded by the third rib above, the seventh rib below, the parasternal line anteromedially, and the midaxillary line posterolaterally. A prolongation of the gland often extends into the axillary fold. The mammary gland is supplied with blood by the following arteries:

1. Perforating branches from the internal thoracic (mammary) artery. Although the internal thoracic artery gives off branches to the upper six intercostal spaces, only two (occasionally only one) of these supply the breast. They may be any combination of two of the upper four branches (Fig. 16–13). These branches penetrate the intercostal and pectoralis major muscles in the parasternal line and then pass laterally in the subcutaneous position to the gland, converging toward the nipple.

2. Branches from the thoracicoacromial branch of the axillary artery or directly from the axillary artery itself. These perforate the pectoralis major and minor (to which they give off branches) to obtain a superficial position just below the clavicle, and then descend vertically toward the nipple.

3. Branches from the lateral thoracic branch of the axillary artery. These turn around the axillary border of the pectoralis major muscle to pass either directly forward upon the gland or to descend first along its lateral margin.

Every arterial branch to the mammary gland has an accompanying vein.

The gland is thought to be innervated by the fourth, fifth, and sixth intercostal nerves with their autonomic components.

From the above description it can be seen that on the deep surface of the mammary gland there are no vessels or nerves of appreciable size, so with an incision made at the inferior breast margin the entire mammary mass may be dissected upward away from the thoracic wall without difficulty and with minimal disturbance to its vascular supply.

The posterior surface of the chest wall is covered by the following muscles:

The *trapezius* is a large, triangular muscle which overlies the upper part of the back (see Fig. 16–3). It arises above from the superior nuchal line and external occipital protuberance and passes thence along the ligamentum nuchae and the spinous processes of the seventh cervical and all the thoracic vertebrae, together with the supraspinous ligaments. Its upper fibers pass downward and outward, the middle ones directly outward, and the lower ones upward and outward, to be inserted into the outer third of the posterior border of the clavicle, the inner border and upper surface of the acromium process, the upper border of the spine of the scapula, and the tubercle at the base of the scapular spine. Its inferolateral edge is free. The trapezius muscle is innervated by the spinal accessory nerve and by the third and fourth cervical nerves. The fibers of a portion of the muscle must be transected when making the posterior portion of an upper thoracotomy incision.

The *latissimus dorsi* muscle covers the lower portion of the posterior and lateral chest walls. It also is triangular in shape and arises from the spinous processes of the lowest six thoracic vertebrae and the intervening interspinous ligaments beneath the origin of the trapezius, from the lumbodorsal fascia, from the posterior portion of the crest of the ilium, and by fleshy digitations from the outer surfaces of the lower three or four ribs. Its fibers pass upward and laterally over the inferior angle of the scapula, from which an additional slip is usually added to the muscle. It then curves around the lower border of the teres major to insert, ventrally to that muscle, into the crest of the inner tuberosity of the humerus.

The latissimus dorsi is innervated by the long subscapular nerve from the sixth, seventh, and eighth cervical nerves. Its muscle fibers must be transected in making most thoracotomy incisions for exposing the esophagus.

The *levator scapulae* is an elongated muscle on the lateral surface of the neck. It arises from the transverse processes of the upper four cervical vertebrae and passes

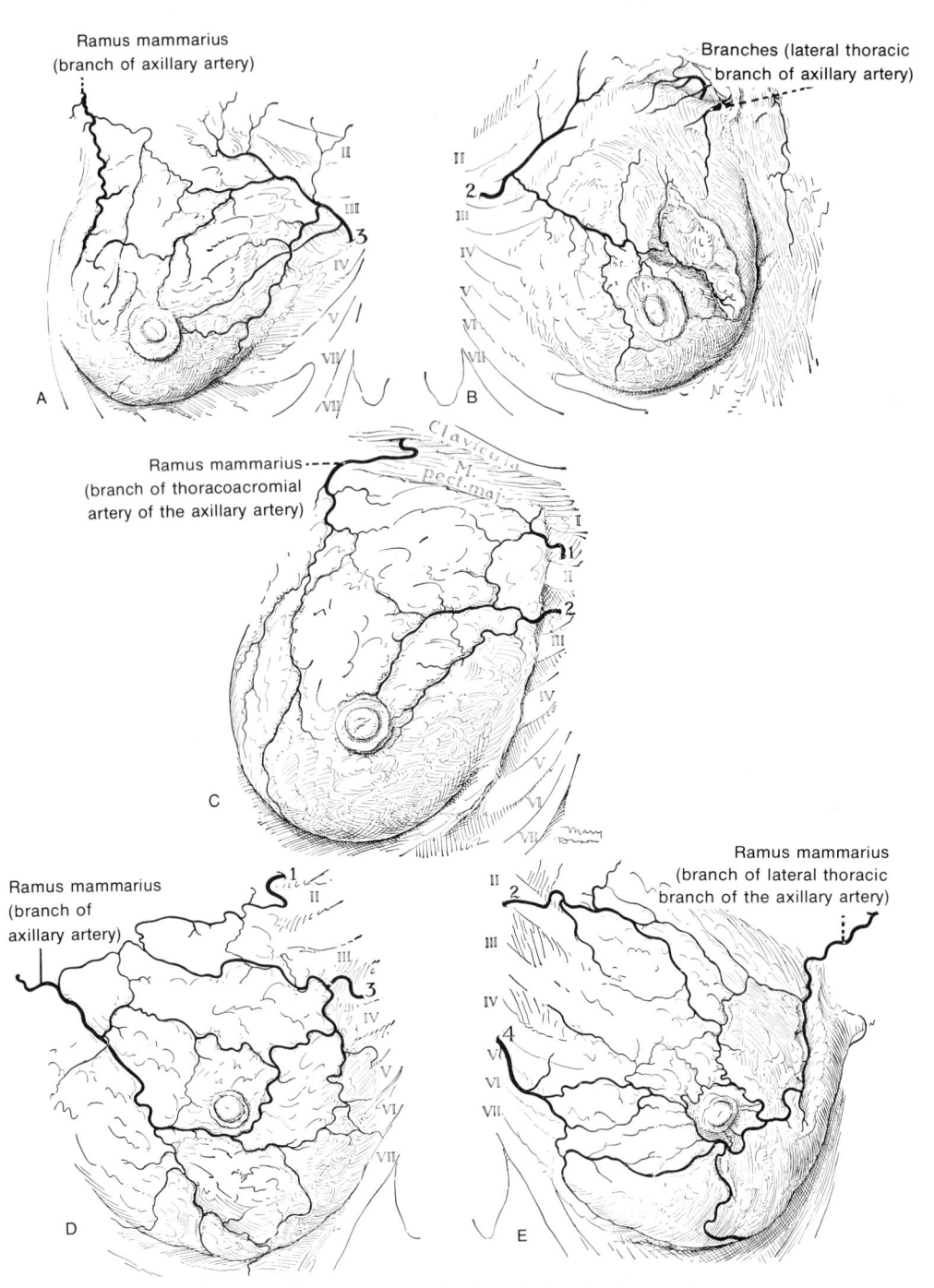

Figure 16–13. Arterial supply of the mammary gland; variations in the source, and anastomotic pattern of the vessels.

downward, forward, and laterally to be inserted into the medial (superior) angle of the scapula (see Fig. 16–3). It is innervated by the dorsal scapular nerve from the fifth cervical nerve. This muscle is not disturbed in approaching the thoracic esophagus.

The *rhomboideus minor* is a bandlike muscle which lies immediately inferior to the levator scapulae and which arises from the lower part of the ligamentum nuchae and from the spinous process of the last cervical vertebra. It passes laterally and downward to be inserted into the upper portion of the vertebral border of the scapula.

The rhomboideus major muscle lies immediately inferior to the rhomboideus minor and is a quadrilateral muscular sheet which arises from the spinous processes of the four upper thoracic vertebrae. Its fibers run downward and laterally to insert into the lower two-thirds of the vertebral border of the scapula. Its inferior margin is free.

Both the rhomboideus major and minor are innervated by the dorsal scapular nerve from the fifth cervical nerve. The dorsal scapular nerve runs downward along the vertebral border of the scapula beneath the rhomboideus muscles. When dividing whatever portion of these muscles is necessary to displace the scapula for adequate exposure, the division should be made well away from the vertebral border of the scapula to protect the nerve from injury. The amount of the rhomboideus muscles to be divided will depend upon the level of the thoracotomy incision. A thoracotomy incision made at or below the level of the eighth rib will avoid the necessity of their division.

The serratus posterior superior is a quadrangular, flat muscle which is situated deep to the rhomboids and arises by a flat tendon from the lower part of the ligamentum nuchae and from the spinous processes of the seventh cervical and upper two or three thoracic vertebrae. Its fibers are directed downward and laterally to be inserted into the outer surface of the second to the fifth ribs, lateral to their angles (Fig. 16-14). It is innervated by the first to fourth thoracic nerves.

It is encountered and severed only in incisions placed high on the posterior part of the chest wall.

The serratus posterior inferior muscle arises by a broad but thin tendon from the posterior layer of the lumbodorsal fascia from about the level of the second lumbar to that of the tenth or eleventh thoracic vertebrae (Fig. 16-14). Its fibers are directed upward and laterally and are inserted into the outer surfaces of the lower four ribs. It is innervated by the ninth to twelfth thoracic nerves. This muscle is encountered in incisions requiring removal of the posterior portions of the four lower ribs to which it is attached.

The *scapula* with its embracing musculature is not a part of the thoracic wall but overlies a considerable portion of the upper posterior chest and must be considered in planning a posterior or posterolateral approach to the thoracic esophagus. The scapula is a triangular-shaped flat bone (Fig. 16-15A). Its posterior (vertebral) border is the longest, and in the resting position it runs vertically, parallel and about 4 cm. lateral to the spinous processes of the vertebrae. The superior angle of the vertebral border is about on the level of the upper edge of the second rib, while the inferior angle is on the level with the seventh intercostal space. These palpable points are valuable landmarks in selecting the site for a thoracotomy incision or a thoracentesis.

When the arms are raised and the shoulders brought forward, the vertebral border of the scapula is elevated and changes direction so that it now runs from above obliquely downward and laterally, its inferior angle being displaced upward and laterally for a variable distance. This mobili-

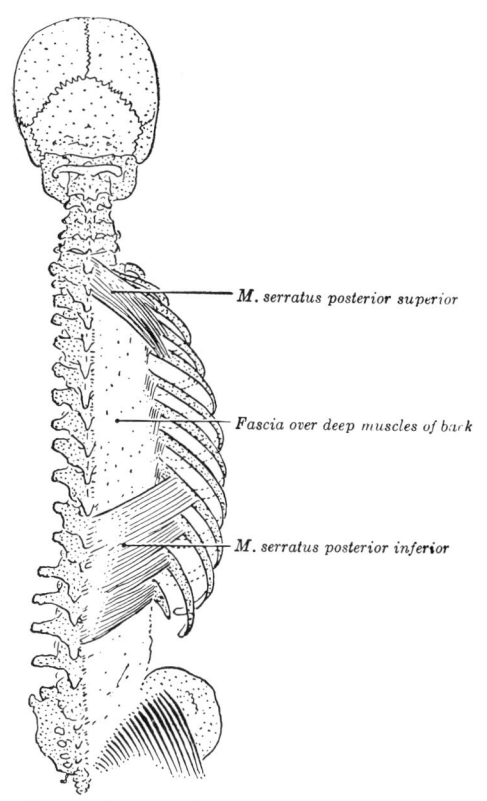

Figure 16-14. The serratus posterior muscles (Marshall-Lazier: An Introduction to Human Anatomy.)

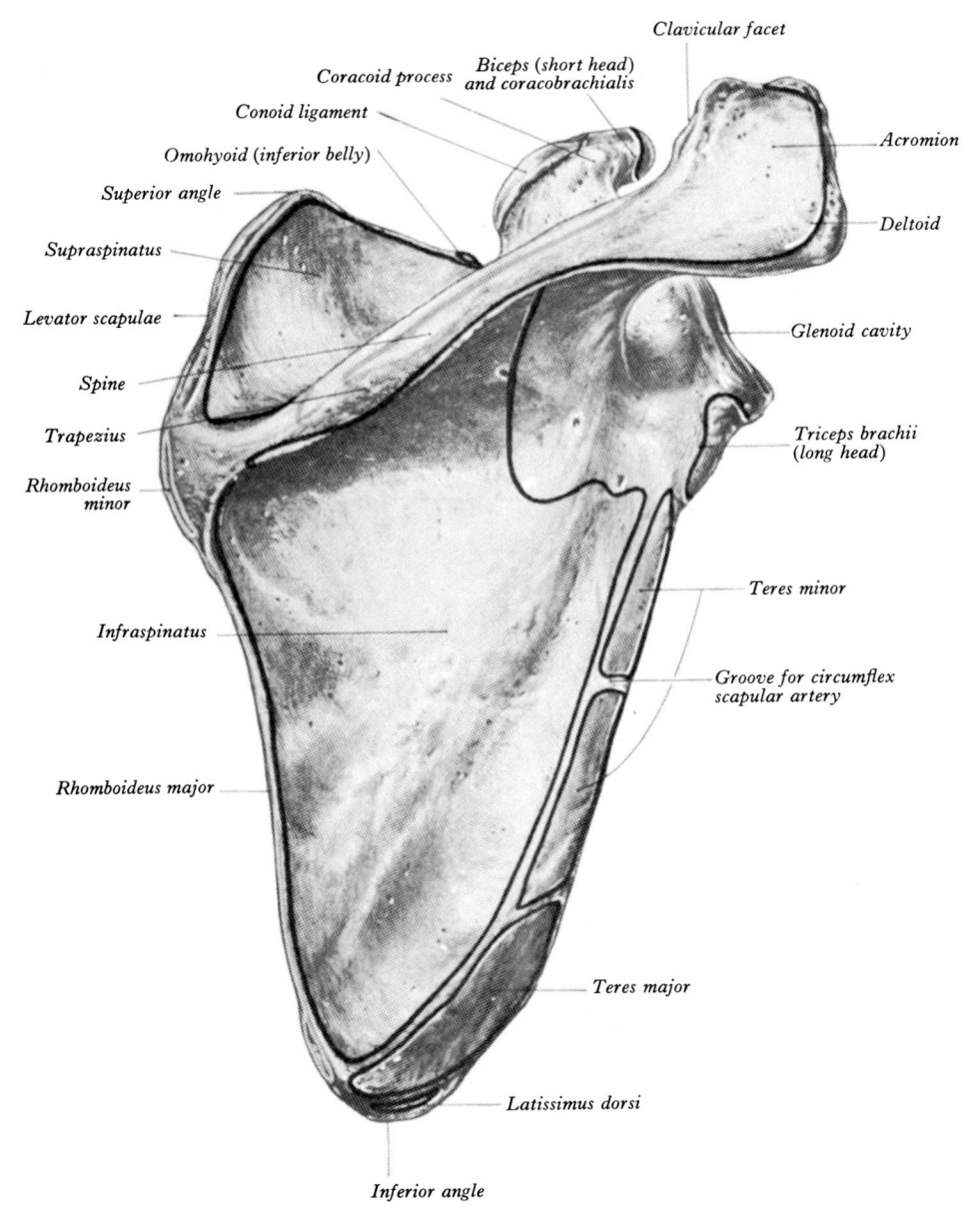

Figure 16-15. A, The right scapula. Dorsal aspect.

Illustration continued on opposite page

ty of the scapula should be taken advantage of in positioning the patient on the operating table in a way that will provide the greatest exposure with the minimal division of muscles.

The other two borders of the scapula are the superior and the axillary, which play no part in exposures of the esophagus.

The *anterior (ventral, costal, or deep)* surface of the scapula is concave and filled by the *subscapularis muscle* (Figs. 16-10 and 16-15B), which arises from that surface, its fibers passing laterally to insert into the lesser tuberosity of the humerus. This muscle is innervated by the upper and lower subscapular nerves from the fifth and sixth cervical nerves. The subscapularis muscle does not attach to the chest wall and is not disturbed in approaching the esophagus, during which it is encountered only when

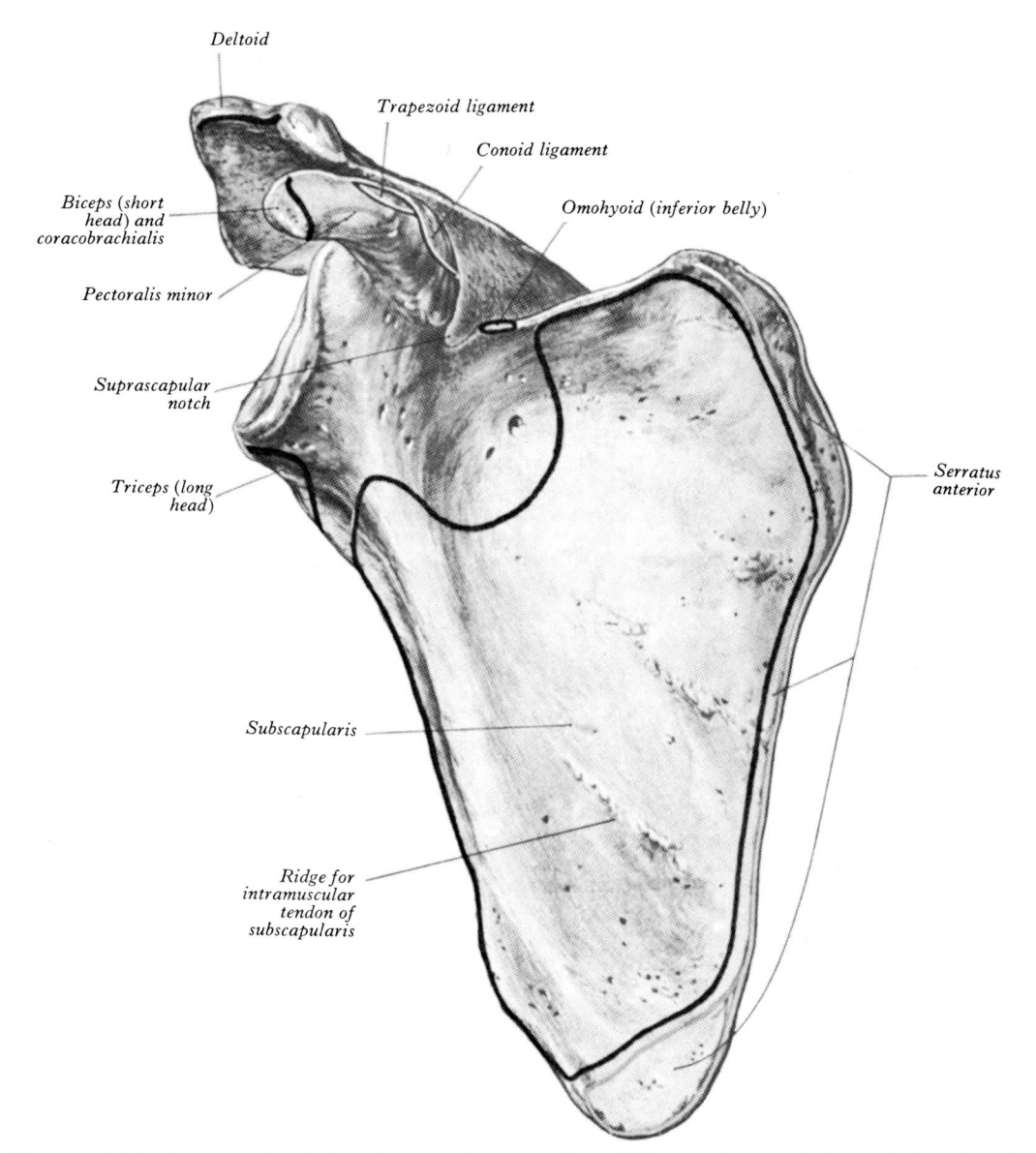

Figure 16–15. *Continued.* *B*, Anterior (costal) aspect. (From Williams, P. L., and Warwick, R. (eds.): Gray's Anatomy, 36th Br. ed. Philadelphia, W. B. Saunders, 1980.)

necessary to displace the scapula upward, in which case it is felt and seen on the undersurface of the scapula.

The *posterior (dorsal)* surface of the scapula is divided by a spine (scapular spine) which extends upward and laterally from the vertebral border opposite the third thoracic spinous process to become continuous with the acromion. The scapular spine is palpable and serves as a surface landmark. The posterior surface of the scapula above the spine is occupied by the *supraspinatus*, and that below the spine, by the *infraspinatus* muscle (Figs. 16–15A and 16–16). These muscles arise from the posterior scapular surface, and pass laterally to insert into the greater tuberosity of the humerus. They have no attachment to the chest wall and are not encountered when making an incision to approach the esophagus. Both

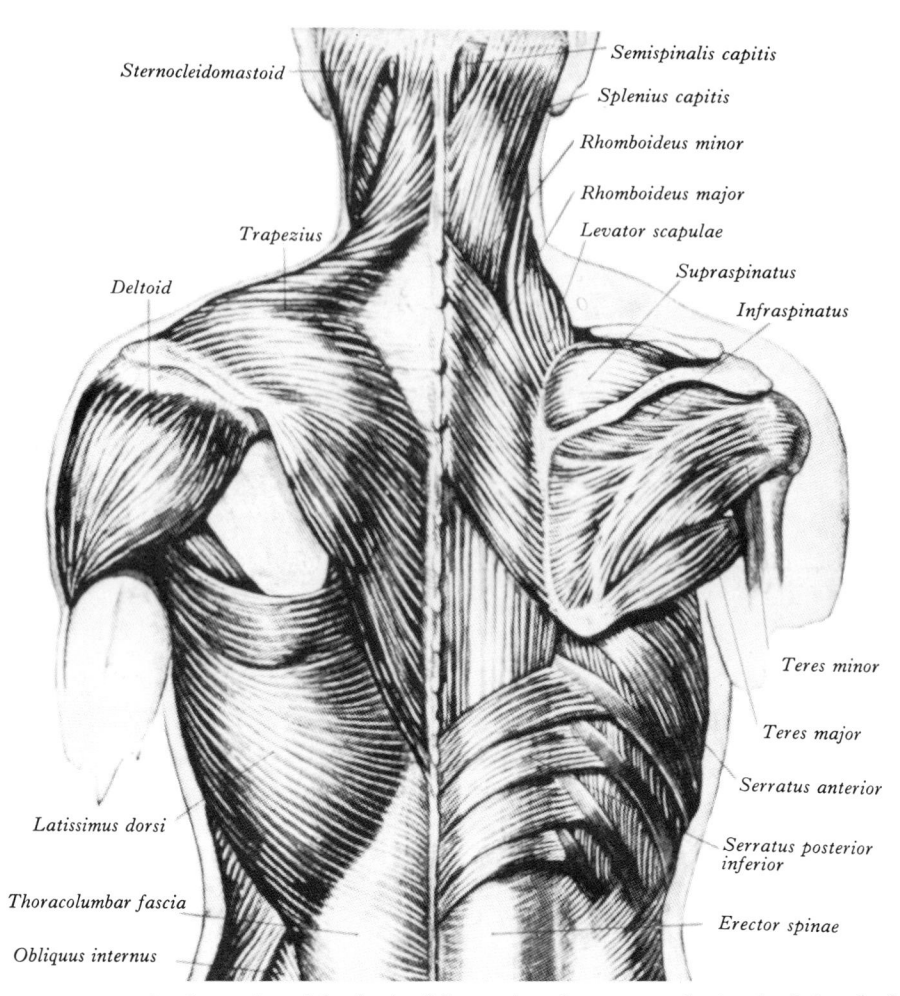

Figure 16–16. Superficial muscles of the back of the neck and upper trunk. On the left only the skin and superficial and deep fasciae have been removed; on the right, the sternocleidomastoid, trapezius, latissimus dorsi, deltoid, and obliquus externus abdominis have been dissected away. (Modified from Warwick, R., and Williams, P. L.: Gray's Anatomy, 35th Br. ed. Philadelphia, W. B. Saunders Company, 1973.)

muscles are innervated by the suprascapular nerve from the fourth, fifth, and sixth cervical nerves.

To displace the scapula upward and laterally, it is necessary to divide the latissimus dorsi muscle, and a part of the rhomboideus muscles. The lower border of the scapula can then be lifted outward and upward, laterally exposing the posterior parts of the upper ribs which it previously covered (Fig. 16–16). The fibers of the anterior serratus muscle may or may not require division, depending upon the level and extent of the exposure needed.

FASCIAE OF THE THORACIC WALL

The *superficial pectoral fascia* is continuous above with the superficial cervical fascia and below with the superficial abdominal fascia. It covers the entire anterior and lateral wall of the thorax, contains a considerable amount of fat, and has embedded in it the mammary gland.

The *deep (pectoral) fascia* attaches above to the clavicle, mesially to the sternum, and laterally to the axillary fascia in the floor of the axilla, and to the fascia covering the deltoid. This layer encloses the pectoralis major muscle and is continuous below with the fascial covering of the serratus anterior and external oblique muscles.

Beneath the deep (pectoral) fascia lies the *clavipectoral fascia*. This is attached above to the clavicle, encloses the subclavius muscle, and continues downward to the upper border of the pectoralis minor muscle. Here it divides into two sheets, which enclose this muscle and at its lower margin reunite to form a single sheet. This becomes continuous with the axillary fascia close to the lower border of the pectoralis major muscle. The portion of this fascia that intervenes between the clavicle and the subclavius muscle and the upper border of the pectoralis minor is termed the *coracoclavicular* fascia or *costocoracoid membrane*, which is prolonged laterally along the upper border of the pectoralis minor, over the upper portion of the axillary vessels, to the coracoid process, its outer portion being thickened to form the *costocoracoid ligament*.

It can be seen that most of the muscles of the thoracic wall are covered or invested by one or more layers of fascia. It is these fascial coverings that make it possible for sutures to hold when transected muscles are repaired. Transected muscles should be repaired in accurate layers.

THORACIC CAVITY AND ITS CONTENTS

The interior of the thorax consists of a large space which is subdivided into two pleural cavities with the mediastinal space between. The anterior, lateral, and posterior limits of each pleural cavity are bounded by the bones of the thorax. Their medial boundaries are the lateral margins of the mediastinum. Inferiorly they are bounded by the diaphragm and superiorly both pleural cavities end as a small dome-shaped projection of the pleura which extends just above the level of the first rib for a short distance into the neck (Fig. 16–17).

The thoracic cavity contains three complete serous sacs: the right and left pleurae and the mediastinum.

Pleurae. The pleurae are two serous membranes which form independent closed sacs. Into each sac at its mesial aspect is invaginated the respective lung. Hence two layers are present: one applied over and adherent to the inner surface of the walls of the thorax, called the parietal layer; and the other, intimately applied over the surface of the invaginated lung, called the visceral or pulmonary layer.

The *visceral pleura* is thin and so intimately applied to the lung surface that it dips into the interlobar fissures and cannot be detached without lacerating the lung. At the root of the lung it is continuous with the pleura over the mediastinum.

The *parietal pleura*, for descriptive purposes, can be divided into four portions: costal, diaphragmatic, mediastinal, and cervical.

The *costal portion* of the parietal

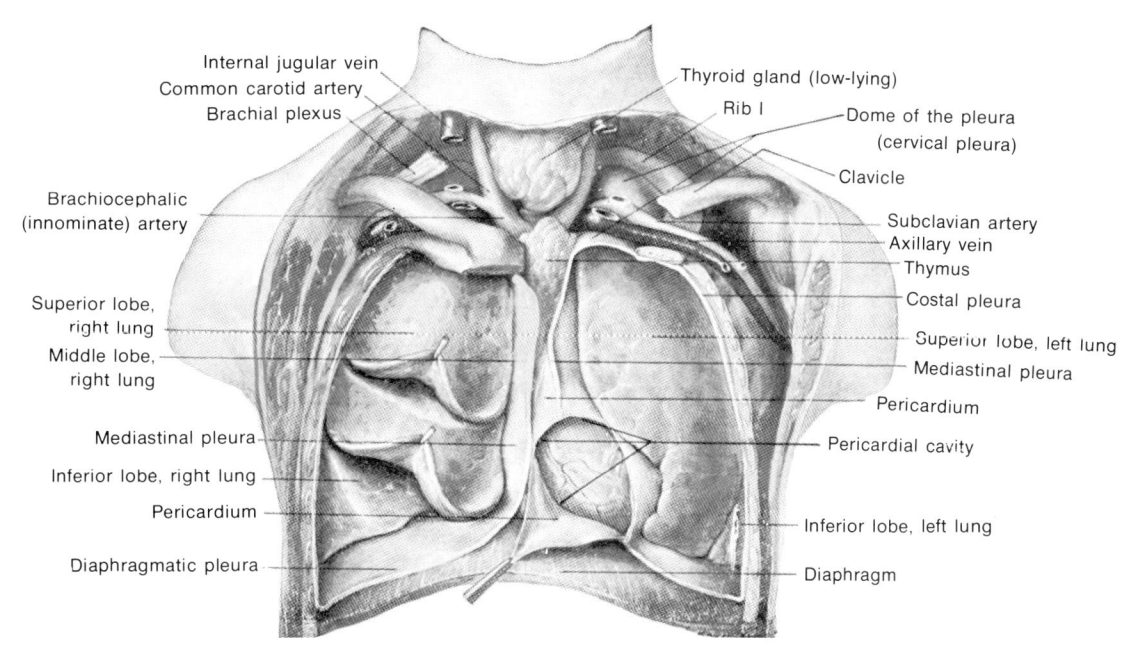

Figure 16–17. Lungs and their relations to the pleurae and mediastinum.

pleura is in contact with the ribs, the intercostal spaces, and the thin endothoracic fascia that lines the inner surface of the thoracic cage. Because of its toughness and relatively loose attachment to the endothoracic fascia it can be easily separated from the chest wall. It continues anteriorly into the anterior mediastinal pleura and also posteriorly into the posterior mediastinal pleura. It is the costal pleura that is incised to enter the pleural cavity when making a thoracotomy incision.

The *diaphragmatic portion* of the parietal pleura spreads over and is adherent to the diaphragm, covering all of that muscle not covered by the diaphragmatic pericardium. It does not extend quite to the line of attachment of the diaphragm to the chest wall but is separated from it by a small interval containing fatty areolar connective tissue.

The *mediastinal portion* of the parietal pleura lies loosely over the structures, including the esophagus, against which it rests and from which it can easily be stripped. In the upper part of the chest cavity on each side the mediastinal pleura extends without interruption from the sternum to the spine, but below it is reflected from the pericardium over the root of the lung and becomes continuous with the pulmonary (visceral) pleura. This reflection of mediastinal pleura over the inferior margin of the lung root is the *inferior pulmonary ligament* to which reference is made in operations that expose the lower portion of the thoracic esophagus.

The *cervical pleura* (dome of the pleura) ascends into the neck over the apex (cupola) of the lung. The pleura extends downward to reach the vertebral column at the level of the twelfth thoracic spine about 1 cm. inferior to the head of the twelfth rib. The dome (superior border) of the pleura extends upward into the neck to a level just above the first rib.

If one enters the pleural cavity through a transthoracic approach to the alimentary tract the lung will be encountered. Normally it is not adherent to the parietal pleura and can be retracted out of the operative field. When adherent, its adhesions are freed as is described on page 446. When freeing the posteromedial portion of the lung or incising the posterior mediastinal pleura over the lower esophagus, care must be taken not to dissect so high as to injure the inferior pulmonary vein, which is the most inferior structure of the hilum of the lung.

MEDIASTINUM. The mediastinum, or central compartment of the chest cavity, is the space bounded laterally by pleural membrane. It is bounded anteriorly by the posterior aspect of the sternum, posteriorly by the anterior surface of the spine, and inferiorly by the diaphragm. Superiorly it is in continuity with the deep subfascial spaces of the neck. The mediastinum lies more to the left of rather than precisely in the midline. It is shut off from the abdominal cavity except at the aortic opening posteriorly, the esophageal hiatus, and a narrow opening anteriorly between the sternal and costal attachments of the diaphragm. This opening is filled with loose connective tissue. It communicates freely above with the subfascial spaces of the neck.

The mediastinum contains such important structures as the heart with its great blood vessels and pericardium; the trachea and bronchi; the esophagus; the aorta; important nerves; mediastinal lymph glands; and the thymus gland. It may contain abnormally placed thyroid or parathyroid glands or both.

Although the mediastinum is a single space, for descriptive purposes it may be arbitrarily divided into *superior* (upper) and *inferior* (lower) compartments. A horizontal plane passing from the manubriosternal joint to the inferior surface of the fourth thoracic vertebra separates the superior from the lower compartment. The inferior compartment can be further subdivided into *anterior*, *middle*, and *posterior* mediastinal portions (Fig. 16–18).

The superior mediastinum contains the thymus gland; the brachiocephalic veins forming the superior vena cava; the aortic arch; the brachiocephalic and left common carotid arteries; the vagus, phrenic, and left recurrent laryngeal nerves; the thoracic duct; esophagus; trachea; and the brachiocephalic, paratracheal, and tracheobronchial lymph nodes. These structures are not usually encountered in operations on the alimentary tract except when the upper part of the thoracic esophagus is exposed through a left thoracotomy incision, in which case the arch of the aorta presents difficulties. It is for this reason that a right-sided approach to this area seems preferable (Fig. 16–19).

The anterior mediastinum is a narrow

EXPOSURE OF THE THORACIC ALIMENTARY TRACT

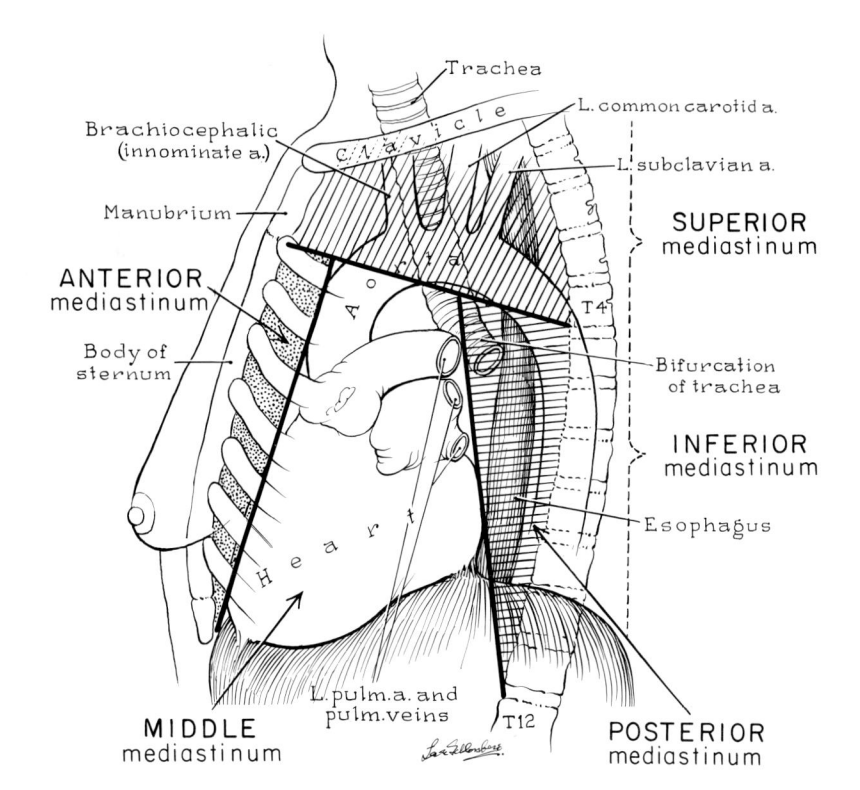

Figure 16–18. Anatomic divisions of the mediastinum.

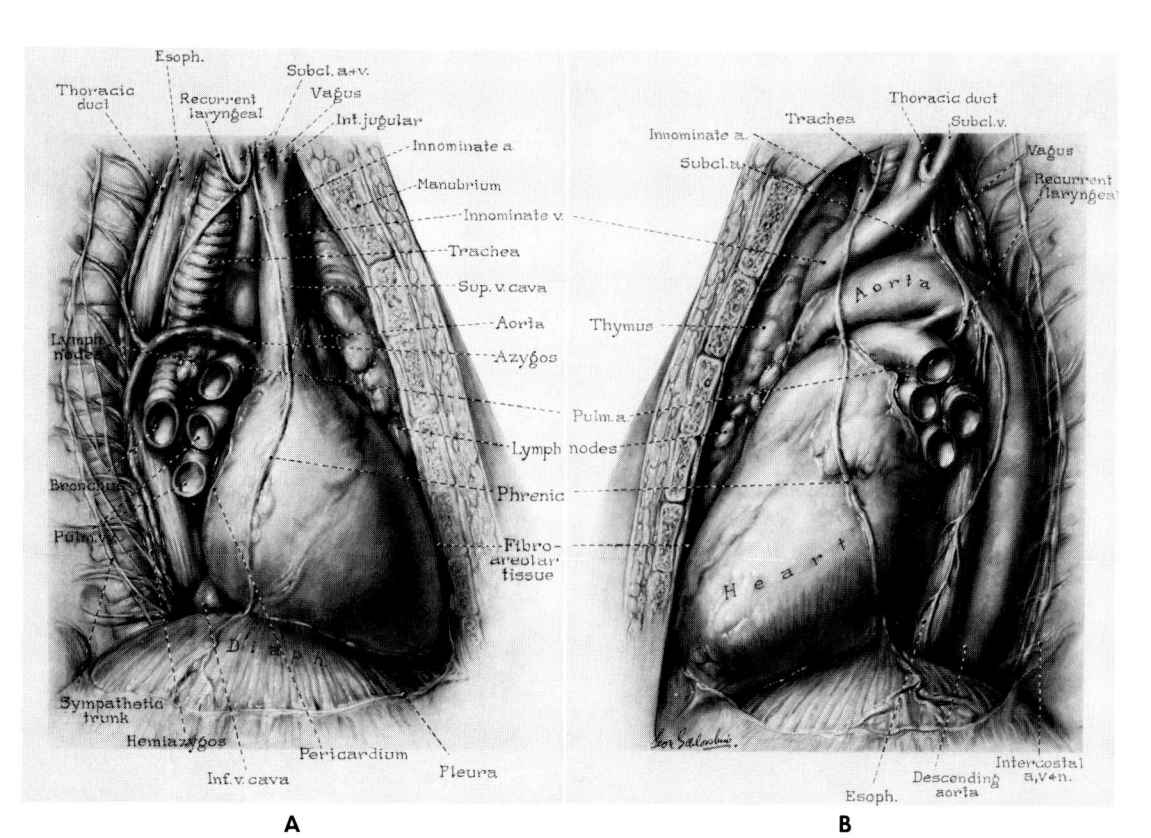

Figure 16–19. Anatomic structures of the mediastinum as seen from the right side (A) and from the left side (B). (From Sabiston, D. C., Jr., and Spencer, F. C. (eds.): Gibbon's Surgery of the Chest. Philadelphia, W. B. Saunders Company, 1976.)

compartment, which lies between the sternum and the pericardium. It contains some lymphatic and adipose tissue and can contain a portion of the thymus gland (see Figs. 16–18 and 16–19B).

The middle mediastinum contains the pericardium and the heart. The pericardium is a closed fibroserous sac within which the heart and the proximal portion of its great vessels are enclosed. It consists of a visceral and a parietal layer between which lies the pericardial cavity. The posterior surface of the parietal pericardium overlies and is in intimate relationship with the anterior surface of the lower esophagus, but can be separated intact from it by blunt dissection. Better exposure is obtained if the patient is positioned on the table with the side to be operated upon somewhat elevated when operating upon this portion of the alimentary tract. The pericardium is also in contact on both sides with the parietal pleura and inferiorly with the diaphragm. It can usually be separated by blunt dissection from these structures for a variable distance. The heart is not exposed in operations on the alimentary tract unless the pericardium is opened. The middle compartment also contains the tracheal bifurcation, bifurcation of the bronchus, the pulmonary trunk, the right and left pulmonary arteries and veins, and the phrenic nerve (Figs. 16–18 and 16–19).

The posterior mediastinum contains the thoracic esophagus, descending part of the thoracic aorta, thoracic duct, vagus nerve, sympathetic ganglion trunk, azygos and hemiazygos vein, and an abundant amount of areolar tissue (Figs. 16–18 and 16–19).

The anatomy of the esophagus and its relation to the above structures is described in Volume 1 (pp. 6–24).

DIAPHRAGM

The diaphragm also is described in Volume 1 (pp. 11–13).

APPROACHES TO THE THORACIC ESOPHAGUS

The thoracic portion of the esophagus can be exposed through a right or a left thoracotomy incision, through a posterior extrapleural approach, or through a thoracicoabdominal approach.

At present, a posterior extrapleural approach is used chiefly for repairing congenital tracheoesophageal fistulas or draining a posterior mediastinitis.

A right posterolateral thoracotomy incision provides the best access to all portions of the thoracic esophagus and can be used for all operations on the esophagus that do not require the use of the stomach for anastomosis to the proximal end of the esophagus.

When a segment of the esophagus is to be removed and replaced by an esophagogastric anastomosis, a left posterolateral thoracotomy incision is used to facilitate mobilization of the stomach (or jejunum in rare cases). If a long segment of the esophagus is to be removed and replaced by an esophagogastric (or esophagojejunal) anastomosis, a standard left thoracotomy incision is made and either enlarged upward by posterior division of the adjacent ribs, or it is supplemented by another left thoracotomy incision through the bed of the fourth rib, which is removed. Some surgeons prefer to mobilize the stomach or jejunum through an abdominal incision and then carry out the esophageal resection and anastomosis through a separate thoracotomy incision.

A more satisfactory approach for lesions of the midportion or higher of the thoracic esophagus requiring resection followed by esophagogastric anastomosis is a right thoracicoabdominal incision. The chest is entered through a right thoracotomy incision made through the bed of the removed right seventh rib. This incision is continued across the costal cartilage and midepigastrium to enter the abdominal cavity.

Lesions requiring removal of the portion of the thoracic esophagus situated in the superior mediastinum above the arch of the aorta are exposed by a cervical incision combined with a separate upper thoracotomy incision.

The short abdominal segment of the esophagus can be approached by an upper abdominal incision; a standard left thoracotomy incision through the eighth intercostal space or bed of the ninth rib, along with an incision through the dome of the left diaphragm; or through a left thoracicoabdominal incision.

Although a right-sided approach provides the most satisfactory exposure for most benign lesions, such as congenital or inflammatory tracheoesophageal fistulas, benign tumors to be removed by local excision, and in patients who do not require the use of the stomach for anastomosis, it is obvious that when any esophageal lesions present predominantly on one side the incision should be made on the presenting side.

MINOR THORACOTOMY INCISIONS

Minor thoracotomy incisions are inadequate for exposing the alimentary tract but are employed for complications of lesions involving that tract or following operations upon it. Hence they may be used to drain a pleural empyema, a lung abscess, a liver abscess, or a subdiaphragmatic abscess.

SELECTION OF INCISIONS

The incision is made over the estimated or predetermined area occupied by the collection of pus, and, if possible, so as to drain the most dependent portion of the abscess.

The relation selected between the inclination of the ribs and the direction of the incision through the skin, fat, and muscles should depend upon the purpose for which the incision is to be used. Furthermore, the relation between the actual direction of a skin incision and the direction of its underlying ribs will vary according to whether the incision is placed in the posterior, middle, or anterior portion of the chest wall, and whether it is in the upper or lower portion of the thorax, because of the difference in obliquity of the ribs at different levels and of their curved course.

It has been pointed out that for drainage of an empyema an important consideration is to have the drainage tube at the bottom of the cavity. If the lowermost level can be determined accurately before operation, the incision through the soft parts is made in the direction of the rib that is to be resected. When there is uncertainty as to the lowermost level of the pus-containing cavity, the incision through the soft tissues is preferably made vertically so as to cross

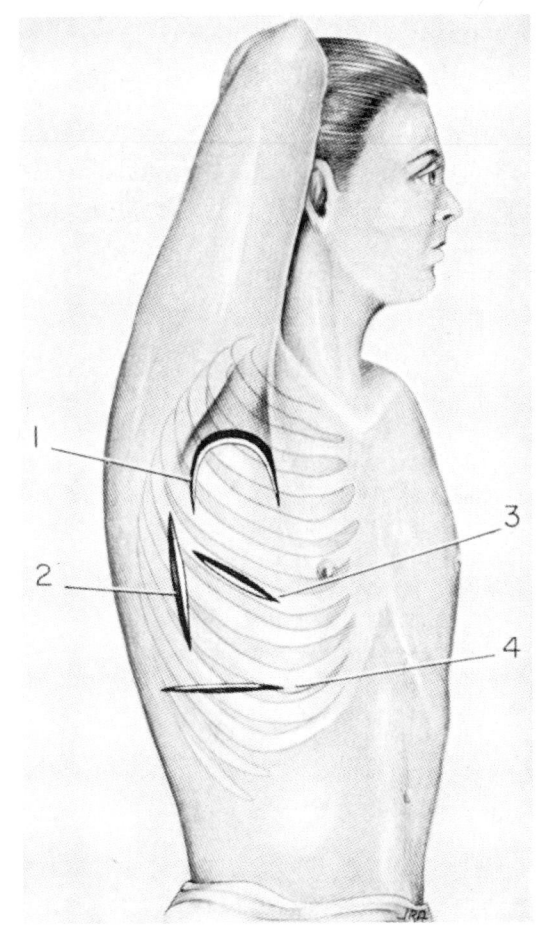

Figure 16–20. Minor thoracotomy incisions for drainage of empyema and lung abscess. 1. Inverted U-shaped axillary incision for drainage of abscesses in the upper lobe of the lung. 2, Vertical incision over two or more adjacent ribs for drainage of empyema or abscess in the apex of the lung. For the latter it must be made between the medial border of the scapula and the spine. 3, Oblique incision in the direction of a rib used in certain cases of empyema or pulmonary abscess where localization is accurate. 4, Transverse incision used in transpleural drainage of subdiaphragmatic or liver abscesses. (From Sweet, R. H.: Thoracic Surgery, ed. 2. Philadelphia, W. B. Saunders Company, 1954.)

the direction of the underlying ribs. Then if the rib chosen for resection is found to be too high, the same incision can be extended downward and used for resecting the next rib below it. Needle aspiration of the area will help define the lowest extent of the empyema cavity.

The location and extent of empyema can usually be determined preoperatively with sufficient accuracy that the incision through the soft parts is usually made parallel to the direction of the portion of rib to be

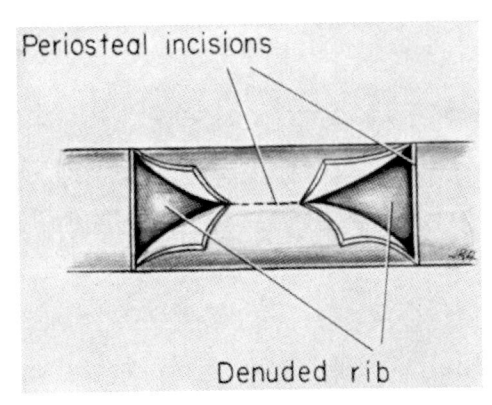

Figure 16–21. Technic of rib resection. Correct placement of incisions in the periosteum to avoid necrosis of rib ends in empyema or abscess cases. (From Sweet, cited in previous figure.)

resected. If the empyema is in the anterior or posterior segment of the upper lobe and presents in the axilla, an inverted U-shaped incision (Fig. 16–20) may be preferable to a linear incision that is vertical or parallel to the direction of the ribs.

Transthoracic drainage of a subdiaphragmatic or hepatic abscess is usually carried out through an incision made transversely across the lower chest wall so that a segment of rib anterior or posterior to that originally selected for resection can be excised. The lowermost ribs run a more oblique course than do those at a higher level.

TECHNIC

In the selected direction and location a short incision (7 to 14 cm. in length) is made through the skin, fat, and muscles down to the rib. The edges of the incision through the soft parts are retracted so that the bared rib surface is exposed. The periosteum covering the presenting (external) surface of the rib is incised in the direction of the rib for a distance equal to the length of rib that is to be excised.

At each end of this incision the periosteum should be incised transversely across the rib (Fig. 16–21) to prevent leaving a V-shaped portion of bone bared of periosteum with potential later for necrosis and sequestration. The leaves of the divided periosteum are stripped off the rib with a periosteal elevator around the entire rib circumference. The rib is transected at the edge of the transverse incision in the external periosteum at each end of its bared segment, and the resected portion is removed.

An incision is then made through the deep periosteal layer and pleura that lie under the resected portion of the rib. This completes the incision.

COMMENTS

Since this type of thoracotomy is usually employed for drainage, no closure is required. It is advisable, however, to clamp, cut, and ligate the adjacent intercostal artery, vein, and nerve at each end of the incision. The intervening portion of intercostal nerve and vessels is removed. This step will prevent later hemorrhage from pressure necrosis of these vessels caused by drains and will minimize the pain produced by the same cause.

A thoracotomy incision to be used for prolonged drainage of an empyema or abscess should be made larger than would at first seem necessary because of the tendency of these openings to contract and later produce difficulties caused by inadequate drainage.

In those patients in whom it is desired to enlarge the opening by resecting a segment of an adjacent rib or ribs so as to unroof an abscess cavity, not only is the portion of the rib removed but also the intervening costal muscles, intercostal nerve and vessels, and underlying deep periosteum and pleura are excised.

MAJOR THORACOTOMY INCISIONS

In surgery of the alimentary canal, major thoracotomy incisions are employed for a wide exposure of and operations upon the structures contained in the thoracic portion. A number of different types have been utilized and will be discussed. The choice of the position and direction of the incision will depend upon the location of the lesion and the extent of the alimentary tract that requires exposure. It also will be influenced somewhat by the physical build of the patient. In individuals with a long, narrow chest it is important to center the incision as close to the lesion as possible, while in short individuals the thoracotomy wound need not be placed as accurately. Furthermore, in a patient with a long chest the incision should be much more oblique than in a short, broad-chested individual, in whom the incision should be more transverse.

In young women some, though secondary, consideration should be given to cosmetic appearance in the selection of an incision. When possible, in these patients, incisions that are carried transversely across the chest above the breast should be avoided. This can be accomplished in those individuals requiring a high exposure by making the anterior portion of the incision below the breast or in the submammary fold and retracting the breast and pectoral muscle upward while the thoracotomy incision is made. When possible, the upward extension of the posterior end of a thoracotomy incision should not be carried too close to the shoulder where its unsightliness will be exposed by some types of clothing.

Major thoracotomy incisions can be divided into two general types: those in which the thoracic cavity is entered through an intercostal space without removal of the rib, and those in which the thoracic cavity is entered through the bed of a rib that has been resected. The former has the advantage in that (1) it can be made and closed more rapidly, and (2) it is less likely to cause structural abnormalities in the chest of growing children. In older adults, ribs become relatively inelastic and brittle, and intercostal incisions are frequently complicated by the fracture of adjacent ribs produced by opening the rib spreader to obtain better exposure. This complication can be prevented by transecting the rib below the intercostal space and, if more exposure is needed, cutting the rib above the intercostal space through which the thoracic cavity is entered.

Standard (Posterolateral) Thoracotomy Incision

This incision is employed on either the right or the left side, and may be used at any level from the third to the tenth ribs. The level of the seventh or eighth ribs provides the widest exposure. It is the incision most commonly used for operations on the thoracic portion of the esophagus and for the transthoracic repair of diaphragmatic hernias or transthoracic operations on the stomach. The incision preferably may be made as an intercostal one without rib resection, or the chest may be entered through the bed of a removed rib.

TECHNIC

The patient is placed on his or her side on the operating table with the side to be incised uppermost (Fig. 16–22). The arm on

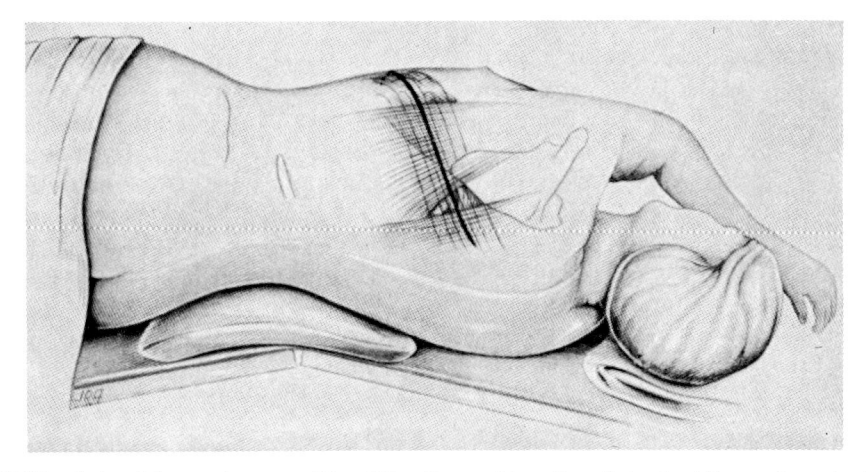

Figure 16–22. Lateral thoracotomy position. Direction and location of standard thoracotomy incision over the seventh rib shown by dark line. Scapula and important muscles are shown in outline. Note the angulation of the table with pillow beneath the patient to arch the side of the operation so as to widen the intercostal spaces. The head is lower than pelvis. (From Sweet, cited in Figure 16–20.)

this side is carried forward and upward so as to displace the scapula upward out of the way. The patient is maintained in this position by wide adhesive tapes attached to each side of the table, the lower one passing over the hips and the upper one over the shoulder. The ribs can be identified by palpation through the skin, counting upward from the twelfth rib.

A long incision is made over the rib to be resected or the intercostal space to be entered (usually the seventh or eighth). This incision begins anteriorly at the nipple line and extends obliquely posteriorly parallel to the direction of the ribs almost to the vertebral column. The incision is deepened through the skin and subcutaneous tissues to expose the underlying muscles. Two fingers are inserted beneath the latissimus dorsi muscle in the posterior portion of the incision to press upward and minimize bleeding while this muscle is transected along the course of the incision and its vessels clamped. As this muscular layer is incised posteriorly, the lateral fibers of the trapezius muscle and of the rhomboideus muscles are divided in a similar way if the incision is at the level of the seventh rib or higher. The latter two muscles are not usually encountered if the incision is made at a level lower than the seventh rib. All three of these posterior muscles have no costal attachments so that the fingers can easily be passed beneath them before their division, and their line of division need not be precisely placed. Before dividing the muscles of the anterior thoracic wall, the rib to be resected or the intercostal space to be entered must be identified because of the insertion of the anterior muscles into the ribs. Identification of the ribs at this stage can be made by inserting a finger beneath the inferior margin of the scapula which has been freed by division of the latissimus, palpating the flat-shaped first rib and counting the ribs downward.

At this point the decision is made as to whether the thoracotomy incision is to be an intercostal one or made through the bed of a resected rib.

INTERCOSTAL METHOD. If the thoracic cavity is to be entered through an intercostal space, the serratus anterior and external oblique muscles are divided at a point where their attachments to the rib to be resected can be avoided.

The intercostal muscles occupying the chosen intercostal space are now exposed. The anesthetist is notified that the chest cavity is about to be opened. A short preliminary incision is made through the intercostal muscles midway between the adjacent ribs at any suitable point, and the pleura is exposed. The pleura is carefully incised, care being taken to avoid injury to the underlying lung. As soon as the pleura is opened, the lung, if not adherent, will fall away from the thoracic wall. If the lung is adherent it is bluntly dissected away from the pleura; a finger is placed ahead of the advancing knife or scissors used to lengthen the incision so that it extends from beyond the costochondral junction anteriorly to the neck of the rib posteriorly. The posterior portion of this incision should be made close to the superior margin of the inferior rib to avoid cutting the intercostal vessels of the rib above as they cross the intercostal space to reach its lower margin (see Fig. 16–7). Care is also taken not to extend the incision sufficiently far anteriorly to injure the internal thoracic (mammary) vessels. If either the intercostal or internal thoracic vessels are injured they must be ligated. Their ligation is harmless.

During the process of making this long pleural incision, several small branches of the intercostal vessels will be encountered and may require ligation. One is situated in the anterior portion of the wound close to the sternum and another occurs posterior to the angle of the rib, while several are placed at points between these two. The incision must traverse the full length of the intercostal space to obtain adequate exposure with an intercostal type of thoracotomy.

After the incision has been completed for its full length and the lung freed from any adhesions to this portion of the thoracic wall, a Finochietto rib retractor is inserted, and the wound edges are separated by cranking the blades apart. The latter part of this separation should be done slowly to prevent the ribs from fracturing. After maximum separation appears to have been obtained at first, it will be found that after a delay the retractor blades can be even further separated later in the operation. If more exposure is required, the rib adjacent to the intercostal space can be divided.

RIB RESECTION METHOD. If the chest is to be entered through the bed of a resected rib, the insertions into the rib of the serratus anterior and external oblique mus-

MAJOR THORACOTOMY INCISIONS

tance without injuring the pleura. A rib stripper can now be passed beneath and around the rib, which is then easily stripped for its full length (Fig. 16-23). The rib is then transected anteriorly through the costal cartilage almost at the costochondral junction and again posteriorly through the neck of the rib. The rib is removed.

The anesthetist is notified that the pleural cavity is about to be entered. The pleural cavity is entered through a short incision made through the periosteal bed of the resected rib, and the lung is allowed to fall away from the chest wall. A finger is then placed inside the pleural cavity, and the pleural incision is lengthened throughout the entire length of the resected rib (Fig. 16-24). If the underlying lung is found to be adherent, each cut edge of the pleura is retracted with a clamp by an assistant while the surgeon presses the lung away to put the adhesions on stretch and thereby facilitate their division.

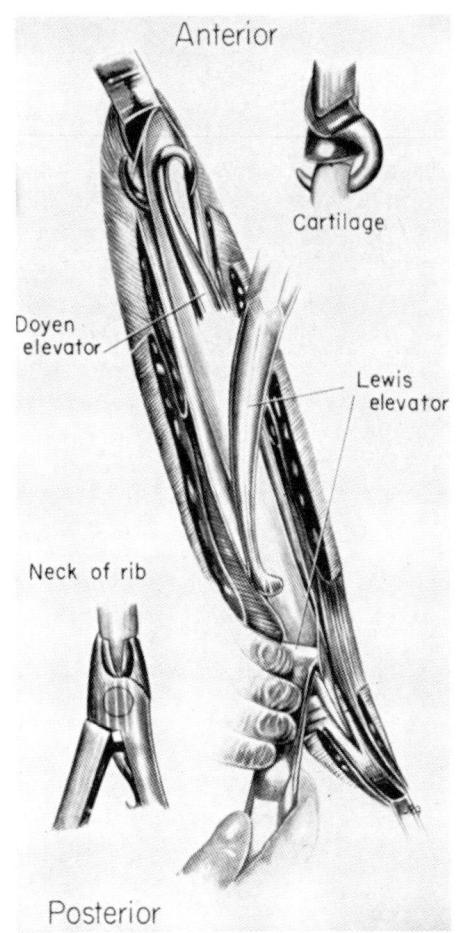

Figure 16-23. Standard thoracotomy incision (rib resection technic). Muscles are completely divided. Three phases of the elevation of the periosteum are shown, using the Lewis elevator to strip the outer aspect of the rib and to free the edges, and the Doyen elevator to strip the inner surface of the rib. Inserts show the technic of transection of the neck of the rib posteriorly and the cartilage anteriorly. (From Sweet, cited in Figure 16-20.)

cles are divided. The presenting surface of the rib periosteum is incised from the anterior costochondral junction to the neck of the rib posteriorly. The periosteum is stripped off the outer, superior, and inferior surfaces of the rib with a periosteal elevator for the entire length of the rib. Because of the direction of the intercostal muscle fibers inserting into the margins of the rib, the superior edge can be freed most easily by passing the instrument from back to front, while the inferior margin is more easily cleared by passing the instrument from front to back. Using a blunt periosteal elevator, the deep periosteum is separated from the deep surface of the rib for a short dis-

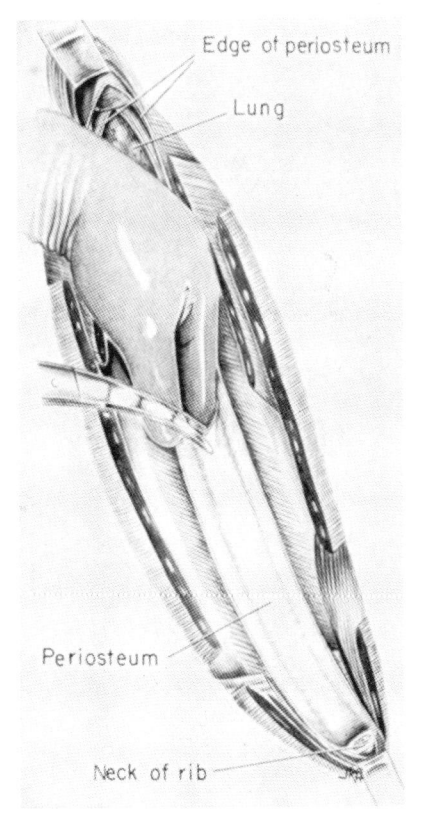

Figure 16-24. Standard thoracotomy incision (rib resection technic). Incision of the periosteum and parietal pleura. The fingers of the surgeon's left hand are inserted to hold the lung away from the points of the scissors. (From Sweet, cited in Figure 16-20.)

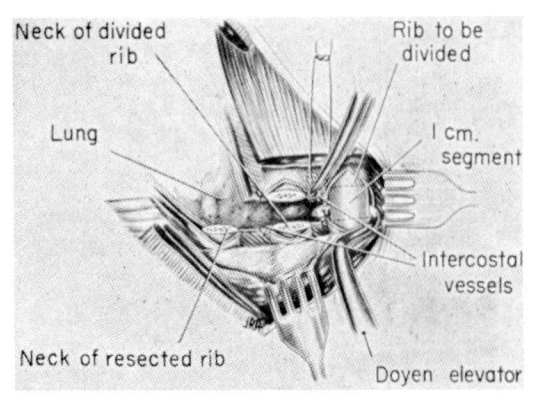

Figure 16-25. Standard thoracotomy incision (rib resection technic). Method of enlarging the incision posteriorly by cutting adjacent ribs. (From Sweet, cited in Figure 16-20.)

The wound margins are then spread with a Finochietto rib retractor. This should be done gradually to minimize the possibility of fracturing the ribs, particularly in older patients.

ENLARGEMENT OF THE INCISION. Either an intercostal or a rib resection type of standard thoracotomy incision can be enlarged to increase the exposure by one of two methods:

1. By dividing posteriorly the rib adjacent above or below the incision or both (Fig. 16-25). When this is necessary, it is advisable to excise a 1- or 2-cm. segment of the posterior portion of the rib or ribs that are transected in order to eliminate the cut edges rubbing against each other during the postoperative period. It is also advisable to divide and ligate the accompanying intercostal vessels and nerve.

2. By cutting across the costochondral arch and continuing the thoracotomy incision across the upper portion of the oblique abdominal muscles if better exposure anteriorly is desired. The incision can stop without an opening being made into the abdominal cavity or it can be continued into the abdominal cavity to convert the thoracic incision into a thoracicoabdominal one.

One of these methods of enlarging the incision is more frequently required with an intercostal thoracotomy than with a rib resection–type.

CLOSURE OF INCISIONS

The lung is fully expanded by the anesthetist before the closure is begun.

The first step in closing an intercostal incision consists of inserting a row of pericostal heavy chromic, polyglycolic acid, or polyglactin 910 sutures through the intercostal spaces above and below the two ribs that were separated so as to encircle these ribs. None are tied until all have been placed (Figure 16-26). The ribs are then approximated by a rib approximator or bone holding forceps or by traction on suitably placed towel clips. The sutures are then tied so as to hold the ribs in this approximated position. Nonabsorbable suture material should not be used for pericostal sutures. Occasionally one heavy wire suture may be used to help reapproximate the ribs.

After the pericostal sutures have been tied, the cut edges of the deep fascial investment of each divided layer are united, preferably with running or interrupted 2-0 chromic, polyglactin 910 or polyglycolic acid sutures. The muscle layers are all closed in anatomic fashion. If the patient is very muscular, both the posterior and anterior fasciae of each muscle layer will have to be closed.

The subcutaneous layer of thoracic fascia is closed preferably with running or interrupted 2-0 chromic synthetic absorbable sutures. The skin is closed with running or interrupted sutures of 4-0 nylon or stainless steel staples.

In closure of a *rib resection type* of thoracotomy incision, pericostal sutures are not necessary but may be used if desired. The separated ribs are brought closer together by a rib approximator (Fig. 16-27).

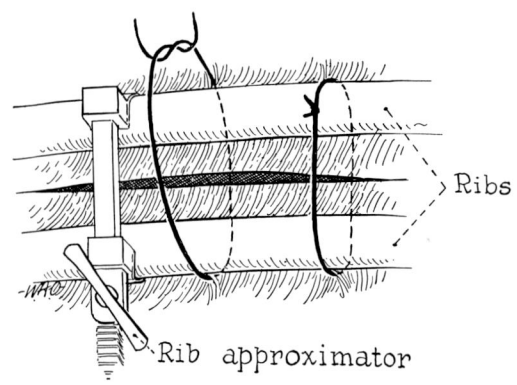

Figure 16-26. First step in closure of intercostal incision: a row of sutures inserted through the intercostal spaces above and below the two ribs that have separated so as to encircle them. No suture is tied until all have been placed.

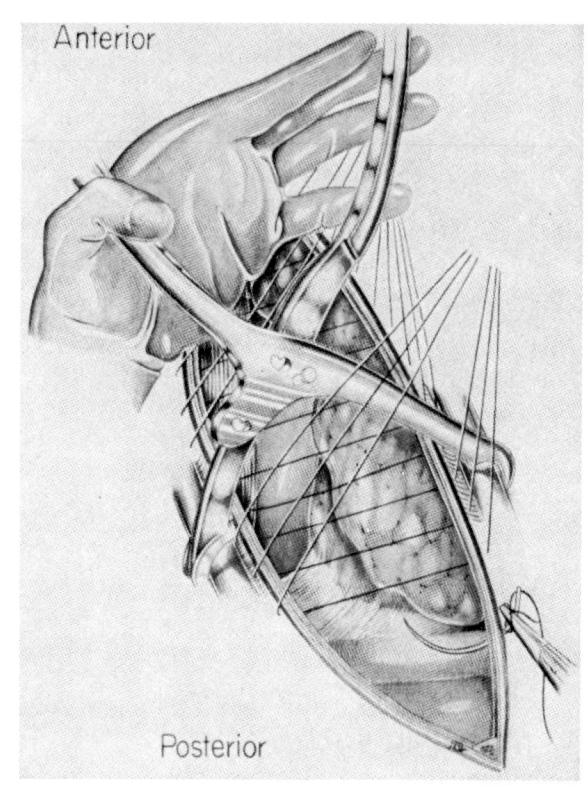

Figure 16-27. Standard thoracotomy incision (rib resection technic). Closure of incision using Lambotte bone-holding forceps as a rib approximator. Sutures (all but the last) in place ready for tying. (From Sweet, cited in Figure 16-20.)

The divided edges of the muscles are sutured together in two layers (deep and superficial fascial investment layers), and the subcutaneous fascia and skin are closed as described above for the intercostal type of thoracotomy.

It will be noted that it is not necessary, indeed it is usually impossible, to suture the cut edges of the pleura together as a separate layer. It also should be pointed out that the deep row of sutures should be placed so as to avoid including the intercostal nerve, a factor in minimizing postoperative pain. It is for this same reason that pericostal sutures should be of absorbable rather than nonabsorbable material.

When a thoracotomy tube for drainage is left in a chest cavity it is brought to the outside through a separate stab wound.

Before closing a thoracotomy incision, it is advisable to inspect the entire length of the two retracted ribs for evidence of a fracture. If a fracture has occurred and the ends of the fragments are jagged, these pointed projections should be removed with a bone rongeur, so as to avoid later injury to the lungs or intercostal vessels. The adjacent intercostal vessels should also be inspected, and, if they have been injured, they should be ligated.

Special measures to reduce postoperative pain by excising a portion of the intercostal nerve or injecting it with a long-lasting anesthetic have not appeared to be worthwhile.

Anterolateral Thoracotomy Incision

This approach may be useful for repairing a hiatal hernia or hernia through the right or left leaf of the diaphragm, or for performing some operations on the lower third of the esophagus. It may be employed on either the right or the left side, the choice depending upon which side the lesion presents. Hiatal hernias, hernias through the left diaphragm, and lesions of the lower esophagus that do not present on the right are approached through the left side of the chest. Today the anterolateral thoracotomy incision is used mostly for cardiac operation. Most surgeons tend to prefer the posterolateral approach for most types of esophageal surgery.

An anterolateral thoracotomy incision provides a more limited exposure than does a posterolateral one and frequently must be enlarged by cutting across the anterior chondral portions of the separated ribs.

TECHNIC

The patient is placed supine on the operating table with the shoulder and chest of the side to be operated upon elevated about 30 degrees on sandbags so as to permit extension of the incision posteriorly to the posterior axillary line. The arm on this side is held in 90-degree abduction by an extension board.

In the female, the breast is retracted upward.

An incision is made through the skin and subcutaneous tissue overlying the sixth or seventh rib and extending from close to the midline in front to the posterior axillary line behind (Fig. 16-28).

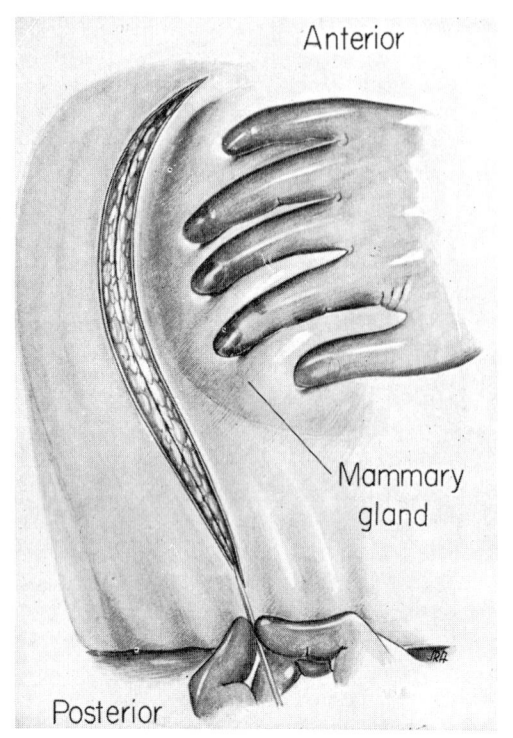

Figure 16-28. Anterolateral intercostal incision. First step: Skin incision beneath the breast with lateral extension posteriorly. (From Sweet, cited in Figure 16-20.)

The pectoralis major, serratus anterior, and sometimes a portion of the latissimus dorsi muscles are divided and retracted, exposing the ribs and intercostal spaces (Fig. 16-29). The chest is usually entered through an intercostal space without resecting a rib. The appropriate intercostal space is selected (usually the sixth or seventh for an operation on the diaphragm or lower esophagus) and the thoracic cavity is entered through this space by the technic already described for a posterolateral intercostal thoracotomy (p. 446). In completing the anterior part of this incision care must be taken to avoid injury to the internal thoracic (mammary) vessels, which run beneath the lateral margin of the sternum. If injured, or if the incision is to be extended across them, they must be divided and ligated.

If additional exposure is desired, the costal cartilages of the ribs to be separated are divided close to their sternal insertions. When this is done, the corresponding intercostal vessels and nerves must be clamped, cut, and ligated. If necessary, the incision can be extended into a thoracicoabdominal one by cutting across the costal margin.

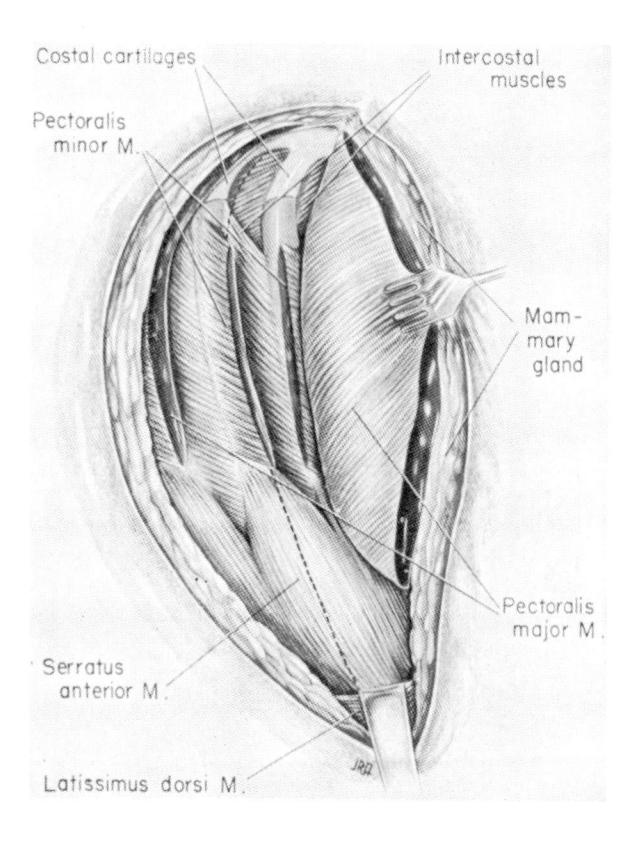

Figure 16-29. Anterolateral intercostal incision. Pectoral muscles divided and retracted, revealing the ribs and intercostal muscles beneath. (From Sweet, cited in Figure 16-20.)

MAJOR THORACOTOMY INCISIONS

Figure 16–30. Posterior extrapleural thoracotomy. Right parascapular incision. (After Potts, W. J.: Deformities of the esophagus. Surg. Clin. North Am. *31*:97, 1951.)

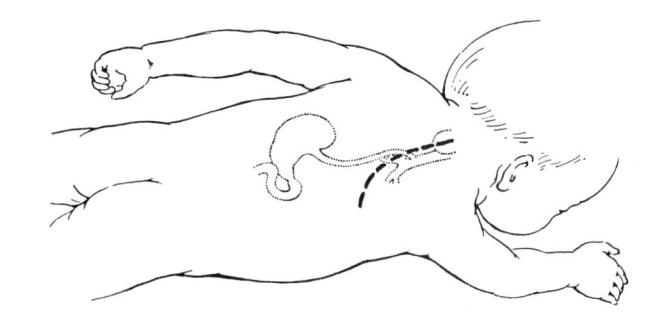

After completion of the incision, its margins are spread with Finochietto rib retractors.

This type of incision is closed in the same way as described for a posterolateral intercostal thoracotomy incision, using perichondral absorbable sutures and approximating the cut edges of the muscles with absorbable sutures.

If the anterior costal cartilages were cut across, the cut edges should be reunited with sutures of No. 30 stainless steel wire inserted through the ends of the cartilages and tied. This is essential because of the great mobility of the thoracic cage in this area.

Posterior Extrapleural Thoracotomy Incision

This approach provides a more limited exposure of the esophagus than does a transthoracic intrapleural approach. Some surgeons believe this is better tolerated (particularly by children) than an intrapleural approach, a debatable issue. The extrapleural approach does provide the advantage of draining purulent material or a fistulous tract extrapleurally without having to enter the intrapleural thoracic cavity. Realistically, even in the extrapleural thoracotomy the pleural space is frequently entered.

The posterior extrapleural thoracotomy incision is used chiefly for repairing congenital atresia of the esophagus associated with tracheoesophageal fistula but has also been employed for drainage of a posterior mediastinal abscess, esophagotomy, esophagostomy, and other operations on the thoracic esophagus. This approach to the esophagus is made from the right side to avoid the aorta.

TECHNIC

The patient is placed on the operating table in the prone position and with the right arm abducted and extended so as to draw the scapula away from the posterior midline.

A right parascapular incision is made through the skin and subcutaneous tissue. This incision begins at the right of the seventh cervical vertebra and runs downward along the vertebral border of the abducted scapula to curve around its inferior angle (Fig. 16–30). It is deepened through the subcutaneous tissue until the trapezius muscle is exposed. This muscle is divided in the direction and length of the incision. The upper portion of the latissimus dorsi muscle may also be divided. The exposed rhomboideus muscles are now divided in a vertical direction. The scapula can now be displaced laterally so that the posterior part of the ribs can be seen.

At this point there is a choice of procedures. A short posterior segment of the second, third, fourth, and fifth ribs can be subperiosteally resected (Fig. 16–31), or the greater part of the third or fourth rib can be removed. Potts (1951) found the latter to be far more satisfactory. The rib is resected subperiosteally. With a spatula or finger the pleura is carefully dissected from the ribs and vertebra, displacing it medially until the azygos vein and esophagus are exposed. If the pleura is torn during this maneuver it is immediately repaired, or the opening is covered with a moist gauze pad. The part of the azygos vein that passes forward over the lateral wall of the esophagus may be divided and ligated to increase the exposure of the esophagus.

After the operation has been completed and any required drains placed, the lung is expanded by the anesthetist, and the pleura is allowed to resume its normal position.

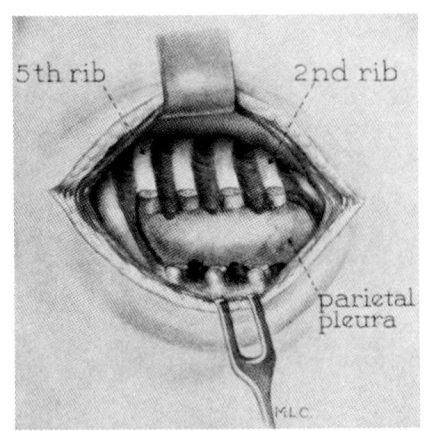

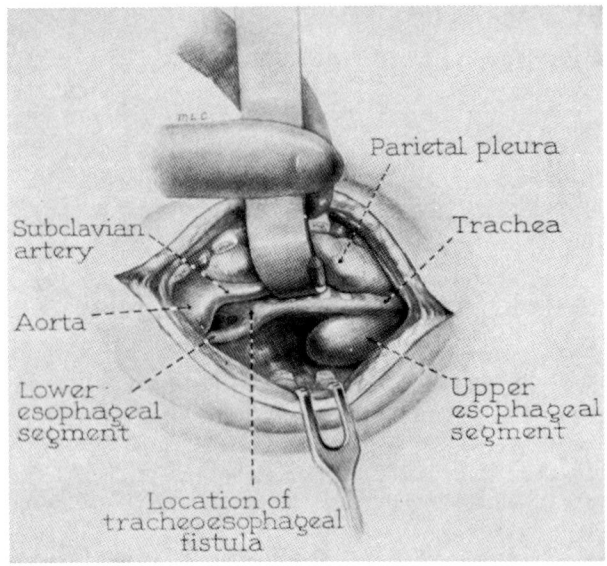

Figure 16–31. Posterior extrapleural thoracotomy *(continued).* A, Extent of costal resection. B, Exposure of esophageal anomaly. (From Haight, C., and Towsley, H. A.: Congenital atresia of esophagus with tracheoesophageal fistula; Extrapleural ligation of fistula and end-to-end anastomosis of esophageal segments. Surg. Gynecol. Obstet. 76:672, 1943.)

The severed muscles are approximated accurately in anatomic layers, preferably with running or interrupted sutures of 2–0 chromic, polyglycolic acid, or polyglactin 910 sutures. No perichondrial sutures around the ribs are necessary. The subcutaneous tissues are closed with running or interrupted sutures of 4–0 or 3–0 chromic, polyglycolic acid, or polyglactin 910 materials. The skin is closed with interrupted or running 4–0 nylon sutures.

Thoracicoabdominal (Abdominothoracic) Incision

This incision can be made on either the left or the right side. When made on the left, it provides excellent exposure of the lower portion of the esophagus, the left half of the diaphragm, the cardiac portion of the stomach, and the spleen. When made on the right it provides excellent exposure of the lower portion of the esophagus, the right half of the diaphragm, the cardiac portion of the stomach, the liver, the gallbladder, common bile duct, portal vein, hepatic artery, and inferior vena cava.

A thoracicoabdominal (abdominothoracic) incision not only provides excellent exposure of the field of operation but permits the great convenience in some operations of working both above and below the diaphragm at the same time.

The disadvantages of the incision are:

1. It opens both the pleural and abdominal cavities and, therefore, compared with an abdominal or thoracotomy incision alone, it is more shocking, is less well tolerated and exposes two cavities instead of one to the possibility of infection.

2. The incision is more tedious to close than either a thoracotomy or abdominal incision alone.

Thoracicoabdominal incisions are seldom necessary or desirable in infants or children.

A left thoracicoabdominal incision is useful for resecting a carcinoma of the lower esophagus, a total gastrectomy, elective splenectomy with an enlarged spleen, and splenorenal shunt. It may also facilitate the exposure of pancreatic cysts and removal of retroperitoneal tumor.

A right thoracicoabdominal incision is used for difficult operations on the common bile duct, portacaval shunt, and right hepatic lobectomy. It is used by some surgeons for resecting a portion of the thoracic esophagus followed by an esophagogastric anastomosis. Excellent exposure of the liver is afforded by this incision so it is used to treat major hepatic injuries.

MAJOR THORACOTOMY INCISIONS

TECHNIC

The position into which the patient is placed on the operating table will depend somewhat on the operative procedure contemplated.

For resections of the lower esophagus or upper stomach, the patient is placed on the right side.

For splenectomy or operations for hiatal hernia or splenorenal anastomosis, the patient is placed supine on the table with the left side of the chest elevated on a sandbag so as to be somewhat higher than the right (Fig. 16–32).

A right thoracoabdominal incision for portacaval anastomosis or operations on the common bile duct is usually made with the patient supine on the table with the right side elevated on a sandbag so as to be somewhat higher than the left.

An incision is made over the eighth intercostal space (see Figs. 16–1 and 16–32), extending from the midscapular line behind to pass forward to the anterior midline of the epigastrium or beyond. The latissimus dorsi, serratus anterior, and external oblique muscles are divided to expose the ribs and intercostal space and the peritoneum. The chest cavity may now be entered through an intercostal thoracotomy incision made through the seventh or eighth intercostal space (see p. 446) or by resecting the eighth or ninth rib and entering the chest through its periosteal bed. On the left side an intercostal thoracotomy incision is usually employed, but if the incision is on the right the entire eighth or ninth rib is usually resected to permit the liver to be more easily displaced upward into the right thoracic cavity and better expose the bile ducts, portal vein, and vena cava.

In either case the chest cavity is first entered near the midaxillary line so as to avoid injury to the diaphragm. The thoracotomy incision is carried forward, and the eighth and ninth or ninth costal arches are cut across to continue the incision into the peritoneal cavity. The diaphragm is divided radially toward the esophageal hiatus for as far as is necessary to provide the desired exposure. It may be extended into the esophageal hiatus if desired (Fig. 16–33).

After the operation has been completed, the incision in the diaphragm is closed by interrupted sutures of heavy No. 1 black silk, polyglycolic acid, or polyglactin 910,

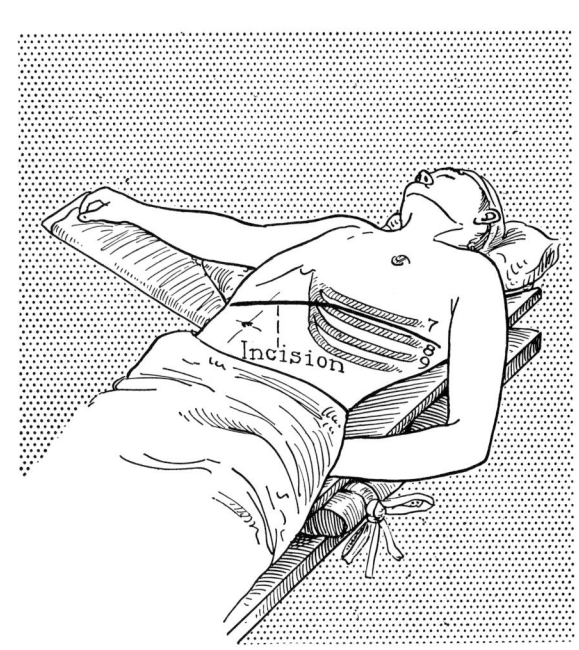

Figure 16–32. Position of the patient on the operating table for repair of esophageal hiatal hernia, splenorenal anastomosis, or total gastrectomy when the abdominothoracic approach is indicated. (From Hood, R. T., Jr., and Kirklin, J. W.: Usefulness of abdominothoracic incision. Surg. Clin. North Am. 33:1447, 1953.)

reconstructing the hiatus if it was divided. The part of the diaphragm adjacent to the costal margin cannot be closed until the costal arch is reconstructed, so the outermost two of the three diaphragmatic sutures are placed with their ends in the abdominal side of the diaphragm but are not tied until later. A separate stab wound is made in the ninth intercostal space in the posterior axillary line, and through this a chest tube is placed. If an intercostal thoracotomy incision was used, about three pericostal sutures of heavy chromic catgut, polyglycolic acid, or polyglactin 910 are placed around the ribs immediately above and below the incised intercostal space. The cut ends of the costal arches are reapposed with No. 30 stainless steel wire. The ribs are approximated with the rib approximator by the pericostal sutures, and the sutures to the costal arch are tied. The end-tied diaphragmatic sutures are now tied. Again, the lung should be expanded by the anesthesiologist.

If the incision was an intercostal one, the pleura and the intercostal muscles are closed as previously described. If a rib was removed, the cut edges of the intercostal

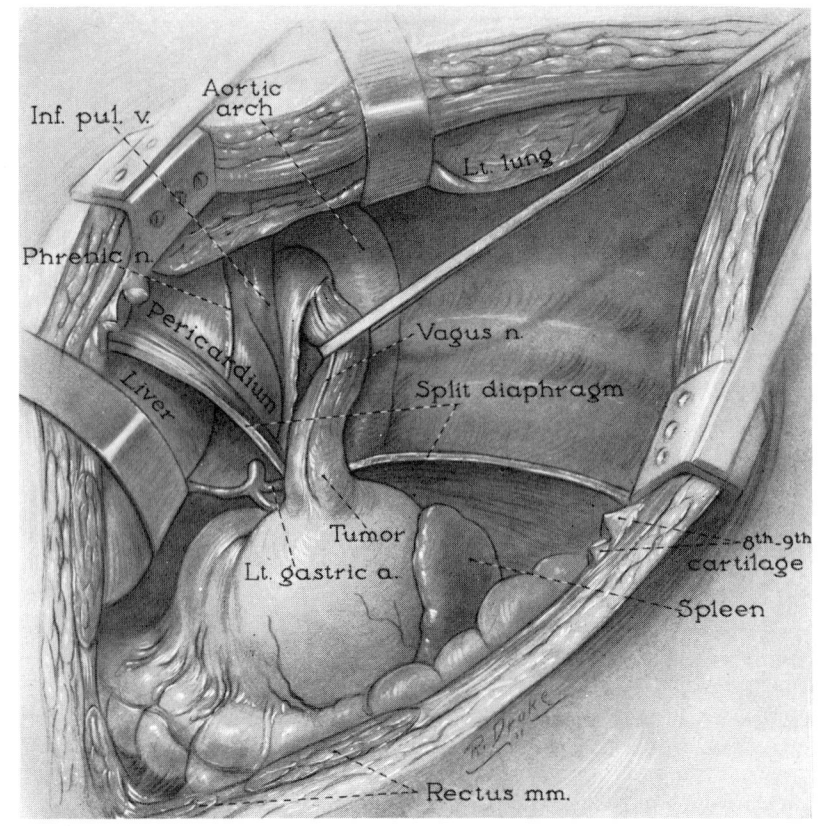

Figure 16–33. Exposure obtained through an abdominothoracic incision for performance of esophagogastrectomy for carcinoma of the lower part of the esophagus. (From Hood and Kirklin, cited in previous figure.)

muscles, periosteum, and pleura are approximated as one layer, preferably with running or interrupted sutures of 2–0 chromic, polyglycolic acid, or polyglactin 910. The cut edges of the external oblique, serratus anterior, and latissimus dorsi muscles are reapproximated in an anatomic fashion, with the deep and superficial row of preferably running or interrupted sutures of 2–0 chromic, polyglycolic acid, or polyglactin 910 sealing over the thoracic portion of the incision.

The peritoneal opening is closed with a continuous suture of 2–0 plain catgut. The anterior sheath of the rectus muscle is closed with interrupted sutures of No. 30 stainless steel wire or 0 prolene. The subcutaneous tissue and the skin of the entire thoracicoabdominal incision are closed with either running or interrupted sutures of 3–0 or 4–0 chromic, polyglycolic acid, or polyglactin 910. The skin is closed with a running or interrupted 4–0 nylon suture or stainless steel staples.

Chapter 17

EXPOSURE OF THE STOMACH AND DUODENUM

Good exposure is essential for operations on the stomach and duodenum. An upper midline incision from the xiphoid to the umbilicus offers a highly satisfactory and versatile approach for the common operations on the stomach and duodenum. It can be easily extended into an abdominothoracic incision when desired for total gastrectomy or operations upon the cardiac end of the stomach. This is accomplished by extending the incision laterally to the left at the upper end of the vertical incision (Fig. 17-1), cutting across the ninth costal cartilage and incising laterally the eighth intercostal space into the left thoracic cavity. The diaphragm can then be divided down to the esophageal hiatus. This gives an excellent exposure of the lower esophagus (Fig. 17-2), the full length of the stomach, and the proximal duodenum. Another method that may be used to extend a midline incision upward is to split the lower sternum in the midline upward to the level of the fourth or fifth intercostal space, taking care not to enter either pleural cavity (Fig. 17-3).

A right or left upper paramedian incision is also satisfactory for most operations upon the stomach or duodenum. A right transrectus incision provides adequate exposure for these procedures but has the serious defect of destroying much of the nerve and blood supply to the rectus muscle, resulting too frequently in postoperative hernia.

An upper abdominal transverse incision is used by many for operations on the stomach and pancreas. It is the incision of choice for the latter, but does not provide a comfortable exposure for operations that involve the upper portion of the stomach.

After the peritoneal cavity is entered, the stomach is identified by its relation to the inferior surface of the liver, its continuity with the anterior layer of the gastrohepatic omentum, its thick wall, the direction of its blood vessels (Fig. 17-4), its lack of longitudinal taenia and haustrations, and by its pinkish-white color and absolute opacity. The stomach and the transverse colon have

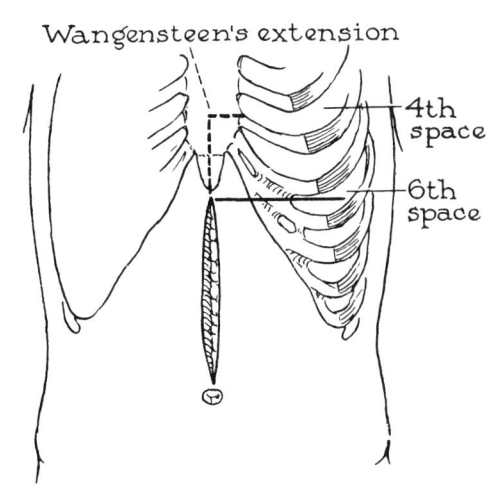

Figure 17-1. Midline incision which may be extended by splitting the sternum upward as high as the fourth intercostal space (Wangensteen) or by extending the incision laterally through the sixth intercostal space.

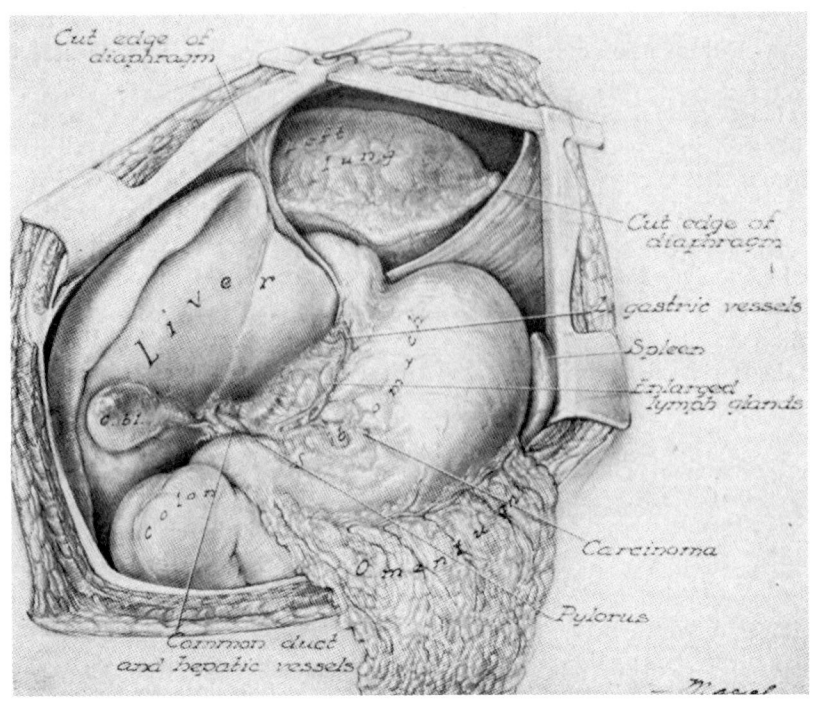

Figure 17–2. The exposure of the stomach obtained by a combined thoracicoabdominal incision. (From Carter, B. N., and Helmsworth, J. A.: Some observations on use of combined thoracicoabdominal incision. Ann. Surg. *131*:687, 1950.)

been mistaken for each other. The anterior gastric wall lies in the greater peritoneal cavity, and the posterior wall in the lesser cavity. Each is accessible by an approach through its respective cavity.

The duodenum is the first portion of the small intestine and is in distal continuity with the pylorus. Its proximal end is identified by palpating the pyloric sphincter and seeing the pyloric vein of Mayo (Fig. 17–4), which is small, runs vertically across the pylorus, is usually visible externally, and marks the gastric side of the pylorus. It is quite constant and is particularly helpful in distinguishing a gastric from a duodenal ulcer.

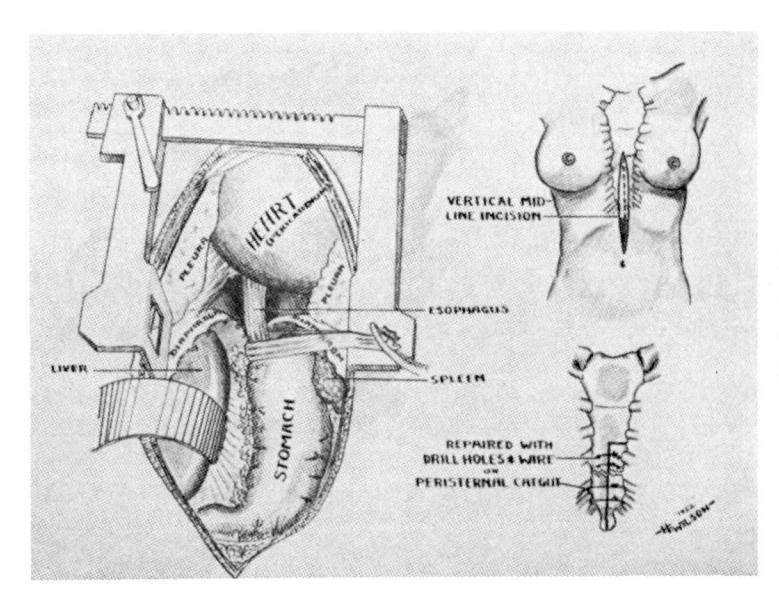

Figure 17–3. Large figure on left represents exposure for gastroesophageal resection or for repair of hiatal hernia. (From Miller, H. I.: Sternum-splitting incision for upper abdominal surgery. Arch. Surg. *65*:876, 1952.)

EXPOSURE OF THE STOMACH AND DUODENUM

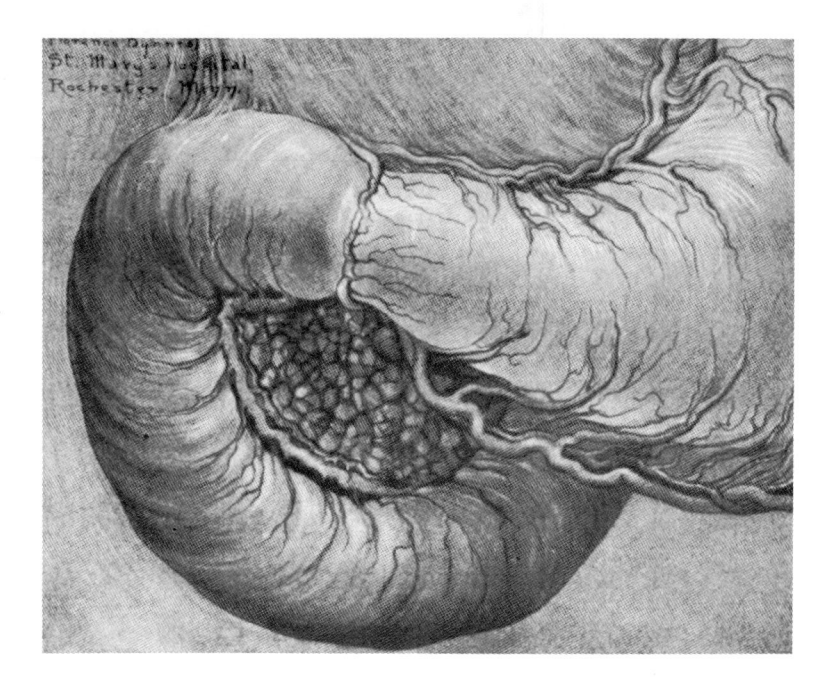

Figure 17-4. Blood vessels about the pyloric end of the stomach and duodenum, with special reference to the pyloric vein.

In humans, all of the duodenum except part of the first portion ultimately is anchored to the primitive posterior parietal peritoneum. Variations in its fusion to the posterior abdominal wall account for variations in mobility. The right colic flexure and the fixed portion of the transverse mesocolon anchor the duodenum still more firmly and render it doubly retroperitoneal.

The cap or *first portion* of the duodenum passes backward and upward toward the neck of the gallbladder for 5 cm. Its first 2.5-cm. half is surrounded by peritoneum and is quite mobile, which facilitates plastic

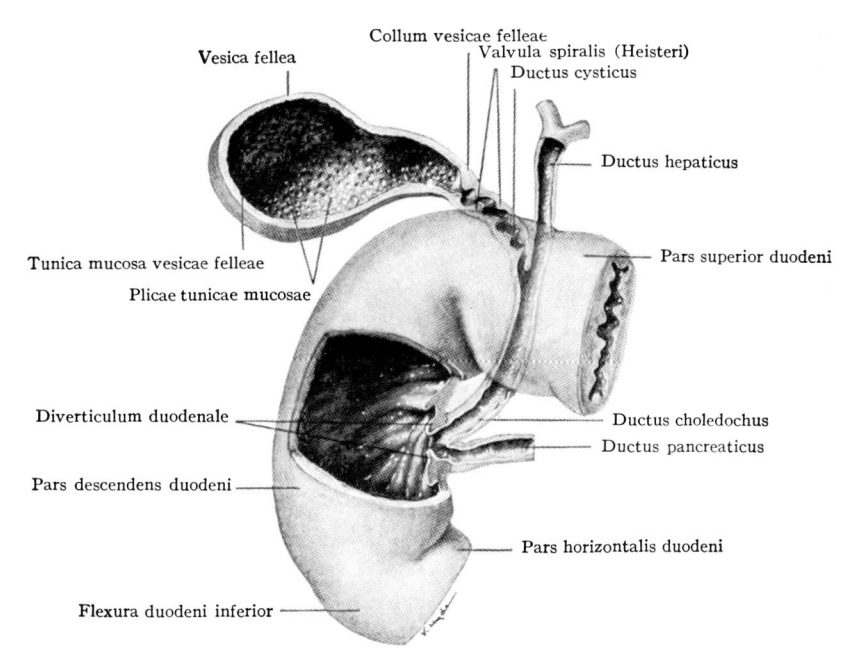

Figure 17-5. The duodenum, showing the superior, descending, and transverse portions with the relationship to the gallbladder and bile ducts.

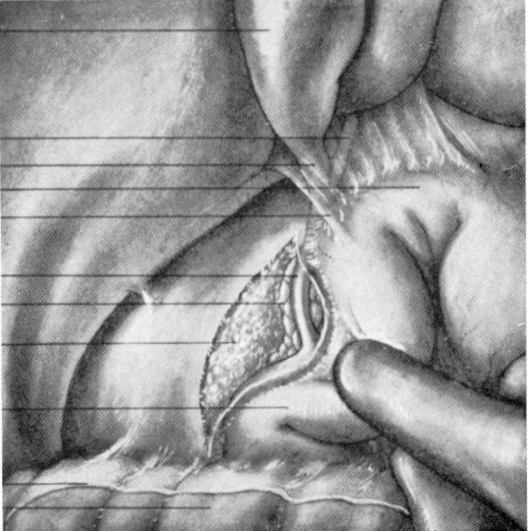

Figure 17-6. Surgical mobilization of the descending duodenum completed.

operations upon the pylorus and duodenum, but its distal 2.5 cm. part is covered only in front by peritoneum, so mobility here depends upon the elasticity of the peritoneal coat.

The *descending* (vertical) or *second portion* of the duodenum forms an acute angle (Fig. 17-5) with the first portion and is fixed in position by fusion of its lateral visceral peritoneum to the parietal peritoneum of the lateral abdominal wall. By dividing the peritoneum at the lateral edge of the upper half of the vertical segment (Kocher's maneuver, Fig. 17-6), the descending duodenum can be mobilized medially so as to render surgically accessible the retroduodenal, intrapancreatic, and intraduodenal portions of the common duct. After mobilization, the duodenum can be turned forward, downward, and to the left to bring it into position for anastomosis with the part of the stomach left after partial gastrectomy (see Billroth I partial gastrectomy with gastroduodenostomy, p. 296, or Finney pyloroplasty, p. 377).

The third or *transverse portion* of the duodenum, 12.5 cm. in length, runs horizontally to the left in front of the ureter, the inferior vena cava, lumbar spine, and aorta, and ends at the left of the third lumbar vertebra. Near its termination it is crossed by the root of the mesentery of the jejunoileum. The superior mesenteric artery runs downward over the anterior surface of the transverse duodenum to enter the root of the mesentery (Fig. 17-7). Tight stretching of the artery over this segment may cause duodenal obstruction. The pancreas is separated from the upper border of the segment by a groove in which lies the inferior pancreaticoduodenal artery (Fig. 17-7).

The *fourth* or *ascending portion* of the duodenum runs upward and slightly to the left for 2.5 cm. along the left side of the spine, to the duodenojejunal angle at the root of the transverse mesocolon. At the left of the second lumbar vertebra, the terminal part of the duodenum bends sharply downward, forward, and to the left to form the *duodenojejunal flexure*, at which point the ligament of Treitz is attached (Fig. 17-8). This is a readily recognized landmark that is found by passing a hand backward to the posterior abdominal wall behind the greater omentum and palpating upward along the left of the spine until the flexure is located.

Although more difficult to expose than the first and second portions, the third and fourth portions of the duodenum can be exposed satisfactorily by the method of Cattell and Braasch (1960), which is based on raising the mesentery of the small bowel and right half of the colon along the line of fusion of the mesentery of the right half of the colon to the posterior parietes (Figs. 17-9 and 17-10). The initial dissection is started by severing the lateral attachments

EXPOSURE OF THE STOMACH AND DUODENUM

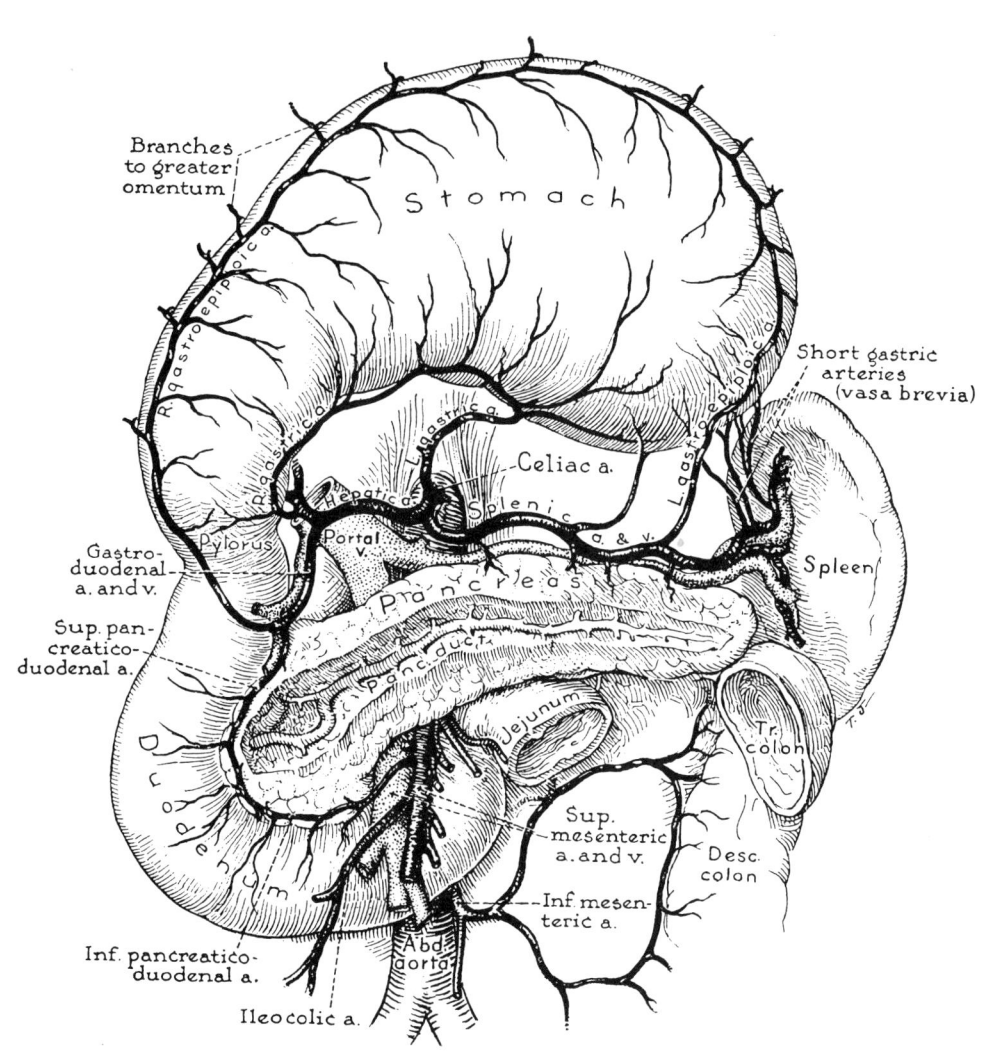

Figure 17-7. Blood supply of the stomach, duodenum, spleen, and pancreas. The stomach is shown reflected upward and the pancreatic duct is exposed. (Jones and Shepard: A Manual of Surgical Anatomy.)

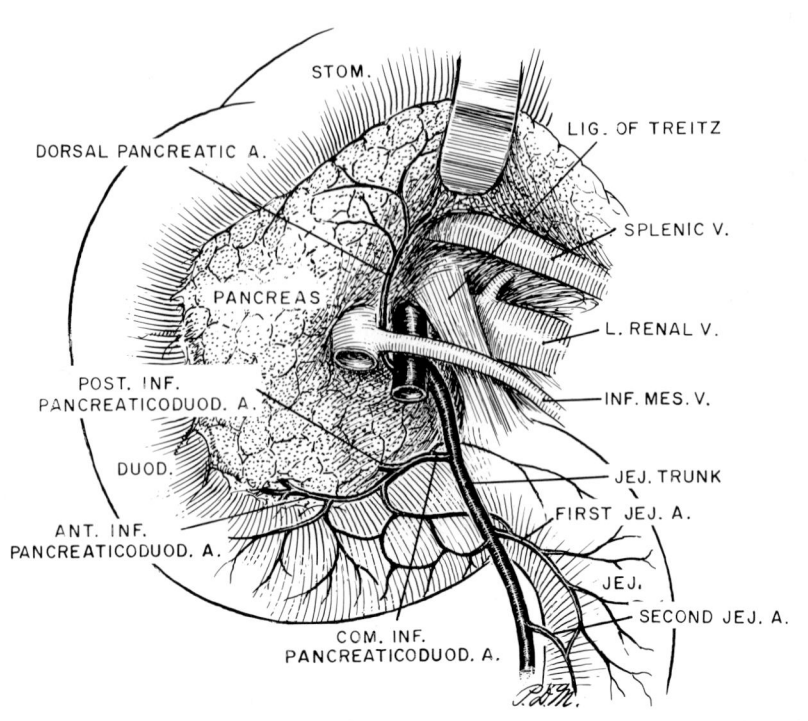

Figure 17–8. The duodenojejunal junction. The superior mesenteric vein and artery have been removed to show the detail of arterial supply to the bowel. The artery gives off an anomalous branch to the pancreas and a special jejunal trunk. (From Edwards, E. A., Malone, P. D., and MacArthur, J. D.: Operative Anatomy of Abdomen and Pelvis. Philadelphia, Lea and Febiger, 1975, p. 133.)

of the cecum and right half of the colon (Fig. 17–9A). This line of cleavage is developed (see Fig. 17–9B, which shows the planned retroperitoneal dissection) until the cecum and ascending colon and the mesentery of the small intestine, along with the superior mesenteric artery and vein, are mobilized completely and turned up like an apron. Figure 17–10 shows exposure after mobilization is completed; complete exposure of the third and fourth portions of the duodenum is obtained. The superior mesenteric vessels are clearly seen as they cross the duodenum. If desired, the duodenojejunal junction can be mobilized by dividing the suspensory ligament of Treitz while avoiding injury to the nearby inferior mesenteric vein which crosses it (see Fig. 17–8). After Treitz's ligament is divided, the terminal duodenum can be pushed to the right under the superior mesenteric vessels. The blood supply for the duodenum to the left of the mesenteric artery is derived from that vessel and enters anteromedially.

Although the duodenum here can be separated from the pancreas, the inferior pancreaticoduodenal vessels must be avoided. Cattell and Braasch (1960) warned that "if resection of portions of the duodenum is required, the surgeon must safeguard the short branches of the first portion of the superior mesenteric artery which supply the proximal portion of the jejunum." For this reason, any dissection for removal of portions of the duodenum should be performed close to the duodenal wall. They reported one patient in whom the third portion of the duodenum was resected and continuity successfully restored by end-to-end anastomosis; they found this maneuver for exposure and direct visualization to be useful for dealing with neoplasm, ulceration, or perforation occurring in the third and fourth portions of the duodenum.

We have also successfully performed a segmental resection of a portion of the second portion of the duodenum for an arteriovenous malformation causing upper gastrointestinal bleeding in a 68-year-old woman.

The operation is concluded by replacing the right half of the colon and the small intestine in their normal positions within the abdominal cavity. No effort is made to

EXPOSURE OF THE STOMACH AND DUODENUM 461

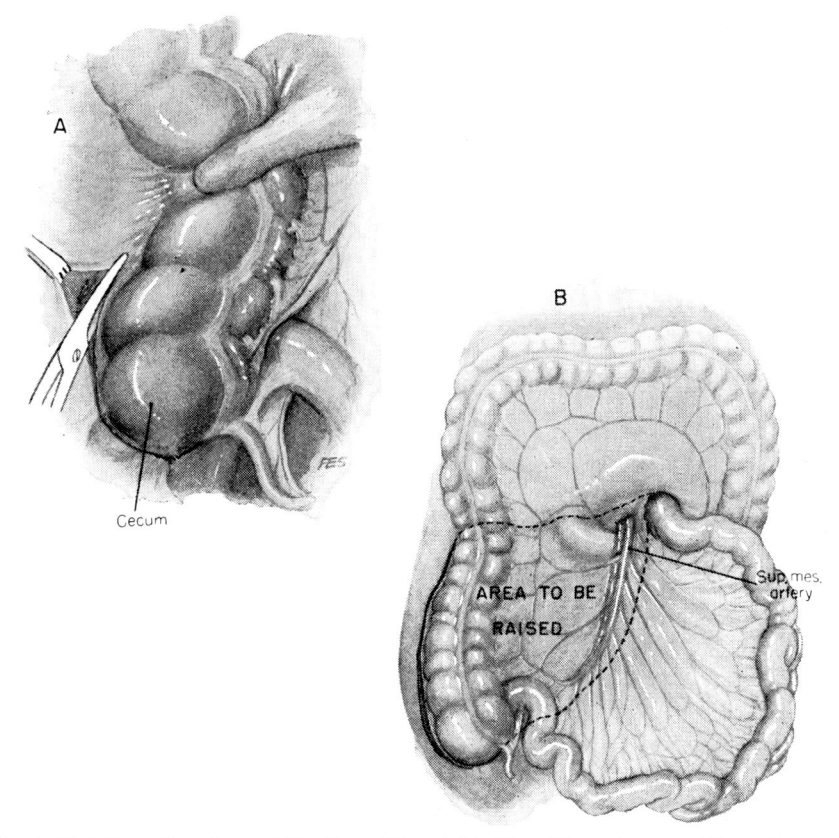

Figure 17-9. Initial dissection for mobilization of the right side of the colon, small intestine, and mesentery. (From Cattell, R. B., and Braasch, J. W.: A technique for the exposure of the third and fourth portions of the duodenum. Surg. Gynecol. Obstet. *111*:380, 1960.)

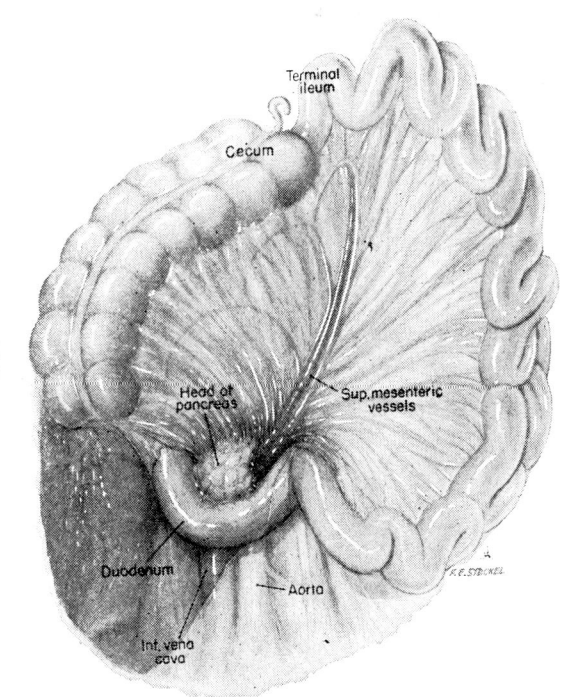

Figure 17-10. Exposure obtained of the third and fourth portions of the duodenum. (From Cattell and Braasch, cited in previous figure.)

GASTROTOMY

Opening of the stomach by incision, followed by its closure at the same operation, is termed "exploratory gastrotomy."

INDICATIONS

Gastrotomy may be performed for exploration of the interior of the stomach; removal of foreign bodies from the stomach or from the lower end of the esophagus; repair of stomach wounds; control of gastric hemorrhage; treatment of gastric ulcer; removal of pedunculated gastric tumors; dilation of an esophageal or pyloric stricture; and operation upon the posterior wall of the stomach. Technically speaking, any procedure that involves opening of the stomach necessitates gastrotomy.

Recently Schwartz (1976) introduced an additional indication for gastrotomy: for treating serious cases of drug poisoning in which the swallowed drug has formed a drug-containing mass persisting in the stomach. Delayed absorption produces continued worsening of the patient's condition despite treatment with the usual supportive methods, gastric lavage, hemodialysis, and peritoneal dialysis. When gastroscopy shows the drug-containing mass to be too large and gelatinous for removal with the gastroscope, gastrotomy is indicated.

Schwartz reported a 56-year-old woman brought to the emergency department 4 hours after ingesting 36 g. of meprobamate. Initially she was lethargic, with a blood pressure of 130 mm. Hg and a pulse rate of 112 per minute. She rapidly became comatose. An oral endotracheal tube was inserted. Gastric lavage returned cloudy liquid. After lavage with 10 liters of physiologic saline, 30 g. of activated charcoal and a cathartic were instilled. Controlled mechanical ventilation maintained arterial blood gases in the normal range. Two hours after admission, frequent premature ventricular contractions developed, which were treated with lidocaine and resolved after 2 hours. Infusions of physiologic saline and dopamine were necessary to maintain blood pressure and urinary output over the next 24 hours.

Sixteen hours after admission, the patient was still deeply comatose and the meprobamate level was 11.4 mg./dl. Gastroscopy showed a large mass of gelatinous material in the stomach, some of which adhered to the endoscope after withdrawal.

Eighteen hours after admission, hemodialysis was performed for 11.5 hours, and the coma lightened. The meprobamate level decreased to 8.4 mg./dl. Coma deepened over the next 4 hours, and the serum meprobamate level rose to 12.6 mg./dl.

A second gastroscopy showed no decrease in the size of the mass. Forty hours after admission, a tarry mass weighing 140 g. was removed by gastrotomy. The tarry mass was dried and 24.9 g. of meprobamate were eluted from it, demonstrating that large amounts of the drug may remain in the stomach. Eight hours after the operation and a 6-hour hemodialysis, the meprobamate level fell to 2.1 mg./dl., the patient began to respond to verbal stimuli, and the endotracheal tube was removed. Pneumonia and anemia ensued but resolved without further complications. The patient was transferred to the psychiatric service.

Schwartz pointed out that most patients with meprobamate intoxication can be treated with the usual supportive measures; however, in addition to hemodialysis and gastroscopy, surgical removal of a drug-containing mass from the stomach may be necessary in those in whom the clinical condition, drug levels, and endoscopy point to the persistence of such a mass. Drugs other than meprobamate may cause the same problem and also require gastrotomy.

TECHNIC

General inhalation, local infiltration, or regional anesthesia may be used.

Adequate exposure of the stomach for simple gastrotomy may be obtained via an upper median or a right or left paramedian abdominal incision. After the peritoneal cavity is opened, the stomach is identified. The general peritoneal cavity is packed off with gauze pads.

The stomach can be opened transversely or longitudinally. Incision in the long axis of the stomach gives better exposure of the

GASTROTOMY

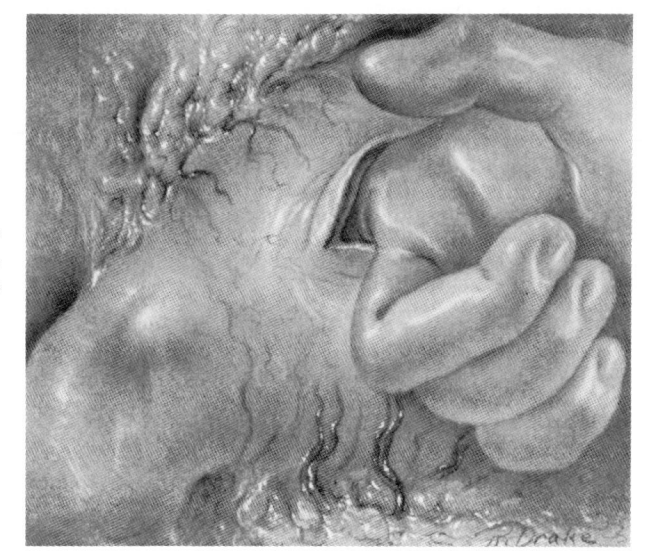

Figure 17-11. Digital exploration of the duodenum. (From Eusterman, G. B., and Balfour, D. C.: The Stomach and Duodenum. Philadelphia, W. B. Saunders Company, 1935.)

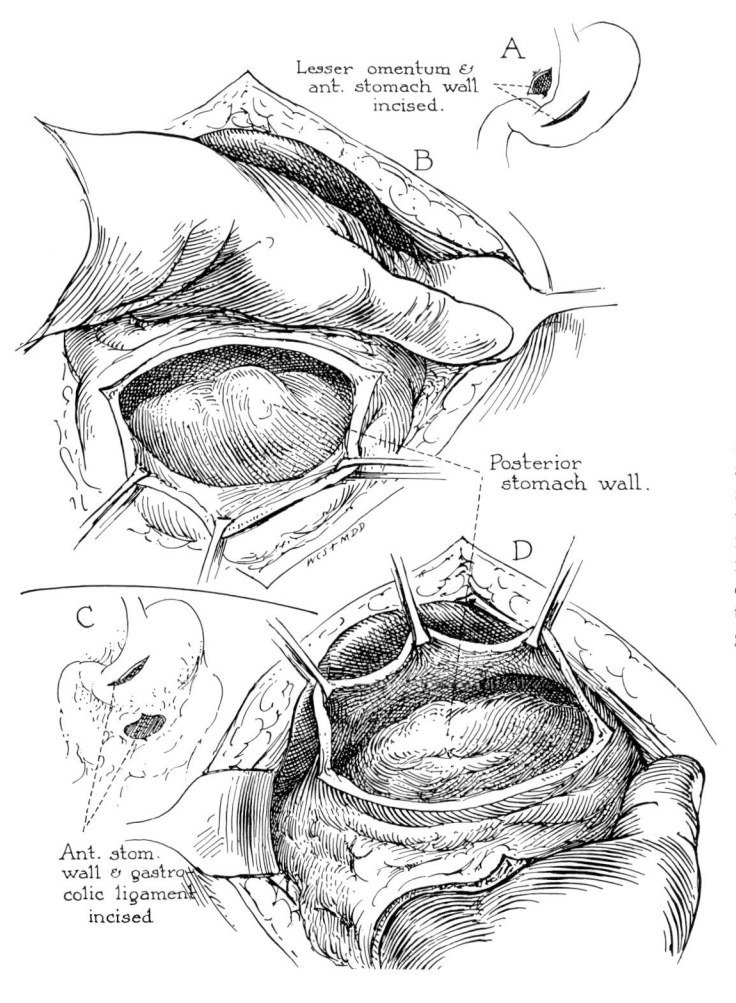

Figure 17-12. Examination of stomach mucosa through an anterior axial incision. *A* and *B*, The posterior stomach wall is pressed up into the retracted anterior incision with the fingers inserted posteriorly through an opening in the lesser omentum. *C* and *D*, Further examination is facilitated by inserting the fingers through an opening in the gastrocolic ligament.

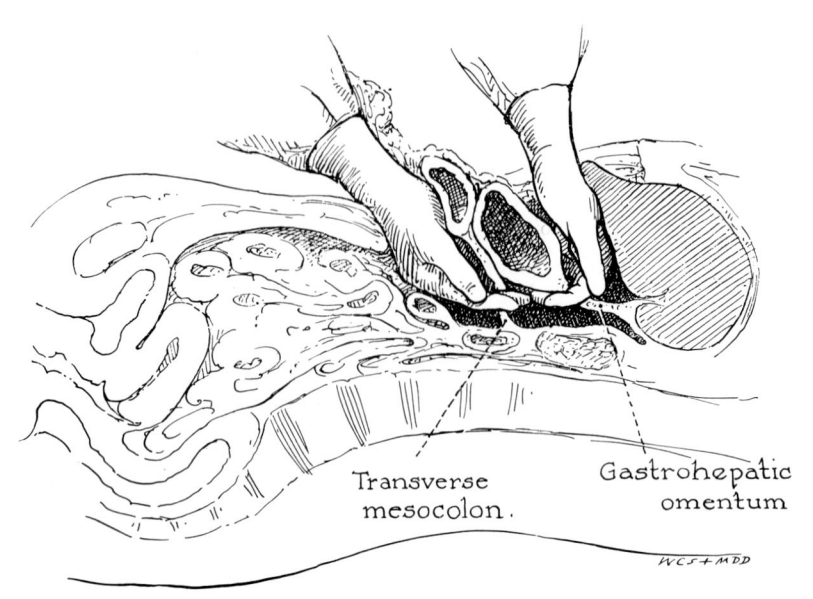

Figure 17-13. Bimanual palpation of the posterior wall of the stomach. The fingers of the left hand are shown passing through the gastrohepatic omentum, and those of the right hand through the transverse mesocolon. The fingers meet upon the posterior stomach wall within the lesser peritoneal cavity.

interior than does a transverse incision, but causes more bleeding. Selection of the site and the direction and length of the gastrotomy incision depend upon the purpose of the operation and the exposure desired.

The portion of the anterior gastric wall to be incised is held in an exposed position within the area of the retracted abdominal wound by use of a traction suture or Babcock clamp grasping the gastric wall at each end of the intended gastrotomy incision. With these ends under traction in opposite directions, an opening large enough to admit an exploring finger is made through all the coats of the stomach into its lumen, avoiding large vessels. Immediately a traction suture or Babcock forceps is placed on each lip of the stomach to be explored, for retraction of its walls. A suction tube is inserted and the gastric contents are aspirated through the small opening, the edges of which are elevated by forceps to prevent the escape of gastric contents. Any material left behind is then removed with sponges.

The stomach opening then is enlarged to the required size. Bleeding vessels in the wound margins must be ligated carefully. The interior is explored by introducing a finger (Fig. 17-11) or by retracting the edges of the incision with a pair of small retractors. To better inspect the posterior wall it is often helpful to pass two sponge sticks, each containing a small sponge, through the incision and to flatten out the posterior wall between them. If only a small portion of the interior of the stomach is to be treated through the gastrotomy opening, that part can be isolated by two compression clamps applied across the stomach through the gastrocolic ligament from the greater to the lesser curvature.

Examination of the mucosa of much of the stomach can be accomplished by passing two fingers through an incision in a comparatively bloodless part of the gastrocolic ligament just below the stomach or in the gastrohepatic ligament above the stomach (Fig. 17-12) and pressing the posterior stomach wall up through the incision in the anterior stomach wall. The abdominal esophagus may be difficult to locate from within the stomach because its orifice is concealed in folds of mucous membrane.

If adhesions within the lesser sac are not extensive, a very thorough palpation of the posterior wall of the stomach can be made by inserting the fingers on one hand through an incision in the gastrohepatic omentum and those of the other hand through an incision in the transverse mesocolon. The fingers meet upon the posterior wall of the stomach (Fig. 17-13).

After the purpose of the operation is accomplished, the stomach wall is closed.

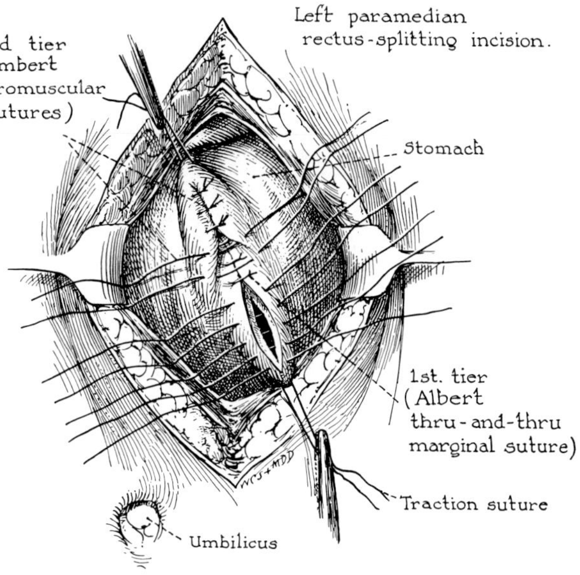

Figure 17-14. Transverse closure of a longitudinal gastrotomy incision. A traction suture was placed centrally on each of the superior and inferior margins of the longitudinal incision, and traction on them has converted the incision into a transverse one.

TECHNIC OF CLOSURE OF GASTROTOMY INCISION

The incision is usually closed transversely to the long axis of the stomach, but may be closed longitudinally if located in a wide part of the stomach. A traction suture (Fig. 17-14) is placed on each of the superior and inferior edges of the incision so that traction on them converts the incision into a transverse one.

The mucosae are then inverted and approximated by a continuous Connell suture (see Fig. 22-11) of 2-0 plain catgut swaged on a noncutting-edge atraumatic intestinal needle. This suture is tied at each end and the ends left uncut to serve as traction sutures. The traction sutures originally placed are then removed.

A Marshall U-stitch (see Fig. 22-13) of silk is placed at each angle extending beyond the Connell suture in such a way that the angles and the knots of the uncut ends of the Connell suture are cut and the U-sutures are tied, thus burying the knots of the Connell suture and snugly inverting the dangerous angles of the incision.

The closure is completed by placing a second tier of silk sutures beginning beyond the U-suture at one end of the incision and finishing just beyond the U-suture at the other end of the incision. This suture may be continuous or interrupted. If continuous it may be a Cushing suture or a running Lembert suture (see Fig. 22-3). If interrupted sutures are used, a row of Lembert stitches or Halsted mattress sutures should be used. After this row of sutures has been completed and tied, a small part of the greater omentum may be sutured loosely over the closure for additional security.

If preferred the opening may be closed by the use of an appropriate TA (thoracoabdominal) stapler (see p. 583). After closure by either method the stomach is then dropped back into place. Intraperitoneal drainage is unnecessary. The abdominal wound is closed tightly except, if desired, for a soft Penrose drain placed beneath the muscle and fascia down to the peritoneal layer. If a drain is left, it may be removed in 48 hours. Postoperatively, a Levin nasogastric tube is left indwelling in the stomach. Through it the stomach contents are removed by gentle suction and later are allowed to siphon into a bedside receptacle. Nothing other than plain water is permitted by mouth until peristalsis returns. Then the tube is removed and oral feeding commenced.

GASTRORRHAPHY

Gastrorrhaphy is the closure of a wound of the stomach. Its chief object is to prevent leakage of stomach contents into the peritoneal cavity. Wounds of the stomach may be caused by trauma, disease, or a planned surgical operation; hence, gastrorrhaphy is a part of all operations upon the stomach.

Openings into the stomach are more safely closed than openings in any other part of the gastrointestinal tract, for the following reasons:

1. The stomach is mobile and therefore it is relatively easy to expose all parts of it, excepting possibly the cardiac end, and to approximate incised edges without tension.

2. Its walls are thick and sutures are easy to place and may include substantial bites of tissue without penetrating into the lumen.

3. The stomach has a profuse blood supply so that the danger of ischemic necrosis is minimal.

4. Visceral peritoneum which quickly adheres to itself and seals over the anastomosis covers the stomach.

5. The bacterial flora of the stomach is either minimal or absent so that infection is not likely to occur.

6. The gastric lumen is so wide that there is little danger of obstruction resulting from a constriction caused by its repair by suture except at the pyloric and cardiac ends.

Wounds of the stomach should be closed in two layers. Before beginning the repair, damaged nonviable margins should be excised back to normal healthy tissue.

In repairing wounds or incisions into the stomach, there are three fundamental aims:

(1) to insure a watertight closure;
(2) to insure hemostasis; and
(3) to avoid obstruction or stenosis of the gastric lumen.

To accomplish this, one must make certain that all the mucosa is inverted into the gastric lumen. If any mucosa projects through the suture line to the outside of the stomach wall, leakage will occur with resulting fistula formation or peritonitis.

Every effort should be made to approximate the gastric mucosa by suture in all wounds of the stomach. If not sutured, the gastric mucosal edges retract, thus exposing the underlying submucosal blood vessels which become eroded and may cause subsequent hemorrhage simulating that of acute peptic ulceration.

Nonabsorbable sutures should not be used to penetrate all the layers of the stomach and remain exposed within its lumen. Leakage may occur along the suture tract from within the lumen through the stomach wall and cause local irritation and infection. For these reasons absorbable material (for example, 2-0 chromic catgut or Dexon) is used for any suture that will remain within the lumen of the stomach, such as the suture approximating the mucosa. The mucosal suture is usually continuous, as continuous sutures are more watertight and hemostatic than are interrupted sutures. The weakest period in any gastrointestinal suture consisting of catgut is from the sixth to the tenth day. By the sixth day the catgut is beginning to weaken while organic union is not appreciable before the tenth day. Synthetic polyglycolic sutures are absorbable and more durable than catgut, so are often used for the mucosal suture.

In addition, relatively broad surfaces of the serosal coat should be approximated, as serosal surfaces quickly heal adherent to each other and seal over the closure. This is accomplished by a second (outer) layer of either continuous or interrupted Lembert seromuscular silk sutures, thus completing the two-layer closure of the stomach.

Before closing the abdomen the completed gastric closure should be examined carefully for evidence of bleeding, leakage, or obstruction in the pyloric and cardiac areas so that such flaws can be corrected and their occurrence as postoperative complications prevented. A nasogastric tube is left in place for postoperative decompression until healing has occurred and peristalsis has returned. The need for abdominal drainage varies with individual cases.

Gastrorrhaphy may be performed by hand-suturing as described above, or by stapling, the technics of which are described in the section on mechanical suturing. The former is more adaptable to unforeseen anatomic circumstances and is the more widely used.

Chapter 18

ABDOMINAL INCISIONS

The abdominal portions of the alimentary tract lie within the abdominal cavity and are usually approached through incisions made in the abdominal wall.

A large variety of abdominal incisions have been devised for operations upon the abdominal portion of the alimentary tract. In order to discuss their relative merits and demerits, it is essential to describe the anatomy of the abdominal wall.

ANATOMY

Layers of the Abdominal Wall

The abdominal wall consists of seven layers (Fig. 18–1) of tissue, of which the fourth or middle layer, the muscle-bone layer, is the most important. These layers will be considered in the order in which

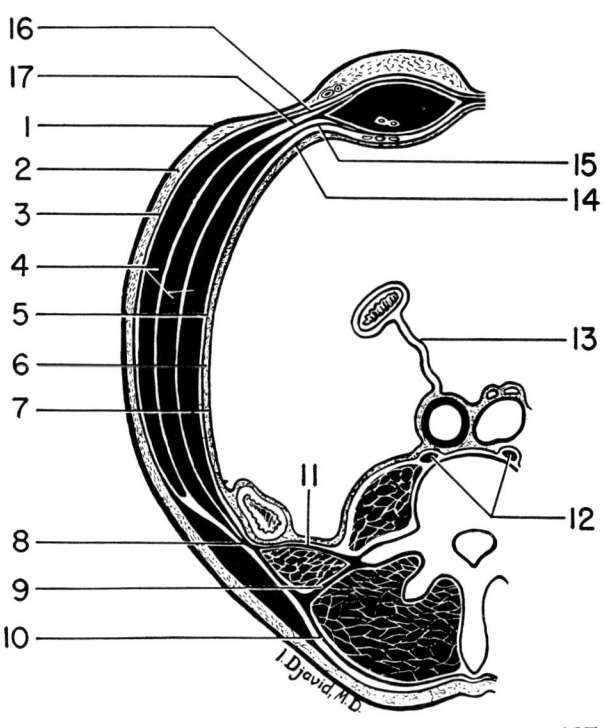

Figure 18–1. Cross section of seven layers of abdominal wall. 1, Skin — first layer. 2, Superficial fascia — second layer. 3, Deep fascia — third layer. 4, External oblique, internal oblique, transversus abdominis muscles of the fourth or muscle-bone layer. Each muscle has fascial layer on superficial and deep aspects. 5, Transversalis fascia — fifth layer. 6, Extraperitoneal or subserous fat of sixth layer. 7, Peritoneum — seventh layer. 8, Fusion point of three layers of lumbodorsal fascia. 9, Middle layer of lumbodorsal fascia. 12, Right and left sympathetic trunks behind inferior vena cava and aorta, respectively. 13, Peritoneum reflected off posterior abdominal wall as mesentery of intestine. 14, Transversalis fascia — also lines abdominal cavity but is not reflected onto viscera. 15, Aponeurosis of transversus abdominis fusing to posterior rectus sheath. 16, Aponeurosis of external oblique fusing to anterior rectus sheath. 17, Aponeurosis of internal oblique splitting to form anterior and posterior rectus sheath.
(From Lampe, E. W.: Surgical anatomy of the abdominal wall. Surg. Clin. North Am. 32:545, 1952.)

467

they are encountered while progressing from without inward.

1. SKIN

The skin is the outermost layer. The course of the connective bundles of the corium forms lines of tension (Langer's lines of cleavage) in the skin. Over the anterior abdomen these lines of cleavage run in a more or less transverse direction (Fig. 18–2). Skin incisions made parallel to these lines of cleavage result in much finer scars than do those that cut across the lines of cleavage. This factor is not of primary importance in selecting an abdominal incision, but it may be taken into consideration if other factors are equal and for those patients in whom the cosmetic result is important.

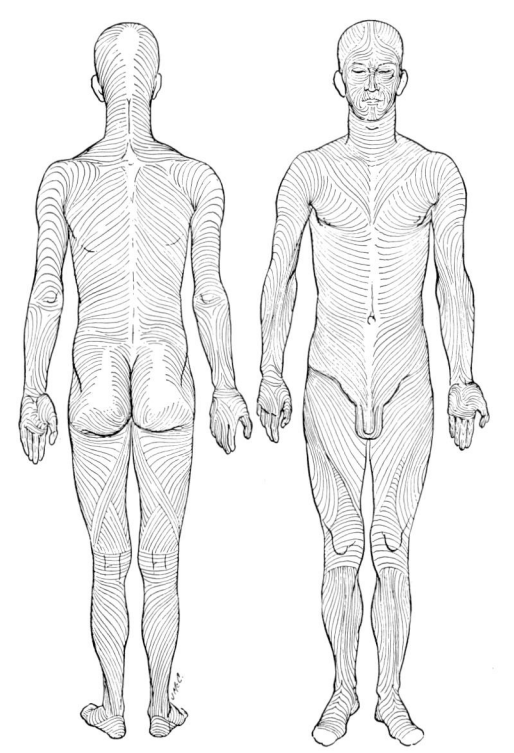

Figure 18–2. Lines of tension of the skin (Langer). The general course of the connective tissue bundles of the corium determines the direction of these linear clefts. Whenever possible, incisions should follow these lines, since there will then be little gaping of the wound and a subsequent fine scar. Broader scars follow incisions across the lines.

2. SUBCUTANEOUS TISSUE

This consists of fat, which is variable in amount, contained within fibrous compartments. The more superficial portion of the subcutaneous fat contains much less fibrous tissue than does the deeper portion. This is called Camper's fascia. It continues beneath the skin to envelop the body. The deeper portion of the subcutaneous tissue of the abdominal wall contains more fibrous elements and forms a membranous fascial layer (Scarpa's fascia), which is separated from the underlying deep fascia by areolar tissue. Scarpa's fascia extends a few centimeters below the inguinal ligament to fuse with the deep fascia (fascia lata) of the thigh. This more superficial fascia continues over the penis and the surface of the spermatic cord and eventually forms the dartos layer. In the midline, Scarpa's fascia fuses with the deep fascia to form the fundiform ligament of the penis.

These inferior attachments of Scarpa's fascia explain why urine extravasated from a ruptured urethra often extends upward toward the costal margin rather than downward over the thigh, and also why femoral hernias tend to progress up over the inguinal ligament rather than down toward the knee.

Both Camper's and Scarpa's fasciae have a relatively poor blood supply, which causes them to heal slowly and to become easily infected. Scarpa's fascia is the only one of the two layers that is sufficiently strong and well defined to be readily sutured.

3. DEEP FASCIA

The deep fascia of the abdominal wall is an ill defined, thin, and unimportant layer consisting of loosely formed fibrous tissue. It can be demonstrated more easily on the muscular part of the external oblique muscle than on its aponeurosis where it is quite firmly adherent. It is connected loosely to the overlying Scarpa's fascia by areolar tissue.

The deep fascia extends along the spermatic cord to form the external spermatic fascia, and along the penis where it is called Buck's fascia.

4. MUSCLE-BONE LAYER

This is the most important of the seven layers, consisting of nine muscles, with their fasciae and aponeuroses on each side of the midline, and the five lumbar vertebrae situated posteriorly. This layer will be described in more detail.

On either side of the anterior midline (linea alba) of the abdomen are situated the right and left rectus abdominis and pyramidalis muscles (Fig. 18–3). These muscles form the anterior group. Their fibers run in a vertical direction and are enveloped between the anterior and posterior rectus sheaths, formed by a splitting of the aponeuroses of the internal oblique muscles (see Fig. 18–1).

Lateral to the anterior group are the external oblique, internal oblique, and

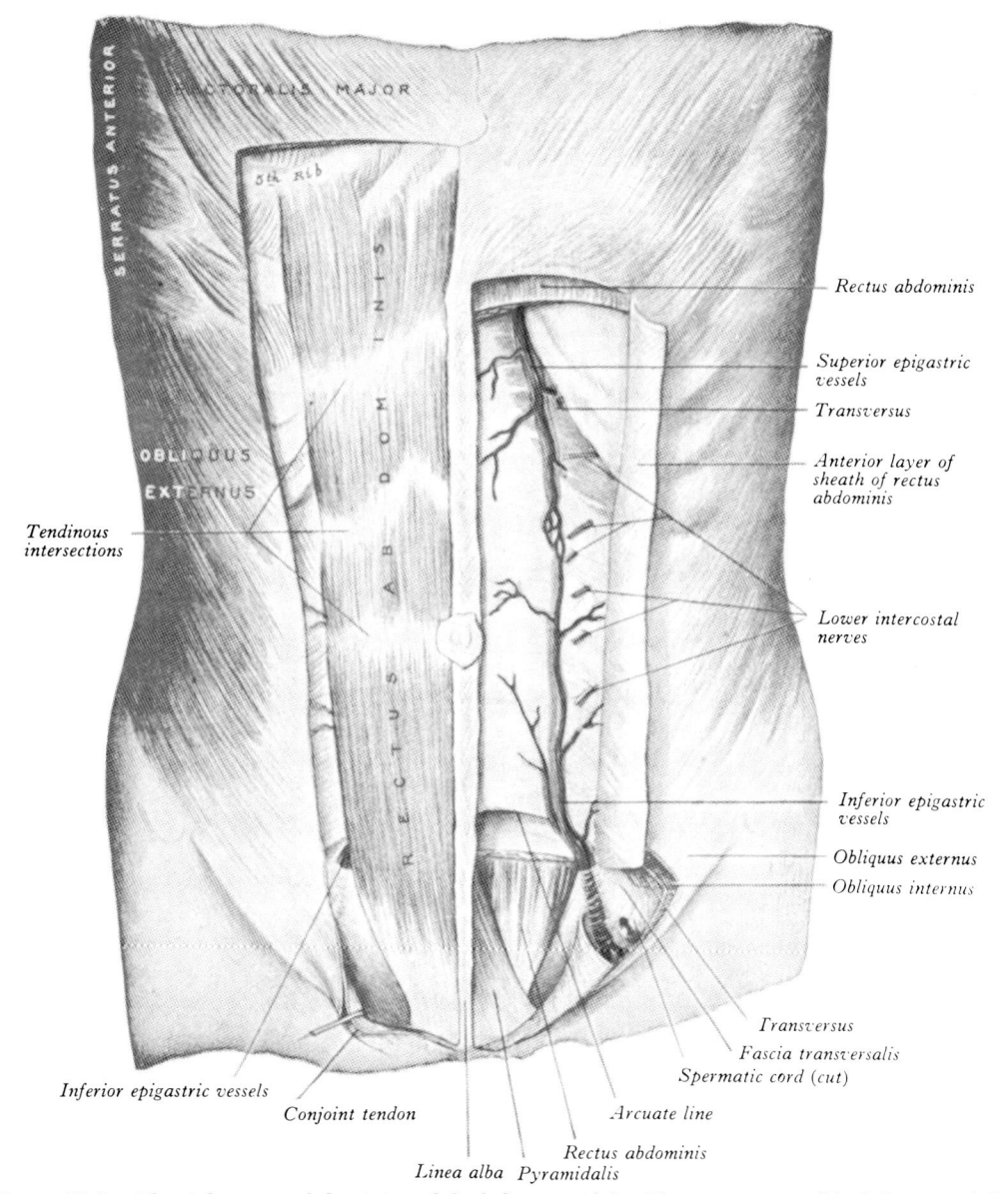

Figure 18–3. The right rectus abdominis and the left pyramidalis. The greater part of the left rectus abdominis has been removed to show the superior and inferior epigastric vessels. (From Williams, P. L., and Warwick, R. (eds.): Gray's Anatomy, 36th Br. ed. Philadelphia, W. B. Saunders Compnay, 1980.)

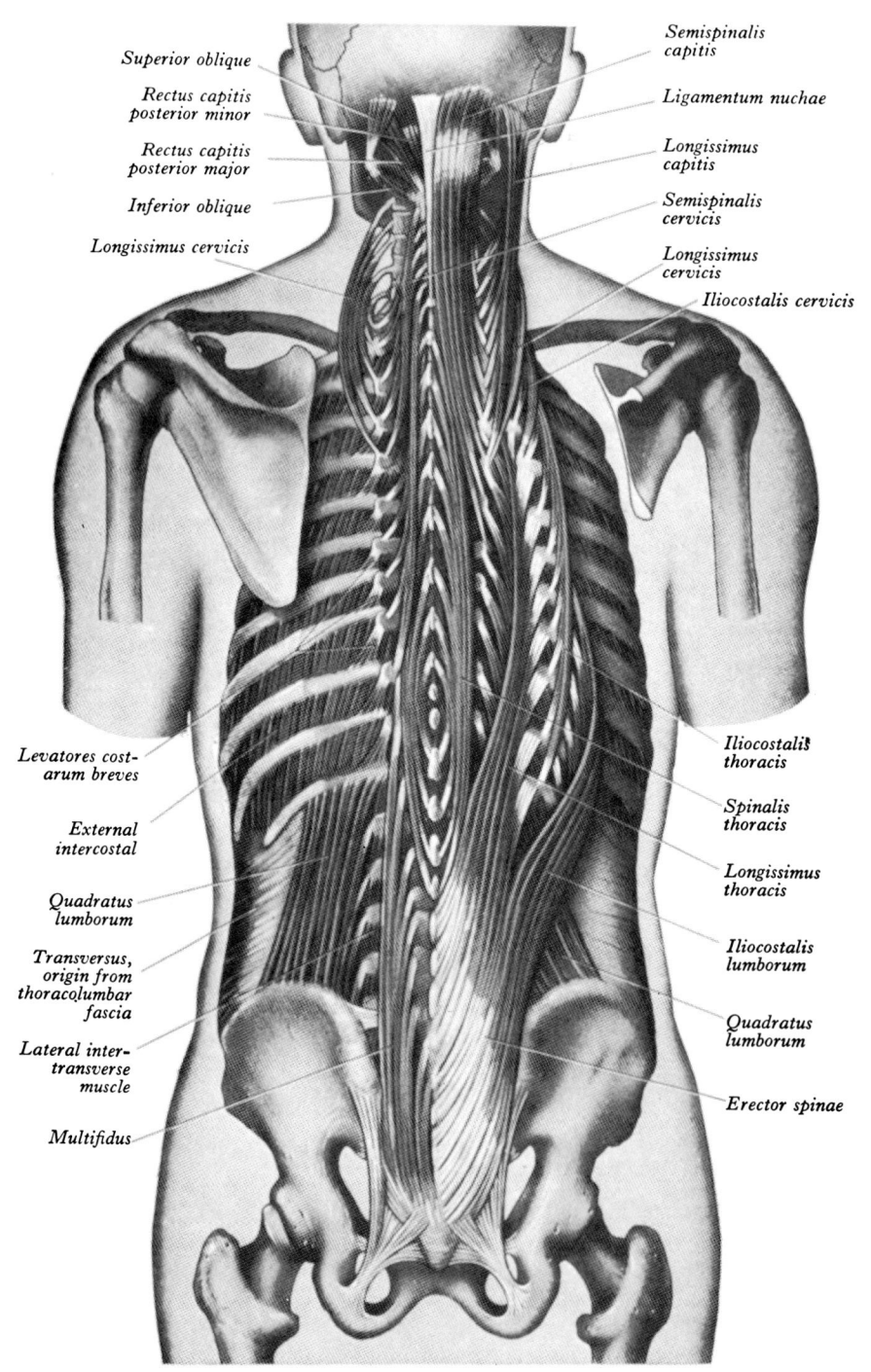

Figure 18–4. The deep muscles of the back. On the left side the erector spinae and its upward continuations (with the exception of the longissimus cervicis, which has been displaced laterally) and the semispinalis capitis have been removed. (From Williams and Warwick, cited in preceding figure.)

transversus abdominis muscles with their fasciae and aponeuroses (see Figs. 18-3 and 18-5). These three muscles form the flat or oblique group, extending laterally and posteriorly from the lateral border of the rectus abdominis practically to the lateral border of the posteriorly situated quadratus lumborum muscle. The direction of their fibers is closer to transverse than to vertical.

The posterior portion on each side of the posterior midline of this muscle-bone layer consists of the quadratus lumborum, the psoas major, the sacrospinalis (erector spinae), and the lower portion of the latissimus dorsi muscles. These four muscles comprise the posterior group, and the direction of their fibers is vertical (see Fig. 16-16, p. 438, and Fig. 18-4).

The posterior midline of this layer is formed by the lumbar vertebrae with their transverse processes.

These structures will now be described individually in greater detail.

Anterior and Lateral (Oblique) Abdominal Muscles and Related Structures

The paired *rectus abdominis muscle* (one on each side) is attached below to the os pubis and ligaments of the symphysis pubis, while superiorly it is attached to the xiphoid cartilage and the anterior surfaces of the fifth, sixth, and seventh ribs. The superior attachment is three to four times as broad as the pubic insertion, hence the muscle is thick and narrow below the umbilicus while it is thin and wide in its upper portion. As a result, an upper abdominal transverse incision may extend laterally almost to the anterior axillary line without passing beyond the lateral margin of the rectus muscle.

The rectus muscle is crossed by three transverse tendinous intersections, one of which is located at or near the level of the umbilicus. The other two are about equally spaced between it and the costal margin. Occasionally a fourth intersection is present a short distance below the umbilicus, but more often there are none below the navel. These tendinous insertions are intimately fused with the anterior sheath of the rectus but occupy only the anterior half of the muscle, so they are not attached to the posterior rectus sheath. This attachment of the upper portion of the rectus muscle to the anterior sheath while it is free from the posterior sheath is of practical importance for the following reasons:

1. When a transverse incision is made in the upper abdomen, the tendinous intersections prevent the cut ends of the rectus muscle fibers from retracting too far for later approximation. As a result, sutures uniting the transversely cut edges of the anterior rectus sheath will approximate the cut ends of the muscle fibers sufficiently for them to heal with the formation of a new tendinous intersection. A transverse incision across the lower abdomen, where tendinous intersections are absent, may result in too great retraction of the cut muscle ends, hence it may be advisable to place several muscle-sheath transfixing sutures just above and below the transverse incision of the anterior sheath before dividing the muscle, in order to decrease the degree of muscle retraction. There is a difference of opinion about the necessity or desirability of this maneuver.

2. The lack of attachment of the tendinous intersections to the posterior rectus sheath permits the muscle belly to be retracted so that a paramedian incision can be made.

The rectus abdominis muscle receives its nerve supply from the lower six or seven costal nerves (ventral rami of the thoracic spinal nerves) equally spaced throughout its length.

The *pyramidalis muscles* are triangular in shape and lie anterior to the rectus muscles within the lowermost portion of the rectus sheath. They consist entirely of muscle fibers that are attached below to the os pubis and insert above into the linea alba midway between the symphysis pubis and the umbilicus (see Fig. 18-3). They may be absent. These muscles play little part in the making or closing of abdominal incisions. They may, however, be helpful guides in locating the midline while making a low midline incision in an obese patient. By identifying the lateral margin of the pyramidalis muscle on one side it can be followed upward and medially until it meets its fellow of the opposite side. The midline lies between the two. The pyramidalis muscles are innervated by the twelfth thoracic spinal nerve.

The *external oblique muscle* (one on

each side) (Fig. 18–5) arises from the anterolateral aspects of the lower six ribs. Its fibers run downward and medially, the most lateral portion running almost vertically to insert into the anterior half of the crest of the ilium without becoming aponeurotic. The posterior border of the muscle is free and forms the anterior border of Petit's triangle (Fig. 18–6).

The more medial fibers run in a more medial direction; the upper ones are almost transverse while the lower ones are progressively more oblique. They become apo-

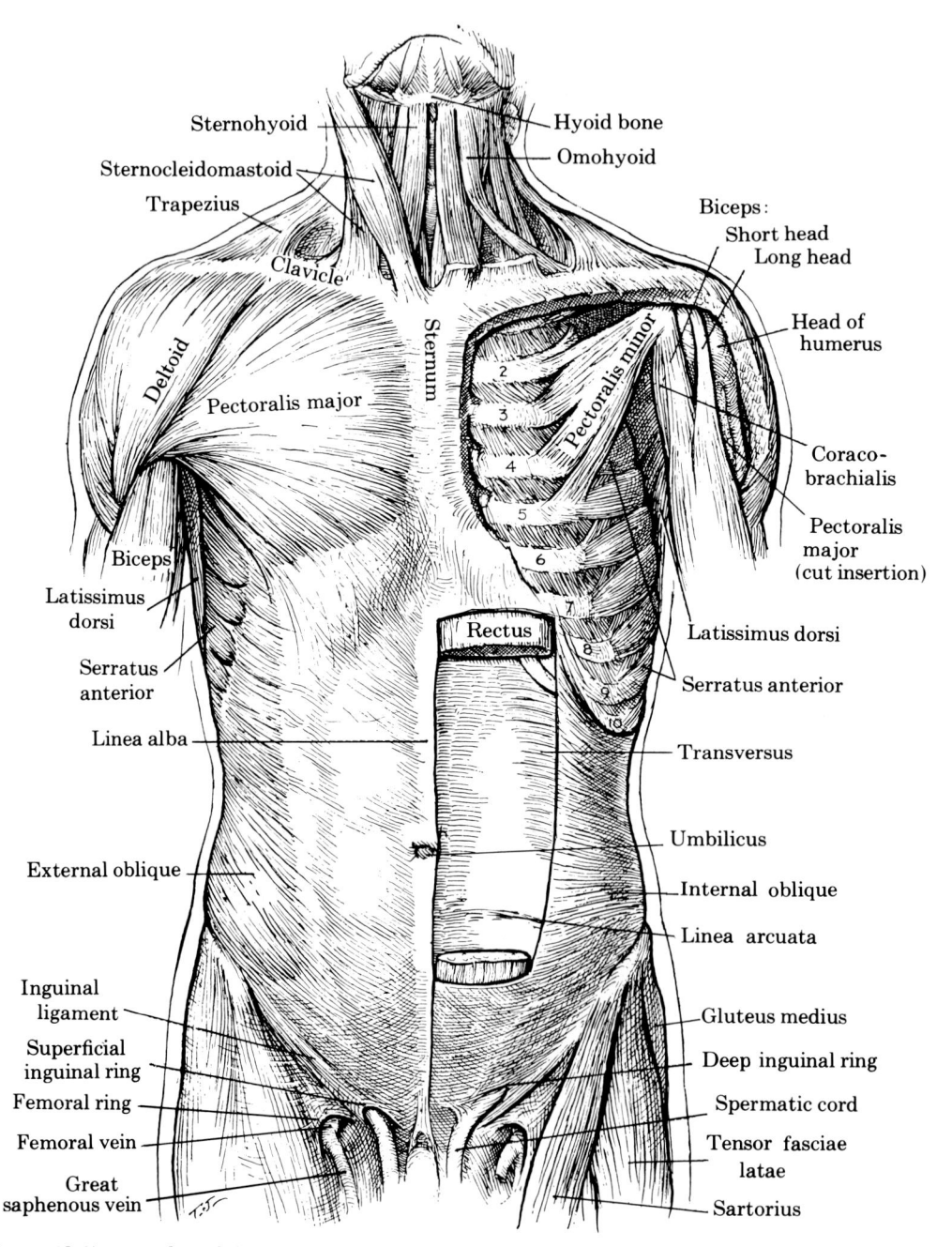

Figure 18–5. Muscles of the trunk, anterior view. The left sternocleidomastoid, pectoralis major, external oblique, and a portion of the deltoid have been removed to show underlying muscles. A portion of the rectus abdominis has been cut away to expose the posterior part of its sheath. (From Dorland's Illustrated Medical Dictionary, 26th ed. Philadelphia, W. B. Saunders Company, 1981.)

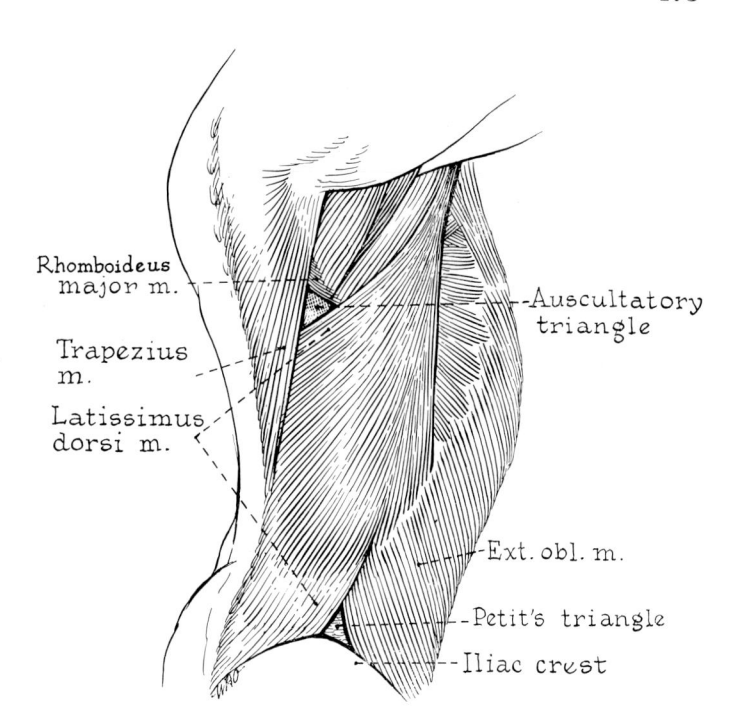

Figure 18-6. Boundaries of Petit's triangle and the triangle of auscultation.

neurotic about two to four fingerbreadths below the costal margin. These aponeurotic fibers fuse with the anterior fibers of the internal oblique aponeurosis to form the anterior sheath of the rectus muscle, and thence to insert into the linea alba throughout its length. Coller and MacLean (1949) point out, however, that this fusion of the aponeurosis of the external and internal oblique muscles does not occur at the lateral border of the rectus muscle but further medially, so that the fibers of the external oblique, particularly below the umbilicus, can be separated from those of the internal oblique for a variable distance toward the midline over the rectus muscle (see Fig. 18-3). This makes it possible to make a relaxation incision through the anterior portion of the internal oblique muscle forming the anterior sheath of the rectus at a point lateral to its fusion with the external oblique, so that the incision is deep to the external oblique which will cover the exposed rectus muscle. Inferiorly, the external oblique muscle takes a part in forming the inguinal (Poupart's) ligament.

It has been pointed out that the usual subcostal cholecystectomy incision is placed two to three fingerbreadths below and parallel to the costal margin, transecting the muscular or adjacent aponeurotic portion of the external oblique muscle. As a result the upper portion of the muscle usually retracts above the costal margin under the superficial fascia so that it may be overlooked and not included in the sutures during closure of the incision. Occasionally in a transverse abdominal incision the internal oblique and transversus abdominis muscles can be split in the direction of their fibers more easily if the overlying and transversely divided external oblique aponeurosis is also incised upward and downward about 1 cm. lateral to its fusion with the anterior rectus sheath. This forms superior and inferior flaps of the external oblique muscle, which can be retracted to facilitate division of the underlying muscles. The maneuver causes no nerve injury. The external oblique aponeurosis is reattached to the anterior rectus sheath when the incision is closed.

The *internal oblique muscle* (one on each side) arises from the lumbodorsal fascia, the anterior half of the iliac crest, and the lateral half of the inguinal (Poupart's) ligament. It lies immediately beneath the external oblique muscle, and its muscle fibers run upward and inward, about at right angles with those of the overlying external oblique muscle (Fig. 18-7). The lowermost and most medial fibers that arise from the inguinal ligament arch upward and then downward to become aponeurotic and fuse with the aponeurotic fibers of the transversus abdominis muscles to form the conjoined tendon which inserts into the pubic tubercle. Sometimes these fibers form a very high arch, leaving Hesselbach's triangle relatively unsupported, an anatomic condition that is thought to favor the formation of a direct inguinal hernia. The upper and most posterior fibers of the internal oblique muscle run upward without becoming aponeurotic and insert into the costal margin (lower six ribs). All the remainder of the fibers from the inguinal ligament and iliac crest run transversely in the lower abdomen and upward and medially in the upper abdomen to become aponeurotic at the lateral border of the rectus throughout its length.

These aponeurotic fibers almost immediately split into two lamellae. The anterior lamella passes in front of the rectus muscle and fuses with the aponeurosis of the external oblique muscle to form the anterior

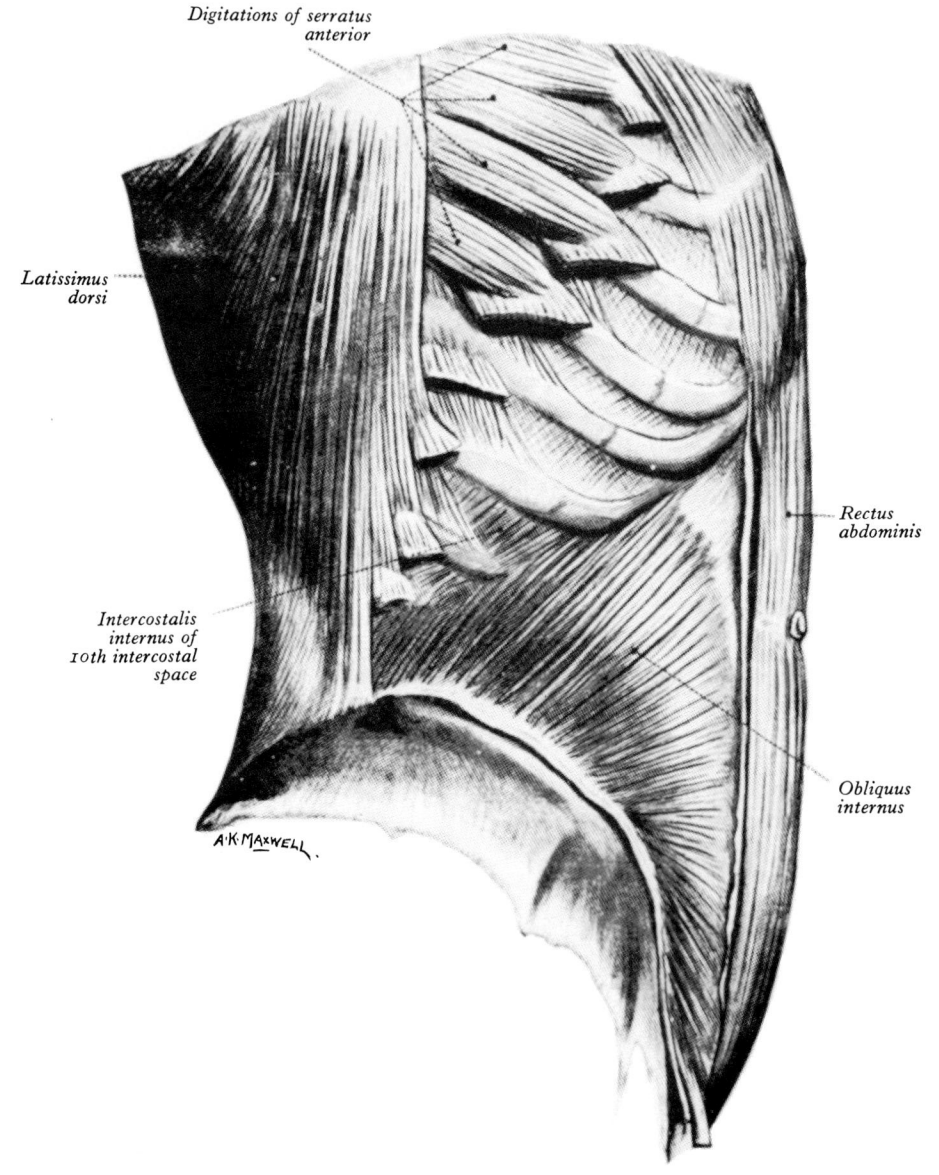

Figure 18–7. Muscles of the right side of the trunk. The external oblique has been removed to show the internal oblique, but its digitations from the ribs have been preserved. The sheath of the rectus abdominis has been opened and its anterior lamina removed. (From Warwick, R., and Williams, P. L.: Gray's Anatomy, 35th Br. ed. Philadelphia, W. B. Saunders Company, 1973.)

sheath of the rectus muscle, which fuses with its fellow of the opposite side to form the linea alba, which extends from the xiphoid process to the pubic symphysis. The posterior lamella passes behind the rectus muscle to fuse with the aponeurotic fibers of the transversus abdominis and form the posterior sheath of the rectus which also inserts into the linea alba. The uppermost fibers of the posterior lamella insert into the seventh, eighth and ninth costal cartilages.

From a point about midway between the umbilicus and the symphysis pubis down to the pubis, all of the internal oblique and transverse abdominis aponeurotic fibers pass anterior to the rectus muscle, leaving no posterior rectus sheath in this area. This point of cessation of the posterior rectus sheath is called the arcuate line (semicircular line of Douglas) (see Figs. 18–3 and 18–8) and is present at variable levels above the symphysis in different individuals.

Thus the posterior rectus sheath extends from the costal margin above to the arcuate line, while the anterior rectus sheath extends from the fifth costal cartilage above to insert into the pubic crest below. Both sheaths insert into the linea alba medially. The direction of the multitude of small aponeurotic fibers forming the anterior and posterior rectus sheaths is transversely toward the linea alba into which they insert.

The line along which the aponeurotic fibers of the internal oblique muscle split into anterior and posterior lamellae is called the *linea semilunaris* and is at the lateral margin of the rectus muscle from the pubic tubercle to the tip of the ninth costal cartilage. It is along this line that the intercostal and lumbar vessels and nerves enter the rectus sheath, and it is through these openings that spigelian hernias, which are rare, occur.

The *transversus abdominis muscle* (one on each side) lies deep to the internal oblique. Like the latter muscle it arises inferiorly from the lateral third of the inguinal (Poupart's) ligament and the anterior three-fourths of the crest of the ilium. Its mid-portion arises from the lumbodorsal fascia, while its upper portion arises from the inner surface of the lower six ribs where it interdigitates with the attachments of the diaphragm (see Fig. 18–3).

The lowermost fibers of this muscle pass downward and medially to arch over the spermatic cord and to fuse with those of the internal oblique muscle and form the conjoined tendon. The remainder of the transversus abdominis muscle fibers pass transversely to become aponeurotic before fusing with the posterior lamella of the internal oblique muscle to form the posterior rectus sheath. The fibers of the transversus abdominis muscle become aponeurotic at distances from the linea alba that vary with the level of the abdominal wall of these fibers, thus (1) at the end below the

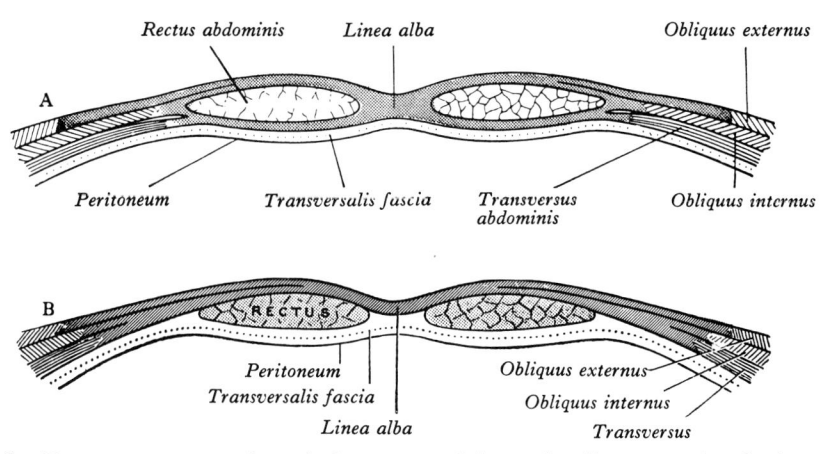

Figure 18–8. Transverse sections through the anterior abdominal wall. A, Immediately above the umbilicus. B, Below the arcuate line. Note the extent to which the external oblique aponeurosis remains as a separate entity, passing medially, ventral to rectus, before blending with the other aponeuroses; these have already fused, lateral to rectus. (From Warwick and Williams, cited in preceding figure.)

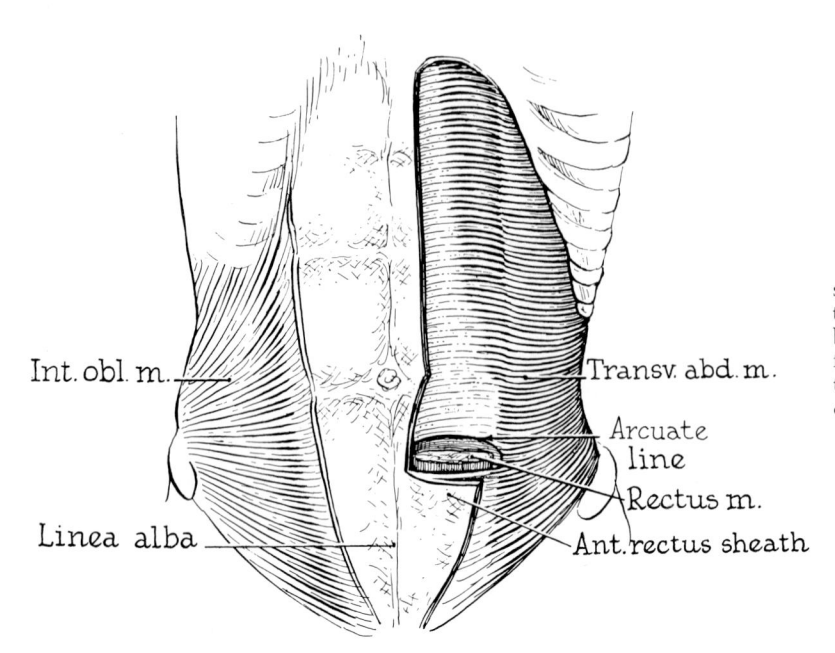

Figure 18–9. Illustration showing that the fibers of the transversus abdominis muscle become aponeurotic at distances from the linea alba that vary with the level on the abdominal wall of the fibers.

umbilicus the muscle fibers become aponeurotic at the lateral border of the rectus muscle, and (2) at the xiphoid process the muscle fibers do not become aponeurotic until they have passed to within 2 to 4 cm. from the linea alba (Fig. 18–9). From this level downward the point of transition from muscle fiber to aponeurosis passes progressively more laterally until at the level of the umbilicus the fibers become aponeurotic at the lateral border of the rectus.

Coller and MacLean (1949) point out that this variation in point of transition from muscle fiber to aponeurosis has some importance in the selection of incisions. They state: "It may readily be seen then that, above the umbilicus, the lateral portion of the posterior rectus sheath is formed only by the posterior lamella of the internal oblique aponeurosis; this deficiency produces an inherent weakness in closure of incisions in this region, particularly those which pass vertically through the lateral rectus sheaths."

The aponeurotic fibers of the transversus abdominis muscle pass behind the rectus muscle to fuse with the posterior lamella of the internal oblique muscle and insert into the linea alba, forming the posterior rectus sheath, except below the arcuate line where the fibers pass anterior to the rectus muscle to insert into the linea alba, since no posterior rectus sheath is present in this area.

The *nerve supply* of the rectus abdominis, external oblique, internal oblique, and transversus abdominis muscles comes by way of the lower six or seven intercostal and first lumbar nerves (by the iliohypogastric nerve, which is formed by the twelfth thoracic and first lumbar nerves, and by the ilioinguinal nerve, which arises from the first lumbar). The intercostal nerves run deep to the inferior margin of their corresponding ribs. Rees and Coller (1943) have shown that in this location each nerve exists not as a single trunk, but as two or three branches. These branches communicate with each other within the same intercostal space and communicate also with the intercostal nerve above and the one below, by connections that run beneath the rib. At the anterior end of the intercostal space the divisions of an intercostal nerve gather into a single trunk. The sixth, seventh, eighth, and ninth trunks then pass beneath the costal arch to enter the abdominal wall between the transversus abdominis and internal oblique muscles (Fig. 18–10). The trunks of the tenth, eleventh, and twelfth intercostal nerves pass forward beyond the free ends of their corresponding ribs to enter the same layer of the abdominal wall.

The anterior division of the iliohypogastric nerve penetrates the internal oblique muscle about 2 cm. medial to the anterior superior spine of the ilium (Fig.

18–10) and then runs forward and downward beneath the external oblique aponeurosis. It is frequently injured in lower abdominal incisions.

The ilioinguinal nerve runs close and parallel to the iliohypogastric but nearer the iliac crest. However, unlike the iliohypogastric, it passes through the inguinal canal with the spermatic cord or round ligament of the uterus to reach a more superficial level.

As the nerves run forward and medially between the transversus abdominis and internal oblique muscles of the abdominal wall, the intercostal nerves anastomose freely with each other (Fig. 18–11), and also the twelfth intercostal nerve anastomoses frequently with the iliohypogastric. When the nerves reach the lateral border of the rectus sheath, they pierce the sheath and fan out transversely beneath the muscle to be distributed to its deep surface. Coller and MacLean (1949) comment that "because of the rich anastomosis between the intercostal nerves, both in the intercostal spaces and in the abdominal wall, it is possible to cut two, and sometimes even three, of the nerves without noticeable loss of function. It is apparent, however, that the nearer to the spinal cord the nerve is cut, the greater is the chance of function being taken over by adjacent nerves through distal anastomoses. It is also worthy of note that, once the nerves have reached the lateral border of the rectus muscle, little if any anastomosis occurs. For this reason any incision that passes vertically through the rectus muscle or through its lateral border must denervate that portion of the muscle medial to the incision."

In their course across the abdominal wall the nerves can be retracted upward or downward for variable distances without being injured.

The anterolateral abdominal wall receives its *arterial blood supply* from the last six intercostal and the four lumbar arteries (which run roughly in a transverse direction with a segmental distribution), together with the superior and inferior epigastric and the deep circumflex iliac arteries (which run roughly in a vertical direction).

All except the uppermost two posterior *intercostal arteries* (which are not concerned with the abdominal wall) arise from the aorta and pass forward and medially with their corresponding intercostal nerve to anastomose with their corresponding anterior

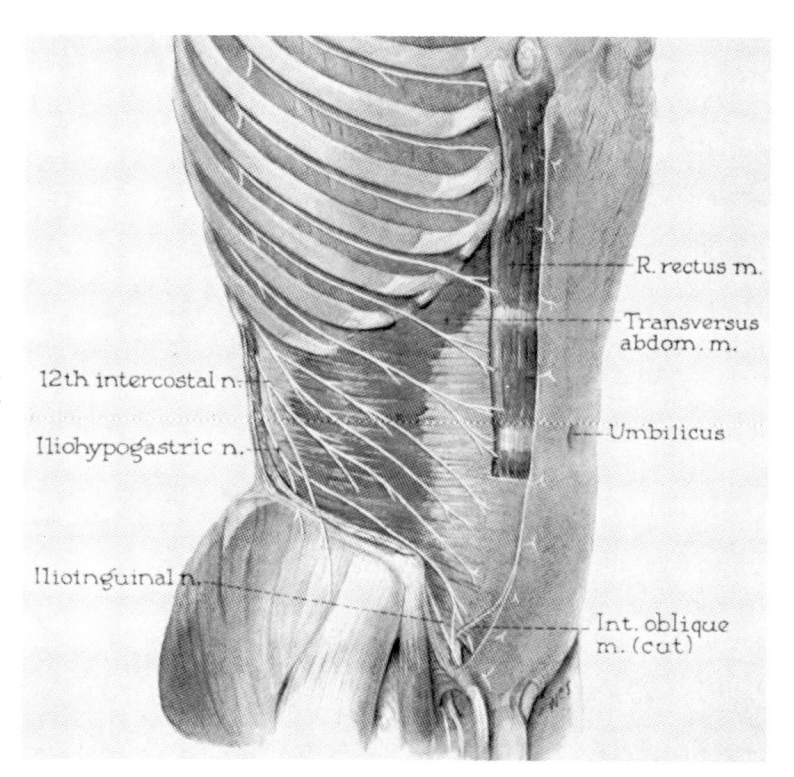

Figure 18–10. The abdominal wall. Course of the right intercostal nerves below the fourth rib.

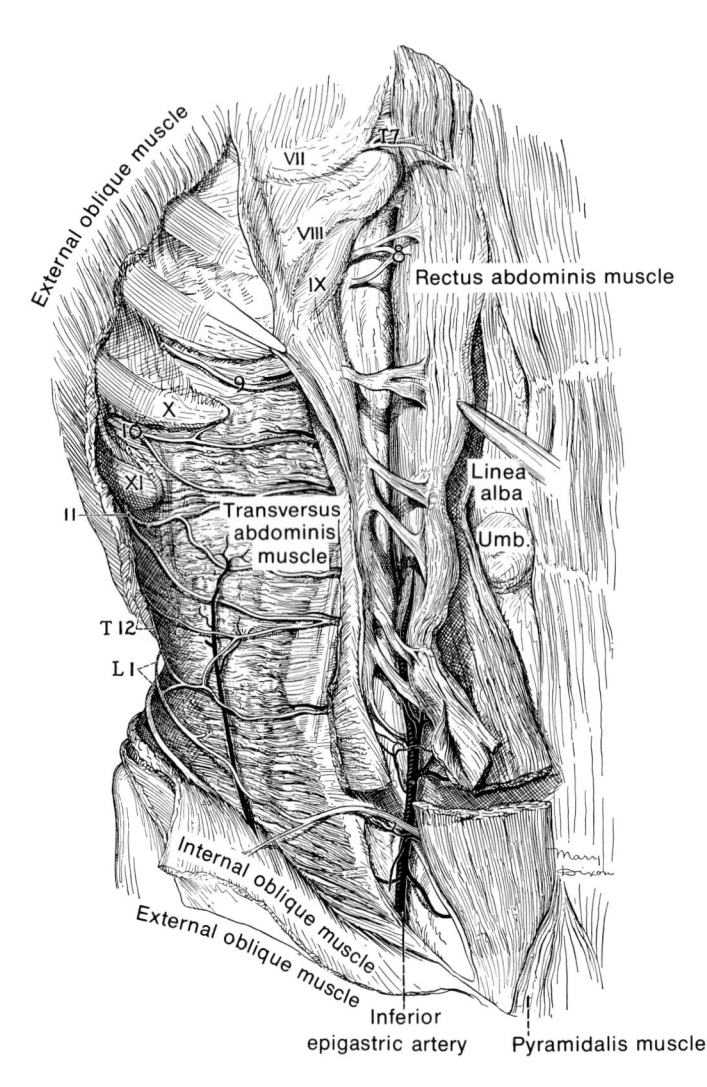

Figure 18–11. Abdominal plexus of the thoracic nerves. The nerves are exposed by removal of the external and internal oblique muscles and by reflection of the rectus muscle. The seventh through the twelfth thoracic nerves, and the first lumbar, are shown as they anastomose after emergence from the intercostal spaces. (From Bishop, W. E., Carr, B. W., Anson, B. J., et al.: Parietal intermuscular plexus of thoracic nerves. Quart. Bull. Northwestern Univ. M. School *17*:209, 1943.)

intercostal artery, which is a branch of the internal mammary or superior epigastric artery, thus forming arterial arches between the aorta and the internal thoracic superior-inferior epigastric systems. In addition, in its course each intercostal artery anastomoses freely with the artery immediately above and below it. Likewise, the lumbar arteries progress forward and medially across the same plane of the abdominal wall as the nerves and anastomose with the superior and inferior epigastric arteries as well as with each other (Fig. 18–12).

The *internal thoracic (mammary) artery* arises from the subclavian artery and passes vertically downward (one on each side) parallel and approximately 1.25 cm. lateral to the lateral margin of the sternum (giving off anterior intercostal branches at the lower margin of each rib). It lies deep to each rib that it crosses and is separated from the pleural cavity by the parietal pleura. One of its terminations passes beneath the costal arch (through the costoxiphoid opening in the diaphragm) to enter the abdominal wall where its continuation downward is called the *superior epigastric artery*. It continues downward within the rectus sheath and deep to the rectus muscle on a line situated about 3 cm. lateral to the anterior midline of the abdomen, to anastomose freely with the inferior epigastric artery at the level of the umbilicus. Throughout its course it gives off branches, which anastomose directly with the intercostals and other branches that are distributed to the rectus muscle, rectus sheath, and overlying integument.

The *inferior epigastric artery* arises from the external iliac just proximal to the

ANATOMY

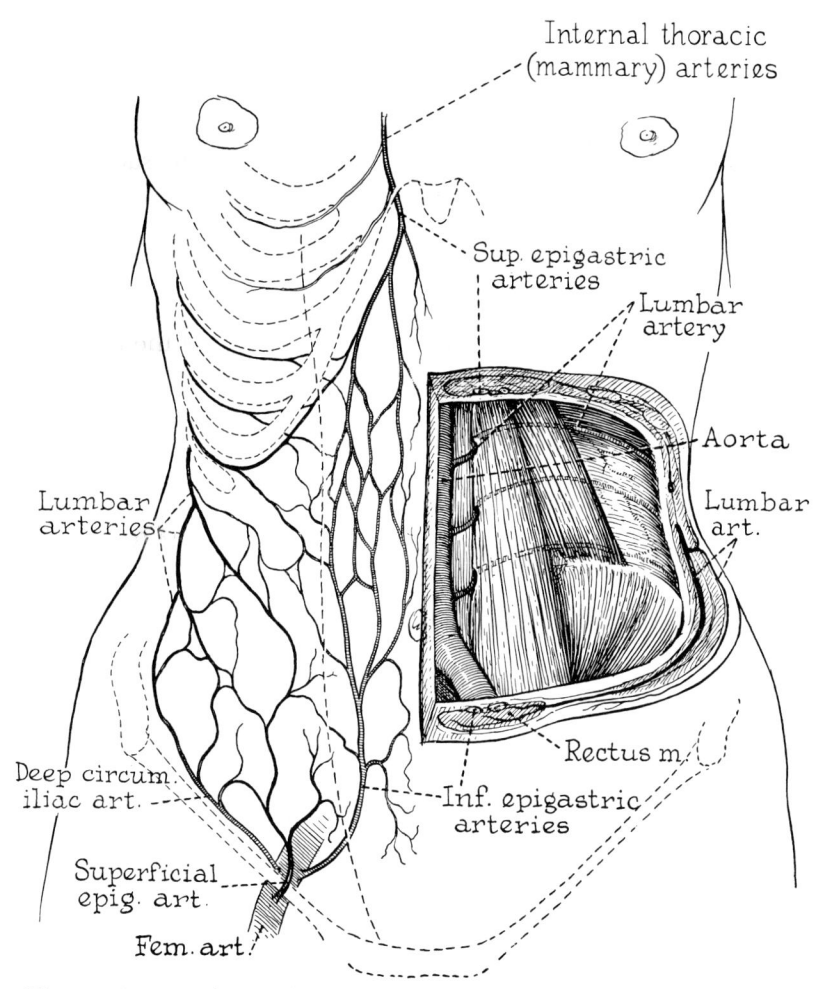

Figure 18–12. Scheme of blood supply to the anterolateral abdominal wall.

inguinal ligament and ascends across the posterior wall of the inguinal canal to pass obliquely, superiorly and medially toward the umbilicus. It pierces the transversalis fascia to enter the rectus compartment by passing in front of the arcuate line (semicircular line of Douglas) and passes vertically upward in a line situated about 3 cm. lateral to the anterior abdominal midline to anastomose with the superior epigastric artery. In its course it lies deep to the rectus muscle and gives off branches to anastomose with the intercostal and lumbar arteries, and to nourish the overlying muscle, rectus sheath, and integument.

The superior and inferior epigastric arteries anastomose only sparsely with their fellows of the opposite side, therefore the linea alba is a relatively avascular area and has a poor blood supply.

The lateral branches of the epigastric arteries penetrate the lateral margin of the rectus sheath in the linea semilunaris to anastomose with the intercostal or lumbar arteries. The arteries accompanied by their satellite veins pass through the same opening as the corresponding intercostal or lumbar nerve. Occasionally one of these openings may be or become large enough for a spigelian or lateral ventral hernia to occur.

In incisions through the rectus muscles — whether or not they are muscle-splitting — the epigastric vessels must be considered, as they may be the source of troublesome bleeding.

The *deep circumflex iliac artery* arises from the lateral aspect of the external iliac at a point opposite the origin of the inferior epigastric artery. It passes upward and laterally to a point just above the iliac crest near the anterior superior spine. Here it gives off a sizeable ascending branch, which may be injured in making a McBurney incision (Fig. 18–12).

Posterior Abdominal Muscles and Related Structures.

These muscles, along with the vertebrae, comprise the posterior portion of the muscle-bone layer of the abdominal wall. They play a smaller part in the making and closing of abdominal incisions than do the anterior and lateral groups previously described. However, they serve as important landmarks and should be mentioned.

The *quadratus lumborum muscle* extends from the posterior third of the crest of the ilium to the medial half of the twelfth rib (see Fig. 18–4). It is contained within the fibrous compartments formed by the middle and anterior lamellae of the lumbodorsal fascia and is separated from the transversalis fascia by the anterior lamella.

The *psoas major muscle* arises from the twelfth thoracic and all five lumbar vertebrae and occupies the gutter between the bodies and transverse processes of the lumbar vertebrae (Fig. 18–13). It passes downward and laterally along the margin of the pelvic brim to have its tendon fuse with that of the iliacus and insert into the lesser trochanter of the femur. The psoas is an important landmark for locating the lumbar sympathetic ganglia.

The *iliacus muscle* arises from the iliac fossa (Fig. 18–13). The quadratus lumborum and iliopsoas muscles are innervated by the upper three lumbar nerves.

The *sacrospinalis (erector spinae) muscle* lies in the groove along the spinous processes from the sacrum to the base of the skull and is attached to the vertebrae throughout its length. It is a large, thick muscle, about a palmbreadth in width. It occupies the aponeurotic compartment formed by the dorsal and middle layers of the lumbodorsal fascia (see Fig. 18–4). Lateral fasciculae of the costal part of the muscle extend as far as the angles of the ribs, and some of these must be cut or elevated with a periosteal elevator to permit exposure and removal of the posterior part of a rib or ribs.

The lateral fibers of the muscle occasionally require transection to increase exposure. If the medial ones also must be cut one should remember that there are blood vessels near either side of the roots of the vertebral spines, which extend vertically from the base of the skull to the sacrum. It is

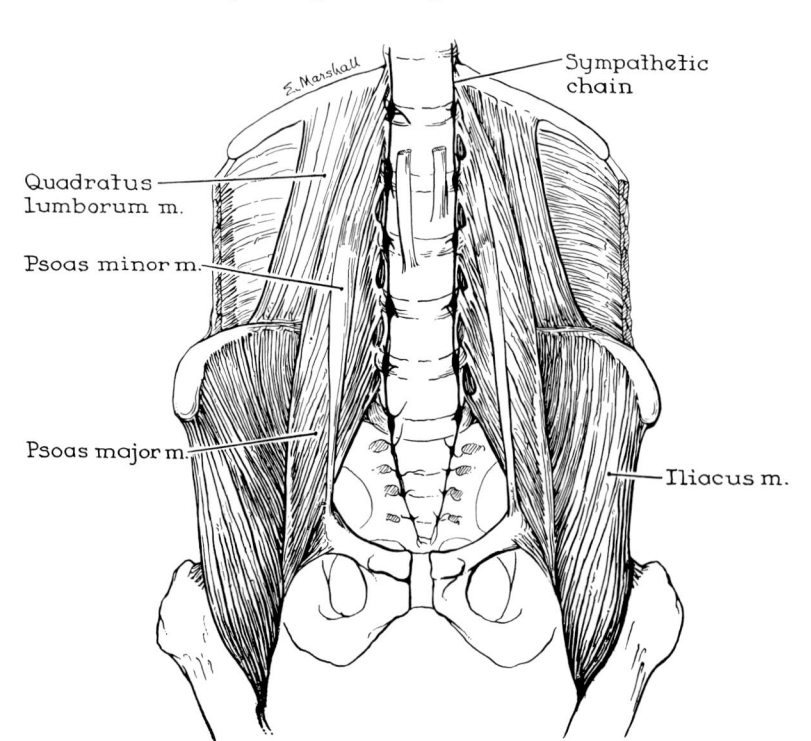

Figure 18–13. Lumbar muscles, vertebrae, and sympathetic ganglia. Anterior view.

to avoid injury to these vessels, with troublesome hemorrhage, that the sacrospinalis is freed and retracted laterally by cleaving closely to the spinous processes and lamina while performing an operation of the spine. The sacrospinalis is innervated by the posterior divisions of the sacral, lumbar, intercostal and cervical nerves.

The *latissimus dorsi muscle* arises from the posterior half of the crest of the ilium, from that part of the dorsal leaf of the lumbosacral fascia that is attached to the dorsum of the sacrum, and from the lumbar and lower six thoracic spines (see Fig. 18–6). Its uppermost fibers arise from the inferior angle of the scapula, where they form the lower boundary of the *auscultatory triangle,* the trapezius forming the medial superior while the medial border of the scapula forms the laterosuperior boundaries. The latissimus fibers converge superiorly and laterally to attach by a flat tendon into the bicipital groove of the humerus.

The lateral and inferior border of the latissimus dorsi is free and its lower portion forms the posterosuperior boundary of the inferior lumbar triangle of Petit. The base of this triangle is a portion of the iliac crest, its superolateral boundary is the external oblique muscle, and its floor is the internal oblique muscle (see Fig. 18–6). This triangle is variable in size.

The latissimus dorsi muscle is innervated by the thoracodorsal nerve, which is derived from the sixth, seventh, and eighth cervical nerves. This nerve, accompanied by an artery, vein, and lymphatics, runs vertically down along the deep surface of the muscle from the subclavian region.

The latissimus dorsi must frequently be transected in making thoracic, thoracicoabdominal, or abdominal incisions. It can easily be done by passing two fingers beneath its posterior free edge and cutting between them. The cut edges should be accurately reapproximated when the incision is being closed.

The *lumbodorsal fascia* consists of three layers, which form two investing compartments (Figs. 18–1 and 18–14) on each side of the spinous processes.

The *posterior* or *external layer* attaches to the tips of the lumbar spines and supraspinous ligaments and forms the dorsal part of the fascial compartment that invests the sacrospinalis muscle (Figs. 18–1 and 18–14). This is by far the thickest lamella of the lumbodorsal fascia. It is covered externally by the latissimus dorsi and the serratus posterior inferior muscles, to which it partly gives origin.

The *middle layer* of the lumbodorsal fascia is attached to the posterior surfaces and tips of the transverse processes (see Fig. 18–1). It lies in front of the sacrospinalis muscle and behind the quadratum lumborum. At the lateral margin of the sacrospinalis muscle the middle and posterior layers fuse to enclose this muscle in a dense aponeurotic compartment. In its upper portion the middle layer is strengthened by the *lumbocostal ligament,* which runs from the transverse processes of the first and second lumbar vertebrae to the outer margin of the lowest rib (twelfth, if present, or, when not, to the eleventh). This ligament has a sharp, recognizable edge, and marks the inferior line of pleural reflection. Its division will usually result in inadvertently opening the pleura, and for this reason it should be avoided.

The *anterior* or *internal layer* of the lumbodorsal fascia arises from the anterior surfaces of the lumbar transverse processes and their bases (see Fig. 18–1), and lies anterior to the quadratum lumborum muscle. The anterior is the weakest of the three layers. In its upper portion it is strengthened by the *lumbocostal (external arcuate) ligament,* which lies anterior and lateral to the posterior lumbocostal ligament. It is the origin of some of the posterior fibers of the diaphragm (Fig. 18–15) and is in intimate relation to the pleura. The anterior layer joins with the fusion aponeurosis of the posterior and middle fascial layers at the lateral margin of the quadratus lumborum, forming a fascia compartment for this muscle. At this point all three layers fuse to form a single broad lumbar aponeurosis, which runs laterally and serves as part of the origin of the internal oblique and transversus abdominis muscles. Through this broad aponeurosis lateral to the quadratus lumborum muscle, access can be gained to the retrorenal spaces.

Lampe (1952) points out that:

"An incision parallel to and about two fingerbreadths below the lateral half of the twelfth rib and extending a variable distance toward the anterior superior iliac spine will pass through the fusion point of the three layers of lumbodorsal fascia and make it easier to split the posterior parts of the internal oblique and transversus ab-

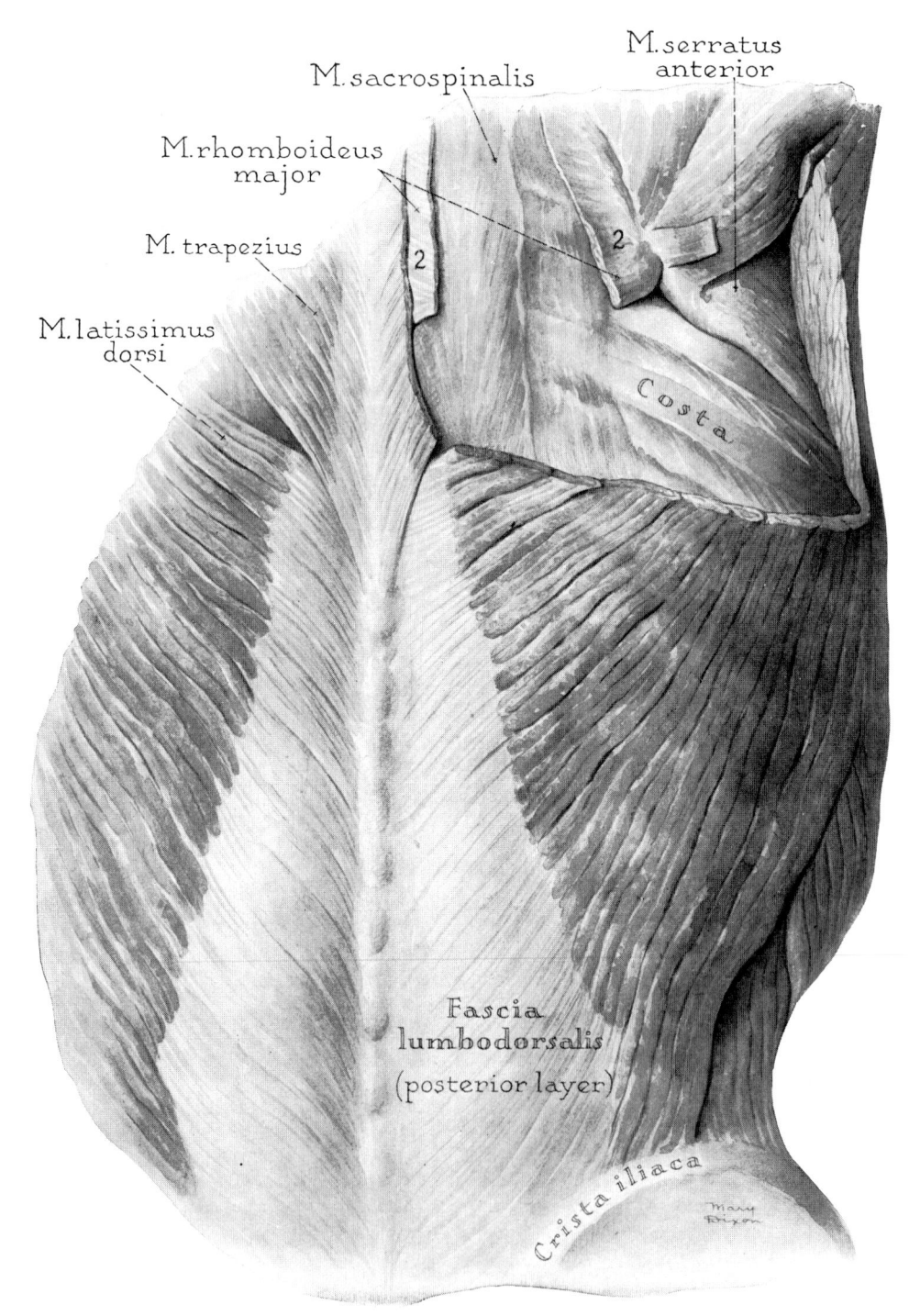

Figure 18–14. Muscles of the back; first and second layers. The trapezius muscle has been removed; triangular segment has been cut from the cranial portion of the latissimus dorsi. The rhomboideus major (at 2), one of the three constituents of the second layer of flat muscles of the back, has been removed in its middle half to expose the column of long muscles.

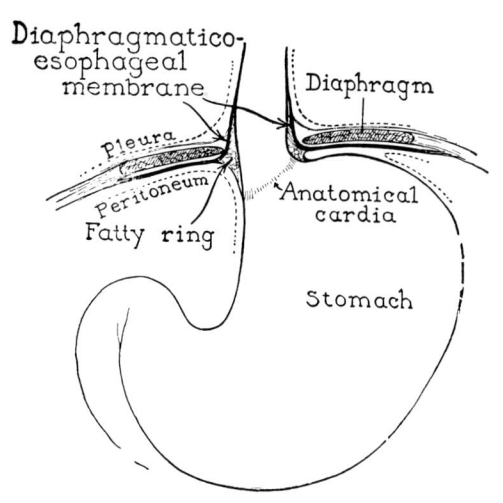

Figure 18–15. Normal anatomic relationship between lower end of esophagus, cardiac end of stomach, and esophageal hiatus, showing the relationship of the diaphragmatico-esophageal membrane of these structures. (Harrington: J. Thoracic Surg., Vol. 8.)

dominis muscles in the direction of their fibers. In cutting through the fusion area of the lumbodorsal fascia, the first lumbar nerve is usually encountered. With slight modifications, this incision can serve as an approach to the kidney, upper ureter, lumbar sympathetic chain, and the inferior vena cava on the right side and abdominal aorta on the left side. It is also low enough to prevent injury to the pleura, which frequently extends as far as a fingerbreadth below the medial half of the twelfth rib — a point to be remembered, if one is attempting to do an extraperitoneal drainage of a posterior subphrenic abscess (Ochsner approach)."

5. FIFTH LAYER OR TRANSVERSALIS FASCIA

The fifth layer of the abdominal wall is the transversalis fascia, which lines the abdominal cavity somewhat like the peritoneum, with the important difference that it is not reflected onto and over the abdominal viscera (see Fig. 18–1), except for a partial reflection onto the viscera of the pelvic cavity (Fig. 18–16). This is discussed in more detail in the section on the anatomy of the rectum (Volume 3). The portion of transversalis fascia beneath the rectus muscle is so intimately attached to the overlying posterior rectus sheath and underlying peritoneum that the three layers (posterior rectus sheath, transversalis fascia, and peritoneum) are sutured together as one layer in closing the peritoneal layer of the incision.

Lateral to the posterior rectus sheath the transversalis fascia is loosely attached to the transversus abdominis, quadratus lumborum, and psoas major muscles so that it can be freed from them with ease and, along with its underlying peritoneum and the upper portion of the ureter and kidney, can be reflected medially to expose the lumbar sympathetic chain and vena cava or aorta extraperitoneally.

The transversalis fascia is appreciably thicker in the lower half of the abdomen, particularly below the level of the arcuate line (of Douglas), where the posterior rectus sheath is absent. In the inguinal region it is

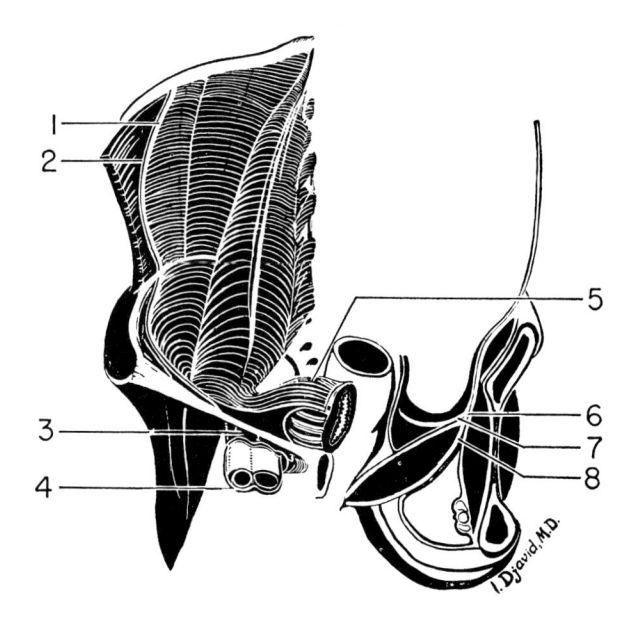

Figure 18–16. Disposition of transversalis fascia. 1, Peritoneum. 2, Transversalis fascia. 3, The three compartments of the femoral sheath. Lateral compartment contains femoral artery; middle compartment, the femoral vein; and the medial compartment forms the femoral canal, containing the gland of Cloquet. Femoral hernia extends into the canal. 4, Femoral sheath formed by femoral prolongation of transversalis fascia. 5, Peritoneum and transversalis fascia overlying bladder. 6, Tendinous arch where transversalis fascia splits to form superior (7) and inferior (8) pelvic diaphragmatic fascia. Note visceral fascia arising from superior pelvic diaphragmatic fascia.

(From Lampe, E. W.: Surgical anatomy of the abdominal wall. Surg. Clin. North Am. 32:545, 1952.)

also relatively strong and fuses with the aponeurosis and fasciae of the transversus abdominis muscle to form most of the posterior wall of the inguinal canal. In this area the inferior epigastric vessels lie deep to the transversalis fascia, which must be incised to bare those vessels.

The transversalis fascia is attached below to the inner lip of the iliac crest, the outer half of the inguinal (Poupart's) ligament, the lacunar ligament (of Gimbernat), and the pubic crest. This fascia is continued downward behind the mesial half of the inguinal ligament and over the femoral vessels to pass into the thigh, forming the *femoral sheath.*

It is considered important to close the divided transversalis fascia in repairing incisions for inguinal or femoral hernias, for lower rectus-splitting or paramedian incisions where the posterior rectus sheath is absent, and in lower transverse abdominal or McBurney muscle-splitting incisions. In those incisions in which the peritoneum has been opened, the transversalis fascia is included in the peritoneal suture. If the peritoneum has not been opened, the transversalis fascia is closed as a separate layer or is included in the stitches closing the transversus abdominis muscle or the transversus abdominis and internal oblique combined in one layer. In this connection, Lampe (1952) states:

"If, in the making of a *McBurney incision,* the surgeon separates gently the fibers of the external oblique, internal oblique, and transversus abdominis muscles and gently elevates the separated edges of the transversus abdominis, he reveals a substantial transversalis fascia. If this procedure is done roughly, the points of the scissors or clamp or the fingers actually tear through the transversalis fascia, creating a rent whose edges retract under the transversus abdominis muscle and are very apt not to be included in the suture that closes the peritoneum. Whenever a surgeon notices, in closing the peritoneum in a McBurney incision, that the peritoneum seems 'very thin' and not much stronger than wet tissue paper, chances are that he has torn a sufficiently large rent in the transversalis fascia to have its edges retract out of sight under the edges of the transversus abdominis muscle and thus not be included in the so-called peritoneal suture. Obviously, this weakens the abdominal closure; may weaken the abdominal wall; and even lay the groundwork for a future hernia.

If it is important to close the transversalis fascia in a hernia repair in the nearby inguinal region, why is it not logical to close the transversalis fascia in the 'peritoneal closure' of a McBurney incision?"

6. SIXTH OR EXTRAPERITONEAL FAT LAYER

This layer consists of loose areolar fibrous tissue containing variable amounts of fat and lies between the overlying transversalis fascia and underlying parietal peritoneum. Its thickness is varied in different parts of the abdominal wall. Subdiaphragmatically and posterior to the upper half of the posterior rectus sheaths except the area occupied by the falciform ligament, and also laterally to the midaxillary line, the sixth layer contains very little fat. As a result, in incisions in these areas the posterior rectus sheath, transversalis fascia, extraperitoneal layer, and peritoneum can be included in one suture line. For the same reason, in a McBurney incision the transversalis fascia, extraperitoneal layer, and peritoneum can be closed in one suture line.

Upper right rectus-splitting, upper right paramedian, or upper midline incisions will encounter the *falciform ligament* which is a fold of the parietal peritoneum that lines the anterior wall of the abdomen and partially encloses the extraperitoneal ligamentum teres of the liver. It also contains extraperitoneal fat and paraumbilical blood vessels which may cause annoying hemorrhage. This ligament runs from the umbilicus upward just to the right of the midline to the liver and when encountered its extraperitoneal fat often obscures the peritoneal layer. In these cases the peritoneal layer can be more easily identified and safely incised to the right or to the left of the ligament. When the falciform ligament and its ligamentum teres is transected, the cut ends should be reapproximated by tying them together just prior to closing the incision.

7. SEVENTH LAYER – PERITONEUM

The parietal peritoneum is the smooth, serous layer that bounds the peritoneal cavity and is reflected onto the various viscera to form the visceral peritoneum as well as ligaments, mesenteries, and folds, which are described elsewhere in the specific areas under discussion.

The parietal peritoneum is the portion concerned in abdominal incisions. The peritoneum has characteristics important to the surgeon in that it heals quickly with a smooth surface and for this reason its cut edges should be approximated whenever possible in closing an abdominal incision. Peritoneum stretches easily and has little strength so that it requires the support of its overlying muscles and fascia to maintain the normal boundaries and shape of the abdominal cavity. Furthermore, it tears easily so that sutures cannot be placed through it under tension unless they also include bites of tougher overlying transversalis fascia or even muscle fibers to strengthen their bite.

The peritoneum is the innermost, seventh, and final layer of the abdominal wall.

Linea Alba

The linea alba extends in the anterior midline of the abdomen (see Figs. 18–3 and 18–17) from the xiphoid to the symphysis. It is divided by the umbilicus into supraumbilical and infraumbilical segments of about equal length. The linea alba consists of a band of dense, criss-cross fibers of the aponeuroses of the broad abdominal muscles (Fig. 18–17).

At the linea alba, the aponeurosis of the external oblique muscle and the anterior lamella of the internal oblique muscle, which have formed the anterior sheath of the rectus muscle, fuse with the posterior rectus sheath. The latter consists of the posterior lamella of the internal oblique

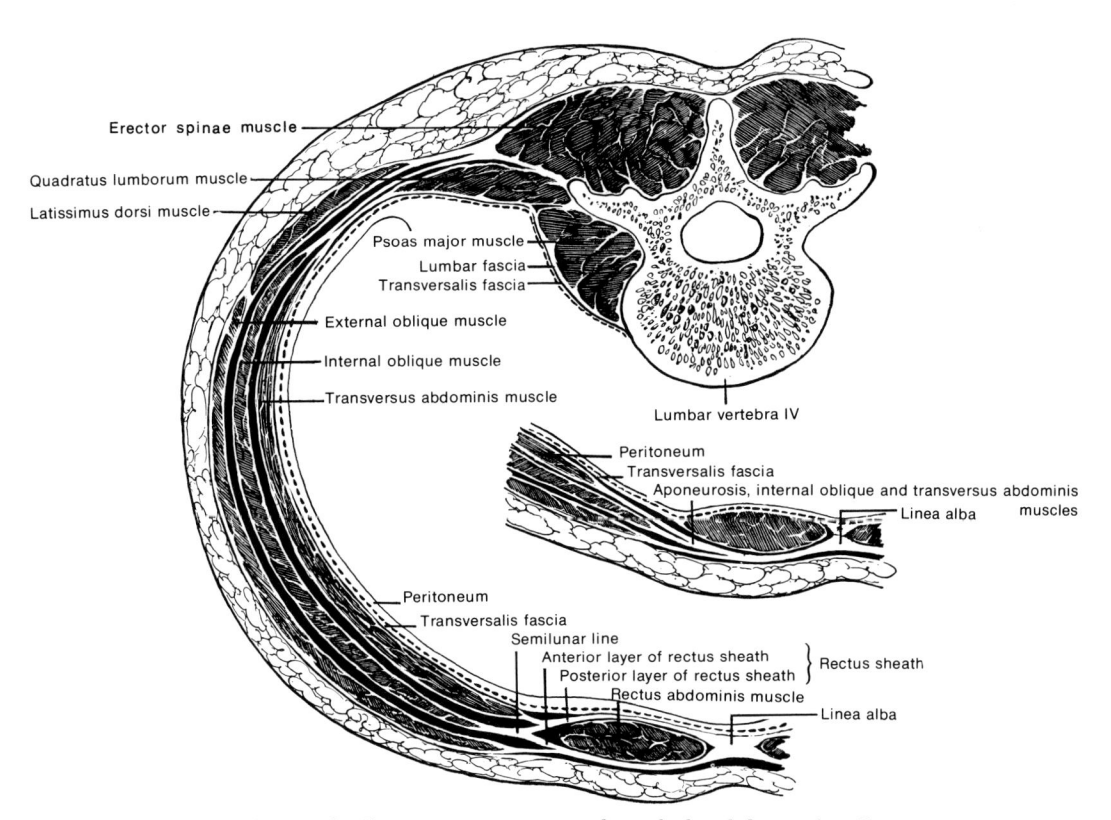

Figure 18–17. Transverse section through the abdominal wall.

muscle, which has previously fused with the aponeurosis of the transversus abdominis muscle to close the medial margin of the rectus compartment. All these layers form a dense fibrous band which unites with a similarly formed fibrous band from the opposite side to create the linea alba. Above the umbilicus it widens out, but below that level it is narrow and sometimes difficult to recognize. In the broad supraumbilical portion of the linea alba small openings are present, through which the perforating vessels and nerves pass and through which an epigastric hernia may occur. Since the branches of the epigastric arteries anastomose very sparsely across the midline, the blood supply of the linea alba is less copious than in other areas.

Since the linea alba represents a fusion of all the layers forming the anterior and posterior rectus sheaths, an incision made along its midline will not open up the rectus compartment on either side, nor will it expose the separate aponeurotic layers. As a result, the peritoneum and transversalis fascia can be closed with one row of sutures; all the other aponeurotic layers are closed with another row of sutures without the necessity of a time-consuming closure in separate layers. Furthermore, an incision made in the midline is through a relatively avascular layer, with minimal attendant bleeding, and does not destroy the innervation of any part of any muscle. It is believed, however, to be more prone to postoperative herniation than are incisions in other locations, because of its relatively meager blood supply.

Umbilicus

The umbilicus (Fig. 18–5) is the fibroaponeurotic scar formed within the central portion of the linea alba. This represents the embryonic defect in the abdominal wall through which the vitellointestinal duct, omphalomesenteric vessels, and urachus pass, but under normal conditions these structures atrophy into fibrous cords, and the umbilical ring is obliterated by fibrous tissue intimately covered by skin epithelium. This process will be detailed in the section on umbilical hernia. As a result of this obliterative process, the umbilicus is a point at which all the layers of the anterior abdominal wall are fused and cannot be separated.

The umbilicus is important only in that an incision should avoid it by skirting it or by excising it entirely. When closing an incision, if the needle enters umbilical tissue the dense scar will make its penetration difficult.

TYPES AND CHOICE OF INCISIONS

Abdominal incisions can be divided roughly into three general types: (1) vertical incisions, (2) transverse incisions, and (3) special incisions. In many instances any one of the three types will provide satisfactory exposure for the procedure contemplated, and there is considerable difference of opinion, particularly when the choice lies between a vertical and a transverse incision, as to which incision should be selected.

Abdominal incisions have a marked effect on pulmonary physiology. The upper abdominal incisions are more significant in their effect upon respiration. Breathing patterns are changed, the respiratory rate increases, and tidal volume and vital capacity are reduced. Patients tend to become hypoxemic. Forced expiratory volume at 1 second (FEV_1) is reduced.

In the 1940s it was noted that pulmonary complications occurred four times more frequently in the patient with a vertical rather than a transverse abdominal incision. Despite very few reports, some of which conflict, it appears now that transverse incisions may not impair respiration as much as vertical incisions. The severely obese person appears to have better postoperative pulmonary function when a transverse instead of a vertical upper abdominal incision can be used.

Rees and Coller (1943) and Coller and MacLean (1949) expressed a strong preference for transverse incisions over vertical ones for abdominal operations, and pointed out these advantages:

1. The skin incision parallels Langer's lines of skin cleavage and gives a better cosmetic result than does a vertical incision.

2. Transverse incisions are closed in a

TYPES AND CHOICE OF INCISIONS

direction that places only one-thirtieth as much tension on the suture line as is exerted on the suture line of a vertical incision. This is due to the lateral force exerted by the oblique abdominal musculature during breathing, coughing, vomiting, and defecation.

3. Transverse incisions run more or less parallel to and do not transect the fibers of the muscle aponeuroses, so that when the involved muscles are tensed the edges of the transverse wound tend to be approximated while the edges of a vertical wound are strongly separated.

4. Transverse incisions facilitate closure of the peritoneum and posterior rectus sheath, an important factor in minimizing postoperative adhesions.

5. Transverse incisions run almost parallel to the direction of the neural and vascular supply and therefore destroy fewer nerves and blood vessels than do vertical transrectus incisions, or vertical incisions made along the lateral margin of the rectus muscles.

6. Transverse incisions can be extended vertically in the midline, either up or down, when further exposure is required.

7. The blood supply to the region of a transverse incision is better than that to a vertical midline incision, and therefore healing of a transverse incision should be more rapid.

These arguments should be balanced against the advantages of vertical incisions:

1. Compared with transverse incisions, vertical midline or paramedian incisions are more quickly made and more quickly closed. They pass through fewer tissue layers and require less suturing for closure. If an emergency arises they can be closed with one through-and-through row of sutures.

2. Vertical midline or paramedian incisions destroy few if any nerves or blood vessels supplying the tissues.

3. Vertical midline or paramedian incisions are made through a relatively avascular field and give less troublesome bleeding than do transverse incisions.

4. In some areas vertical midline or paramedian incisions provide better exposure or are more easily extended than transverse incisions. This is particularly true for operations on the cardiac end of the stomach or the rectosigmoid.

It also should be pointed out again that transverse incisions made well below the umbilicus may be followed by such great retraction of the severed rectus muscle fibers that their cut ends cannot be well approximated at the time of closure. This is due to the frequent absence of the transverse tendinous intersections in that area.

There is a place for both vertical and transverse incisions. When vertical incisions are used they should be in the midline or paramedian and middle or lateral transrectus in exceptional circumstances. Special incisions also have a place for special specific operations.

An incision should be selected with the following qualifications in mind:

1. It must give ready and direct access to the source of trouble and provide adequate exposure for the operation contemplated.

2. It should be extensible in the direction that probably would be required by any increase in the magnitude of the operation.

3. It should injure the fewest possible number of motor nerves, preferably not more than one.

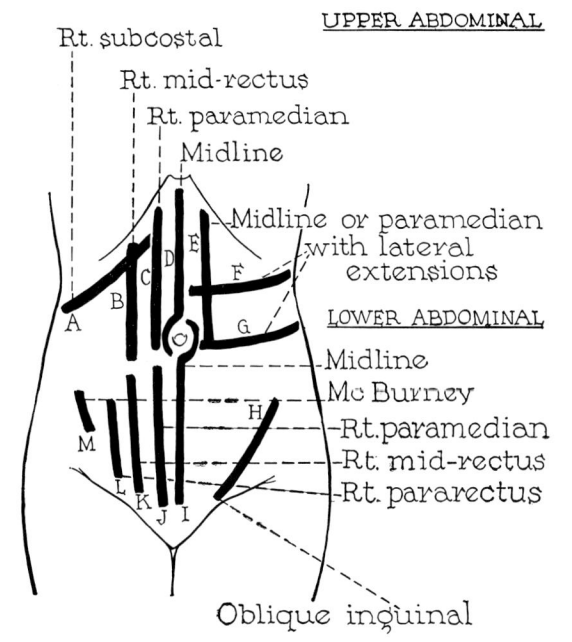

Figure 18–18. Principal vertical abdominal incisions. These may be made on either side, depending upon the site of the surgical lesion.

Figure 18-19. Principal transverse abdominal incisions. These are preferred by an increasing number of surgeons in recent years, and are usable on either side, depending upon the site of the surgical lesions.

4. It should be capable of being securely repaired so as to leave the abdominal wall at least as strong after the operation as before.

5. It should provide an acceptable cosmetic result when possible.

It is important that an abdominal incision be made long enough to provide an adequate visualization of the operative field and uncrowded conditions for the necessary manipulations. Although it is true that wounds heal across the line of incision and therefore are not affected by the length, there is no point in making incisions longer than necessary to obtain the exposure desired.

With these objectives in mind, specific abdominal incisions (Figs. 18-18 and 18-19) will be described.

Upper Midline Incisions

This is the incision preferred by many surgeons for exploration of and most operations upon the stomach. It provides excellent exposure for partial gastrectomy and can easily be extended upward to or into the chest for total gastrectomy or operations on the lower esophagus or diaphragm. It can be extended downward around the navel for as far as necessary and, when required, can be extended laterally as a T or L incision. An upper midline incision destroys no nerves, and can be quickly made and easily closed. It is thought to be more vulnerable to postoperative herniation because of its relatively meager blood supply.

TECHNIC

An incision is made through the skin and subcutaneous tissue from the tip of the

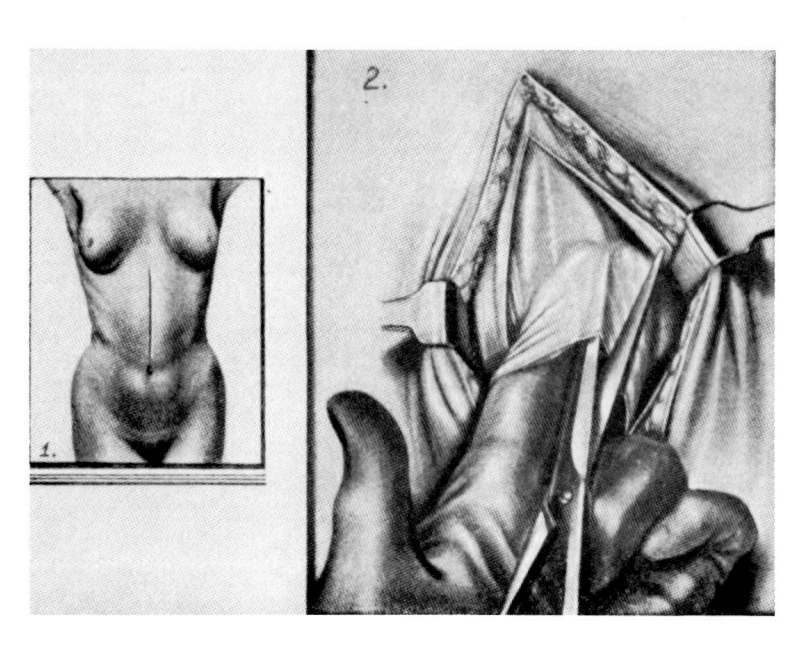

Figure 18-20. Midline vertical epigastric incision. 1, The line of the incision extends from the xiphisternum to the umbilicus. 2, Method of opening the peritoneal cavity. (From Maingot, R.: Abdominal Operations, ed. 2. New York, Appleton-Century-Crofts, 1948.)

xiphoid downward in the midline to a point about 3 cm. proximal to the umbilicus. If a longer incision is desired, it is extended downward to curve around either the right or left side of the umbilicus to continue in the lower midline.

The shiny white linea alba and anterior rectus sheath are cleared of fat laterally for about 2 cm. on each side. The linea alba and transversalis fascia are divided exactly in the midline, exposing the extraperitoneal fat. Since the extraperitoneal fat may be abundant and vascular in the upper part of the incision and since it contains the ligamentum teres of the liver, which runs just to the right of the midline, it is advisable to avoid cutting through it by opening the peritoneal layer at a point well left of the midline, beneath the belly of the left rectus muscle and in the lower portion of the incision. After the peritoneal cavity has been opened, a finger is slipped beneath it, and the peritoneum is divided over the finger as it is advanced (Fig. 18–20) upward and downward, protecting underlying viscera from injury. If the ligamentum teres interferes with exposure, it should be divided between clamps and the cut ends ligated.

After the operation has been completed, the incision is closed.

There are many acceptable ways to close an abdominal incision. The method of closure should be chosen so as to produce the fewest wound complications: dehiscence, incisional hernia, and infection. One should select the method of closure that is best for the patient and is well performed by the surgeon.

Wound Closure in Layers

In the patient whose condition is good and in whom rapid closure is not imperative, the wound can be approximated in layers in the following manner:

1. If the ligamentum teres of the liver has been severed, the two cut ends are reapposed with a catgut, synthetic absorbable, or silk ligature.

2. The cut edges of the peritoneum, transversalis fascia, and posterior rectus sheath are approximated with a row of sutures (see Fig. 18–30A). For this, one may prefer to employ a continuous over-and-over suture of 2–0 plain catgut, 2–0 chromic, or synthetic absorbable. Others prefer interrupted sutures of the same materials or of silk. In placing these sutures, if the peritoneum is so friable as to permit the sutures to cut through, a few muscle fibers and the deep and medial portion of the rectus muscle should be included in each bite to provide firmer anchorage.

3. The cut edges of the linea alba are approximated with interrupted sutures. This is the most important and strength-giving portion of the closure and must be performed with care. A variety of suture materials and types of suture have been employed. Nonabsorbable suture material is best for this purpose. One could employ 0-nylon, 0-polypropylene, or No. 30 stainless steel wire suture in patients in whom the intestinal tract has been opened, or drainage is instituted. For clean wounds one could use 2–0 silk or any of the above sutures. Some surgeons prefer to use absorbable suture material for this layer. No. 1 chromic catgut, or synthetic absorbable 0-polyglycolic or polyglactin 910 has been used successfully.

The method of suturing the linea alba with nonabsorbable suture may vary. In the average patient, when there is little or no tension a row of simple, interrupted, over-and-over sutures placed through the linea alba at least 1 cm. lateral to the cut edge on each side, and including a few underlying fibers of the rectus muscle in each side, is used. Each stitch is tied immediately. The tied long ends can be cut or can be left long and held for traction until the next suture has been placed.

When the cut edges of the linea alba can be approximated only with tension, one can close with interrupted far-near sutures. These penetrate the rectus sheath about 3 cm. lateral to the cut edge, pass beneath it through the anterior fibers of the rectus muscle to cross the wound and emerge through the anterior rectus sheath 0.5 cm. from its cut edge on the other side, cross over the wound to penetrate the original side of the anterior sheath from superficial to deep at a point 0.5 cm. lateral to its cut edge, recross the wound, and pass through the superficial rectus fibers beneath the rectus sheath of the other side to emerge about 3 cm. lateral to the edges (Fig. 18–21A). When these sutures are pulled taut and tied, any tension is distributed to four

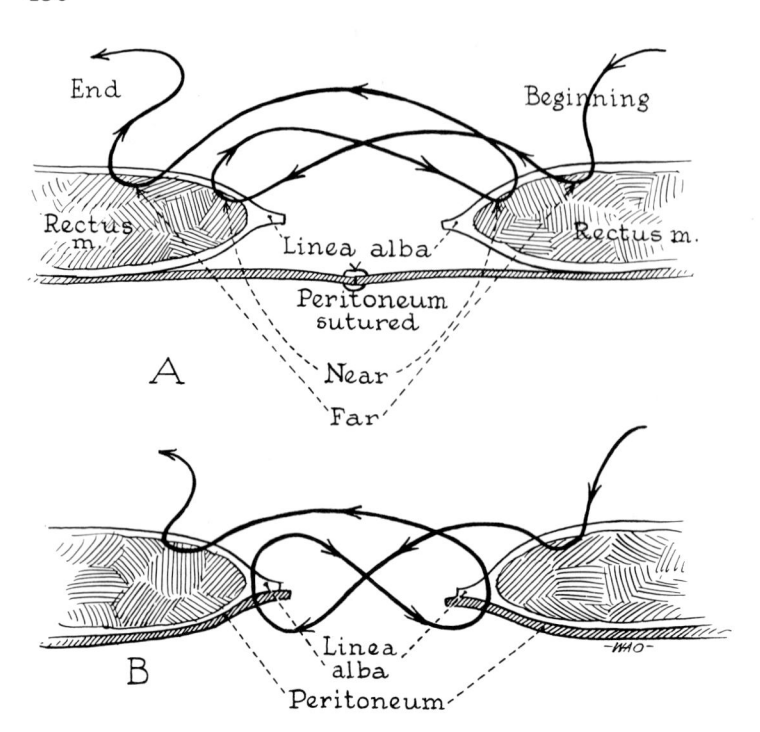

Figure 18-21. *A*, Scheme of interrupted far-near suture used when linea alba can be approximated only with tension; *B*, same type of suture used to close the linea alba and peritoneum. (Modified from Maingot, cited in previous figure.)

points instead of only two and a stronger closure results, although more time is consumed in its performance.

This type of suturing is also helpful when there is difficulty in approximating the cut edges of the peritoneum. In such a subject a few peritoneal sutures are placed and then covered over with near-far sutures placed in the rectus sheath as just described. This more closely approximates the portion of the wound just above so that more peritoneal sutures can be placed above to be covered in turn by the rectus sheath. Progressing in this way, a peritoneal layer which previously seemed impossible to close can often be approximated satisfactorily. In some instances suturing of the rectus sheath alone will approximate the peritoneal edges without the necessity of the edges being sutured separately, but for most patients a separate peritoneal closure would be preferred.

The same type of technic can be used to close the peritoneum and linea alba with one row of stainless steel wire or 0-polypropylene sutures (Fig. 18-21). This is a particularly valuable method when the peritoneal layer cannot be separated from the overlying layers.

When closing either the peritoneal or linea alba layer, the suturing should begin at the lower end of the incision and progress upward toward the xiphoid. Sutures should be placed about 1 cm. apart, and, at the conclusion of the closure, there should be no space between them wide enough to admit the tip of a little finger.

4. After the linea alba has been firmly closed, the subcutaneous fat and fascia are approximated with a row of fine sutures. For this layer, one may use 4-0 plain catgut, 3-0 or 4-0 polyglactin 910, polyglycolic acid or 4-0 silk, placed as simple over-and-over interrupted sutures. Silk should never be used in possibly contaminated wounds.

5. The skin is closed with 3-0 or 4-0 nylon or 4-0 silk by one of the methods described under skin sutures (p. 544). Continuous or interrupted sutures are used for this layer. Stainless steel staples also can be used. If the wound is suspected of possible contamination, one should use interrupted sutures. These sutures are removed on the fifth to seventh postoperative day.

METHODS OF UPWARD EXTENSION

An upper midline incision easily can be extended to provide greater exposure upward by removing the xiphoid process, by extrapleural division of the costal arch, by abdominothoracic extension, or by splitting

TYPES AND CHOICE OF INCISIONS

the sternum. Note that these methods either open a thoracic cavity intentionally or carry the risk of doing so unintentionally.

By Removing the Xiphoid Process

LeFevre (1946) recommended this method of extending the incision for improving the exposure in performing total gastrectomy, and Saint and Braslow (1953) have pointed out its usefulness also for such operations as subdiaphragmatic vagotomy, splenectomy, and repair of a diaphragmatic hernia through the abdominal approach.

It is executed as follows:

The abdominal cavity is entered and explored through a conventional upper midline incision, as previously described. When additional exposure is desired the incision is extended upward through the skin and superficial fascia to a point about 2 cm. above the xiphosternal junction. The linea alba, which passes upward over the lower edge of the xiphoid to attach to the upper half of its anterior surface, is incised. The anterior and posterior surfaces as well as the lateral margins of the xiphoid are freed of their attachments by the use of a blunt periosteal elevator. The sternal origin

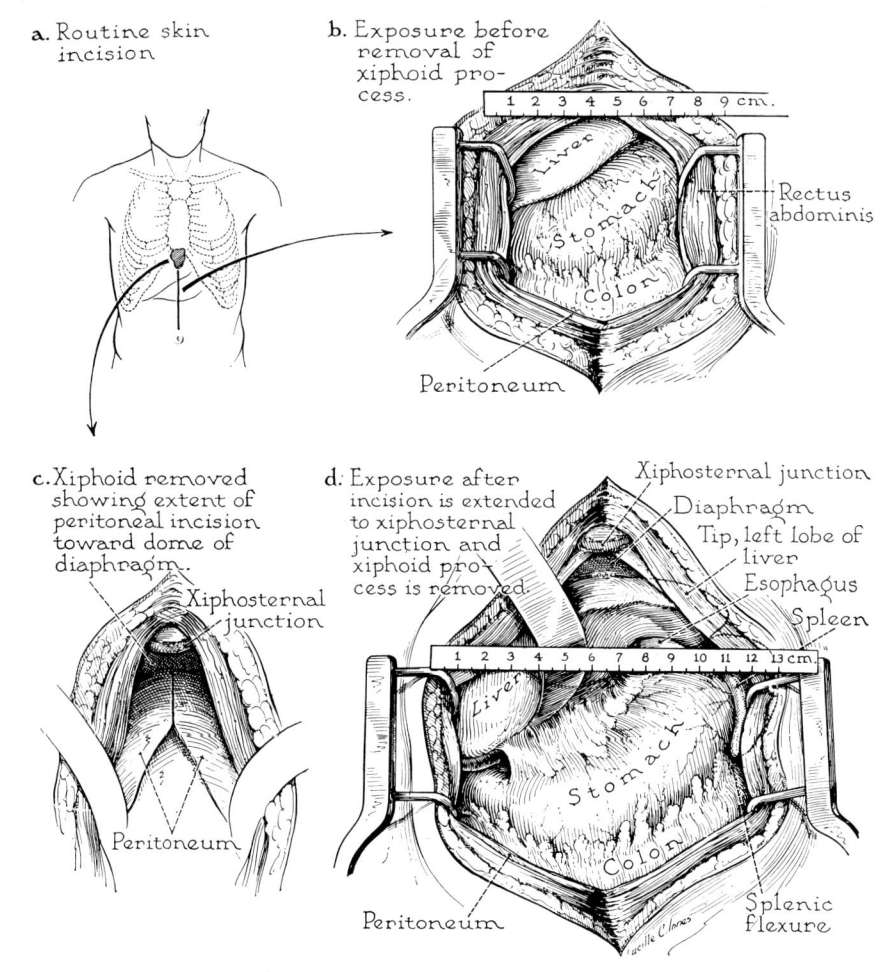

Figure 18–22. Upper abdominal midline incision; enlargement of the operative field resulting from the removal of the xiphoid process and the upward extension of the peritoneal opening made possible by this procedure. (From photographs taken at operation.) (From Saint, J. H., and Braslow, L. E.: Removal of the xiphoid process as an aid in operations on the upper abdomen. Surgery 33:361, 1953.)

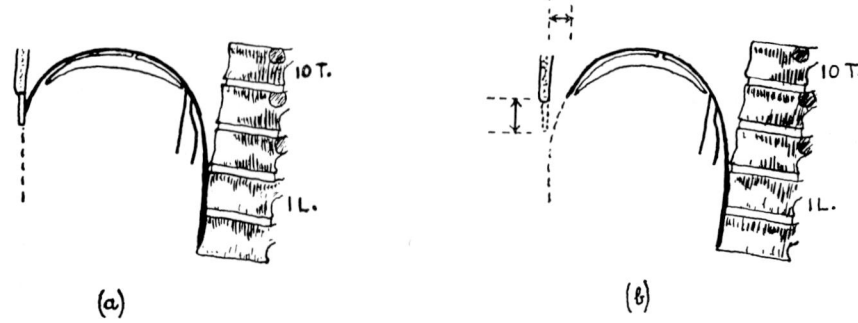

Figure 18-23. Diagrams in sagittal plane showing upper midline incision before (A) and after (B) removal of the xiphoid process. Note in B the upward extension of the peritoneal incision and the resultant decrease in anteroposterior depth of the wound. (From Saint and Braslow, cited in previous figure.)

of the diaphragm attaches to the posterior surface of the xiphoid, and its release permits this portion of the diaphragm to fall backward, carrying with it its covering peritoneum. The bared xiphoid is now removed by piecemeal excision with a bone rongeur. The diaphragm can now be incised upward in its midline for 4 to 5 cm. (Fig. 18-22).

These steps increase the length of the exposure to reach almost the top of the diaphragmatic dome, facilitating the approach to structures attached to its inferior surface. They also increase the width of the exposure by permitting the edges of the incision to be retracted about one-half again as much as was previously possible (Fig. 18-22). Furthermore, the depth of the wound is decreased, with the result that the structures are more accessible to manipulations. This is due to the fact that the upper edges of the incised diaphragm and peritoneum have dropped posteriorly after their attachments to the xiphoid have been severed (Fig. 18-23).

After the operation has been completed, this incision is closed in the way described for closing a conventional upper midline one, except for its upper end. After the peritoneal opening has been closed, the upper portion of the incised linea alba is closed with three or four nonabsorbable sutures which include a bite in the previously retroxiphoid margin of the diaphragm. When these sutures are tied the diaphragm becomes reattached to the abdominal midline, and the dead space left by removal of the xiphoid is obliterated.

One should be aware that the patient can develop a pneumothorax from a very small tear along the diaphragmatic attachment.

By Extrapleural Division of the Costal Arch

This method is useful to gain 3 to 5 cm. additional exposure upward in performing a subdiaphragmatic vagotomy, high subtotal gastrectomy, or repair of a diaphragmatic hernia through an abdominal approach.

The technic is as follows:

A conventional upper midline incision is made and exploration completed. If a few centimeters of additional exposure upward are desired, the upper end of the incision is extended laterally to either the right or the left (usually the left) at the level of the tip of the xiphoid for about 6 cm. The incision will encounter the costal arch (forward extension of the seventh costal cartilage). The arch is scraped bare around its entire circumference for a distance of about 6 cm. with a periosteal elevator, and its bared area is cut through with a scalpel (one can cut through the costal arch at each end of the bared area and remove the intervening segment [Fig. 18-24]). If the accompanying intercostal vessels are injured, they should be ligated. The same is true of the superior epigastric vessels. Care is taken not to open the pleura. After the costal arch has been divided, a retractor placed on that side will retract the wound edge appreciably farther than hitherto had been possible and may change the exposure from one that was crowded to one that is comfortable.

After the operation has been completed the incision is closed as previously described for an upper midline incision. If the

TYPES AND CHOICE OF INCISIONS

Figure 18–24. Method of extending an upper midline incision. *A*, Lateral extension (dotted line) of conventional upper midline incision. *B*, Exposure of costal arch; the cartilage has been scraped bare around its entire circumference. Incisions either to reflect or resect the costal arch are indicated.

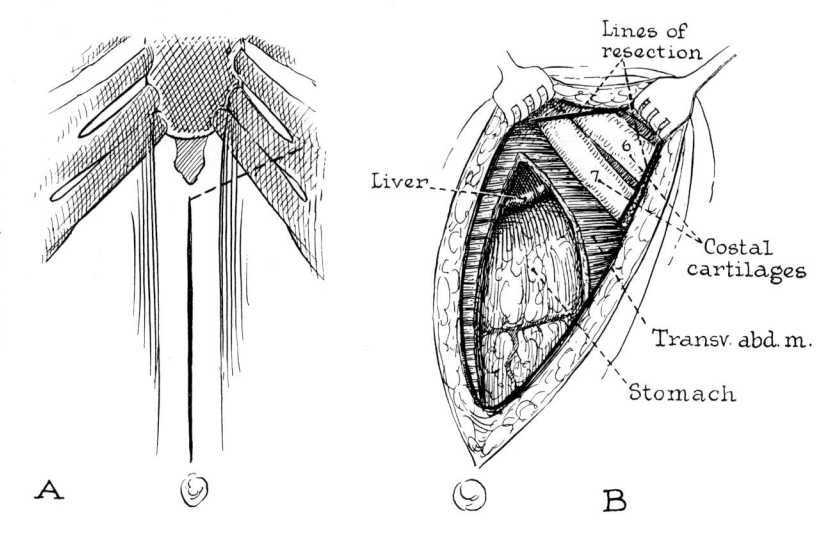

costal arch was only divided without removing a segment, the cut ends of the cartilage are reapproximated with a single suture of No. 1 silk, 0–1 nylon, polyglactin 910, or No. 26 stainless steel wire. If a short segment of the arch was removed, this step is unnecessary as the cut ends need not be sutured.

This method is useful to gain small amounts of additional exposure with minimal effort in appropriate cases.

By Abdominothoracic Extension (Garlock)

This method of extending an upper midline incision upward is useful for performing a total gastrectomy, high subtotal gastrectomy, or resection of the lower portion of the esophagus. It provides an exposure similar to the thoracoabdominal incision of Carter (p. 452), but has the advantage in that the abdominal exploration is first carried out through a midline abdominal incision and the chest is not opened until after the decision to proceed with the operation has been made.

Its technic is described:

A conventional upper midline incision is made and the abdomen explored to determine the nature and operability of the lesion and the extent of the exposure that will be required.

The upper end of the incision is then extended upward and laterally to the left, across the left costal arch, to pass along the seventh intercostal space to the posterior axillary line (Fig. 18–25).

The eighth costal cartilage is bared of attachments around its entire circumference for about 4 cm. by the use of periosteal

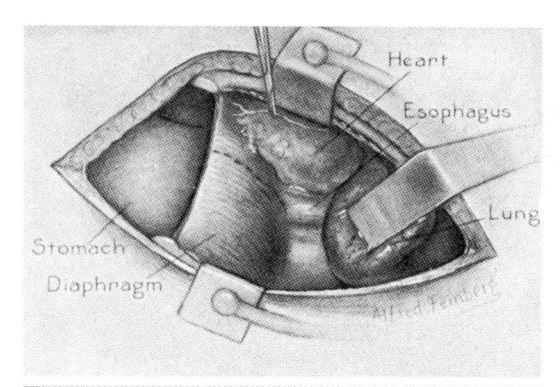

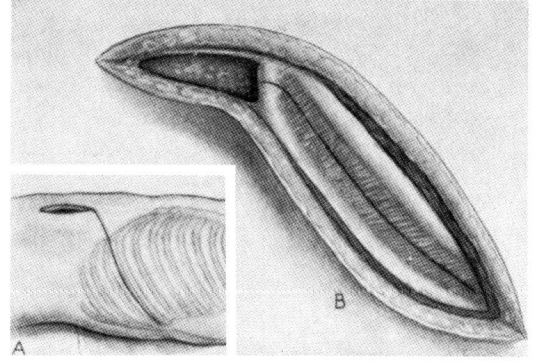

Figure 18–25. Garlock combined abdominothoracic approach to lower end of esophagus and cardia of stomach. A 12.5-cm. left pararectus incision begins just below the costal arch between the left eighth and ninth ribs. The incision is swung upward and outward in the eighth rib intercostal space as far as the vertebral border of the scapula. The costal arch is divided along the line of incision between the eighth and ninth ribs. (From Garlock, J. H.: Combined abdominothoracic approach for carcinoma of cardia and lower esophagus. Surg. Gynecol. Obstet. 83:737, 1946.)

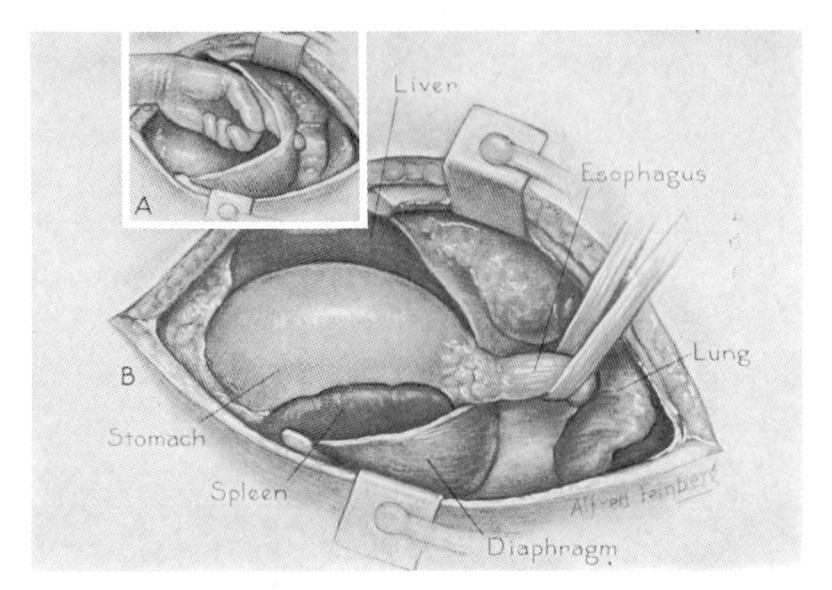

Figure 18-26. Garlock combined abdominothoracic incision (*continued*). Diaphragm divided in direction of skin wound from its peripheral attachment to the esophageal hiatus. Rib edges retracted and excellent exposure of gastric cardia and lower esophagus obtained. (From Garlock, cited in previous figure.)

elevator and is transected with a knife. The superior epigastric (internal mammary) and the eighth intercostal vessels are clamped, cut, and ligated where they emerge from beneath the transected portion of the costal cartilage. The pleural cavity is entered through the seventh intercostal space (as described for an intercostal thoracotomy, p. 446), and the seventh and eighth ribs are spread with a Finochietto retractor. The left half of the diaphragm is divided from the point of transection of the costal cartilage radially toward and through the esophageal hiatus (Fig. 18-26). This provides an excellent exposure of the gastric cardia and lower esophagus.

In those patients in whom the esophagus requires mobilization as high as the inferior margin of the lung hiatus, it is preferable to extend the upper midline abdominal incision upward along the left side of the xiphoid to the xiphosternal junction and then carry it to the left along the fifth intercostal space to the posterior axillary line. It is necessary to transect both the seventh and sixth costal arches, and the pleural cavity is entered in the fifth intercostal space. This modification provides a better exposure of the junction of the middle and lower thirds of the thoracic esophagus while providing a similar exposure of abdominal viscera as obtained when the seventh intercostal space is entered.

After the operation has been completed, the incision in the diaphragm is closed with interrupted No. 1 silk sutures, 0-1 polyglactin 910, or polyglycolic acid or braided polyester, the rib retractors being relaxed as the outermost of these sutures is tied. The peritoneal layer of the abdominal portion of the incision is closed with a continuous 0 plain catgut suture or 0 polyglactin 910 or polyglycolic acid. A separate stab wound is made in the posterior axillary line in the most dependent part of the chest, and through it a thoracotomy drainage catheter is positioned in the left thoracic cavity. The separated ribs are approximated with several perichondral sutures of No. 1 chromic catgut. The cut ends of the costal cartilages are sutured together with No. 1 silk or No. 30 stainless steel wire sutures. The lung is fully expanded by the anesthetist. The incised muscles and fascia of the thoracic incision are approximated with interrupted sutures of 2-0 polyglactin 910, or polyglycolic acid, or 2-0 silk. The linea alba of the abdominal portion of the incision is repaired, using the same type of sutures. The subcutaneous tissues are approximated. The skin incision is closed.

This incision provides excellent exposure, but its closure is tedious.

By Splitting the Sternum (Wangensteen)

This method of extension provides excellent exposure for operations on the lowermost portion of the esophagus, gastric cardia, diaphragm, spleen, and left lobe of the liver. Somewhat higher portions of the esophagus are obscured by the heart, and for them the abdominothoracic approach of Garlock is better.

The procedure is executed as follows:

A conventional upper midline incision is made from the xiphoid to just above the umbilicus, and through this the abdominal exploration is carried out. If extension of this incision upward is desired, a small incision is made in the tissues just posterior to the xiphoid, and a finger is inserted into the anterior mediastinum just under the sternum. Care is taken not to enter either pleural cavity. The sternum and xiphoid are split. At the uppermost portion of the division of the sternum the incision may or may not be carried diagonally across the sternum to the intercostal space without entering the pleural cavity. Care is taken to avoid injuring the internal thoracic (internal mammary) vessels. If they are injured their cut ends must be ligated (Fig. 18–27). A short Finochietto retractor is inserted, and the split edges of the sternum are gradually spread apart. The diaphragm is divided between successive Kelly clamps radially toward the esophageal hiatus for as far as desired. The length of its division will vary with the operative procedure to be performed. Suture ligatures are placed through the diaphragm beneath each hemostat to control bleeding, and their ends are left long to serve for traction and to facilitate later closure of this structure. The pericardium can usually be separated from the superior surface of the diaphragm with ease, although Miller (1952) has pointed out that it will be more difficult in a secondary operation on this area.

When the operative procedure has been completed the cut edges of the diaphragm are reunited with interrupted sutures of No. 1 silk, No.1 polyglactin 910, or polyglycolic acid, care being taken to re-form the esophageal hiatus to a suitable size if it had been divided. The divided sternum may be approximated either by drilling holes in each side through which No. 30 stainless steel wire sutures are passed and tied across the incision, or by the use of peristernal sutures of No. 1 chromic catgut or No. 1 polyglactin 910. In either method, care is taken to avoid injuring the internal thoracic vessels or the pleura on either side.

The abdominal portion of the incision may be closed as described for the closure of an upper midline incision.

This procedure provides an excellent exposure for the esophago-gastric-diaphragmatic area and does so without opening into a pleural cavity.

EXTENSION BY LATERAL TRANSVERSE ABDOMINAL INCISION

Occasionally an exploration through an upper midline incision will reveal a lesion in a lateral portion of the abdominal cavity

Figure 18–27. Large figure on left represents exposure for gastroesophageal resection or for repair of hiatal hernia. (From Miller, H. I.: Sternum-splitting incision for upper abdominal surgery. Arch. Surg. 65:876, 1952.)

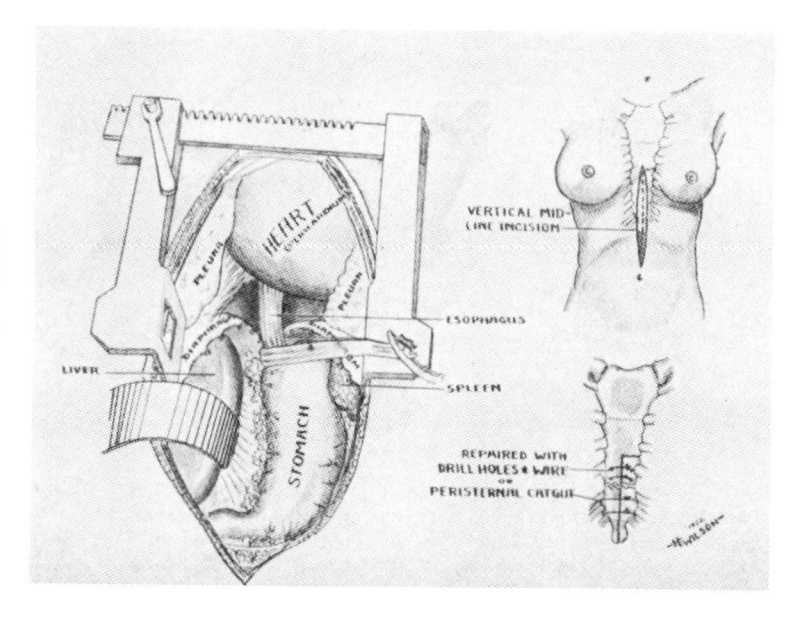

which cannot be exposed satisfactorily through the original incision. In this case the midline incision can be extended laterally to either side by making a transverse incision through the abdominal wall at the appropriate level to join the midline incision. Thus if the lateral incision joins the midportion of the midline incision, it forms a T-shaped incision, or if it joins the midline incision at its lowermost point, it forms an L-incision.

The T- or L-shaped incision is useful in patients in whom the spleen or liver is found to be ruptured and better exposure is required for its removal or repair; in those with tumors extending further laterally than anticipated, particularly tumors involving the kidney or the splenic or hepatic flexures of the colon.

This type of incision should seldom be planned in advance as transverse abdominal incisions alone will usually suffice, but it is most useful when exploration reveals the need for greater exposure laterally.

The technic is as follows:

Abdominal exploration is carried out through an upper midline incision.

When lateral extension is desired, the skin and subcutaneous tissues are incised laterally at the desired level for as far as is considered necessary. The anterior rectus sheath is incised transversely from the midline to its lateral margin. The upper and lower corners of the rectus sheath are each marked with a traction suture to identify them and facilitate their approximation at the time of closure. The median free margin of the rectus muscle is identified and raised, and two fingers are passed deep to the rectus fibers but superficial to the posterior rectus sheath. The rectus muscle is transected over these fingers from its medial to its lateral edge (Fig. 18–28A). The superior epigastric vessels on that side are clamped, cut, and ligated.

The fibers of the aponeurosis of the external oblique muscle are severed from their attachment to this portion of the anterior rectus sheath upward and downward for about 4 cm. in each direction. The external oblique muscle can then be divided in the direction of its fibers as far laterally as desired and retracted enough to provide adequate exposure despite the upward obliquity of the fibers' course (Fig. 18–28B). This simple step, although not essential, saves cutting across the external oblique fibers, minimizes bleeding, and facilitates the subsequent closure. Innervation is preserved.

Two fingers are passed laterally beneath the peritoneum and over these fingers the posterior sheath and peritoneum are divided laterally (the upper and lower corners of the peritoneum are tagged with a suture to facilitate their later identification and approximation). While the edges of the external oblique muscle are retracted, the incision is continued laterally to divide the internal oblique and the transversus ab-

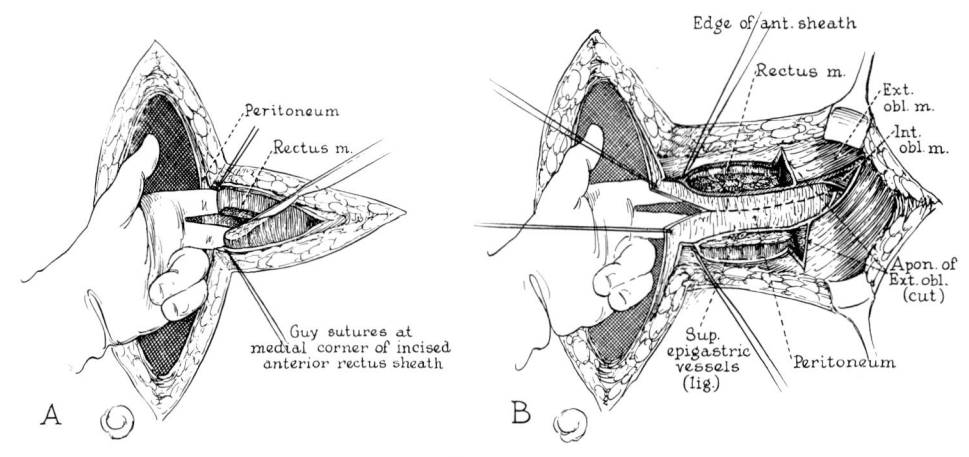

Figure 18–28. T-shaped extension of upper midline incision. A, Transection of rectus muscle over two fingers placed deep to the muscle and anterior to the posterior sheath. B, Fibers of external oblique aponeurosis severed upward and downward at attachment to anterior rectus sheath; oblique muscles split in direction of fibers, preserving innervation; lateral division over fingers of posterior rectus sheath and peritoneum.

dominis muscles in the direction of their fibers and to incise the underlying transversalis fascia and peritoneum for as far as necessary to obtain the exposure desired. Bleeders are clamped and tied as they are cut. This incision, if made transversely, nearly always cuts across one intercostal nerve, occasionally two, but rarely is long enough to sever three. Paralysis of the abdominal muscles following the use of this technic is rarely observed.

After the operation has been completed, the incision is closed in the following manner:

The sutures identifying the upper and lower corners of the peritoneum at the point where the midline incision was T'd are tied together to approximate those corners and delineate the vertical and transverse components of the peritoneal layer of the incision. The peritoneal layer of the transverse portion of the incision is closed with a continuous 2-0 plain catgut, polyglactin 910, or polyglycolic acid suture. The peritoneum and posterior rectus sheath of the vertical portion of the incision are closed with another continuous suture of the same material. The divided edges of the internal oblique and transversus abdominis muscles are approximated by interrupted sutures of 2-0 silk, polyglactin 910, or polyglycolic acid passed through their investing fasciae, closing the deeper muscular layer of the transverse part of the incision. The superficial muscular part is closed by suturing together the divided edges of the external oblique muscle with the same material, care being taken to reattach the portion that was detached from the anterior rectus sheath. The sutures marking the corners of the divided rectus sheath are tied together, delineating the transverse incision of that sheath. This incision is closed with interrupted sutures of doubled 2-0 silk or No. 30 stainless steel wire, or a nylon or polypropylene suture.

The vertical incision through the linea alba is closed with interrupted sutures of the same material.

The subcutaneous tissue of the vertical and also of the transverse portions of the incision is approximated with interrupted sutures of 4-0 silk, polyglactin 910, or polyglycolic acid. The transverse portion of the skin incision is approximated with a continuous 4-0 nylon or silk suture, and the vertical portion with another but similar suture.

Interrupted sutures can be used for the skin. Rapid closure can be accomplished by using stainless steel skin stapling devices. if preferred, but are more time-consuming.

This incision is a tedious one to close, but a strong closure usually can be obtained, and the occurrence of a subsequent incisional hernia has seemed little if any more frequent than with more conventional incisions of the same magnitude.

Lower Midline Incision

This incision is commonly employed by gynecologists for operations on the female pelvic organs. It is also frequently used for operations on the rectosigmoid and other viscera in the lower abdomen or pelvis. The technic differs slightly from that of an upper midline incision. When this incision is contemplated one should make certain that the urinary bladder has been emptied just prior to the operation.

TECHNIC

An incision is made through the skin and subcutaneous tissue in the midline from a point just below the umbilicus to the crest of the symphysis pubis.

The surface of the anterior sheath of the rectus is cleared of fat for about 2 cm. lateral to the midline on each side for the entire extent of the incision (Fig. 18-29A). Doing this at this time will greatly facilitate the subsequent exposure.

The linea alba is narrow below the umbilicus and may be difficult to identify. When its exact location is in doubt, the anterior rectus sheath should be incised carefully just above the symphysis pubis, where the direction of the fibers of the pyramidalis muscle on either side will lead upward to the midline. Once its location is identified, the linea alba is incised at the upper end of the incision, and this incision is carried down to the symphysis pubis (Fig. 18-29B,C,D).

The right and left rectus sheaths, with their contained rectus muscles, are retracted laterally, exposing the underlying transversalis fascia, urachus cord, and peritoneum.

The peritoneal layer is carefully

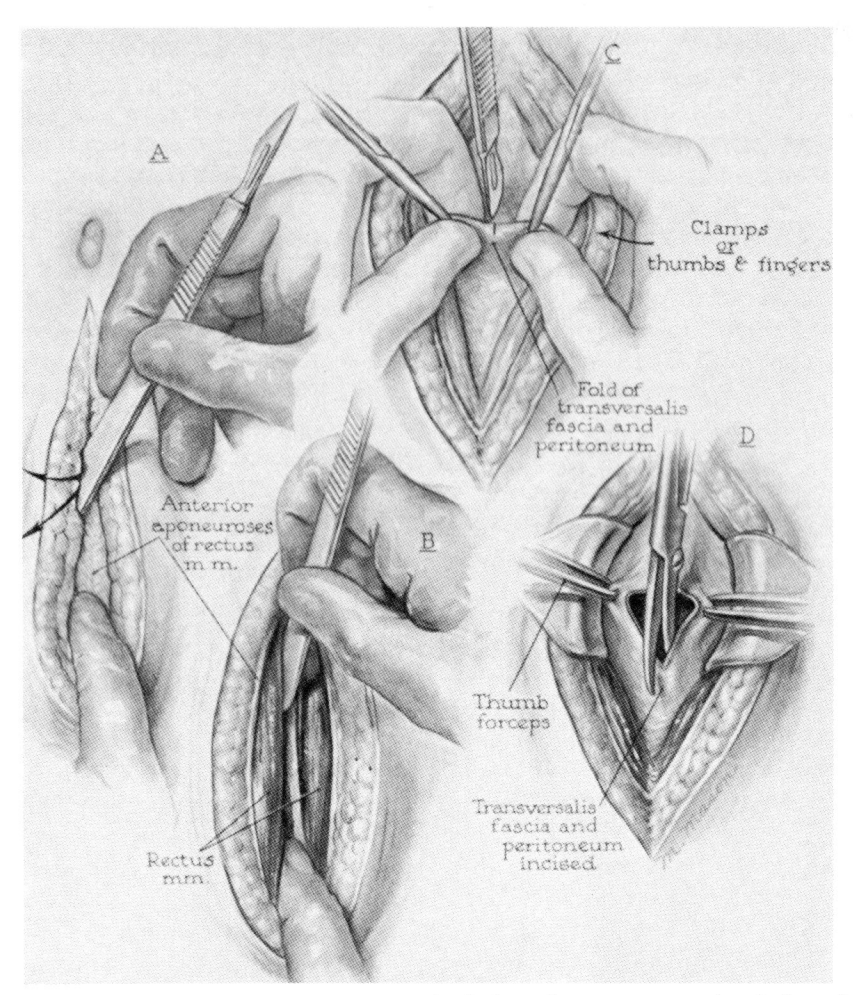

Figure 18–29. Lower midline incision. *A*, Clearing the fat from the anterior recti sheaths lateral to the midline; *B*, the linea alba has been incised and the muscle compartments opened; *C* and *D*, incision of the transversalis fascia and peritoneum with scissors.

opened about 4 cm. below the umbilicus and, before it is divided further, two fingers are inserted into the peritoneal cavity and passed downward to palpate the upper limits of the urinary bladder. With the fingers pushing the peritoneum anteriorly, the transversalis fascia is divided vertically downward by blunt dissection with the handle of the knife to the symphysis pubis. This maneuver will strip any upward extension of the bladder downward out of harm's way. The thin peritoneum can now be incised vertically with relatively safety for the entire length of the abdominal incision.

After the operative procedure has been completed, the peritoneal and transversalis fascial layers are closed together with a continuous suture of 2–0 plain catgut, or polyglactin 910, or polyglycolic acid suture (Fig. 18–30). The anterior rectus sheath is closed using the technic employed to close the upper midline incisions.

COMMENT

A low midline incision is easily made, provides good exposure of the lower abdomen and pelvis, and is easily and quickly closed. It destroys no nerves.

METHODS OF EXTENSION

A low midline incision cannot be extended downward.

TYPES AND CHOICE OF INCISIONS 499

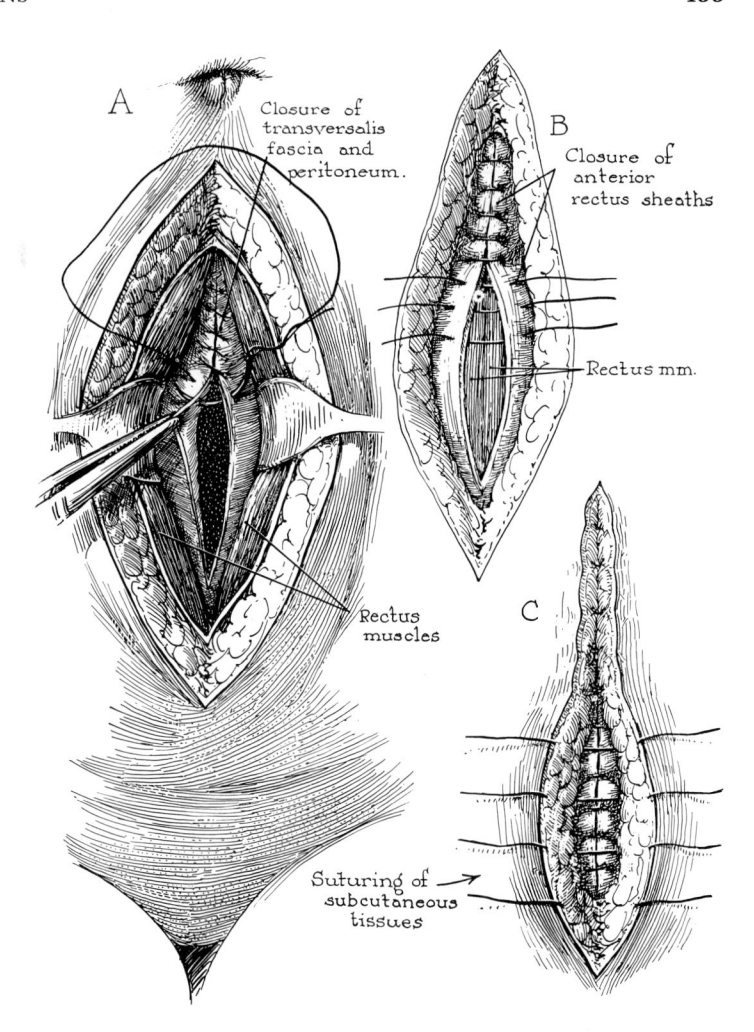

Figure 18-30. Closure of lower midline incision. *A*, Suture of the transversalis fascia and peritoneum; *B*, suture of linea alba (anterior rectus sheaths); *C*, suture of the subcutaneous tissues. The skin edges are approximated with interrupted sutures.

It can be extended upward by curving the incision around either side of the umbilicus (preferably the left so as to avoid the falciform ligament) to continue in the upper midline for as far as desired.

It can be extended laterally by adding a transverse abdominal component to form a T or an L, as described for the lateral extension of an upper midline incision (p. 495). In this instance the transverse portion of the incision should be placed in the upper portion of the lower abdomen, nearer the umbilicus than the symphysis, to minimize the amount of retraction of the cut rectus fibers.

Paramedian Incision

A paramedian incision can be made on either the right or the left side of the midline and in the upper, middle, or lower portions of the abdomen, or it can be extended vertically from one to the other. In an upper paramedian incision, the greater part of the incision extends upward above the level of the umbilicus, in a middle paramedian incision the center of the incision is to the right or left of about the level of the umbilicus, and in a low paramedian incision the greater portion of the incision extends below the umbilicus. Paramedian, like midline, incisions do not destroy the nerve supply to any muscles, hence they can be made as long as required without creating irreparable damage. They are thought to heal more rapidly than midline incisions because of their more abundant blood supply and are believed to provide stronger healing because an intact rectus muscle overlies and supports the suture line in the posterior rectus sheath and peritoneum.

The paramedian incision is a very popular one for many operative procedures, and many surgeons consider it the incision of choice for operations in which it provides adequate exposure. Hence a right upper paramedian is used by some for operations on the liver, gallbladder, or common duct. A left upper paramedian is used for a partial or total gastrectomy.

Low paramedian incisions on the left are used for operations on the left colon and rectosigmoid and on the right are used for operations on the female pelvic organs or right colon or for the removal of an uncertainly diagnosed pathologic appendix.

TECHNIC

At the desired level and for the desired length, a vertical incision is made about 2 cm. lateral and parallel to the anterior midline of the abdomen. The anterior sheath of the rectus muscle is bared of fat for a width of about 3 cm. and is incised vertically about 2 cm. lateral to the abdominal midline (Fig. 18–31). The cut edge of the medial flap of rectus sheath is held forward while the surgeon employs the handle of the scalpel to locate and free the medial edge of the rectus muscle from any attachment to its sheath or to the midline. In so doing, any transverse tendinous intersections encountered should be severed from their medial attachment to the linea alba with a knife. The rectus muscle is now retracted laterally, carrying the epigastric vessels out of harm's way with it.

The posterior sheath of the rectus muscle (there is no posterior sheath below the arcuate line), the transversalis fascia, and the peritoneal layer are now carefully incised as one layer at a point 2 cm. lateral to the midline. After the peritoneal cavity has been opened, two fingers are inserted between the peritoneum to protect the underlying viscera while this layer is incised upward and downward for the desired distance.

After the operation has been completed, the peritoneum, transversalis fascia, and posterior rectus sheath (when present) are closed as a single layer by a continuous suture of 2–0 plain catgut, polyglactin 910, or polyglycolic acid. The rectus muscle is allowed to fall medially into its normal position which overlies the peritoneal suture line. Any tendinous intersections that had their medial attachment divided are rettached to the linea alba with a single suture for each. This step is not essential but makes a neater and possibly stronger closure (Fig. 18–32). The anterior sheath of the rectus muscle is closed with interrupted sutures of 0 nylon or polypropylene or No. 1 silk or No. 30 stainless steel wire. In addition, other techniques previously described can be used.

After the anterior rectus sheath has been sutured, the subcutaneous tissue is approximated with interrupted sutures of 4–0 silk, plain catgut, polyglactin 910, or polyglycolic acid, and the skin is closed with continuous or interrupted sutures of 4–0 nylon.

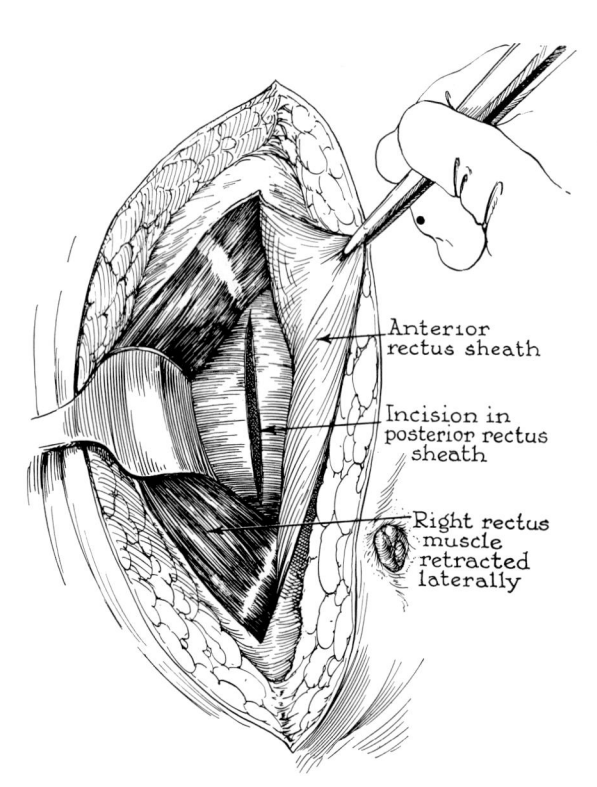

Figure 18–31. Paramedian incision. Right side. The anterior rectus sheath has been incised 2 cm. lateral to the abdominal midline. A medial flap of the sheath is raised from the rectus muscle and the latter retracted laterally from its compartment, exposing the posterior sheath. The posterior sheath is incised.

METHODS OF EXTENSION

A paramedian incision can be extended upward or downward by simply continuing

TYPES AND CHOICE OF INCISIONS

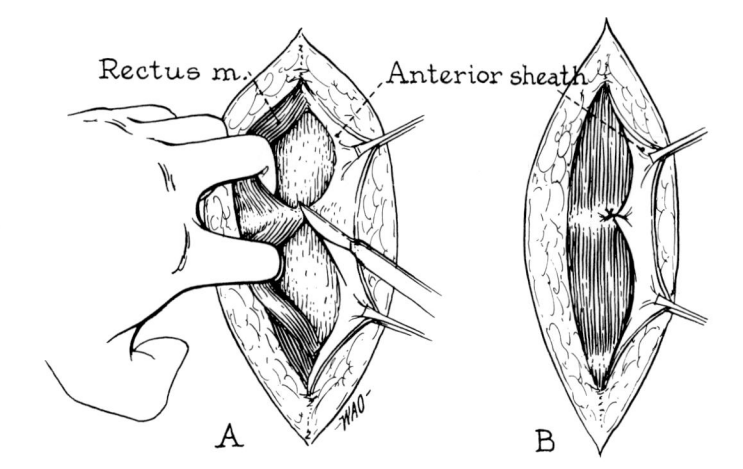

Figure 18–32. Dissection (*A*) and reattachment (*B*) of tendinous intersections of rectus muscle to anterior rectus sheath.

the incision in the appropriate direction for the distance desired. Since the incision severs no nerves, its length is limited only by the pubis below and the costal margin above. It can also be extended upward to continue into the chest by any of the methods described for enlarging an upper midline incision (p. 490) to be converted into an abdominothoracic incision.

A paramedian incision can be extended

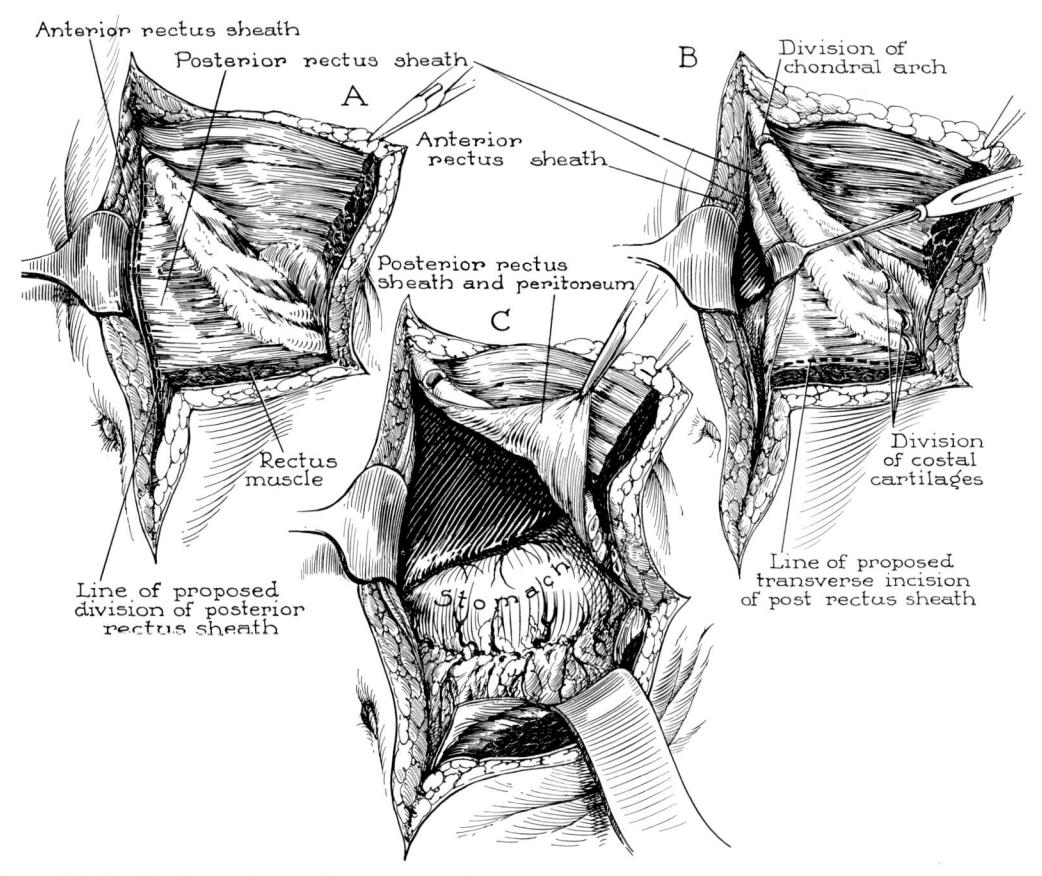

Figure 18–33. Technic of extending a paramedian incision by dividing the rectus muscle and the costal cartilages extraperitoneally. *A*, Reflection as a flap of the upper segment of the divided rectus muscle with its overlying subcutaneous tissues and skin. *B*, Division of chondral arch and cartilages of three ribs; vertical division of the posterior rectus sheath and lateral division of same indicated. *C*, Exposure through paramedian incision extended laterally.

laterally by a transverse abdominal component just as described for the lateral extension of a midline incision (p. 495), dividing the costal cartilages extrapleurally if necessary to obtain more extensive exposure (Fig. 18-33).

Midrectus (Transrectus) Incision

A midrectus (transrectus) incision may be made to the right or left of the midline and may be situated in the upper, middle, or lower part of the abdominal wall. The incision is a vertical one which splits the rectus muscle in the direction of its fibers and destroys at least part of the innervation to the medial portion of the divided muscle. It is used for the same procedures mentioned for a paramedian incision. When there is a choice, the paramedian incision is by far the better of the two. Midrectus incisions should seldom be used.

When making a midrectus incision, the rectus muscle should not be divided more than 2 cm. lateral to its medial border in order to minimize the amount of the muscle that is denervated. For the same reason the incision should be restricted in length, thus decreasing the number of nerves that are transected.

TECHNIC

A vertical incision of appropriate length is made about 3 cm. lateral to the anterior abdominal midline and is situated at the desired level on the abdominal wall.

The surface of the anterior rectus sheath is cleared of subcutaneous fat for a width of about 3 cm. for the length of the incision.

The anterior sheath of the rectus muscle is incised vertically for the desired length. Using blunt dissection, the underlying rectus muscle is split in the direction of its fibers for the length of the incision. In doing this, the transversely running tendinous intersections should be divided between clamps and ligated as they usually contain bleeders. Furthermore, the line of division of the muscle fibers should be placed medial to the course of the epigastric vessels, for if placed immediately over them the vessels will be repeatedly torn and cause troublesome bleeding that will require a considerable amount of clamping and ligating. The divided portions of the rectus muscle are retracted (Fig. 18-34), and the posterior rectus sheath (when present), transversalis fascia, and peritoneum are incised carefully as one layer to enter the abdominal cavity. Two fingers are inserted deep to the peritoneum to proect the abdominal viscera while the peritoneal layer is incised upward and downward for the full length of the abdominal incision.

After the surgical procedure has been completed the peritoneum, transversalis fascia, and posterior sheath of the rectus muscle (when present) are closed as one layer with a continuous suture of polyglactin 910, polyglycolic acid, or 2-0 plain catgut. No sutures are used to appose the separated rectus muscle fibers. The anterior sheath of the rectus muscle is closed with interrupted sutures of 0 nylon or polypropylene, No. 1 silk, or No. 30 stainless steel wire. Closing the anterior rectus sheath also reapproximates the separated rectus muscle fibers. If the rectus sheath is closed with absorbable sutures such as catgut, stay sutures should be employed as described for a paramedian incision closed with catgut (Fig. 18-34). The subcutaneous tissues are approximated with interrupted sutures of polyglactin 910, polyglycolic acid, 4-0 silk, or catgut, and the skin is closed with continuous or interrupted sutures of 4-0 nylon or stainless steel staples.

METHODS OF EXTENSION

An upper midrectus incision either on the right or on the left can be extended upward in one of the ways described for upward extension of an upper midline incision (see p. 490).

Other midrectus incisions can be extended upward or downward (as far as the pubis) by simply continuing the incision in the appropriate direction. It should be remembered, however, that a midrectus incision is a muscle-splitting one which interrupts the nerve supply to the more medial portion of the muscle, hence the incision should not be made into an unusually long one so as to minimize the amount of muscle that is denervated.

TYPES AND CHOICE OF INCISIONS

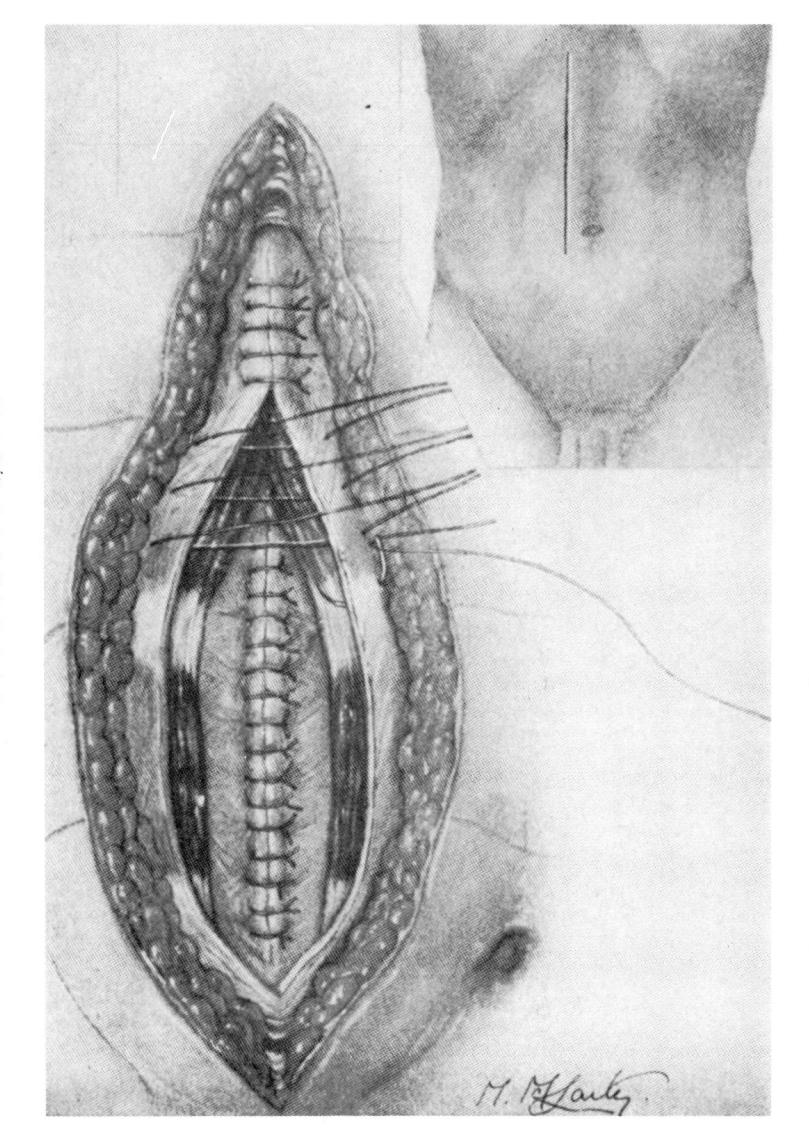

Figure 18–34. Upper vertical transrectal (muscle-split) incision. This wound may be closed in the manner depicted, with a series of closely applied interrupted sutures. There is no need to insert any special sutures to draw the muscle edges themselves together as the muscle margins fall together when the anterior sheath of the rectus muscle is approximated. (From Maingot, R.: Abdominal Operations, ed. 2. New York, Appleton-Century-Crofts, 1948.)

Midrectus incisions can be extended laterally in the same way as described for the lateral extension of a midline incision.

Pararectus Incision (Kammerer-Battle)

A pararectus incision can be made on either the right or left side of the abdominal midline, and can be placed at any level, but has usually been used in the lower abdomen. The incision is made along the lateral border of the rectus muscle; to be of a useful length it must transect or widely stretch two or more intercostal nerves, interrupting the innervation to the portion of the rectus muscle supplied by them. For this reason a pararectus incision should not be used when other nonnerve-cutting incisions will provide an adequate exposure for the contemplated procedure.

TECHNIC

A vertical incision of the desired length (it should not exceed about 10 cm.) is made through the skin, subcutaneous tissue, and anterior rectus sheath about 1 cm. medial to the lateral border of the rectus muscle. The lateral flap of the divided rectus sheath is held forward while the lateral margin of the

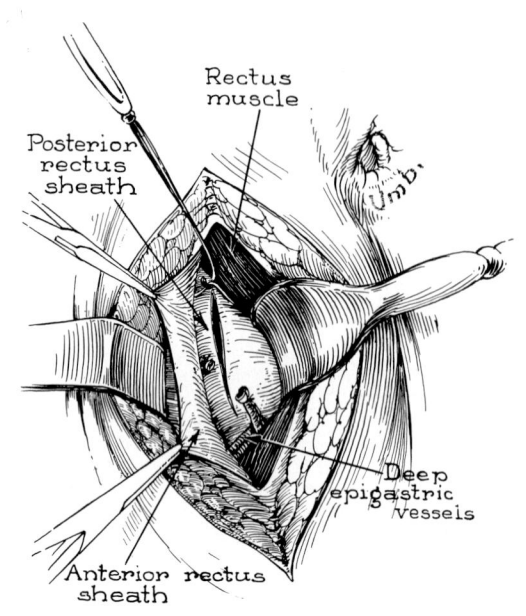

Figure 18–35. Technic of pararectus incision in the lower abdomen (Kammerer-Battle). A vertical incision is made through the skin, subcutaneous tissues, and anterior rectus sheath, 1 cm. medial to the lateral border of the rectus muscle. The lateral flap of the anterior sheath is held forward and the rectus muscle retracted medially after having been freed by ligation and division of its vascular attachments. The intercostal nerve encountered is shown uncut. The posterior rectus sheath of the transversalis fascia and the peritoneum are incised.

rectus muscle is identified and freed from its attachments (Fig. 18–35). In so doing it will be necessary to divide and ligate one or two or more intercostal nerves and vessels as they enter the lateral border of the rectus sheath to be distributed to the rectus muscle. The intact rectus muscle is then retracted medially while the posterior rectus sheath (when present), transversalis fascia, and peritoneum are carefully incised as one layer about 1 cm. medial to the lateral border of the rectus muscle. The abdominal cavity is entered and two fingers are placed beneath the peritoneum to protect the underlying viscera while the peritoneum is incised over them for the full length of the incision.

After the surgical procedure has been completed the peritoneum, transversalis fascia, and posterior rectus sheath (when present) are closed as one layer with a continuous suture of polyglactin 910, polyglycolic acid, or 2-0 plain catgut. The intact rectus muscle is allowed to resume its normal position so that its lateral portion overlies the peritoneal closure. The anterior sheath of the rectus muscle is closed with interrupted suture of 0 nylon, polypropylene, or No. 1 silk or No. 30 stainless steel wire sutures. Other methods of closure previously described can also be used. After the anterior rectus sheath has been sutured the subcutaneous tissue is approximated with interrupted sutures of polyglactin 910, polyglycolic acid, 4-0 silk, or catgut, and the skin with interrupted or continuous suture of 4-0 silk or nylon or stainless steel staples.

METHODS OF EXTENSION

A pararectus incision can be extended upward or downward by simply continuing the incision in the appropriate direction. However, this should be carried out for only a limited distance for reasons that have already been given.

A pararectus incision may be extended laterally or medially by adding a transverse abdominal component to the incision. This should be avoided when possible because the denervation of the rectus muscle produced by the vertical portion of the incision produces at least partial paralysis of that muscle and, when combined with an additional transverse incision, is likely to result in a later incisional hernia.

Because of its many disadvantages, a pararectus incision is best avoided when possible.

Transverse Abdominal Incisions

Transverse abdominal incisions may be used at any level on the abdominal wall and may be made on the right or on the left, or so as to extend on both sides of the midline. They require a longer time to make and are more tedious to close than vertical incisions but have advantages that have been mentioned previously.

UPPER ABDOMINAL TRANSVERSE INCISION

This incision is used by many for operations on the stomach and pancreas. For

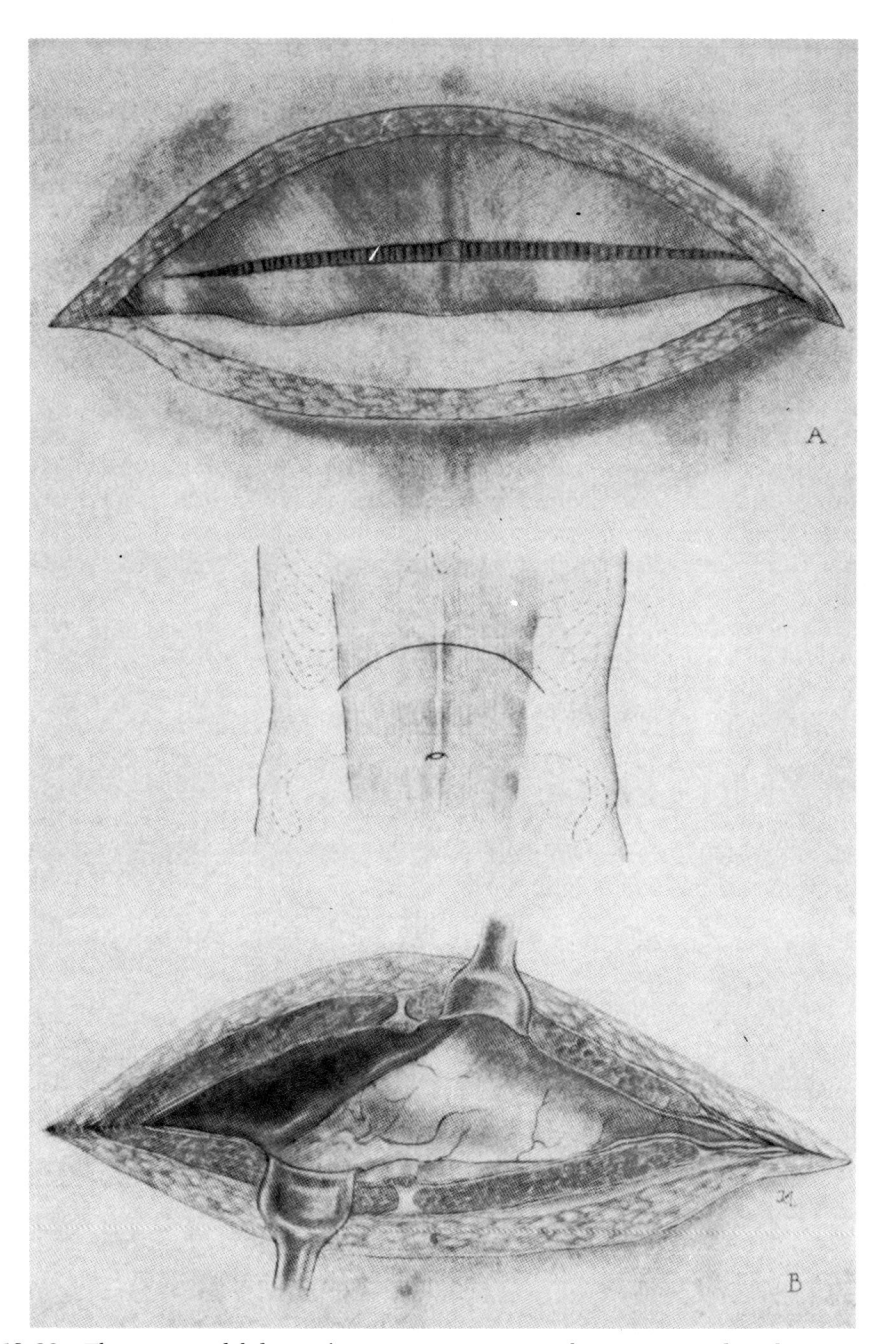

Figure 18–36. The upper midabdominal transverse incision. *A*, Skin incision made and anterior rectus sheaths incised transversely. *B*, Rectus muscles transected and the incision completed. Note that the rectus muscles do not retract beneath the sheath. (From Coller, F. A., and MacLean, K. F.: *In* Cole, W. H.: Operative Technic in General Surgery. New York, Appleton-Century-Crofts, 1949.)

many surgeons it is the incision of choice for the latter, but does not provide a comfortable exposure for operations that involve the upper portion of the stomach. It is usually made so as to extend an equal distance on both the right and left sides of the midline but may be made asymmetric when indicated.

Technic

The skin incision is made transverse in patients with a wide costal angle and is curved slightly upward toward the xiphoid in patients with a narrow costal angle. In either type of patient it is placed so as to pass inferior to both the right and left costal margins and to extend to the lateral border of both rectus sheaths. In most instances this places the incision at a point midway between the xiphoid process and the umbilicus (Fig. 18-36). The skin and subcutaneous tissue are incised down to the anterior sheath of the rectus muscle.

Both the right and left anterior rectus sheaths are exposed and incised transversely from one lateral border to the other. Both rectus muscles are freed at their medial borders sufficiently for a finger to be passed beneath them. With a finger beneath to tent the muscle anteriorly, the fibers of each rectus muscle are cut across over the finger and the blood vessels clamped, cut, and ligated as they are exposed. The posterior rectus sheath, linea alba, transversalis fascia, and peritoneum are carefully incised transversely, avoiding injury to the underlying viscera. The ligamentum teres of the liver is divided between clamps, and its cut ends are ligated to control bleeding from its accompanying vessels.

After the surgical procedure has been completed the wound is closed in the following way:

The ligamentum teres is reconstructed by tying its two cut ends together in a single ligature of 2-0 silk, catgut, or synthetic absorbable suture. This is considered important because obstruction may occur later if the ends are left free to dangle in the peritoneal cavity. The peritoneum, transversalis fascia, and posterior rectus sheaths are closed together as one layer with a continuous suture of 2-0 plain catgut or synthetic absorbable suture. The cut edges of the anterior rectus sheaths and linea alba are approximated with interrupted sutures of No. 1 silk, synthetic absorbable, or No. 30 stainless steel wire or 0 polypropylene. The subcutaneous tissue is approximated with running or interrupted sutures of 4-0 plain catgut or synthetic absorbable.

The skin is closed with continuous or interrupted sutures of 4-0 nylon or stainless steel staples.

Methods of Extension

An upper abdominal transverse incision may be extended laterally on either or both sides by continuing the incision in the desired direction or directions to split the external oblique, internal oblique, and transversus abdominis muscles for a short distance in the direction of their fibers. The length of this extension will be limited by the costal margins on each side in patients with a deep and narrow costal margin.

The incision can be extended upward or downward by a vertical incision in the desired direction through the abdominal midline. This causes no harm but requires a more time-consuming closure than does a lateral extension.

MODIFIED UPPER ABDOMINAL TRANSVERSUS INCISION BY RETRACTING INSTEAD OF SEVERING THE RECTUS MUSCLES (SANDERS)

This incision requires more tedious dissection and provides a more limited exposure than does the conventional type of upper transverse abdominal incision described above. It is less than satisfactory for most operations in this area.

Technic

A transverse incision is made through the skin and subcutaneous tissue from one lateral border of the rectus muscle to the other at the desired level on the abdominal wall (Fig. 18-37). Both anterior rectus sheaths are exposed and incised transversely from the lateral margin of one to the lateral margin of the other. The medial borders of both rectus muscles are freed for as far as possible up and down by severing the medial attachment of the linea transver-

TYPES AND CHOICE OF INCISIONS

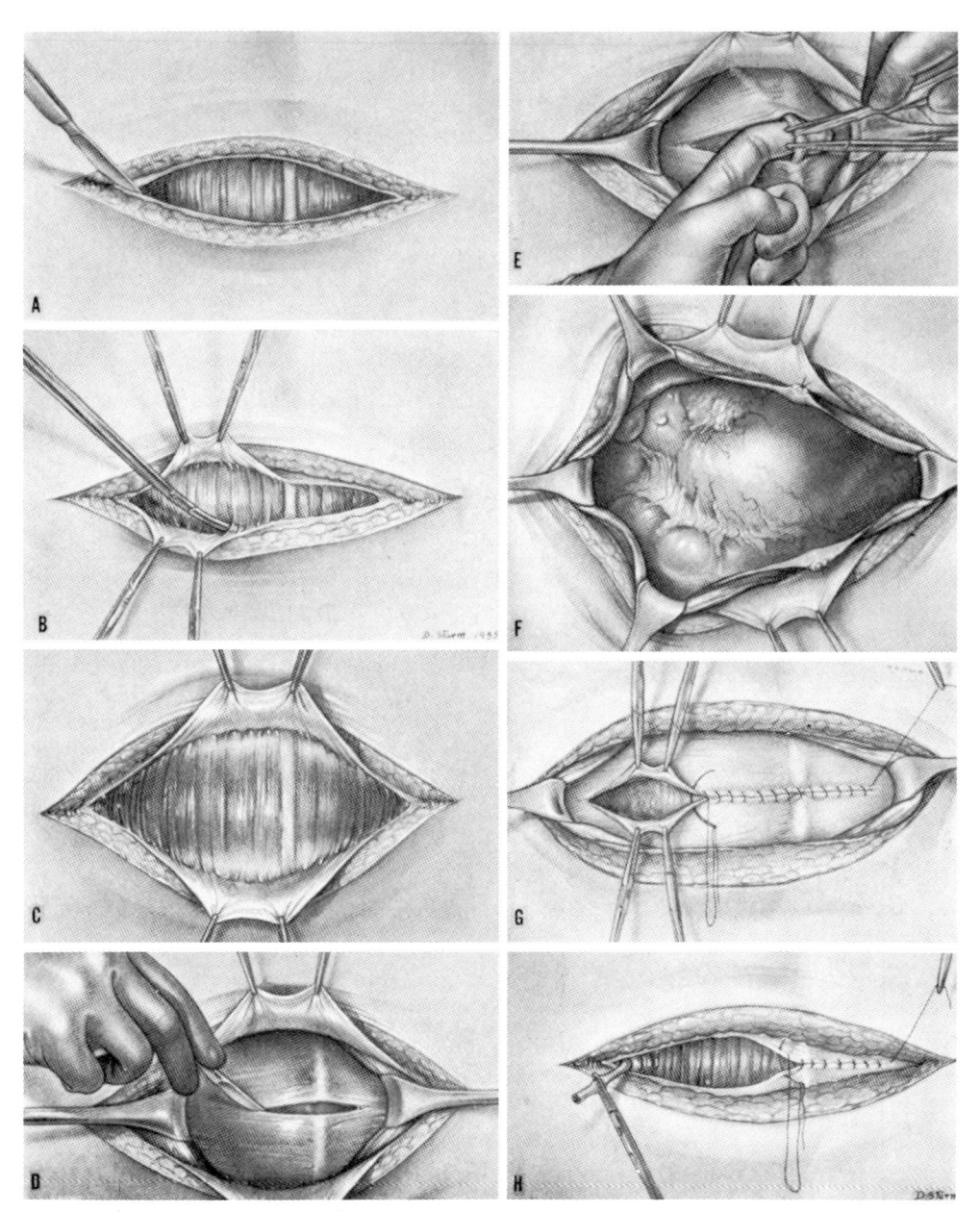

Figure 18–37. Modified upper abdominal transverse incision by retracting instead of severing the rectus muscles (R. L. Sanders). *A*, Incision through skin, subcutaneous tissues, and anterior rectus sheaths about 3 cm. above the umbilicus. *B* and *C*, Anterior sheaths dissected from attachments to lineae transversae of rectus muscles and retracted. *D*, Lateral retraction of rectus muscles and transverse incision of the posterior sheaths and peritoneum. *E*, Division of the round ligament of the liver between clamps. *F*, Round ligament ligated; margins of incision retracted, exposing the adjacent abdominal viscera. *G*, Suture of the peritoneum and posterior rectus sheaths. *H*, Suture of the anterior rectus sheath. Interrupted sutures are preferred by many surgeons to approximate the cut edges of the anterior sheaths.

sa from the linea alba. Each intact rectus muscle is now retracted laterally, exposing the posterior rectus sheaths. The posterior rectus sheaths, transversalis fascia, linea alba, and peritoneum are carefully incised and the abdominal cavity is entered without injuring the underlying viscera. The ligamentum teres is transected between clamps; its cut ends are ligated.

When the surgical manipulations have been completed, the wound is closed in the same way as described for an upper abdominal transverse incision.

Comments

Sloan (1927) preserved the rectus muscles in a transverse type of incision by making a vertical midline incision through the skin and subcutaneous tissue of the upper abdomen. Both anterior rectus sheaths were then incised vertically near their median borders. The median margins of the rectus muscles were freed and retracted laterally. The posterior rectus sheaths, linea alba, transversalis fascia, and peritoneum were then incised transversely to enter the abdominal cavity.

Singleton (1931) modified Sloan's incision by using a transverse skin incision and incising the left anterior rectus sheath transversely.

None of these incisions is as widely used as the transverse incision made through all the layers, including the rectus muscles, as described above.

LATERAL UPPER ABDOMINAL TRANSVERSE INCISION (SINGLETON)

This incision, when made on the right side, may be used for operations on the biliary tract. When made on the left side it may be used for a splenectomy. It is not widely used, as other incisions are preferable for these procedures.

Technic

When made on the right, the incision starts at the linea alba midway between the xiphoid and the umbilicus, but when made on the left for a splenectomy the incision is made slightly lower, about 7 cm. above the umbilicus; otherwise the technics are identical.

An incision is made through the skin and subcutaneous tissue, beginning at the midline of the abdominal wall and proceeding downward and laterally on the appropriate side to a point that is just posterior to the anterior superior spine of the ilium and just superior to the iliac crest. The anterior rectus sheath and external oblique aponeurosis are incised in the line of the skin incision. This divides the rectus sheath obliquely downward and transects the muscle fibers of the external oblique muscle almost at right angles to their course. The lateral border of the rectus muscle is freed and retracted medially (Fig. 18–38). The posterior rectus sheath and peritoneum are carefully incised transversely to enter the abdominal cavity. This incision is continued downward and laterally, splitting the internal oblique muscle in the direction of its fibers and cutting across the fibers of the transversus abdominis muscle.

When making this incision on the right, the ninth and tenth intercostal nerves are identified as they enter the lateral margin of the rectus sheath and are retracted or cut if necessary. On the left the eleventh intercostal nerve is cut while the tenth and twelfth are retracted out of harm's way.

Closure is effected by suturing the peritoneum, transversalis fascia, and posterior rectus sheath with a continuous 2–0 plain catgut suture or a synthetic absorbable suture.

The divided fibers of the internal oblique muscle are approximated with interrupted sutures of 2–0 catgut or 2–0 synthetic absorbable sutures. The intact rectus muscle is allowed to resume its normal position. The anterior sheath of the rectus and the external oblique muscle are closed with interrupted sutures of No. 30 stainless steel wire, 0 polypropylene, or 2–0 silk.

The subcutaneous tissue is approximated with interrupted sutures of 4–0 catgut or synthetic absorbable material, and the skin is closed with continuous or interrupted sutures of 4–0 nylon or stainless steel staples.

Methods of Extension

A lateral transverse abdominal incision can be extended medially or to the other

TYPES AND CHOICE OF INCISIONS

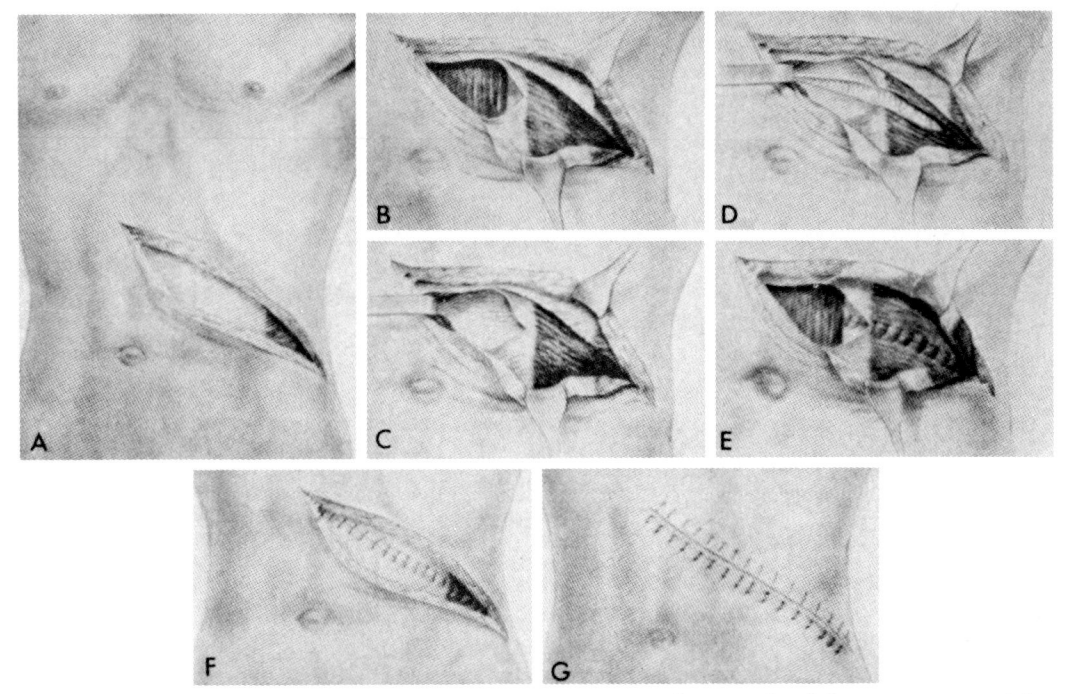

Figure 18-38. *A*, Skin incision. *B*, Anterior sheath of rectus muscle incised and the incision carried through fascia of the external oblique until muscle fibers are reached. Incised fascial margins are shown retracted, exposing the rectus and internal oblique muscles. *C*, Medial retraction of the rectus muscle preparatory to division of the posterior rectus sheath and entering the abdominal cavity. *D*, Lateral and downward continuation of the incision, splitting the fibers of the internal oblique and cutting across the fibers of the transversus abdominis and through the peritoneum. *E*, *F*, and *G*, Progressive steps of closure of the fascial, muscular, and skin layers. (From Singleton, A. O.: Splenectomy. Surg. Gynecol. Obstet. 70:1051, 1940.)

side of the abdomen by cutting across the ipsilateral or both rectus muscles and the linea alba.

It can be extended upward or downward by cutting across the ipsilateral rectus muscle to the midline and then extending the incision vertically in the linea alba in the desired direction.

TRANSVERSE MIDABDOMINAL INCISION

This incision is usually made on either the right or the left side only, depending upon the location of the contemplated field of operation, but it can be extended across both sides of the abdominal wall to provide an almost terrifyingly wide exposure.

A transverse midabdominal incision is widely used for operations on the right transverse (including hepatic and splenic flexures), descending and upper sigmoid colons. It is used for some for operations on the small intestine, such as for intestinal obstruction. The incision is attaining increasing and deserved popularity.

Technic

The skin incision begins at the abdominal midline at a point about 2 cm. above or 2 cm. below the umbilicus, according to the level of the lesion. It is extended in an exact transverse direction for as far laterally as is estimated to be required for the contemplated surgery. The incision is deepened through the subcutaneous fat to expose the anterior rectus sheath and aponeurosis of the external oblique muscle. The anterior rectus sheath is incised transversely, and this incision is extended upward and laterally to split the external oblique muscle in the direction of its fibers (Fig. 18-39) as far as desired. A finger is passed beneath the lateral border of the rectus and the fibers of

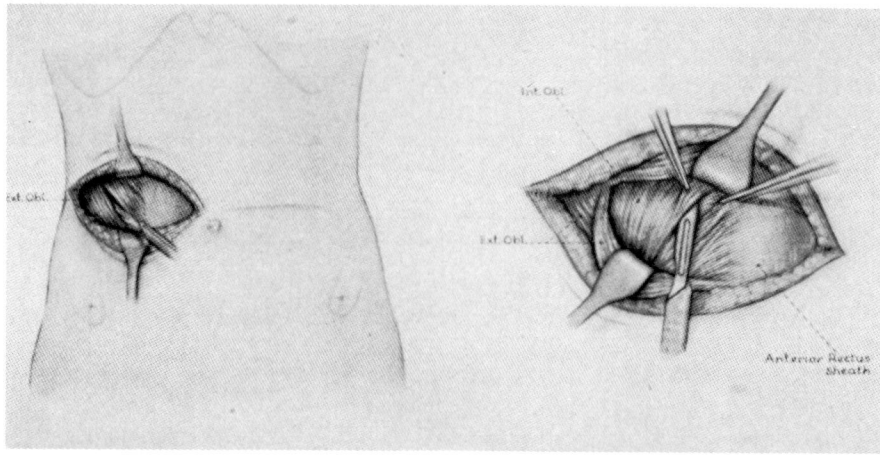

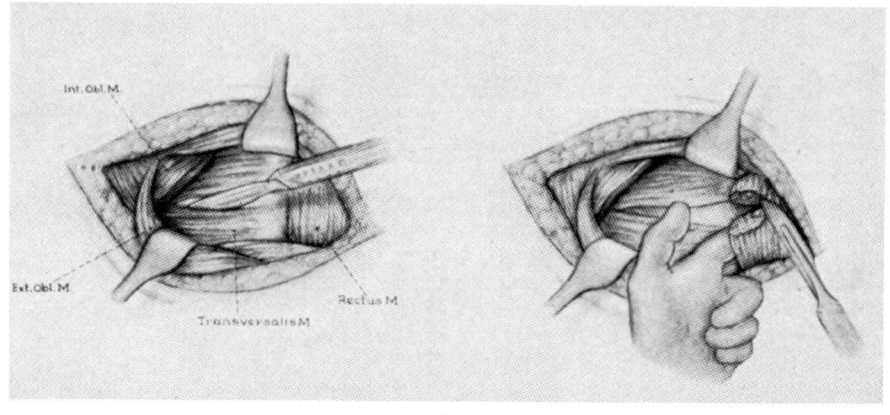

Figure 18–39. *A*, Incision used for right colectomy. External and internal oblique muscles split in direction of their fibers. Left healed transverse scar used for ileotransverse colostomy. *B*, Transversalis muscle split in direction of its fibers and rectus muscle cross cut in part or in whole, depending upon exposure needed. (From Coller, F. A., and Vaughan, H. H.: Treatment of carcinoma of colon. Ann. Surg. *121*:305, 1945.)

this muscle are cut across over it. Bleeders, including the epigastric vessels, are clamped, cut, and ligated. The ninth intercostal nerve (above the umbilicus) or the eleventh intercostal nerve (below the umbilicus) is identified as it runs over the posterior rectus sheath, and retracted upward. The posterior rectus sheath and peritoneum are carefully incised transversely to open the peritoneal cavity. From the lateral border of the rectus muscle, the internal oblique and transverse abdominis muscles are split in the direction of their fibers by blunt dissection with the fingers. The muscle fibers of the external oblique, internal oblique, and transversus abdominis muscles are retracted upward and downward while the incision through the posterior rectus sheath, transversalis fascia, and peritoneum is carried as far laterally into the flank as is desired. The amount of exposure can be varied by the length of the incision.

After the operation has been completed, the peritoneum, transversalis fascia, and posterior rectus sheath are reapproximated in one layer by a continuous 2–0 plain or chromic gut or synthetic absorbable suture. The cut edges of the anterior sheath of the rectus muscle are approximated with inter-

TYPES AND CHOICE OF INCISIONS

rupted sutures of No. 1 silk, No. 30 stainless steel wire, or 0 polypropylene. The transversus abdominis muscle is usually too attenuated for suturing in a separate layer, but the divided fibers of the internal oblique muscle are approximated by a row of interrupted sutures of 2-0 silk or chromic or synthetic absorbable suture. Likewise the divided fibers of the external oblique muscle are approximated by a row of similar sutures. The subcutaneous tissues are apposed by a row of 3-0 continuous or interrupted chromic or synthetic absorbable sutures. The skin is approximated by continuous or interrupted sutures of 4-0 nylon or stainless steel staples.

Methods of Extension

As previously mentioned, this incision can be extended across to the other side of the abdomen by cutting across the other rectus sheath and rectus muscle to continue laterally into the other flank just as performed on the original side. Extension to the other side provides vast exposure.

Extension upward or downward can be obtained quite easily by making a vertical incision upward and downward through the linea alba (skirting either to the right or the left side of the umbilicus) for as far as necessary in the desired direction.

TRANSVERSE LOW ABDOMINAL INCISION

This incision is employed by some gynecologists for operations on the female pelvic organs. For this purpose it is not as widely used as a vertical low midline incision, for it does not provide quite as satisfactory an exposure. It also has the disadvantage that in the lower abdomen the absence of tendinous intersections permits the transected fibers of the rectus muscles to retract further than in the upper abdomen, at times sufficiently far to make reapposition of their cut ends difficult.

Technic

An incision is made transversely through the skin at the level of the junction of the middle and lower thirds of a line running from the umbilicus to the symphysis pubis. The incision extends from one lateral border of the rectus muscle to the other and is deepened through the subcutaneous tissue to expose the anterior sheaths of both rectus muscles. Both anterior rectus sheaths and the linea alba are divided transversely. Both rectus muscles are transected across a finger inserted beneath them and the inferior epigastric vessels, which run vertically beneath the medial third of each muscle, are clamped, cut, and ligated. Since there is usually no posterior rectus sheath at this level the transversalis fascia is thus exposed. This fascia and the peritoneum are carefully incised transversely to enter the peritoneal cavity.

After the operation has been completed the peritoneum and transversalis fascia are closed by one row of sutures, the anterior sheath of the rectus by another row, the subcutaneous tissue by a third row, and the skin by a fourth row. The type of suture and the material used are the same as just described for a transverse midabdominal incision.

Methods of Extension

The incision can be extended laterally by splitting the oblique and transversus abdominis muscles in the direction of their fibers on one or both sides, as described for a transverse midabdominal incision.

It can be extended upward or downward by a vertical incision through the linea alba in the desired direction.

Pfannenstiel Incision

This incision may be used for some operations on the female pelvic organs.

It is designed to produce the maximum cosmetic effect by placing the subsequent scar within the area covered by the pubic hair. It provides a relatively crowded exposure. It usually is employed only when the cosmetic result is of more than average importance and the contemplated operative procedure will not be extensive and will be readily accessible.

If this incision is contemplated, the urinary bladder should be emptied by catheterization just prior to operation.

TECHNIC

A skin incision is made along the slightly curving interspinous crease of the lower abdominal wall. This incision curves transversely across the lower abdomen, lies wholly within the area of pubic hair, and is about 12 cm. long, with its center situated about 5 cm. above the symphysis pubis (Fig. 18–40). It is deepened through the subcutaneous tissue to expose both rectus sheaths.

Both rectus sheaths and the linea alba are divided transversely for the entire length of the incision. Hemostats are placed on the upper and lower edge of the cut rectus sheaths, which are then widely separated above as far toward the umbilicus as possible, and below to the pubis from the underlying rectus muscle. The rectus muscles are separated and each is retracted laterally. There is no posterior rectus sheath in this area. The transversalis fascia and peritone-

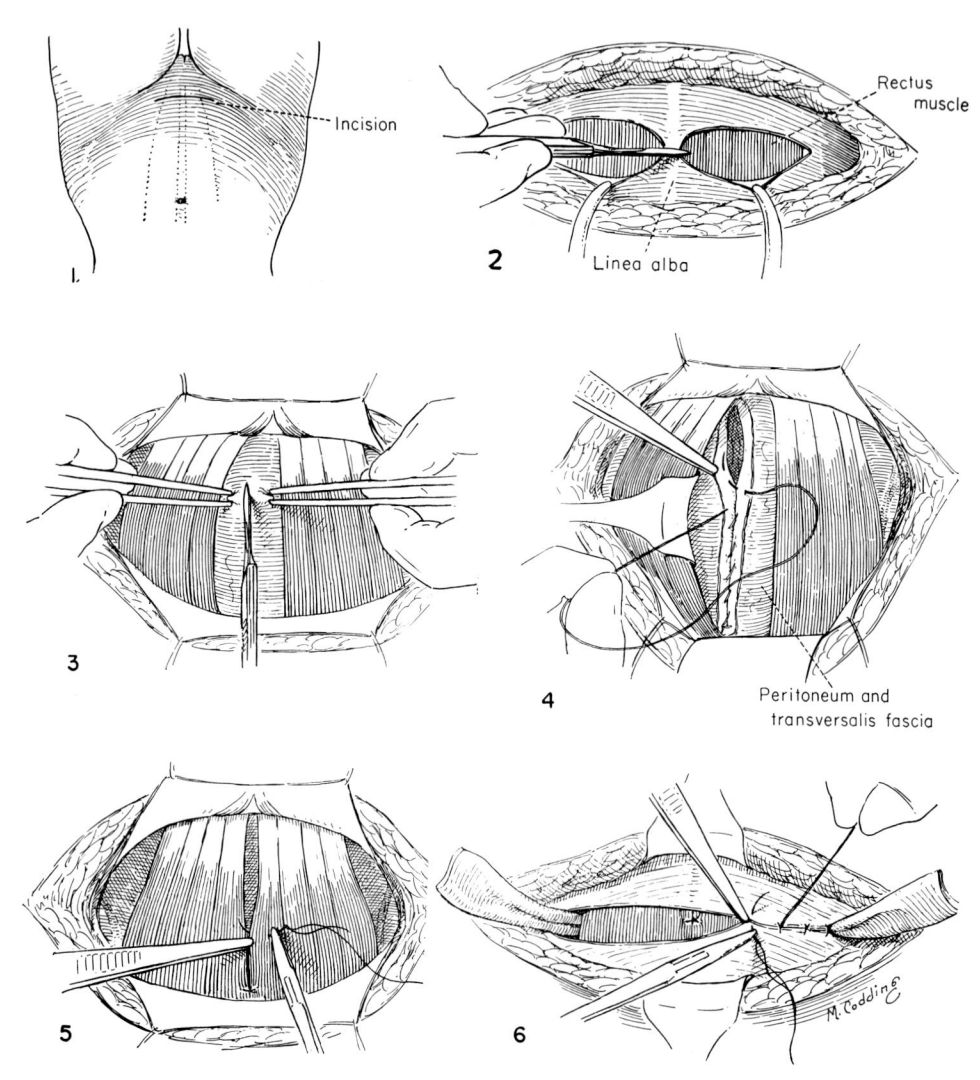

Figure 18–40. Pfannenstiel incision. 1, Curved incision just above pubic hairline, extending beyond lateral borders of rectus muscles; 2, fascial covering of recti incised; 3, transversalis fascia and peritoneum incised between tissue forceps. Closure: 4, Suture of transversalis fascia and peritoneum approximating serosal surfaces of peritoneum; 5, approximation of median borders of rectus muscles with interrupted stitches; 6, suture of anterior fascial defect. (From Parsons, L., and Ulfelder, H.: Atlas of Pelvic Operations. Philadelphia, W. B. Saunders Company, 1968.)

um are incised vertically in the midline, care being taken not to injure the bladder at the lower end of this incision.

After the surgery has been completed, the peritoneum and transversalis fascia are closed with a continuous 2–0 catgut or synthetic absorbable suture. The rectus muscles are allowed to resume their normal position but require no suturing.

The cut edges of the anterior sheath of the rectus muscle are approximated with interrupted sutures of No. 1 silk or No. 30 stainless steel wire or 0 polypropylene.

The subcutaneous tissue is apposed with interrupted sutures of 2–0 catgut or synthetic absorbable suture, and the skin with continuous or interrupted sutures of 4–0 nylon or stainless steel sutures.

METHODS OF EXTENSION

The incision may be extended laterally on one or both sides by one of two methods.

1. By dividing the tendinous attachments of the rectus muscle or muscles (Cherney) to the pubis (Figs. 18–41 and 18–42), reflecting them upward and incising the transversalis fascia and peritoneum laterally in the desired direction. If necessary, the incision in the anterior sheath of the rectus muscle can be extended on one or both sides to split the external oblique aponeurosis in the direction of its fibers.

2. By strongly retracting the rectus muscle *medially* on the side requiring further lateral exposure, dividing and ligating

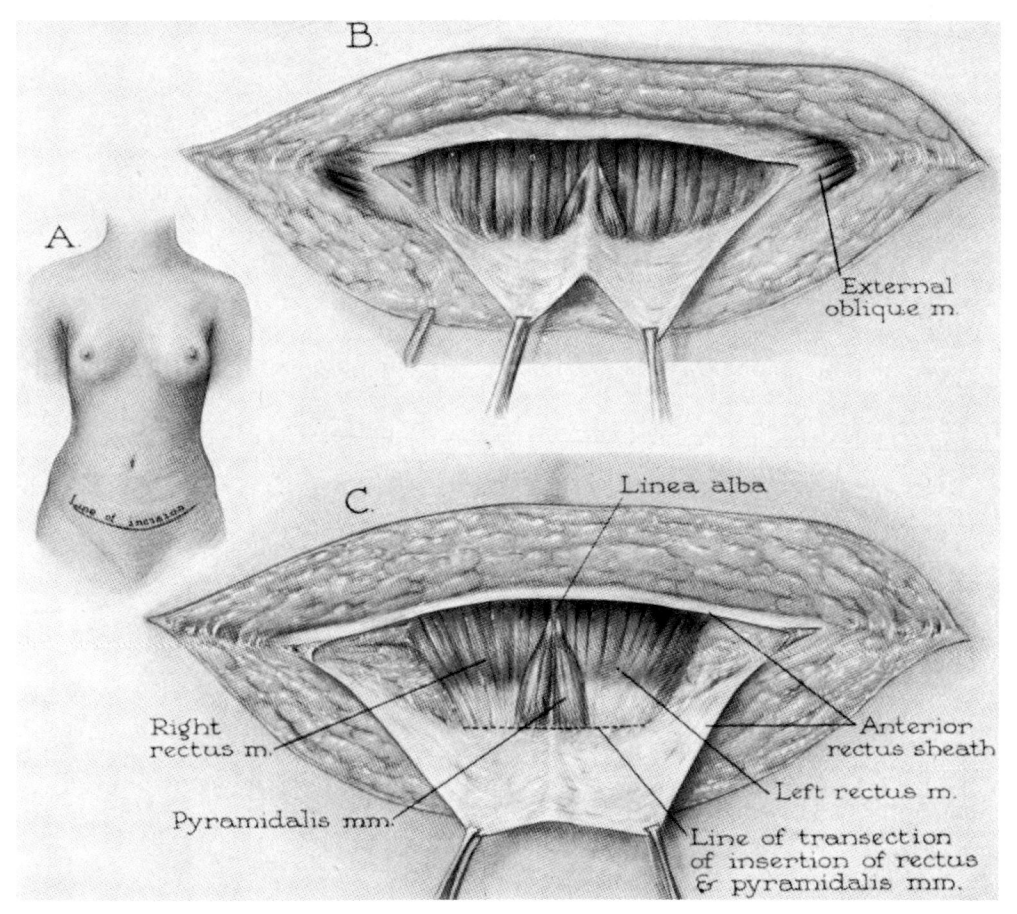

Figure 18–41. Method of extending a Pfannenstiel incision (Cherney). *A*, Transverse skin incision; *B* and *C*, aponeurosis incised and line of transection of rectus and pyramidalis muscles at their insertion to pubis.

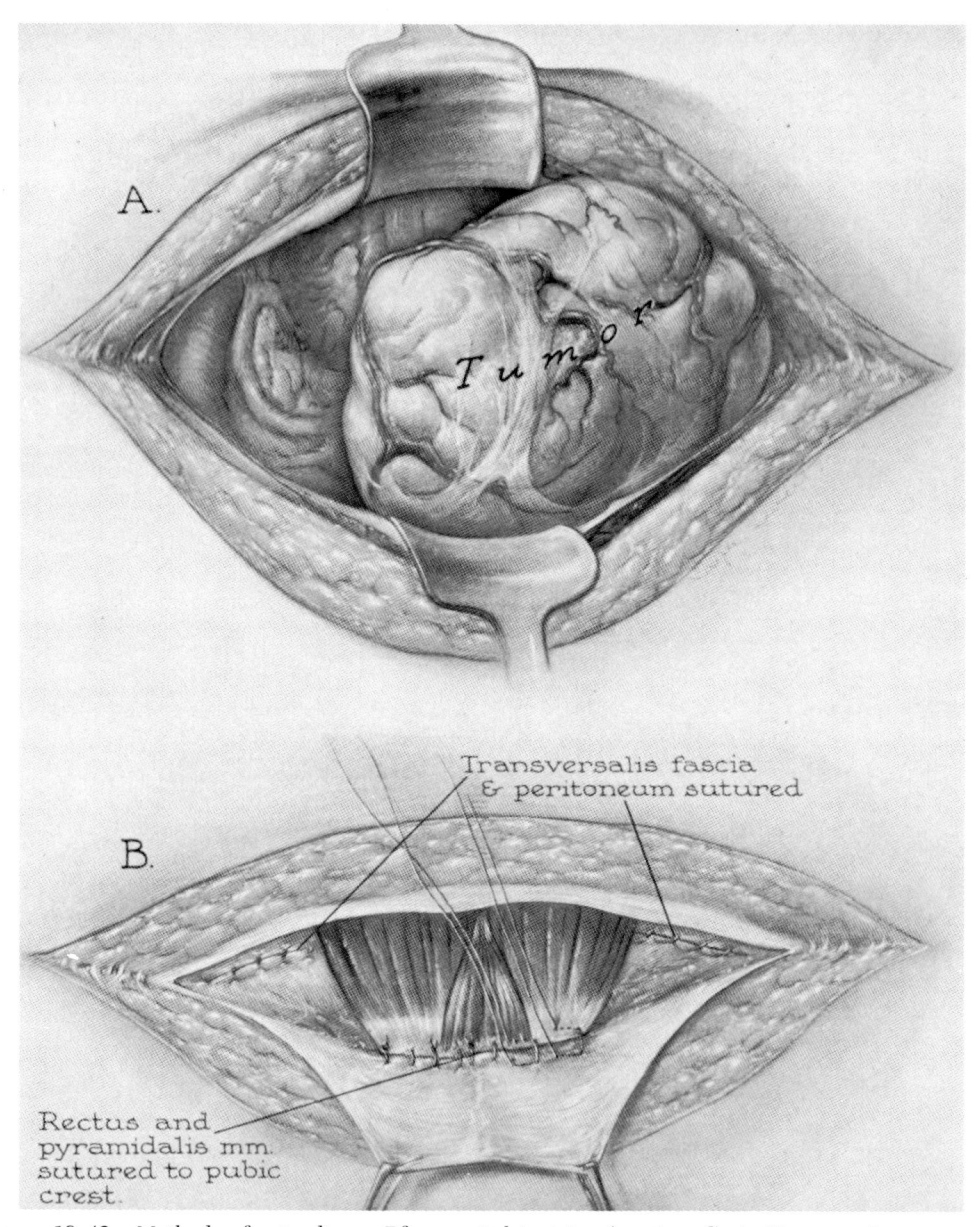

Figure 18–42. Methods of extending a Pfannenstiel incision *(continued)*. *A*, Exposure by retraction after incision of the transversalis fascia and peritoneum. *B*, Suture of deep fascial and serosal layers; suture of transected muscles to pubic crest.

TYPES AND CHOICE OF INCISIONS

the inferior epigastric vessels, carrying the transverse incision in the anterior sheath laterally to split the fibers of the external oblique, and incising the transversalis fascia and peritoneum transversely in the desired direction.

A Pfannenstiel incision can be extended upward by vertically incising the linea alba in that direction.

Left Transverse Incision for Abdominoperineal Excision of Rectum (Coller)

Coller and MacLean (1949) employed this incision (Fig. 18–43) for the abdominal portion of combined abdominoperineal resections and found it of equal value for low sigmoid resections, with or without end-to-end anastomosis. It has given excellent exposure, closes readily, and heals firmly. Like other transverse incisions, it is less painful postoperatively than are vertical incisions.

TECHNIC

The skin incision is begun either at or immediately to the right of the midline, 2.5 cm. above the symphysis, and is extended transversely to the lateral border of the left rectus sheath, where it is carried upward in the line of the fibers of the external oblique muscle to terminate just above and usually about 5 cm. medial to the anterosuperior spine.

An alternative skin incision may be used if desired. This incision is begun 2.5 cm. above the symphysis and is extended in a straight line to terminate 5 cm. above and medial to the spine.

After either skin incision is made, the aponeurosis of the external oblique muscle is split in the line of its fibers, and the iliohypogastric nerve is isolated beneath it and retracted downward. Extending the aponeurotic incision, the anterior rectus sheath and linea alba are incised transversely. After the rectus muscle is freed at its lateral border, a finger is placed beneath it over which it is transected. The inferior epigastric vessels running upward and medially beneath the rectus muscle are isolated, transected, and ligated. The internal oblique and transversus abdominis muscles are freed by blunt dissection as far as their attachment at the iliac wing. The transversalis fascia and peritoneum are opened in the line of the aponeurotic incision.

If more exposure is required, the transverse limb of this incision can be extended across the linea alba and the right rectus muscle, or the incision may be duplicated on the right.

The incision is closed in the way described for the closure of a midabdominal transverse incision (p. 510).

Oblique Incisions

SUBCOSTAL INCISION (KOCHER)

This incision can be made on either the right or the left side.

When made on the right, it provides an excellent exposure of the gallbladder and common duct and is probably the incision of choice for operations on these structures in obese patients who have a wide costal margin.

On the left it provides an excellent exposure for performing the average splenectomy or for forming a splenorenal venous anastomosis.

A bilateral subcostal incision crossing the midline has been used for operations on the stomach.

Technic

The skin incision begins exactly in the midline at a point about one-third the distance from the tip of the xiphoid process to the umbilicus (Fig. 18–44). It is carried laterally and downward parallel and about 5 cm. inferior to the costal margin, toward a point midway between the twelfth rib and the iliac crest, usually terminating at about the anterior axillary line. It should not be extended farther than this unnecessarily, to avoid injuring the many nerves.

The incision is deepened through the subcutaneous tissue. The surface of the anterior sheath of the rectus muscle and the surface of the external oblique muscle are cleared of subcutaneous tissue for a width of about 4 cm. for the length of the incision.

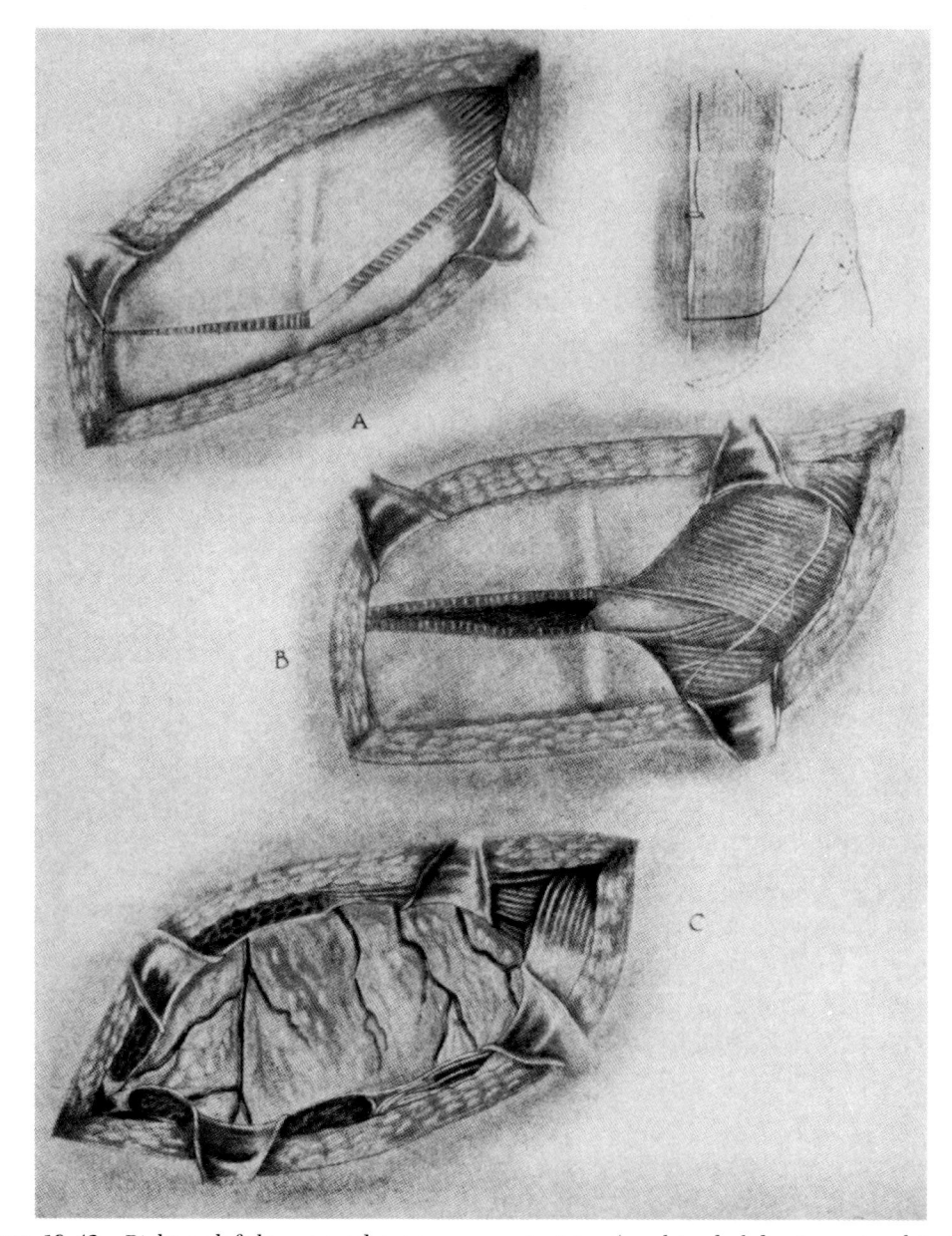

Figure 18–43. Right or left lower quadrant transverse incision (combined abdominoperineal incision). *A*, Anterior rectus sheath incised transversely and external oblique fibers split. *B*, External oblique retracted. Internal oblique and transversus abdominis split clear to the pelvic wall. *C*, Rectus muscle transected, and the incision is completed. Note retraction of the iliohypogastric nerve. (From Coller, F. A., and MacLean, K. F.: *In* Cole, W. H.: Operative Technic in General Surgery. New York, Appleton-Century-Crofts, 1949.)

TYPES AND CHOICE OF INCISIONS

The anterior sheath of the rectus muscle can be incised transversely (which is preferred) or obliquely in the line of the skin incision. The lateral border of the rectus muscle is freed, and a finger is passed beneath it over which all the fibers of the rectus muscle are cut across and the superior epigastric vessels are divided and ligated (Fig. 18–45). The small eighth and large ninth intercostal nerves may be seen entering the lateral border of the rectus muscle. The former may be sacrificed with impunity, but an

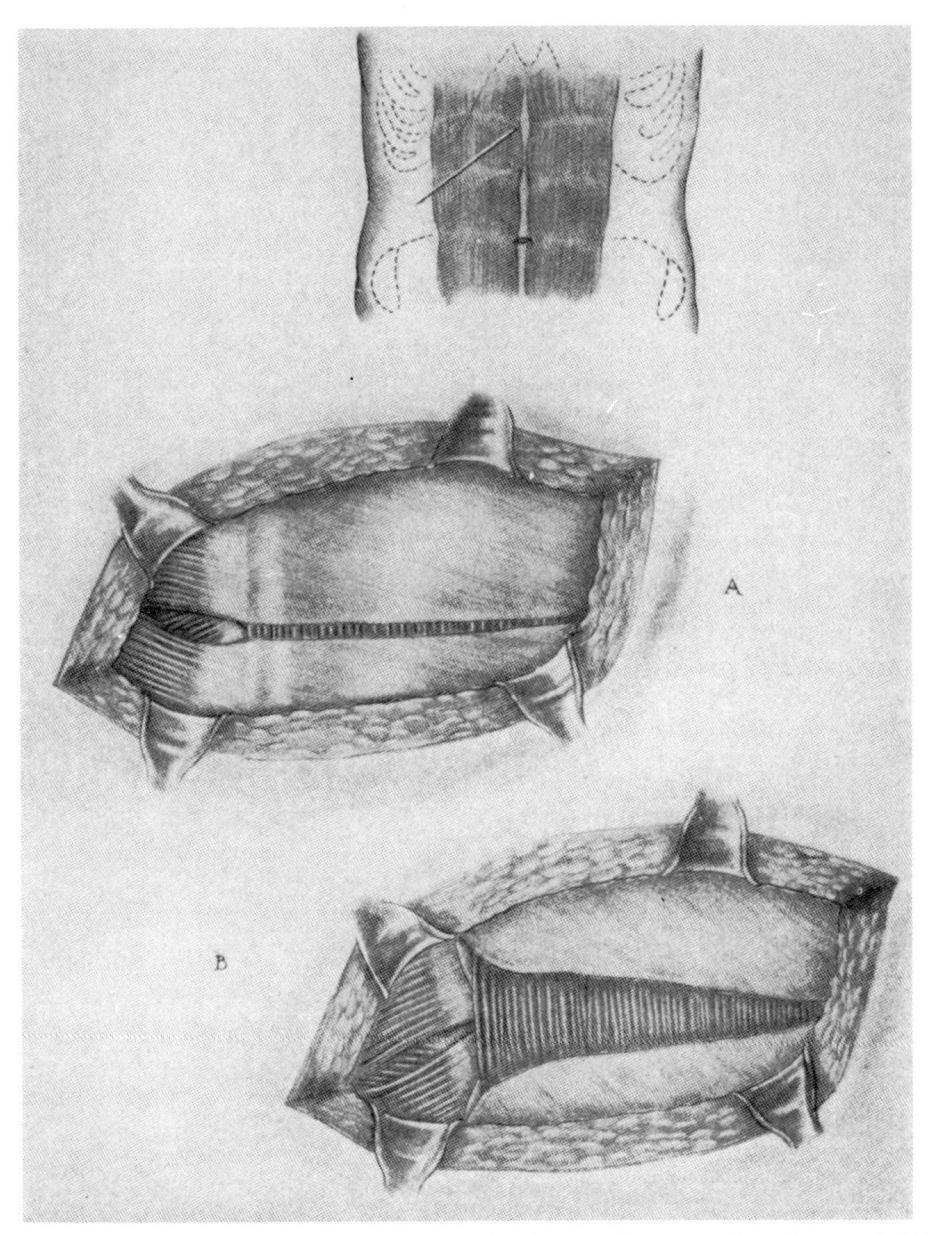

Figure 18–44. Oblique incision. A, Anterior rectus sheath incised transversely and external oblique fibers split. B, Rectus muscle freed at lateral border and external oblique retracted. Used primarily for biliary operations on the right and splenectomy on the left. (Coller and MacLean: Abdominal Incisions, in Cole [ed.]: Operative Technic. Courtesy Appleton-Century-Crofts, Inc.) (From Coller and MacLean, cited in previous figure.)

effort should be made to retract the latter out of harm's way and preserve its integrity.

The posterior rectus sheath, transversalis fascia, and peritoneum are now carefully incised in a transverse direction. This incision is continued laterally through the linea semilunaris. In some subjects the rectus muscle may be so wide that the incision need not extend lateral to the rectus sheath. In the majority of patients, however, further lateral extension is required. To accomplish this the external oblique muscle is divided in the direction of its fibers upward and laterally to the rib margin. These margins are retracted upward and downward. The internal oblique and transversus abdominis muscles are di-

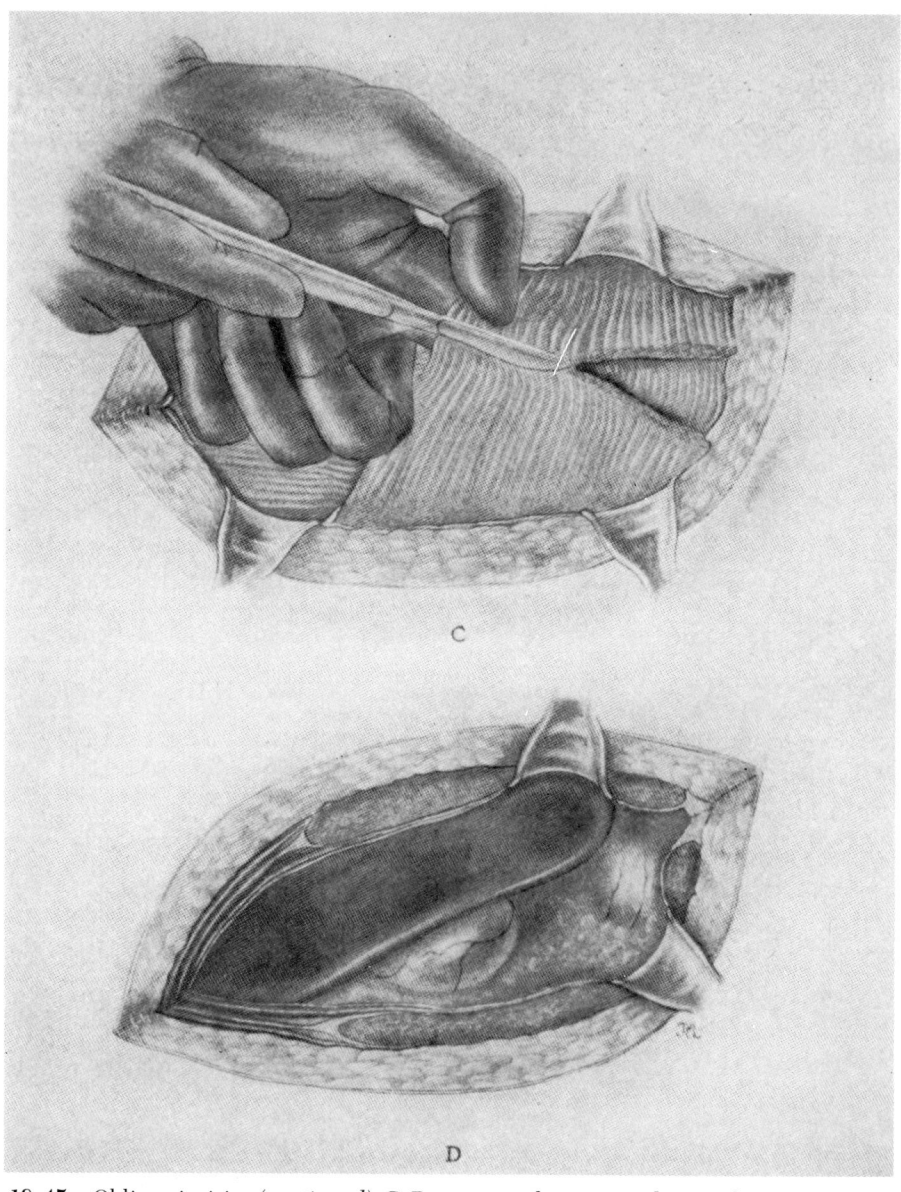

Figure 18–45. Oblique incision *(continued).* C, Rectus muscle transected over a finger inserted beneath it. D, Incision completed. (From Coller and MacLean, cited in Figure 18–44.)

vided in the direction of their fibers while avoiding unnecessary injury to the ninth and other intercostal nerves, which run transversely on the anterior surface of the transversus abdominis muscle.

In some patients it is preferred or necessary to extend the incision lateral to the lateral margin of the rectus sheath by cutting downward and laterally across the external oblique muscle fibers at their attachment to the rectus sheath, instead of dividing them in the direction of their course, but such a small portion of them is transected that no harm results. However, when closure is performed one must remember to reapproximate the cut ends because otherwise the upper flap may be contracted up under the costal margin and be overlooked. Even though it is necessary to transect the external oblique muscle, the internal oblique and transversus abdominis muscles can usually be split in the direction of their fibers with the sacrifice of only one intercostal nerve. The divided edges of the muscles are retracted and the peritoneal incision is continued laterally for the desired distance.

If the operating table is broken upward to hyperextend the patient, the exposure is improved.

After the surgery has been completed the wound is closed in layers, as previously described for the closure of a midabdominal transverse incision.

Methods of Extension

A subcostal incision can be extended to the other side of the abdomen by continuing the upper and medial end of the incision transversely across the linea alba and other rectus sheath and muscle, transecting the ligamentum teres between clamps, and ligating its cut ends. If still further extension is needed, the incision can be continued laterally and downward, parallel and inferior to the costal margin, forming an identical subcostal incision on the other side. This maneuver provides excellent exposure.

A subcostal incision can be extended upward by dividing the linea alba and peritoneum vertically upward in the midline to the tip of the xiphoid. If further extension is needed, this incision can be continued obliquely upward and laterally to transect the costal arch on the ipsilateral side without entering into the pleural cavity. This increases the exposure greatly, but, if still more is needed, after the cartilage has been transected the incision can be continued laterally to enter the thoracic cavity in the sixth or fifth intercostal space to form an abdominothoracic incision.

A subcostal incision can be extended downward by incising the linea alba and midline of the peritoneum downward for the desired distance, skirting the ipsilateral side of the umbilicus if necessary to extend the opening to or below that level.

McBURNEY GRIDIRON INCISION

The McBurney incision was devised for performing an appendectomy. It is made in the right lower quadrant of the abdomen. It is the incision of choice for carrying out a predetermined appendectomy. It is also useful for performing a cecostomy.

An identical incision made in the left lower quadrant is useful for performing a sigmoidostomy. A McBurney incision affords a limited exposure and does not permit an extensive intra-abdominal exploration.

An oblique skin incision is made two fingerbreadths (about 3 cm.) superomedial to the anterosuperior spine of the ileum and across a line running from the anterosuperior spine to the umbilicus. The upper third of the incision lies above this line and the lower two-thirds below it. The incision runs downward and medially, paralleling the direction of the fibers of the underlying external oblique muscle, for about 8 cm. It is deepened through the subcutaneous tissue, and its edges are retracted to expose the external oblique muscle. The aponeurosis of the external oblique muscle is divided in the direction of its fibers for the extent of the skin incision. This usually means that in its upper third the incision separates the muscular fibers of the external oblique muscle, while in its lower two-thirds the aponeurotic fibers of this muscle are separated. The external oblique muscle is retracted, and by blunt dissection the internal oblique muscle is divided in the direction of its fibers (Fig. 18–46) and retracted. The transversus abdominis muscle is then bluntly

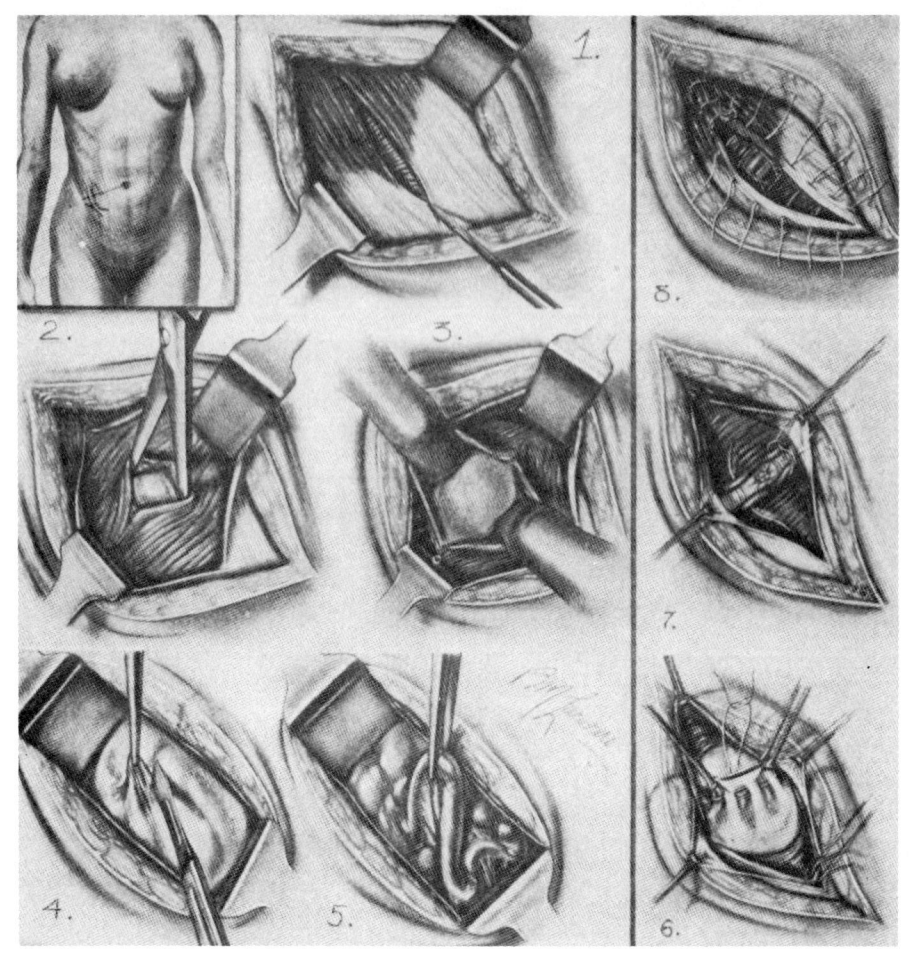

Figure 18–46. McBurney or gridiron incision, as employed for appendectomy. (From Maingot, R.: Abdominal Operations, ed. 2. New York, Appleton-Century-Crofts, 1948.)

divided in the direction of its fibers and retracted. A finger is swept around the entire circumference of the wound deep to the transversus abdominis muscle. This loosens the attachments of the transversalis fascia and allows it and its underlying peritoneum to bulge up into the wound where they can be incised more satisfactorily. This maneuver is particularly valuable in patients with a thick abdominal wall. The transversalis fascia and peritoneum are carefully incised in the direction of the skin incision, care being taken to avoid injury to the underlying cecum or other viscera.

After the operation has been completed, the peritoneum and transversalis fascia are closed with a continuous suture of 2–0 catgut or synthetic absorbable suture. The divided edges of the transverse abdominis and internal oblique muscles may be reapproximated with one row of about three interrupted sutures of 2–0 catgut or synthetic absorbable sutures. However, this step is not necessary. The edges of the external oblique muscle are reapposed with a row of interrupted sutures of 2–0 silk or chromic, or synthetic absorbable sutures or 2–0 polypropylene. The subcutaneous tissues are approximated with interrupted sutures of 4–0 catgut or synthetic absorbable sutures. The skin is closed with continuous or interrupted sutures of 4–0 nylon or stainless steel staples.

Methods of Extension

A McBurney incision may be extended upward and laterally for several centimeters

TYPES AND CHOICE OF INCISIONS

without cutting across the muscles, by simply enlarging the incision.

It can be extended medially by transversely dividing the ipsilateral or both rectus sheaths and muscles for the desired distance, provided the cut inferior epigastric vessels are ligated. In any case it is advisable to avoid injury to the iliohypogastric nerve.

As a general rule, if abdominal exploration or a considerably wider operative field is indicated, it is wiser to close the McBurney incision rather than extend it and immediately make a right paramedian or other more suitable incision.

ROCKEY-DAVIS INCISION

This incision is a popular substitute for the McBurney incision just described.

Technic

A transverse skin incision is made so as to cross the junction of the lower and middle thirds of a line extending from the anterosuperior iliac spine to the umbilicus (Fig. 18–47). The medial end of this incision is at the lateral border of the rectus muscle while its lateral end is about 3 cm. superior and medial to the anterosuperior iliac spine.

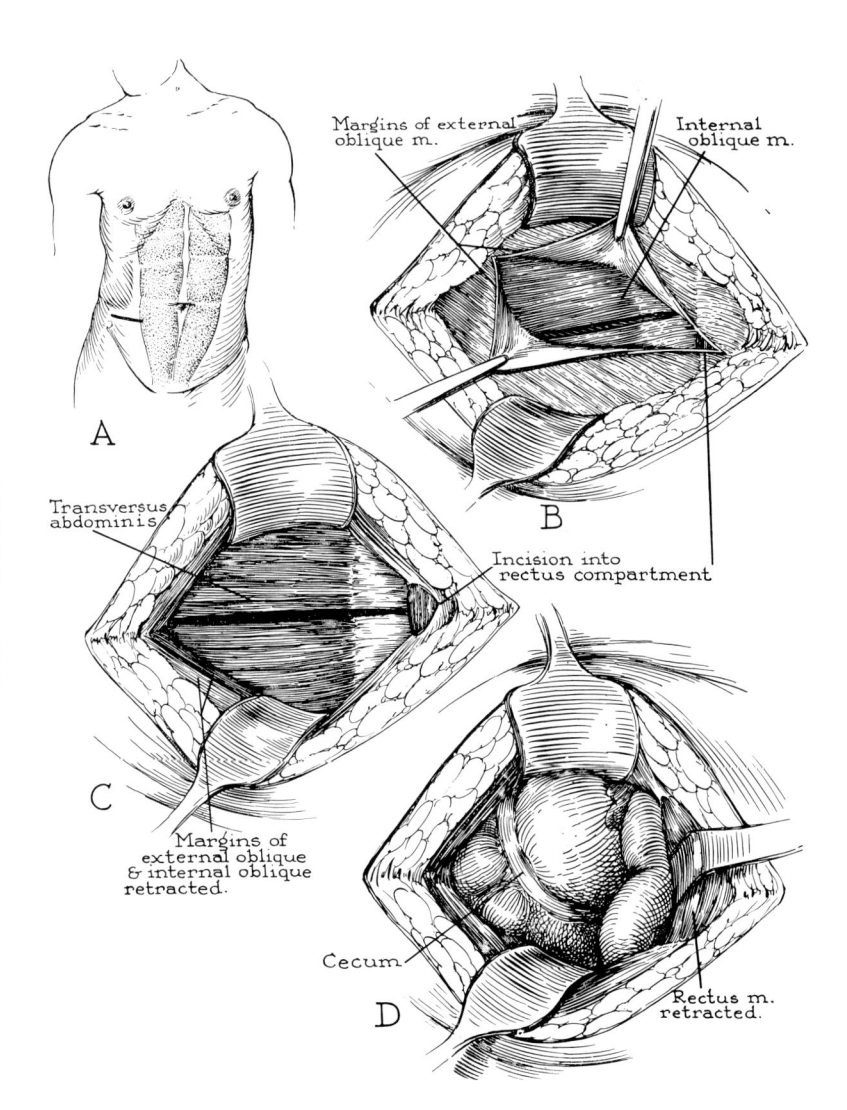

Figure 18–47. Rockey-Davis incision in the right lower quadrant. A, Transverse incision through skin and subcutaneous tissues. B, External oblique split and retracted; split fibers of internal oblique indicated. C, Transversus abdominis split; rectus compartment incised. D, Retracted wound.

The incision is deepened to expose the aponeurosis of the external oblique muscle which is split in the direction of its fibers, continuing the split medially onto the rectus sheath. The aponeurotic junction of the internal oblique and transversus abdominis muscles is incised transversely at the linea semilunaris and then bluntly extended laterally to divide those muscles in the direction of their fibers. The lateral border of the rectus sheath is incised for about 0.5 cm., but the rectus muscle is not disturbed (Weir or Harrington's medial extension, which may also be used in a

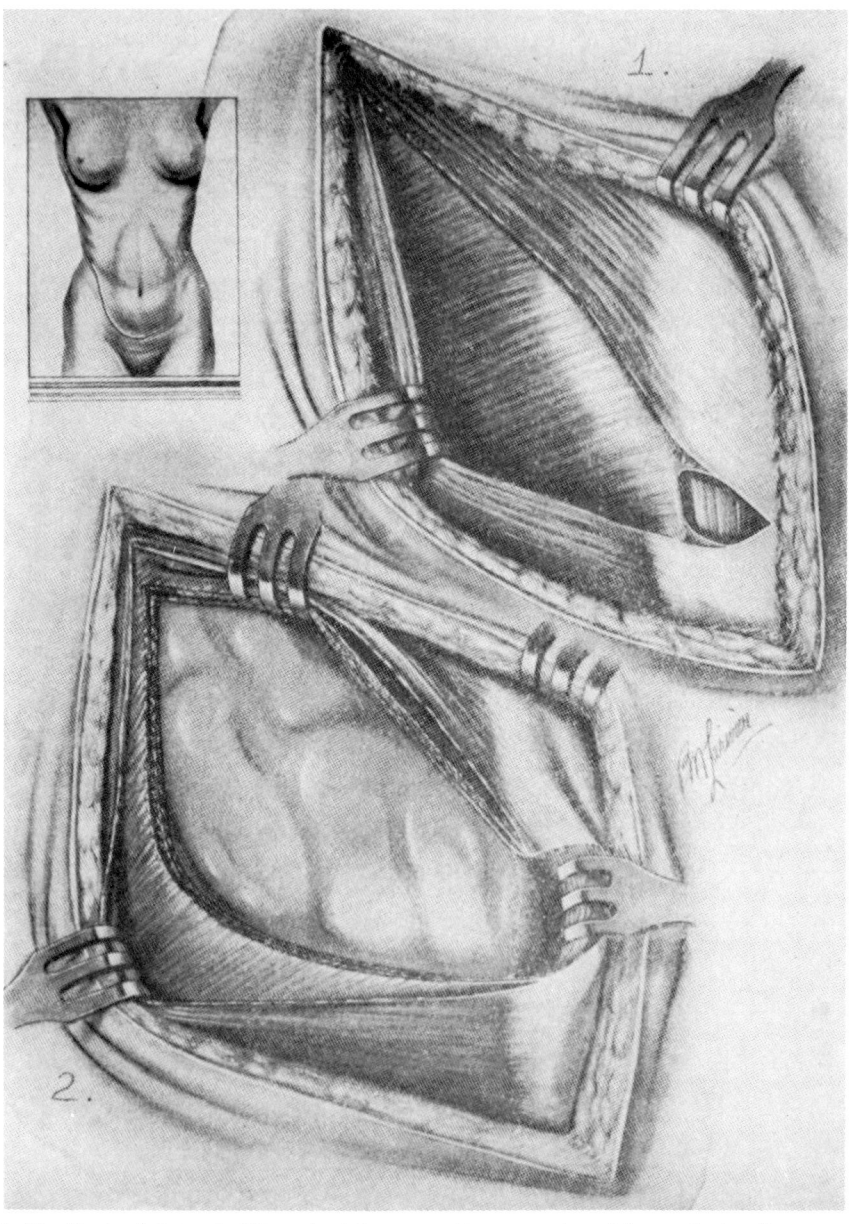

Figure 18–48. Kocher's lateral oblique incision, sometimes employed for exploring the ascending colon in patients with carcinoma. (From Maingot, R.: Abdominal Operations, ed. 2. New York, Appleton-Century-Crofts, 1948.)

TYPES AND CHOICE OF INCISIONS

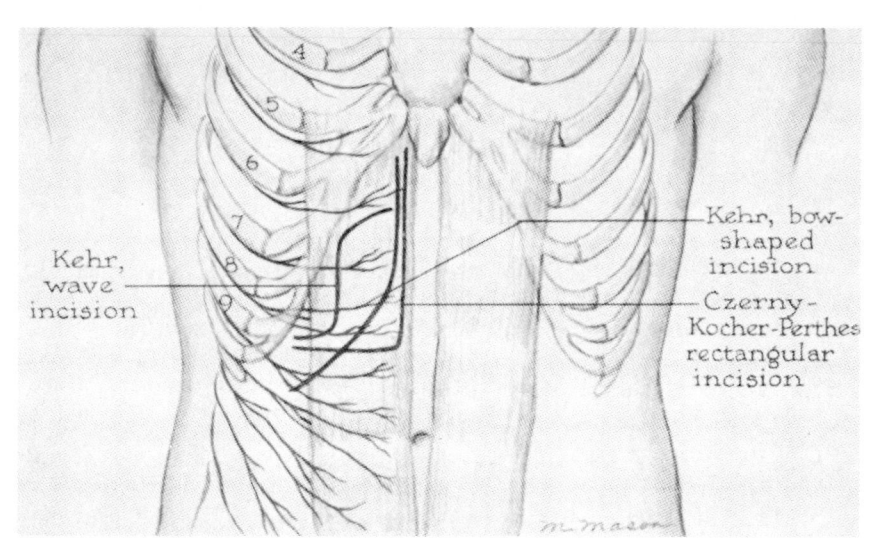

Figure 18–49. Combined vertical and transverse incisions in the right upper quadrant shown in relationship with the course of the intercostoabdominal nerves.

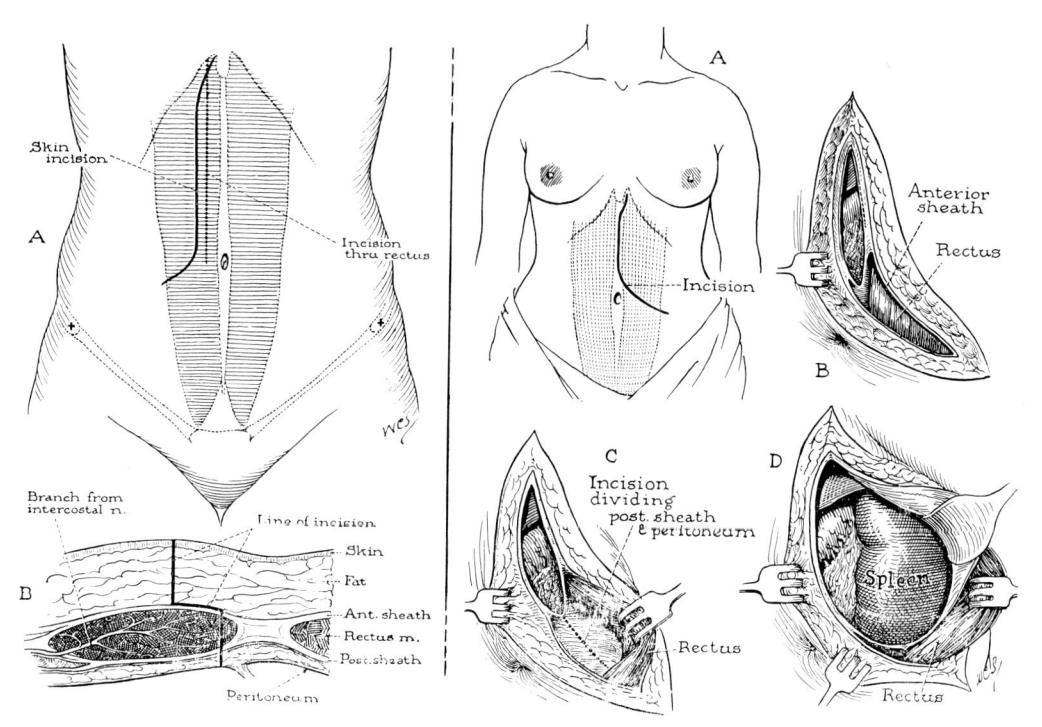

Figure 18–50. Bevan nerve-conserving incisions in the upper abdominal quadrants.

McBurney incision). The transversalis fascia and peritoneum are incised transversely.

The incision is closed in layers, as described for a McBurney incision, except that the nick in the rectus sheath is closed with one or two sutures.

The Rockey-Davis incision is the same as a McBurney incision except that the direction of its skin incision is transverse. It can be extended by the same methods as described for a McBurney incision.

LATERAL OBLIQUE ABDOMINAL INCISION WITH DIVISION OF MUSCLES IN SAME DIRECTION AS SKIN INCISION (KOCHER)

This incision can be used in either the right or the left lower quadrants. It is employed on the right by some surgeons for operations on the cecum and ascending colon, and on the left for operations on the descending and sigmoid colon. It provides good exposure for these procedures, heals firmly, and rarely is followed by an incisional hernia.

Technic

The patient is placed on the operating table with the side to be incised elevated about 15 degrees by sandbags.

The skin incision begins at the tip of the tenth rib (Fig. 18-48). It proceeds obliquely downward and medially, to terminate just above the pubic crest. The incision is deepened through the subcutaneous tissue to expose the external oblique muscle and its aponeurosis. The external oblique, internal oblique, and transversus muscles are divided in line with the skin incision. The lower and medial portion of this incision nicks the lateral border of the rectus sheath but leaves the rectus muscle intact. Since this roughly parallels the direction of the nerves, very little of the muscle is denervated. The peritoneum is divided in the same direction.

When the operation has been completed, the peritoneum and transversalis fascia are repaired with a continuous suture of 2-0 plain catgut or synthetic absorbable suture. The cut edges of the internal oblique and transversus abdominis muscles are approximated with one row of interrupted sutures of 2-0 silk or No. 30 stainless steel wire or 2-0 polypropylene. The edges of the external oblique muscle are approximated with another row of the same type of sutures. The subcutaneous tissue is approximated with interrupted sutures of 3-0 catgut or synthetic absorbable sutures and the skin with a continuous or interrupted row of 4-0 nylon sutures or stainless steel staples.

Methods of Extension

This incision may be extended medially at its lower end by cutting transversely across the rectus sheath and tendinous attachment of the rectus muscle to the pubic crest.

Extensions in other directions are difficult. This is a disadvantage of the incision.

COMMENTS ON ABDOMINAL INCISIONS

A large variety of other incisions have been devised, but their description has been omitted here either because of ignorance, because they are obsolete or little used, or because they are modifications of those described.

Complicated incisions also have been omitted as they seem less desirable than the simpler ones described (Figs. 18-49 and 18-50).

Incisions for repairing hernias and for performing sacral, perineal and anal operations are discussed with the specific operative procedures.

Closure of incisions is most conservatively handled by using nonabsorbable suture material when strength is desired. A clean wound in a healthy patient can frequently be closed using absorbable synthetic sutures instead of wire, silk, or polypropylene.

Chapter 19

DRAINAGE OF ABDOMINAL WOUNDS

The use of drains in abdominal surgery can be for either therapeutic or prophylactic reasons. Therapeutic drainage occurs when there is an intra-abdominal collection of pus or the extravasation of such material as bile or pancreatic juice. Therapeutic drainage will be successful only in an area where an abscess cavity has been established or when there is a continuous flow of fluid. Prophylactic drainage is used after an operative procedure when there is a probability of leakage of a physiologic fluid that would be better drained than allowed to wall off and create other problems (Tanner, 1964).

The principles for the use of drains are quite clear. Drains should take the shortest practical route from the area to be drained to the skin surface. The drain should be carefully placed so it will be at a site where the fluid to be drained will collect. As a general policy, drains should not be brought out through the operative incision. The exiting of even a Penrose drain through the abdominal incision instead of through a separate adjacent stab wound increases the incidence of infection from 2.4 to 4 per cent. An even more marked increase in wound infection rate is seen in cholecystectomy incisions. Here the incidence of infection with a separate stab incision is 1.8 per cent. When the drain is brought out through the primary incision, the incidence rises to 9.9 per cent (Cruse and Foord, 1973).

The material used to construct abdominal drains must exhibit certain physical and chemical properties. It should be soft and pliable. The drain should elicit only mild-to-no tissue reaction. It should be composed of a stable material that will not readily decompose. Drains should be carefully placed so as to adequately drain the area. The possibility of erosion into a vessel or organ should be minimized by careful placement of the drain.

Several methods are commonly used to drain the peritoneal cavity. Perhaps the most common is the latex rubber drain known as the Penrose or cigarette drain (Fig. 19–1A). The Penrose drain establishes a tract and provides drainage by overflow of

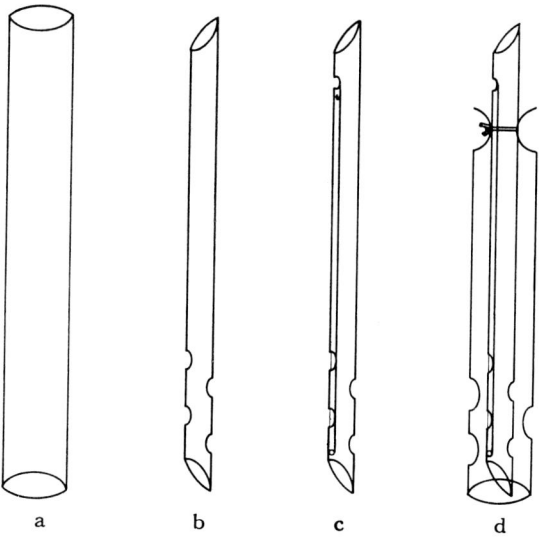

Figure 19–1. Four types of drains for peritoneal drainage. *a*, Penrose drain; *b*, tube drain; *c*, sump drain; and *d*, sump-Penrose drain. (From Hanna, E. A.: Efficiency of peritoneal drainage. Surg. Gynecol. Obstet. *131*:983, 1970.)

fluid through its lumen. Its drainage is affected by position, gravity, small pressure differences, and capillary action. Effective drainage cannot be accomplished by a small stab wound for the Penrose drain; one must be able to insert at least one finger through all layers into the peritoneal cavity (Tanner, 1964; Hanna, 1970).

The tube drain also is a simple method of drainage. It is an overflow drain and acts like a Penrose drain. The tube drain tends to be rigid and, if not placed carefully, can erode adjacent viscera. The holes in a tube drain can be occluded by intraperitoneal surfaces, fat, or organs. Another method of drainage is a rubber or plastic tube and an indwelling catheter (Fig. 19–1B).

A modification of the tube drain is the closed-tube suction drain (Fig. 19–2). A perforated tube is inserted by trochar through the abdominal wall into the abdominal cavity and correctly positioned. The suction–drainage collection apparatus is then hooked to the catheter or catheters. System failure is usually due to improper positioning of the catheter, inadequate diameter of the catheter, the loss of negative pressure on the catheter, or the formation of clots within the drainage tubes. Most of the commercially obtained closed-suction drainage systems are made with fairly stiff plastic drainage tubes. Some surgeons have substituted softer rubber tubes in order to milk out clots and debris (Hanna, 1970; Garcia-Rinaldi, 1975). Closed-suction drainage is theoretically the ideal form of drainage. Not only does it eliminate dead space but it also continuously removes any accumulation of fluid.

Another commonly used form of drainage is the sump drain. A smaller tube is incorporated into the drain, which allows air to be sucked through the larger tube. This permits the larger tube to remain patent and prevents adjacent structures from being sucked into the openings of the outer tube (Fig. 19–1C). Many types of sump drains are available. Some of these products have a bacterial filter in the air inlet tube into the sump drain. As long as the suction is kept at low levels (120 mm. Hg) rather than high, there appears to be no difference in rate of wound contamination. Whether or not the filter is present, high-level suction

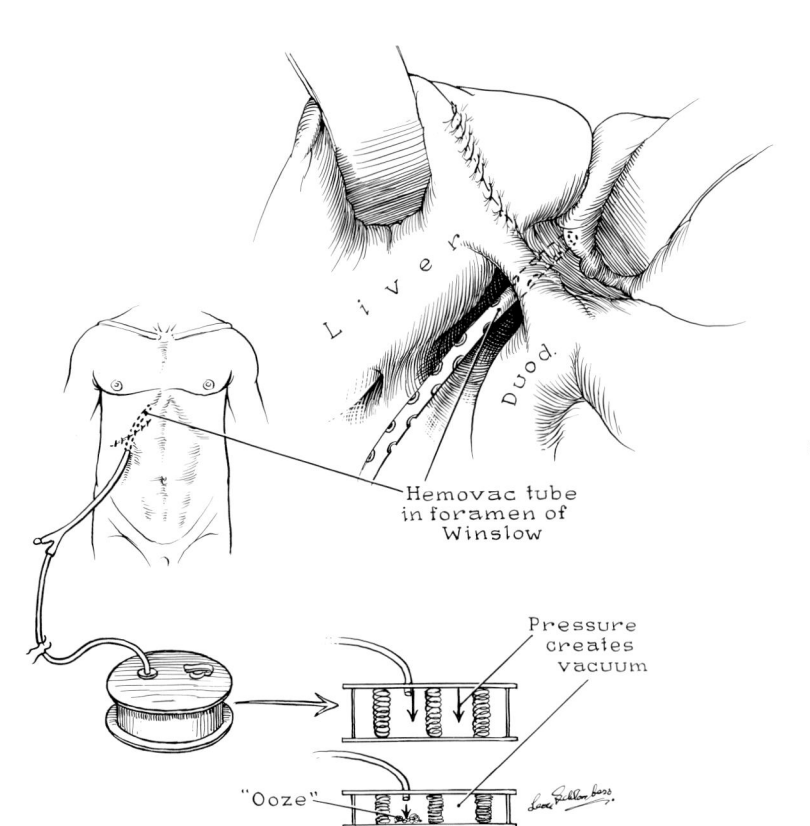

Figure 19–2. Closed-tube suction drain.

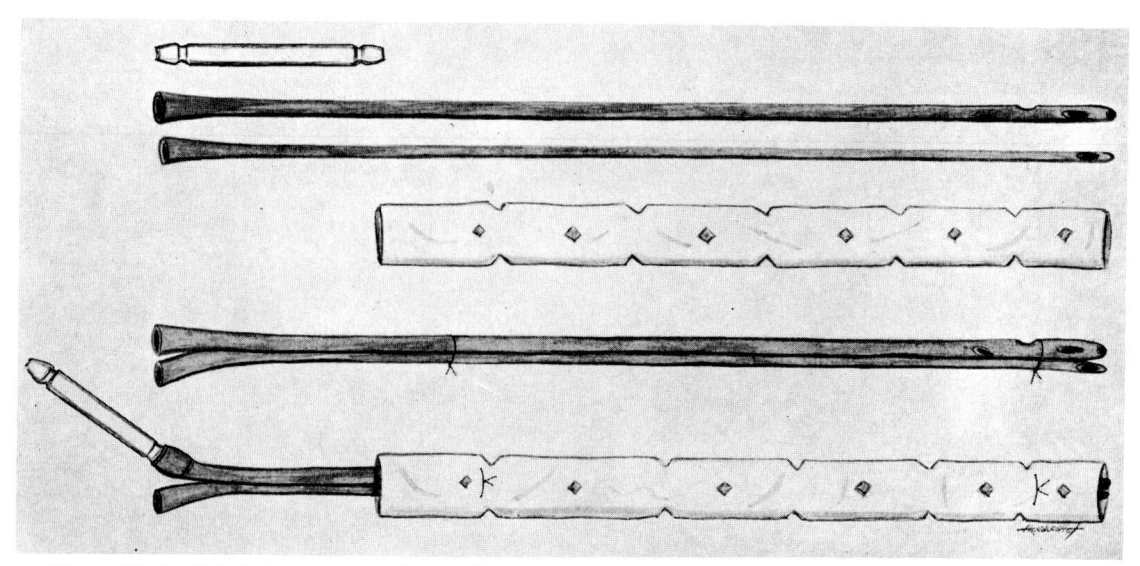

Figure 19–3. Triple-lumen sump drain. A longer rubber urethral catheter connected to suction and tied side-by-side to a smaller catheter, inserted into the lumen, sutured to the wall of a large Penrose drain, with multiple perforations over the entire length. (From Water, N. G., Walsky, R., Kasdan, M. L., et al.: The treatment of acute hemorrhagic pancreatitis by sump drainage. Surg. Gynecol. Obstet. *126*:963, 1968.)

will lead to an increase in the rate of wound infection (Baker and associates, 1977). Sump drains have also been modified to provide a third lumen for irrigation (Abramson, 1970; Formeister and Elias, 1976).

Another common drain is the Penrose sump or Waterman drain, a triple-lumen sump drain. It is usually composed of a large Penrose drain and a No. 20 (or larger) and a No. 12 rubber urethral catheter. This drain apparently does not clog easily, works well in abscess cavities, and commonly does not erode (Fig. 19–3) (Waterman and associates, 1968). Modification to prevent erosion has been suggested (Fig. 19–4) (Ranson, 1973).

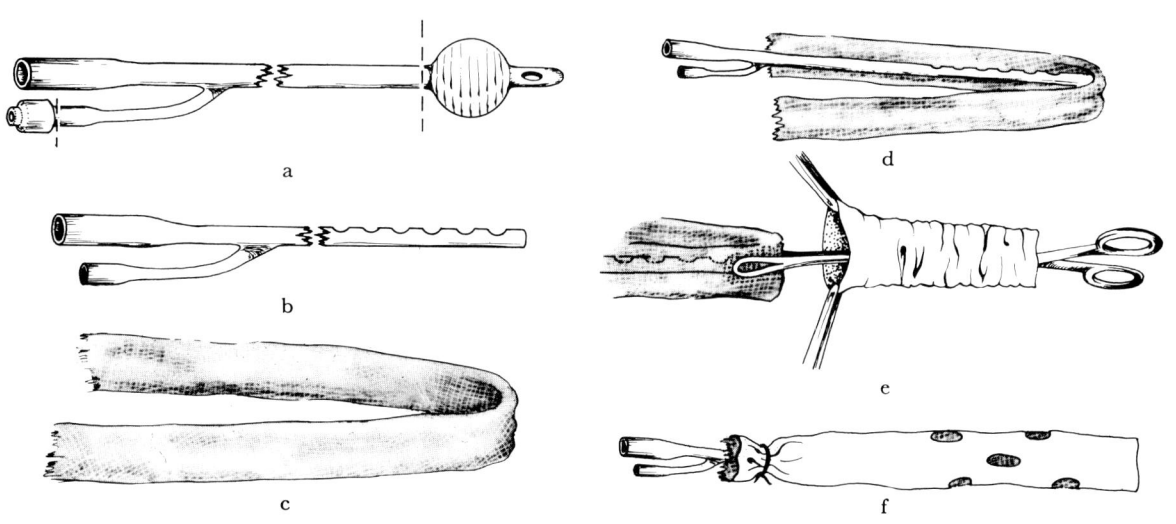

Figure 19–4. Sump drain construction. *a*, No. 22 F. Foley urethral catheter. *b*, The balloon tip and inlet seal are cut from the Foley catheter. Holes are also cut on the side of the large outlet catheter. *c*, Vaginal or plain gauze packing. *d*, The sump catheter is completely enclosed in gauze packing. *e*, The Penrose drain is introduced over the gauze-covered sump. *f*, A heavy tie fixes the catheter, gauze, and Penrose drain. Holes are cut in the side of the Penrose drain.

(From Ransom, J. H. C.: Safer intraperitoneal sump drainage. Surg. Gynecol. Obstet. *137*:841, 1973.)

There are other, less frequently used drains, such as the corrugated latex or plastic drain that is at least as effective as the Penrose drain. All drains should be fixed to the skin to prevent accidental removal. Indications for use and removal of drains will be discussed with specific diseases. In general, a drain that has stopped draining or is clotted should be removed.

Chapter 20

COMPLICATIONS OF INCISION

CONTAMINATED WOUNDS

Contamination in surgical wounds causes a significant increase in both morbidity and mortality. Hospitalizations are prolonged. In one study major complications developed in 10.5 per cent of patients with contaminated wounds, while individuals with clean wounds had a complication rate of 1 to 2 per cent.

The identification of the obviously contaminated wound is not a problem. An incision where surfaces are in contact with pus or an infective fluid during an operative procedure is considered highly contaminated. Wounds that are exposed to feces are highly contaminated. Moderate contamination occurs when a patient is subjected to a cholecystectomy. Trauma is one of the more obvious producers of wound contamination. The wound is not only exposed to unsterile foreign debris and bacteria, but soft tissue damage and the subsequent injury to tissue vascularity may cause more tissue necrosis than is readily apparent at initial examination and treatment (Conolly, Hunt, and Dunphy, 1969).

The concentration of bacteria in tissue can be quantified. The critical concentration of bacteria in a wound ranges from 10^5 to 10^6 bacteria per gram of tissue. If the count exceeds this level, the wound will become grossly infected. When available, quantitative bacteriology can play an important part in wound management. The "rapid slide" technique for quantifying bacterial concentration has been developed. Even though it is most frequently used in burn patients, it can be utilized in any wound. This method has a 95 per cent accuracy compared with results obtained from routine quantitative bacterial cultures (Krizek and Robson, 1975).

Moderately contaminated wounds may create management problems. Fortunately, most heal without developing gross infection. However, many factors can cause a moderately contaminated wound to develop gross infection. One example is impaired immunologic response. Pre- or coexisting diseases requiring chemotherapy or immunosuppressive drugs alter immune response as does the malnutrition that is associated with many diseases.

A healing wound requires an intact circulation to supply nutrients and oxygen for collagen synthesis and wound repair and in addition to remove metabolites and provide cellular defense mechanisms. The use of vasoconstricting drugs, hypovolemia, shock, or any condition causing decreased perfusion to the wound is associated with an increased incidence of wound infection. Tissue tension is important. When tissue planes are approximated under stress with heavy sutures, the circulation along the suture line may be compromised by edema. The resultant inadequate tissue perfusion will provide the environment for wound infection.

Tissue trauma, either prior to or during the operative procedure, markedly enhances the chances of wound infection. The use of meticulous technique to decrease tissue destruction during an operation is an important factor. Devitalized tissue within the operative field must be kept at a minimum. Wound hematomas provide the environment for infection. It has been reported that 20 to 30 per cent of wound infections are associated with wound hematomas. The prevention of faulty hemostasis, adequate drainage, and minimal dead space within the wound will minimize this problem.

The attainment of adequate hemostasis is sometimes difficult, but poor hemostasis frequently is the result of poor operative techniques. When small vessels are transected by a sharp scalpel they will usually retract and provide their own hemostasis after the application under pressure of moist packs. Hot packs are to be avoided since they cause vasodilation and heat destruction of tissue. Blood vessels that are larger or continue to bleed should be ligated or electrocoagulated. Vessels should be ligated with the minimum of surrounding tissue, using the smallest size suture that can be safely tied around the bleeding vessel. The use of electrocautery so as to coagulate or "burn" large amounts of tissue to obtain hemostasis is deplored.

Bacterial concentration in a wound can be markedly reduced but not eliminated. Gross contamination by spillage of infected material can be prevented by careful handling of tissue and organs. Mechanical protection can be provided by discarding contaminated drapes, gloves, and instruments. Plastic drapes can be used to cover wounds and isolate the operative field in order to reduce contamination (Conolly, Hunt, and Dunphy, 1969). Plastic drapes do not necessarily reduce the bacterial concentration on the skin.

The use of preoperative antibiotics as prophylaxis against wound infection has been shown to be effective, especially in stomach, biliary, and large bowel surgery (Stone and colleagues, 1976). Antibiotics are not a substitute for careful debridement and good technique. Topical antibiotics have been applied to wounds to reduce bacterial activity. Ideally, the antibiotics should have a wide range of activity against both gram-negative and gram-positive organisms and should not be tissue irritants. Topical antibiotics may be used as a powder or in irrigation fluid. The topical application of antibiotics will not sterilize a wound that contains blood, sera, foreign body, or devitalized disease. Even though the topical antibiotics may reduce the incidence of wound infection under certain circumstances, the value of routine use is questionable. It is practical to use topical antibiotics in a heavily contaminated wound or when debridement must be delayed (Conolly, Hunt, and Dunphy, 1969).

Irrigation of a wound will markedly reduce the bacterial concentration. The most effective method is high-pressure pulsatile irrigation. Pulsatile water is very effective in cleaning the debris from a wound, although it has been reported that continuous high pressure irrigation is equally effective (Rodeheaver and associates, 1975). Pulsatile irrigation produces less irritation and edema than scrubbing with a brush. Normal saline will lyse cells, and irrigation with saline could cause irritation of wound tissue. Ringer's lactate is less irritating to tissue (Brown and associates, 1978).

Other factors are associated with increased susceptibility to wound infection. Previous irradiation of tissue appears to make tissue very susceptible to wound infection. Irradiated tissue should be handled very carefully during an operative procedure.

DELAYED CLOSURE

One good technique for reducing the incidence of postoperative wound infection is to use delayed closure, even when there is only the slightest possibility of bacterial contamination. One could quantitate the concentration of pathogens by the "rapid slide" technique and delay closure on those wounds that exceed 10^5 organisms per gram of tissue (Robson, Shaw, and Heggers, 1970). All suspected or grossly heavily contaminated wounds should not be closed primarily but instead delayed closure is indicated.

Contaminated wounds should not be closed with silk, cotton, or any other nonabsorbable multifilament material tending to harbor infection or cause persistent sinus drainage. Nonabsorbable monofilament suture should be used to close the fascial layers. Either No. 30 stainless steel wire or 0 polypropylene may be used. The peritoneum, muscle, and aponeurotic (fascial) layers are closed in the usual manner. The wound is copiously irrigated. Far-near nylon sutures or large mattress sutures are

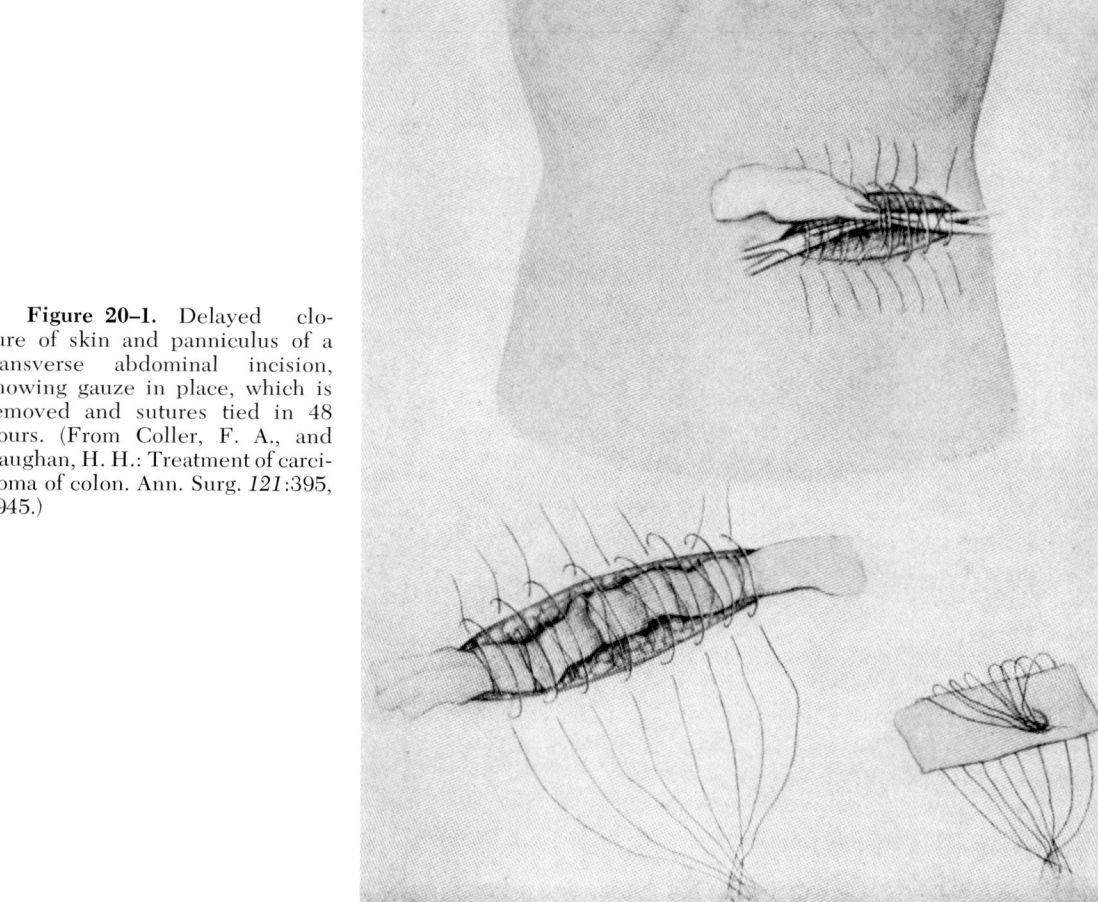

Figure 20–1. Delayed closure of skin and panniculus of a transverse abdominal incision, showing gauze in place, which is removed and sutures tied in 48 hours. (From Coller, F. A., and Vaughan, H. H.: Treatment of carcinoma of colon. Ann. Surg. *121*:395, 1945.)

placed in the skin and subcutaneous tissues (Fig. 20–1) but are not tied. The subcutaneous cavity beneath the skin sutures is filled with gauze soaked in povidone-iodine or impregnated with nitrofurazone or other antibacterial agents or with sterile gauze. This dressing should be changed at least twice a day, and more frequently in a heavily contaminated wound. The incision should not be closed until the concentration of bacteria in the wound is less than 10^5 organisms, or the wound appears to be clean and is exhibiting a healthy granulation response.

Experimental studies demonstrate that only 3 per cent of wounds that are closed secondarily on or after the fourth postoperative day will develop infection. It is easiest to place skin sutures at the time of the original surgical procedure (Edlich and associates, 1969). If this is not done, one may have to use local anesthesia to complete the secondary closure. Steri-strips are useful in delayed closure, and many times will approximate the skin edges successfully. A good cosmetic result is usually observed in patients who undergo delayed closure of an incision.

It is possible that delayed primary closure need not be used in all patients who are at risk of developing wound infections. Patients who undergo operations upon the gastrointestinal tract could have the abdominal incision closed primarily and have indwelling closed-suction catheters left in the incision for the purpose of continuous suction with intermittent antibiotic irrigation. This method is not used in the presence of gross contamination. It also requires some special attention by the nursing staff (McIlrath, 1976).

OTHER COMPLICATIONS

DISRUPTION

This dreaded complication most commonly occurs between the sixth to tenth postoperative day. It is particularly common after operations performed upon patients with malignant disease or who are cachectic for other reasons, or upon those who have had severe distention, coughing, vomiting, wound infection, or wound hematoma during the postoperative period. Obstruction may result from herniation of the bowel through the disrupted area.

Disruption is often heralded by the appearance of serosanguinous drainage on the dressings about the sixth postoperative day. When this occurs one should inspect the wound and have the patient strain gently to observe any unusual protrusion *while having in hand a sterile towel to quickly hold back the intestine if it shows signs of eviscerating.*

Often the first recognition of wound disruption is the sudden occurrence of evisceration.

As soon as wound disruption is diagnosed, regardless of how small it may be, there is no virtue in procrastinating by employing conservative measures of treatment.

A sterile towel should be strapped over the wound with adhesive, to serve as a tampon to retain the viscera while the patient is immediately taken to the operating room and anesthetized. The wound is opened as widely as is necessary and the viscera are replaced in the abdominal cavity. The wound is then closed with through-and-through sutures of stainless steel wire or polypropylene, utilizing previously described techniques.

WOUND INFECTION

This complication is usually heralded on or after the third postoperative day by a daily rise in the patient's temperature. When inspected the wound is found to be tender and possibly indurated in one area. Some localized edema and redness may be present.

As soon as the presence of pus is recognized or suspected, drainage should be promptly instituted. The skin sutures in that portion of the wound should be removed. With a sterile clamp the wound edges can be gently separated until the collection of pus is encountered and drainage is established. The wound should be cultured and a sample of the pus Gram-stained. Anesthesia is usually unnecessary. Hot moist compresses are applied and nothing further is necessary at this time. If the incision had been closed with silk or cotton, it is possible that a draining sinus may persist and require removal of the infected silk suture. This is not necessary when wire, polypropylene, catgut, or synthetic absorbable suture has been used.

WOUND HEMATOMA

A collection of blood may accumulate in the depth of the incision. Its presence is usually manifested by a patient's low-grade fever and more tenderness in the wound than is usual after four or five postoperative days have elapsed. A hematoma is often difficult to recognize. Usually it can be diagnosed by palpating a tender, indurated mass, which is generally situated in the lower part of the wound, the position determined by gravitational forces. There may be ecchymosis of varying degree over the hematoma.

A hematoma should be evacuated as soon as it is recognized because of the danger that it will cause separation of the wound edges. If it is superficial, the skin edges over it can be parted with a hemostat until the collection of blood is encountered and allowed to escape. If the hematoma is more deeply situated, the skin over its site can be infiltrated with a local anesthetic and the blood aspirated with a needle and syringe.

If the blood is clotted, under some form of anesthesia of the patient the wound will have to be opened down to the clot and the hematoma manually evacuated. The opened part of the wound is reclosed around a drain placed in the space formerly occupied by the hematoma. This drain is not removed until drainage has ceased. At the time of evacuating the hematoma, it is advisable to seek and ligate any source of bleeding that might have been its cause.

Part 4
SUTURES

Chapter 21

CLOSURE OF WOUND

THE GENESIS OF SUTURING

The use of sutures to close wounds dates far back into antiquity (MacKenzie, 1973). Bone needles with eyes were invented between 50,000 and 30,000 B.C. India appears to have been the most advanced of the early civilizations in the skills of surgery. The Egyptians, Babylonians, and Arabians probably acquired much of their knowledge of surgery from contact with early Indian peoples. An early text, Compendium of General Medicine, written by the Indian physician Súsruta (circa 600 B.C.), describes sutures made from flax, hemp, leather strips, horse hair, animal tendons, and bark fibers from the Ashmántaka tree. As early as 1000 B.C. the heads of large ants were used to close incisions. Later, antheads were used to anastomose small intestine. The Edwin Smith papyrus, written about 1600 B.C., first records the use of suture closure for the treatment of a shoulder laceration.

Aurelius Cornelius Celsus (circa A.D. 30) is credited as the first to write that hemostasis could be obtained by suture ligation. Celsus also described what is now known as a Michel clip. The suturing of severed tendons in gladiators was reported by Galen of Pergamon (circa A.D. 150). Galen made the first known reference to catgut. From his writings, it is apparent that catgut had been in use for many years. Galen also advocated the use of stronger suture material such as silk.

For centuries the term catgut has been used to describe suture made from the intestines of herbivorous animals, most commonly sheep. The term appears to be derived from kitgut or kitstring, the string used on a kit, an early musical instrument. Confusion probably results from the use of "kit," a term describing a young cat.

An Arabian physician, Rhazes of Baghdad (A.D. 852), was the first to describe the use of catgut (harpstrings) for abdominal closure. Another Arabian physician, Avicenna, first used monofilament suture. Avicenna realized that in the presence of gross infection most of the suture materials used at that time tended to break down rapidly. In an attempt to find a more durable material, he used pig bristle, the first example of a monofilament suture.

Henri de Mondeville (1260–1320) advocated the practices of attaining hemostatically dry wounds and using sharp, clean needles to prevent wound infection. He was one of the first to demand that more attention be given to anatomy.

When Islam began to decline, the Christian West began to establish its foundation in the surgical sciences. Guy de Chauliac (1300–1367) described an inverted stitch for the closure of intestines. Leonardo Bertapaglia of Padua (15th century) recognized the superiority of the technic of isolated suture ligation over en masse ligation of tissue. He is credited as the first to describe the practice of suture ligating a blood vessel.

Ambrose Paré (1517-1590) reintroduced many of the practices used by earlier surgeons. He popularized the use of ligatures, rather than indiscriminate cauterization, for hemostasis. He was among the first to advocate closure of all dead space in a wound. Hieronymus Fabricius ab Aquapendente (1537-1619) introduced gold wire suture material. He discovered that wire sutures were more flexible and possessed less tissue-cutting properties than did catgut.

For many centuries one of the most persistent problems was the infection that inevitably accompanied sutured wounds (Edlich and associates, 1973). Surgeons had for the most part dismissed the use of gut suture and were using nonabsorbable suture material for wound closure. It was perceived that one solution to reducing the incidence of wound infection would be the use of absorbable sutures for closure. In 1840, Luigi Porta demonstrated that catgut was a strong material and appeared to be a superior suture. Catgut became widely used for wound closure. Despite the fact that it was an absorbable suture, the problems of wound infection and sepsis persisted. In 1867, Joseph Lister developed the antiseptic gut ligature. Later he treated catgut with chromic salts in order to delay its dissolution into tissue. Nevertheless, sepsis in wounds closed with catgut was still a persistent problem. (Actually it was in the 1930s that processes were finally developed to render catgut sterile. Until that time, spore-forming organisms had resisted sterilization and were the probable etiology of so many of the catgut suture, closed wound infections.)

The inability to successfully close vesicovaginal fistulas with catgut or silk caused J. Marion Sims to seek other materials. He used silver wire for suture material and finally obtained a successful result. Thereafter he used silver wire in all of his operative procedures (Goldenberg, 1959).

The frequency of infection in wounds closed with catgut finally persuaded Theodor Kocher to change to silk sutures. The incidence of wound infection in his patients decreased markedly. Impressed by Kocher's results, William Halsted began to use silk sutures in 1882. In 1913, after publishing several reports on surgical technic, Halsted concluded that silk was the best available suture material. After 20 years of controversy, the superiority of silk was generally accepted.

In the past several decades, other materials such as cotton and linen have been reintroduced. Steel alloy drawn into wire was introduced in 1934 by W. W. Babcock. In the past few years synthetic nonabsorbable sutures, for example, nylon and polypropylene, have come into general use. Recently the first absorbable synthetic sutures were put into general use for ligature and wound closure.

ABSORBABLE AND NONABSORBABLE SUTURES

The United States Pharmacopeia (U.S.P.) classifies and standardizes surgical suture material. Suture materials capable of being digested or hydrolyzed are classified as absorbable sutures. Nonabsorbable sutures are composed of materials resistant to any enzymatic digestion or hydrolysis. In general, absorbable sutures are either obtained from natural collagen or are synthetic copolymers of lactide and glycolide or a homopolymer of glycolide. The absorption of suture material is determined by several factors: the size and composition of sutures, the condition of the tissues being reapposed, and the general health and nutritional status of the patient (Postlethwait and associates, 1959).

Surgical gut and synthetic suture can be used in the presence of infection, although these materials are more rapidly decomposed under these conditions. Plain gut tends to be quickly digested. It may be used in tissues that heal quite rapidly and require minimal support (Lawrie, 1959; Lawrie, Angus, and Reese, 1959; Jenkins and associates, 1974). Chromic gut and synthetic absorbable sutures may be used in tissues that tend to heal more slowly and require some degree of support during the healing (Van Winkle and associates, 1975). Synthetic absorbables can be used in many instances when chromic gut previously had been the suture of choice. Of the two synthetic absorbable sutures presently obtainable, the polyglactin 910, a copolymer of lactide and glycolide, appears to better maintain its tensile strength and absorb

ABSORBABLE AND NONABSORBABLE SUTURES

Table 21-1. Absorbable Suture Material

Suture	Type	Raw Material	Properties	Frequent Uses	Knot Pull Lbs.—U.S.P. Size 0	2-0	3-0	4-0
Surgical gut	Plain	Collagen obtained from submucosal layer of sheep or serosa of beef intestine	Digested rather rapidly by body tissue enzymes. Complete absorption by 10–14 days. Most marked inflammatory response. After 5 to 7 days will have lost up to 90% of tensile strength*	Ligate superficial blood vessels; suture subcutaneous tissue; suture rapidly healing tissue that requires minimal support. Ophthalmology	8.4	5.7	3.9	2.4
	Chromic	Collagen source, same as plain gut. Treated with chromic salt solutions	Digestion is slowed by chromic salt treatment. May see suture remnants for 50 to 70 days. Less inflammatory reaction than plain gut. Maintains substantial tensile strength at least for 14 days*	Tissues that heal slowly and need support—fascia and peritoneum; very versatile, can be used in practically all tissues. Ophthalmology	8.4	5.7	3.9	2.4
Polyglactin 910	Braided	Synthetic—copolymer of lactide and glycolide	Slowly absorbed by hydrolysis. Minimal tissue reaction. At two weeks still has 55% of original tensile strength. By three weeks has approximately 20% of original tensile strength.* Complete absorption by 60 to 90 days	Ligation or suturing of tissues where absorbable suture is desired. Not recommended for approximation under prolonged stress. Polyglycolic acid suture tends to be absorbed more quickly and has less tensile strength	8.8	6.2	3.9	2.4
Polyglycolic acid	Braided	Synthetic—homopolymer of glycolide						

*Studies performed in rats.

Table 21-2. Nonabsorbable Suture Material

Suture	Type	Raw Material	Properties	Frequent Uses	Knot Pull Lbs – U.S.P. Size				
					0	2-0	3-0	4-0
Surgical silk	Braided	Raw silk, a natural protein fiber spun by a silkworm	Very slowly absorbed, encapsulated; moderate inflammatory response. Loses 50% tensile strength in one year. No tensile strength present after two years	Most body tissues for ligating and suturing, general surgery, ophthalmology and plastic surgery	6.8	5.0	3.1	2.1
Surgical cotton	Twisted	Long staple cotton fibers that are combined, aligned, and twisted	Nonabsorbable, remains encapsulated; moderate inflammatory response. Loses 50% of tensile strength in 6 months; has 33% of tensile strength at end of two years	Same use as silk, weakest of nonabsorbable materials, no real advantages over silk	6.3	4.0	3.1	2.1
Nylon	Monofilament	Synthetic polyamide polymer	Nonabsorbable, remains encapsulated. Very little inflammatory response.	Skin closure, retention sutures, plastic surgery, ophthalmology	8.2	6.5	4.3	2.9
	Braided	Synthetic polyamide polymer	Loses 25% of tensile strength over 2-year period; very little tissue reaction	Most body tissues for ligating and suturing general closure; neurosurgery	7.0	4.8	3.5	2.3
Polyester fiber	Braided	Synthetic polymer (Dacron)	Nonabsorbable, remains encapsulated; very little tissue reaction; tends to maintain tensile strength	Cardiovascular and plastic surgery	9.2	6.0	4.1	1.9
Coated polyester fiber	Braided	Polyester fiber coated with surgical lubricant (polybutilate)		Cardiovascular, plastic surgery, general closures	8.7	6.5	4.0	2.8
Polypropylene	Monofilament	Polymer of propylene	Nonabsorbable, remains encapsulated; little tissue inflammatory response; tends to maintain tensile strength	General, plastic, and cardiovascular surgery	7.8	5.8	3.8	2.3

B&S Gauge for Wire

Suture	Type	Raw Material	Properties	Frequent Uses	26	28	30	32/34
Surgical steel	Monofilament	Low carbon iron alloy	Nonabsorbable, remains encapsulated	General and skin closure, retention sutures, tendon repair, orthopedic, neurosurgery	15.7	10.7	6.2	4.1/3.2
	Multifilament	Low carbon iron alloy			20.8	13.1	7.9	5.2/3.7

more slowly than the polyglycolic acid polymer (Aston and Rees, 1977).

Tables 21–1 and 21–2 provide a comparison of sutures, both absorbable and nonabsorbable.

Nonabsorbable sutures are classified by the U.S.P. into three groups. Class 1 sutures are composed of silk or synthetic fibers. They may be of monofilament, twisted, or braided configuration. Class 2 sutures are composed of cotton, linen, and coated natural or synthetic fibers. Class 3 sutures are composed of monofilament or multifilament steel alloy wire (Postlethwaite, 1970).

The most widely used suture material is surgical silk, which is considered a nonabsorbable suture. However, silk will absorb slowly over a long period of time. Surgical cotton is used by some surgeons in place of silk. It tends to be the weakest of the nonabsorbable sutures. If it is moistened prior to use it gains some increase in tensile strength. Even though it is used in place of silk, it offers no advantages. Linen suture, made from twisted flax fibers, is occasionally used by some surgeons in gastrointestinal procedures. Its tensile strength is markedly inferior to that of the other nonabsorbable suture materials.

Stainless steel suture material has very high tensile strength and very low reactivity in tissue. Unfortunately, the material is sometimes difficult to handle; it kinks easily. Wire sutures placed improperly or tied too tightly can cut and tear tissues. Nevertheless, when used in careful fashion, wire is an acceptable material for general closure, retention sutures, and tendon repairs. Some surgeons use fine wire for esophageal or gastrointestinal anastomoses.

One of the best-known of the synthetic nonabsorbable suture materials is nylon. Nylon has a very high tensile strength. It tends to degrade quite slowly and slowly lose its tensile strength. A main disadvantage of nylon is its elasticity, for it requires at least 3 knots or a double square knot to prevent slippage of the knot. Nylon suture material also can be made into a multifilament suture that handles like silk. Polyester fiber sutures are also synthetic polymers and can be made into a multifilament suture strand. Many of the polyester sutures, either coated or uncoated, are used in cardiothoracic surgery. Polypropylene is synthetic suture material that is extruded as a monofilament suture. It may be used in general, cardiovascular, and plastic surgery. Like surgical gut and stainless steel, it can be used in the presence of infection because it has the properties of a noncapillary monofilament strand. The synthetic materials have the property of "memory," leading to knots slipping and untying. Extra care must be taken to properly "lay down" each portion of a knot and add extra "throws" to it.

MONOFILAMENT AND MULTIFILAMENT SUTURES

Suture materials can be grouped according to whether they are monofilament or multifilament. All surgical gut tends to act like a monofilament suture despite large sizes made from several ribbons of sheep intestinal mucosa and beef intestinal serosa (Lawrie and Angus, 1960). Multifilament sutures are generally easier to handle and tie more easily than monofilament sutures. Surgical steel is a monofilament requiring careful placement of the suture. The knot must be tied in a very meticulous fashion to prevent kinking of the suture. If tied too tightly, it will cause cutting of tissues.

INFECTION

The selection of the type of monofilament suture depends upon many factors. One controversial subject is the question of what suture material should be used in surgical wounds that are or could be infected. The incidence of infection in staphylococcal-contaminated tissue has been studied under controlled conditions in the laboratory rat. Polypropylene, nylon, and the absorbable suture material polyglycolic acid were observed to have the lowest incidence of infection. In vitro studies have demonstrated that degradation products of nylon and polyglycolic acid appear to have antibacterial properties. The biological inertness of polypropylene probably accounts for its success. Naturally occurring fibers such as silk and cotton elicited the most pronounced infection. Stainless steel, which one would think inert, potentiated wound infection but less so than did cotton or silk. Wire sutures are stiff and with time undergo degradation and break. The lack of pliability of steel suture means that upon movement there may be mechanical irritation, with tissue damage that could impair local tissue resistance to infection.

Monofilament or absorbable sutures should be used in wounds that have potential for infection. Regardless of what material is used, there will always be an increased incidence of infection in a contaminated wound. Ideally, the contaminated wound should contain no suture. In order to reduce this wound complication, the use of an inert monofilament suture is the most practical solution. However, one should use meticulous technic, taking care to be as atraumatic as possible, close or drain dead space, and remove all obvious nonviable tissue before closing the incision (Van Winkle and Hastings, 1972).

PRINCIPLES OF SUTURE SELECTION

The basic principles of suture selection are well summarized in a monograph published by Ethicon, Incorporated (Suture Use Manual, 1976).

1. When a wound has reached maximal strength, sutures are no longer needed. Therefore:
    a. Tissues that ordinarily heal slowly such as skin, fascia, and tendons should usually be closed with nonabsorbable sutures.
    b. Tissues that heal rapidly such as stomach, colon, and bladder may be closed with absorbable sutures.
2. Foreign bodies in potentially contaminated tissues may convert contamination to infection. Therefore:
    a. Avoid multifilament sutures, which may convert a contaminated wound into an infected one.
    b. Use monofilament or absorbable sutures in tissue with potential for contamination.
3. Where cosmetic results are important, close and prolonged apposition of wounds and avoidance of irritants will produce the best result. Therefore:
    a. Use the smallest inert monofilament suture materials, such as nylon or polypropylene.
    b. Avoid skin sutures and (whenever possible) close subcuticularly.
    c. Under certain circumstances, to secure close apposition of skin edges, skin closure tape may be used.
4. Foreign bodies in the presence of fluids containing high concentrations of crystalloids may act as a nidus for precipitation and stone formation. Therefore:
    a. In the urinary and biliary tracts, use rapidly absorbed sutures.
5. Regarding suture size:
    a. Use the finest size commensurate with the natural strength of the tissue.
    b. If the postoperative course of the patient may produce sudden strains on the suture line, reinforce it with retention sutures. Remove them as soon as the patient's condition is stable.

ANATOMIC CONSIDERATIONS

Peritoneum

The peritoneal layer should be exactly approximated when possible to minimize the occurrence of postoperative adhesions to the line of the incision.

When the peritoneal layer is separated from the overlying muscles and fascia, then the peritoneum, transversalis fascia, and (when present) the posterior sheath of the rectus muscle should be closed as one layer. In so doing the peritoneal surfaces should be everted so that their serosal surfaces are in contact. A continuous 2-0 or 0 plain or chromic catgut or synthetic absorbable suture is passed back and forth through the cut edges or placed as a lock-stitch. Some surgeons prefer interrupted sutures, but the placing of these is time-consuming, and does not provide as smooth an approximation of the serosal surfaces as does a continuous suture.

In some incisions, previous operations have made it impossible to isolate the peritoneal layer. In such cases, since separate suturing of the layer is impossible, the wound is closed by sutures placed through the fascia, muscle, and peritoneum. These should be of nonabsorbable material, and can be simple, through-and-through sutures, or far-near pulley sutures. Great care must be taken while they are being placed and tied to prevent bowel from being caught in or injured by them. The same is true of through-and-through sutures, usually wire, placed through all the layers of the abdominal wall, including the skin, when repairing a dehiscence.

Muscle Layers

The suturing of muscle layers depends upon the location of the incision and

ANATOMIC CONSIDERATIONS

whether the muscle fibers are cut across or divided in the direction of their course.

Muscle tissue does not hold sutures well. Muscles that have been separated in the direction of their fibers can be approximated by interrupted sutures. When the fibers have been cut across they cannot be approximated by suture unless the muscle contains or is invested by sufficient fibrous tissue to hold the suture. Muscle suturing is performed primarily to obliterate dead space. It provides little strength.

In contaminated wounds, muscle sutures should be of catgut or synthetic absorbable suture. In clean wounds, catgut, silk, or synthetic absorbable suture may be used.

Aponeuroses

The aponeurotic layer provides the strength to the successful wound closure. It should be approximated with great care under little or no tension and without ischemia. Nonabsorbable sutures may be employed for closure. If the wound has been contaminated, one should use interrupted sutures of No. 30 stainless steel wire or 0 polypropylene. For clean wounds, interrupted sutures of No. 30 stainless steel wire, No. 1 silk, 0 polypropylene, cotton, catgut, or synthetic absorbable suture are used.

There are a number of different ways of placing these sutures. A simple end-over suture in the average wound with good tissues easily approximates edges. If these conditions are absent, then a far-near pulley type of suture approximates the edge more strongly because any tension is distributed to the four points of tissue penetrated rather than to only two. The aponeurotic layer should not be apposed with a continuous suture.

Subcutaneous Tissues

This layer is mostly fatty, with weak fascial strata, and its repaired area has no strength. It is sutured with 4-0 silk (clean wounds) or catgut or synthetic absorbable suture that bites Scarpa's fascia on each

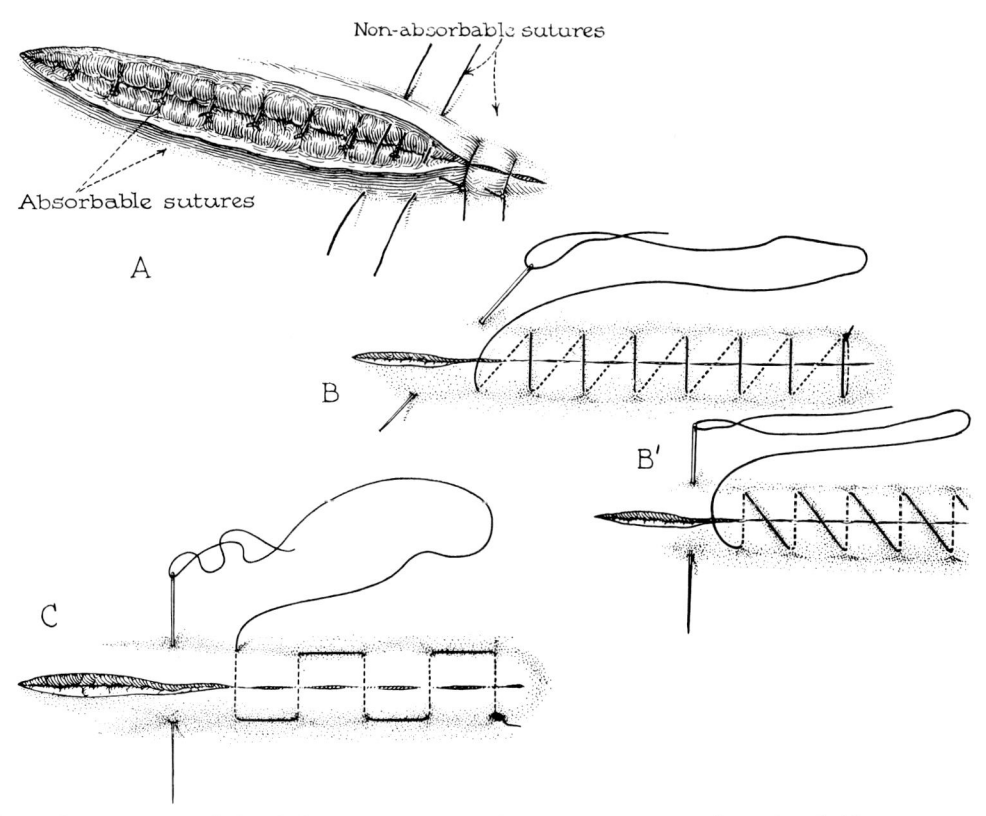

Figure 21–1. *A*, Buried absorbable sutures in the subcutaneous tissues and nonabsorbable sutures to approximate the skin margins. *B* and *B'*, Continuous sutures applied obliquely and transversely. *C*, Mattress (quilt) or right-angle suturing of the skin.

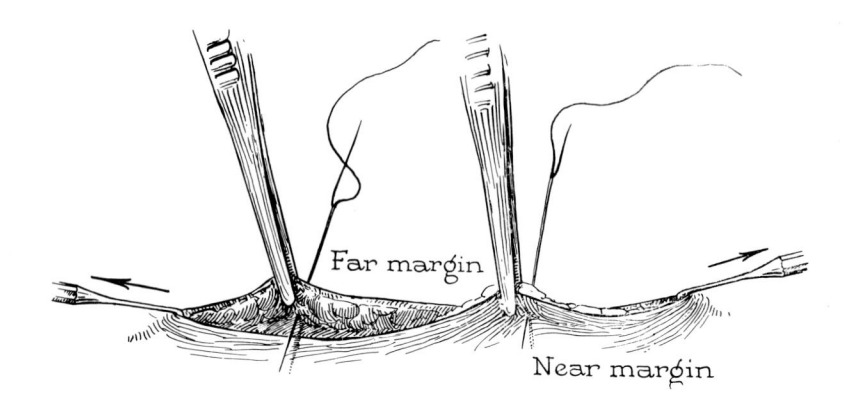

Figure 21-2. Everting the skin edge sharply so that the suture penetrates at the same distance from the edge on both deep and superficial surfaces.

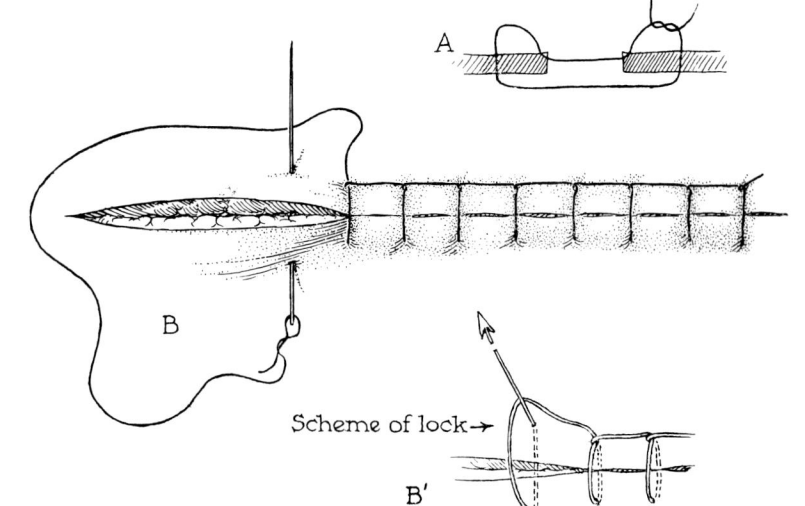

Figure 21-3. *A*, End-on interrupted mattress suture. *B* and *B'*, Continuous lock-suture.

ANATOMIC CONSIDERATIONS

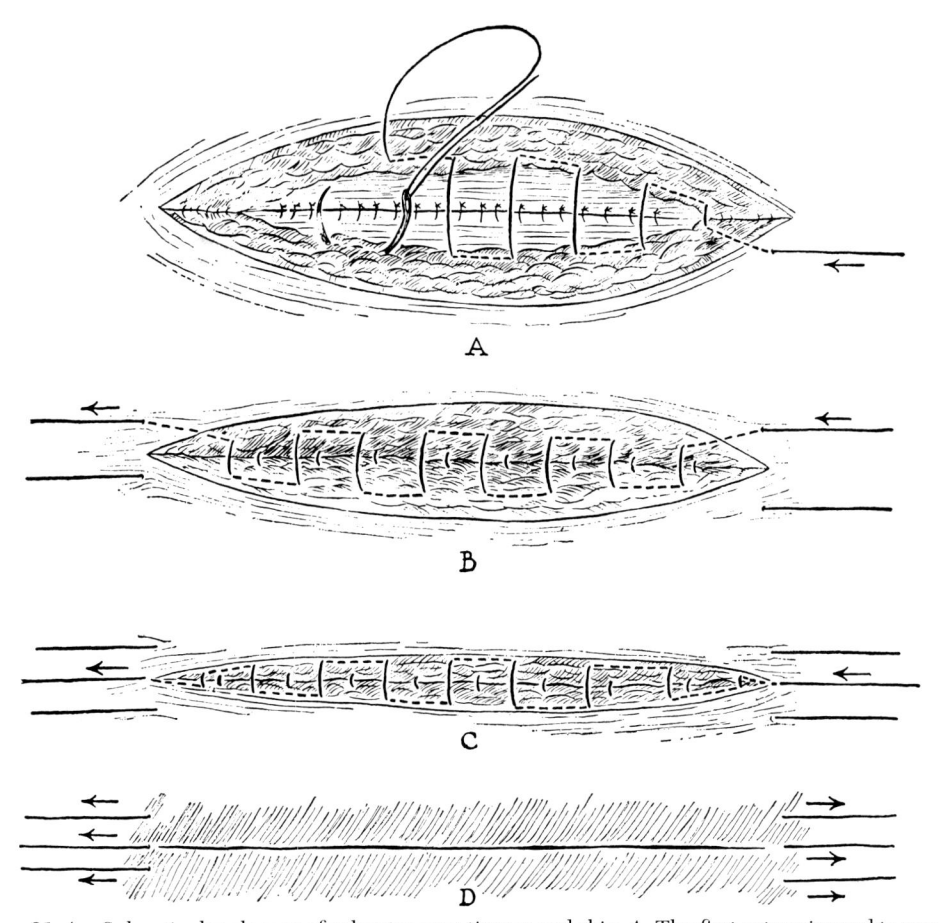

Figure 21–4. Subcuticular closure of subcutaneous tissues and skin. *A*, The first suture is used to approximate the deep fat and includes Scarpa's fascia. *B*, Second suture closes intermediate fat layer. *C*, Third suture runs immediately beneath the skin and approximates it. *D*, Closure completed. As indicated by arrows, the sutures are run back and forth to assure that they are free and can be easily removed. Either stainless steel wire, nylon, or polypropylene may be used for this closure. (From Coller, F. A., and MacLean, K. F.: *In* Cole, W. H. [ed.]: Operative Technic in General Surgery. New York, Appleton-Century-Crofts, 1949.)

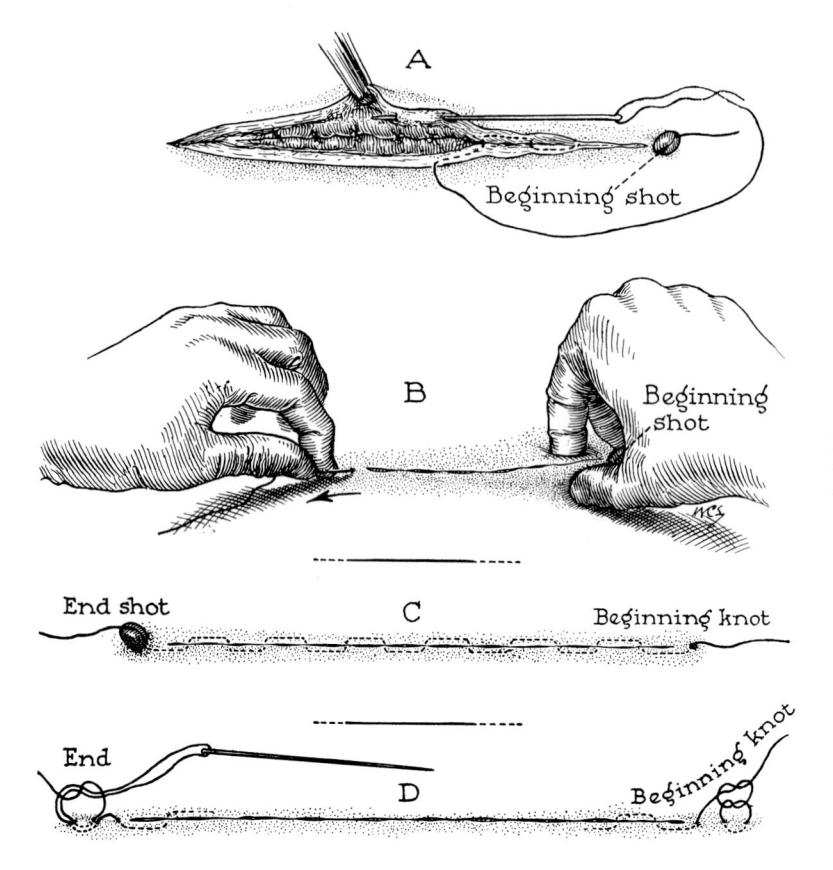

Figure 21-5. Method of placing a subcuticular suture and a variety of methods of fixing its ends.

side, obliterating dead space and taking some of the tension off the skin suture line.

Skin

The skin edges are always approximated with a nonabsorbable suture material, usually nylon (Fig. 21-1). The methods of suturing the skin are legion. One good method is a simple over-and-over suture (continuous in clean wounds and interrupted in contaminated wounds). In placing these stitches the skin edge is sharply everted at the time each penetrates its deeper surface so that the suture will be the same distance lateral to the edge on both the deep and superficial surface of the skin (Fig. 21-2).

Some prefer interrupted or continuous end-on mattress sutures (Fig. 21-3A), which are thought to provide a better cosmetic result but take longer to place. Others prefer a continuous over-and-over lock-stitch (Fig. 21-3B). Still others employ a subcutaneous suture of stainless steel wire (Fig. 21-4) or of silk (Fig. 21-5).

Many surgeons now use stainless steel clips to close the skin. Clips save a great deal of time in skin closure. The scar is not adversely affected by the use of clips. Removal is not difficult nor uncomfortable if the proper instrument is used to remove them.

Skin sutures are usually removed on the sixth to eighth postoperative day.

TYPES OF WOUND CLOSURES

Single Row of Interrupted Sutures

Successful closure of a wound can be obtained by buried monofilament stainless steel retention sutures. The incidence of wound disruption using this technique has been reported to be as low as 0.4 per cent. After carefully obtaining hemostasis, the abdomen is closed using No. 28 stainless steel monofilament wire.

The single suture is passed through the fascial-muscular layers and peritoneum (Fig. 21-6). The margins of the incision are carefully apposed. Care is taken not to tie

TYPES OF WOUND CLOSURES

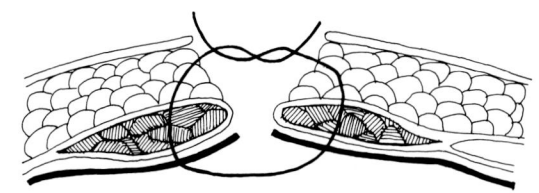

Figure 21–6. Method of closure of the abdominal wall with stainless steel wire. (From Halevy, A., Oland, Y., and Adam, Y. G.: Stainless steel wire for closure of abdominal operative wounds. Am. Surg. 44:342, 1978.)

too tightly. Too much tension can lead to strangulation of muscle and fascia. Wire "tails" are carefully buried (Fig. 21–7). One could substitute 0 polypropylene for wire and expect similar results. Subcutaneous tissue is approximated as previously described.

Single Row of Sutures Through All Layers

If the patient's condition has deteriorated so that a rapid closure of the wound is desirable, when the wound is contaminated, when chest complications associated with heavy coughing are present, or when a disrupted wound is being closed, a satisfactory method of closure is with a simple row of through-and-through wire sutures which pass through all the layers of the abdominal wound (Fig. 21–8). Very heavy wire, as thick as No. 23 stainless steel monofilament, is used. Heavy nylon, No. 2 or heavier, could be substituted.

Through-and-through wire sutures are most safely placed by arming each end of the suture with a large, curved, cutting-edge needle. The needle on one end is then passed from within the peritoneal cavity outward through the peritoneum and all the layers of the abdominal wall, emerging through the skin at a point about 4 to 5 cm. lateral to the incision on one side. The needle on the other end of the suture is likewise passed through the abdominal wall at the same distance on the other side of the incision. Both needles are removed from the suture, but the suture is not twisted until all the others have been placed. During the placing of these sutures the intestine is protected by being covered with a gauze or rubber pad. The sutures are placed about 2 cm. apart.

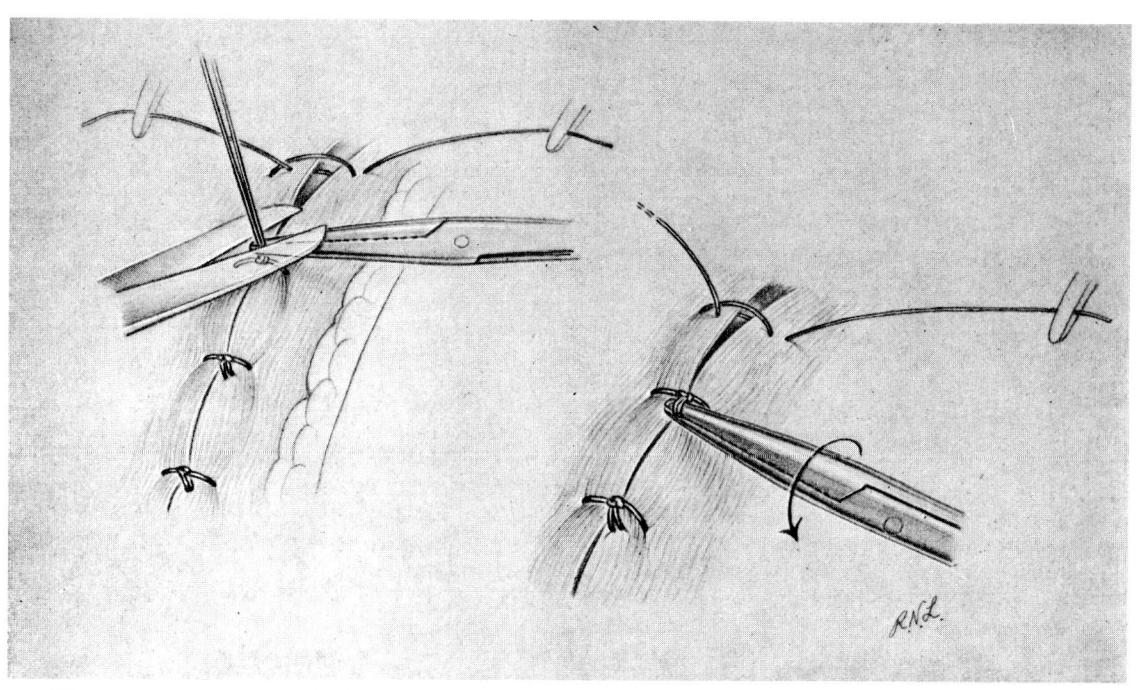

Figure 21–7. Method of dealing with "tails" of wire at knots. *A*, After the knot has been tied, the tails are held taut vertically and clipped with the point of a pair of artery forceps as close as possible to the knot. The wire is then cut flush with the forceps. *B*, Before the forceps is removed, it is rotated 180° to turn the short tails into the tissues and away from the skin. (From Goligher, J. C., Irvin, T. T., Johnston, D., et al.: A controlled clinical trial of three methods of closure of laparotomy wounds. Br. J. Surg. 62:823, 1975.)

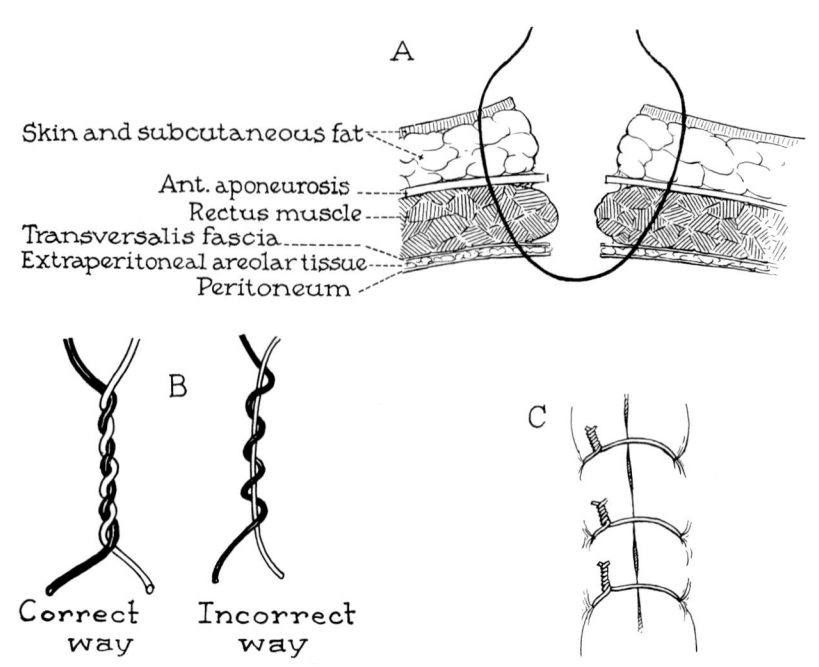

Figure 21–8. *A*, Through-and-through wire suture. *B*, Correct and incorrect way of twisting wire ends. *C*, Wire sutures placed and secured.

After all the sutures have been placed the lowermost one is drawn taut by an assistant while the operator places a finger beneath that portion of the wound to make certain that intestine or omentum is not caught in the loop and at the same time to evert the abdominal wall so that the peritoneal surfaces are in contact. The assistant tenses and twists the ends of the wire around each other (Fig. 21–8) (this is better than attempting knots with wire of this heavy caliber) for six to eight turns. The ends of the wire are cut off with a wire cutter just distal to the last twist.

Each succeeding suture is drawn taut and secured in the same manner, the pad protecting the intestine being removed just prior to securing the uppermost two sutures. A thick layer of gauze is placed alongside the suture line, and the cut ends are bent over into it to prevent them from sticking into the wound.

If speed is essential, the sutures can be placed by having only one end armed with a needle and passing the needle from the outside through the skin and all the layers of the abdominal wall into the peritoneal cavity. Here it crosses the wound to the other side and passes out through all the layers of the abdominal wall. In using this method the abdominal wall must be held outward so the needle can be passed under direct vision, to be certain that the intestine is not inadvertently injured.

With either method, another great danger is that intestine or omentum will bulge into the wire loop as the loop is tensed and secured. It is emphasized that the surgeon must keep a finger beneath each suture as it is drawn taut and twisted.

The method of wound closure with wire sutures passed through all layers is rapid and gives a strong closure. There is some danger that the sutures will be drawn so tightly as to strangulate the blood supply of the involved portion of the abdominal wall and produce a slough. A large slough rarely occurs, but it is advisable to inspect the wound daily. If the sutures appear too tight they can be loosened by untwisting them for a turn. One or two sutures may cut entirely through the skin and require removal, but all the sutures should not be removed until after the fourteenth to eighteenth postoperative day.

Incisional hernias are said to be uncommon after this type of wound closure.

Continuous Suture

Fascial closure by the technique of continuous suture is a timesaver. The theoretical advantage of this closure is the equal distribution of tension over the entire

TYPES OF WOUND CLOSURES

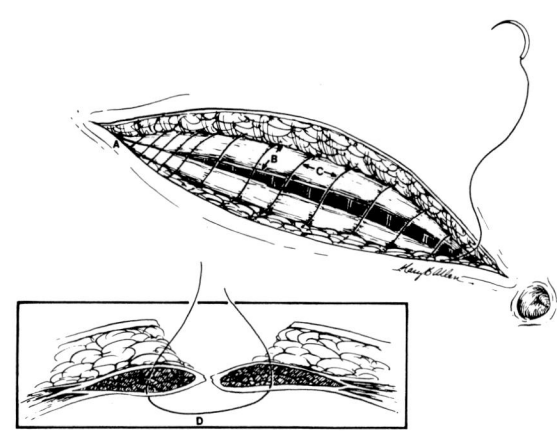

Figure 21-9. Continuous suture. *A,* initial knot tied intraperitoneally. *B* and *D,* Large tissue inclusion 2.5 to 4.0 cm. from incision. *C,* Suture advancing 1 to 1.5 cm. (From Martyak, S. N., and Curtis, L. E.: Abdominal incision and closure. Am. J. Surg. *131*:476, 1976.)

length of the closed fascial layer. In some reports, the risk of dehiscence is less than with interrupted closure. The amount of suture material in the wound is much less than with interrupted closure. Less time is spent in closing the incision. A disadvantage is that if the suture breaks, the entire wound can separate. A monofilament No. 2 nylon (or 0 polypropylene) may be used (Fig. 21–9). The initial suture is placed, tying the knot intraperitoneally. The continuous suture is then "run," placing the needle so the suture enters tissue at least 2.5 cm. from the margin of the incision and keeping the stitches about 1.0 to 1.5 cm. apart. Subcutaneous tissues are closed or left open, depending on the thickness of the tissue layer.

Tom Jones Far-and-Near Sutures

The fascial-muscular layers and parietal peritoneum are approximated by a single

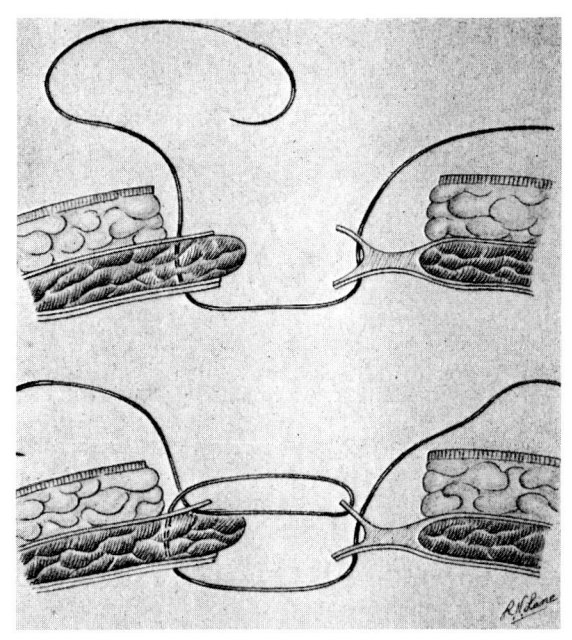

Figure 21-10. The two components of the Tom Jones far-and-near mass suture of the musculoaponeurotic layers and parietal peritoneum. (From Goligher, J. C., Irwin, T. T., Johnston, D., et al.: A controlled clinical trial of three methods of closure of laparotomy wounds. Br. J. Surg. *62*:823, 1975.)

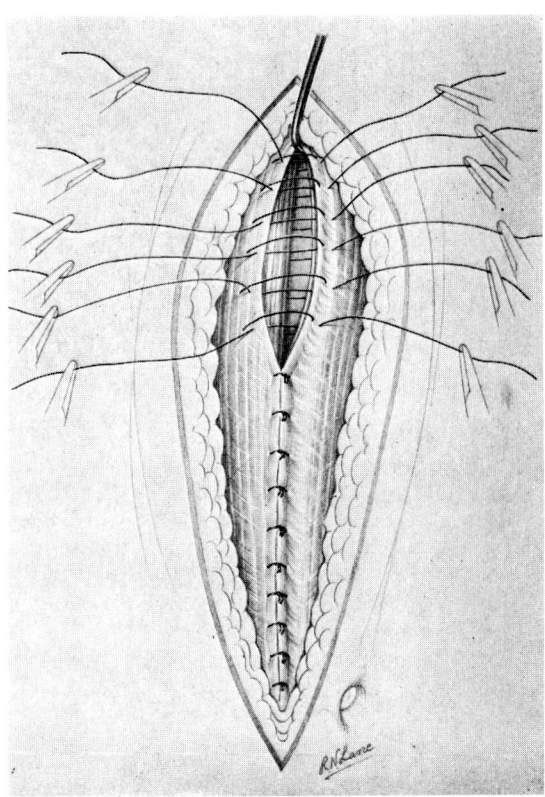

Figure 21-11. The wire suture technic in practice. First, five or six sutures were placed in the upper part of the wound and left untied, while the lower two-thirds of the wound was brought together with sutures that were tied as they were inserted. The protecting "flat fish" of rubber, which had been put on the surface of the loops of intestine before the closure was begun, was then removed, and the upper end of the wound was elevated by upward traction on a Langenbeck retractor while the loose-lying remaining sutures were tied. (From Goligher, et al., cited in previous figure.)

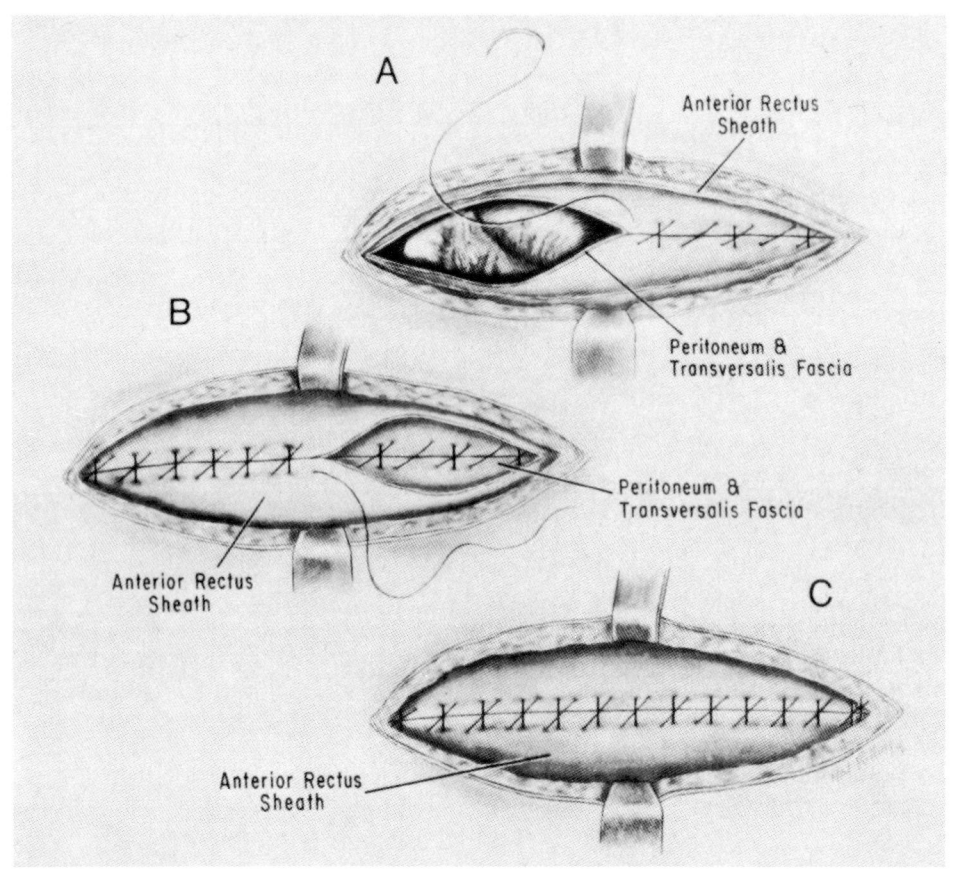

Figure 21–12. *A*, *B*, and *C*, Abdominal wall closure with polyglycolic acid basting suture reinforced with fascial staples. (From Elliott, T. E., Albertazzi, V. J., and Danto, L. A.: A new technique for abdominal wall closure. Surg. Gynecol. Obstet. *145*:425, 1977.)

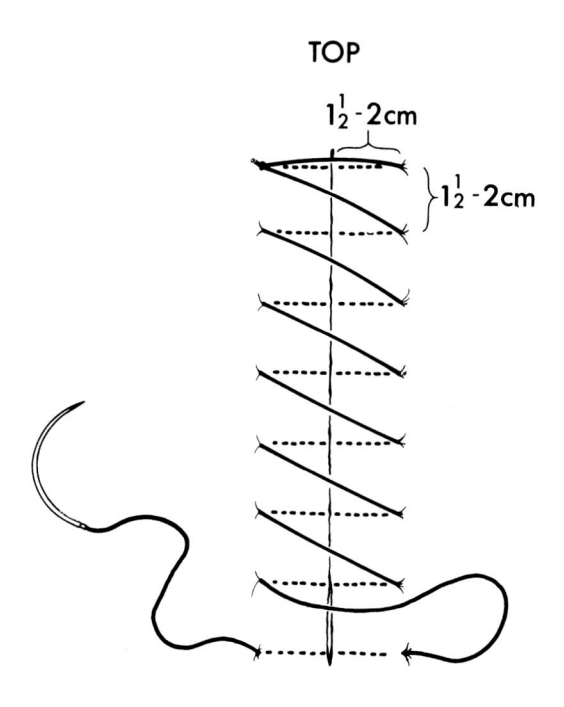

Figure 21–13. Continuous synthetic absorbable suture is placed 1.5 to 2 cm. back from cut edge of wound and 1.5 to 2 cm. apart. (From Murray, D. H., and Blaisdell, F. W.: Use of synthetic absorbable sutures for abdominal and chest wound closure. Arch. Surg. *113*:477, 1978.)

row of No. 28 stainless steel monofilament wire sutures. One could substitute 0 polypropylene for wire. A large atraumatic needle is passed through one side of the incision, passing through the anterior rectus sheath, the rectus muscle, the posterior rectus sheath, and the parietal peritoneum, about 2.5 to 3 cm. from the edge of the incision, entering the peritoneal cavity. The needle and suture are then passed through the same layers on the opposite side of the wound. The distance from the edge is identical. However, the needle passes from the parietal peritoneum through the anterior rectus sheath. The needle is then reinserted and a suture is passed in the same plane and direction, but it is passed through close to the incised edge of the anterior rectus sheath. If one is closing a midline incision, the suture passes through the cut edge along the linea alba (Figs. 21–10 and 21–11). The subcutaneous tissue and skin are closed as previously described. With the use of stainless steel monofilament wire suture, Goligher reported a dehiscence/incisional hernia incidence of 0.9 per cent. The far-and-near stitch appears to be superior in mechanical strength.

Absorbable Sutures

Synthetic absorbable sutures have been used successfully to close abdominal incisions. A continuous or basting 0 or 00 polyglycolic acid or polyglactin 910 suture is used to close the peritoneum and the transversalis fascia. Many surgeons do not close these layers in an upper midline incision. However, other abdominal incisions can be better closed by approximating either one or both of these layers (Fig. 21–12). The anterior rectus sheath, major fascial layers, or the linea alba is closed using 0 or 1 polyglycolic acid or polyglactin 910 continuous running sutures. The suture should be followed so as to have uniform tension. Suture line tension should be adequate to firmly approximate the fascial edges. The sutures should be placed 1.5 to 2 cm. from the edge of the incision and about 1.5 to 2 cm. apart in order to have ample "bite." The large bite will make far less tension along the suture line (Fig. 21–13). A variation is to close the major fascial layer with the continuous basting suture and then reinforce the suture line with stainless steel staples (Fig. 21–12). The incidence of wound dehiscence/evisceration and infection is very low for either technic.

Some surgeons still prefer to use absorbable No. 1 chromic catgut to approximate the linea alba. If chromic catgut is used, retention stay sutures also should be used.

Retention Sutures

A retention suture is a reinforcing suture for abdominal wounds, utilizing exceptionally strong material like braided silk, stainless steel, or silkworm gut, and including a large amount of tissue in each stitch. It is intended to relieve pressure on the primary suture line and prevent postoperative disruption (Fig. 21–14).

Nonabsorbable suture materials are used for retention sutures. Probably the most popular material is No. 2 nylon. However, 0 or 1 polypropylene and No. 23 to No. 28 stainless steel wire are commonly used for retention sutures.

Many technics are employed to place retention sutures. The simplest is to place the suture lateral to the wound so as to pass through the skin, subcutaneous tissues, anterior sheath, and rectus muscle on one side and then pass the suture deep to the rectus muscle (but superficial to the peritoneal layer) to cross the incision and penetrate outward through the rectus muscle, anterior sheath, subcutaneous tissue, and skin at a corresponding distance lateral to the other side of the wound (Fig. 21–15). These stay sutures are placed before the anterior sheath is sutured. They are not tied until the skin suturing has been completed. They are then tied so loosely that a finger can be easily placed beneath them.

A disadvantage of this method is that one may inadvertently go too deep and damage the small bowel. To prevent this, the extraperitoneal suture is placed under direct vision before closing the peritoneum (Fig. 21–16A). Then the surgeon pulls up on the retention suture and closes the peritoneum (Fig. 21–16B).

A persistent problem is that the retention sutures may be tied too tightly and the tissue becomes edematous, compromising the blood supply and resulting in tissue death and slough. Rubber bridges are used to prevent tying the suture too tightly. As

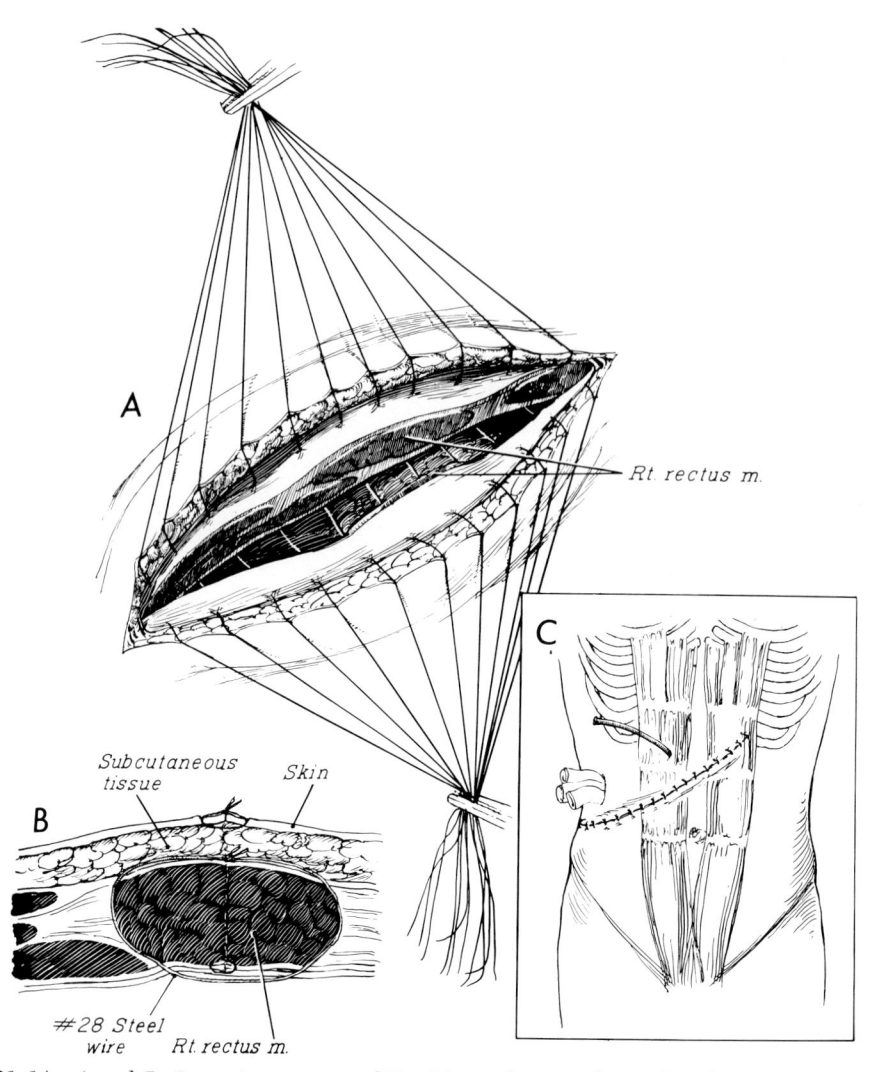

Figure 21–14. *A* and *B*, Retention sutures of No. 28 stainless steel are placed to include all layers of the abdominal wall except the skin and subcutaneous tissue. Sutures are kept taut while the peritoneum and posterior sheath are closed. *C*, The sutures are then tied to be snug but not so tight as to cause tissue edema and vascular impairment. (From Cooper, P. (ed.): The Craft of Surgery, 2nd ed. Boston, Little, Brown, and Company, 1971, p. 1283.)

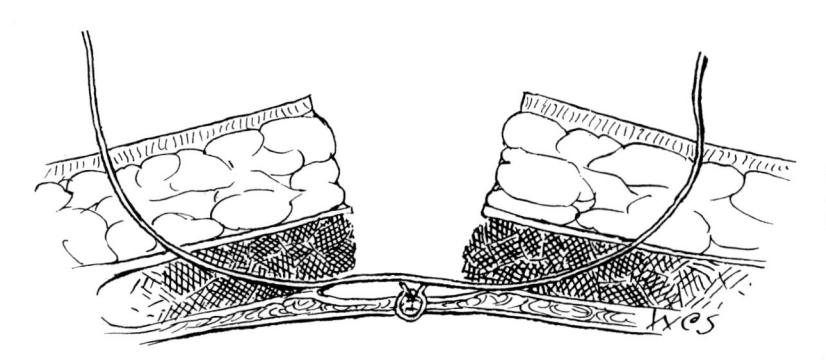

Figure 21–15. Stay suture, including rectus muscle, anterior sheath, subcutaneous tissue, and skin.

TYPES OF WOUND CLOSURES

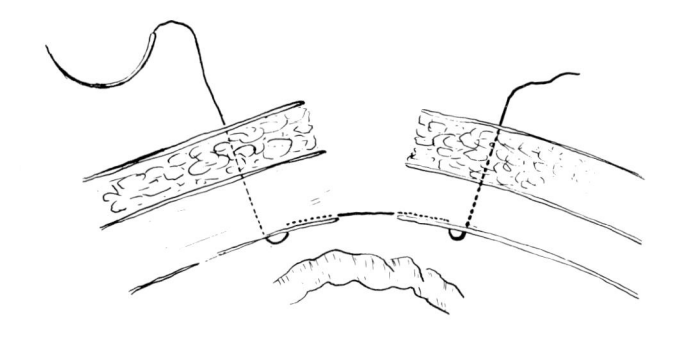

Figure 21-16. *A*, Extraperitoneal retention suture. *B*, Closure of the peritoneum when the retention sutures are pulled up. (From Vysal, T.: Extraperitoneal retention sutures. Am. J. Surg. *131*:389, 1976.)

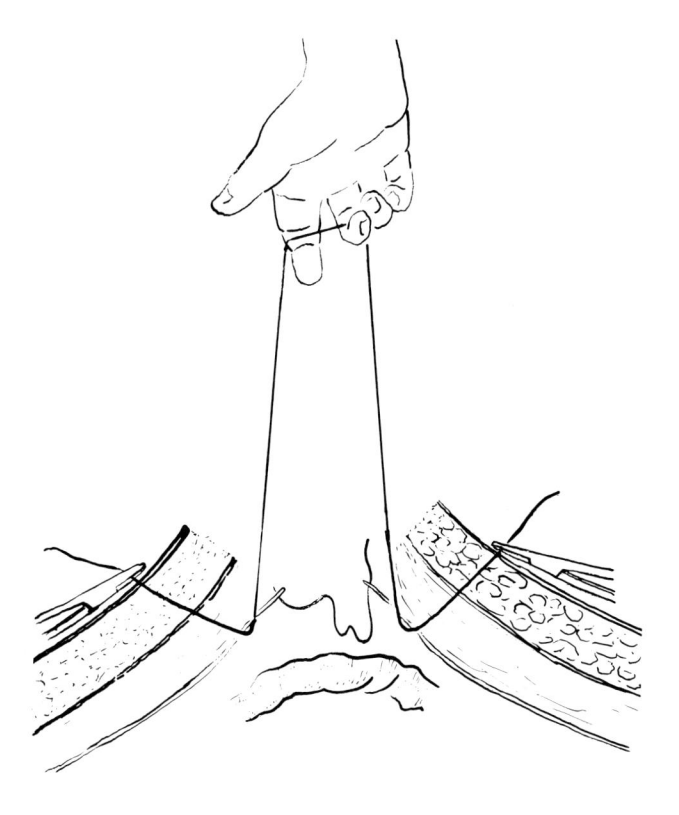

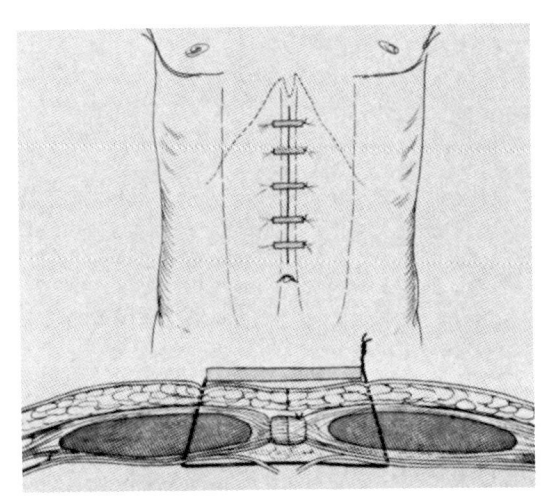

Figure 21-17. The use of wire retention sutures traversing all layers of the abdominal wall and entering the skin somewhat closer to the incision than they exit through the deep fascia. The linea alba has been approximated. (From Hubbard, T. B., and Rever, W. B.: Retention sutures in the closure of abdominal incisions. Am. J. Surg. *124*:378, 1972.)

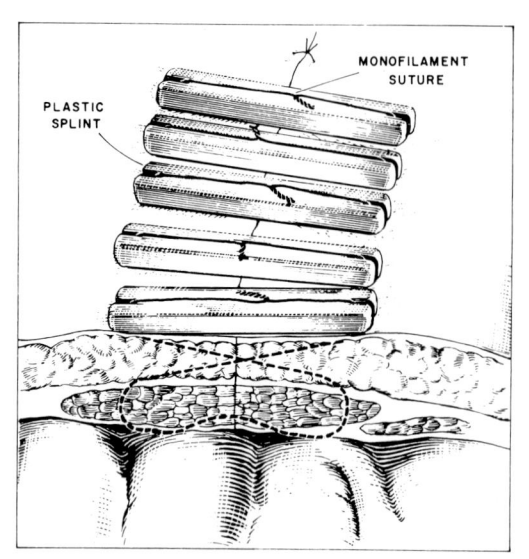

Figure 21–18. Figure-of-8 through-and-through monofilament abdominal wall closure with wound splints. (From Dennis, C., and Aka, E.: The figure-of-8 through-and-through monofilament abdominal wound closure with wound splints: Elimination of evisceration in poor-risk wounds over 25 years. Surgery 73:171, 1973.)

shown in Figure 21–17, the wire or nylon traverses all layers of the abdominal wall. The suture at the surface should be closer to the incision than to where it exits into the peritoneal cavity. This helps to better distribute and minimize the tension.

Various forms of wound splints have been used with retention sutures to prevent pressure necrosis (Figs. 21–18 and 21–19). One method uses figure-of-8 monofilament sutures. The suture can be either stainless steel or one of the more inelastic monofilaments. The retention suture also can be tied down over a gauze bolster wrapped in waterproof plastic. Figure 21–20 is a good example of this technic utilizing a "double-loop mass closure." The suture material is No. 2 nylon.

A polyvinyl retention bar has been successfully used to better distribute the pressure (Fig. 21–21). The bar has a lateral flange that allows for outward retraction and also keeps the bar from rolling in toward the center, since the sutures are passed through the lateral flange.

Figure 21–22 illustrates what one can do when presented with a large, fat, flabby abdomen and a wound that has suffered dehiscence. Deep mattress sutures are tied over firm rubber tubes that parallel the incision. The tubes are about 6 to 7 cm. from the margin of the incision. The sutures are

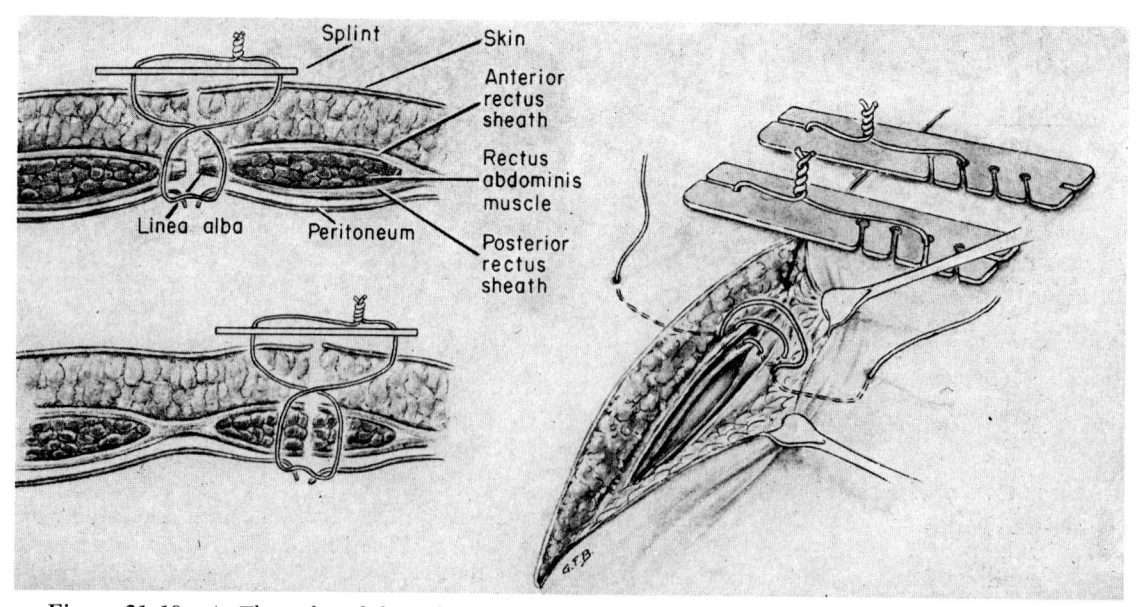

Figure 21–19. *A,* Through-and-through suture technic employing external splints for midline and rectus muscle–splitting incisions, respectively. As in *B,* the deeper limbs of the sutures should be shown taking much wider bites of tissue. *B,* An operative view of a midline abdominal incision being closed by the technic discussed. (From Broaddus, C. A., Jr.: A technique for rapid one-layer abdominal closure. Surg. Gynecol. Obstet. *124*:359, 1967.)

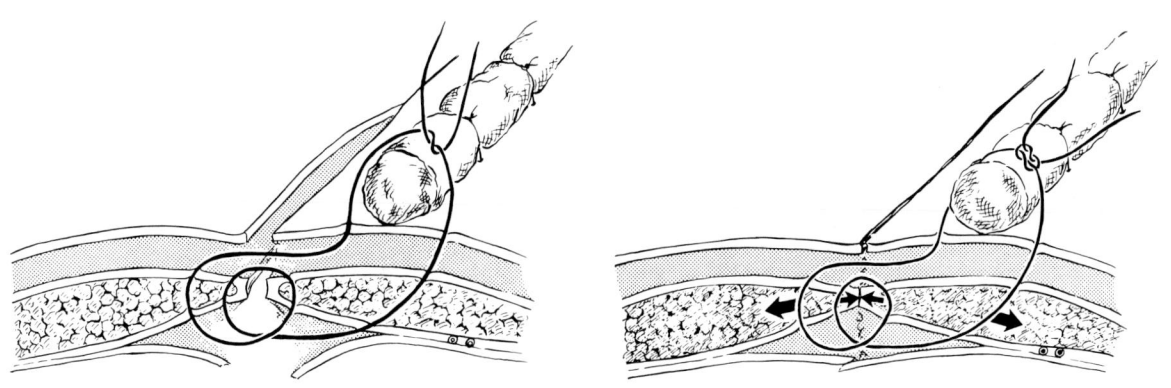

Figure 21-20. *Left*, Double-loop mass closure suture. Both loops encompass full thickness of abdominal wall, and both suture ends exit on the same side of the incision. *Right*, Double-loop mass closure. Inner loop is tightened and approximates midline when outer loop is distracted by contraction of the abdominal wall muscle. (From Burleson, R. L.: Double loop mass closure technique for abdominal incisions. Surg. Gynecol. Obstet. *147*:414, 1978.)

Figure 21-21. A retention bar, which permits even distribution of pressure on the skin and prevents "retention suture necrosis." (From Lary, B. G.: Retention bars. Am. Surg. *36*:355, 1970.)

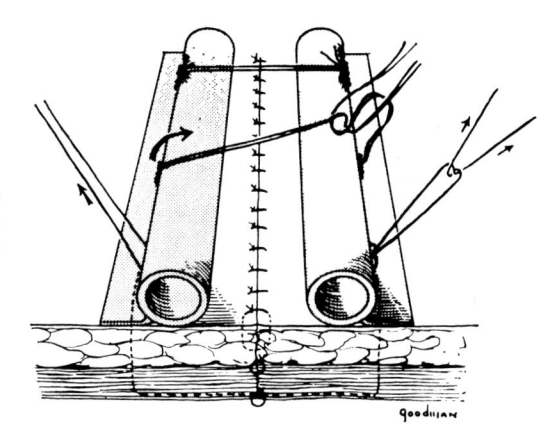

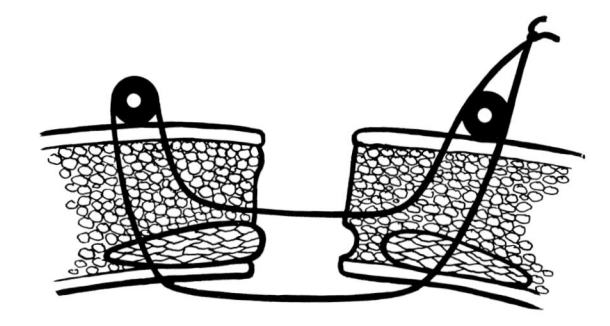

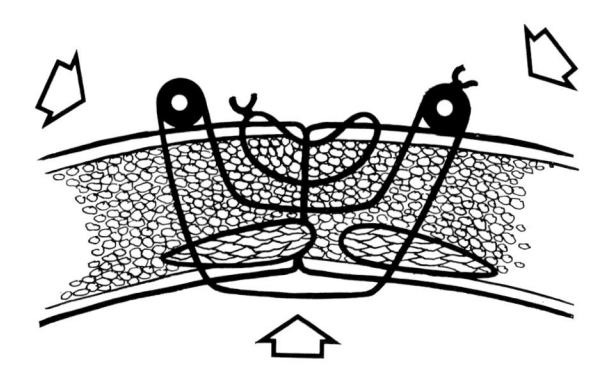

Figure 21-22. *A*, Cross section showing details of suture insertion. *B*, Cross section showing final position of sutures. (From Young, D.: Repair of burst abdominal incisions. Br. J. Surg. *61*:456, 1974.)

553

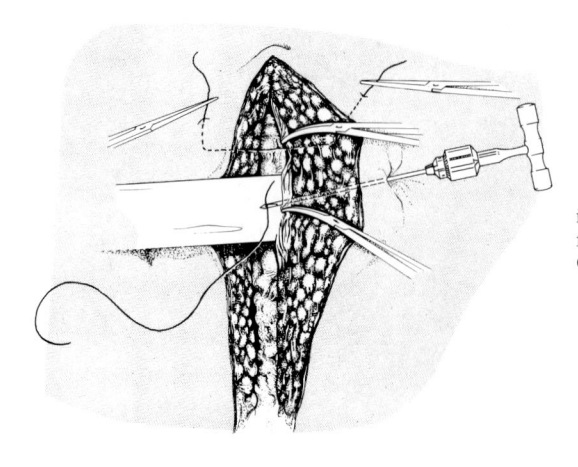

Figure 21-23. Technic for placing retention sutures in the morbidly obese. (From Charters, A. C.: Technique for placing retention sutures in the morbidly obese. Surg. Gynecol. Obstet. *137*:839, 1973.)

Figure 21-24. Retention sutures over buttons. The needle is passed around the wire suture, which brings the wire retention suture snug against the peritoneum. The wires in the suture appear to be apart in the illustration; actually, the wires are close together since they go in the same needle tract in the abdominal wall. (From Ponce, L. C., and Morgan, M. W.: A safer wire retention suture. Am. Surg. *36*:509, 1970.)

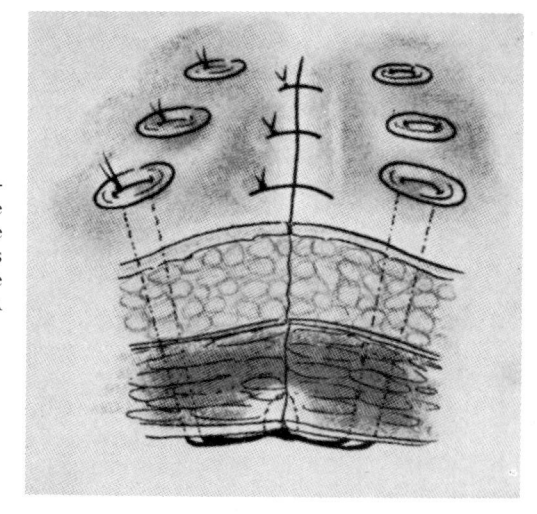

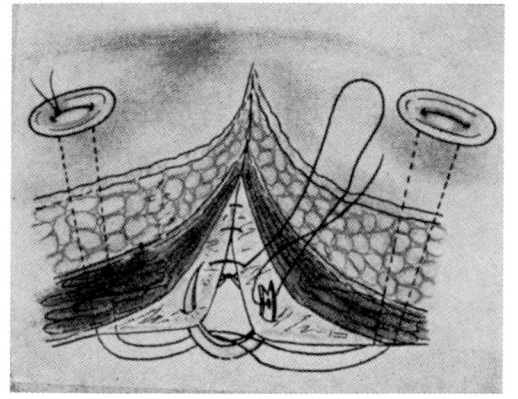

Figure 21-25. Retention sutures over buttons (*continued*). The wire suture is pulled tightly against the peritoneum, avoiding the possibility of injury to the intestine. (From Ponce and Morgan, cited in previous figure.)

TYPES OF WOUND CLOSURES

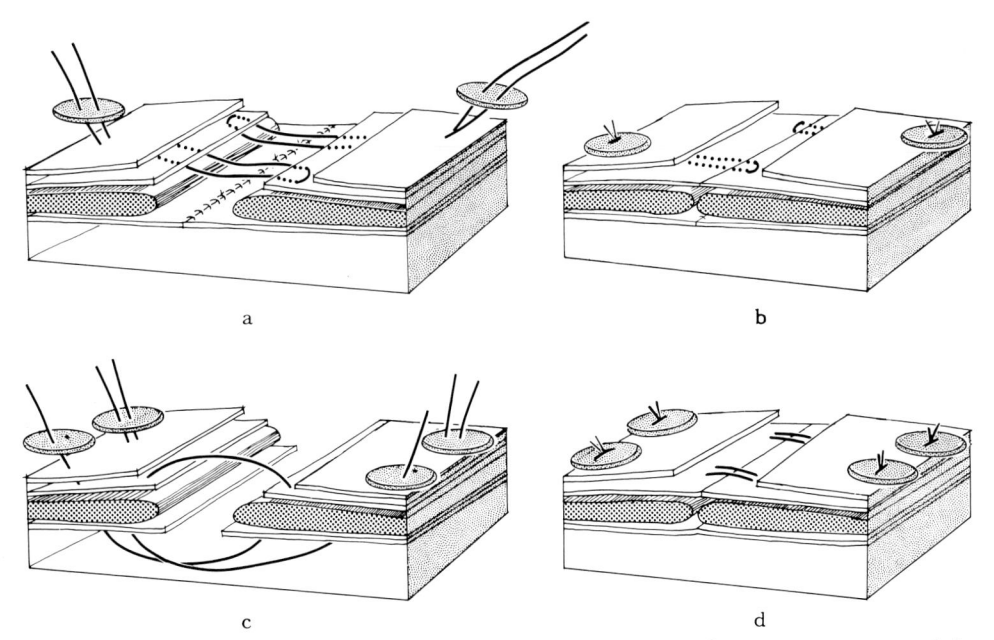

Figure 21–26. Retention suture technics using buttons. *A*, Insertion of retention sutures with buttons as prophylaxis against wound disruption. *B*, As retention sutures are tied, the fascial layers are approximated. *C*, Retention sutures using buttons for secondary closure of wound disruption. *D*, Approximation of fascial layers, using retention sutures with buttons for wound disruptions. (From Goldbach, M., and Currie, D. J.: Retention suture technique using buttons. Surg. Gynecol. Obstet. *141*:931, 1975.)

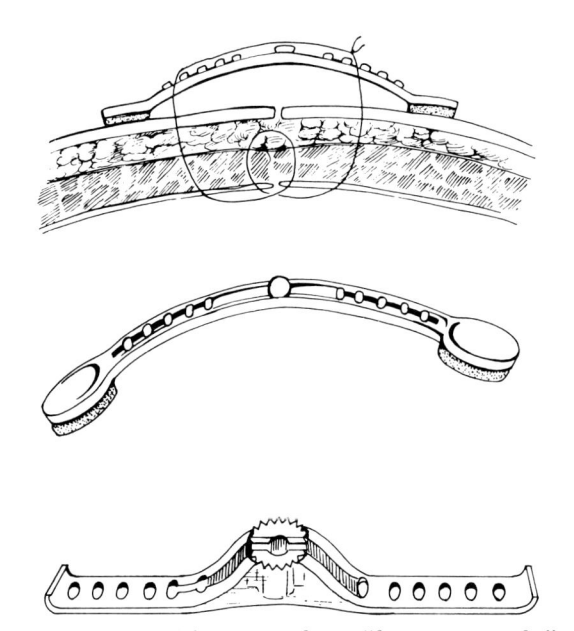

Figure 21–27. *A*, One-layer "far near, near far" closure. *B*, Retention sutures. *Top*, The wound span bridge. *Bottom*, The retention suture bridge. (From Barrer, S., Paulides, C. A., and Matsumoto, T.: Ideal laparotomy closure: Comparison of retention suture with new retention bridging devices. Am. Surg. *42*:582, 1976.)

placed about 2 cm. apart. Heavy braided nylon suture was used originally; monofilament suture also could be used.

The placing of retention sutures on an obese person can be quite difficult. A practical method is to drill a hole in the end of a Steinmann pin and secure the pin in a hand chuck. The pin is then passed through the abdominal wall, and the suture is threaded in the hole in the pin and pulled back through the tissue. A small incision is made in the skin to get the pin through the skin (Fig. 21–23).

Wire and nylon sutures have been started over buttons with good results (Figs. 21–24, 21–25, and 21–26). Other devices also have been manufactured specifically to be used as suture bridges (Fig. 21–27).

Most retention sutures are removed at 10 to 14 days postoperatively or when the patient has stabilized to the point at which these sutures are no longer needed. Retention sutures can be buried and left permanently. If the wound becomes infected, it can be opened without the risk of dehiscence.

Chapter 22

GASTROINTESTINAL SUTURING

Proper suturing is essential for gastrointestinal surgery. Getzen (1969) published an excellent history of the development of gastrointestinal suturing. Further discussion of suture material appears in Chapter 21 of this volume.

As long ago as 1812, Travers wrote that primary closure of intestinal wounds could be obtained by suture. He thought that the particular type of suture was unimportant, provided secure closure and close contact of the divided ends were achieved.

In 1826, Lembert showed that serosal apposition was essential for secure union and that mucosal eversion was likely to result in leakage. The purpose of the *seromuscular* Lembert stitch was to produce inversion and appose the peritoneal coats (see Fig. 22–3).

In 1887, Halsted pointed out that this stitch should penetrate deeply enough to take a good bite of the submucosa, which is the toughest layer of the gastrointestinal wall. He also counseled against too much inversion and emphasized the importance of preventing pouting of mucosa through the suture line to the exterior. Since then it has become almost universal practice to perform a two-layer, inverting, serosa-to-serosa anastomosis using (1) an inner Czerny stitch to roughly appose the cut edges and secure hemostasis, which is particularly important in the stomach; and (2) an outer Lembert stitch to produce inversion and serosal apposition (see Fig. 22–17).

In 1966, Getzen, Roe, and Holloway reported that experiments in dogs had shown that an inverted anastomosis had a weaker union than an everted anastomosis, and that an anastomosis formed by a single row of interrupted silk sutures placed so as to evert the anastomosis (Fig. 22–1) was better than the conventional two-layer inverting technic. It was easier and quicker to perform, they stated; it maintained a wider lumen of the anastomotic stoma; healing was more secure, as determined histologically and by studies of tensile strength at various stages after operation; and the resulting mortality was no higher than with the inverting technic. This report stimulated a number of other investigators to test the validity of these surprising claims. Results of the tests were controversial.

The principal attraction of the everting anastomosis is that the risk of narrowing the anastomotic stoma is slight with it. With an inverting anastomosis, whether or not the anastomotic stoma is greatly or slightly narrowed depends upon how much tissue is inverted by the technic in the individual case.

Canalis and Ravitch (1968) showed that dogs will survive just as well with an everting as with an inverting anastomosis. However, partial isolation of the anastomosis from the peritoneal cavity by loose wrapping with Silastic gauze almost invariably resulted in leakage, abscess, peritonitis, and death. This was true regardless of the manner in which the anastomosis had been performed — inverting or everting, open or closed — and regardless of antibiotic preparation.

In 1975, at the annual meeting of the Society for Surgery of the Alimentary Tract, Goligher, (1976), in his guest oration, reviewed the effect of various modifications in suture technic on healing of anastomoses in various parts of the alimentary tract, as shown by controlled clinical comparisons made by himself and by other investigators. He concluded that:

1. The principle of avoiding mucosal eversion appears to have been firmly established, but whether it is necessary to use the conventional two-layer inverting technic of suture seemed debatable.

2. In small bowel anastomoses and in colonic and colorectal anastomoses in which both participating stumps have a peritoneal coat, an inverting suture has been found to be more secure than an everting technic, but no significant difference has been demonstrated between the classic two-layer inverting technic and a one-layer inverting technic. However, for low anterior resections in which the distal stump has no peritoneal coat, the one-layer, end-on, slightly inverting technic (Fig. 22–2) has been shown to be followed by significantly fewer anastomotic dehiscences than the two-layer technic.

For anastomosis between the stomach and the intestine and for small bowel anastomosis, there were no convincing comparative studies to show the superiority of either method, but the weight of surgical experience thus far favors the two-layer technic, which is also preferred by Goligher and by us. It provides better gastric hemostasis. However, Belsey (1965) and Collis (1971) have each reported a large series of esophagogastric, esophagojejunal, or esophagocolonic anastomoses in which a one-layer, end-on, slightly inverting suture technic was used, with wire instead of silk. Their results were amazingly good in operative mortality and avoidance of anastomotic dehiscence.

In 1976, Matheson and Irving reported that they had routinely used a single layer of interrupted, nonabsorbable No. 00 braided nylon sutures, incorporating all layers except mucosa, in 205 elective anastomoses of stomach to duodenum, of small intestine, of colon, and of colorectum. Clinically apparent leakage did not occur except in one of the 52 patients who had undergone colorectal anastomosis.

Getzen (1969) published an excellent history of the development of intestinal anastomotic procedures and made the following observations.

Patent anastomoses can be created safe-

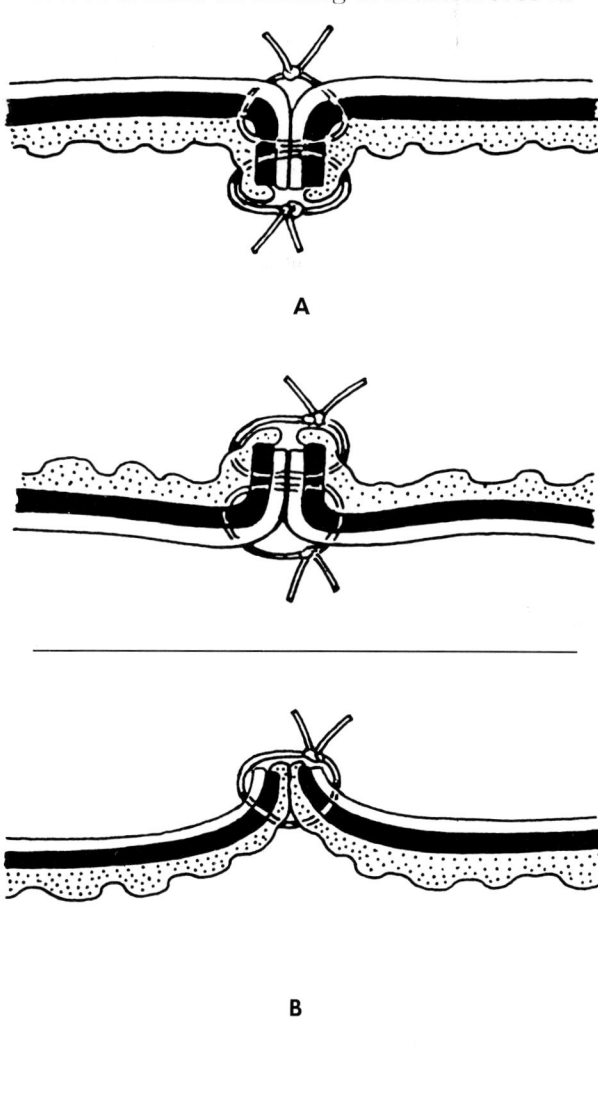

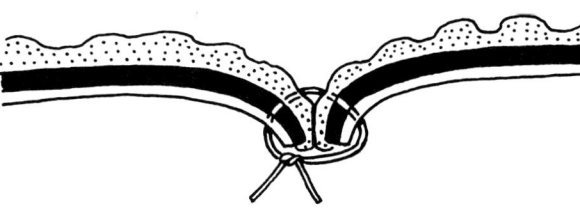

Figure 22–1. *A,* Conventional two-layer inverting technic of intestinal anastomosis. *B,* One-layer everting technic of intestinal anastomosis. (From Goligher, J. C.: Visceral and parietal suture in abdominal surgery. Am. J. Surg. *131*:130, 1976.)

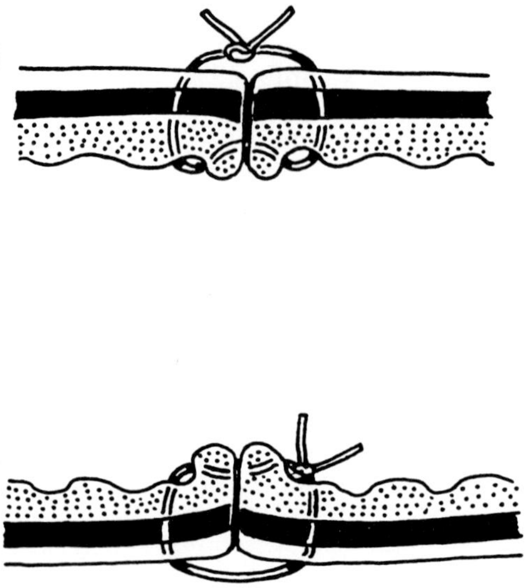

Figure 22–2. Technic of intestinal anastomosis with one-layer, end-on, slightly inverting suture. (From Goligher, cited in previous figure.)

ly by a one-layer interrupted or continuous suture, multiple rows of either interrupted or continuous sutures, or a combination thereof. The bowel will remain coapted if maintained without significant tension. For maximal strength the submucosa must be included in each suture. Whether or not the suture pierces the mucosa does not appear to alter the wound healing. Anastomotic disruptions usually are associated with leaks, due to either local avascular necrosis or a misplaced suture and tension on the anastomosis. Another cause of anastomotic disruption is the metabolic state of the patient. An anastomosis in a hypoproteinemic, chronically ill patient is more likely to disrupt than one in a patient who is in good health and nutrition. Healing of a well-constructed anastomosis of any type depends more on the preoperative nutritional state of the patient, the intra-abdominal inflammatory reaction at the time of the surgical procedure, and the vascular supply of the anastomosis than on the particular type of anastomosis performed.

End-to-end anastomoses heal satisfactorily whether the approximated bowel wall is inverted or everted, with or without a stent, and with or without telescoping. An everted anastomosis is less likely than an inverted anastomosis to be followed by anastomotic obstruction, both initially and in the subsequent months of observation, and apparently there is no adverse effect from mucosal eversion.

End-to-end anastomoses are preferable to end-to-side or side-to-side anastomoses.

Halsted demonstrated in 1887 that intestinal anastomotic wound healing required only one row of sutures, but each of these sutures must include the submucosa in order to secure good union. Sutures through the mucosa, muscularis, or serosa have no significant holding power. A second or third row of sutures provides no additional strength to the anastomosis.

A single row of sutures is less likely to impair the blood supply to the anastomosis and also is less likely to cause postoperative anastomotic obstruction than when two or three rows are used to construct the anastomosis. Although recently there has been an upsurge in the usage of a single row of sutures in alimentary tract anastomoses most surgeons still prefer a two-row anastomosis.

Before antibiotics were available, closed (aseptic) anastomotic technics were tried in an attempt to control infection, but these technics produced a greater incidence of postoperative obstruction at, and bleeding from, the anastomotic suture line than had occurred with open anastomoses. The latter are preferred now that antibiotics are available to provide some protection against infection, and closed anastomoses are rarely, if ever, used today.

Adequate suturing technics have been developed for closure of a lateral opening in the alimentary tract, for the end of a divided segment, for anastomosing the openings in two segments, and for making a permanent communication between a gastric or intestinal opening and the body surface (formation of an external fistula).

Certain conditions militate against satisfactory suture in the alimentary tract: when the intestinal contents are infected and stitches passed through the entire thickness of the bowel wall are constantly in contact with this infectious material. Gas, fluids, and solid feces propelled by peristaltic movements in the intestine place a real strain on the suture line joining two segments.

In spite of these unfavorable influences, gastrointestinal suturing usually is dependable because the walls of the stomach and bowel are pliable and resistant. Mechanically they are very good material to work with. The all-important fact is that serous surfaces, when brought into close apposition, adhere rapidly and solidly. A well-performed gastrointestinal suture is remarkably secure within a week, the serous surfaces having united firmly.

The purpose of a gastrointestinal suture is to provide a watertight closure of a viscus or its anastomosis with another viscus. The most reliable, time-tested technic for accomplishing this is by inverting the mucous membrane within the lumen of the viscus, with wide apposition of the serosal surfaces of the gut at the site of suture. If any mucous membrane everts to the outside through the suture line, leakage of gastrointestinal contents will occur with resulting peritonitis or fistula formation.

Definite objectives to be sought in every gastrointestinal suture are:

1. A watertight, leakproof closure by the careful placement of sufficient, closely spaced sutures.

2. Prevention of any portion of the mucous membrane from extruding through the suture line.

3. Broad apposition of serous surfaces to form a tight union as quickly as possible, but avoiding inversion of too much tissue.

4. Control of hemorrhage from the incised intestinal wall.

5. Approximation of the cut edges of the mucosa to prevent cicatricial narrowing.

6. Avoidance of tension on the suture line.

Many suture methods meet these demands, and any of the well-tested procedures yield good results in skilled hands.

If a gastrointestinal suture is placed so as to penetrate from the outer surface of a viscus completely through its wall into its lumen, gross leakage may occur along that suture, resulting in peritonitis, unless it is covered by a second nonpenetrating tier of sutures apposing the serosal surfaces over it.

The greatest advance over the through-and-through intestinal suture is the interrupted or continuous, seromuscular stitch which passes through the serous and muscular coats of the bowel into the submucosa but does not penetrate the mucosa. This stitch approximates apposed serous surfaces (not margins), the union of which is very strong. The seromuscular suture may be the only suture used in closure, but more often it is used to reinforce some through-and-through forms of suturing. Theoretically the seromuscular suture does not penetrate all the coats of the intestine, but frequently it does so accidently.

The strength of a gastrointestinal suture depends upon its grasp of the submucous fibromuscular layer. Its watertight closure depends to a considerable degree upon the approximation of the serous layers at the site of the suture line. Apposed serosal surfaces of the gastrointestinal tract adhere rapidly and quickly seal over the line of suture.

MATERIALS

SUTURE MATERIAL

In gastrointestinal surgery, various suture material is used for various specific reasons. The material may be absorbable or nonabsorbable.

Absorbable material is used for sutures that will remain within the lumen of the gastrointestinal tract where it is exposed to the contents of the alimentary canal; hence it is used for the inner tier of sutures approximating the mucous membranes in a two-layer anastomosis or closure of the gastrointestinal tract.

Plain or chromicized catgut prepared from the collagen of animal intestine is the absorbable suture that has long been the one most commonly used for this purpose. It should be swaged on the end of a noncutting needle to reduce the size of the hole made in the gut wall. In 1937 Rhoads, Hottenstein, and Hudson published an excellent review of the development of catgut sutures and reported their studies on the decline in the strength of the different types of catgut after exposure to living tissues.

Although catgut has served surgeons well for many years it has several faults: it has variable strength and unpredictable absorption in tissue; its tensile strength and absorption rate are singularly affected by secretions and tissue enzymes; the cellular reaction of the tissue to catgut may be severe enough to impede healing; it is a good growth medium for bacteria so is seldom used for skin closure; it tends to fray when handled and weakens after knotting. Despite these faults, catgut continues to be used by surgeons with satisfactory results.

Because of these faults, in 1960 search began for a synthetic substance that could be absorbed or degraded in living tissue within a reasonable time, would be nontoxic and capable of fabrication into a strong fiber with acceptable knotting and handling qualities, and could withstand sterilization without damage to any of its physical and biologic properties. Not until 1970 was the first synthetic absorbable surgical suture, a polyglycolic acid polymer (Dexon), introduced for clinical use. Extensive premarket experimental use in animals and in clinical trials showed this suture to have behavior characteristics almost identical to those of chromic catgut, without catgut's undesirable tissue reactivity and with improvements such as resistance to enzymatic action, uniformity of tissue response, strength, and rate of absorption.

In 1974, a second synthetic absorbable suture, polyglactin (Vicryl) was introduced. The chemical structure of the two materials differs only slightly; they have virtually identical characteristics and working qualities.

In 1977, Laufman and Rubel published an excellent collective review of the development of synthetic absorbable sutures and summarized the reported experiences with its clinical and experimental use. They reported that synthetic absorbable sutures have been approved by the F.D.A. for almost all surgical uses except certain cardiovascular and neurosurgical procedures and suturing a prosthesis to tissue, where nonabsorbable sutures are mandatory. They have been used in thousands of surgical operations of many types in place of the catgut traditionally used in these cases. Moreover, because of their retained strength and low tissue reactivity, synthetic absorbable sutures are being used in place of nonabsorbable sutures in some procedures, permitting the surgeon to use one synthetic absorbable suture in different sizes, instead of different suture materials for an entire operation. Laufman (1977) editorialized, "Now that we have two synthetic absorbable sutures with proved advantages over catgut, is catgut obsolete?" The reply to this question is "not yet."

For a two-layer anastomosis or closure of the gastrointestinal tract, chromic catgut is still widely used for the inner row of absorbable sutures that penetrates the mucosa. It is pliable, easy to handle, and is less expensive. Nonabsorbable silk sutures are used for the outer, seromuscular, reinforcing layer. Although many surgeons continue this practice, there is a strong trend for using a synthetic suture instead of catgut for the inner layer, and some use synthetic sutures for both layers.

Postlethwaite (1975) tested the rate of breaking strength/loss of absorbable sutures in vivo in the stomach of dogs. Each animal underwent gastrotomy through which 2-0 plain catgut, chromic catgut, and Dexon and Vicryl sutures were placed in the posterior wall of the stomach and tied loosely, with the ends left long and lying within the gastric cavity, exposed to the acid-pepsin secretions. The gastrotomy and abdomen were closed in a routine manner. The dogs were allowed a liquid diet and then sacrificed respectively in 24 hours, 48 hours, and 3, 4, 5, 6, 7, 10 and 14 days. Any remaining suture material was recovered and its breaking strength was determined. No plain gut was recovered in 24 hours; chromic catgut was found as long as 48 hours after implantation, but its breaking strength was reduced markedly. Dexon and Vicryl lost strength slowly in a curve similar to the loss after implantation in other tissues.

Deveney and Way (1977) performed studies in dogs to determine whether the synthetic absorbable sutures would be preferable to catgut for use in the gastrointestinal tract. Dissolution times of plain and chromic catgut were compared with those of Dexon and Vicryl sutures exposed to gastrointestinal contents in vitro and in vivo. Strength and healing of gastric, jejunal, and colonic anastomoses performed with each suture were compared. Catgut sutures were susceptible to rapid proteolytic digestion throughout the gastrointestinal tract, whereas Dexon and Vicryl were well preserved. The type of suture did not affect microscopic healing in the stomach, jejunum, or colon. However, gastric anastomoses of Dexon were stronger at 4 and 7 days and jejunal anastomoses of Dexon and Vicryl were stronger at 7 days than anastomoses of catgut.

The investigators concluded that Dexon and Vicryl may be superior to catgut for use in gastrointestinal anastomoses, but they do not advocate one-layer anastomoses for situations in which two-layer anastomoses are routinely performed. They pointed out that whether the greater strength that can be provided by the synthetic sutures is really important in two-layer anastomoses has not been directly answered by this experiment, but it has demonstrated that the fate of synthetic sutures differs from that of catgut sutures in a way that could be advantageous.

Nonabsorbable sutures are employed to approximate seromuscular layers of the gastrointestinal tract in which the suture does not enter into the lumen. They should form the outermost layer of sutures of any multilayered gastrointestinal anastomosis or closure. When only a single layer of sutures is utilized, the material should be nonabsorbable.

Silk and cotton, particularly the former, have long been the most commonly used nonabsorbable suture materials. Formerly steel wire sutures were not used for gastrointestinal work because of their relative rigidity and concern that the sharp-pointed ends might cause intestinal perforation. Very thin pliable steel wire sutures are now available, however, and have been used with satisfaction and success for single-layer end-on alimentary tract anastomoses by Belsey, Collis, and others.

As noted, some surgeons use synthetic absorbable sutures in place of nonabsorbable sutures in some procedures.

The ultimate fate of intestinal sutures differs according to their location. Absorbable sutures that penetrate the mucosa undergo rapid disintegration. Nonabsorbable sutures that penetrate all the coats, or become exposed within the lumen of the bowel during healing, eventually are cast off into the intestinal canal. Nonabsorbable sutures that do not enter the bowel lumen usually remain partially or entirely buried, according to the method of suturing. Absorbable sutures behave like nonabsorbable sutures until absorption begins, at which time an inflammatory reaction occurs and persists until the suture is absorbed. Monofilament sutures are the least reactive.

In 1972, Van Winkle and Hastings published a collective review, "Considerations in the Choice of Suture Material for Various Tissues," and emphasized that suture materials should be chosen on the basis of known biologic properties of the suture and the particular clinical situation to be dealt with.

Sutures should be at least as strong as but need not be stronger than the normal tissue through which they are passed; so, above the limits of the strength of the tissue, no advantage is gained by using a larger or stronger material to hold the wound edges together.

NEEDLES

Any needle used for intestinal suturing should be round in its body and toward the point. It should taper gradually so that it will push away, rather than cut, the intestinal tissue it passes through. A sharp-edged needle makes a small incision, which the suture material enlarges when the knot is tied. Round needles are preferable to triangular cutting ones because the round hole made by such a needle is closed securely by the suture material. The round needle, in contrast to the cutting needle, cannot harm previously placed sutures. Both straight and curved needles should be available. The needle should not be thicker than the thread it carries, so the thread will fill entirely the hole made by the needle.

Although the needle may be no larger than the single thread, the part of the thread which is doubled increases the size of the needle hole in the bowel during the time of its passage. Generally this is not a practical consideration because the swelling about the needle puncture quickly closes around the wound made by the needle and thread. Needles to which sutures are swaged (end-on) are a definite refinement in intestinal suturing. All varieties of suture material swaged to all varieties of needles are available. This solves the problems of disparity between the size of the needle and the suture material and the difficulties of needle-threading, and eliminates the time loss attending the escape of suture material from the needle's eye.

Fundamental Forms of Simple Suturing

Sutures are of two fundamental types: *interrupted*, in which each suture is a separate thread, and *continuous*, in which the entire suture line is completed with one thread.

Interrupted sutures are safer than continuous sutures, for in the latter the integrity of the entire suture line depends upon one knot which may become untied. In the former, if one suture becomes untied the wound edges will still be coapted by the intact sutures on both sides of the faulty one. Other advanges of interrupted sutures are that tension on each suture can be adjusted, there is less interference with the blood supply of the edges of the intestine, and some lateral expansion of the suture line can occur — impossible with a continuous suture, which tends to have a pursestring effect and constrict the anastomotic stoma.

The advantages of continuous sutures over the interrupted variety are that the closure may be made more rapidly, the suture line is more watertight, there is less chance of mucosal eversion, and hemostasis is better.

Experience has shown that postoperative hemorrhage and narrowing of the anastomotic stoma by inversion of too much tissue occurs far less frequently if an anastomosis of the gastrointestinal tract is performed by the open technic, with ligation of the individual bleeders of the cut edges of the stomach and intestine, than when the closed, so-called aseptic method is used. For this reason, the open technic is preferred.

Standards for Satisfactory Intestinal Suturing

When utilizing the optimal technique for suturing, two broad peritoneal surfaces are brought into contact; closure is tight enough to hold water; the mucous membrane is not penetrated by the suture that is intended to pass through only the seromuscular coat; when only one tier of suturing is used, the mucous membrane is not included in the stitch bite; the suturing is not tight enough to strangulate the edges of the intestinal wound; the method of suturing is simple enough to be carried out easily and rapidly; the suture takes a sufficiently firm hold in the intestine to resist tearing out under considerable tension; the seromuscular sutures that pass through the serous and muscular layers must engage part or all of the strong submucous coat; and the suture material is durable and nonirritating.

Suturing is often expedited by placing two or four temporary traction sutures of silk through the serous and muscular coats in such positions as to draw into parallel ridges the two edges of the intestines to be apposed.

TYPES OF SUTURES

The sutures to be described may be used in any part of the gastrointestinal tract.

Interrupted Lembert Suture

This is the most important and fundamental suture in gastrointestinal surgery. It is illustrated in Figure 22–3. The needle is inserted from the outside and 2.5 mm. lateral to the incision. It is directed downward toward the cut edge of the incision to penetrate first the serosa and then the muscularis down to, but not through, the submucosal layer. It then is directed superficially so that it emerges from the viscus wall through the muscularis and serosa quite close to the edge of the incision. It is reinserted close to the incision's edge, passing laterally through the serosa and muscularis

TYPES OF SUTURES

down to *but not through* the muscularis, and again is brought up through the muscularis and serosa. *At no time does it penetrate into the lumen of the viscus.* The sutures are placed 3 to 5 mm. apart. The knots are not tied tightly enough to strangulate tissue, and the ends are cut close to the knots.

By this suture method the serosal surfaces are approximated to each other, while the mucous membrane is inverted, and the fibromuscular layer is well grasped. Furthermore, there is a minimal strangulation of tissue as only that thin line directly pressed upon by the single strand of the suture has tension placed upon it. For these reasons the interrupted Lembert suture is the safest and most useful stitch in gastrointestinal surgery. It is used chiefly to approximate the outer layer in any multiple-layer closure of an anastomosis or opening in the gastrointestinal tract or other hollow viscus. It is also used for a one-layer closure of an anastomosis or opening in the gastrointesti-

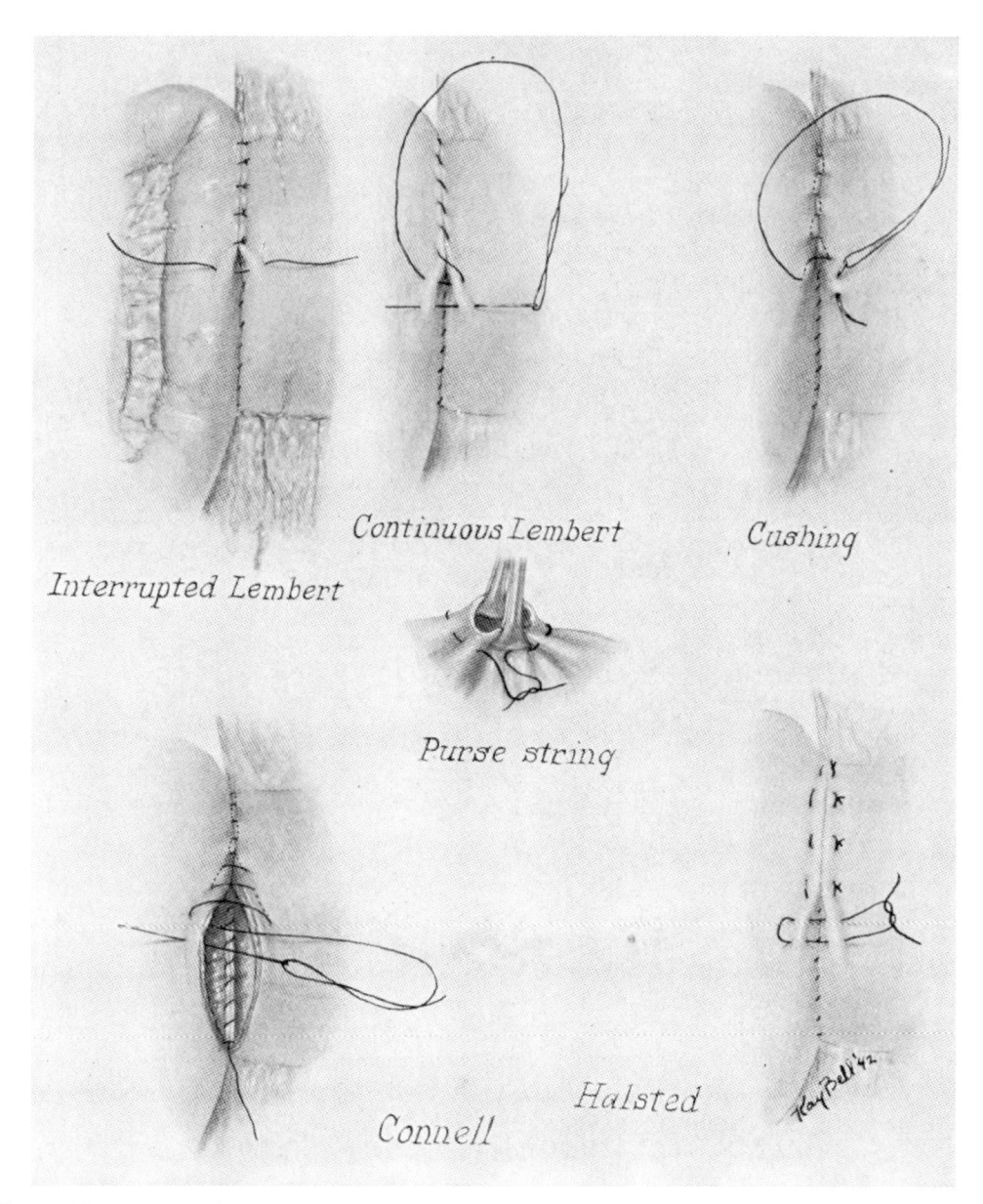

Figure 22–3. Types of intestinal sutures in common use. (From Orr, T. G.: Operations of General Surgery, 2nd ed. Philadelphia, W. B. Saunders Company, 1949.)

nal tract. This is particularly true in the colon where the arterial blood supply is less abundant than elsewhere in the stomach and intestines. Its material should always be nonabsorbable when it is used for the purposes just described.

Although a carefully placed single layer of interrupted Lembert sutures can be used successfully in an emergency, these sutures are not sufficiently secure to be used routinely for this purpose.

The objections to the interrupted Lembert sutures are that, in comparison with continuous sutures, they take more time for placing and tying, and they must be positioned closer together to ensure a watertight closure.

Continuous Lembert Suture

This is placed exactly as the interrupted Lembert suture (see Fig. 22–3) except that it is a continuous suture. Some surgeons place the stitches slightly oblique to the wound margins. The spacing is similar to that of the interrupted Lembert suture. The continuous suture is tied to itself at its proximal end and again at its distal end.

It is used to approximate the outer layer of a multiple-layer anastomosis or closure of the gastrointestinal tract, and its material, when so used, should be nonabsorbable. It is also utilized in a buried layer in a multiple-layer anastomosis or closure of the gastrointestinal tract, in which case it may be of either absorbable or nonabsorbable material.

It should not be used for a single-layer closure or anastomosis of the gastrointestinal tract except under exceptional circumstances.

The continuous suture requires less time than does the interrupted one as the time consumed in individual knot-tying is eliminated. It is probably more watertight and also more strangulating than the interrupted suture.

Halsted Interrupted Quilt (Mattress) Suture

The Halsted interrupted quilt or mattress suture is a modification of the Lembert seromuscular stitch (see Fig. 22–3). It consists of an ordinary quilt (mattress) suture so applied that the loop end is on one side of the wound and the two free ends are on the other. In its manner of application, each quilt suture should be regarded as two parallel Lembert sutures united by a loop. When each knot is tightened, the fold on the side of the wound held by the loop and the fold on the side of the wound held by the knot are brought into contact.

This suture takes a strong hold, approximates the parts very accurately, and compresses the tissues very little. A series of mattress sutures is especially serviceable in friable tissues where other sutures tear out.

A suture line of mattress stitches is stronger than one composed of Lembert stitches but probably strangulates the blood supply more than an interrupted Lembert suture. It can be used to close an intestinal wound without placing a subjacent marginal tier of suturing, though this is not recommended as a routine practice.

Pursestring Suture

This is essentially a continuous Lembert suture placed in a circle around a circular opening, except that neither end is tied until the entire suture is placed (see Fig. 22–3).

After being placed, the first phase of a square knot is tied loosely in the two untied ends and equal traction upward is exerted while the opening in the gut is inverted into it. It is of considerable help in obtaining good inversion to have an assistant use an Allis clamp to grasp that part of the pursestring suture exactly opposite the knot (Fig. 22–4) and to exert like traction upward on this portion of the suture. When the gut is satisfactorily inverted, the Allis clamp is released, the pursestring is drawn tight, gathering in the wall of the gut, and the knot is tied in all its phases.

Like all Lembert-type sutures, this stitch does not penetrate into the lumen of the gut, or, if it does, it is covered over by another tier of sutures.

Pursestring sutures may be of nonabsorbable or absorbable material, but the outer layer of sutures should be nonabsorbable.

TYPES OF SUTURES

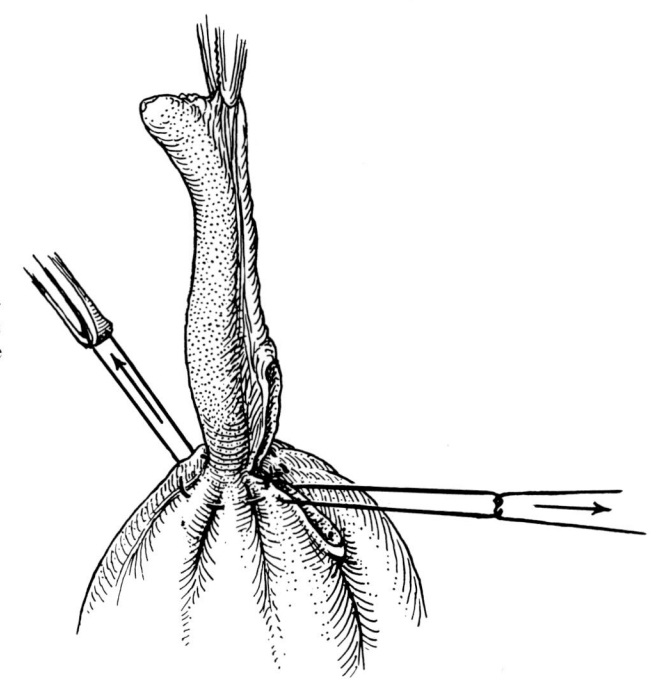

Figure 22-4. Method of facilitating pursestring inversion. A stitch of the pursestring is grasped with an Allis clamp directly opposite the knot to be tied and counter traction applied.

This suture is used to close circular openings such as to invert the stump of an amputated appendix or diverticulum, a small perforation of the gastrointestinal tract, or the open end of a transected small or large intestine. When so used it is usually reinforced by a second tier of either pursestring, mattress, or Lembert sutures.

When applicable, a pursestring suture is the simplest and safest method of closing a circular opening into the gastrointestinal tract. It is useful for closing an opening around an indwelling tube. Its disadvantage is the large amount of gut wall that it inverts. For this reason, if it is used to close the severed proximal end of the duodenum, one should avoid inverting so much duodenal wall that it impinges upon and obstructs the opening of the common duct into the duodenum.

However, it should be pointed out that the pursestring suture is unsatisfactory for closing perforating wounds of the stomach because the suture does not include the gastric mucosa. Hence the mucosa edges retract, exposing the underlying submucosal blood vessels, which erode and bleed. It is advisable to enlarge transversely small circular wounds of the stomach, so that the mucosa can be exposed and accurately sutured and hemostatis secured. (See Missile Wounds of the Stomach, p. 206.)

Cushing Suture

In this method of continuous suturing, the thread is carried along in its onward progress exactly parallel with the edges of the wound (see Fig. 22-3) in the gut, and, when the wound is crossed, the crossing is always directly at right angles to the course of the wound. The suture penetrates through the serosa and muscularis to but *not through* the submucous layer of the wall of the viscus, hence the gastrointestinal lumen is not entered. The suture is tied to itself at its proximal and again at its distal end. It is buried throughout its course except where it crosses the wound, and even this portion is buried by the invagination of the lips of the wound when the suture is drawn tight.

It inverts the mucosa and approximates the serosal surfaces, so it can be used in approximating any layer in gastrointestinal repair or anastomosis. If it is to be used to close the final and outer layer, it should be of nonabsorbable material. It is not hemostatic in occluding bleeding from the cut edges of the mucosal layer, as is the Connell stitch.

Connell Suture

Each segment of the Connell or U-shaped continuous suture is passed 4 to 5 mm. from, and parallel to, each wound edge (see Fig. 22–3). This suture pierces all the layers of the gut wall with an "in-and-out-on-the-same-side" or "loop-on-the-mucosa" type of stitch. In placement, it resembles the Cushing right-angled continuous suture but is composed of through-and-through bites instead of bites through the seromuscular layers only.

The suture is tied after its first stitch is taken, the knot being placed either within or without the gastrointestinal wall, depending upon the site of origin of the suture. After the knot is tied the needle is passed from without to the inside of the intestinal wall. It then is advanced about 0.3 cm. and is reinserted from within to the outside of the gut wall, after which it is brought across the incision to penetrate the opposite wall from without inward, and so forth. The suture is tied again at the far end. It is important to remember that *the suture crosses the incision only from the outside of one wall to penetrate the outside of the opposite wall. It penetrates from the inside to the outside only on the same side on which the previous stitch ended.*

This suture is hemostatic in that it compresses all the layers of the gut wall. It is used to approximate the first layer in the repair of an incision into the gastrointestinal tract, the first layer in closure of the anterior wall of a gastrointestinal anastomosis, and the first layer in the closure of an open end of resected gut. It should be of catgut or synthetic absorbable suture and is always reinforced by an outer layer of nonabsorbable sutures that buries it and does not penetrate through all the layers of the gastrointestinal wall into the lumen.

Parker-Kerr Stitch

This stitch (Figs. 22–5 and 22–6) is a Cushing stitch, advancing parallel to the cut edges of the gut but crossing to the other wall over a clamp that holds the edges in apposition. Neither end is tied, and, after the suture has advanced the full length of the opening, the two ends of the suture are pulled in opposite directions (Fig. 22–6) as the clamp is slowly withdrawn from beneath the suture, allowing the gut walls to invert as they appose each other. After the clamp has been entirely removed and the suture drawn as tight as possible, the needle end of the suture is brought back as a second-layer Cushing suture, inverting further the first layer and ending at its origin to which it is tied. This stitch is used to close the open ends of resected gut. It may be of absorbable or nonabsorbable material. It is always reinforced by another layer of nonabsorbable sutures, and each angle should be reinforced by a Marshall U-stitch.

Through-and-Through U-Stitch

This stitch inverts more securely the angles at the ends of any through-and-through suture line. It differs from the Marshall U-stitch in that the latter penetrates the seromuscular layers only. The suture material utilized should be of the absorbable variety.

The stitch begins (Fig. 22–7) at one angle of the incision. It starts from the outside and penetrates through all the coats of one wall to within the lumen. It then penetrates both walls of the septum between the two viscera being anastomosed, to enter the lumen of the viscus apposing that originally entered, after which it penetrates the angle of the second viscus from within its lumen to the outside, where it is tied to its original end. When tied, this mattress-type suture inverts and secures the angle, which is the most dangerous point of leakage in a suture line.

After the knot is made, the suture material may be utilized to form a continuous lock-stitch or other type of suture (Fig. 22–8) to appose the two walls of the septum. At the far end of the incision the angle is inverted by the same series of steps used for inversion of the first angle (Figs. 22–9 through 22–12), and suturing is continued back to the point of origin by placing an anterior row of Connell stitches. This series

Text continued on page 571

TYPES OF SUTURES 567

Figure 22–5. Parker-Kerr method of inverting the ends of the bowel. (From Partipilo, A. V.: Surgical Technique and Principles of Operative Surgery. Philadelphia. Lea & Febiger, 1949.)

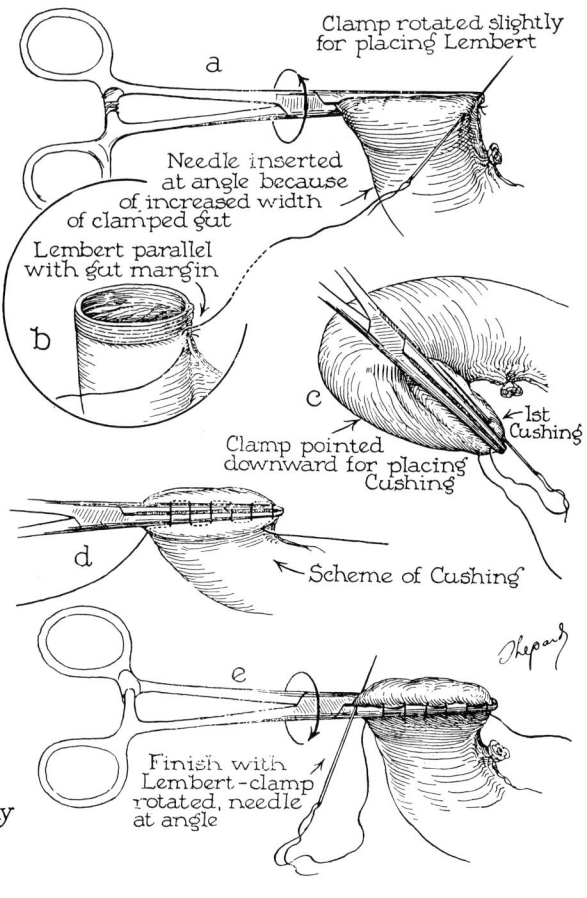

Figure 22–6. Continuation of the Parker-Kerr stitch. *a*, *b*, and *c*, Method of inversion; *d* and *e*, second row of Cushing stitches to reinforce the inner row. (From Partipilo, cited in previous figure.)

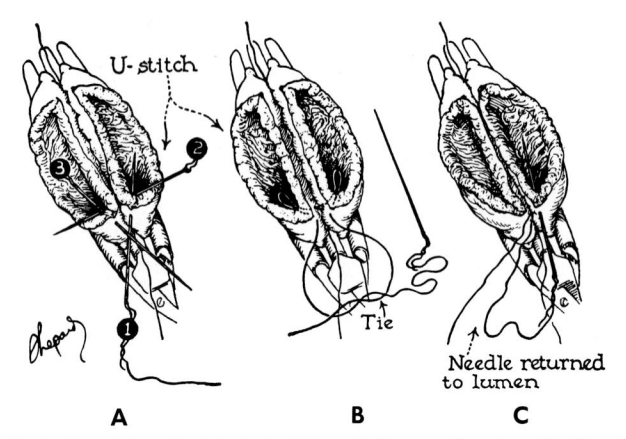

Figure 22–7. *A*, Method of applying the U-stitch; (1) starts from without and is directed inward; (2) through the septum; and (3) out again. *B*, U-stitch completed and ready for tying. *C*, After tying the U-stitch, the needle re-enters the lumen. (From Partipilo, cited in Figure 22–5).

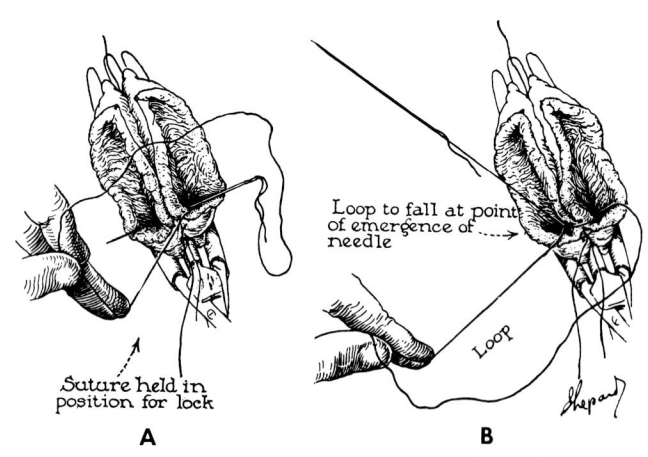

Figure 22–8. *A*, The septum is sutured with a continuous lock stitch. *B*, The suture is held so that the loop will fall at the point of emergence of the needle. (From Partipilo, cited in Figure 22–5.)

TYPES OF SUTURES 569

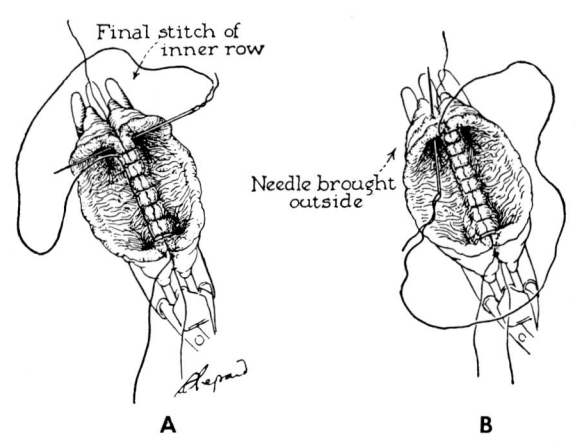

Figure 22–9. *A,* Final stitch at the septum. *B,* Beginning to invert the corner. (From Partipilo, cited in Figure 22–5.)

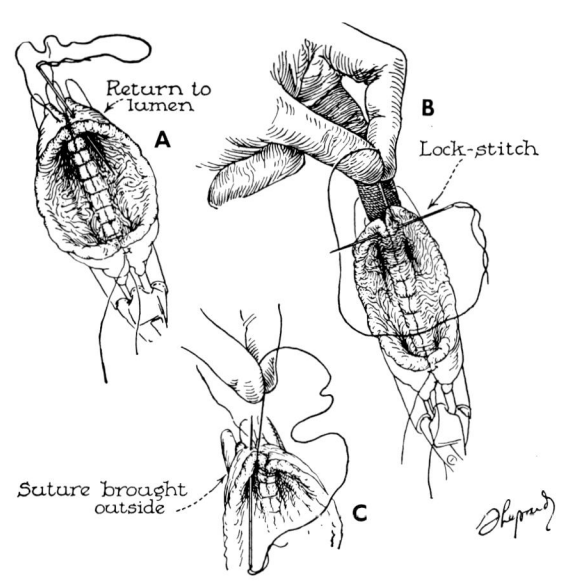

Figure 22–10. *A,* Completing the inversion of the corner, the needle re-enters the lumen. *B,* After the corner has been inverted, the angle is reinforced by a lock stitch. *C,* The needle is carried from within and is directed outward, and the anterior edges are then inverted. (From Partipilo, cited in Figure 22–5.)

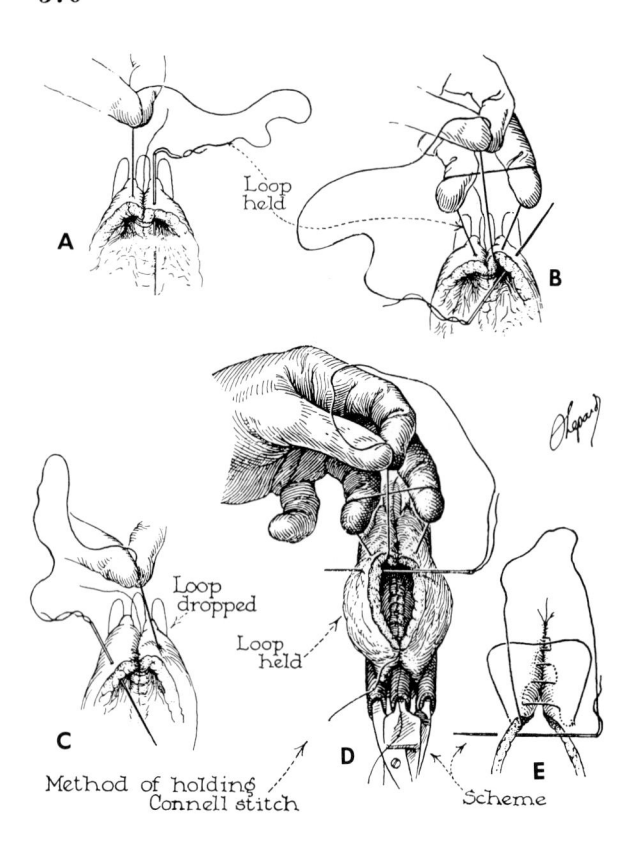

Figure 22–11. Inverting the anterior edges with a Connell suture. *D* illustrates Partipilo's method of holding the suture. (From Partipilo, cited in Figure 22–5.)

Figure 22–12. Method of applying terminal stitches at the angle. *A* and *B*, Terminal stitches applied; *C*, thumb pressure before the sutures are pulled tightly; *D* and *E*, the long end is tied to the short end. (From Partipilo, cited in Figure 22–5.)

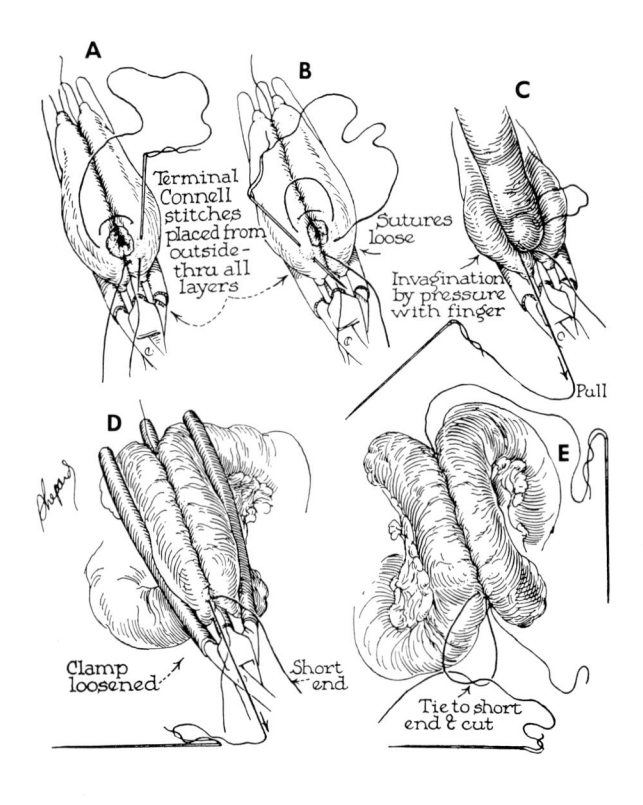

of stitches is used for the inner row of sutures in a gastrointestinal anastomosis or closure.

Each angle should be reinforced later by a Marshall U-stitch.

Marshall U-Stitch

This is an interrupted mattress stitch of silk which penetrates the seromuscular layers only and does not enter the lumen (Fig. 22–13). It is placed at the angle of any anastomosis or closure of the cut intestine.

The suture begins in the wall of one viscus about 1 cm. from the angle and passes toward the angle, emerging distal to the tied end of the inner row of sutures. It then passes to the wall of the other viscus involved in the anastomosis and penetrates the seromuscular layer to emerge opposite its origin. When tied, it further inverts that angle. The tied ends may then be cut or the needle end of the material used to form a continuous Lembert or Cushing suture.

Furrier Suture

The first stitch of the furrier continuous marginal suture (Fig. 22–14) passes through all the intestinal coats and is knotted on the outside. The suturing progresses by piercing alternately opposite margins of the bowel incision from within outward. The amount of serosa on the two sides brought into contact is proportional to the width of margin included in the stitches. Absorbable material is used for this suture.

The furrier-stitch suture line always is reinforced by a layer of overlying seromuscular sutures, because this suture penetrates into the intestinal lumen and leakage along the suture line is possible. This suture method is seldom used at present as the stitches cross from the outside of one wall of the gut to the inner surface of the other wall, and hence there is danger of leakage. Other methods are preferred.

Simple Overhand Continuous or Interrupted Suture (Albert)

This suture (Fig. 22–15) penetrates, in the order named, the serosa and muscularis of the gut wall on one side and then crosses to the other side of the incision to penetrate the opposite wall deeply, entering the muscularis and emerging through the serosa (Fig. 22–16).

Sometimes it is used to penetrate all the coats of the gut. When such is the case, the material should be of the absorbable variety. If the suture does not penetrate into the lumen, its substance can be either absorbable or nonabsorbable.

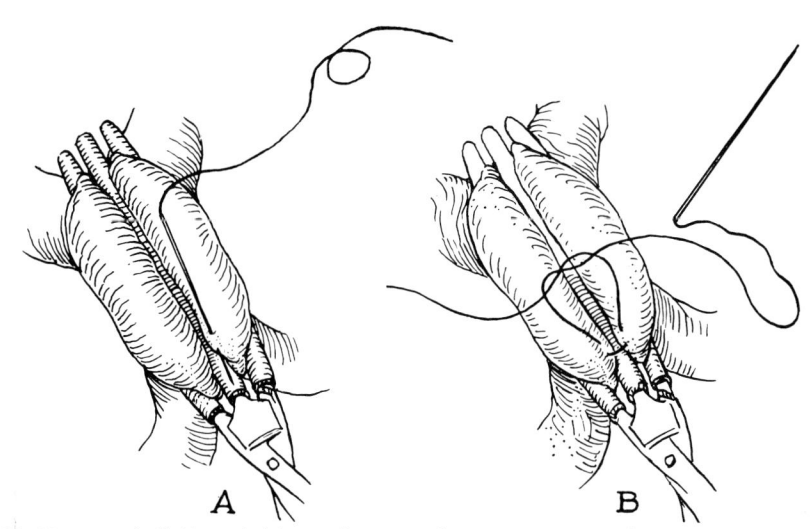

Figure 22–13. Marshall U-stitch (shown here as a beginning to a Cushing approximation suture).

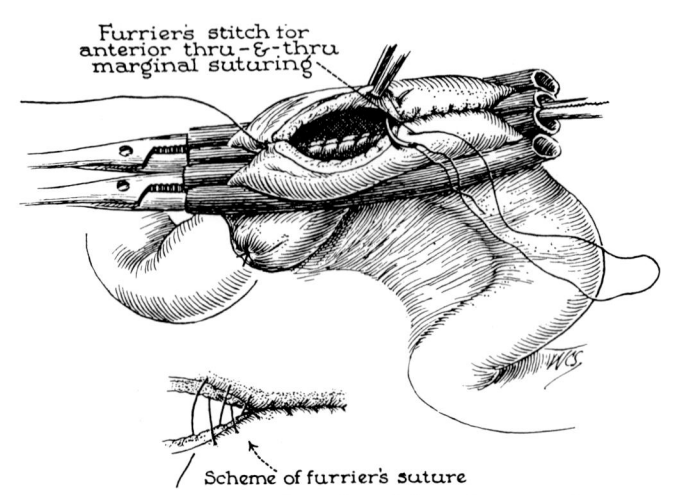

Figure 22-14. Furrier through-and-through marginal suture.

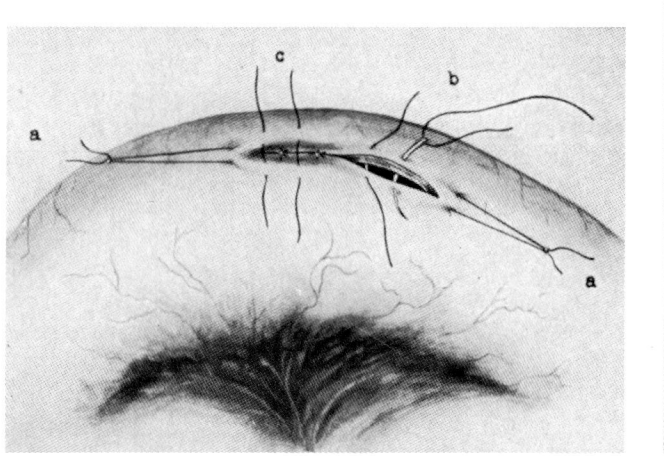

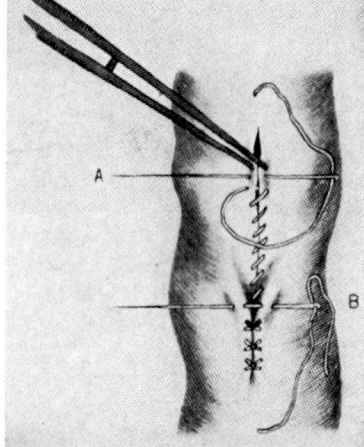

Fig. 22-15.

Fig. 22-16.

Figure 22-15. Enterorrhaphy by the combined Albert-Lembert sutures. *a*, Nonpenetrating traction sutures to tauten and make parallel and prominent the margins of the wound; *b*, through-and-through marginal sutures of all the coats; *c*, reinforcing Lembert sutures of the seromuscular submucosal coats.

Figure 22-16. Enterorrhaphy by combined overhand continuous suture of all the coats, followed by interrupted Lembert sutures of the other coats. *A*, Continuous overhand marginal suture; *B*, interrupted Lembert sutures.

This stitch is used to form a first row of sutures in anastomosis or repair of openings in the gastrointestinal tract, but its suture line is usually inverted by a second layer of Lembert-type stitches. It may also be used to form the outer row of sutures, in which case it should not enter the lumen of the gut.

Lock-Stitch (Glover Stitch)

This stitch is hemostatic and is commonly used to approximate the posterior septum in a gastrointestinal anastomosis. It can be used for the anterior row of stitches as well, but the Connell suture is preferred for making that closure.

The suture begins as a U-stitch (see Fig. 22–7A). After this stitch is tied, the needle returns into the lumen of the gut (see Fig. 22–7C) and penetrates all the layers of the posterior septum (see Fig. 22–8), which is sutured with a continuous over-and-over lock-stitch. In the application of the stitch the loop is made to fall at the point of emergence of the needle (see Fig. 22–8B) so that the needle comes up through the loop, forming a self-locking stitch when pulled taut. When the entire posterior row has been placed, the suture line is inspected for bleeding. Any bleeding found is controlled by placing a mattress suture at the bleeding point.

After hemostasis is obtained, the suturing is continued (see Fig. 22–9A) by inverting the angles. The corners are inverted by passing the needle from within outward (see Fig. 22–9B), over to the other side, and again bringing it into the lumen (see Fig. 22–10A). This maneuver is repeated without going through the septum, until the corner is inverted adequately (see Fig. 22–10B and C). After the corner is locked the needle is brought to the outside and the anterior edges are inverted with a Connell suture (see Fig. 22–3).

Czerny Interrupted Sutures

The Czerny sutures are placed so that all the knots fall within the bowel lumen

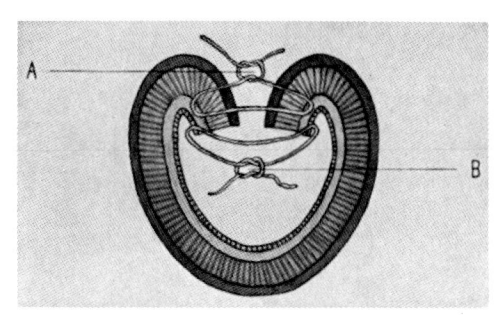

Figure 22–17. Enterorrhaphy by the Czerny-Lembert interrupted suture. *A,* Interrupted Lembert suture through serous, muscular, and part of submucous coats — applied from without. *B,* Interrupted Czerny suture through mucous and part of submucous coats — applied from within. The latter is applied first.

(Fig. 22–17). Catgut or synthetic absorbable material is used for these sutures. With a fine thumb-forceps, the mucosa of one side of the wound is drawn forward and slightly everted. A curved needle then is passed from the mucosal surface outward through the mucosa and the submucous coat. The mucous membrane of the opposite edge of the wound is picked up with the forceps, and the needle is passed from without inward through the submucous coat and the mucosa. The two ends of each suture are tied within the bowel lumen. For two-thirds of the distance in linear enterorrhaphy, the Czerny sutures are applied easily. The last few sutures are difficult to place. When the last one or two knots of the Czerny sutures are tied, the knots are pressed into the lumen with the blunt end of the probe.

An outer or reinforcing layer of *Lembert sutures* of silk should completely enclose the layer of Czerny suture (Fig. 22–17).

This combination of sutures is not used as much now as formerly, but it is still the only combination of stitches in which the inner layer penetrates the inner coats; the outer layer, the outer coats; and neither layer, all the coats.

Continuous Through-and-Through Marginal (Albert) Suture and Interrupted Gould Inverted Mattress Suture for Enterorrhaphy

This type of enterorrhaphy is performed by placing a through-and-through

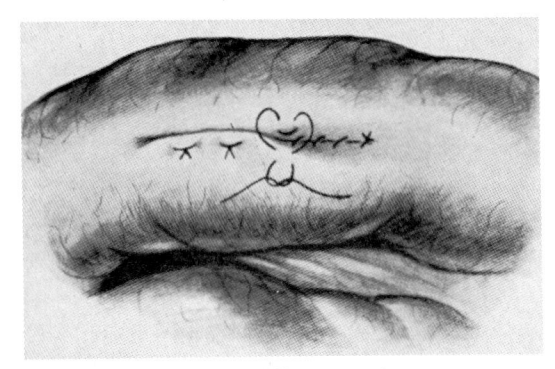

Figure 22-18. Gould's inverted mattress suture overlying the through-and-through marginal suture.

Albert continuous marginal suture and reinforcing it with a layer of interrupted Gould inverted mattress sutures (Fig. 22-18). This closure is especially applicable in friable tissue, in which single-strand sutures tear out under tension. The Gould reversed mattress sutures are applied so that the loop of each stitch is inverted and lies toward, rather than away from, the sutured margin.

The Gould stitch takes longer to apply than does the ordinary mattress suture and is not often used.

Three-Layer Suture Line

This is seldom the method of choice. The first row of sutures includes all layers of the margins of the bowel. The Albert stitch (see Fig. 22-16), the Connell stitch (see Fig. 22-3), or the lock-stitch (see Fig. 22-8) may be used for this row of stitches. The two reinforcing rows are some variety of seromuscular suturing.

The method apposes broad areas of the surfaces and seals the ends of the wound firmly. However, too much infolding of the wound margins, with resulting impairment of the blood supply to the sutured area, is often seen. The technic is used only when there is doubt as to the security of the routinely applied two-tier suturing. Actually, a few reinforcing interrupted seromuscular sutures, applied where weak areas are thought to exist in two-row suturing, are as effective as an entire third row of suturing.

Gambee Single-Layer Open Intestinal Anastomosis

This is an interrupted inverting suturing of the full thickness of the bowel walls, using a single row of nonabsorbable sutures. Gambee (1951) introduced the procedure, described the technic, and reported that the method had proved most satisfactory in his and his colleagues' hands over a period of years under a variety of circumstances. They used it in repairing the small as well as the large intestine, and for anastomosing the gallbladder to the open end of

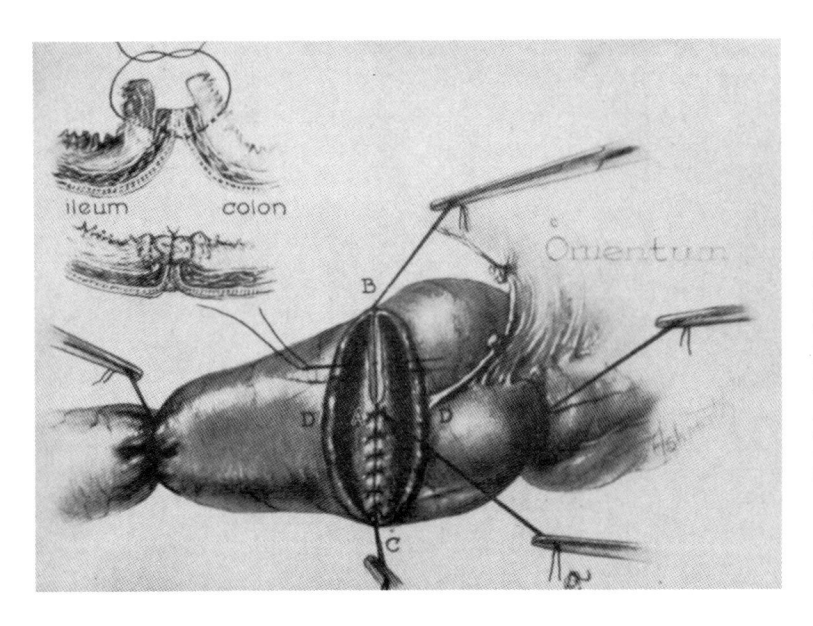

Figure 22-19. The sutures in the first half of the anastomosis are placed from within the lumen, as shown. Slight tension on guy sutures (*B* and *C*) facilitates inversion of the edges. The proximal and distal occlusive ligatures are placed before dividing the bowel. (From Gambee, L. P., Garnjobst, W., and Hardwick, C. E.: Ten years' experience with a single layer anastomosis in colon surgery. Am. J. Surg. 92:222, 1956.)

TYPES OF SUTURES

the jejunum and the esophagus to the duodenum.

Prior to beginning the open anastomosis, fecal spillage is controlled by heavy occlusive ligatures tied around the intestine several inches from the divided ends. Since these ligatures do not compress the mesenteric vessels, as rubber-shod clamps might, they permit continuous assessment of the adequacy of the vascular supply, after division of the bowel, and also allow manipulation of the cut ends with minimal trauma. The cut ends are approximated, a lateral guy traction suture is placed at what will be each angle of the anastomosis, and inversion of the bowel walls is supplied by slight tension on the lateral guy sutures. The posterior halves of the intestinal circumferences are sutured from within the lumen by interrupted sutures that penetrate the full thickness of the walls and are tied with the knot remaining within the lumen (Fig. 22–19).

The remaining anterior half of the anastomosis is completed by inverting "Gambee" sutures, placed as shown in Figure 22–20. These characteristic Gambee sutures enter the serosal surface of the efferent bowel 6 to 8 mm. from its cut edge, penetrate through the mucosa, immediately re-enter the mucosa, and exit the serosa on the same side 2 to 3 mm. from the edge. They then cross to the efferent bowel and enter its serosal surface 2 to 3 mm. from the edge, penetrate through the mucosa, immediately re-enter the mucosa 5 to 6 mm. from the edge, and exit through the serosa on the same side and are tied on the serosal surface of the bowel. Additional sutures are added whenever necessary to provide inversion and sealing. Gambee used silk or cotton for the suture material.

In 1956, Gambee, Garnjobst, and Hardwick reported their ten years' experience with this single-layer anastomosis in colon surgery. One hundred sixty-three large bowel anastomoses had been performed by the described technic, after resection for various indications. There were five fatalities, due directly or indirectly to anastomotic failure with leak — a mortality rate of 3 per cent. "Eight other postoperative deaths occurred in the series. In five of these, autopsy showed the anastomosis to be intact and patent. In the remaining three there were no clinical suspicions of anastomotic complication" (and no autopsy).

Nine nonfatal anastomotic complications occurred, so the incidence of all types of anastomotic complications was 8.6 per cent. Anastomotic obstruction occurred in only two cases, symptomatic stenosis in none. Symptomatic leaks occurred in only two cases without pre-existing complications.

The investigators stated that the advantages of this procedure are its simplicity and ease of performance even under relatively adverse conditions. It is particularly valuable in anastomosing bowel ends that are uneven in diameter, and a single row of sutures results in a narrow flange of turned-

Figure 22–20. The anastomosis is completed by interrupted inverting sutures, placed as shown. (From Gambee, Garnjobst, and Hardwick, cited in previous figure.)

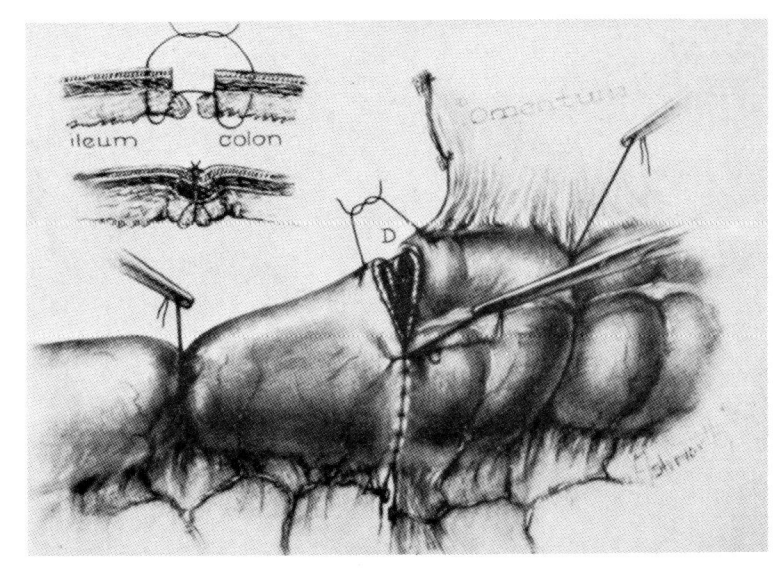

in tissue so there is little likelihood of obstruction and of impairment of the blood supply to the anastomotic area.

This report, presented before the Pacific Coast Surgical Association, was discussed by Dr. Robert Scarborough. In the preceding 10 years, he and his colleagues used the conventional two-layer technic for large bowel anastomoses and had mortality and morbidity rates from anastomotic complications about one-third (mortality, 1 per cent; morbidity, 3 per cent) those just reported with this single-layer anastomosis.

Initially there was great enthusiasm for the Gambee single-layer open intestinal anastomosis and it was widely used, but it is our undocumented impression that its popularity is waning in favor of a two-layer technic.

Probably the most widespread use of the Gambee suture is in Weinberg's and associates (1956) modification of the Heineke-Mikulicz pyloroplasty with one-row suture technic that, combined with vagotomy, is very popular for treating duodenal ulcer. This operation is discussed and

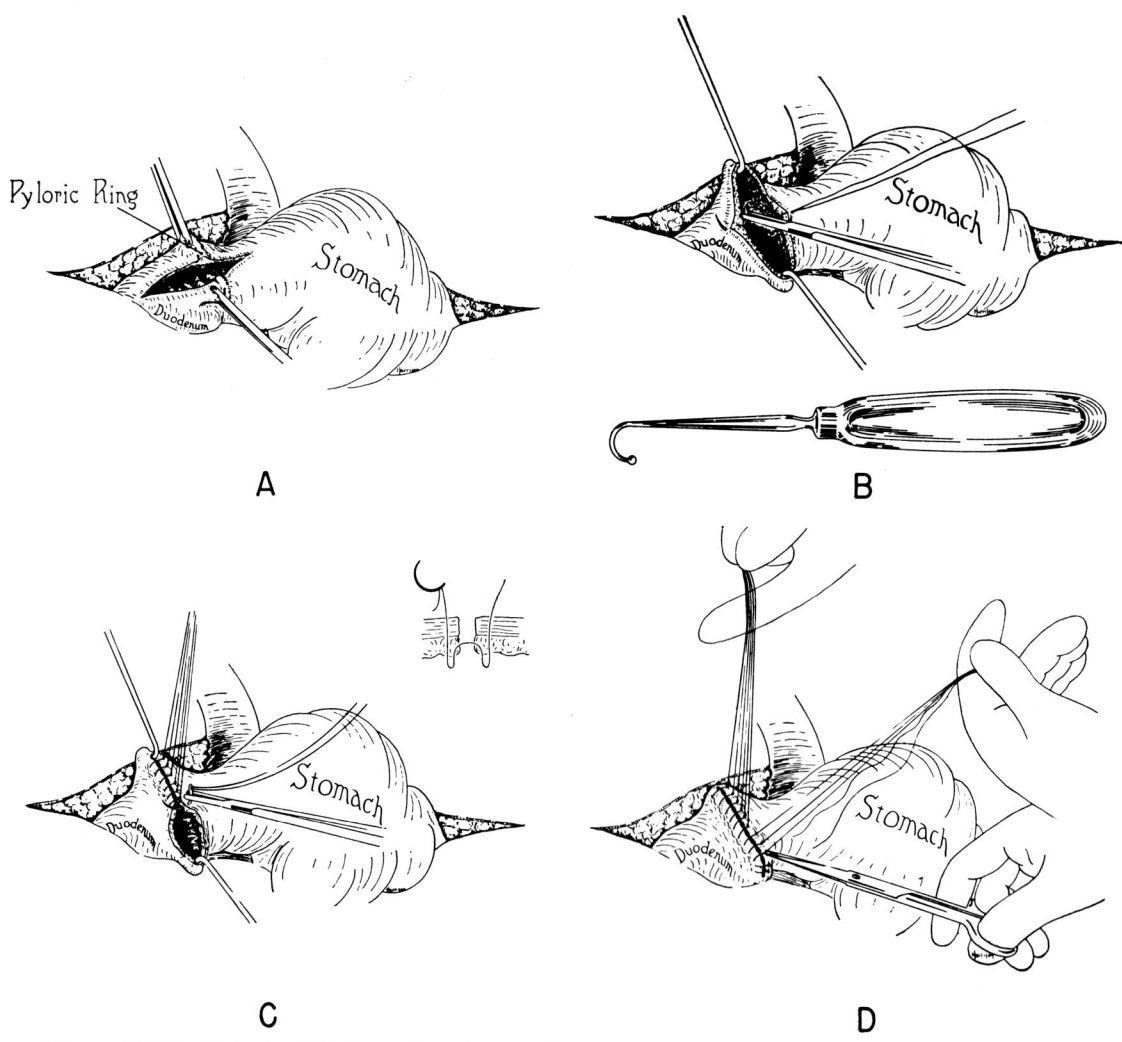

Figure 22–21. Heineke-Mikulicz pyloroplasty with one-row suture technic. *A*, Longitudinal incision across pyloric ring extending through all layers, including mucosa. *B*, Pyloroplasty retractors convert wound by lateral traction and at the same time provide exposure for accurate placement of sutures. *C*, Insert shows Gambee stitch, which aligns mucosa to mucosa. *D*, Completion of pyloroplasty. (From Weinberg, J. A.: Vagotomy and pyloroplasty for duodenal ulcer. Am. J. Surg. 92:203, 1956.)

described in the section on pyloroplasty and is illustrated in Figure 22–21.

Navy Single-Layer Everting Anastomosis

In 1964 Getzen, Roe, and Holloway, at the surgical research laboratory of the U.S. Naval Hospital in San Diego, introduced a one-row through-and-through everting intestinal anastomosis, which, in dogs, was secure, quickly and easily performed, and produced no luminal narrowing. It has been termed the "Navy" anastomosis. Getzen (1966) published their clinical experience with this technique in 136 gastrointestinal anastomoses. One anastomotic leak resulted in death.

Hamilton (1966), in experiments on dogs, compared four methods for gastrointestinal anastomoses then in use. The methods studied (Fig. 22–22) were (1) the double-row inverting anastomosis most commonly used and therefore termed the "standard"; (2) the Halsted single-row inverting stitch which catches only the submucosa; (3) the Navy single-row through-and-through everting anastomosis; and (4) the Gambee single-row through-and-through inverting stitch. All four methods were performed in each of 29 dogs and studied for anastomotic defects, associated adhesions, gross and histologic edema and inflammation at the suture line, amount of inverted anastomotic cuff, operating time, and air inflation leak test.

Hamilton reported that these experiments, together with a limited clinical experience, showed that the more time-consuming and difficult double-row standard anastomosis is less secure than the Gambee and turns in a larger cuff. The Halsted is slightly stronger than the Gambee but has nearly as great an obstructing inverted cuff as the standard. "The Navy anastomosis, though simple and quickly performed and devoid of obstructing cuff, has such low leak pressure with air inflation that we hesitate to use it for any critical anastomosis, especially of colon or esophagus. In short, our investigations and clinical experience seem to show the Gambee to be superior to other anastomoses tested and is becoming our procedure of choice."

Hamilton's report was presented at the annual meeting of the Southern Surgical Association. Bronwell, Rutledge, and Dalton (1966) reported a study of 327 patients

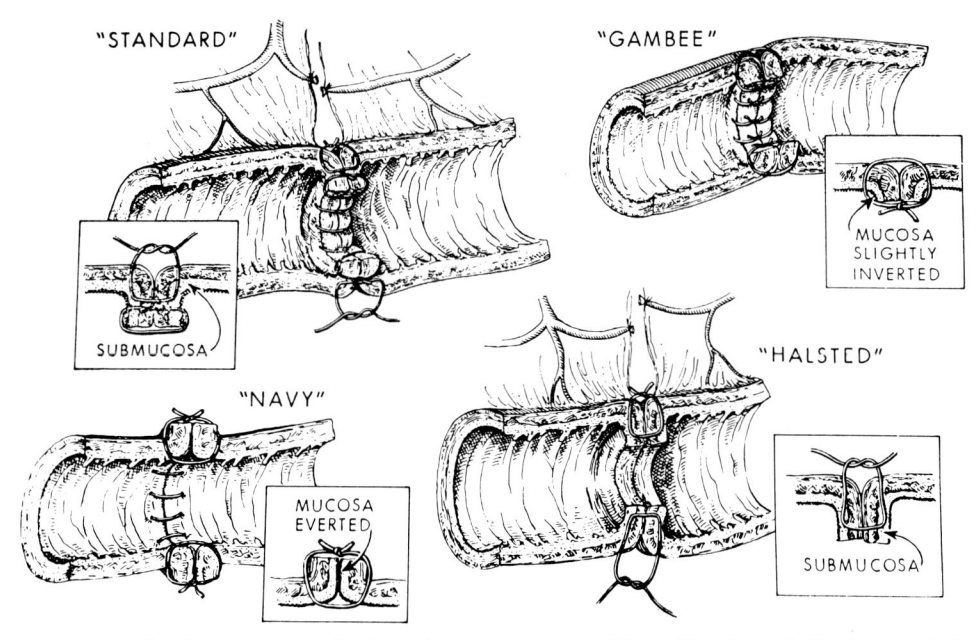

Figure 22–22. The four suture methods under investigation. (From Hamilton, J. E.: Reappraisal of open intestinal anastomoses. Trans. South. Surg. Assoc. 78:273, 1966.)

in which single-layer was compared with multiple-layer anastomoses in two groups of patients — 136 with colon anastomoses and 191 with gastrojejunal anastomoses. In anastomoses at both sites, patients with single-layer closures tolerated food and passed flatus and stools 24 hours earlier than those with multiple-layer closures. There were no anastomotic leaks and no deaths in the single layer series. In the multiple-layer anastomoses of the colon, three patients had leaks at the anastomotic site, and one died. None of the multiple-layer closures of the gastrojejunal region leaked. They concluded that "single-layer anastomoses can be accomplished with less morbidity, and with comparable mortality to multiple-layer closures."

In subsequent discussion, Dr. George Sanders stated that the Gambee stitch has less gripping power than a through-and-through stitch penetrating first the serosa, then all coats of the bowel into the lumen, and exiting out again through the serosa, in other words, a perforating Lembert or a perforating Halsted mattress suture, which he has used exclusively in 129 anastomoses. Three anastomotic leaks occurred, all in low colorectal anastomoses, and no fistulas or abscesses. The only death was due to an extraneous medical complication 4 weeks later. However, he has found brisk bleeding from the gastrojejunal suture line, so he has returned to a two-layer anastomosis for gastrojejunal anastomoses only.

Bronwell commented that when doing gastrojejunal anastomoses it is necessary to meticulously ligate the submucosal blood vessels prior to the anastomosis in order to prevent postoperative hemorrhage. When this has been done, he has found no problem with postoperative bleeding. In colon anastomoses, it has not been necessary to ligate the vessels as the suture will control the hemorrhage from the submucosal blood vessels.

Chapter 23

MECHANICAL SUTURES

Mechanical sutures of the gastrointestinal tract represent a fundamental departure from traditional manual techniques by virtue of certain basic features, such as the everting suture of transected and tangentially opened bowel, resulting in mucosa-to-mucosa closures; the use of metal sutures; the application of a mechanical device producing standardization and uniformity in the reconstructive phase of an operation, in which surgeons have felt the need for and were even proud of exercising minute differences in technique; and, finally, the speed with which nearly "closed" anastomoses can be performed, drastically reducing the duration of open bowel exposed in the operative field and the potential for contamination and sepsis.

THE HEALING OF INTESTINAL WOUNDS

Over 150 years ago, Lembert (1826) emphasized the importance of inversion of the bowel and serosa-to-serosa approximation, although it is noteworthy that at the same time he pointed out that excessive inversion invited intestinal obstruction. His drawings do show a very considerable inverted flange. Since that time the cardinal principle of intestinal anastomoses, namely, inversion with serosa-to-serosa closure, was established firmly. It was believed equally firmly that mucosa-to-mucosa closures could not heal, and acceptance of everting sutures has been most difficult for surgeons to this day.

However, at the time of Lembert's publication the work by Benjamin Travers (1812), Astley Cooper's great pupil, had already appeared, in his treatise "An Inquiry into the Process of Healing and Repairing Injuries of the Intestines." In this publication Travers gave very explicit directions for performing an everting anastomosis, mucosa-to-mucosa. Lembert himself commented upon Travers' "lovely experiments," and almost every writer on the subject of intestinal healing mentions the treatise of Benjamin Travers; however, all of them appear to have paid very little attention to what Travers actually said. His illustrations show everting anastomoses and, in his experimental animals, they healed. He commented that too much had been made of the technique of anastomosis and that if the sutures were placed properly, by whatever technic, the anastomosis would heal.

Interest in the mucosa-to-mucosa anastomosis persisted and in the year of Lembert's publication, Henroz (1826), in his doctoral thesis, reported the use of two jointed rings containing alternating needles and holes, which could be placed outside the bowel to snap together through the everted flanges of the two bowel ends, producing an everting mucosa-to-mucosa anastomosis that was successful in his animal experiments. Henroz's instrument is truly the first mechanical suture device and is a precursor of Murphy's (1892) button. This button consisted of two hollow, telescoping cylinders with a perforated mushroom cap at either end, so that each end of the bowel could be pursestringed around the mushroom cap and the cylinders telescoped, compressing the mushroom edges together. This produced an inverting anastomosis which depended upon the compression necrosis of the two inverted diaphragms to produce a slough, with ultimate discharge of the button into the bowel lumen.

Halsted (1887) made a major contribution to intestinal surgery, almost three-quarters of a century after Lembert: for secure intestinal anastomosis the suture had to pass through the tough submucosa. Halsted stressed the fact that penetration through the mucosa into the lumen would invite infection of the suture line and hence should be avoided. He noted, with some scorn, that it seemed to be a matter of no concern to Lembert whether his needle punctured the mucosa or not. Halsted, like Nicholas Senn (1893) and all the other students of intestinal suturing and healing, insisted upon an inverting serosa-to-serosa anastomosis (Otis, 1876).

It should be no great surprise that mucosa-to-mucosa closure could heal. The fact has long been recognized for the bronchus, and mucosa-to-mucosa closure of the bronchus has become standard practice, after brief and unsuccessful early flirtations with inversion of the bronchial stumps. Rienhoff, Gannon and Sherman (1942) showed in the bronchus, as we have in the bowel, that the healing actually takes place at the viable cut end and not at the juxtaposed mucosal surfaces. The raw, perfused, and viable cut end of the bowel beyond the suture line heals together, just as does the cut end of the bronchus.

Getzen (1966), with his Navy stitch, demonstrated that a one-layer, partially everting, partially inverting anastomosis in the bowel is as reliable as an inverted suture line.

MECHANICAL SUTURES IN THE HEALING OF INTESTINAL WOUNDS

Wire sutures made of bronze, silver, steel, aluminum, tantalum — monofilament and braided — and in every size and range of ductility and tensile strength have been used by several generations of surgeons. Except for the suture manufacturers, we are long past the day of heated debate over the relative virtues of sutures of animal, vegetable, mineral, or petrochemical origin, recognizing the various virtues and deficiencies of each. Steel used in modern staples is relatively reactionless in the tissues, does not corrode, and possesses the appropriate physical properties so that the staple will maintain its shape. It is not deformed by mechanical forces of peristalsis and distention, and it is not weakened by the process of closure so that there might be any risk of breakage or fragmentation of the formed staple.

The instruments used to place and shape the staples into the B-form do not crush or devitalize the bowel. The B-form of the staples allows vessels to pass through the openings in the staples and between them so that the transected and stapled duodenal stump or gastric or colonic cut end is viable beyond the line of staples out to its very edge. The cut and stapled end can be seen to ooze a little fresh blood, which is of no consequence except to prove that the very edge of tissue is viable; occasionally there may even be a frank arterial bleeder which then has to be clamped and tied or coagulated. We have demonstrated that if the staples are driven across the stomach or duodenum, which is then bypassed by an anastomosis proximal to the stapling line, the mucosa is not crushed but remains intact and viable.

Healing of the transected bowel end, stapled mucosa-to-mucosa with a double row of staggered staples, occurs securely without the necessity for inversion or covering with adjacent tissues and without the formation of dense adhesions. Nutrition of the stapled bowel ends and healing across these raw ends are provided by the intrinsic circulation of the bowel wall, not by adjacent tissues.

Mechanical suture technics do not release the surgeon or the patient from the basic rules of surgery or the penalties for their violation. Bowel deprived of its blood supply or diseased or abused bowel may no more be relied upon to heal when stapled than when sutured with silk. The instruments will not permit surgeons to do what they otherwise could not do manually. They will not permit the safe performance of operative maneuvers by untrained or unskilled personnel, nor do they eliminate the necessity for rigorous surgical training, due regard for tissues, and, of course, training in the various manual technics of resection and anastomosis.

EXPERIMENTAL AND CLINICAL COMPARATIVE STUDIES OF MANUAL AND MECHANICAL SUTURE TECHNICS

Substantially less trauma is inflicted on the bowel by introducing 12 or 32 sutures with a single manipulation of an instrument than by picking up the bowel, inserting the needle, and passing the suture material through the tissues as many times. Gross and microscopic comparison of stapled and manually sewn suture lines shows extraordinarily little edema, hemorrhage, or necrosis with stapled closures and anastomoses in the first week or 10 days, at a time when manual closures and anastomoses show edema, ecchymosis, ragged tags of mucosa and muscularis, and loosened sutures hanging into the lumen. In controlled experiments in dogs, healing of stapled anastomoses has been as reliable as conventional, inverted, two-layer anastomoses of small bowel-to-small bowel, small bowel-to-large bowel, and large bowel-to-large bowel (Brolin and Ravitch, submitted for publication). This remained true when we stimulated intestinal peristalsis with daily doses of prostigmine and of castor oil, beginning immediately after the construction of the anastomosis.

Similarly, we have tested the relative dependability of conventional inverting manual anastomoses and stapled resections and anastomoses in dogs tested by (1) a 24-hour perforative peritonitis, (2) a 48-hour period of ischemia of devascularized small bowel, and (3) a 48-hour intestinal obstruction produced by simple ligation of the terminal ileum. Resection and anastomosis in small bowel in such preparations show slightly greater security with stapling (Kolter and Ravitch, unpublished data).

Satisfactorily controlled, comparative studies of stapled and manual resection and anastomosis in humans have not yet been reported. Chassin's (1978) substantial study seems to show no difference in results of manual and stapled anastomoses in the same hospital, in the same period of time, by the same surgeons, when the only difference in the clinical material was that substantially more of the stapled patients had peritonitis, perforative trauma, or other conditions requiring emergency operation under possibly unfavorable circumstances. Our own experience in comparing small-to-large and large-to-large bowel anastomoses operated on in a nonrandomized fashion in the same hospital, over the same period of time, by resident surgeons led us to the conclusion that stapling is at least as reliable as manual suturing although (as in Chassin's study) stapling technics were used essentially on the sicker emergency patients at night, whereas manual anastomoses were used on the less critically ill patients during the daytime (Thompson, Stremple, and Steichen, submitted for publication).

In another study, of ileal bladders created in the same university center, by the same surgeons, over the same period of time, in which the only difference was a functional end-to-end stapled anastomosis of the small bowel compared with a manual anastomosis, significant differences were found in the duration of operation, postoperative ileus, and hospital stay, as well as postoperative fever and wound infection, all favoring the use of staplers (Karamcheti and associates, 1978).

In a consecutive series of 64 jejunoileal shunts in which the jejunum and ileum were each transected and closed with a stapler, the bypassed bowel was anastomosed to the colon with the stapling machine, and the jejunoileal anastomosis was performed with the stapling machine, no cases of peritonitis, intra-abdominal abscess, fecal fistula, or operative deaths from any cause occurred (Ravitch and Brolin, in press).

HISTORY OF STAPLING INSTRUMENTS

The principle of stapling the gastrointestinal tract is best known to surgeons as embodied in the widely used von Petz instrument. Aladar von Petz, in 1921, at the

Eighth Congress of the Hungarian Surgical Society, presented what was, in essence, a giant Payr clamp, in which two rows of rather gross staples of German silver were loaded by hand and sequentially driven in by a bar advanced by the turning of a wheel (von Petz, 1924, 1927). In fact, the use of staples in surgery originated with von Petz's professor, Humer Hültl (1909, 1910) of Budapest. At the Second Congress of the Hungarian Surgical Society, in 1908, he presented an instrument for use in the resection of distal gastric lesions. The instrument was massively heavy (3.5 kg.) and laborious to assemble and load. However, it placed two double rows of fine steel-wire staples (similar to those in use today) so that the stomach and duodenum could be transected, leaving a double row of staples on either side of the section. The staples were closed in the B-shape that has been standard ever since. Hültl — and for that matter von Petz and all their successors — employed the instrument only for temporary closure of the transected viscus, the stapled end of which was then inverted in the conventional way. Hültl's instrument seems to have been fairly widely known at that time. Willie Meyer (1915), for instance, in New York, referred to using it for the construction of a Beck-Jianu gastric tube for replacement of the thoracic esophagus, apparently thinking that mention of the Hültl apparatus required no particular exposition.

A substantial advance was contributed by Friedrich of Ulm (1934). Although he, too, used German silver staples, which formed in the familiar B-shape, the staples could be preloaded by hand into interchangeable cartridges, allowing for repeated use of the same instrument in the same operation. A squeeze of the handles closed down the two parallel jaws and gradually compressed the tissues to be stapled. A second compression of the handles, after release of a catch, drove in the staples. Sandor (1936), Tomoda (1937a, 1937b), and others contributed minor modifications to the Hültl and von Petz instruments. Nakayama simplified von Petz's instrument by removing the wheel and the advancing bar. The staples were loaded into slots in the jaws of the instrument; the instrument was closed and the staples were driven home with a huge pair of pliers to press down the housing that held the staple pushers.

The operation of surgical stapling instruments, from Hültl's time on, requires two steps. In the first step, the tissues are approximated to the degree required for appropriate penetration and formation of the staples. There is no violent compression, as with a desk stapler, for instance. In the second step, the staples are driven through the tissues, which are held so that they do not slide or tear on the sharpened points of the staples. In the same step the staples are driven through the tissues and formed on the anvils of the lower jaw into the proper B-shape. Neither the instrument nor the staples crush tissue, which is viable out to the cut end.

The development of surgical stapling instruments received an enormous impetus as a result of the work done in Moscow at the Scientific Research Institute for Experimental Surgical Apparatus. The first instrument appears to have been that of Gudov (1950) for vascular anastomosis. An entire family of extremely complicated vascular staplers was developed, sharply limited in their utility because they were applicable only to normal vessels and required longer free segments than those needed in a manual anastomosis (Androsov, 1956). On the other hand, they produced mathematically precise everting anastomoses without the slightest constriction. Next, instruments were devised for closure of the gastrointestinal tract: for mucosa-to-mucosa anastomosis with a subsequent inversion and for serosa-to-serosa anastomosis of adjacent loops of bowel; a ponderous but ingenious instrument for stapling the cut end of the stomach in one operation and then inverting the cut end with the machine in a second step; and even a mechanically ingenious but technically unsatisfactory instrument for inverted end-to-end anastomoses of bowel (Kalinina, 1964a, 1964b, 1967).

Our experience with stapling began some 20 years ago with the Russian instruments and has continued progressively with development of the American instruments (Ravitch and associates, 1964; Ravitch and associates, 1966; Ravitch and Rivarola, 1966; Ravitch and Steichen, 1972; Ravitch, Ong, and Gazzola, 1974; Ravitch and Steichen, 1979; Steichen, Talbert, and Ravitch, 1968; Steichen, 1968; Steichen and Ravitch, 1973; Steichen, 1977). The Russian instruments are finished by hand so that parts are not interchangeable and they must be hand-loaded, a process that requires a partial disassembling of some of the instruments in order to replace the expended cartridge. Additionally, multiple fine moving parts are incorporated in the basic instrument, creating difficulties in cleaning and maintenance and when breakage occurs. Each instrument can take only a single size of cartridge or arrangement of staples, so an impressive array of individual instruments must be available at every operation. Instruments that contained permanent knife edges obviously suffered from the inevitable dulling of the knife.

The American instruments are characterized by functional construction, better balance, and the provision of preloaded, presterilized, disposable, color-coded cartridges that can be inserted in the instruments without disassembling them at all. Fine moving parts and knife blades have been incorporated in the disposable cartridges, leaving the basic instrument a relatively simple, trouble-free, controlled-compression device.

THE CONTEMPORARY AMERICAN INSTRUMENTS

Four basic stapling instruments are currently available for use in operations upon the gastrointestinal tract. The *TA instruments (thoracoabdominal)* consist of two nesting Ls; the long vertical arms slide upon each other when a wing nut at the end is turned. The short horizontal jaws approximated by this maneuver contain in the upper jaw the removable staple cartridge and in the lower jaw the removable anvil for forming the staples. The jaws are approximated until verniers on the two vertical members of the Ls indicate that the tissues to be sutured have been compressed to the required degree. A squeeze of the handle now drives in two staggered rows of staples, 30, 55, or 90 mm. long, depending upon the instrument. They are used to produce terminal or tangential mucosa-to-mucosa closures (and, in the special instance of the Kock continent ileostomy pouch, a serosa-to-serosa closure). Color coding indicates staples of 3.8 or 4.5 mm. height to be used for bowel of varying thickness. The very fine white cartridge fits in the 30 mm. instrument, for closure of bowel in children, for occlusion of the portal vein, or closure of the pulmonary vein or artery.

The *instrument of gastrointestinal anastomosis (GIA)* consists of two long, slender limbs, for carrying the disposable staple cartridge and disposable anvil, respectively. The disposable activating assembly consists of two bars and a central blade. The two outer bars drive in two rows of staples, and the central cutting blade follows at a distance of a staple and a half behind them. When the two halves of the instrument are mated and locked and the assembly pressed home, two double, staggered rows of staples are introduced, suturing the two limbs of bowel together, while the knife divides the tissue between the two middle rows, creating the anastomotic opening, with a double row of staples on either side of the cut (see Figs. 23–5 and 23–7). Placed across the bowel, the instrument divides the bowel, simultaneously stapling both ends (Fig. 23–1). Inserted through stab wounds in two apposed bowel loops, the instrument staples them together and creates an anastomosis at the same time. The orifice made for the insertion of the instrument remains to be closed mucosa-to-mucosa by application of the TA instrument, or conventionally by manual suturing (see Fig. 23–6).

The instrument is supplied with two sizes of staples, for adults and for children. Supplied without a knife blade, the instrument inserts four rows of staples for use in special situations, for example, the control of varices, by stapling first the anterior and then the posterior walls of the stomach below the esophagogastric junction (Rinecker and Danek, 1975), or ensuring the persistence of the nipple in the Kock ileostomy by placing one limb of the instrument from within the pouch into the lumen of the nipple and the other, still from within the pouch, on the outside of the nipple, applying this three or four times around the nipple circumference (Steichen, 1977).

The *LDS (ligating and dividing stapler) instrument* places two clips of stainless steel on either side of the dividing blade, thus simultaneously ligating and dividing tissues picked up in its U-curved tip. The instrument contains 15 pairs of staples for repetitive use. The U-shaped staples used in this instrument encircle the structures to be ligated and are then compressed into a semi-lunar curve, appearing as little curved radiopacities in the abdominal film (Fig. 23–2A).

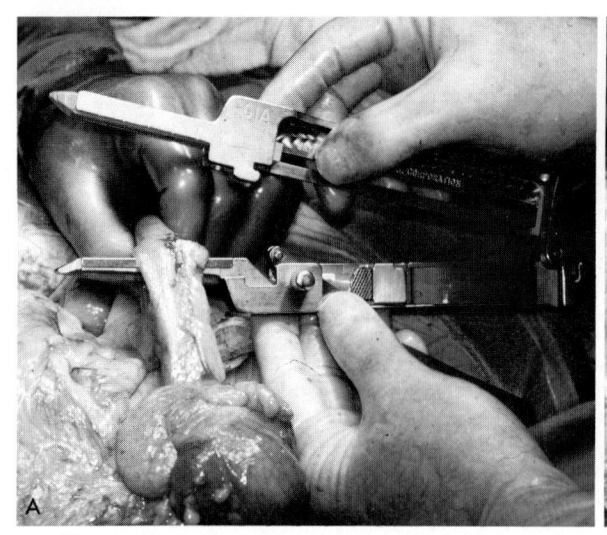

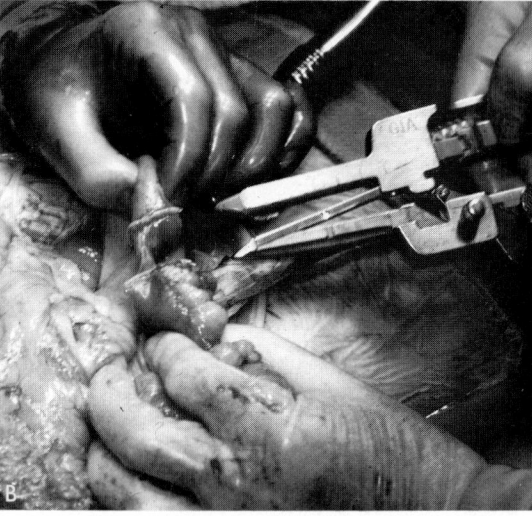

Figure 23–1. *Simultaneous transection and closure of bowel.* A, The bowel is placed between the arms of the GIA instrument. The instrument halves are then mated and closed, and the pusher-knife assembly is activated. B, The GIA instrument is being removed, showing the transection of the bowel and the closure of both bowel ends with a double, staggered row of staples. (Reprinted with permission of U.S. Surgical Corporation, Stamford, Conn. © U.S. Surgical Corporation 1974, all rights reserved.)

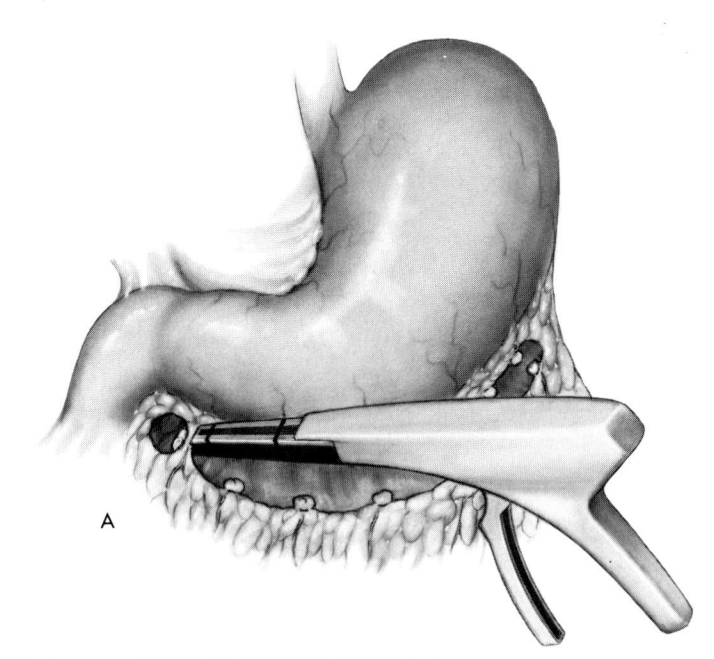

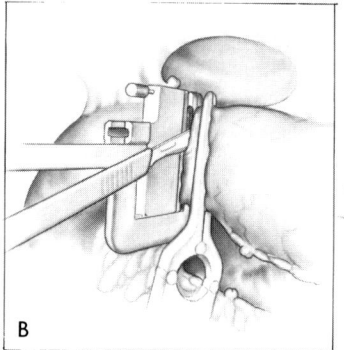

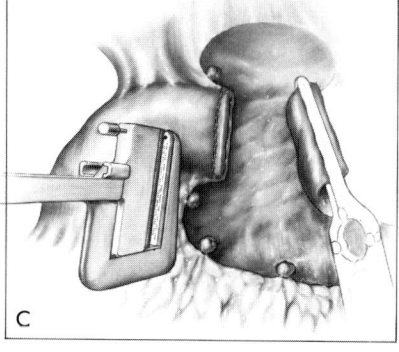

Figure 23–2. Billroth II gastrectomy. A, The greater curvature is liberated with the LDS instrument. Reasonable bites of tissue are developed by the assistant, who passes a curved Rankin clamp through the gastrocolic ligament under the vessels. (This part of the procedure is not shown in the drawing.) As the clamp is withdrawn the operator follows it back with the lower lip of the LDS and the freed tissue is then held in the hooklike tip of the instrument. As the instrument is activated, two clips of stainless steel are introduced on either side of a dividing blade, and the vessels and surrounding fat are transected and ligated on both sides of this section.

The duodenum is closed with the use of the TA-55 stapler, just distal to the pylorus. The duodenum is then transected between the stapler and a Payr clamp applied to the pylorus. C, The double, staggered row of staples closing the duodenal stump is clearly visible. This suture line is not reinforced by any manual sutures. D, Next the antrectomy is completed by transecting the stomach between a row of staples introduced with the TA-90 instrument and a large Payr clamp. The specimen is removed.

Illustration continued on opposite page

MECHANICAL SUTURES

Figure 23-2 *Continued.*

E, Gastrointestinal continuity is then re-established by performing a gastroenterostomy using the GIA instrument. One arm of the instrument is introduced through a stab wound in the posterior wall of the stomach near the greater curvature, some 2 cm. proximal to the gastric closure line. The other arm of the instrument is introduced through a stab wound in the jejunum. By activating the pusher-knife assembly of the GIA instrument, the septum represented by the gastric and jejunal walls is transected while a double row of staples is introduced on either side of this transection. The knife is shorter than the staple line by 1.5 staples. This insures a safe suture at the far end of the gastroenterostomy.

F, The GIA instrument is removed; stay sutures are introduced to approximate both corners and the mid-portion of the now common GIA introduction site. The TA-55 stapler is used to close the opening made for the introduction of the GIA instrument.

G, The gastroenterostomy is completed. Great care should be taken that the entire circumference of the GIA opening is visible beyond the jaws of the TA instrument in order to insure complete and safe closure of the opening. The excess tissue is resected, again using the TA blade as a guide. The narrow band of posterior gastric wall situated between the gastric closure and the gastroenterostomy has not been a problem in large numbers of operations performed by this technic.

(Reprinted with permission of U.S. Surgical Corporation, Stamford, Conn. © U.S. Surgical Corporation 1974, all rights reserved.)

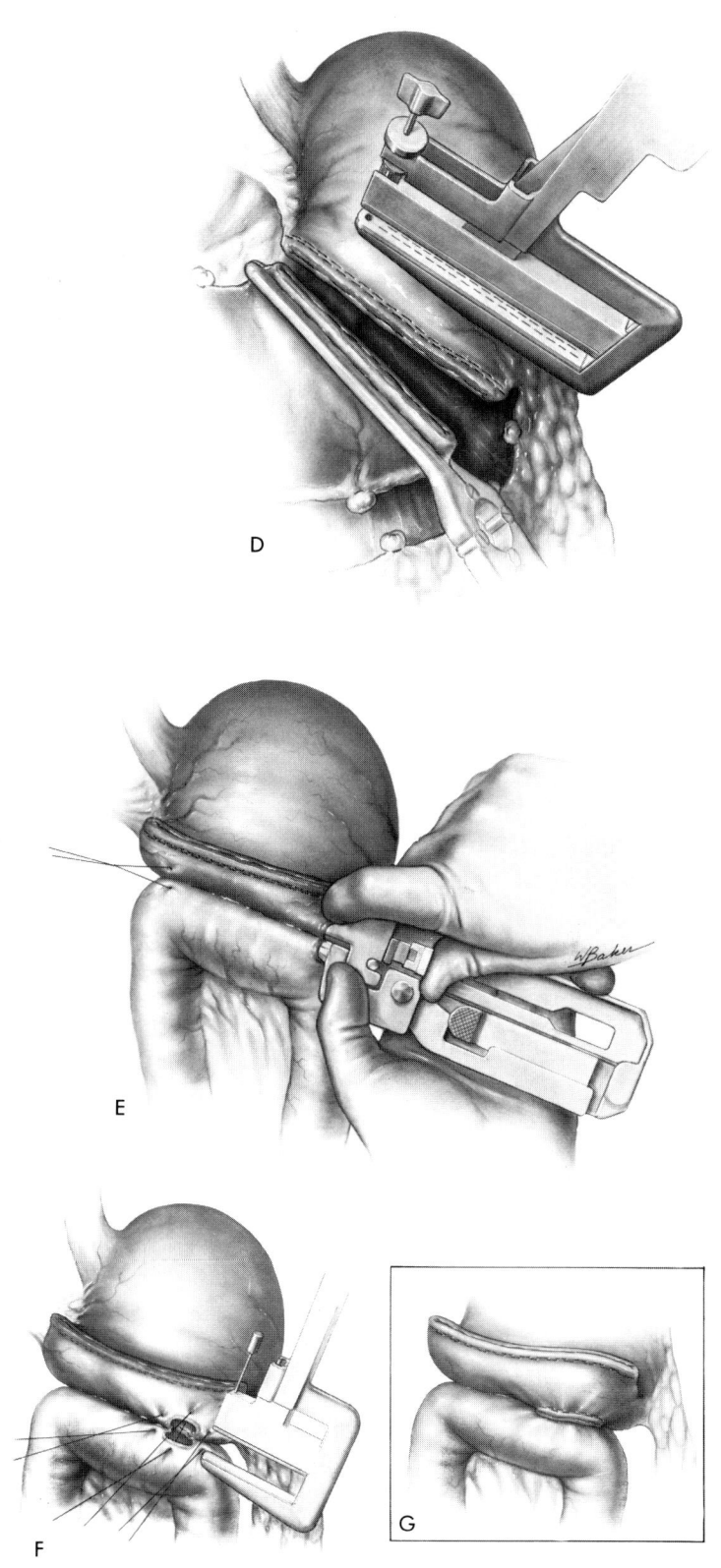

The *EEA (end-to-end anastomosis) instrument*, a tubular instrument much like a sigmoidoscope, has at one end a handle for activating the instrument, and a wing nut for separating or approximating the staple and anvil halves of the disposable cartridge. At the other end, the disposable cartridge consists of a cylinder capped by a hemispheric nose cone. The cylinder contains the cartridge with two staggered rows of staples, the pushers to drive the staples forward, and a circular knife just within the ring of staples. The nose cone contains the anvil for formation of the staples, and within it a heavy plastic ring against which the circular knife cuts out the double diaphragm of bowel. For a low anterior resection the instrument is passed through the anus (see Fig. 23–9); for an esophagogastric anastomosis, it is passed into the esophagus through a gastrotomy; for a Billroth II gastrojejunostomy, it is passed into the stomach through a gastrotomy, as shown in Figure 23–3E and F for a Billroth I.

The segments to be anastomosed are drawn up by pursestrings around the nose cone and around the proximal portion of the cartridge and approximated by turning the wing nut. Compression of the handle simultaneously drives in the double staggered rows of staples and the circular knife, which cuts off the double diaphragm formed by the two pursestring bowel ends, creating an instantaneous inverting end-to-end anastomosis. The instrument is supplied with cartridges having outside diameters of 31, 28.6 and 25 mm., which produce anastomoses 21, 18, and 15 mm. in internal diameter, respectively. The largest cartridge is readily accommodated by the adult rectum and the smaller ones will usually be accommodated by the adult esophagus.

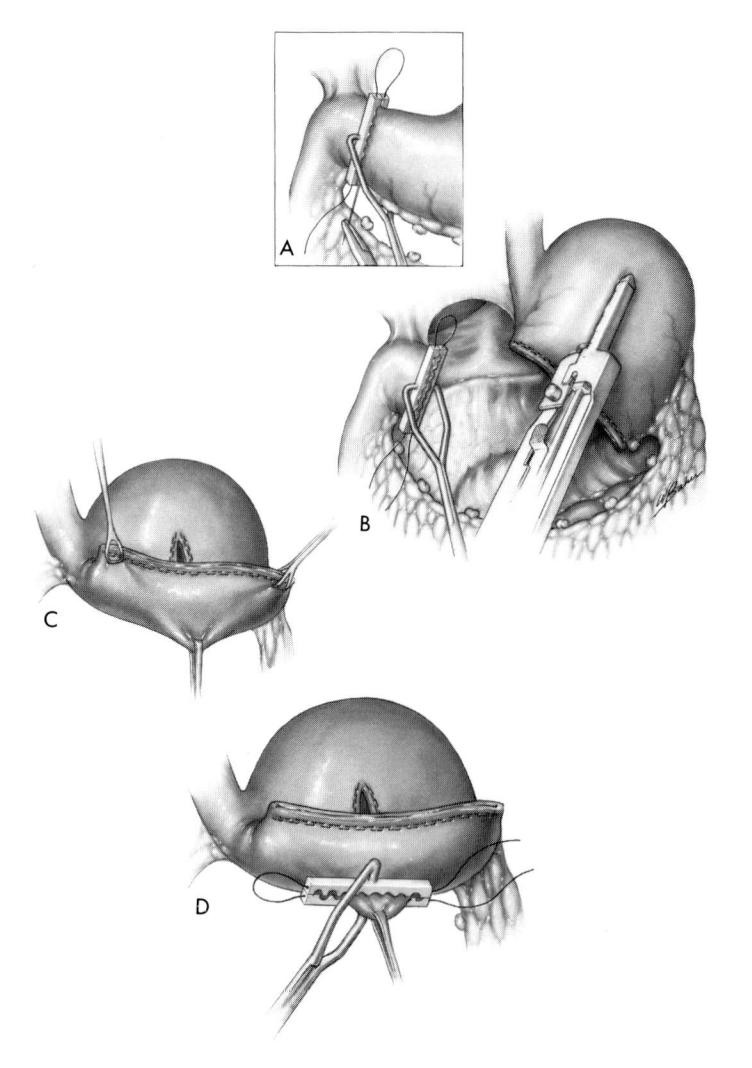

Figure 23–3. *Billroth I gastrectomy using the EEA instrument. A,* After liberating the greater and lesser curvatures and the first portion of the duodenum, the modified Furniss clamp is applied immediately distal to the pylorus. The serrations of the modified Furniss clamp have been cut so as not to digitate. When the needle is passed through in one direction and returned in the other, it grasps only one wall of the bowel on each side.

B, The antrectomy has been completed by transecting the duodenum proximal to the Furniss clamp and the stomach distal to a row of sutures placed with the TA-90 stapler on the gastric side. Through a small stab wound on the anterior wall of the stomach, approximately 3 cm. proximal to the gastric closure, the GIA stapler loaded with the SGIA cartridge is introduced and activated.

C, The anterior gastrotomy has been accomplished with the use of the SGIA staples. The clean gastrotomy is bordered by a double row of staggered staples that produce perfect hemostasis, thus avoiding the bothersome bleeding so often associated with a gastrotomy. The gastric closure line is pulled upward and the posterior wall of the stomach — future site of the anastomosis to the duodenum — is pulled inferiorly with an Allis clamp.

D, The Furniss clamp is applied on the posterior wall, 2 cm. proximal to the gastric closure. The pursestring suture is again applied by passing a straight needle carrying a monofilament nylon suture back and forth. The portion of gastric wall pulled through the jaws of the Furniss clamp is excised.
Illustration continued on opposite page

Figure 23–3 *Continued.*

E, The EEA instrument carrying the cartridge but not the anvil is introduced through the anterior gastrotomy, and the central rod of the instrument is pushed out through the center of the pursestring suture, surrounding the opening created previously in the posterior wall of the stomach. The anvil is now attached to the central rod, and the pursestring suture is tightened.

F, The anvil, separated from the EEA cartridge, is introduced into the lumen of the duodenum, and the duodenal pursestring suture is tied around the central rod. The anvil and the cartridge are brought together by turning in a clockwise direction the wing nut at the end of the EEA instrument. The instrument handle is squeezed, and this maneuver drives in a double, staggered, circular row of staples and advances a circular knife inside the ring of staples, cutting the double diaphragm made by the two pursestrings of stomach and duodenum, respectively.

G, The EEA instrument is then disengaged from the gastroduodenostomy. It is removed from the stomach, and the gastrotomy is closed with the TA-55 instrument. The anastomosis between stomach and duodenum, placed on the posterior wall of the stomach, is clearly visible by transparency.

H, At the end of the operation, the gastroduodenostomy shows a decumbent position, and the previous gastric closure is displaced upward, onto what becomes now the anterior wall of the stomach. The EEA introduction site is again visible. Because of excellent blood supply, various suture lines in the stomach heal well, and so far in an important series of cases the relative proximity of various suture lines has not been a problem.

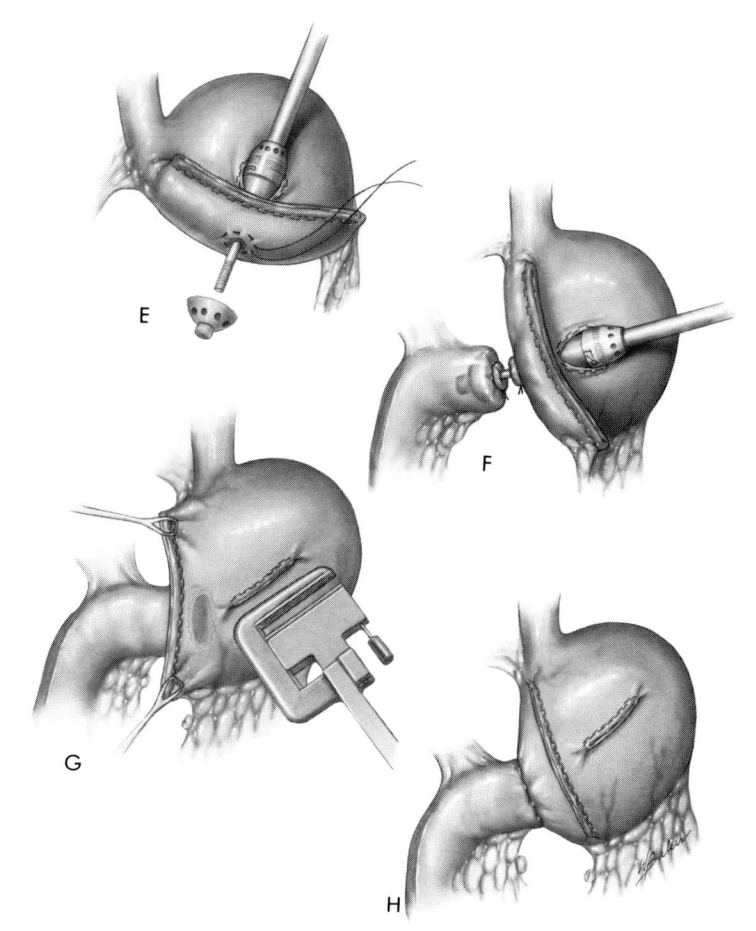

(Reprinted with permission of U.S. Surgical Corporation, Stamford, Conn. © U.S. Surgical Corporation 1974, all rights reserved.)

The *SFM (skin and fascia) stapler*, with the fascia stapler load is used for closing the linea alba in midline incisions. The skin staples produce clean skin closures and no cross hatching, such as may be observed in skin closures with other suture materials; there is essentially no reaction, and the staples are easily removed with a special disposable device. This is the single instrument thus far that is also provided in a totally disposable form.

SURGICAL TECHNICS WITH STAPLING INSTRUMENTS

The instruments of the TA series are employed to close the cut ends of transected bowel or the edges of incised bowel (Fig. 23–3G, H). In transecting the duodenum, one jaw of the instrument is placed under the duodenum, the retaining pin inserted, the instrument closed down, the staples driven home, and the duodenum proximal to the instrument transected with a knife running along the instrument's edge (see Fig. 23 2B). A Zenker's pharyngeal diverticulum, or Meckel's diverticulum with a small base, is conveniently drawn through the instrument, which is placed down to the base; the instrument is activated and the diverticulum excised peripheral to the instrument. In the resection of a mural lesion of the stomach, a bowel leiomyoma, a sessile polyp, or a nodule of ectopic pancreas, the portion of the viscus containing the lesion is merely pulled through the jaws of the clamp which is then operated to provide a secure closure. The full-thickness portion

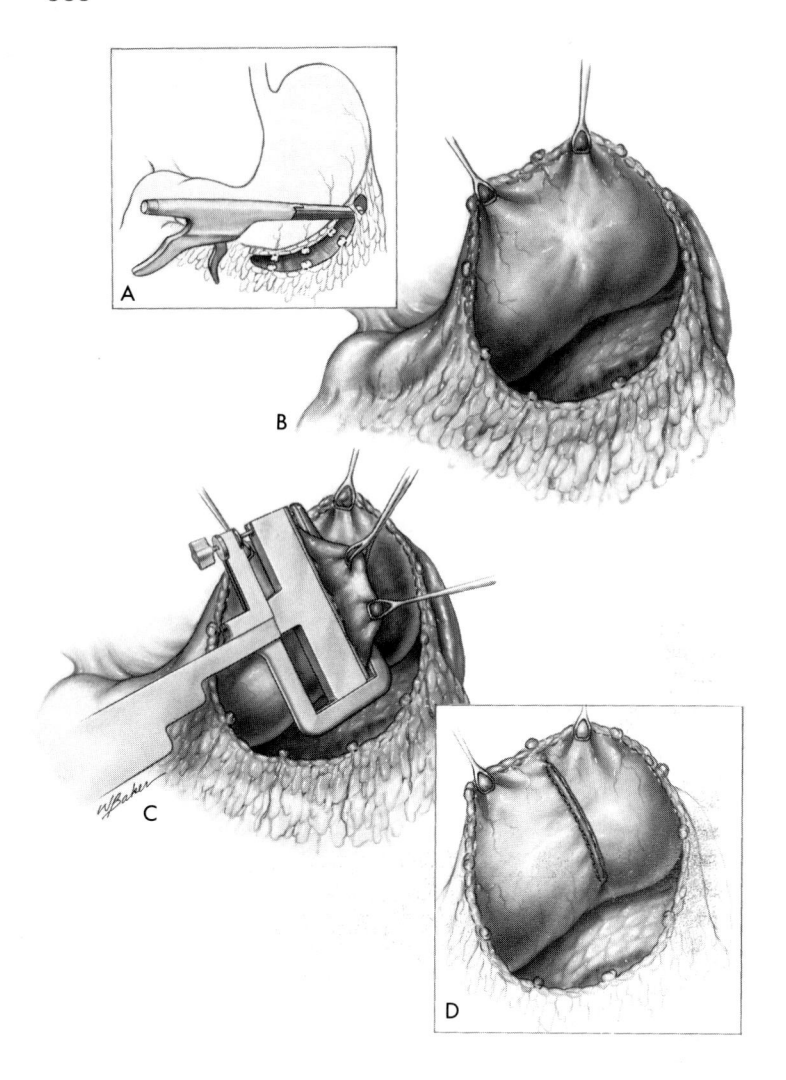

Figure 23-4. *Resection of a mural lesion of the stomach. A,* To expose a nodule of ectopic pancreas on the posterior wall of the stomach, the greater curvature is liberated with the LDS instrument, applied repeatedly to the gastrocolic ligament. *B,* The stomach is rotated along its long axis and the mural lesion on the posterior wall of the stomach is clearly visible.

C, The portion of the gastric wall containing the lesion is pulled through the jaws of the TA-90 instrument, which is applied at right angle to the long axis of the stomach. The instrument jaws are approximated, the staples are placed, and the full thickness of the gastric wall containing the lesion is resected, using the jaws of the TA instrument to guide the scalpel. *D,* Removal of the TA stapler shows a nice and secure closure. The specimen is sent to the pathology department for frozen section; further operative maneuvers will depend on the histology of the specimen that was removed. In this patient, no further operative treatment was needed.

(Reprinted with permission of U.S. Surgical Corporation, Stamford, Conn. © U.S. Surgical Corporation 1974, all rights reserved.)

of the viscus wall containing the lesion is resected, using the jaws of the TA instrument to guide the scalpel (Fig. 23-4).

The Heineke-Mikulicz pyloroplasty is easily closed transversely with the TA-55 stapler if the duodenum is not too edematous, and a duodenotomy made for exposure of the ampulla of Vater is readily closed with the same TA instrument. These suture lines are not reinforced or inverted, and this practice appears to be widely, if not universally, used by American surgeons employing staples. The TA instrument is advantageously used in dismantling humanly created anatomic changes or pathologic fistulous communications. Thus, in taking down a gastroenterostomy, the jaws of the instrument are slid onto the stomach as far to the gastric side of the anastomosis as required. The stomach is stapled and cut away, requiring no further attention so far as this portion of the operation is concerned. The jejunum then can be transected proximal and distal to the gastroenterostomy with the GIA instrument that is described in the next paragraph.

The transection of the small and large bowel is almost invariably performed by slipping the bowel between the jaws of the GIA instrument; operating the instrument transects the bowel and leaves both cut ends with a staggered, double row of staples, regardless of whether further steps of the operation will require one or both ends to be anastomosed, resected, or brought out as ileostomy or colostomy. There is no need to leave dangling Kocher clamps on bowel loops or to cover the ends with rubber gloves or laparotomy pads. The substantial advantage of both the TA and GIA instruments for transecting and sealing the cut end of bowel is that one need clear only a bare centimeter of bowel of its mesentery to operate the instruments safely. This avoids the risk, in manual anastomoses, of devascularizing the bowel in order to perform a careful anastomosis under direct vision. Nor is it necessary to leave mesenteric fat close to the cut edge to prevent ischemia, so that it is difficult to place the sutures securely at the mesenteric border.

For gastrointestinal anastomoses, the GIA instrument is inserted either through the excised antimesenteric corners of the stapled closures of the bowel or through cautery or knife punctures in the intact bowel. Operation of the instrument staples two loops together and provides an opening between them, the edges of which are bordered by a double row of staggered staples. It is necessary then only to close the fused GIA insertion wounds, and this is usually done mucosa-to-mucosa with a TA instrument of appropriate size (Figs. 23–5, 23–6, and 23–7).

The Finney and Jaboulay pyloroplasties are nicely performed with the GIA instrument, depending upon whether it is inserted downward from a duodenal opening for the Finney pyloroplasty (Fig. 23–8) or upward from separate openings in the duodenum and greater curvature of the stomach for the Jaboulay pyloroplasty. In either case, the single opening remaining after withdrawal of the GIA instrument is closed either manually or with the TA instrument. Practice varies as to reinforcement of staple suture lines with silk. For a Jaboulay pyloroplasty, we do place a single suture at the lower angle to avoid excess tension by possibly atonic and overfilled stomach, and many surgeons place a suture between the loops at the level of the tips of the GIA prongs. By the same token, in a low

Text continued on page 593

Figure 23–5. *Posterior gastroenterostomy.* A, Following liberation of the greater curvature, the posterior wall of the stomach, near the pylorus, is pulled through an incision in the avascular portion of the transverse mesocolon.

B, The anterior and posterior lips of the mesocolic opening are sutured to the gastric wall anteriorly and posteriorly. Sufficient wall is kept free to allow for the comfortable introduction of one arm of the GIA instrument into the gastric lumen through a small stab wound. Similarly, through a small stab wound in the jejunum, near the ligament of Treitz, the other arm of the GIA is introduced into the jejunal lumen. The instrument is matched, locked, and activated, creating an instantaneous gastroenterostomy.

C, Following removal of the GIA instrument, the now common opening is closed in an everting fashion with a TA-55 instrument. Care is taken to keep the ends of the GIA suture lines apart.

(Reprinted with permission of U.S. Surgical Corporation, Stamford, Conn. © U.S. Surgical Corporation 1974, all rights reserved.)

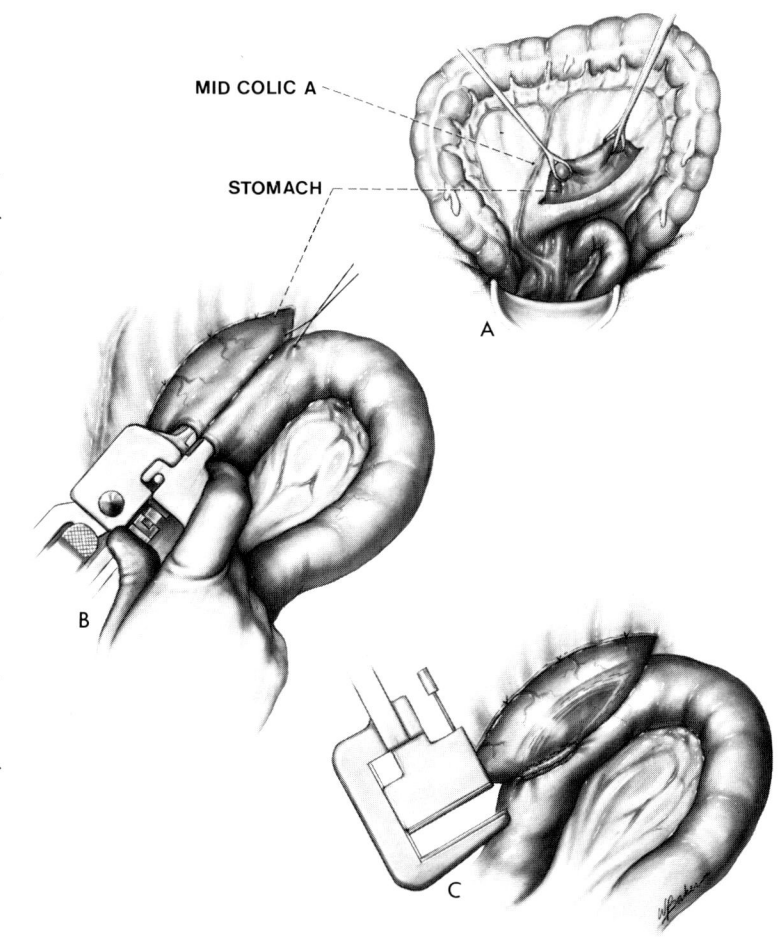

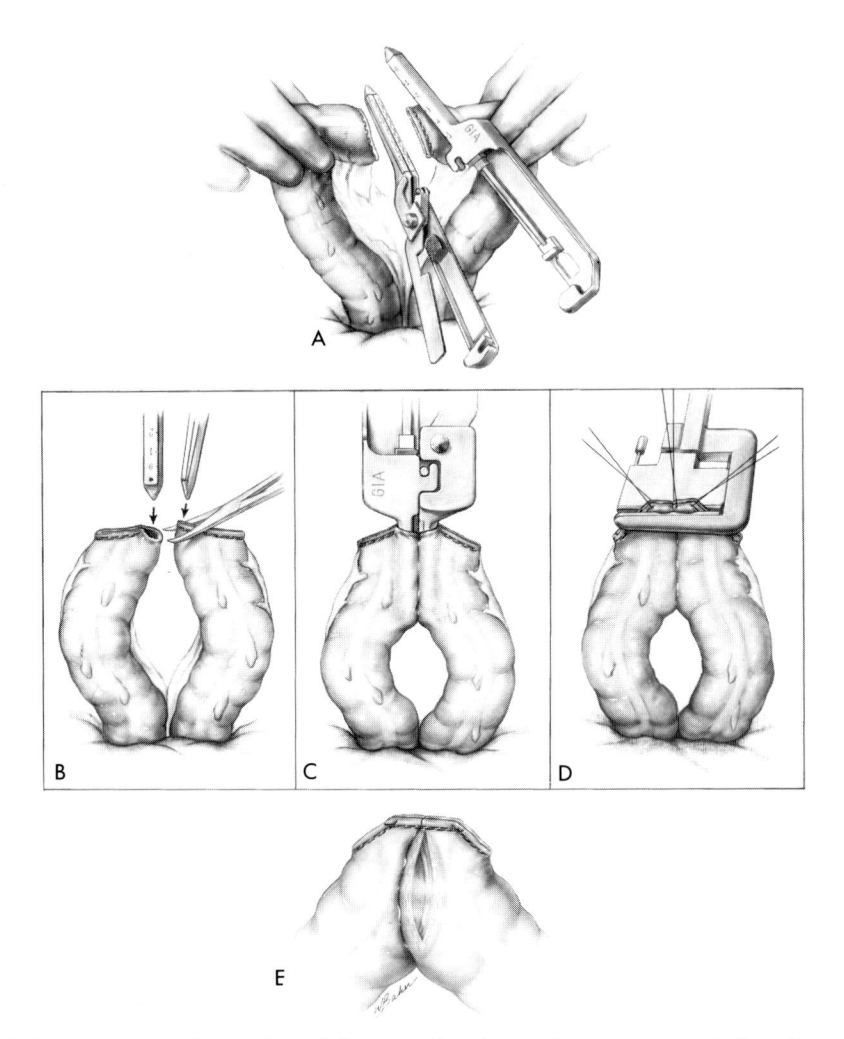

Figure 23–6. *Anatomic side-to-side and functional end-to-end anastomosis.* A, Bowel transection is performed proximal and distal to the lesion to be resected, using the GIA instrument as illustrated in Figure 23–1A and B. B, Following removal of the specimen, the proximal and distal closed bowel segments are approximated in a shotgun fashion and the antimesenteric or antimesocolic corners of bowel are excised. C, One arm of the GIA instrument is placed into each bowel lumen. The instrument is matched and locked. The pusher-knife assembly is advanced, and an instantaneous side-to-side anastomosis is created.

D, The now common GIA introduction opening is closed with the application of the TA-55 instrument. Again, great care is taken that the total circumference of the GIA opening be visible beyond the jaws of the TA-55 stapler. E, The excess tissue from the GIA introduction site has been removed, using the TA-55 as a guide. Because of the construction of this anastomosis, avoiding any blind ends, it does function as an end-to-end anastomosis.

(Reprinted with permission of U.S. Surgical Corporation, Stamford, Conn. © U.S. Surgical Corporation 1974, all rights reserved.)

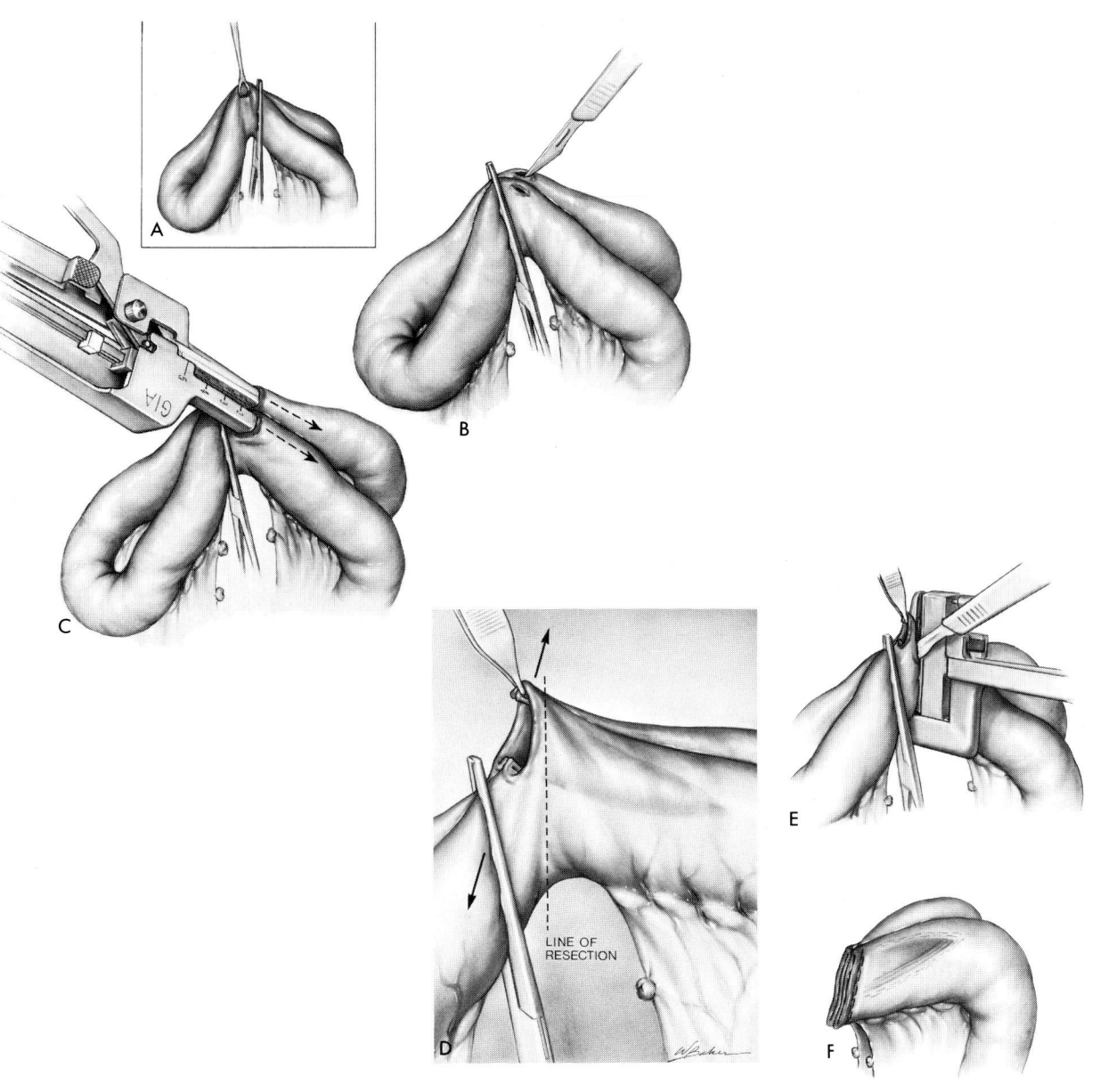

Figure 23–7. *Modified functional end-to-end anastomosis. A,* With this technic, transection of the bowel and removal of the specimen are performed after the anatomic side-to-side anastomosis has been established. In this particular case, resection of a small bowel loop is illustrated. The extent of the resection is defined first, and the bowel to be resected is freed with its corresponding mesentery. As the planned extent of resection is completed, the future afferent and efferent loops are brought together in a parallel fashion and held by a Kocher clamp placed across all four bowel walls.

B, Stab wounds are produced in both the afferent and efferent loops proximally, respectively, distal to the Kocher clamp.

C, The GIA instrument is then positioned, with one arm of the instrument going into each one of the bowel loops. The instrument is activated, and an anatomic side-to-side anastomosis is created, with the specimen still attached to the anastomosis.

D, After the anastomosis has been accomplished, the specimen will now be resected along the line shown in this drawing. In this fashion all four walls of the bowel will be stapled, the angles of the GIA application will stay separated, and the GIA orifice will be closed simultaneously.

E, The TA-55 instrument has been applied, bringing together all four walls of small bowel. The instrument has been activated and the specimen containing the GIA introduction orifice is removed, using the TA instrument as a convenient guide for the transection.

F, The final status of the anastomosis is clearly seen. Again this type of an anastomosis functions in an end-to-end fashion. There have been no problems with that part of the bowel that is situated peripheral to the TA-55 suture line despite the fact that this suture line is placed through four and not two thicknesses of bowel wall.

(Reprinted with permission of U.S. Surgical Corporation, Stamford, Conn. © U.S. Surgical Corporation 1974, all rights reserved.)

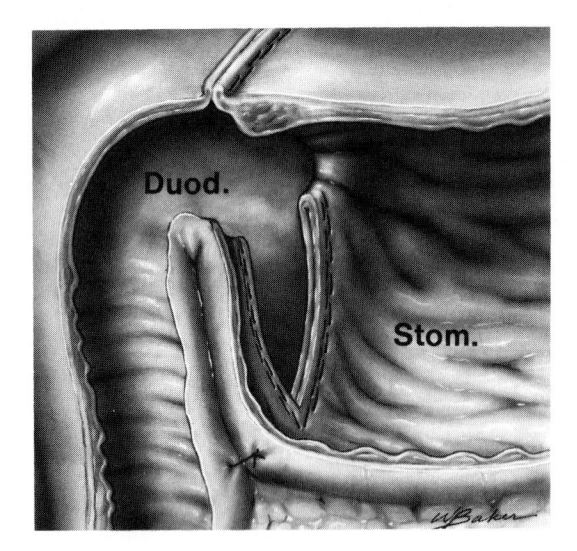

Figure 23–8. *Finney pyloroplasty.* The final result obtained in the creation of a Finney pyloroplasty. The GIA instrument was introduced in this patient through a stab wound of the pylorus. One arm of the GIA instrument is positioned in the stomach and the other arm in the first portion of the duodenum. The instrument is activated, and an instantaneous gastroduodenostomy is created. A single silk suture is placed at the lower angle, to avoid excess tension by possibly atonic or overfilled stomach. The GIA introduction site is closed transversely with a TA-55 stapler. (Reprinted with permission of U.S. Surgical Corporation, Stamford, Conn. © U.S. Surgical Corporation 1974, all rights reserved.)

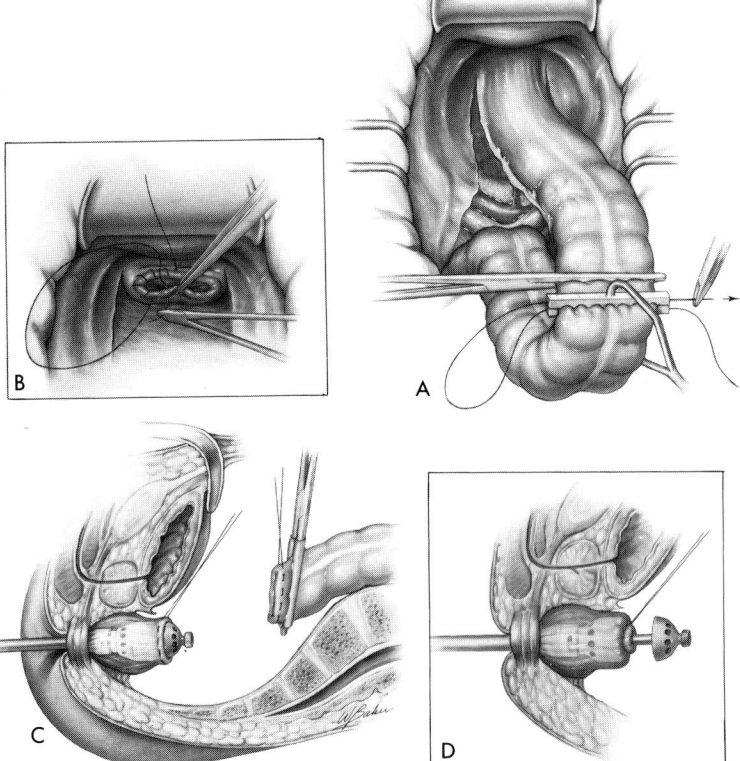

Figure 23–9. *Low rectal anastomosis using the EEA instrument. A,* The proximal pursestring suture is shown being placed with the help of a modified Furniss clamp. Since the serrations of the clamp do not digitate, as the needle is passed in a to-and-fro fashion, only the anterior and the posterior walls of the bowel, respectively, are penetrated by the needle and the suture.

B, In a narrow male pelvis, for instance, especially if the anastomosis will be very low, it is difficult to use the Furniss clamp satisfactorily. We therefore use an over-and-over pursestring suture with strong, smooth, monofilament material. A pursestring made in this fashion also avoids the introduction of excessive bowel wall into the limited space within the EEA cartridge.

C, The EEA instrument, with the anvil closed against the cartridge, is introduced through the rectum. As the anvil penetrates into the pelvis and is seen beyond the rectal pursestring, the rectal suture is held tight, and the anvil is separated from the cartridge.

D, With the anvil separated from the cartridge, the rectal pursestring suture is tied very precisely around the central rod. Great care is taken to make sure that this pursestring encompasses the complete circumference of the bowel as the knot is brought down.

Illustration continued on opposite page

SURGICAL TECHNICS WITH STAPLING INSTRUMENTS

anterior rectal anastomosis performed with the GIA we place a single manual suture at the lowest end.

The GIA instrument has been accepted by pediatric surgeons as providing the ideal technic for dividing the common colorectal wall in the performance of the Duhamel operation for Hirschsprung's disease (Steichen, Talbert, and Ravitch, 1968).

The LDS instrument has apparently required more skill, familiarity, and practice than have the others, and a bit of experience-bred dexterity may be required for its use. We find it secure; an enormous time-saver in the ordinary resection of bowel. It is not useful in patients with an extremely fat or thickened mesentery. The assistant passes a closed, curved, Rankin clamp through the mesentery under the vessel and, as the clamp is withdrawn, the operator follows it back with the lower lip of the LDS (see Fig. 23–2A). Tissues must not be on tension when stapled. The instrument has a fail-safe mechanism, which prevents it from being activated when the last staple load has been discharged.

It will be perceived readily that, in a single operation, several or most of these instruments may be applied, most particularly in such extensive procedures as replacement of the esophagus by reversed gastric tube or segment of colon, replacement of the stomach by jejunal pouch, and construction of a continent (Kock) ileostomy.

In extremely low rectal anastomoses, the EEA instrument, which produces an inverting, direct, end-to-end, circular anastomosis with a double staggered row of staples, comes closest to making it possible for an experienced surgeon to do what might not be possible manually (Goligher and associates, 1979). The anastomosis can be made within easy reach of the finger (and the inversion is so minimal that the anastomotic line is barely palpable) (Fig. 23–9).

Figure 23–9 *Continued.* *E*, The proximal colon is now brought over the anvil, and the proximal pursestring suture is tied around the central rod. By turning the wing nut in a clockwise fashion, both segments of bowel are apposed.

F, The proximal colon and the rectum have now been approximated in a precise fashion. The handle of the instrument is squeezed, and this drives in a double, staggered, circular row of staples and advances at the same time a circular knife, cutting out the double diaphragm made by the two apposed pursestring bowel ends.

G, By rotating the wing nut at the end of the instrument in a counterclockwise fashion, anvil and cartridge are separated.

H, After separating the anvil and cartridge, the instrument is rotated and gently maneuvered up and down to disengage it from the anastomosis. With the surgeon gently pulling the anterior rim of the anastomosis over the flat, dome-shaped anvil (like removing a tire from a bicycle rim), the entire instrument can be removed from the anastomotic site with great ease.

(Reprinted with permission of U.S. Surgical Corporation, Stamford, Conn. © U.S. Surgical Corporation 1974, all rights reserved.)

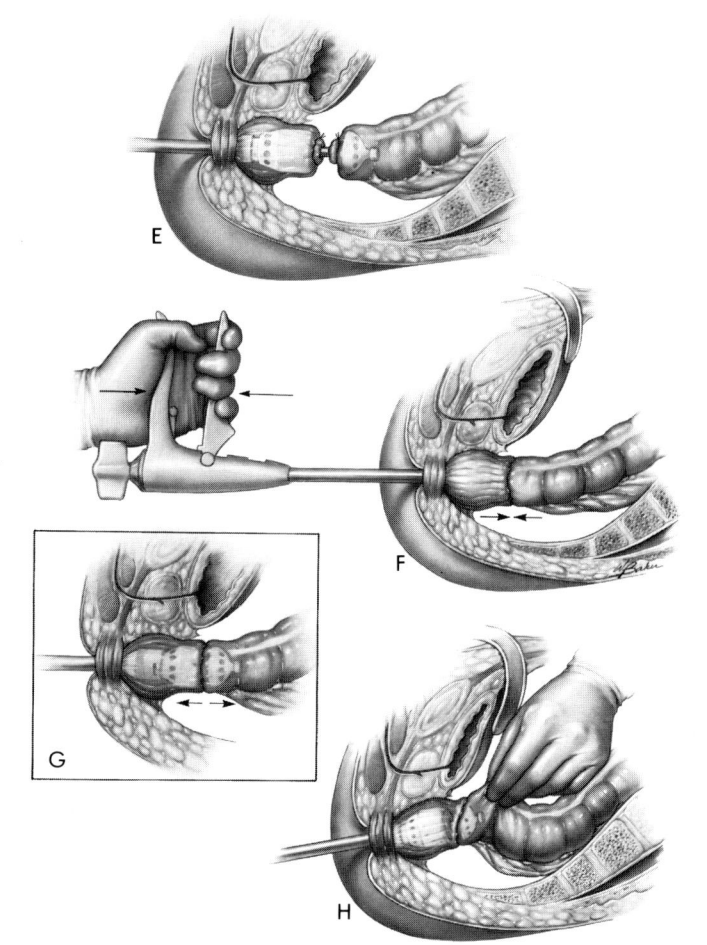

The other principal use we have envisaged for the EEA instrument (Vankemmel, 1972; Ravitch and Steichen, 1979) was for esophagogastrostomy or esophagojejunostomy, in which the instrument could be inserted from below through a gastrotomy, or through the still open end of a jejunal loop, or up through the side opening made for the subsequent enteroenterostomy, completing the Roux-Y. Since the anastomoses obtained with the GIA instrument have been so easy and safe to construct and their function has been uniformly satisfactory, it seems unlikely that merely providing an inverting end-to-end anastomosis would justify use of the EEA instrument in situations in which an additional enterotomy or gastrotomy would be necessary.

However, the instrument does lend itself readily that way to the performance of a Billroth I gastroduodenostomy or a Billroth II gastrojejunostomy, at the small cost of either closing an additional gastrotomy or leaving the transected stomach partially or completely open until the anastomosis has been performed. In addition, Nance (1979) recently reported use of the instrument for end-to-end small bowel and colorectal anastomoses from above, through a separate enterotomy.

The advantages of the instruments, as we have seen them, lie in their precision, the decreased risk of intraoperative contamination or bleeding, and in the minimal manipulation and trauma to the viscera, since a single application may insert 32 sutures, or staples. The saving of time, of course, is substantial and may be significant to the patient in some of the extensive reconstructive procedures mentioned. The decreased operative time may at times represent a significant contribution to the patient's welfare, and in this day of concern for hospital costs, the decreased cost of operating room utilization and the decreased anesthesia charge may more than compensate for the cost of the cartridges employed in the operation.

PRECAUTIONS AND SAFEGUARDS

Mishaps, of course, are inherent in the use of devices, as they are in all other aspects of surgery. At a national meeting, a speaker reported that he had seen the common duct stapled as well as the duodenum and that in another instance the staples had not been placed across the entire end of the stomach, which had leaked from the unstapled portion (Wassner, Yohai, and Heimlich, 1977). We have already marked that the instruments do not permit the surgeon to ignore basic rules. We have experienced, or heard of, or conceived of some or all the following errors in or complications with the use of the instruments.

TA Instruments

(1) Failure to insert the pin that aligns the upper and lower jaws, which assures perfect formation of the staples and prevents compressing the bowel out beyond the line of staples;
(2) failure to employ an anvil, or using the anvil from a different type of cartridge, which results in malformed staples that will not hold;
(3) using an empty cartridge;
(4) forgetting to compress the handle and fire the staples;
(5) transecting the viscus on the patient side of the instrument rather than on the specimen side.

It is reassuring to see oozing from the cut end, but very rarely a spurting vessel requires suture or coagulation. We have never seen or heard of intraperitoneal bleeding attributable to staples. Vigorous bleeding, when the instrument is removed, almost invariably means that mesentery and a mesenteric vessel have been included in the jaws of the instrument. The TA instruments cannot be relied upon for control of vessels in the mesentery or omentum.

GIA Instruments

(1) Forcing the instrument halves together improperly. The halves must be properly mated. If the driving assembly is not easily advanced, the instrument has probably been incorrectly locked together;
(2) failure to use an anvil;
(3) positioning of the activating assembly so that two of the three elements are in one slot, with the result that the knife will cut out one suture line;
(4) in transecting the bowel, failure to make certain that all the bowel to be transect-

ed is within the area of graduations marking the position of the staples.

In anastomoses with the GIA instrument, we usually look inside the anastomosis and if there appears to be bleeding, we pack it with a sponge for 2 minutes. Occasionally, it is necessary to put in a fine suture or two. Bleeding from bowel transected with the GIA instrument is usually minimal. Profuse bleeding, like the similar situation with the TA instrument, means that the mesentery inappropriately was seized up in the tissue to be transected.

We have seen a single instance, and heard of others, in which the cut and stapled edges of a GIA anastomosis very largely healed to each other — a theoretic possibility since the edges are completely viable. This need not happen if, in closing an anastomosis, the TA clamp is applied so that the ends of the GIA suture line are held apart rather than compressed together.

EEA Instruments

(1) Failure to tie the pursestring suture tightly enough around the shaft, with the result that an intact disc of full-thickness bowel from both ends is not obtained;
(2) placing the pursestring suture too far back from the edge, so that an unacceptably large mass of tissue must be compressed within the cavity of the closed cartridge;
(3) forcing the largest-size cartridge into esophagus or bowel too small for it;
(4) jeopardizing the completed anastomosis by rough withdrawal of the instrument;
(5) failure to push the handle all the way; this will advance the staples but not the circular knife, and hence the instrument cannot be disengaged.

LDS Instruments

(1) Pulling upward on the tissue to be cut, which may allow it to slip out as the staples are closing;
(2) attempting to include too large a mass of tissue in the instrument;
(3) catching a staple on a roughly withdrawn Mikulicz pad, which can displace it.

All the instruments are long, and their weight is great enough that the leverage of force that can be exerted at the business end with a relatively small movement of the handle can be significant. One must learn to avoid this.

REPORTED EXPERIENCE WITH AUTOSUTURE INSTRUMENTS

In 1973, Steichen and Ravitch reported their overall experience with autosuture instruments during the period 1967 to 1971. A total of 218 patients (69 gastric, 60 intestinal, 15 esophageal, 49 pulmonary, 14 vascular, 8 gynecologic, and 3 miscellaneous) underwent 222 operations, which included 477 individual staple procedures. Postoperative complications occurred in 17 cases; in 13 they were stapler-related but in the remaining 4 their stapler relation was questionable. The single death followed a pulmonary operation.

Included in this series were 147 gastrointestinal procedures. Postoperative anastomotic bleeding occurred in five of these patients, three of whom required reoperation. Five other patients had suture line leaks: one had breakdown of a duodenal closure; a 10-day-old baby had an anastomotic leak after resection of the ascending colon and was found later to have Hirschsprung's disease, hence the anastomosis had been made proximal to a mechanical obstruction. Another patient who had a total esophagectomy and one-stage esophagocologastrostomy had a small temporary discharge of saliva through the neck incision. Two colonic leaks were reported, one in irradiated bowel and one after a difficult colorectal anastomosis. In summary, postoperative stapler-related complications occurred in 10 (6.8 per cent) of the 147 gastrointestinal procedures.

Ravitch and colleagues have published at least three other valuable papers on stapling instruments and their use (Ravitch and associates, 1966; Ravitch and associates, 1972; Steichen, 1977). Others also have published valuable contributions to the literature on mechanical suturing.

Latimer and associates (1975) reiterated the history of the development of staplers and described the different machines. They also reported their experience with 104 patients in whom gastrointestinal surgery was performed partly or wholly with the autosuturing devices by technics similar to those described by Ravitch and Steichen (1972). A total of 112 operations was performed on these 104 patients — 1 esophageal, 29 gastric, 23 small intestinal, 56 large intestinal, and 3 miscellaneous; 256 stapling procedures were performed.

Eighteen complications occurred, 13 of which were nonstapler-related. Three were questionably stapler-related, and two were definitely stapler-related. Of the four deaths in the series, two were nonstapler-related, and two were stapler-related.

The overall complication rate was 17.3 per cent, and the mortality was 3.8 per cent. If only stapler-related complications and deaths are considered, the mortality decreases to 1.0 per cent and the complication rate to 1.9 per cent.

McGinty (1979) reported one colonic anastomotic leak in a series of 38 patients; Painter, Park, and Hochberg (1974) reported two complications in 63 patients, one bleeding from a gastrojejunostomy that required reoperation, and the other a fistula from a side-to-side ileocolostomy.

Awe and Loehden (1973) described one case of massive hemorrhage after gastrojejunostomy, but at reoperation a bleeding site could not be found. The two colonic anastomoses in which they used the triangulation method leaked and required reoperation.

Halloran (1975) reported that in 275 patients with antrectomy and Billroth II anastomoses, suture line bleeding occurred in 6, stomal dysfunctions in 2, and duodenal leaks in 5. A leak occurred in one patient who had an intestinal bypass for obesity; two others had bleeding of the gastrointestinal tract. No stapler-associated deaths occurred in his series.

Latimer and associates (1975) reviewed their stapler-related complications. Three patients had anastomotic dysfunction; in two, gastroscopy showed the anastomosis was open. In the three patients, stomal dysfunction resolved with nonoperative management. In one other patient stomal dysfunction developed secondary to dense external adhesions, and reoperation was required. They pointed out that stomal dysfunction is not uncommon and has been reported in 4.7 per cent of patients with hemigastrectomy and vagotomy (Hardy, 1980). Getzen (1966) reported an incidence of 5 per cent in inverted, hand-sutured anastomoses.

Causes of stomal dysfunction have included adhesions, gastrojejunal intussusception, retrogastric hernia, and stomal edema. It may occur without obstruction seen on x-ray films or gastroscopy. Latimer (1975) suggested that a possible source of stapled stomal dysfunction is the potentially ischemic area that occurs between the gastric closure and retrogastric gastrojejunostomy (Fig. 23–10). Such a case has been

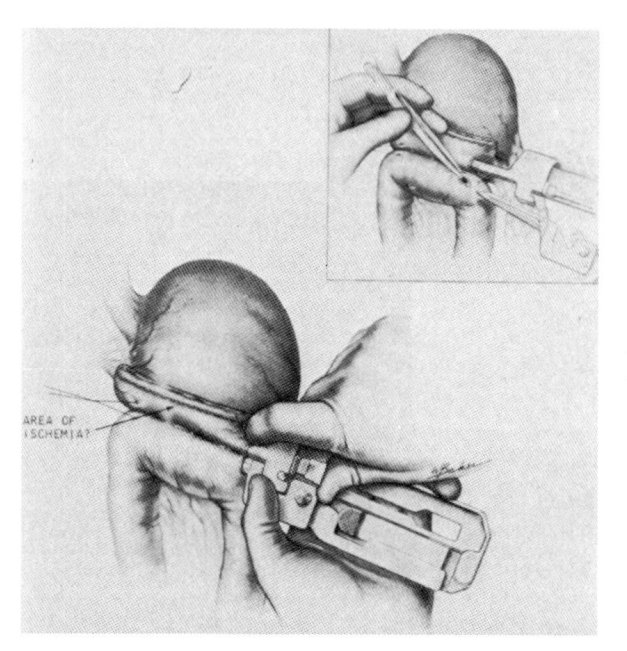

Figure 23–10. Potential area of ischemia that develops with use of the GIA stapler for gastrojejunostomy. (From Latimer, R. G., Doane, W. A., McKittrick, J. E., et al.: Automatic staple suturing for gastrointestinal surgery. Am. J. Surg. *130*:766, 1975.)

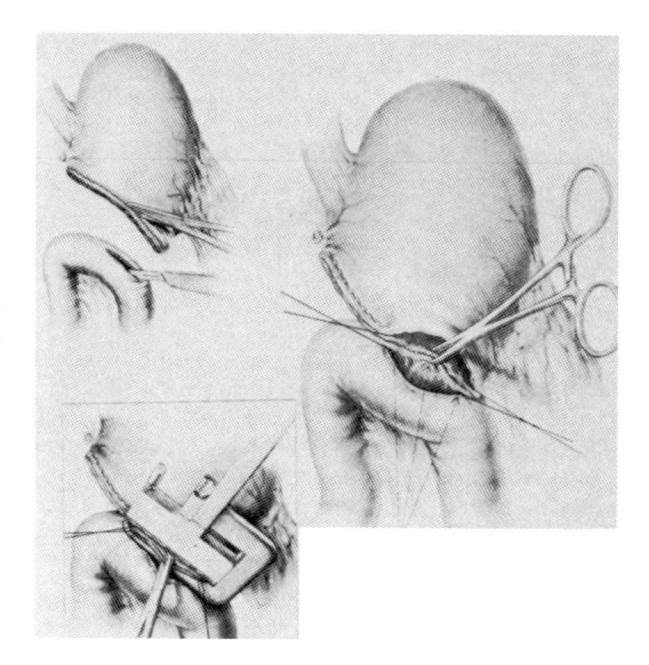

Figure 23–11. Alternative method for a stapled gastrojejunostomy. (From Latimer et al., cited in previous figure.)

reported by Dickman (1971). To avoid this complication, a portion of the stapled closure is amputated and a triangulation end-to-side anastomosis formed (Fig. 23–11). Another patient with previously irradiated small bowel developed an enterocutaneous fistula from a decompression enterotomy.

One patient had an intramural hematoma with abscess after sigmoid colotomy with polypectomy. This complication was considered to be a technical error that could have been avoided if the stapled base of the polyp as well as the colotomy had been examined more carefully for bleeding and electrocoagulated or sutured.

Of the four deaths in the series, two were secondary to carcinoma associated with chemotherapy and small bowel obstruction and were not related to staple failures. One of the deaths occurred in a 76-year-old man who had a total gastrectomy, cholecystectomy, and esophagojejunostomy. He died from septicemia, presumably due to dehiscence of a stapled suture line. The second stapler-related death occurred in an 80-year-old woman with obstructive jaundice secondary to ampullary carcinoma, who was treated by a GIA-stapled cholecystojejunostomy. This was complicated by bleeding from the suture line, which required reoperation to oversew the suture line. Progressive hepatorenal failure developed, and she died.

Latimer and colleagues noted that Dickman (1971) had reported a 3.4 per cent incidence of anastomotic bleeding in stapled gastric anastomoses and had recommended routine oversewing of all GIA anastomoses. The necessity for this in all cases is debatable, but certainly all GIA anastomoses should be inspected carefully for bleeding before closing the anastomosis.

From this series of patients Latimer and associates (1975) concluded that (1) automatic staplers provide a rapid, sure method for closure, transection, and anastomosis of the stomach, small intestine, and colon; (2) mortality and complication rates do not exceed those for the same hand-sutured technics; (3) all closures, particularly by the GIA instrument, should be inspected carefully. Because of the B-shaped staple that preserves blood supply, failure to inspect can lead to the complication of anastomotic hemorrhage; and (4) surgical judgment should choose between the stapler and hand-suturing technics.

Fischer (1976) described three patients with massive bleeding after stapler-performed intestinal anastomoses. Two patients required secondary operation for control. The cause was mechanical instrument failure. He recommended periodic in vitro testing as a preventive measure.

Elliott, Albertazzi, and Danto (1977) presented two cases of anastomotic stenosis after the use of the GIA autosuture stapler as examples of a potential problem that exists in using this instrument. They mentioned the possible causes and outlined suggestions for eliminating this complication.

Wassner, Yohai, and Heimlich (1977) reported the intraoperative and postoperative complications that had occurred in 132 patients who had undergone gastrointestinal operations performed with use of TA or GIA stapling devices, evaluated the relationship of these complications to the staple-suture technic, and suggested methods for avoiding staple-related complications. Fifty-five procedures involved the colon and 77 gastrointestinal procedures were exclusive of the colon. A variety of complications, such as infection, did not seem related to the stapling technic. Of seven deaths, only one was associated with use of a stapling instrument.

The following complications were considered to be stapler-related:

1. *Bleeding.* Significant staple-related bleeding occurred in nine instances, and in many of the patients additional sutures were required for hemostasis. In three gastroenterostomies and one enterocolostomy, bleeding from the anastomotic line was excessive and necessitated special effort to gain control. In three other gastroenterostomies, significant postoperative bleeding ceased with conservative measures. Excessive bleeding occurred in two colocolostomies, one of which was oversewn at operation; the other was diagnosed after operation and required reoperation.

Bleeding from the cut edge of a resected viscus — for example, stomach or duodenum — that was stapled with the TA instrument was mentioned in many reports and required additional sutures or oversewing the staple line. The investigators believe that the complication of bleeding from the anastomotic line is directly attributable to the technic.

2. *Technical failure of stapling instruments.* Malfunction of the instrument occurred in five cases. In one, the mechanism of the stapler became locked, making removal from the bowel difficult. A pelvic abscess developed subsequently and was drained. In another, excessive bleeding prompted careful inspection of the gastrojejunal suture line and it was discovered that many of the staples were not engaged. Manual sutures were placed. Subsequently the patient showed delayed function of the anastomosis and upper gastrointestinal bleeding, both of which responded to conservative measures. Nonfiring of some staples was observed in one other patient, so sutures were inserted. In two instances the cause of malfunction was not stated, but the surgeon abandoned the instrument and used standard hand-suturing.

3. *Inadequate approximation of tissues.* In two instances of duodenal closure, at operation it was noted that a portion of the cut edge of the duodenum had not been approximated by the staples, and the instrument was reapplied. Similarly, in one case the full extent of the lesser curvature of the stomach was not included in the stapler, and sutures were used to close the defect. Postoperative duodenal stump leak occurred in three other patients, all of whom recovered. In one a Penrose drain had been inserted at operation, the second drained through the wound, and the third required reoperation. A disrupted colonic anastomosis contributed to the death of one patient operated on for perforated carcinoma.

4. *Lack of visualization of pathology and adjacent structures.* Two instances of bleeding from an unresected duodenal ulcer necessitated reoperation. Use of the stapler had prevented visualization of the bleeding ulcer within the duodenum. In another case, following resection of a Meckel's diverticulum with the stapler, the pathologist found ectopic gastric mucosa at the margins of the specimen.

Jaundice caused by inadvertent stapling of the common duct followed a total gastrectomy and required reoperation for biliary bypass in one case.

Wassner and colleagues pointed out that many surgeons placed silk sutures to invert the staple line, and there is clinical and experimental evidence that although the inverting layer is not always necessary, the addition of this simple precaution is justified.

They warned that it is essential that the surgeon not only be familiar with the instrument but also, at operation, be alert to its mechanical integrity because several of the complications mentioned were related to malfunctioning of the device. Also, before discharging the staples, special attention should be given to the position of the instrument because mishaps, particularly with the GIA device that incises the bowel as it inserts staples, could be difficult to correct. Furthermore, as pointed out by Ravitch and Steichen (1972), the staples are not designed to control bleeding from mesenteric or omental vessels so the line of transection must be cleared of any vasculature beforehand, and all stapled anastomoses should be inspected before final closure of the viscus. Also all the edges of the tissue intended for closure should be visualized to be certain that they lie within the jaws of the stapler, particularly in closure of a pyloroplasty, or of the duodenum, and in closure of the stab wounds made in the bowel to insert the jaws of a GIA instrument.

Bleeding complications were due in part to the fact that, with the use of staplers, duodenal disease was not visualized. For convenience and to avoid contamination, surgeons may be tempted to staple and transect the duodenum without inspecting the pathology. Usually, during subtotal gastrectomy for acute bleeding, the ulcer should be exposed and resected or oversewn before applying a stapler for duodenal closure.

Hardin (1977) reported his experience with the use of surgical stapling instruments in over 300 gastrointestinal operations, of which 60 were gastric resections. Duodenal ulcer with all types of its complications was the indication for operation in 32, over half, of these patients. Gastric ulcer was the indication for resection in 19 patients. The remaining cases were more complicated types of resection.

After antrectomy or hemigastrectomy, Billroth II anastomosis was performed in 40 of these 60 cases. A Billroth I anastomosis was performed with staplers in only one case. Complicated gastrectomy was done in 16 of the patients, with either radical subtotal resection or total resection with reconstruction of a gastric pouch. Vagotomy and gastrojejunostomy were done in only three patients.

Operating time was significantly reduced by using mechanical staplers. Review of 55 procedures (excluding the five cases of pancreatectomy with gastric reconstruction) revealed that operating time varied from 50 to 290 minutes. Three resections required less than 1 hour, 15 required 1 to 2 hours, 22 required 2 to 3 hours, 10 required 3 to 4 hours and 5 required 4 to 5 hours. Additional experience with the technic has reduced the operating time so that gastric resections can be done in approximately 60 to 90 minutes.

Another advantage of using mechanical staplers is the rapidity with which gastrointestinal recovery occurs postoperatively. In several of these patients, the nasogastric tube was removed the first postoperative day; in the majority it was removed either the second or third day, with an average of 2.6 postoperative days. A liquid diet was begun, on the average, by the fourth postoperative day and a regular diet 6.1 days after operation. All these patients were on regular diets before discharge from the hospital, which averaged 11.8 days after operation. All patients in the hospital beyond 14 days remained because of general medical problems and not because of delayed intestinal recovery. Radiographic studies showed the anastomosis was patent almost immediately after operation in these patients.

Suture line bleeding was negligible after anastomoses done with the GIA instrument. No reoperation was necessary because of continued suture line bleeding. Only one patient developed a postoperative wound infection. There was complete absence of direct stapler-related complications. There were no anastomotic or duodenal stump leaks and no reoperations because of anastomotic bleeding.

Three indirect, nonstapler-related complications occurred. The first was in a patient who developed volvulus of the efferent loop after a Billroth II anastomosis and required reoperation about six months after resection for gastric carcinoma. After the volvulus had been reduced surgically, the patient's recovery was uneventful. A second complication occurred in a patient who required reoperation on the seventh postoperative day because of abdominal tenderness and a possible leaking duodenal stump. At reoperation, a leak was found in the area of the gastroenterostomy, where the stab wounds in the stomach and jejunum had been closed by manual suturing. Another patient developed delayed emptying of the stomach and required regression from a regular diet to a liquid diet for 3 weeks while edema in the gastric remnant resolved, after which he remained well.

All 60 patients who had gastric surgery using autosutures had been followed for 6 to 40 months. The results were satisfactory in

50. The ten unsatisfactory results were due to problems with malignancy or general medical problems. One patient died from pulmonary emboli in the immediate postoperative period after total gastrectomy. No unsatisfactory result was related to the use of staplers.

Hardin also mentioned having used staplers in approximately 240 other gastrointestinal operations. These included pancreatic surgery, either for gastrointestinal continuity after partial or total pancreatectomy or for suturing the pancreas in cases of distal pancreatectomy; multiple bypasses for malignancy and chronic pancreatitis; cholecystojejunostomy; and jejunostomy and gastrojejunostomy for obstructive jaundice. No fistulas developed after pancreatic surgery in which staplers were used.

The small intestine was particularly suitable for stapling. Resections were done for inflammatory bowel disease, trauma, malignancy, and Meckel's diverticula; and palliative bypasses for cancer and obesity.

Nearly all types of colon surgery, including sigmoid resection, right hemicolectomy, low anterior colon resection, total colectomy with ileorectal anastomosis, total proctocolectomy with permanent ileostomy, and abdominoperineal resection, were performed with staplers. Hardin found the instruments convenient in resecting the right or transverse colon, but inconvenient in the pelvis because of their bulkiness.

In several cases cholecystectomy and incidental appendectomy were done using staplers. Also, in some cases other procedures were being performed and the cholecystectomy or appendectomy was incidental. In retrospect, Hardin concluded that it did not seem worthwhile routinely to perform either of these procedures with the staplers. However he is convinced that the use of autosuture surgical instruments for gastrointestinal surgery reduces the operating time, produces good results, has wide application, and has proved its safety.

COMMENTS

The use of stapling instruments has been firmly established as an acceptable method for suturing in many operations on the gastrointestinal tract. It is now widely used and is increasing in popularity. Newer instruments that increase capabilities and usage are being made available.

Mechanical suturing has mortality and morbidity rates that do not exceed the rates for the same procedures performed by hand-suture technic. It shortens the operating time. The staples are placed with a uniform degree of compression and spacing, unlike hand-placed sutures. Anastomoses made with staplers have a narrower flange, and therefore a wider stoma, so begin to function earlier after operation than do hand-sutured anastomoses. The use of staplers reduces tissue manipulation and tissue handling.

Most surgeons agree that it is unnecessary to oversew the stapler line routinely, but it is extremely important to inspect the staple line of all closures, because of the B-staple configuration that preserves blood supply. Failure to inspect can lead to the complication of anastomotic hemorrhage.

Mechanical suture instruments cannot be used in all circumstances or in all patients or for all operations or for all lesions in the gastrointestinal tract.

Whether to use these instruments or hand suturing should be determined by surgical judgment and the surgeon's experience and familiarity with each of these technics.

Before considering the use of mechanical suturing, the surgeon should become thoroughly familiar with the instruments and several alternative technics for their use, by practice in animals and automobile tire inner tubes. Seminars are available for those desiring to learn to use these instruments.

The United States Surgical Corporation has published an invaluable, and superbly done, atlas of stapling technics in general surgery, a copy of which is delivered with each autosuture stapler purchased.

Stapling instruments are expensive to buy and also to maintain. Hence they are not available in every hospital in which surgery is performed. Manual suturing equipment is far cheaper to purchase and to maintain and is universally available. Each method has its advantages and disadvantages for performing various surgical procedures; it is advisable, therefore, for surgeons to be familiar with, and surgical residents to be trained in, the use of both methods.

BIBLIOGRAPHY

Abramson, D. J.: A new, soft, triple lumen, overflow and suction drain. Am. J. Surg. 120:414, 1970.

Adnopoz, A., and Fortuna, A. B.: Retroperitoneal rupture of the duodenum; Report of a case with subcutaneous emphysema of the neck. Arch. Surg. 83:937, 1961.

Aguirre, A., Fisher, J. E., and Welch, C. E.: The role of surgery and hyperalimentation in therapy of gastrointestinal-cutaneous fistulae. Ann. Surg. 180:393, 1974.

Akin, J. T., Jr., Gray, S. W., and Skandalakis, J. E.: Vascular compression of the duodenum: Presentation of ten cases and review of the literature. Surgery 79:515, 1976.

Albo, R., De Lorimier, A. A., and Silen, W.: Spontaneous rupture of the stomach in the adult. Surgery 53:797, 1963. Cited in Gue, 1970.

Albot, G., and Magnier, F.: Arch. Mal. App. Dig. 44:1162, 1955. Cited in Rowling, 1959.

Alday, E. S., and Goldsmith, H. S.: Small intestine control of gastric secretion. Surg. Gynecol. Obstet. 136:185, 1973.

Alden, J. F.: Gastric and jejunoileal bypass. Arch. Surg. 112:799, 1977.

Alder, R. L., and Terry, B. E.: Measurement and standardization of the gastric pouch in gastric bypass. Surg. Gynecol. Obstet. 144:762, 1977.

Allen, H. M., Block, M. A., and Schuman, B. M.: Gastroduodenal endoscopy. Management of acute upper gastrointestinal hemorrhage. Arch. Surg. 106:450, 1973.

Allen, R., Thoshinsky, M., Stallone, R., et al.: Corrosive injuries of the stomach. Arch. Surg. 100:409, 1970.

Altemeier, W. A.: Discussion of Moore, S. W., and Erlandson, M. E.: Intramural hematoma of the duodenum. Ann. Surg. 157:798, 1963.

Althausen, T. L., Deamer, W. C., and Kerr, W. J.: The false "acute abdomen," Henoch's purpura, and abdominal allergy. Ann. Surg. 106:242, 1937. Cited in Jones, et al., 1971.

Anderson, W. C., Vivit, R., Kirsch, I. E., et al.: Arteriomesenteric duodenal compression syndrome; Its association with peptic ulcer. Am. J. Surg. 125:681, 1973.

Andrews, E.: Duodenal hernia: A misnomer. Surg. Gynecol. Obstet. 37:740, 1923.

Androsov, P. I.: New method of surgical treatment of blood vessel lesions. Arch. Surg. 73:902, 1956.

Appel, M. F.: Endoscopic removal of gastric and duodenal polyps. South. Med. J. 69:593, 1976.

Appel, M. F., and Bentlif, P. S.: Endoscopic removal of bleeding Brunner gland adenoma. Arch. Surg. 111:301, 1976.

Appel, M. F., Bentlif, P. S., and Dickson, J. H.: Arteriomesenteric duodenal compression syndrome: Comparison of methods of treatment. South. Med. J. 69:340, 1976.

Arey, L. B.: Developmental Anatomy, rev. 7th ed. Philadelphia, W. B. Saunders Company, 1974.

Asch, M. J., and Sherman, N. J.: Gastric volvulus in children. J. Pediatr. Surg. 12:1059, 1977.

Ascherman, S. W., Bednarz, W. W., and Olix, M. L.: Gastric volvulus: Special reference to hepatodiaphragmatic interposition of colon. Arch. Surg. 76:621, 1958.

Aston, S. J., and Rees, T. D.: Vicryl sutures. Aesthet. Plast. Surg. 1:289, 1977.

Atkinson, M., and Ferguson, R.: Fiberoptic endoscopic palliative intubation of inoperable esophagastric neoplasms. Br. Med. J. 1:266, 1977.

Awe, W. C., and Loehden, O. L.: Automatic stapling devices. Am. Surg. 39:475, 1973.

Bagley, C. M., Jr., Thomas, L. B., Johnson, R. E., et al.: Diagnosis of liver involvement by lymphoma: Results in 96 consecutive peritoneoscopies. Cancer 31:840, 1973.

Baglio, C. M., and Fattal, G. A.: Spontaneous rupture of the stomach in adults. Am. J. Dig. Dis. 7:75, 1962.

Baker, M. S., Borchardt, K. A., Baker, B. H., et al.: Sump tube drainage as a source of bacterial contamination. Am. J. Surg. 133:617, 1977.

Baker, M. S., Fisher, J. H., Van der Reis, L., et al.: The endoscopic diagnosis of an aortoduodenal fistula. Arch. Surg. 111:304, 1976.

Ballard, H. S., Fame, B., and Hartsock, R. J.: Familial multiple endocrine adenoma–peptic ulcer complex. Medicine 43:481, 1964.

Bariety, M., Poulet, J., and Courtois-Suffit, M.: Diaphragme muqueux prepylorique et cancer bronchique primitif. Presse Med. 65:785, 1957. Cited in Gray, et al., 1972.

Barner, H. B., and Sherman, C. D., Jr.: Vascular compression of the duodenum: Collective review. Int. Abstr. Surg. 117:103, 1963.

Barnett, W. O., and Wall, L.: Megaduodenum resulting from absence of the parasympathetic ganglion cells in Auerbach's plexus. Ann. Surg. 141:527, 1955.

Barone, R. M.: Reconstruction after total gastrectomy: Construction of a Hunt-Lawrence pouch using auto suture staples. Am. J. Surg. 137:578, 1979.

Barreros, R. E., and Donaldson, R. M., Jr.: Gastric secretion during hypercalcemia in man. Gastroenterology 50:881, 1966.

Bartlett, M. K., Wang, C., and Williams, W.: The surgical management of paraduodenal hernia. Ann. Surg. 168:249, 1968.

Beard, R. J., Lee, E. C., Haysom, A. H., et al.: Non-carcinomatous tumors of the stomach. Br. J. Surg. 55:535, 1968.

Beaudin, D. J., Da Costa, L. R., Prentice, R. S., et al.: Duodenoscopy in diagnosis of upper gastrointestinal disease. Can. Med. Assoc. J. 108:565. 1973.

Beck, C., and Carrel, A.: Demonstration of specimens illustrating a method of formation of prethoracic esophagus. Ill. Med. J. 7:463, 1905.

Becker, J. M., Schneider, K. M., and Fischer, A. E.: Pyloric atresia. Arch. Surg. 87:71, 1963.

Begg, A. S.: The anomalous persistence in embryos of parts of peri-intestinal rings formed by vitelline veins. Am. J. Anat. 13:103, 1912.

Belber, J. P.: Endoscopic examination of duodenal

bulb: Comparison with X-ray. Gastroenterology 61:55, 1971.
Bell, M. J., Ternberg, J. L., Keating, J. P., et al.: Pyloric gastric antral web: A puzzling epidemic. J. Pediatr. Surg. 13:307, 1978.
Belsey, R.: Reconstruction of the esophagus with left colon. J. Thorac. Cardiovasc. Surg. 19:33, 1965.
Bender, H.: Spontaneous Rupture of the Small Intestine in the Newborn. Delivered before the Society for Clinical Surgery, April, 1964.
Benedict, E. B.: Endoscopy. Baltimore, Williams & Wilkins, 1951.
Bennett, R. J.: Atresia of the pylorus. Am. J. Dig. Dis. 4:44, 1937.
Benson, C. D.: Prepyloric and pyloric obstruction. In Mustard, W. T., et al. (eds.): Pediatric Surgery, 2nd ed. Chicago, Year Book Medical Publishers, 1969.
Benson, C. D., and Coury, J. J.: Congenital intrinsic obstruction of the stomach and duodenum in the newborn. Arch. Surg. 62:856, 1951.
Benson, C. D., and Lloyd, J. R.: Duodenal obstruction of congenital origin. Am. J. Surg. 101:610, 1961.
Berci, G. (ed.): Endoscopy. New York, Appleton-Century-Crofts, 1976, p. 115.
Berci, G., Morgenstern, L., Shore, J. M., et al.: A direct approach to differential diagnosis of jaundice; Laparoscopy with transhepatic cholecystocholangiography. Am. J. Surg. 123:372, 1973.
Berci, G., Shore, J. M., Parrish, L., et al.: Evaluation of a new peritoneoscope as a diagnostic aid to the surgeon. Ann. Surg. 178:37, 1973.
Berg, J.: Zwei Fälle von Axendrehung des Magens. Nord Med. Ark. 19:1, 1897. Cited in Gosin and Ballinger, 1965.
Berg, R. B., Schuster, S. R., and Colodny, A. H.: The use of gastrostomy in feeding premature infants. Pediatrics 33:287, 1964.
Berggren, O. G. A.: Littre's hernia as complication of laparoscopy. Nord. Med. 72:1150, 1964.
Berman, J. K., and Ballenger, F.: Prepyloric membranous obstruction. Q. Bull. Indiana U. Med. Center 4:14, 1948.
Bernardo, J. R., Soderberg, C. H., and Migliaccio, A. V.: Gastric ulcer; Surgery of the Rhode Island Hospital cases in the ten year period 1946–1955. Surgery 44:804, 1958.
Berne, C., Donovan, A., White, E., et al.: Duodenal diverticulization for duodenal and pancreatic injury. Am. J. Surg. 127:503, 1974.
Berne, T. V., and Shore, E. H.: Appraisal of the traumatized abdomen. Surg. Clin. North Am. 48:1197, 1968.
Berti, A.: Singolare attortigliamento dell'esofago col duodeno sequito da rapido morte. Gazz. Med. Ital. 9:139, 1866.
Bishop, H. D., and Koop, C. E.: Surgical management of duplications of the alimentary tract. Am. J. Surg. 107:434, 1964.
Bisla, R. S., and Louis, H. J.: Acute vascular compression of the duodenum following cast application. Surg. Gynecol. Obstet. 140:563, 1975.
Bitar, D. E., and Holmes, T. W., Jr.: Polybezoar and gastrointestinal foreign bodies in the mentally retarded. Am. Surg. 41:497, 1975.
Bivins, B. A., Sachatello, C. R., Daugherty, M. E., et al.: Diagnostic peritoneal lavage is superior to clinical evaluation in blunt abdominal trauma. Am. Surg. 44:637, 1978.

Blair, E. L.: The question of release of histamine by gastrin. In Grossman, M. I. (ed.): Proceedings of Conference. Los Angeles, University of California Press, 1966.
Blair, P.: An account of the dissection of a child, communicated in a letter to Dr. Brook Taylor, Royal Society Secretary. Philos. Trans. R. Soc. Lond. (I) 30:631, 1717. Cited in Gray and Skandalakis, 1972.
Blank, E., and Chisolm, A. J.: Congenital microgastria; Case report. Pediatrics 51:1037, 1973.
Block, M. A., and Zikria, E. A.: Preduodenal portal vein causing duodenal obstruction associated with pneumatosis cystoides intestinalis. Ann. Surg. 153:407, 1961.
Bloodgood, J. C.: Acute dilatation of the stomach: Gastromesenteric ileus. Ann. Surg. 46:736, 1907.
Bloom, G. P., Fromm, D., Rosenberg, S., et al.: Attempted retrograde cannulation of the ampulla: A probable cause of mass in pancreas. Ann. Surg. 183:107, 1976.
Bockus, H. L.: Duodenal ulcer. In Gastroenterology, 2nd ed. Vol. 1. Philadelphia, W. B. Saunders Company, 1963.
Bockus, H. L.: Gastroenterology, 3rd ed., Philadelphia, W. B. Saunders Company, 1976, p. 1052.
Bockus, H. L., and Bank, J.: Upper gastrointestinal disease associated with syphilis. J.A.M.A. 90:175, 1928 and Am. J. Syphilis 13:30, 1929.
Bolt, D. E., and Hennessy, W. B.: Rupture of the stomach complicating gastric hemorrhage. Lancet 2:485, 1955.
Borchardt, M.: Zur Pathologie und Therapie des Magenvolvulus. Arch. Klin. Chir. 74:243, 1904.
Bornside, G. H., Reese, R., Bornside, B., et al.: Microbial flora of the diseased stomach at resection. Am. Surg. 44:196, 1978.
Bowden, T. A., Jr.: Fiberoptic endoscopy of the stomach after gastrectomy. Am. Surg. 43:287, 1977.
Bowen, J. C., Fleming, W. H., and Thompson, J. C.: Increased gastrin release following penetrating central nervous system injury. Surgery 75:720, 1974.
Bower, R. J., and Ternberg, J. L.: Preduodenal portal vein. J. Pediatr. Surg. 7:579, 1972.
Boyden, E. A., Cope, J. G., and Bill, A. H., Jr.: Anatomy and embryology of congenital intrinsic obstruction of the duodenum. Am. J. Surg. 114:190, 1967.
Boyle, J. D., and Goldstein, H.: Management of pyloric obstruction. Med. Clin. North Am. 52:1329, 1968.
Brady, P. G., and Johnson, W. F.: Removal of foreign bodies: The flexible fiberoptic endoscope. South. Med. J. 70:702, 1977.
Braun, P., Collin, P. P., and Ducharme, J. C.: Preduodenal portal vein: a significant entity? Report of two cases and review of the literature. Can. J. Surg. 17:316, 1974.
Braun, P., and Cuendet, A.: Preduodenal portal vein. Prog. Pediatr. Surg. 3:121, 1971.
Brawley, R. K., Cameron, J. L., and Zuidema, G. D.: Severe upper abdominal injuries treated by pancreaticoduodenectomy. Surg. Gynecol. Obstet. 126:516, 1968.
Brea, C. A., Jr., Albites, V. R., and Otenasek, F. J.: Spontaneous rupture of the stomach and duodenum in a patient with a brain tumor: Report of a case. Am. Surg. 29:23, 1963.
Brolin, R. E., and Ravitch, M. M.: Security of stapled and sutured intestinal anastomoses in the face of

stimulated peristalsis. (Submitted for publication.)
Bronwell, A. W., Rutledge, R., and Dalton, M. L., Jr.: Single-layer open gastrointestinal anastomosis. Trans. South. Surg. Assoc. 78:281, 1966.
Brown, L. L., Shelton, H. T., Bornside, G. H., et al.: Evaluation of wound irrigation by pulsatile jet and conventional methods. Ann. Surg. 187:170, 1978.
Brown, R. P., and Hertzler, J. H.: Congenital prepyloric gastric atresia. Am. J. Dis. Child. 97:857, 1959.
Brühl, W.: Incidence and complications during laparoscopy and liver puncture under vision: Results of a survey. J.A.M.A. 199:168, 1967.
Buchanan, J.: Volvulus of the stomach. Br. J. Surg. 18:99, 1930.
Buckwalter, J. A.: Clinical trial of surgery for morbid obesity. South. Med. J. 71:1370, 1978.
Buckwalter, J. A., and Herbst, C. A.: Complications of gastric bypass for morbid obesity. Am. J. Surg. 139:55, 1980.
Bunch, W., and Delaney, J.: Scoliosis and acute vascular compression of the duodenum. Surgery 67:901, 1970.
Burrus, G. R., Howell, J. F., and Jordan, G. L., Jr.: Traumatic duodenal injuries: An analysis of 86 cases. J. Trauma 1:96, 1961.
Butler, E., and Carlson, E.: Pain in the testicles: Symptoms of retroperitoneal traumatic rupture of the duodenum. Am. J. Surg. 11:118, 1931.
Caffey, J.: Pediatric X-ray Diagnosis, 3rd ed. Chicago, Year Book Medical Publishers, 1956. Cited in Gray and Skandalakis, 1972.
Calder, J.: Two examples of children born with preternatural conformations of the guts. M. Essay Obst. Soc. Edinburgh 1:203, 1733.
Camblos, J. F. B.: Acute volvulus of the stomach. Am. Surg. 35:505, 1969.
Campbell, J. B., and Davis, W. S.: Neonatal gastric volvulus. Presented at the 19th Annual Meeting of the Society for Pediatric Radiology, Washington, D.C., September, 1976.
Campbell, J. R., and Sasake, T. M.: Gastrostomy in infants and children. Am. Surg. 40:505, 1974.
Canty, T. G.: Retrograde esophageal dilatation in children; An alternative to the indwelling string. Am. J. Surg. 132:422, 1976.
Carr, G. C., and Heimlich, H. J.: Circle tie to prevent removal of nasogastric tube by patient. Surg. Gynecol. Obstet. 134:317, 1972.
Carter, D. C., Dozois, R. R., and Kirkpatrick, J. R.: Gastric secretory response to insulin infusion in vagotomized subjects. Br. J. Surg. 60:702, 1973.
Cattell, R. B., and Braasch, J. W.: A technique of the exposure of the third and fourth portions of the duodenum. Surg. Gynecol. Obstet. 111:378, 1960.
Cauldwell, E. W., and Anson, B. J.: The visceral branches of the abdominal aorta; Topographical relationships. Am. J. Anat. 73:27, 1943. Cited in Akin, Gray, and Skandalakis, 1976.
Cave, H. W.: Wounds of the duodenum (118 casualties). In Surgery in World War II. Vol. 2: General Surgery. Washington, D. C., Office of the Surgeon General, Dept. of the Army, 1955.
Challa, V. R., Jona, J. Z., and Markesberry, W. R.: Ultrastructure observations of the myenteric plexus of the pylorus in idiopathic hypertrophic pyloric stenosis. Am. J. Pathol. 88:309, 1972.
Chassin, J. L.: Stapling technic for esophagogastrostomy after esophagogastric resection. Am. J. Surg. 136:399, 1978.
Chinn, A. B., Weckesser, E. C.: Acute hemorrhage from peptic ulceration: An analysis of 322 cases. Ann. Intern. Med. 34:339, 1951.
Chong, G., Beahrs, O., and Payne, W.: Management of corrosive gastritis due to ingested acid. Mayo Clin. Proc. 49:861, 1974.
Christiansen, J., Rehfeld, J. F., and Stadil, F.: Interaction of calcium and magnesium on gastric acid secretion and serum gastrin concentration in man. Gastroenterology 68:1140, 1975.
Christiansen, P., Amdrup, E., Fenger, C., et al.: Gastric ulcer. II. Non-surgical treatment. Acta Chir. Scand. 139:466, 1973.
Chung, R. S. K., and DenBesten, L.: Fiberoptic endoscopy in treatment of corrosive injury of the stomach. Arch. Surg. 110:725, 1975.
Chung, R. S. K., Safaie-Sherazi, S., and DenBesten, L.: Dilation of esophageal strictures: A new technique controlled by fiberoptic endoscopy. Arch. Surg. 111:795, 1976.
Classen, M., and Demling, L.: Endoskopische Sphinkterotomie der Papilla Vateri und Steinextraktion aus dem Ductus Choledochus. Dtsch. Med. Wochenschr. 99:496, 1974.
Classen, M., and Safrany, L.: Endoscopic papillotomy and removal of gallstones. Br. Med. J. 4:371, 1975.
Cleveland, H. C., and Waddell, W. R.: Retro-peritoneal rupture of the duodenum due to non-penetrating trauma. Surg. Clin. North Am. 43:413, 1963.
Cocke, W. M., Jr., and Meyer, K. K.: Retroperitoneal duodenal rupture: Proposed mechanism, review of literature and report of a case. Am. J. Surg. 108:834, 1964.
Code, C. F.: Reflections on histamine, gastric secretion and the H2 receptor. N. Engl. J. Med. 296:1459, 1977.
Cohen, D. H.: Proc. Paediatric Surg. Congress, Melbourne 1:205, March 1970.
Cohen, M. M.: Treatment and mortality of perforated peptic ulcer: A survey of 852 cases. Can. Med. Assoc. J. 105:263, 1971.
Colcher, H.: Current concepts: Gastrointestinal endoscopy. New Engl. J. Med. 293:1129, 1975.
Colcher, H.: Reply to question whether general anesthesia for gastroscopy is contraindicated in an excited patient. J.A.M.A. 237:158, 1977.
Cole, B. C., and Dickinson, S. J.: Acute volvulus of the stomach in infants and children. Surgery 70:707, 1971.
Coleman, M., Lightdale, C. J., Vinciguerra, V. P., et al.: Peritoneoscopy in Hodgkin disease: Confirmation of results by laparotomy. J.A.M.A. 236:2364, 1976.
Coller, F. A., and MacLean, K. F.: In Cole, W. H. (ed.): Operative Technic in General Surgery. New York, Appleton-Century-Crofts, 1949, pp. 314–358.
Collis, J. L.: Surgical treatment of carcinoma of the oesophagus and cardia. Br. J. Surg. 58:801, 1971.
Connar, R. G., and Sealy, W. C.: Gastrostomy and its complications. Ann. Surg. 143:245, 1956.
Connehaye, P., Coupris, L., Labour, P. E., et al.: Ann. Chir. Infant. 16:45, 1975.
Conolly, W. B., Hunt, T. K., and Dunphy, J. E.: Management of contaminated surgical wounds. Surg. Gynecol. Obstet. 129:593, 1969.
Corley, R. D., Norcross, W. J., and Shoemaker, W. C.:

Traumatic injuries to the duodenum: A report of 98 patients. Ann. Surg. *181*:92, 1975.
Cornell, W. P., Ebert, P. A., and Zuidema, G. D.: X-ray diagnosis of penetrating wounds of the abdomen. J. Surg. Res. *5*:142, 1965.
Cotton, P. B.: *In* Truelove, S., and Trowell, J. (eds.): Topics in Gastroenterology. Philadelphia, J. B. Lippincott Company, 1975, p. 11.
Cotton, P. B., Chapman, M., Whiteside, C. G., et al.: Duodenoscopic papillotomy and gallstone removal. Br. J. Surg. *63*:709, 1976.
Cotton, P. B., Rosenberg, M. T., Axon, A. T. R., et al.: Diagnostic yield of fibre-optic endoscopy in the operated stomach. Br. J. Surg. *60*:629, 1973.
Cox, A. G., and Williams, J. A.: After Vagotomy. London, Butterworths, 1969.
Cox, W. D., and Gillesby, W. F.: Gastrostomy in postoperative decompression: Indications and methods. Am. J. Surg. *113*:298, 1967.
Craven, D. E., Goodman, D., and Carter, J. H.: Familial multiple endocrine adenomatosis: Multiple endocrine neoplasia, type I. Arch. Intern. Med. *129*:567, 1972.
Cremin, B. J.: Neonatal pre-pyloric membrane. South Afr. Med. J. *41*:1076, 1967.
Crooks: Estomac se terminant en cul-de-sac. Arch. Gen. Med. *17*:264, 1828. Cited in Gray and Skandalakis, 1972.
Cruse, P. J., and Foord, R.: A five-year prospective study of 23,649 surgical wounds. Arch. Surg. *107*:206, 1973.
Curtiss, L. E., Simmon, S., Buerk, C. A., et al.: Evaluation of the effectiveness of controlled pH in management of massive upper gastrointestinal bleeding. Am. J. Surg. *125*:474, 1973.
Czeizel, A.: Birthweight distribution in congenital pyloric stenosis. Arch. Dis. Child. *47*:978, 1972.
Dalgaard, J. B.: Volvulus of the stomach. Acta Chir. Scand. *103*:131, 1952.
Darby, R. E., Johnson, H. F., and Till, E. W.: Preoperative diagnosis of intramural hematoma. J. Pediatr. *72*:393, 1968.
Davenport, H. W.: Gastric secretion. *In* Physiology of the Digestive Tract, 3rd ed. Chicago, Year Book Medical Publishers, 1971.
Davies, W. T., Griffith, G. H., Owen, G. M., et al.: The effect of drainage operations on the rate of gastric emptying in duodenal ulcer patients. Br. J. Surg. *61*:590, 1974.
Davis, D. A., and Douglas, K. R.: Congenital pyloric atresia, a rare anomaly. Ann. Surg. *153*:418, 1961.
Davis, D. R., and Thomas, C. Y.: Intramural hematoma of the duodenum and jejunum. Ann. Surg. *153*:394, 1961.
Davis, J. M.: Preduodenal portal vein. N.Y. State J. Med. *76*:2038, 1976.
Davis, Z., Verheyden, C. N., Van Heerden, J. A., et al.: The surgically treated chronic gastric ulcer: An extended follow-up. Ann. Surg. *185*:205, 1977.
Deitel, M., and McIntyre, J.: Torsions of the stomach. Ann. R. Coll. Surg. Can. *3*:72, 1970.
Delaney, J. P.: The paucity of arteriovenous anastomoses in the stomach. Surgery *78*:411, 1975.
DeMatteis, R. A., and Hermann, R. E.: Vagotomy and drainage for obstructing duodenal ulcers. Importance of adequate drainage. Am. J. Surg. *127*:237, 1974.
Dent, T. L.: The surgeon and fiberoptic endoscopy. Surg. Gynecol. Obstet. *137*:278, 1973.

Derrick, J. R., and Fahdi, H. A.: Surgical anatomy of the superior mesenteric artery. Am. Surg. *31*:545, 1965. Cited in Akin, Gray, and Skandalakis, 1976.
DeSpirito, A. J., and Guthorn, P. J.: Recovery from meconium peritonitis associated with diaphragm-like obstruction of the prepyloric mucosa. J. Pediatr. *50*:599, 1957.
Deveney, C. W., Deveney, K. S., Jaffe, B. M., et al.: Use of calcium and secretin in the diagnosis of gastrinoma (Zollinger-Ellison syndrome). Ann. Intern. Med. *87*:680, 1977.
Deveney, C. W., Deveney, K. S., and Way, L. W.: The Zollinger-Ellison syndrome — 23 years later. Ann. Surg. *188*:384, 1978.
Deveney, K. S., and Way, L. W.: Effect of different absorbable sutures on healing of gastrointestinal anastomoses. Am. J. Surg. *133*:86, 1977.
Devroede, G. J., Tirol, F. T., LoRusso, V. A., et al.: Intramural hematoma of the duodenum and jejunum. Am. J. Surg. *112*:947, 1966.
Dickman, R. W.: Improved technics using the bowel stapling clamps in nineteen consecutive gastric resections. Am. J. Surg. *121*:628, 1971.
Diethrich, E. B., and Regan, W. J.: Antral mucosal diaphragm associated with esophageal hiatus hernia: Case report and review of the literature. Am. J. Surg. *110*:482, 1965.
Dineen, J. P., and Redo, S. F.: Pyloric obstruction due to mucosal diaphragm. Surgery *53*:674, 1963.
Dodge, J. A.: Maternal factor in infantile hypertrophic pyloric stenosis. Arch. Dis. Child. *49*:825, 1974.
Donovan, A. J., and Hagen, W. E.: Traumatic perforation of the duodenum. Am. J. Surg. *111*:341, 1966.
Dorph, M. H.: The cast syndrome. N. Engl. J. Med. *243*:440, 1950.
Douglass, H. O., Jr.: Levarterenol irrigation: Control of massive gastrointestinal bleeding in poor-risk patients. J.A.M.A. *230*:165, 1974.
Doutre, L. P., Quinton, A., and Gratadour, P.: L'endoscopie per operatoire en chirurgie digestive. Nouv. Presse Med. *3*:1217, 1974.
Dragstedt, L. R.: Vagotomy for gastroduodenal ulcer. Ann. Surg. *122*:973, 1945.
Dragstedt, L. R.: Physiology of the gastric antrum. *In* Thompson, C. M., et al. (eds.): The Stomach. New York, Grune & Stratton, 1967.
Dragstedt, L. R.: Duodenal inhibition of gastric secretion. Am. J. Surg. *117*:841, 1969.
Dragstedt, L. R., Camp, E. H., and Fritz, J.: Recurrence of gastric ulcer after complete vagotomy. Ann. Surg. *130*:593, 1949.
Dragstedt, L. R., de la Rosa, C., Woodward, E. R., et al.: The mechanism for gastrin release. Arch. Surg. *97*:816, 1968.
Draser, B. S., Shiner, M., and McLeod, G. M.: Studies of intestinal flora in healthy and achlorhydric persons. Gastroenterology *56*:71, 1969. Cited in Yeo and McNamara, 1973.
Dunkerley, R. C., Schull, H. J., Jr., Avant, G. R., et al.: Fiberendoscopic removal of large foreign bodies from the stomach. Gastrointest. Endosc. *21*:170, 1975.
Dunphy, J. E., Way, L. W., et al. (eds.): Current Surgical Diagnosis and Treatment. Los Altos, Cal., Lange Medical Publications, 1973.
Dupont, J. B., Jr., Lee, J. R., Burton, G. R., et al.: Adenocarcinoma of the stomach; Review of 1,497 cases. Cancer *41*:941, 1978.

Duthie, H. L., and Kwong, N. K.: Vagotomy or gastrectomy for gastric ulcer. Br. Med. J. 4:79, 1973.

Duthie, H. L., Moore, K. T. H., Bardsley, D., et al.: Surgical treatment of gastric ulcers. Br. J. Surg. 57:784, 1970.

Duthie, H. L., and Smith, G. H.: A comparison of vagotomy plus pyloroplasty with Billroth I gastrectomy in the treatment of gastric ulcer. J. R. Coll. Surg. Edinb. 13:324, 1968.

Dwyer, H. M., Yellin, A. E., Craig, J., et al.: Gastric hemostasis by laser phototherapy in man: A preliminary report. J.A.M.A., 236:1383, 1976.

Eade, G. G., Metheny, D., and Lundmark, V. O.: An evaluation of the practice of routine postoperative nasogastric suction. Surg. Gynecol. Obstet. 101:275, 1955.

Eaton, H., and Tennekoon, G. E.: Squamous carcinoma of the stomach following corrosive acid burns. Br. J. Surg. 59:382, 1972.

Edelson, Z.: Preduodenal portal vein. Am. J. Surg. 127:599, 1974.

Edkins, J. S.: On the chemical mechanism of gastric secretion. Proc. R. Soc. Lond. 76:376, 1905.

Edkins, J. S.: The chemical mechanism of gastric secretion. J. Physiol. 34:133, 1906.

Edlich, R. F., Panek, P. H., Rodeheaver, C. T., et al.: Physical and chemical configuration of sutures in the development of surgical infection. Ann. Surg. 177:679, 1973.

Edlich, R. F., Rogers, W., Kasper, G., et al.: Studies in the management of the contaminated wound. I. Optimal time for closure of contaminated open wound. II. Comparison of resistance to infection of open and closed wounds during healing. Am. J. Surg. 117:323–329, 1969.

Edwards, E. A., Malone, P. D., and MacArthur, J. D.: Operative Anatomy of Abdomen and Pelvis. Philadelphia, Lea & Febiger, 1975.

Edwards, F. C., and Coghill, N. F.: Clinical manifestations in patients with chronic atrophic gastritis, gastric ulcer, and duodenal ulcer. Q. J. Med. 37:377, 1968.

Eiseman, B., and Heyman, R. L.: Stress ulcers — a continuing challenge. N. Engl. J. Med. 282:372–374, 1970.

Eisenberg, H., and Steer, N. L.: The non-operative treatment of massive pyloroduodenal hemorrhage by retracted clot embolization. Surgery 79:414, 1976.

Eisenberg, R. L., Margulis, A. R., and Moss, A. A.: Giant duodenal ulcers. Gastrointest. Radiol. 2:347–353, 1978.

Elliott, T. E., Albertazzi, V. J., and Danto, L. A.: Stenosis after stapler anastomosis. Am. J. Surg. 133:750, 1977.

Ellison, E. H., and Wilson, S. D.: The Zollinger-Ellison syndrome: Re-appraisal and evaluation of 260 registered cases. Ann. Surg. 160:512, 1964.

Emanuel, B., Gault, J., and Sanson, J.: Neonatal intestinal obstruction due to absence of intestinal musculature: A new-entity. J. Pediat. Surg. 2:332, 1967.

Emergency War Surgery, first United States revision of NATO Handbook (Whelan, T. J., Jr. [ed.]). Washington, D.C., U.S. Government Printing Office, 1975.

Ernst, N. P.: A case of congenital atresia of the duodenum treated successfully by operation. Br. Med. J. 1:644, 1916.

Evans, C. H.: Atresias of the gastrointestinal tract. A collective review. Surg. Gynecol. Obstet. 92:1, 1951.

Evans, D. S.: Acute dilatation and spontaneous rupture of the stomach. Br. J. Surg. 55:940, 1968.

Evarts, C. M., Winters, R. B., and Hall, J. E.: Vascular compression of duodenum associated with treatment of scoliosis. J. Bone Joint Surg. 53A:431, 1971.

Fahrländer, H.: Laparoscopy in acute abdominal disease. Dtsch. Med. Wochenschr. 94:890, 1969.

Farris, J. M., and DeLaria, G. A.: Jaboulay method of pyloroplasty (lateral gastroduodenostomy); A modification. Surg. Tech. Illus. 1:69, 1976.

Farris, J. M., and Smith, G. K.: An evaluation of temporary gastrostomy: A substitute for nasogastric suction. Ann. Surg. 144:475, 1956.

Farris, J. M., and Smith, G. K.: Long-term appraisal of the treatment of gastric ulcer in situ by vagotomy and pyloroplasty. Am. J. Surg. 126:292, 1973.

Feggetter, S.: A review of the long-term results of operations for duodenal atresia. Br. J. Surg. 56:68, 1969.

Feldman, E. J., and Isenberg, J. I.: Effects of metiamide on gastric acid hypersecretion, steatorrhea and bone-marrow function in a patient with systemic mastocytosis. N. Engl. J. Med. 295:1178, 1976.

Feliciano, D. V., and Van Heerden, J. A.: Pyloric antral mucosal webs. Mayo Clin. Proc. 52:650, 1977.

Felson, B., and Levin, E. J.: Intramural hematoma of the duodenum; A diagnostic Roentgen sign. Radiology 63:823, 1954.

Fenger, C., Amdrup, E., Christiansen, P., et al.: Gastric ulcer. I. Analysis of 701 patients. Acta Chir. Scand. 139:455, 1973.

Ferguson, L. K.: Simplicity in surgery. Surg. Gynecol. Obstet. 88:539, 1949.

Filpi, R. G., Massoud, M., and Lo Presti, J. M.: Reversible gastric stricture following iron ingestion. South. Med. J. 66:845, 1973.

Finney, J. M. T.: A new method of pyloroplasty. Bull. Johns Hopkins Hosp. 13:155, 1902.

Finney, J. M. T.: Gastromesenteric ileus. Boston Med. Surg. J. 155:107, 1906a.

Finney, J. M. T.: The relation of dilatation of the duodenum to gastric disturbances. Bull. Johns Hopkins Hosp. 17:37, 1906b.

Finney, J. M. T.: A new method of gastroduodenostomy, end-to-side; With illustrations. Trans. South. Surg. Assoc. 36:576, 1924.

Fischer, M. G.: Bleeding from stapler anastomosis. Am. J. Surg. 131:745, 1976.

Fish, J. C., and Johnson, G. L.: Rupture of duodenum following blunt trauma: Report of a case with avulsion of papilla of Vater. Ann. Surg. 162:917, 1965.

Fleischer, D., and Samloff, M.: Cimetidine therapy in a patient with metiamide-induced agranulocytosis. N. Engl. J. Med. 296:342, 1977.

Fordtran, J. S., and Grossman, M. I.: Third symposium on histamine H_2-receptor antagonists: Clinical results with cimetidine. Gastroenterology 74:338, 1978.

Formeister, J. F., and Elias, E. G.: Safe intraabdominal and efficient wound drainage. Surg. Gynecol. Obstet. 142:415, 1976.

Foster, J. H., Hall, A. B., and Dunphy, J. E.: Surgical management of bleeding ulcers. Surg. Clin. North Am. 46:387, 1966.

Frederick, P. L., and Osborne, M. P.: The development of surgical procedures for the treatment of peptic ulceration of the stomach and duodenum. Surgery 58:884, 1965.

Freeark, R. J., Corley, R. D., Norcross, W. J., et al.: Intramural hematoma of the duodenum. Arch. Surg. 92:463, 1966.

Freeman, J. B., and Burchett, H. J.: A comparison of gastric bypass and gastroplasty for morbid obesity. Surgery 88:433, 1980.

Fricke, F. J., and Niewodowski, M. A.: Hazardous gaseous distention of intestinal balloons. J.A.M.A. 235:2611, 1976.

Friedman, I. H., and Wolff, W. I.: Laparoscopy: A valuable adjunct to the abdominal surgeon's armamentarium. Am. J. Surg. 135:160, 1978.

Friedrich, H.: Ein neues Magen-Darm-Nähapparat. Zentralbl. Chir. 9:504, 1934.

Friesen, S. R.: Effect of total gastrectomy on the Zollinger-Ellison tumor: Observations by second-look procedures. Surgery 62:609, 1967.

Fruhmorgen, P., et al.: Clinical results of laser coagulation in gastrointestinal bleeding. Dtsch. Med. Wochenschr. 101:1305, 1976.

Fullen, W. D., Hunt, J., and Altemeier, W. A.: Prophylactic antibiotics in penetrating wounds of the abdomen. J. Trauma 12:282, 1972.

Fullen, W. D., Selle, J. G., Whitley, D. H., et al.: Intramural duodenal hematoma. Ann. Surg. 179:549, 1974.

Gadacz, T. R., and Zuidema, G. D.: Bile acid composition in patients with and without symptoms of postoperative reflux gastritis. Am. J. Surg. 135:48, 1978.

Gaisford, W. D.: Gastrointestinal polypectomy via the fiberendoscope. Arch. Surg. 106:458, 1973.

Gallagher, M. W., Tyson, K. R., and Ashcroft, K. W.: Gastrostomy in pediatric patients: An analysis of complications and techniques. Surgery 74:536, 1973.

Gambee, L. P.: A single layer open intestinal anastomosis applicable to the small as well as the large intestine. West. J. Surg. 59:1, 1951.

Gambee, L. P., Garnjobst, W., and Hardwick, C. E.: Ten years' experience with a single layer anastomosis in colon surgery. Am. J. Surg. 92:222, 1956.

Gandhi, R. K., and Robarts, F. H.: Hour-glass stricture of the stomach and pyloric stenosis due to ferrous sulphate poisoning. Br. J. Surg. 49:613, 1962.

Garcia-Rinaldi, R., Defore, W. W., Jr., Green, Z. D., et al.: Improving the efficiency of wound drainage catheters. Am. J. Surg. 130:372, 1975.

Gerbeaux, J., Couvreur, J. Vialas, M., et al.: Absence congénitale d'estomach. Ann. Pediatr. (Paris) 18:349, 1971.

Gerber, A.: An appraisal of paralytic ileus and the necessity of postoperative gastrointestinal suction. Surg. Gynecol. Obstet. 117:294, 1963.

Gerber, A.: Gastrointestinal distention in the infant. J. Pediatr. 46:67, 1955.

Gerber, A., Rogers, F. A., and Smith, L. L.: The treatment of paralytic ileus without the use of gastrointestinal suction. Surg. Gynecol. Obstet. 107:247, 1958.

Gerber, B. C., and Aberdeen, S. D.: Prepyloric diaphragm: An unusual abnormality. Arch. Surg. 90:472, 1965.

Getzen, L. C.: Clinical use of everted intestinal anastomosis. Surg. Gynecol. Obstet. 123:1027, 1966.

Getzen, L. C.: Intestinal suturing. I. The development of intestinal sutures. II. Inverting and everting intestinal sutures. Curr. Prob. Surg., August, September, 1969.

Getzen, L. C., Roe, R. D., and Holloway, C. K.: Intestinal Anastomosis: Inverted and Everted; A Gross and Microscopic Comparative Study. Exhibit, American College of Surgeons Congress, Chicago, 1964.

Getzen, L. C., Roe, R. D., and Holloway, C. L.: Comparative study of intestinal anastomotic healing in inverted and everted closures. Surg. Gynecol. Obstet. 123:1219, 1966.

Gibbon, J. H., Jr., Nealon, T. F., Jr., and Greco, V. F.: A modification of Glassman's gastrostomy with results in 18 patients. Ann. Surg. 143:838, 1956.

Gilbertson, V. A., and Knatterud, G. L.: Gastric analysis as a screening measure for cancer of the stomach. Cancer 20:127, 1967.

Glass, G. C.: Hemorrhage in a newly born infant causing intestinal and biliary obstruction. Am. J. Dis. Child. 54:1052, 1937.

Glassman, J. A.: A new aseptic double-valved tubogastrostomy. Surg. Gynecol. Obstet. 68:789, 1939.

Golden, R.: Functional obstruction of efferent loop of jejunum following partial gastrectomy. J.A.M.A. 148:721, 1952.

Goldenberg, I. S.: Catgut, silk, and silver — the story of surgical sutures. Surgery 46:908, 1959.

Goligher, J. C.: Visceral and parietal sutures in abdominal surgery. Guest Oration. 16th Annual Meeting, Society for Surgery of the Alimentary Tract, San Antonio, Texas, 1975. Am. J. Surg 131:130, 1976.

Goligher, J. C., Irvin, T. T., Johnston, D., et al.: A controlled clinical trial of three methods of closure of laparotomy wounds. Br. J. Surg. 62:823, 1975.

Goligher, J. C., Lee, P. W. R., Macfie, J., et al.: Experience with the Russian Model 249 suture gun for anastomosis of the rectum. Surg. Gynecol. Obstet. 148:517, 1979.

Goligher, J. C., Pulvertaft, C. N., Irvin, T. T., et al.: Five- to eight-year results of truncal vagotomy and pyloroplasty for duodenal ulcer. Br. Med. J. 1:7, 1972.

Gomez, C. A.: Gastroplasty in the surgical treatment of morbid obesity. Am. J. Clin. Nutr. 33:406, 1980.

Gosin, S., and Ballinger, W. F.: Recurrent volvulus of the stomach. Report of a case with recurrence after simple decompression. Am. J. Surg. 109:642, 1965.

Graham, R. R.: A technic for total gastrectomy. Surgery 8:257, 1940.

Gray, S. W., and Skandalakis, J. E.: Embryology for Surgeons: The Embryological Basis for the Treatment of Congenital Defects. Philadelphia, W. B. Saunders Company, 1972.

Greenberg, M.: Mercury-weighted nasogastric tube: Its danger in intestinal surgery. South. Med. J. 65:1154, 1972.

Greene, J. F., Jr., Sawicki, J. E., and Doyle, W. F.: Gastric ulceration: A complication of double-lumen nasogastric tubes. J.A.M.A. 224:338, 1973.

Greenlee, H. B., Vivit, R., Paez, J., et al.: Bacterial flora of the jejunum following peptic ulcer surgery. Arch. Surg. 102:260, 1971.

Griffen, W. O., Young, V. L., and Stevenson, C. C.: A

BIBLIOGRAPHY

prospective comparison of gastric and jejunoileal bypass procedures for morbid obesity. Ann. Surg. 186:500, 1977.

Grimson, K. S., Randles, R. W., Baylin, G. T., et al.: Vagotomy; Observation during four years. Surgery 27:49, 1950.

Gross, K. E., and Durham, M. W.: Pyloric antral mucosal diaphragm. Radiology 61:368, 1953.

Gross, R. E.: The Surgery of Infancy and Childhood. Philadelphia, W. B. Saunders Company, 1953.

Gross, R. E.: An Atlas of Children's Surgery. Philadelphia, W. B. Saunders, 1970.

Grossman, M. I.: The Veterans Administration Cooperative Study on Gastric Ulcer. Chapter 10: Resume and Comment. Gastroenterology 61:635, 1971.

Gudov, V. F.: A method for the application of vascular sutures by mechanical means. Khirurgiia 12:58, 1950.

Gue, S.: Spontaneous rupture of stomach: A rare complication of inguinal hernia. Br. J. Surg. 57:154, 1970.

Guernsey, J. M., and Conolly, J. E.: Acute, complete gastric volvulus: Collective review and report of two cases. Arch. Surg. 86:423, 1963.

Gustafson, J. R.: Videofluorographic observations on various types of pyloroplasty. Am. Surg. 33:546, 1967.

Guyton, A. C.: Textbook of Medical Physiology, 6th ed. Philadelphia, W. B. Saunders Company, 1981.

Haggie, S. J., Fermont, D. C., and Wyllie, J. H.: Treatment of duodenal ulcer with Cimetidine. Lancet 1:983, 1976.

Haley, J. C., and Peden, J. K.: The suspensory muscle of the duodenum. Am. J. Surg. 59:546, 1943.

Haley, J. C., and Perry, J. H.: Further study of the suspensory muscle of the duodenum. Am. J. Surg. 77:590, 1949.

Hall, L. W.: The cast syndrome incognito. Am. J. Surg. 127:371, 1974.

Hall, W. H., and Hodges, S. C.: Effect of fluoroscopic tube placement on basal gastric secretion collections. South. Med. J. 69:164, 1976.

Hallenbeck, G. A.: Elective surgery for treatment of hemorrhage from duodenal ulcer. Gastroenterology 59:784, 1970.

Hallenbeck, G. A., Gleysteen, J. J., Aldrete, J. S., et al.: Proximal gastric vagotomy: Effects of two operative techniques on clinical and gastric secretory results. Ann. Surg. 184:435, 1976.

Haller, J. A., Jr., and Cahill, J. L.: Combined congenital gastric and duodenal obstruction: Pitfalls in diagnosis and treatment. Surgery 63:503, 1968.

Halloran, L. G.: Personal communication to Latimer, Doane, McKittrick, et al., 1975.

Halnagyi, A. F.: A critical review of 125 patients with upper gastrointestinal hemorrhage. Surg. Gynecol. Obstet. 130:419, 1970.

Halsted, W. S.: Circular suture of the intestine. An experimental study. Am. J. Med. Sci. 99:463, 1887.

Hamilton, J. E.: Reappraisal of open intestinal anastomoses. Trans. South. Surg. Assoc. 78:273, 1966.

Hancock, B. D., Bowen-Jones, E., Dixon, R., et al.: The effect of posture on the gastric emptying of solid meals in normal subjects and patients after vagotomy. Br. J. Surg. 61:945, 1974.

Handelsman, J. C.: Telephone communication, September, 1976.

Handelsman, J. C., Bloodwell, R., Bender, H., et al.: An unusual cause of neonatal intestinal obstruction: Congenital absence of the duodenal musculature. Surgery 58:1022, 1965.

Hanna, E. A.: Efficiency of peritoneal drainage. Surg. Gynecol. Obstet. 131:983, 1970.

Hanselman, R. C., and Meyer, R. H.: Complications of gastrointestinal intubation; Collective review. Int. Abstr. Surg. 114:207, 1962. In Surg. Gynecol. Obstet. 114(5).

Hardin, W. J.: Evaluation of autosutures in gastrointestinal surgery. South. Med. J. 70:197, 1977.

Hardy, J. D.: Problems associated with gastric surgery: A review of 604 consecutive patients with annotation. Am. J. Surg. 108:699, 1964.

Hardy, J. D.: Critical Surgical Illness, 2nd ed. Philadelphia, W. B. Saunders Company, 1971.

Harrison, A., Wechsler, R., and Elliott, D.: Gastric analysis in the absence of demonstrable gastric pathology. Am. J. Surg. 123:132, 1972.

Harrison, R. C., and Debas, H. T.: Injuries of the stomach and duodenum. Surg. Clin. North Am. 52:635, 1972.

Hartenstein, P. E., Ziperman, H. H., and Smith, M. L.: Infrapapillary obstruction of the duodenum. Ann. Surg. 154:125, 1961.

Hase, O., Shaw, A., and Gould, H. R.: Duodenal diaphragmatic obstruction with pneumoperitoneum presenting in a 13-year-old girl. Surgery 62:530, 1967.

Hashimoto, S., Tsugawa, C., Horikoshi, R., et al.: Radiologic diagnosis of gastric perforations in neonates. J. Jap. Pediatr. Surg. 13:117, 1977.

Hastings, P. R., Skillman, J. J., Bushnell, L. S., et al.: Antacid titration in the prevention of acute gastrointestinal bleeding. N. Engl. J. Med. 298:1041, 1978.

Hatfield, A. R. W., Slavin, G., Segal, A. W., et al.: Importance of the site of endoscopic gastric biopsy in ulcerating lesions of the stomach. Gut 16:884, 1975.

Haubrich, W. S.: Bilocular stomach. In Bockus, H. L.: Gastroenterology, 3rd ed. Philadelphia, W. B. Saunders Company, 1976, pp. 756–757.

Haws, E. B., Sieber, W. K., and Kiesewetter, W. B.: Complications of tube gastrostomy in infants and children: 15-year review of 240 cases. Ann. Surg. 97:190, 1968.

Hayden, W. F., and Reed, R. C.: A comparative study of Heineke-Mikulicz and Finney pyloroplasty. Am. J. Surg. 116:755, 1968.

Hearn, J. B.: Duodenal ileus with special reference to superior mesenteric artery compression. Radiology 86:305, 1966. Cited by Akin, et al., 1976.

Heilbrun, N., and Boyden, E. A.: Intraluminal duodenal diverticulum. Radiology 82:887, 1964.

Hendry, W. G.: Tubeless gastric surgery. Br. Med. J. 1:1736, 1962.

Henn, R. M., Isenberg, J. I., Maxwell, B. S., et al.: Inhibition of gastric acid secretion by cimetidine in patients with duodenal ulcer. N. Engl. J. Med. 293:371, 1975.

Henroz, J. H. F.: Dissertatio inauguralis critica de methodis ad sananda intestina divisa adhibitis, in qua nova sanationis methodus proponitur. In Universitate Leodiensi Publico Examini Submittit, June 14, 1826.

Henry, E. C.: Acute dilatation of the stomach following operations. Nebraska Med. J. 18:209, 1933.

Herbst, C. A., Jr.: Relationships of gastrin to duodenal

ulcer disease in man and the effects of surgery. Am. J. Surg. 133:619, 1977.
Hermann, R. E.: Obstructing duodenal ulcer. Surg. Clin. North Am. 56:1403, 1976.
Hermreck, A. S., Jewell, W. R., and Hardin, C. A.: Gastric bypass for morbid obesity: Results and complications. Surgery 80:498, 1976.
Herrington, J. L., Jr.: Methods of postoperative gastric decompression, including an experience with the omission of its routine use. Am. J. Surg. 110:424, 1965a.
Herrington, J. L., Jr.: Avoidance of routine use of postoperative gastric suction. Surg. Gynecol. Obstet. 121:351, 1965b.
Herrington, J. L., Jr.: Elimination of routine nasogastric decompression following vagotomy-antrectomy and vagotomy with pyloroplasty or gastroenterostomy. Am. Surg. 33:361, 1967.
Herrington, J. L., Jr.: Iatrogenic marginal ulcer and afferent loop obstructions as sequelae to operation for intramural duodenal hematoma. Am. Surg. 35:326, 1969.
Herrington, J. L., Jr.: Additional experience with elimination of routine nasogastric suction following gastric operations. Surgery 71:132, 1972.
Herrington, J. L.: Telephone communication, June, 1976.
Herrington, J. L., Jr., Edwards, W. H., and Sawyers, J. L.: Elimination of routine use of gastric decompression following operation for gastroduodenal ulcer. Ann. Surg. 159:807, 1964.
Herrington, J. L., Jr., and Sawyers, J. L.: Results of elective duodenal ulcer surgery in women: Comparison of truncal vagotomy and antrectomy, gastric selective vagotomy and pyloroplasty, proximal gastric vagotomy. Ann. Surg. 187:576, 1978.
Hertzer, N. R., and Hoerr, S. O.: An interpretive review of lymphoma of the stomach. Surg. Gynecol. Obstet. 143:113, 1976.
Himal, H. S., Perrault, C., and Mzabi, R.: Upper gastrointestinal hemorrhage: Aggressive management decreases mortality. Surgery 84:448, 1978.
Hinder, R. A., and Kelly, K. A.: Human gastric pacesetter potential: Site of origin, spread, and response to gastric transection and proximal gastric vagotomy. Am. J. Surg. 133:29, 1977.
Hirsch, K.: Ueber Sanduhrmagen. Virchows Arch. Pathol. Anat. 140:459, 1895. Cited in Gray and Skandalakis, 1972.
Hirschowitz, B., Curtis, L., Peters, C., et al.: Demonstration of a new fiberscope. Gastroenterology 35:50, 1958.
Hoag, C. L., and Saunders, J. B.: Jejunoplasty. Surg. Gynecol. Obstet. 68:703, 1939.
Hoile, R. W., and Turner, J. C. D.: Gastric fistula after proximal gastric vagotomy. Br. Med. J. 2:282, 1975.
Holder, T. M., and Gross, R. E.: Temporary gastrostomy in pediatric surgery: Experience with 187 cases. Pediatrics 26:36, 1960.
Holder, T. M., Leape, L. L., and Ashcroft, L. W.: Gastrostomy: Its use and dangers in pediatric patients. N. Engl. J. Med. 286:1345, 1972.
Holgersen, L. O.: Nonoperative treatment of duodenal hematoma in childhood. J. Pediatr. Surg. 12:11, 1977.
Holladay, L. J.: Case report of congenital aplasia of the pylorus. J. Indiana Med. Assoc. 39:350, 1946. Cited in Gray and Skandalakis, 1972.
Holt-Christensen, J., Hart Hansen, O., Pederson, T., et al.: Recurrent ulcer after proximal gastric vagotomy for duodenal and pre-pyloric ulcer. Br. J. Surg. 64:42, 1977.
Hornberger, H. R.: Gastric bypass. Am. J. Surg. 131:415, 1976.
Horseley, J. S.: Surgery of Stomach and Small Intestine. New York, Appleton, 1926, Chap. X.
Hoyt, R. L.: Microgastria. Med. J. Record 119:338, 1924. Cited in Gray and Skandalakis, 1972.
Hudson, C. N.: Congenital diaphragm of the duodenum causing obstruction in an adult. Br. J. Surg. 49:234, 1961.
Hudspeth, A. S., and McWhorter, J. M.: Gastric volvulus causing rupture of the spleen. Arch. Surg. 102:232, 1971.
Hughes, C. E., III, Conn, J., Jr., and Sherman, J. O.: Intramural hematoma of the gastrointestinal tract. Am. J. Surg. 133:276, 1977.
Huguenard, J. R., and Sharples, G. E.: Incidence of congenital pyloric stenosis within sibships. J. Pediatr. 81:45, 1972.
Hültl, H.: II Kongress der ungarischen Gesellschaft für Chirurgie, Budapest, May, 1908. Pester Med.-Chir. Presse 45:108, 121, 1909.
Hültl, H.: Über Pylorektomie. XIV Congrès International de Médecin, Budapest, 1909. Compte-Rendu, Sect. VIIA, Chir., p. 561, Budapest, 1910.
Hurst, A. F., and Stewart, M. J.: Gastric and Duodenal Ulcer. London, Oxford University Press, 1929, p. 339.
Inouye, W. Y., and Evans, G.: Neonatal gastric perforation. Arch. Surg. 88:471, 1963.
Ippoliti, A. F., Isenberg, J. I., Maxwell, V., et al.: The effect of 16,16-dimethyl prostaglandin E2 on meal-stimulated gastric acid secretion and serum gastrin in duodenal ulcer patients. Gastroenterology 70:488, 1976.
Ippoliti, A. F., and Walsh, J. I.: Newer concepts in the pathogenesis of peptic ulcer disease. Surg. Clin. North Am. 56:1479, 1976.
Isbister, W. H.: Is postoperative gastric decompression really necessary? Am. J. Surg. 120:511, 1970.
Ivey, K. J.: Anticholinergics: Do they work in peptic ulcer? Gastroenterology 68:154, 1975.
Ivey, K. J., Baskin, W., and Jeffrey, G.: Effect of cimetidine on gastric potential difference in man. Lancet 2:1072, 1975.
Izant, R. J., Jr., and Drucker, W. R.: Duodenal obstruction due to intramural hematoma in children. J. Trauma 4:797, 1964.
Jaboulay, M.: La gastroenterostomie la jejunoduodenostomie la resection du pylore. Arch. Prov. Chir. (Paris) 1:1, 1892.
Jacobs, E. A., Culver, G. J., and Koenig, E. A.: Roentgenologic aspects of retroperitoneal perforations of the duodenum. Radiology 43:563, 1944.
Jacobson, G., and Carter, R. A.: Small intestinal rupture due to non-penetrating abdominal injury. Am. J. Roentgenol. 66:52, 1951.
Janeway, H. H.: Eine neue Gastrostomie-methode. Münch. Med. Wochenschr. 60:1705, 1913.
Janson, K. L., and Stockinger, F.: Duodenal hematoma. Critical analysis of recent treatment technics. Am. J. Surg. 129:304, 1975.

Jefferiss, C. D.: Spontaneous rupture of the stomach in an adult. Br. J. Surg. 59:79, 1972.

Jenkins, H. P., Hrdina, L. S., Owens, F. M., Jr., et al.: Absorption of surgical gut (catgut). Arch. Surg. 45:74, 1974.

Jennings, K. P., and Klidjian, A. M.: Acute gastric dilatation in anorexia nervosa. Br. Med. J. 2:477, 1974.

Johnson, D.: Operative mortality and postoperative morbidity of highly selective vagotomy. Br. Med. J. 4:545, 1975.

Johnson, H. D.: Gastric ulcer: Classification, blood group characteristics, secretion patterns, and pathogenesis. Ann. Surg. 162:996, 1965.

Johnson, W. C., and Windrich, W. C.: Efficacy of selective splenic arteriography and vasopressin perfusion and diagnosis and treatment of gastrointestinal hemorrhage. Am. J. Surg. 131:481, 1976.

Jona, J. Z., and Belin, R. P.: Duodenal anomalies and the ampulla of Vater. Surg. Gynecol. Obstet. 143:565, 1976.

Jones, S.: Gastrostomy for stricture (cancer of esophagus). Lancet 1:678, 1875.

Jones, T. W.: Paraduodenal hernia and hernias of the foramen of Winslow. In Nyhus, L. M., and Harkins, H. N. (eds.): Hernia. Philadelphia, J. B. Lippincott Company, 1964.

Jones, W. R., Hardin, W. J., Davis, J. T., et al.: Intramural hematoma of the duodenum; A review of the literature and case report. Ann. Surg. 173:534, 1971.

Jordan, G. L., Jr., and DeBakey, M. E.: The surgical management of acute gastroduodenal perforation. Am. J. Surg. 101:317, 1961.

Jordan, P. H., Jr., and Condon, R. E.: A prospective evaluation of vagotomy-pyloroplasty and vagotomy-antrectomy for the treatment of duodenal ulcer. Ann. Surg. 172:547, 1970.

Jordan, P. H., Jr., Hendenstedt, S., Korompai, F. L., et al.: Vagotomy of the fundic gland area of the stomach without drainage: A definitive treatment for perforated duodenal ulcer. Am. J. Surg. 131:523, 1976.

Judd, D. R., Taybi, H., and King, H.: Intramural hematoma of the small bowel. Arch Surg. 89:527, 1964.

Judd, E. S., and Nagel, G. W.: Excision of ulcer of the duodenum. Surg. Gynecol. Obstet. 45:17, 1927.

Kajiwara, T., Tamura, K., and Suzuki, T.: Follow-up study of gastric response after resection of the jejunum and the ileum. Ann. Surg. 186:694, 1977.

Kalinina, T. V.: The use of the apparatuses PKS25 and SK in the Clinic. Moscow, Mechanical Sutures in Surgery of the Gastrointestinal Tract, 1964a.

Kalinina, T. V.: Method of constructing esophagogastric and gastroesophageal anastomoses with the use of the apparatus PKS25. Moscow, Experiences with the Clinical Use of New Apparatus and Instruments, 1964b.

Kalinina, T. V.: Development and clinical use of suturing apparatuses for anastomosis of the gastrointestinal tract. Moscow, Surgical Suturing Apparatus, 1967.

Kaminsky, V. M., and Dietel, M.: Nutritional support in the management of external fistulas of the alimentary tract. Br. J. Surg. 62:100, 1975.

Kampp, M. V., Lundgren, O., and Sjostrand, J.: On the components of the Kr[85] washout curves for the small intestine of the cat. Acta Physiol. Scand. 72:257, 1968.

Karamcheti, A., O'Donnell, W. F., Hakala, T. R., et al.: Autosuture ileal conduit construction: Experience in 110 cases. J. Urol. 120:545, 1978.

Kassner, E. G., Rose, J. S., Kottmeier, P. K., et al.: Retention of small foreign objects in the stomach and duodenum. Radiology 114:683, 1975.

Katsas, A. G., Sapountzis, D. P., and Leoutsakos, B. G.: Unusual cause of intramural hematoma of duodenum. Am. Surg. 36:563, 1970.

Kawai, K., Akasaka, Y., Murakami, K., et al.: Endoscopic sphincterotomy of the ampulla of Vater. Gastrointest. Endosc. 20:148, 1974.

Kawia, K., Murakami, K., and Misaki, F.: Endoscopical observations on gastric ulcers in teenagers. Endoscopy 2:206, 1970.

Keil, P. G., and Landis, S. N.: Peritoneoscopic cholangiography. Arch. Intern. Med. 88:36, 1951.

Kelling, G.: Über Oesophagoskopie, Gastroskopie und Kolioskopie. Münch. Med. Wochenschr. 21 (June 7, 1902).

Kennedy, B. J.: TNM classification for stomach cancer. Cancer 26:971, 1970.

Kennedy, F., MacKay, C., Bedi, B. S., et al.: Truncal vagotomy and drainage for chronic duodenal ulcer disease: A controlled trial. Br. Med. J. 2:71, 1973.

Kennedy, T., Johnson, G. W., Macrea, K. D., et al.: Proximal gastric vagotomy: Interim results of a randomized controlled trial. Br. Med. J. 2:301, 1975.

Kerremans, R. P., Lerut, J., and Pennickx, F. M.: Primary malignant duodenal tumors. Ann. Surg. 190:179, 1979.

Kiefhaber, P., Nath, G., and Moritz, K.: Endoscopical control of massive gastrointestinal hemorrhage by irradiation with a high-power neodymium YAG laser. Prog. Surg. 15:140, 1977.

Klamer, T. W., and Mahr, M. M.: Giant duodenal ulcer: A dangerous variant of a common illness. Am. J. Surg. 125:760, 1978.

Knecht, B. H.: Experience with gastric bypass for massive obesity. Am. Surg. 48:496, 1978.

Knight, H. O.: An anomalous portal vein with its surgical dangers. Ann. Surg. 74:679, 1921.

Knutson, C. O.: Fiberoptic endoscopy: Precise definition of upper gastrointestinal disease. Am. J. Surg. 129:651, 1975.

Koch, H.: Endoscopic papillotomy. Endoscopy 7:89, 1975.

Koga, S., Nishimura, O., Iwai, N., et al.: Clinical evaluation of long-term survival after total gastrectomy. Am. J. Surg. 138:635, 1979.

Kolter, J., and Ravitch, M. M.: Unpublished data.

Konturek, S. J., Kweicien, N., Swierczek, J., et al.: Comparison of methylated prostaglandin Z-E analogs given orally in the inhibition of gastric responses to pentagastrin and peptone meal in man. Gastroenterology 70:683, 1976.

Kothe, W., Poge, A. W., Albert, H., et al.: The quantitative gastric analysis as a foundation for anatomic and physiologic sound gastric surgical procedures. Zentralbl. Chir. 96:529, 1971.

Krais, W.: Kann metallisches Quecksilber vom Magendarm Kanal aus zur Vergiftung; führen? Arch. Toxik. 15:202, 1955.

Kraus, M., Mendeloff, G., and Condon, R. E.: Prognosis of gastric ulcer: twenty-five year follow-up. Ann. Surg. 184:471, 1976.

Kregel, L. A.: Spontaneous rupture of the stomach. Am. Surg. 21:505, 1955.

Kreig, E. G.: Duodenal diaphragm. Ann. Surg. 106:33, 1937.
Kremer, R. M., Lepoff, R. B., and Izant, R. J.: Duplication of the stomach. J. Pediatr. Surg. 5:360, 1970.
Krizek, T. J., and Robson, M. C.: Evolution of quantitative bacteriology in wound management. Am. J. Surg. 130:579, 1975.
Kronborg, O., and Madsen, P.: A controlled, randomized trial of highly selective vagotomy versus selective vagotomy and pyloroplasty in the treatment of duodenal ulcer. Gut 16:268, 1975.
Lahey, F. H.: Experiences with post-operative jejunal ulcer and gastrojejunocolic fistula. Am. J. Dig. Dis. 2:673, 1936.
Lampe, G. W.: Surgical anatomy of the abdominal wall. Surg. Clin. North Am. 32:545, 1952.
Larkworthy, W., Jones, R. T. B., Mahoney, M., et al.: Removal of ingested coins utilizing fibre-endoscopy and special forceps. Br. J. Surg. 61:750, 1974.
Latimer, R. G., Doane, W. A., McKittrick, J. E., et al.: Automatic staple suturing for gastrointestinal surgery. Am. J. Surg. 130:766, 1975.
Laufman, H. (Editorial): Is catgut obsolete? Surg. Gynecol. Obstet. 145:587, 1977.
Laufman, H., and Rubel, T.: Synthetic absorbable sutures; collective review. Surg. Gynecol. Obstet. 145:597, 1977.
Law, D. H., and Ten Eyck, E. A.: Familial megaduodenum and megacystis. Am. J. Med. 33:911, 1962.
Lawrie, P.: A survey of the absorbability of commercial surgical catgut. Br. J. Surg. 46:634, 1959.
Lawrie, P., and Angus, G. E.: The absorption of surgical catgut. II. The influence of size. Br. J. Surg. 47:551, 1960.
Lawrie, P., Angus, G. E., and Reese, A. J. M.: The absorption of surgical catgut. Br. J. Surg. 46:638, 1959.
Lee, C. M.: Transposition of a colon segment as a gastric reservoir after total gastrectomy. Surg. Gynecol. Obstet. 92:456, 1951.
Lee, D., Zacher, J., and Vogel, T. T.: Primary repair in transection of duodenum with avulsion of the common duct. Arch. Surg. 111:592, 1976.
Lee, W. Y.: Evaluation of peritoneoscopy in intra-abdominal diagnosis. Gastroenterology 9:133, 1942.
LeFevre, H.: La gastrectomie totale. Nouvelle technique operatoire. Résultats. Mém. Acad. Chir. 72:580, 1946.
Lembert, A.: Mémoire sur l'entérrhaphie. Rep. Gen. Anat. Physiol. Pathol. 2:101, 1826.
Lemmon, W. T., and Paschal, G. W.: Rupture of the stomach following ingestion of sodium bicarbonate. Ann. Surg. 114:997, 1941.
Lescher, T. J., Teegarden, D. K., and Pruitt, B. A.: The changing spectrum of major gastrointestinal complications in burned patients. Abstract, 27th Congress, Societé Internationale de Chirurgie, Kyoto, Japan, September, 1977, p. 25.
LeVeen, H. H., Falk, G., Diaz, C., et al.: Control of gastrointestinal bleeding. Am. J. Surg. 123:154, 1972.
Levin, A. L.: New gastroduodenal catheter. J.A.M.A. 76:1007, 1921.
Lewis, J. E.: Partial duodenal obstruction with incomplete duodenal rotation. J. Pediatr. Surg. 1:47, 1966.

Liechti, R. E., Mikkelson, W. P., and Snyder, W. H., Jr.: Prepyloric stenosis caused by congenital squamous epithelial diaphragm — resultant infantilism. Surgery 53:670, 1963.
Lilly, J. O., and McCaffery, T. D.: Esophageal stricture dilatation: A new method adapted to the fiberoptic esophagoscope. Am. J. Dig. Dis. 16:1137, 1971.
Llanio, R., Sotto, A., Jimenez, G., et al.: Emergency peritoneoscopy: A study of 1,265 instances. Sem. Hôp. Paris 49:873, 1973.
Lloyd, J. R., and Clatworthy, H. W., Jr.: Hydramnios as an aid to the early diagnosis of congenital obstruction of the alimentary tract: A study of maternal and fetal factors. Pediatrics 21:903, 1958.
Longmire, W. P.: Discussion of Herrington, J. L., Jr., Edwards, W. H., and Sawyers, J. L.: Elimination of routine use of gastric decompression following operation for gastroduodenal ulcer. Ann. Surg. 159:807, 1964.
Longmire, W. P., and Beal, J. M.: Construction of a subsitute gastric reservoir following total gastrectomy. Ann. Surg. 135:637, 1952.
Lucas, C. E., and Ledgerwood, A. M.: Factors influencing outcome after blunt duodenal injury. J. Trauma 15:839, 1975.
Lucas, C. E., Suzawa, C., Riddle, J., et al.: Natural history and surgical dilemma of "stress" gastric bleeding. Arch. Surg. 102:266, 1971.
Lumsten, K., MacLarnon, J. C., and Dawson, J.: Giant duodenal ulcer. Gut 11:592, 1970.
Lundberg, G. D., Mattei, I. R., and Davis, C. J.: Hemorrhage from gastroesophageal lacerations following closed-chest cardiac massage. J.A.M.A. 202:123, 1967.
Lynch, J. D., Jernigan, S. K., Trotta, P. H., et al.: Incidence and analysis of failure with vagotomy and Heineke-Mikulicz pyloroplasty. Surgery 58:483, 1965.
Lynn, H. B.: Duodenal obstruction: Atresia, stenosis and annular pancreas. In Mustard, W. T., et al.: Pediatric Surgery, 2nd ed. Chicago, Year Book Medical Publishers, 1969.
MacGregor, A. B., and Ross, P. W.: Bacterial content of the gastric juice. Br. J. Surg. 59:443, 1972.
MacKenzie, D.: The history of sutures (presented to the Royal College of Surgeons of Edinburgh, 1971). Med. Hist. 17:158, 1973.
Mackenzie, W. C., Lang, A., Friedman, M. H. W., et al.: Congenital atresia of the second portion of the duodenum with associated obstruction of the biliary tract. Surg. Gynecol. Obstet. 110:755, 1960.
Madden, J. L.: Congenital atresia of the esophagus treated by one-stage primary esophagogastrostomy employing a right transpleural approach. J. Thorac. Surg. 21:460, 1951.
Maher, J. W., Wickbom, G., Woodward, E. R., et al.: The effect of vagal stimulation on gastrin release and acid secretion. Surgery 77:255, 1975.
Mahoney, D. H.: Intramural gastric lesion with sudden abdominal pain. J.A.M.A. 230:603, 1974.
Mahour, G. H., Wooley, M. M., Gans, S. L., et al.: Duodenal hematoma in infancy and childhood. J. Pediatr. Surg. 6:153, 1971.
Maimon, H. N., and Milligan, F. D.: Removal of a foreign body from the stomach. A new use of the fiber-esophagoscope. Gastrointest. Endosc. 18:163, 1972.
Mainardi, M., Maxwell, B. S., Sturdevant, R. A. L., et al.:

Metiamide, an H_2-receptor blocker, as inhibitor of basal and meal-stimulated gastric acid secretion in patients with duodenal ulcer. N. Engl. J. Med. 293:371, 1975.

Maingot, R.: Hour-glass deformity. In Abdominal Operations, 5th ed. Vol. I. New York, Appleton-Century-Crofts, 1969, p. 206.

Maingot, R.: Volvulus of the stomach. In Abdominal Operations, 5th ed. New York, Appleton-Century-Crofts, 1969.

Maini, B. S., Blackburn, G. L., and McDermott, W. V.: Technical considerations in a gastric bypass operation for morbid obesity. Surg. Gynecol. Obstet. 145:907, 1977.

Major, J. W., Ottenheimer, E. J., and Whalen, W. A., Jr.: Duodenal obstruction at the ligament of Treitz: Report of a case treated by a plastic procedure. N. Engl. J. Med. 262:443, 1960.

Mann, F. C., and Williamson, C. S.: The experimental production of peptic ulcer. Ann. Surg. 77:409, 1923.

Mansberger, A. R., Hearn, J. B., Byers, R. M., et al.: Vascular compression of the duodenum: Emphasis on accurate diagnosis. Am. J. Surg. 115:89, 1968.

Margolis, I. B., Carnazzo, A. J., and Finn, M. P.: Intramural hematoma of the duodenum. Am. J. Surg. 132:779, 1976.

Markowski, B.: Acute dilatation of stomach. Br. Med. J. 2:128, 1947.

Marshall, S. F., and Knud-Hansen, J.: Gastrojejunocolic and gastrocolic fistulas. Ann. Surg. 145:770, 1957.

Martin, J. W., and Siebenthal, B. J.: Jaundice due to hypertrophic pyloric stenosis. J. Pediatr. 47:95, 1955.

Martin, L. W., and Fultz, C. T.: Use of gastrostomy in pediatric surgery. Arch. Surg. 78:904, 1959.

Martin, T. R., Vennes, J. A., Silvis, S. E., et al.: A comparison of upper gastrointestinal endoscopy and radiology. Gastroenterology 2:21, 1980.

Mason, E. E., and Ito, C.: Gastric bypass: Ann. Surg. 170:329, 1969.

Mason, E. E., Munns, J. R., Kealey, G. P., et al.: Effect of gastric bypass on gastric secretion. Am. J. Surg. 131:162, 1976.

Mason, E. E., Printen, K. J., Barron, P., et al.: Risk reduction in gastric operations for obesity. Ann. Surg. 190:158, 1979.

Mason, E. E., Printen, K. J., Hartford, C. E., et al.: Optimizing results of gastric bypass. Ann. Surg. 182:405, 1975.

Matas, R.: The continued intravenous "drip." Ann. Surg. 79:643, 1924.

Matheson, N. A., and Irving, A. D.: Single-layer anastomosis in the gastrointestinal tract. Surg. Gynecol. Obstet. 143:619, 1976.

Matolo, N. M., Cohen, S. E., Fontanetta, A. P., et al.: Traumatic duodenal injuries: An analysis of 32 cases. Am. Surg. 41:331, 1975.

Maull, K. I., Fallahzadeh, H., and Mays, E. T.: Selective management of post-traumatic obstructing intramural hematoma of the duodenum. Surg. Gynecol. Obstet. 146:221, 1978.

Max, M., and Menguy, R.: Influence of adrenocorticotropin, cortisone, aspirin and phenylbutazone on the rate of exfoliation and the rate of renewal of gastric mucosal cells. Gastroenterology 58:329, 1970.

McCaffery, T. D., Jr., and Lilly, J. O.: The management of foreign affairs of the G.I. tract. Am. J. Dig. Dis. 20:121, 1975.

McCarthy, D. M.: Report on the United States experience with cimetidine in Zollinger-Ellison syndrome and other hypersecretory states. Gatroenterology 74:453, 1978.

McDonald, P. T., Rich, N. M., and Collins, G. J.: Vascular trauma secondary to diagnostic and therapeutic procedures: Laparoscopy. Am. J. Surg. 135:651, 1978.

McDougal, W. S., and Persky, L.: Traumatic and spontaneous pyeloduodenal fistulas. J. Trauma 12:665, 1972.

McGinty, C. P., Kasten, M. C., Kinder, J. L., et al.: Update on stapled bowel anastomosis. Mo. Med. 76: 145, 159, 1979.

McGregor, D. B., Savage, L. E., and McVay, C. B.: Massive gastrointestinal hemorrhage: A twenty-five year experience with vagotomy and drainage. Surgery 80:530, 1976.

McIlrath, D. C., van Heerden, J. A., Edis, A. J., et al.: Closure of abdominal incisions with subcutaneous catheters. Surgery 80:411, 1976.

McInnis, W. D., Aust, J. B., Cruz, A. B., et al.: Traumatic injuries of the duodenum: A comparison of primary closure and the jejunal patch. J. Trauma 15:847, 1975.

McLaughlan, J.: Fatal false aneurysmal tumor occupying nearly the whole of the duodenum. Lancet 2:203, 1838.

McLetchie, N. G. B., Purves, J. K., and Saunders, R. L.: Genesis of gastric and certain intestinal diverticulum and enterogenous cysts. Surg. Gynecol. Obstet. 99:135, 1954.

Meeker, I. A., and Snyder, W. H.: Gastrostomy for the newborn surgical patient: A report of 140 cases. Arch. Dis. Child. 37:159, 1962.

Meissner, W. A.: Leiomyoma of the stomach. Arch. Pathol. 38:207, 1944.

Melchior, E.: Beiträge zur chirurgischen Duodenalpathologie. Arch. Klin. Chir. 125:633, 1923.

Menguy, R.: Gastric mucus and the gastric mucous barrier: A review. Am. J. Surg. 117:806, 1969.

Menguy, R.: The stomach. In Schwartz, S. I., et al.: Principles of Surgery, 2nd ed. New York, McGraw-Hill Book Company, 1974.

Menguy, R.: Surgery of Peptic Ulcer. Philadelphia, W. B. Saunders Company, 1976.

Menguy, R., Gadacz, T., and Zajtchuk, R.: The surgical management of acute gatric mucosal bleeding, stress ulcer, acute erosive gastritis, and acute hemorrhagic gastritis. Arch. Surg. 99:198, 1969.

Mestel, A. L., Trusler, G. A., Thompson, S. A., et al.: Acute obstruction of small intestine secondary to hematoma in children. Arch. Surg. 78:25, 1959.

Metcalfe-Gibson, C.: A case of haemorrhage from volvulus of the gastric fundus. Br. J. Surg. 62:224, 1975.

Metz, A. R., Householder, R., and De Pree, J. F.: Obstruction of the stomach due to congenital double septum with cyst formation. Trans. West. Surg. Assoc. 50:242, 1941.

Metzger, W. H., Cano, R., and Sturdevant, R. A.: Effect of metoclopramide in chronic gastric retention after gastric surgery. Gastroenterology 71:30, 1976.

Meyer, W.: Gastrostomy and inferior oesophagoplasty (Beck-Jianu). Ann. Surg. 61:480, 1915.

Mikulicz, J.: 1886. Cited in Mikulicz, J.: Zur operativen

Behandlung des stenosier enden Magengeschwüres. Arch. Klin. Chir. 37:79, 1888.

Millar, T. McW., Bruce, J., and Paterson, J. R. S.: Spontaneous rupture of the stomach. Br. J. Surg. 44:513, 1957.

Miller, H. I.: Sternum-splitting incision for upper abdominal surgery. Arch. Surg. 65:876, 1952.

Mirsky, S., and Garlock, J. H.: Spontaneous rupture of the stomach; unusual clinical features. Ann. Surg. 161:466, 1965.

Moore, S. W., and Erlandson, M. E.: Intramural hematoma of the duodenum. Ann. Surg. 157:798, 1963.

Moore, T. C.: Congenital intrinsic duodenal obstruction: A report of thirty-two cases. Ann. Surg. 144:159, 1956.

Morgan, Q. G., McAdam, W. A. F., Pacsov, C., et al.: Cimetidine: An advance in gastric ulcer treatment? Br. Med. J. 2:1323, 1978.

Morris, C. R., Ivy, A. C., and Maddock, W. G.: Mechanism of acute abdominal distension. Arch. Surg. 55:101, 1947. Cited in Zer, et al., 1970.

Morton, J. R., and Jordan, G. L., Jr.: Traumatic duodenal injuries: Review of 131 cases. J. Trauma 8:127, 1968.

Moschel, D. M., Walske, B. R., and Neumayer, F.: A new technique for pyloroplasty. Surgery 44:813, 1958.

Moynihan, B. G. A.: Remarks on hour-glass stomachs. Br. Med. J. 1:413, 1904.

Murdfield, P.: Rupture of the stomach from sodium bicarbonate. J.A.M.A. 87:1692, 1926. Cited in Zer, et al. 1970.

Murphy, J. B.: Cholecysto-intestinal, gastro-intestinal, entero-intestinal anastomosis and approximation without sutures; Original research. Chic. Med. Recorder 3:803, 1892.

Mustard, W. T., et al. (eds.): Pediatric Surgery, 2nd ed. Vol. 2. Chicago, Year Book Medical Publishers, 1969.

Nakayama, K.: Personal communication.

Nakayama, K.: Approach to midthoracic esophageal carcinoma for its radical surgical treatment. Surgery 35:574, 1954.

Nance, F. C.: New techniques of gastrointestinal anastomoses with the EEA stapler. Ann. Surg. 189:587, 1979.

Nance, F. C., and Cohn, I., Jr.: Surgical judgment in the management of stab wounds of the abdomen: A retrospective and prospective analysis based on a study of 600 stabbed patients. Ann. Surg. 170:569, 1969.

Neale, A. J.: Case of malformation of stomach. Lancet 1:1057, 1884. Cited in Gray and Skandalakis, 1972.

Netterville, R. E., and Hardy, J. D.: Penetrating wounds of the abdomen. Analyses of 55 cases with problems in management. Ann. Surg. 166:232, 1967.

Newton, W. T.: Radical enterectomy for hereditary megaduodenum. Arch. Surg. 96:549, 1968.

Nicosia, J., Thornton, J., Folk, F., et al.: Surgical management of corrosive gastric injuries. Ann. Surg. 180:139, 1974.

Nielsen, J., Amdrup, E., Christiansen, P., et al.: Gastric ulcer. II. Surgical treatment. Acta Chir. Scand. 139:460, 1973.

Niessen, O. F.: Cascade stomach. In Bockus, H. L.: Gastroenterology, 3rd ed. Philadelphia, W. B. Saunders Company, 1976, p. 1103.

Nyhus, L. M., McDade, W. C., Condon, R. E., et al.: Further experiences with jejunal gastrostomy. Arch. Surg. 83:864, 1961.

Nyhus, L. M., and Wastell, C.: Surgery of the Stomach and Duodenum, 3rd ed. Boston, Little, Brown, & Company, 1977.

O'Donnell, V. A., Lou, S. M. A., Alexander, J. L., et al.: Role of antibiotics in penetrating abdominal trauma. Am. Surg. 44:574, 1978.

Ogbuokiri, C. G., Law, E. J., and MacMillan, B. G.: Superior mesenteric artery syndrome in burned children. Am. J. Surg. 124:75, 1972.

Oglesby, J. E., Smith, D. E., Mahoney, W. D., et al.: Complete duodenal transection in blunt trauma. Am. J. Surg. 116:914, 1968.

Olsen, W. R., and Hildreth, D. H.: Abdominal paracentesis and peritoneal lavage in blunt abdominal trauma. J. Trauma 11:824, 1971.

Oppenheimer, G. D.: Acute obstruction of the duodenum due to submucosal hematoma. Ann. Surg. 98:192, 1933. Cited in Jones, et al., 1971.

Oppolzer, R.: The pathogenesis and surgical therapy of chronic gastric volvulus after paralysis of the diaphragm. Chirurg 28:20, 1957. Cited in Tanner, 1968.

Orr, T. G.: Operations of General Surgery, 2nd ed. Philadelphia, W. B. Saunders Company, 1949, p. 388.

Otis, G. S.: Surgical history. In The Medical and Surgical History of the War of the Rebellion. Vol. II. Washington, D.C., Government Printing Office, 1876.

Pace, W. G., Martin, E. W., Tetirick, T., et al.: Gastric partitioning for morbid obesity. Ann. Surg. 190:392, 1979.

Paine, J. R.: Constant suction by nasal catheter as an adjunct in postoperative treatment. Trans. Minneapolis Surg. Soc., Minn. Med. 1932.

Paine, J. R.: The history of the invention and development of the stomach and duodenum tubes. Ann. Intern. Med. 8:752, 1934.

Painter, R. L., Park, S., and Hochberg, D. T.: One year's experience with the auto-suture stapling device at the Day Kimball Hospital. Conn. Med. 38:59, 1974.

Palmer, W. L.: Hour-glass contracture. In Paulson, M. (ed.): Gastroenterologic Medicine. Philadelphia, Lea & Febiger, 1969, p. 733.

Papp, J. P.: Endoscopic electrocoagulation in upper gastrointestinal hemorrhage: A preliminary report. J.A.M.A. 230:1172, 1974.

Papp, J. P.: Endoscopic electrocoagulation of upper gastrointestinal hemorrhage. J.A.M.A. 236:2076, 1976.

Parrish, R. A., and Cohen, J.: Temporary tube gastrostomy. Am. Surg. 38:168, 1972.

Parrish, R. A., Kavanage, C. B., Wells, J. A., et al.: Congenital antral membrane. Surg. Gynecol. Obstet. 127:999, 1968.

Parrish, R. A., Sherman, H. S., and Moretz, W. H.: Congenital antral membrane. Surgery 59:684, 1966.

Passaro, E., Jr., Basso, N., Sanchez, R. E., et al.: Newer studies in the Zollinger-Ellison syndrome. Am. J. Surg. 120:138, 1970.

Pearsons, S. C., MacKenzie, R. J., and Ross, T.: The use of catheter duodenostomy in gastric resection for duodenal ulcer. Am. J. Surg. 106:194, 1963.

BIBLIOGRAPHY

Pellerin, D., Bertin, P., and Touar, J. A.: Gastroesophageal reflux with hypertrophic pyloric stenosis. Ann. Chir. Infant 15:7, 1974.

Peltier, G., Hermreck, A. S., Moffat, R. E., et al.: Complications following gastric bypass procedures for morbid obesity. Surgery 86:648, 1979.

Perry, J. F., Jr.: Blunt and penetrating abdominal injuries. Curr. Prob. Surg., May, 1970.

Petersen, S. R., and Sheldon, G. F.: Morbidity of a negative finding at laparotomy in abdominal trauma. Surg. Gynecol. Obstet. 148:23, 1979.

Pfeiffer, D. B., and Kent, E. M.: The value of preliminary colostomy in the correction of gastrojejunocolic fistula. Ann. Surg. 110:659, 1939.

Poer, D. H., and Woliver, E.: Intestinal and mesenteric injury due to non-penetrating abdominal trauma. J.A.M.A. 118:11, 1942. Cited in Oglesby, et al., 1968.

Pollock, W. F., Norris, W. J., and Gordon, H. E.: The management of hypertrophic pyloric stenosis at The Los Angeles Children's Hospital: A review of 1,422 cases. Am. J. Surg. 94:335, 1977.

Postlethwait, R. W.: Long-term comparative study of nonabsorbable sutures. Ann. Surg. 171:892, 1970.

Postlethwait, R. W.: Rate of breaking strength loss of absorbable sutures in the stomach. Surgery 78:531, 1975.

Postlethwait, R. W., Schauble, J. F., Dillon, M. L., et al.: Wound healing. II. An evaluation of surgical suture material. Surg. Gynecol. Obstet. 108:555, 1959.

Postlethwait, R. W., Willigan, D. A., and Ulin, L. W.: Human tissue reaction to sutures. Ann. Surg. 181:144, 1975.

Potts, W. J.: Congenital deformities of the esophagus. Surg. Clin. North Am. 31:97, 1951.

Prathikanti, V., and Bhuta, I.: Intramural hematoma of the duodenum. South. Med. J. 69:490, 1976.

Price, W. E., Grizzle, J. E., Postlethwait, R. W., et al.: Results of operation for duodenal ulcer. Surg. Gynecol. Obstet. 131:233, 1970.

Priebe, H. J., Skillman, J. J., Bushnell, L. S., et al.: Antacid versus cimetidine in preventing acute gastrointestinal bleeding. N. Engl. J. Med. 302:426, 1980.

Printen, K. J., and Owensby, M.: Vagal innervation of the bypassed stomach following gastric bypass. Surgery 84:455, 1978.

Pruitt, B.: Discussion at American Surgical Association Meeting, Boca Raton, Fla., 1971, of Wagner, G. R., Miller, R. E., and Eiseman, B.: Duodenal obstruction by the superior mesenteric artery in bedridden combat casualties. Ann. Surg. 174:339, 1971.

Pruksapong, C., Donovan, R. J., Pinit, A., et al.: Gastric duplication. J. Pediatr. Surg. 14:83, 1979.

Puranik, S. R., Keiser, R. P., and Gilbert, M. G.: Arteriomesenteric duodenal compression in children. Am. J. Surg. 124:334, 1972.

Putschar, W. G. J., and Manion, W. C.: Congenital absence of the spleen and associated anomalies. Am. J. Clin. Pathol. 26:429, 1956. Cited in Gray and Skandalakis, 1972.

Pyrtek, L. J., and Bartus, S. H.: *Clostridium welchi* infection complicating gastrointestinal tract surgery. N. Engl. J. Med. 266:689, 1962. Cited in Yeo and McNamara, 1973.

Raffensperger, J., Shakunthala, V., Pildes, R. S., et al.: Feeding gastrostomy in premature infants. Arch. Surg. 97:190, 1968.

Ranson, J. H. C.: Safer intraperitoneal sump drainage. Surg. Gynecol. Obstet. 137:841, 1973.

Rasnicoff, S. A., Morton, J. H., and Block, A. L.: Retroperitoneal rupture of the duodenum due to blunt trauma. Surg. Gynecol. Obstet. 125:77, 1967.

Ravitch, M. M., and Brolin, R. E.: Experimental evaluation of techniques of gastric partitioning for morbid obesity. Ann. Surg. (in press).

Ravitch, M. M., Hirsch, L. C., and Noiles, D.: A new instrument for simultaneous ligation and division of vessels, with a note on hemostasis by a gelatin sponge-staple. Surgery 71:732, 1972.

Ravitch, M. M., Lane, R., Cornell, W. P., et al.: Closure of duodenal, gastric and intestinal stumps with wire staples: Experimental and clinical studies. Ann. Surg. 163:573, 1966.

Ravitch, M. M., Ong, T. H., and Gazzola, L.: A new, precise, and rapid technique of intestinal resection and anastomosis with staples. Surg. Gynecol. Obstet. 139:6, 1974.

Ravitch, M. M., and Rivarola, A.: Enteroanastomosis with an automatic stapling instrument. Surgery 59:270, 1966.

Ravitch, M. M., and Steichen, F. M.: Techniques of staple suturing in the gastrointestinal tract. Ann. Surg. 175:815, 1972.

Ravitch, M. M., and Steichen, F. M.: A stapling instrument for end-to-end inverting anastomoses in the gastrointestinal tract. Ann. Surg. 189:791, 1979.

Ravitch, M. M., Steichen, F. M., Fishbein, R. H., et al.: Clinical experiences with the Soviet mechanical bronchus stapler (UKB-25). J. Thorac. Cardiovasc. Surg. 47:446, 1964.

Rayford, P. L., and Thompson, J. C.: Gastrin; Collective review. Surg. Gynecol. Obstet. 145:257, 1977.

Reeder, D. D., Becker, H. D., and Thompson, J. C.: Effect of intravenously administered calcium on serum gastrin and gastric secretion in man. Surg. Gynecol. Obstet. 138:847, 1974.

Rees, V. L., and Coller, F. A.: Anatomic and clinical study of the transverse abdominal incision. Arch. Surg. 47:136, 1943.

Reid, I. S.: Biliary tract abnormalities associated with duodenal atresia. Arch. Dis. Child. 48:952, 1973.

Rejthar, R.: Spontaneous rupture of the stomach. Br. Med. J. 2:324, 1952.

ReMine, S. G., van Heerden, J. A., Magness, L., et al.: Antecolic or retrocolic anastomosis in Billroth II gastrojejunostomy? Arch. Surg. 113:735, 1978.

Renner, M., Bottger, E., Adolphs, H. P., et al.: Vergleichende Untersuchung über die Diagnosemöglichkeiten der Radiologie und Endoskopie bei Erkrankungen des Magens und des Duodenums. Fortschr. Geb. Roentgenstr. Nuklearmed. 121:744, 1974.

Rhoads, J. E., Hottenstein, H. F., and Hudson, H. F.: The decline in the strength of catgut after exposure to living tissues. Arch. Surg. 34:377, 1937.

Rhodes, J.: Etiology of gastric ulcer. Gastroenterology 63:171, 1972.

Richardson, J. D., and Aust, J. B.: Gastric devascularization: A useful salvage procedure for massive hemorrhagic gastritis. Ann. Surg. 185:649, 1977.

Richardson, W. R., and Martin, L. W.: Pitfalls in the surgical management of the incomplete duodenal diaphragm. J. Pediatr. Surg. 4:303, 1969.

Rienhoff, W. F., Jr., Gannon, J., Jr., and Sherman, I.: Closure of bronchus following total pneumonectomy. Ann. Surg. 116:481, 1942.

Rinecker, H., and Danek, N.: Operative Behandlung blutender Oesophagus-Varicen durch eine subkardiale Blutsperre mittels transmuraler maschineller Klammerung. Chirurg 46:87, 1975.

Ritchie, W. P.: Acute gastric mucosal drainage induced by bile salts, acid and ischemia. Gastroenterology 63:699, 1975.

Rivers, A. B., and Wilbur, D. L.: Syndrome of gastroileostomy and gastroileac ulcer. Surg. Gynecol. Obstet. 54:937, 1932.

Rivilis, J., McArdle, A. H., Wlodek, G. K., et al.: Effect of an elemental diet on gastric secretion. Ann. Surg. 179:226, 1974.

Robbs, J. V., Bark, C., Marks, I. N., et al.: Selection of operation for duodenal ulcer based on acid secretory studies — a reappraisal. Br. J. Surg. 60:601, 1973.

Robson, M. C., Shaw, R. C., and Heggers, J. P.: The reclosure of postoperative incisional abscesses based on bacterial quantification of the wound. Ann. Surg. 171:279, 1970.

Rodeheaver, G. T., Pettry, D., Thacker, J. G., et al.: Wound cleansing by high pressure irrigation. Surg. Gynecol. Obstet. 141:357, 1975.

Roman, E., Silva, Y., and Lucas, C.: Management of blunt duodenal injury. Surg. Gynecol. Obstet. 132:7, 1971.

Rosch, J.: Workshop: Operative endoscopy. Endoscopy 7:156, 1975.

Rota, A. N.: Pyloric obstruction due to mucosal diaphragm. Arch. Pathol. 55:223, 1953. Cited in Gray and Skandalakis, 1972.

Rovelstad, R. A., Maher, F. T., and Adson, M. A.: Gastric analysis. Surg. Clin. North Am. 51:969, 1971.

Rowe, M. I., Buckner, D., and Clatworthy, H. W., Jr.; Wind sock web of the duodenum. Am. J. Surg. 116:444, 1968.

Rowlands, R. P.: A clinical lecture on hourglass contraction of the stomach. Br. Med. J. 2:50, 1931.

Rowling, J. T.: The prepyloric septum: A rare anomaly. Br. J. Surg. 47:162, 1959.

Ruckley, C. V., and Fraser, J.: Gastric volvulus and hiatus hernia. J. R. Coll. Surg. Edinb. 13:217, 1968.

Ruddock, J. C.: Peritoneoscopy. Surg. Gynecol. Obstet. 65:673, 1937.

Ruddock, J. C.: Peritoneoscopy; A critical and clinical review. Surg. Clin. North Am., Oct., 1957, p. 1249.

Rush, B. F., and Ravitch, M. M.: The evolution of total gastrectomy. Int. Abstr. Surg. 114:411, 1962. *In* Surg. Gynecol. Obstet. 114(5).

Russell, G. F. M.: Acute dilatation of the stomach in a patient with anorexia nervosa. Br. J. Psychiatr. 112:203, 1966.

Saint, J. H., and Braslow, L. E.: Removal of the xiphoid process as an aid in operations on the upper abdomen. Surgery 33:361, 1953.

Salzberg, A. M., and Collins, R. E.: Congenital pyloric atresia. Arch. Surg. 8:501, 1960. Cited in Parrish, Sherman, and Moretz, 1966.

Sames, C. P.: Case of partial atresia of the pyloric antrum due to mucosal diaphragm of doubtful origin. Br. J. Surg. 37:244, 1949.

Samloff, I. M., Secrist, D. M., and Passaro, E., Jr.: A study of the relationship between serum group I pepsinogen levels and gastric acid secretion. Gastroenterology 69:1196, 1975.

Sanders, G. B.: Discussion at Southern Surgical Association meeting, Hot Springs, Va., 1963, of Herrington, J. L., Jr., Edwards, W. H., and Sawyers, J. L.: Elimination of routine use of gastric decompression following operation for gastroduodenal ulcer. Ann. Surg. 159:807, 1964.

Sandor, S.: Magen-Darmnaht mit Metallklammern nach Hültl und ein neues Nähinstrument. Zentralbl. Chir. 23:1334, 1936.

Sanfilippo, J. A.: Infantile hypertrophic pyloric stenosis related to ingestion of erythromycin estolate: Report of five cases. J. Pediatr. Surg. 11:177, 1976.

Sauberli, H.: The place of gastrin determination in ulcer surgery. Eur. Surg. Res. 8:269, 1976.

Sawyer, K. C., Hammer, R. W., and Fenton, W. C.: Gastric volvulus as a cause of obstruction. Arch. Surg. 72:764, 1956.

Sawyers, J. L.: Closing discussion at Southern Surgical Association meeting, Hot Springs, Va., 1963, of Herrington, J. L., Jr., Edwards, W. H., and Sawyers, J. L.: Elimination of routine use of gastric decompression following operation for gastroduodenal ulcer. Ann. Surg. 159:807, 1964.

Sawyers, J. L., and Herrington, J. L., Jr.: Perforated duodenal ulcer managed by proximal gastric vagotomy and suture plication. Ann. Surg. 185:656, 1977.

Schatzki, R.: Resorption of duodenal hematoma. Discussion of Felson, B., and Levin, E. J.: Intramural hematoma of the duodenum; A diagnostic Roentgen sign. Radiology 63:823, 1954.

Schiller, K. F. R., Truelove, S. C., and Williams, D. G.: Hematemesis and melena, with special reference to factors influencing the outcome. Br. Med. J. 2:7, 1970.

Schindler, R.: Diagnostic gastroscopy, with special reference to flexible gastroscope. J.A.M.A. 105:352, 1935.

Schnitzler, J.: Über eine Eigentumliche Missbildung mit stenosierung des Magenausganges. Med. Klin. 22:723, 1926.

Scholander, P. F.: Master switch of life. Sci. Am. 209:92, 1963.

Schrock, T. R., and Way, L. W.: Total gastrectomy. Am. J. Surg. 135:348, 1978.

Schroeder, C. M.: Hourglass stomach caused by annular muscular hypertrophy: Report of a case. Ann. Surg. 130:1085, 1949.

Schultz, R. D., and Niemann, F.: Kongenitale Mikrogastrie in Verbindung mit Skelettmissbildungen — ein neues Syndrom. Helv. Pediatr. Acta 26:185, 1971.

Schuster, M. M., and Smith, V. M.: "Pyloric cervix sign" in adult hypertrophic pyloric stenosis. Gastrointest. Endosc. 16:211, 1970.

Schwartz, H. S.: Acute meprobamate poisoning with gastrotomy and removal of a drug-containing mass. N. Engl. J. Med. 295:1177, 1976.

Sedillot, M. C.: Observation de gastrostomie. Gaz d. Hop. 26:160, 1853.

Segal, H. L.: Gastric secretion. *In* Paulson, M. (ed.): Gastroenterologic Medicine. Philadelphia, Lea and Febiger, 1969.

Segal, H. L., Miller, L. L., and Plumb, E. J.: Tubeless gastric analysis with azure A ion-exchange compound. Gastroenterology 28:402, 1955.

Senn, N.: Enterorrhaphy: its history, technique and present status. J.A.M.A. 21:217, 1893.

Sereghy, M., and Von Gyurkovich, T.: Experimentelle

Untersuchungen Über die Einwirkung des Calciums auf die Sekretion und Motilität des Magens. Z. Gesamte Exp. Med. 54:271, 1927.
Shackelford, R. T.: Peritoneoscopy. In Practice of Medicine. Chapter 34, Vol. II. Hagerstown, Md., Harper and Row, 1975.
Shackelford, R. T.: Unpublished directive to U.N.R.R.A. Staff in Hungary about feeding starvation patients. Preventive Medicine in World War II. Vol. 8. Public Health Activities, Office of the Surgeon General, Department of the Army, 1976, p. 357.
Shaftan, G. W.: Indications for operation in abdominal trauma. Am. J. Surg. 99:657, 1960.
Shaker, I. J., Schaefer, J. A., James, A. E., et al.: Aerophagia, a mechanism for spontaneous rupture of the stomach in the newborn. Am. Surg. 39:619, 1973.
Shannon, R.: Traumatic intramural haematoma of the duodenum. Aust. N. Z. J. Surg. 32:28, 1962-3.
Shaw, A., Blanc, W. A., Santulli, T. V., et al.: Spontaneous rupture of the stomach in the newborn: A clinical and experimental study. Surgery 58:561, 1965.
Sheldon, G. F., Gardiner, B. N., Way, L. W., et al.: Management of gastrointestinal fistulas. Surg. Gynecol. Obstet. 133:385, 1971.
Siegler, A. M.: Removal of ectopic intrauterine contraceptive devices aided by laparoscopy: Report of 3 cases and review of the literature. Am. J. Obstet. Gynecol. 42:751, 1973.
Siemens, R. A., and Fulton, R. L.: Gastric rupture as a result of blunt trauma. Am. Surg. 43:229, 1977.
Silen, W.: New concepts of the gastric mucosal barrier. Am. J. Surg. 133:8, 1977.
Silvis, S. E., Nebel, O., Rogers, G., et al.: Endoscopic complications: Results of the 1974 American Society for Gastrointestinal Endoscopy survey. J.A.M.A. 235:928, 1976.
Singleton, A. O.: Improvement in the management of upper abdominal operations, stressing an anatomical incision. South. Med. J. 24:200, 1931.
Skandalakis, J. E., Rowe, J. S., Jr., Gray, S. W., et al.: Identification of vagal structures at the esophageal hiatus. Surgery 75:233, 1974.
Skillman, J. J., Gould, S. A., Chung, R. S. K., et al.: The gastric mucosal barrier: Clinical and experimental studies in critically ill and normal man and in the rabbit. Ann. Surg. 172:564, 1970.
Skoryna, S. C., Dolan, H. S., and Gley, A.: Development of primary pyloric hypertrophy in adults in relation to the structure and function of the pyloric canal. Surg. Gynecol. Obstet. 108:83, 1959.
Sloan, G. A.: A new upper abdominal incision. Surg. Gynecol. Obstet. 45:678, 1927.
Sloop, R. D., and Montague, A. C.: Gastric outlet obstruction due to congenital pyloric mucosal membrane. Ann. Surg. 165:598, 1967.
Smiley, K., Perry, M., and McClelland, R.: Congenital duodenal diaphragm in the adult. Review of the literature and report of a case. Ann. Surg. 165:632, 1967.
Smith, A. D., Jr., Woolverton, W. C., Wiechart, R. F., III, et al.: Operative management of pancreatic and duodenal injuries. J. Trauma 11:570, 1970.
Smith, E. I., Stone, H. H., and Swischuk, L. E.: The importance of Torgersen's muscle in the diagnosis and treatment of infantile hypertrophic pyloric stenosis. South. Pediatr. J. 64:1010, 1971.

Smithwick, W., Gertner, H. R., Jr., and Zuidema, G. D.: Injection of Hypaque (sodium diatrizoate) in the management of abdominal stab wounds. Surg. Gynecol. Obstet. 127:1215, 1968.
Soper, R. T., and Selke, A. C., Jr.: Congenital extrinsic obstruction of the duodenojejunal junction. J. Pediatr. Surg. 5:437, 1970.
Spitz, H., and Zail, S. S.: Serum gastrin levels in congenital hypertrophic pyloric stenosis. J. Pediatr. Surg. 11:33, 1976.
Stabile, B. E., and Passaro, E., Jr.: Recurrent peptic ulcer. Gastroenterology 70:124, 1976.
Stafford, E. S., Ballinger, W. F. 2nd, Zuidema, G. D., et al.: Benign gastric ulcer with life-threatening hemorrhage. Ann. Surg. 165:967, 1967.
Stamm, M.: Gastrostomy: A new method. Med. News 65:324, 1894.
Stammers, F. A. R.: A clinical approach to an analysis and treatment of postgastrectomy syndrome. Br. J. Surg. 49:28, 1961.
Stavely, A. L.: Acute and chronic gastro-mesenteric ileus with cure in a chronic case by duodenojejunostomy. Bull. Johns Hopkins Hosp. 19:252, 1908.
Steichen, F. M.: The use of staplers in anatomical side-to-side and functional end-to-end enteroanastomoses. Surgery 64:948, 1968.
Steichen, F. M.: The creation of autologous substitute organs with stapling instruments. Am. J. Surg. 134:659, 1977.
Steichen, F. M., Efrong, G., Pearlman, D. M., et al.: Radiographic diagnosis versus selective management in penetrating wounds of the abdomen. Ann. Surg. 170:978, 1969.
Steichen, F. M., and Ravitch, M. M.: Mechanical sutures in surgery. Br. J. Surg. 60:191, 1973.
Steichen, F. M., Talbert, J. L., and Ravitch, M. M.: Primary side-to-side colorectal anastomosis in the Duhamel operation for Hirschsprung's disease. Surgery 64:475, 1968.
Steiger, E., and Cooperman, A. M.: Considerations in the managment of perforated peptic ulcers. Surg. Clin. North Am. 56:1395, 1976.
Steinmann, F.: Spontan Magenruptur. Zentralbl. Chir. 44:180, 1917.
Stemmer, E. A.: Discussion of Farris, J. M., and Smith, G. K.: Long-term appraisal of the treatment of gastric ulcer in situ by vagotomy and pyloroplasty. Am. J. Surg. 126:292, 1973.
Stenter, K. L.: Complications of temporary tube gastrostomy. Arch. Surg. 81:103, 1960.
Stephenson, R. H., and Hopkins, W. A.: Volvulus of the stomach complicating eventration of the diaphragm. Am. J. Gastroenterol. 41:225, 1964.
Stern, D. H., and Walsh, J. H.: Gastrin release in postoperative ulcer patients: Evidence for release of duodenal gastrin. Gastroenterology 64:363, 1973.
Stone, H. H.: Prophylactic use of antibiotics in penetrating abdominal trauma. Guest Lecture, Johns Hopkins Surgical Staff Conference, Dec. 15, 1979.
Stone, H. H., and Fabian, T. C.: Management of duodenal wounds. J. Trauma 19:34, 1979.
Stone, H. H., and Fulenwider, T. J.: Renal decapsulation in the prevention of post-ischemic oliguria. Ann. Surg. 186:343, 1977.
Stone, H. H., and Garoni, W. J.: Experiences with the management of duodenal wounds. South. Med. J. 59:864, 1966.

Stone, H. H., Haney, B. B., Kolb, L. D., et al.: Prophylactic and preventive antibiotic therapy. Ann. Surg. 189:691, 1979.

Stone, H. H., Hooper, C. A., Kolb, L. D., et al.: Antibiotic prophylaxis in gastric, biliary, and colonic surgery. Ann. Surg. 184:443, 1976.

Strauch, G.: Influence of previous gastrectomy on major blunt duodenal injury. Am. J. Surg. 124:399, 1972.

Stremple, J. F.: A new operation for the anatomic correction of chronic intermittent gastric volvulus. Am. J. Surg. 125:360, 1973.

Strong, E. K.: Mechanics of arteriomesenteric duodenal obstruction and direct surgical attack upon etiology. Ann. Surg. 148:725, 1958.

Struther, J.: Case of double stomach. Monthly J. Med. Sci. 12:121, 1851. Cited in Gray and Skandalakis, 1972.

Sugawa, C., Werner, M. H., Hayes, D. F., et al.: Early endoscopy. A guide to therapy for acute hemorrhage in the upper gastrointestinal tract. Arch. Surg. 107:133, 1973.

Sunderland, D. A., McNeer, G., Ortega, L. G., et al.: Lymphatic spread of gastric cancer. Cancer 6:987, 1953.

Surgery in World War II. Vol. 2: General Surgery. Washington, D. C., Office of the Surgeon General Department of the Army, 1955.

Sutherland, D. E. R., Miller, I. D., and Najarican, J. S.: Occurrence of both congenital duodenal diaphragm and vascular compression of the duodenum in an elderly patient. Am. J. Surg. 123:351, 1972.

Suture Use Manual: Use and handling of sutures and needles. Somerville, N.J., Ethicon, Inc., 1976.

Swaiman, K. F., Root, J. F., and Raile, R. B.: The coil-spring sign and intramural hematoma of the proximal small intestine. Am. J. Dis. Child. 95:413, 1958.

Swartz, W. T., and Shepard, R. D.: Congenital mucosal diaphragm of the pyloric antrum. J. Ky. Med. Assoc. 54:149, 1956.

Talbot, W. A., and Shuck, J. M.: Retroperitoneal duodenal injury due to blunt abdominal trauma. Am. J. Surg. 130:659, 1975.

Talwalker, V. C.: Pyloric atresia: A case report. J. Pediatr. Surg. 2:458, 1967.

Tan, K.-L., and Murugasu, J. J.: Congenital pyloric atresia in siblings. Arch. Surg. 106:100, 1973.

Tanner, N. C.: Use of drains in the peritoneal cavity and abdominal wall. The Craft of Surgery, 2nd ed. London, J. and A. Churchill, 1964, pp. 918–927.

Tanner, N. C.: Disabilities which may follow the peptic ulcer operation. Proc. R. Soc. Med. 59:362, 1966.

Tanner, N. C.: Chronic and recurrent volvulus of the stomach. Am. J. Surg. 115:505, 1968.

Taylor, H., and Warren, R. P.: Perforated acute and chronic peptic ulcer: Conservative treatment. Lancet 1:397, 1956.

Tedesco, F. J., Goldstein, P. D., Gleason, W. A., et al.: Upper gastrointestinal endoscopy in pediatric patients. Gastroenterology. 70:492, 1976.

Thieme, E. T., and Postmus, R.: Superior mesenteric artery syndrome. Ann. Surg. 154:139, 1961.

Thomas, C. G., and Croom, R. D., III: A method for temporary gastrostoma. Surg. Gynecol. Obstet. 131:292, August, 1970.

Thomas, J. E.: Mechanics and regulation of gastric emptying. Physiol. Rev. 37:455, 1957.

Thompson, A.: Case of traumatic rupture of the duodenum. Edin. Med. J. 1:151, 1855. Cited in Hughes, Conn, and Sherman, 1977.

Thompson, B., Stremple, J., and Steichen, F. M.: A comparison of stapled and hand-sewn colon anastomoses (Submitted for publication).

Thompson, J. B.: Case of spontaneous perforation of the stomach. London Med. Gaz. 30:103, 1842.

Thompson, J. C.: Acute gastric dilatation. In Sabiston, D. C. (ed.): Davis-Christopher Textbook of Surgery, 11th ed. Philadelphia, W. B. Saunders Company, 1972, pp. 938–939.

Thompson, N. W.: Personal communication cited in Benson, C. D.: Prepyloric and pyloric obstruction. In Mustard, W. T., et al.: Pediatric Surgery, 2nd ed. Chicago, Year Book Medical Publishers, 1969.

Thompson, N. W., and Stanley, J. C.: Vascular compression of the duodenum and peptic ulcer disease. Arch. Surg. 108:674, 1974.

Thorek, M.: Tubovalvular gastrostomy, history and technique. J. Mich. Med. Soc. 44:3, 1945.

Threadgill, F. D., and Hagelstein, A.: Duodenal diaphragm in the adult. Arch. Surg. 83:878, 1961.

Tinckler, L.: Nasogastric tube management. Br. J. Surg. 59:637, 1972.

Tobe, T., Chen, S., Henmi, K., et al.: Distribution of gastrin in canine, cat, and human digestive organs. Am. J. Surg. 132:581, 1976.

Toblin, J. J., Schlang, H. A., and James, D. R.: Intramural hematoma of the duodenum associated with per oral small bowel biopsy. J.A.M.A. 198:787, 1966.

Tomoda, M.: Ein neuer Magen-Darmnähapparat. Zentralbl. Chir. 25:1455, 1937a.

Tomada, M.: Eine neue Modifikation der Magenresektionstechnik mit eigenem Magen-Darmnähapparat. Zentralbl. Chir. 27:1584, 1937b.

Tompkins, R. K., Kraft, A. R., and Zollinger, R. M.: Double-lumen gastrojejunostomy tube for simplified postoperative management. Arch. Surg. 105:121, 1972.

Touloukian, R. J.: Gastric ischemia: The primary factor in neonatal perforations. Clin. Pediatr. 12:219, 1973.

Touroff, A. S. W., and Sussman, R. M.: Congenital prepyloric membranous obstruction in a premature infant. Surgery 8:739, 1940.

Travers, B.: An inquiry into the process of healing in repairing injuries of the intestines. London, Longman, Rees, Orme, Brown & Green, 1812.

Traversa, F. P., Nibbi, F., and Bossù, M.: Displasia cistica congenita dell'esofago e dello stomaco. Riv. Chir. Pediatr. 12:212, 1970.

Trimble, C.: Stab wound sinography. Surg. Clin. North Am. 49:1217, 1969.

Trudeau, W. L., and Mcguigan, J. E.: Effects of calcium on serum gastrin levels in Zollinger-Ellison syndrome. N. Engl. J. Med. 281:862, 1969.

Tunell, W. P., and Smith, E. I.: Antral web in infancy. J. Pediatr. Surg. 15:152, 1980.

Turner, F. P.: Fatal *Clostridium welchi* septicemia following cholecystectomy. Am. J. Surg. 108:3, 1964. Cited in Yeo and McNamara, 1973.

Turnipseed, W. D., and Keith, L. M., Jr.: Altered serum gastrin levels in achlorhydric states. Am. J. Surg. 131:175, 1976.

Van Heerden, J. A., Bernatz, P. E., and Rovelstad, R. A.: The retained gastric antrum: Clinical considerations. Mayo Clin. Proc. 46:25, 1971.

BIBLIOGRAPHY

Van Heerden, J. A., Phillips, S. F., Adson, M. A., et al.: Postoperative reflux gastritis. Am. J. Surg. 129:82, 1975.

Van Winkle, W., Jr., and Hastings, C.: Considerations in the choice of suture material for various tissues; Collective review. Surg. Gynecol. Obstet. 135:113, 1972.

Van Winkle, W., Jr., Hastings, J. C., Barker, E., et al.: Effect of suture materials on healing skin wounds. Surg. Gynecol. Obstet. 140:7, 1975.

Vanatta, J. B., Cagas, C. R., and Cramer, R. I.: Superior mesenteric artery (Wilkie's syndrome): Report of three cases and review of the literature. South. Med. J. 69:1461, 1976.

Vankemmel, M.: Anastomoses oeso-gastrique, et deso-jéjunale par agrafes métalliques à l'appareil P.K.S. 25. Lille Méd. 17:850, 1972.

Venables, C. W.: The value of endoscopy and secretion studies in the management of recurrent symptoms after surgery for peptic ulceration. J. R. Coll. Surg. Edinb. 18:297, 1973.

von Petz, A.: Zur Technik der Magenresektion. Ein neuer Magen-Darm-nähapparat. Zentralbl. Chir. 5:179, 1924.

von Petz, A.: Aseptic technique of stomach resection. Ann. Surg. 86:388, 1927.

Von Rokitansky, C.: Cited in Finney, J. M. T.: The relation of dilatation of the duodenum to gastric disturbances. Bull. Johns Hopkins Hosp. 17:37, 1906b.

Walker, W. F., Dewar, D. A. E., and Stephen, S. A.: Congenital intrinsic duodenal stenosis presenting after infancy: A review of recorded cases and report of a case showing duodeno-hepatic reflux. Br. J. Surg. 46:28, 1958.

Wall, L., Jr.: Telephone communication, Sept. 24, 1976.

Wallace, W. A., et al.: Perforation of chronic peptic ulcers after cimetidine. Br. Med. J. 2:865, 1977.

Walsh, J. H., and Grossman, M. I.: Gastrin, Parts I and II. N. Engl. J. Med. 292:1324, 1377, 1975.

Walstad, P. M., and Conklin, W. S.: Rupture of the normal stomach after therapeutic oxygen administration. N. Engl. J. Med. 264:1201, 1961.

Ward, A. S., and Bloom, S. R.: Effect of vagotomy on secretin release in man. Gut 16:951, 1975.

Ward, R.: Apparatus for continuous gastric or duodenal lavage. J.A.M.A. 84:1114, 1925.

Wasch, M. G., and Marck, A.: Radiographic appearance of the gastrointestinal tract during the first day of life. J. Pediatr. 32:479, 1948.

Wassner, J. D., Yohai, E., and Heimlich, H. J.: Complications associated with the use of gastrointestinal stapling devices. Surgery 82:395, 1977.

Wastell, C., and Ellis, H.: Volvulus of the stomach: A review with a report of 8 cases. Br. J. Surg. 58:557, 1971.

Waterman, N. G., Walsky, R., Kasdan, M. L., et al.: The treatment of acute hemorrhagic pancreatitis by sump drainage. Surg. Gynecol. Obstet. 126:963, 1968.

Watts, H. D.: Postemetic hematomas: A variant of the Mallory-Weiss syndrome. Am. J. Surg. 132:320, 1976.

Waye, J. D.: Removal of foreign bodies from the upper intestinal tract with fiberoptic instruments. Am. J. Gastroenterol. 65:557, 1976.

Wayne, E. R., and Burrington, J. D.: Duodenal obstruction by the superior mesenteric artery in children. Surgery 72:762, 1972.

Wayne, E. R., Miller, R. E., and Eiseman, B.: Duodenal obstruction by the superior mesenteric artery in bedridden combat casualties. Ann. Surg. 174:339, 1971.

Weill, J.-P., Monath, C., Kerschen, A., et al.: A study of 210 emergency endoscopies in hemorrhage of the upper digestive tract. Sém. Hôp. Paris 51:1267, 1975.

Weinberg, J. A., Stempien, S. J., Movius, J. J., et al.: Vagotomy and pyloroplasty in treatment of duodenal ulcer. Am. J. Surg. 92:202, 1956.

Weiss, H. D., Anacker, H., Wiesner, W., et al.: Duodenoscopic pancreatography. Radiology 107:33, 1973.

Weiss, W.: Etiology of megaduodenum. Dtsch. Z. Chir. 251:317, 1938.

Welch, C. E., and Rodkey, G. V.: Method of management of duodenal stump after gastrectomy. Surg. Gynecol. Obstet. 98:376, 1954.

Wellman, K. F., Kagan, A., and Fang, H.: Hypertrophic pyloric stenosis in adults. Survey of the literature and report of a case of the localized form. Gastroenterology 46:601, 1964.

Wesdorp, R. I. C., Funovics, J. M., Hirsch, H., et al.: Characteristics of release of duodenal gastrin. Am. J. Surg. 133:280, 1977.

Wesley, J. R., and Mahour, G. H.: Congenital intrinsic duodenal obstruction: A twenty-five year review. Surgery 82:716, 1977.

Wheeless, C. R., Jr.: The Gambee intestinal anastomosis in gynecologic surgery. Obstet. Gynecol. 46:448, 1975.

Wheeless, C. R., Jr., and Thompson, B. H.: Laparoscopic sterilization: Review of 3,600 cases. Obstet. Gynecol. 42:751, 1973.

Whelan, T. J., Jr.(ed.): Emergency War Surgery, 1st U.S. revision of NATO Handbook. Washington, D.C., U.S. Government Printing Office, 1975.

Whitehead, R., Truelove, S. C., and Gear, M. W. L.: The histological diagnosis of chronic gastritis in fiberoptic gastroscope biopsy specimens. J. Clin. Pathol. 25:1, 1972.

Wilkie, D. P. D.: Chronic duodenal ileus. Br. J. Surg. 9:204, 1921

Willett, A.: Fatal vomiting following application of plaster-of-Paris bandage in case of spinal curvature. St. Bartholomew Hosp. Rep. (Lond.) 14:333, 1878. Cited in Bunch and Delaney, 1970.

Willwerth, B. M., Zollinger, R. M., Jr., Izant, R. J., Jr.: Congenital mesocolic (paraduodenal) hernia; Embryologic basis of repair. Am. J. Surg. 128:358, 1974.

Wilson, E. S., Jr.: Neonatal gastric perforations. Am. J. Roentgenog. 103:301, 1968.

Wilson, H., and Sherman, R.: Civilian penetrating wounds of the abdomen. Factors in mortality and differences from military wounds in 494 cases. Trans. South. Surg. Assoc. 62:19, 1960 and Ann. Surg. 153:639, 1961.

Wilson, J. M., Melvin, D. D., Gray, B., et al.: Benign small bowel tumor. Ann. Surg. 181:247, 1975.

Wilson, S. D., Singh, R. B., Kalkoff, R. K., et al.: Does hyperthyroidism cause hypergastrinemia? Surgery 80:231, 1976.

Wilson, W. S., Gadacz, T. R., Olcott, C., et al.: Superficial gastric erosions. Response to surgical treatment. Am. J. Surg. 126:133, 1973.

Wiot, J. F., Weinstein, A. S., and Felson, B.: Duodenal hematoma induced by coumarin. Am. J. Roentgenol. 86:70, 1961.

Wise, L., and Ballinger, W. F.: The elective surgical treatment of chronic duodenal ulcer: A critical review. Surgery 76:811, 1974.

Witzel, O.: Zur Technik der Magenfistelanlegung. Zentralbl. Chir. 18:601, 1891.

Wolf, H. G., and Zwymüller, E.: Angeborener kompletter pylorusverschluss. Kinderheilk. 88:516, 1963.

Wolfe, J. H. N., Behn, A. R., and Jackson, B. T.: Tuberculous peritonitis and role of diagnostic laparoscopy. Lancet 1:852, 1979.

Wolfman, E. F., Jr., Trevino, G., Heaps, D. K., et al.: An operative technic for the management of acute and chronic lateral duodenal fistulas. Ann. Surg. 159:563, 1964.

Womack, N. A.: Blood flow through the stomach and duodenum: Clinical aspects. Am. J. Surg. 117:771, 1969.

Wood, I. J., and Taft, L. I.: Diffuse Lesions of the Stomach. London, Arnold, 1958.

Woolley, M. M., Felsher, B. F., Asch, M. J., et al.: Jaundice, hypertrophic pyloric stenosis and hepatic glucuronyl transferase. J. Pediatr. Surg. 9:359, 1974.

Woo-Ming, M.: Familial relationship between adult and infantile hypertrophic pyloric stenosis. Br. Med. J. 1:476, 1961.

Wuensche, R.: Ein Falle von angeborenen Verschluss des Pylorus. Jahrbuch Kinderheilk. 8:367, 1875. Cited in Gray and Skandalakis, 1972.

Wurtenberger, H.: Gastric atresia. Arch. Dis. Child. 36:161, 1961.

Wychulis, A. R., Priestley, J. T., and Folk, W. T.: A study of 360 patients with gastrojejunal ulceration. Surg. Gynecol. Obstet. 122:89, 1966.

Yamada, K., Holyoke, E. D., and Elias, E. G.: Endoscopy in patients with malignant conditions of the gastrointestinal tract. Surg. Gynecol. Obstet. 141:903, 1975.

Yamamoto, S., and Reynolds, T. B.: Portal venography and pressure measurement in peritoneoscopy. Gastroenterology 47:602, 1964.

Yellin, A. E., Dwyer, R. M., Craig, J. R., et al.: Endoscopic argon-ion laser phototherapy of bleeding gastric lesions. Arch. Surg. 111:750, 1976.

Yeo, C. K., and McNamara, J. J.: Retrograde rupture of duodenum with complicating gas gangrene. Arch. Surg. 106:856, 1973.

Young, H. B.: Addisonian pigmentation due to extreme pyloric stenosis by a mucosal diaphragm. Br. J. Surg. 49:104, 1961. Cited in Gray and Skandalakis, 1972.

Yurko, A. A., and Williams, R. D.: Needle paracentesis in blunt abdominal trauma: A critical analysis. J. Trauma 6:194, 1966.

Zavala, C., Bolio, A., Montalvo, R., et al.: Hypertrophic pyloric stenosis: Adult and congenital types occurring in the same family. J. Med. Genet. 6:126, 1969.

Zer, M., Chaimoff, C., Dintsman, M., et al.: Spontaneous rupture of the stomach following ingestion of sodium bicarbonate. Arch. Surg. 101:532, 1970.

Zimmerman, J. E.: Fatality following metallic mercury aspiration during removal of long intestinal tube. J.A.M.A. 208:2158, 1969.

Zinner, M. J., Turtinen, L. W., and Gurll, N. J.: The role of acid and ischemia in the production of stress ulcers during hemorrhagic shock. Surgery 77:807, 1975.

Zinner, M. J., Zuidema, G. D., Smith, P. L., et al.: The prevention of upper gastrointestinal bleeding in intensive care unit patients: A randomized, prospective, controlled trial comparing the effectiveness of cimetidine and antacids. Surg. Gynecol. Obstet., 1981 (in press).

Zollinger, R. M., and Ellison, E. H.: Primary peptic ulcerations of the jejunum associated with islet cell tumors of the pancreas. Ann. Surg. 14:709, 1955.

Zollinger, R. M., Martin, E. W., Jr., Carey, L. C., et al.: Observations on the postoperative tumor growth behavior of certain islet cell tumors. Ann. Surg. 184:525, 1976.

Zuidema, G. D.: Discussion of Nance, F. C., and Cohn, I., Jr.: Surgical judgment in the management of stab wounds of the abdomen: A retrospective and prospective analysis based on a study of 600 stabbed patients. Ann. Surg. 170:569, 1969.

Zuidema, G. D., Rutherford, R. B., and Ballinger, W. F.: The Management of Trauma, 3rd ed. Philadelphia, W. B. Saunders Company, 1978.

INDEX

Page numbers in *italics* indicate illustrations. The letter *t* following a page number indicates a table.

Abdominal incisions. *See* Incisions, abdominal.
Abdominal muscles, posterior, and related structures, 480–483, *480*, *482–483*
Abdominal plexus, of thoracic nerves, *478*
Abdominal wall, 477
 blood supply to, *479*
 layers of, 467–485, *467*
 transverse sections through, *475*
Abdominal wounds, drainage of, 525–528, *525–527*
Absorbable sutures. *See* Sutures, absorbable.
Accessory nerves, course and distribution of, *416*
Acetylcholine, as gastric secretion stimulant, 25
Acid, intraluminal, in stress ulcer, 266
Acid secretion, duodenal ulcer and, 254–255
 effect of vagotomy on, 368
Acidity, gastric. *See* Gastric acid.
Adam's apple, 403, *405*
Adhesions, of stomach and duodenum, freeing of, 113–114
Aerophagia, in neonatal perforation, 275
Albert suture, 571–573, *572*
 for enterorrhaphy, 573–574, *574*
Alden modification, of gastric bypass, 385
Alimentary tract, cervical, exposure of, 403–422
 thoracic, exposure of, 423–454
Ampulla of Vater, avulsion of, 226–227
Anastomosis(es). *See also* individual operations.
 end-to-end, 558
  versus end-to-side or side-to-side, 558
 everting, single-layer, Navy, 577–578, *577*
 gastrointestinal, complications after, 354–367
  Gambee, 574–577, *574–576*
  materials for, 561
 inverted versus everted, 556–558, *557*, *558*
 mechanical instruments in, *590*, *591*, *592–593*
 splenorenal, patient position in, *453*
Anatomy, in wound closure, 540–544, *541–544*
 of abdominal wall, 467–486
 of duodenum, 38–45
 of stomach, 3–37
  surgical, 6–12, *7–12*
Anesthesia, for peritoneoscopy, 94–95
Angle of Louis, 424, *425*, *427*
Angle of Ludwig, 424
Anomalies, biliary, *139*
 duodenal, *139*
  rotation and fixation, 130
Anorexia nervosa, gastric rupture in, 283, *284*
Ansa cervicalis, *415*, *418*
Antacids, duodenal ulcer and, 256
 gastric ulcer and, 253

Antacids (*Continued*)
 in stress ulcer, 267
  titration regimen for, *268*
Antibiotics, preoperative, as wound infection prophylaxis, 530
Anticholinergics, duodenal ulcer and, 256–257
Antral membrane, congenital, 123–128, *124–125*, *127–128*
Antral mucosal diaphragm, case report of, 126–128, *127–128*
Antral stasis, prevention of, in gastric bypass, 384, *384*, 385
Antral webs, 116–117
Antrectomy, for benign disease, 289
Antrum, of stomach, 7, *7*
Aponeurosis(es), closure of, anatomic considerations in, 541
 intercostal, anterior, 431, *432*
 posterior, 432
Appendectomy, McBurney incision in, *520*
Arcuate ligament, external, 481, *483*
Arcuate line, *469*, *475*, 475, *479*, *483*
Arteriomesenteric duodenal compression syndrome, 155
Arteriomesenteric occlusion, 155
Artery(ies). *See also* names of arteries.
 of abdominal wall, 477–480
 of neck, 412–413, *412*
 of stomach, 10, *11*
 pancreaticoduodenal, 42
Atresia, duodenal, *118*
 biliary tract abnormalities and, 136–141, *137–140*
 cholecystojejunostomy for, *138*
 congenital, 128–141, *132*, *134*
  anesthesia for, 133–134
  clinical course of, 132
  clinical signs of, 131
  diagnosis of, 131–132, *132*, *134*
  embryology of, 129–130, *129*
  pathology of, 130–131, *130*
  preoperative care of, 133
  treatment of, 132–133
   surgical, 135–136, *134–135*
 esophageal, *118*
 intestinal, types of, *130*
 of stomach, 114–128, *115*
  diagnosis of, 117, *118–119*
  history of, 116
  prognosis of, 120
  symptoms of, 117
  treatment of, 119

619

Atropine, as gastric secretion inhibitor, 26
Auscultatory triangle, 473, 481
Autosuture instruments. See Mechanical sutures; Stapling instruments.
Avicenna, 535

Back, muscles of, 482
  deep, 470
Bacterial content, of gastric juice, 17
Balfour-Polya operation, 288, 289
Balfour pyloroplasty, 381, 381–382
Bands, of stomach, division of, 181
Beck-Jianu gastrostomy, 336–337, 338
Beyea's method, of gastropexy, 184, 185
Biliary tract, abnormalities of, duodenal atresia and, 136–141, 137–140
  anomalies of, 139
  peritoneoscopic visualization of, 104
Billroth I operation, 296–297, 297, 298
  history of, 287–289, 288
  mechanical sutures in, 586–587
  modification(s) of, 298
    Horsley, 298
    Kocher, 289, 298, 300–301
    Schoemaker, 297, 298
    Von Haberer, 297–300, 298–300
    Von Haberer-Finney, 298, 301, 302
Billroth I–Von Haberer technic, of gastric resection, 298–300
Billroth II operation, 288, 289, 301–306, 303–305
  duodenal stump leakage following, 362
  mechanical sutures in, 584–585
  modification(s) of, 306–308, 306–308
    Devine exclusion, 306, 307–308
    Finsterer exclusion, 306, 308
    Polya, 304–305
    Polya-Balfour, 306, 306
    Roux-en-Y, 308–309, 308
  recurrent ulcer and, 364
Bilocular stomach, 188–195, 190, 192–195
Biopsy, in peritoneoscopy, 100–101, 100
Bircher's method, of gastric plication, 185, 187
  Moynihan's modification of, 185, 188, 188
  Weir's modification of, 185, 187
Bleeding. See also Hemorrhage.
  gastrointestinal, intubation in, 47–48
  mechanical suturing and, 598, 599
Blood group substances, in gastric juice, 16–17
Blood supply, of abdominal wall, 477, 479. See also individual arteries.
  of duodenum, 11, 459
  of pancreas, 11, 459
  of spleen, 11, 459
Blood vessels, of stomach, 455, 456
  of thorax, 427–430, 428–429
Blunt trauma, of duodenum, 220
  previous gastrectomy and, 230–233, 231, 232
  treatment of, 224–245
  of stomach, 197–205
    diagnosis of, 198–204, 200–204
Braun and Jaboulay operation, 288
Braun reservoir, 329
Bridges, suture, 555, 555
Bullet wounds. See Penetrating trauma.
Burn patients, pediatric, superior mesenteric artery syndrome in, 168–169

Buttons, in wound closure, 554, 555
Bypass, gastric. See Gastric bypass.

Calcium, as gastric secretion stimulant, 25
Camper's fascia, 468
Cantor tube, 46, 50, 54
Carcinoma, gastric, 247–250, 249
  operative treatment of, 248–250, 249
  preoperative treatment of, 248
  staging and classification of, 248
  zonal lymphatic metastases in, 290
Cardia, of stomach, 6–7, 7
Cardiac end, of stomach, 6
Cardiac gland area, of gastric mucosa, 13, 14
Cardiac operation, thoracotomy incision for, 449
Cardiac orifice, of stomach, 7
Carotid arteries, 412–413, 412
Cascade stomach, 195–196, 196
Cast syndrome, 170–171
Catgut, in gastrointestinal suturing, 535, 559–561. See also Suture(s), absorbable.
Cattell and Braasch method of duodenal exposure, 458–460, 461
Celiotomy, for gastric rupture, 285
Celsus, Aurelius Cornelius, 535
Cephalic phase of gastric secretion, 22, 22
Cervical alimentary tract, exposure of, 403–422
Cervical nerve plexus, 418, 419
Cherny method, of extending Pfannenstiel incision, 513, 513
Chest. See Thorax.
Chief cells, of stomach, 14, 15
Children, burned, superior mesenteric artery syndrome in, 168–169
  duodenal hematoma in, 243–245, 243, 244t
  gastric volvulus in, 183
  gastrostomy in, 341–342
  operations in, mechanical instruments for, 593
  peritoneoscopy in, 107–108
  vascular compression of duodenum in, 167–168, 167–168
Cholangiography, peritoneoscopic, technics of, 101–102
Cholangiopancreatography, retrograde, endoscopic, 72–74, 73, 74
Cholecystojejunostomy, for duodenal atresia, 138
CHPS (congenital hypertrophic pyloric stenosis), 277–281
  in adults, 280–281
Chyme, 35–36
Cimetidine, duodenal ulcer and, 257
  gastric ulcer and, 253
  stress ulcer and, 268
  Zollinger-Ellison syndrome and, 265
Closure, delayed, 530–531, 531
  wound. See Wound closure.
Coffey's method, of gastropexy, 184, 185
Colectomy, right, incision for, 509–511, 510
Coller incision for excision of rectum, 515
Colon, ascending, for substitute gastric reservoir, 331, 331
  Gambee anastomosis in, 574–577, 574–576
  peritoneoscopic visualization of, 105–106, 105
  transverse, as substitute gastric reservoir, 331–332
Coloscopy, complications of, 88
Common bile duct, atresia of, 137
  avulsion of, 227–228

INDEX

Complications, after gastric bypass, 391–393, *391–392*
  after gastrointestinal anastomosis, 354–367
    gastric retention, 355
    hematemesis, 354
    jejunal ulcer, 362–363
    jejunoplasty for, 357
    leakage from duodenal stump, 362
    marginal ulcer, 354, 363–364
    obstruction, 357
    repair of gastroileostomy, 367
    rupture of abdominal incision, 362
  after vagotomy, 374
Congenital duodenal atresia, 128–141, *132, 134*
Congenital hypertrophic pyloric stenosis (CHPS), 277–281
  in adults, 281–282
Connell suture, *303, 336, 465, 563, 566*
Contaminated wounds, delayed closure in, 530–531, *531*
Continuous sutures. *See* Suture(s), continuous.
Corrosive injuries of stomach, 217–218
Costal arch, division of, in midline incision, 492–493, *493*
Costal region, of thoracic wall, 424
Costocoracoid ligament and membrane, 439
Cricoid cartilage, arch of, 403, *405*
"Criminal nerve" (nerve of Grassi), 372
"Cup and spill" stomach, 195–196, *196*
Curvoisier operation, *288*
Cushing stitch, 566
Cushing suture, *303, 380, 465, 563,* 565–566
  in Finney pyloroplasty, *380*
Cytology, in gastric ulcer, 252–253
Czerny sutures, 556, 573, *573*

Decompression, gastric, postoperative, 59–65
    critique of, 60–61
  small bowel, long intestinal tubes for, 46–47
Delayed closure, of surgical wounds, 530–531, *531*
Devine exclusion (two-stage partial gastrectomy), 306, *307–308*
Diaphragm, 442
  double, *140,* 141
  eventration of, repair of, 180–181, *181*
  mucosal, antral, case report of, 126–128, *127–128*
  perforate, 123
Diaphragmatico-esophageal membrane, 481, *483*
Diarrhea, postvagotomy, avoidance of, 371
Digastric muscle, *421*
Digestion, 34
  function of stomach in, 32–37, *35*
Dilatation, acute, of stomach, 111–113, *113*
Dilations, esophageal, complications of, 88
Disruption, of incision, 532
Distention, gastric, 282
Dormia-type basket, 87
Double-loop mass closure suture, 552, *553*
Doyen pursestring suture, *294*
Drain(s), cigarette, 525
  in abdominal surgery, 525–528, *525–527*
  latex rubber, 525–526, *525*
  Penrose, 525–526, *525*
  prophylactic, 525
  suction, closed-tube, 526, *526*
  sump, 525, 526–527
    triple-lumen, 527, *527*

Drain(s) (*Continued*)
  sump-Penrose, 525, 527
  therapeutic, 525
  tube, 525, 526
  types of, 525–528, *525–527*
  Waterman, 527, *527*
Drainage, abdominal wound, 525–528, *525–527*
  gastric, intubation in, 46
  minor thoracotomy incisions for, 443–444, *443–444*
Drug poisoning, gastrotomy for, 462
Duodenal diaphragm, SMA syndrome and, 165–166, *166*
Duodenal ulcers. *See* Ulcer(s), duodenal.
Duodenal web, *135*
Duodenal/gastric congenital obstruction, 120–122, *120–122*
Duodenoduodenostomy, for atresia, 134–136, *134–135*
Duodenojejunal flexure, 458, *460*
  as surgical landmark, 40
Duodenojejunal junction, *41*
  obstruction of, 152–155, *153*
Duodenojejunostomy, for duodenal stenosis, 143, *144*
  for megaduodenum, 148–150
Duodenojejunum, transposition of, *168*
Duodenolysis, 113–114
Duodenoscope, 72
Duodenoscopy, 70–72, *72*
  complications of, 88
  through gastrotomy, 89–90
Duodenotomy, for double diaphragm, *140*
  for fenestrated duodenal diaphragm, *138*
  for stenosis, 146–147
Duodenum, adhesions of, freeing of, 113–114
  anatomy of, 38–45
    surgical, 38–45
  anomalies of, 130, *139*
  ascending (fourth) portion of, exposure of, 458, *460*
  associated injuries of, 221–222, 221t, 222t
  atresia of. *See* Atresia, duodenal.
  blood supply of, *11,* 459
  circulation of, *11,* 42–45
  closure of, *294, 295*
    Moynihan, *295*
  coats of, 38
  compression of, 155
  definition of, 38
  descending (second) portion of, exposure of, *457, 458, 458*
    surgical mobilization of, *40*
  digital exploration of, *463*
  divisions of, *11,* 38–40, *39, 457, 458, 458*
  exposure of, 455–466
    Cattell and Braasch method of, 458–460, *461*
  first portion (cap) of, exposure of, 457–458
  fistulas of, 270, 272–273
  fixation of, 40
  foreign bodies of. *See under* Stomach, injuries of.
  hematoma of, 242
    intramural, 233–245
  histology of, 38
  identification of, 456–458, *457–460*
  ileus of, 155
  injuries of, 219–245
    blunt, 220
    corrosive, 217–218
    diagnosis of, 222–224
    penetrating, 220–221, *220*
    treatment of, 224–245
    types of, 219–224

622 INDEX

Duodenum (*Continued*)
 mobilization of, *167*
 obstruction-like disorders of, 184–196
 obstructive disorders of, 111–183
 open, mobilization of, *295*
 physiology of, 45
 rupture of, 224–225
  with ampulla of Vater injury, 226–227
 SMA syndrome operation and, *163*
 stasis of, 155
 stenosis of. *See* Stenosis, duodenal.
 stump of, closure of, *295*, *296*
  leakage from, 362
 transection of, 227–228
 transverse (third) portion of, exposure of, 458, *459*
 tumors of, benign, 247
  malignant, 250
 vascular compression of, 155–156, *156*. *See also* Superior mesenteric artery (SMA) syndrome.
  scoliosis and, 171
Duplication, gastric, 281
 surgical management of, 281
Duret's method, of gastropexy, 184, *187*

EEA (end-to-end anastomosis) stapler, 586, *587*, 592–593
 complications with, 595
 surgical use of, 592–593, 593–594
EGD (esophagogastroduodenoscopy), 68–70, *69*, *71*, 88
Embryo, human, longitudinal section of, *4*
Embryology, of stomach, 3–4, *4*, *5*
Emptying, gastric, 35–37, *35*
Empyema drainage, minor thoracotomy incisions for, 443
Endoscope, *72*, 66–67
 in duodenoscopy, 70
 papillotomy with, 86–88, *86*, *87*
Endoscopic retrograde cholangiopancreatography (ERCP), 72–74, *73*, *74*
Endoscopy, complications of, 88–89
 contraindications of, 68t
 electrocoagulation with, 80–82
 findings in, examples of, *71*
 for Brunner gland adenoma removal, 85–86
 for foreign body removal, 83–85, *83–85*
 for gallstone removal, 86–88, *86*, *87*
 for polyp removal, 82
 for upper GI hemorrhage, 76–77
 illustration of, *69*
 in diagnosis, 75
  of aortoduodenal fistula, 79
 in duodenal ulcer, 256
 in malignant lesions, 79–80
 in palliation of inoperable neoplasms, 80
 in symptomatic postoperative patients, 78–79
 indications for, 69t
 intraoperative, 77–78
 papillotomy with, 86–88
 roentgenography versus, 75–76
 therapeutic procedures with, 80–88
End-to-end anastomosis (EEA) stapler, 586, *587*, 592–593
Enterorrhaphy, sutures for, 573–574, *574*
Epigastric artery, inferior, *478*, 478–479
 superior, *478*, *478*, *479*

ERCP (endoscopic retrograde cholangiopancreatography), 72–74, *73*, *74*
Erector spinae muscle, *470*, 480–481
Esophagoduodenostomy, 329
 and total gastrectomy, 328–332, *331*
 Madden's, 309
Esophagogastrectomy, abdominothoracic incision for, 454
Esophagogastroduodenoscopy (EGD), complications of, 88
 contraindications of, 68, 68t
 in peroral gastroscopy, 68–70
 indications for, 68, 69t
 preparation and procedure in, 68–70, *69*, *71*
Esophagojejunostomy, 329
 gastric reconstruction by, 309–310
 Roux-en-Y, 310
Esophagus, cervical, approaches to, 418–422, *420–422*
  technic of, 420–422, *420–422*
 dilations of, complications of, 88
 surgical mobilization of, *373*
 thoracic, approaches to, 442–443
Evacuation, of intramural hematoma of duodenum, 242
Ewald tube, 47, 59–60
Exalto procedure, in experimental peptic ulcers, 24
Exposure, of cervical alimentary tract, 403–422
 of stomach and duodenum, 455–466
Extension, of lateral oblique abdominal incision, 524
 of lateral upper abdominal transverse incision, 508
 of lower midline incisions, 498
 of McBurney incision, 520
 of midrectus incision, 502
 of paramedian incision, 500
 of pararectus incision, 503
 of Pfannenstiel incision, 513
 of subcostal incision, 519
 of transverse low abdominal incision, 511
 of transverse midabdominal incision, 511
 of upper abdominal transverse incision, 506
 of upper midline incision, 490–495, *491–495*
  abdominothoracic, 493–494, *493*, *494*
  lateral, 495
  upward, 490
  via lateral transverse abdominal incision, 495–497, *496*
Extraperitoneal fat (sixth) layer, of abdominal wall, 484
 incision in, 484

Falciform ligament, 484
Far-and-near sutures, 547–549, *547*
Fascia(e), Buck's, 468
 Camper's, 468
 cervical, deep, *404*, *406*, *408*
  layers of, *404*, 406–408
  superficial, *404*, *406*, *407*
 clavipectoral, 438–439
 coracoclavicular, 439
 deep, 468
 intercostal, external, *431*, *432*
 lumbodorsal, *467*, 481–483, *482*
 pectoral, 438
 Scarpa's, 468
 thoracic wall, 438–439
 transversalis, 483–484, *483*

INDEX

623

Fascia lata, 468
Feeding, gastric secretory response to, 25
Feeding tubes, 47
Femoral sheath, *483*, 484
Fiberendoscopy, upper gastrointestinal, 69. *See also* Endoscopy.
Fiberesophagoscope. *See* Endoscope.
Fiberoptic gastroscopy, description of, 66–67
Fibromas, gastric, 247
Fibromyomas, gastric, 247
Fifth layer (transversalis fascia), of abdominal wall, 483–484, *483*
Figure-of-8 through-and-through monofilament closure, *552*
Finney pyloroplasty. *See* Pyloroplasty, Finney.
finsterer partial gastrectomy, with antral exclusion, 306, 308
Fistula. *See also* Gastrostomy.
   duodenal, 272–273
      causes of, 270
      definition of, 270
      diagnosis of, 273
      treatment of, 273
   gastric, 270–273
      causes of, 270
      definition of, 270
      diagnosis of, 273
      treatment of, 273
   gastrojejunocolic, 271–272, *271*, *272*
      postoperative, 363
   pyeloduodenal, traumatic, 228–230
Food, mixing in stomach of, 34
   propulsion through stomach of, 34
Forceps, foreign body–grasping, *84*
Foreign bodies, of stomach, 216–217
   removal by endoscopy of, 83–85, *83–85*
Fundus, of stomach, 7, *7*
Fundus and body (parietal cell area), of gastric mucosa, 13, *14*
Furrier suture, 571, *572*

Galen of Pergamon, 535
Gallbladder, peritoneoscopic visualization of, 104, *104*
Gallstones, endoscopic removal of, 86–88, *86*, *87*
   postvagotomy, avoidance of, 371
Gambee single-layer open intestinal anastomosis, 574–577, *574–576*
Gambee stitch, in Heineke-Mikulicz pyloroplasty, 377, 576–577, *576*
   Navy anastomosis versus, 577, *577*
Garlock method of abdominothoracic extension, 493–494, *493*, *494*
   closure of, 494
Gas gangrene, duodenal rupture and, 233
Gastrectomy, Billroth I, mechanical sutures in, 586–587
   Billroth II, mechanical sutures in, 584–585
   blunt duodenal injury and, 230–233, *231*, *232*
   duodenal stump leakage following, 362
   extent of, disease and, 289
   for Zollinger-Ellison syndrome, 265
   gastric retention after, 355–361
   incision in, paramedian, 499–502, *500*, *501*
      rupture of, 362
      upward extension of, 491–494, *491–494*

Gastrectomy (*Continued*)
   jejunal ulcer following, 362–363
   partial, 287–309
      Devine exclusion, 306, *307–308*
      Finsterer, 306, 308
      history of, 287–289, *288*
      in idiopathic gastric volvulus, 181–182
      types of, 287
   patient position in, for incision, *453*
   recurrent ulcer following, 363–364
   technic of, 289–296, *290–296*
   total, 309–328
      and reconstruction, 309–328
         technic of, 309–310
      Graham method of, *322–323*, 323
      incision for, *309*
      jejunal interposition in, 328, *328*
      Lahey method of, 315, *315–320*
      Longmire method of, 310–315, *310–314*
      pre- and postoperative care in, 314–315
      Orr method of, 315–316, *321*
      pouch or reservoir reconstruction in, 328, *329*
      Roux-en-Y, *324–327*, *325–328*
         Rienhoff modification of, *325*
      with esophagoduodenostomy, 328–332, *331*
      technic of, 328–331
Gastric. *See also* Stomach.
Gastric acid, augmented histamine test of, 29
   exclusion of, in Mann-Williamson procedure, *24*
   measurement of, 27–28
Gastric analysis, 28–32
   clinical significance of, 30–32
   in duodenal ulcer, 256
   in gastric ulcer, 253
Gastric atresia. *See* Atresia, of stomach.
Gastric bypass, 384–393
   Alden modification of, 385
   complications of, 391–393, *392*
   gastroplasty versus, 396, 400
   jejunoileal bypass versus, 393–394, *393*
   Mason and Ito method of, 384 ff.
   physiologic consequences of, 385–387
   results of, 387–390, *388–390*, 390t
   staples in, 385–388
   technic of, 384–385, *384*, *386*, *388*, *390*
   with short-loop retrocolic gastroenterostomy, 384–385, *384*
Gastric drainage, intubation in, 46
Gastric duplication, 281
   surgical management of, 281
Gastric emptying, 35–37, *35*
Gastric fibromas, 247
Gastric fibromyomas, 247
Gastric fistulas, 270–273
Gastric gland, *15*
Gastric juice, 15–18
   bacterial content of, 17
   nonorganic components of, 17–18
   organic components of, 15
Gastric lesion, resection of by mechanical instruments, 588
Gastric motility, 33
   vagus nerves and, 368
Gastric mucosa, 13–15, *14*, *15*
Gastric mucosal barrier, 15, 18
   renewal of gastric surface epithelium in, 18
Gastric partitioning, in morbid obesity, 394–400, *395–399*
   TA stapler in, 394–400, *395–398*

Gastric plication, technics of, 185–188, *187, 188*
Gastric polyps, 246
Gastric pouch, in gastric bypass, creation of, 384–385, *384, 386, 387, 389*
  measurement of, 387, *389*
Gastric propulsive motor activity, 35
Gastric resection, 287–367. See also Gastrectomy.
  complications of, 354–367
  gastroenterostomy, 343–354
  gastrostomy, 332–341
  pediatric gastrostomy, 341–343
  total gastrectomy and reconstruction, 309–328
  total gastrectomy with esophagoduodenostomy, 328–332
Gastric reservoir, substitute, operations for, 331–332, *331*
Gastric retention, postoperative, 355–361
  diagnosis and treatment for, 356–357
  prevention of, 357
Gastric rupture, celiotomy for, 285
Gastric secretion, cephalic phase of, 22, *22*
  during interdigestive period, 21
  effects of gastric bypass on, 385–386
  gastric phase of, 22, *22*
  gastrin in, 19–21
  inhibition of, 23–25, *24,* 26
  intestinal phase inhibitors of, 23
  of stomach, 13–32
  pharmacologic stimulants of, 25
  phases of, 22–23, *22*
  regulation of, 18–27
  vagal stimulation of, 19
  vagal-antral phase inhibitors of, 23
Gastric secretory response of feeding, 22–23, *22,* 25
Gastric ulcers. See Ulcer(s), gastric.
Gastric volvulus. See Volvulus, gastric.
Gastric washings, in gastric ulcer, 252
Gastric/duodenal congenital obstruction, 120–122, *120–122*
Gastrin, determination of, in duodenal ulcer, 256
  in antral mucosa, 14–15
  in gastric secretion, 19–21
  in Zollinger-Ellison syndrome, 263, 264
  ulcer and, duodenal, 254–255
    recurrent, 364
Gastrinoma (Zollinger-Ellison syndrome), 263–265
Gastritis, 285–286
Gastroduodenostomy, 293, 296, 343, 344, *345–347.* See also Gastroenterostomy.
  infrapapillary, *346–348*
  Jaboulay, 376
  Judd, *383*
  Rienhoff modification of, 344
  terminolateral, *302*
Gastroenterostomy, 343–354
  for gastric fixation, 182
  hemorrhage after, 354–355
  history of, 343–344
  indications for, 344
  mechanical instruments in, 589
  technics of, 344–354
  without vagotomy, 344
Gastrogastrostomy, for hourglass stomach, 192, *192*
Gastroileostomy, repair of, 367
Gastrointestinal anastomosis (GIA) stapler. See GIA stapler.
Gastrointestinal suturing, 556–578, *557*
  materials for, 559–562

Gastrointestinal suturing (*Continued*)
  objectives of, 559
  purpose of, 559
  standards for, 562
  strength of, 559
  types of, 562–578
Gastrojejunostomy, 293, 343, 344, 349, *349, 350.* See also Gastroenterostomy.
  antecolic, *208,* 344, 349, 353
    for duodenal stenosis, 143, *143*
  anterior, 343, 349–352, *350–351*
  antiperistaltic, 349, *349,* 353–354
  Billroth II operation, 288, 289, 301–306, *303–305*
  disconnection of, 364–367
    indications for, 364
    technic of, 364–366, *365–366*
  for duodenal atresia, *138*
  for intramural hematoma of duodenum, 242–243
  GIA stapler for, ischemia with, *596*
  isoperistaltic, 349, *349,* 353–354
  obstruction after, 355–356
    treatment of, 356–357
  posterior, 352–353, *352–353*
  retrocolic, 344, 349, 353, *353*
  stapled, 597
  technic of, essential feature of, 353
  with proximal pouch, for hourglass stomach, 194–195, *195*
Gastrolysis, 113–114
Gastropexy, 184–185, *185–187*
  Beyea's method of, 184, *185*
  Coffey's method of, 184, *185*
  Duret's method of, 184, *187*
  for gastric volvulus, 175–176, *175,* 182
    with colonic displacement, 182–183, *182–183*
  Perthes' method of, 184, *186*
  Rosving's method of, 184–185, *187*
Gastroplasty, for hourglass stomach,
  Kammerer-Finney, 192, *193*
  Heineke-Mikulicz, 192–193, *193*
  gastric bypass versus, 396, 400
Gastroplication, technics of, 185–188, *187, 188*
Gastroptosis, 184
Gastrorrhaphy, 465–466
Gastroscopes, description of, 66–67
Gastroscopy, 66–89
  anterior, through gastrotomy, 89–90
  fiberoptic, description of, 66–67
  gastrotomy in, 89–90
  in gastric ulcer, 252
  peroral, 66–89
    cholangiopancreatography in, 72–75
    definition of, 66
    duodenoscopy in, 70–72
    equipment for, 66–67
    esophagogastroduodenoscopy in, 68–70
    upper GI endoscopy in, 75–89
Gastrostomy, 332–341
  Beck-Jianu, 336–337, *338*
  definition of, 332
  for gastric volvulus, 182
  Glassman's, 337–341, *339–341*
  indications for, 332–333
  Janeway, 334–336, *336–337*
  Kader, 342
  mucosa-lined, 333, 334–341
  pediatric, 341–342
  permanent, 333, 334–341

INDEX 625

Gastrostomy (*Continued*)
  Ssabanejew-Frank, 342–343
  Stamm, 333–334, *333*, *342*, *343*
  types of, 333–341
  Witzel, 333, 334, *335*
Gastrotomy, 462–465, *463–465*
  for gastroscopy, 89–90
  indications for, 462
  technic of, 462
  technic of closure of incision in, 465
G-cell hyperplasia, recurrent ulcer and, 363–364
Getzen, L. C., Navy stitch and, 577, 580
GIA (gastrointestinal anastomosis) stapler, 583, *584*, *589–591*
  complications with, 594
  gastrojejunostotomy with, ischemia with, *596*
  in Finney pyloroplasty, 589, *592*
  in gastric bypass, 385, *387*, *388*
  surgical uses of, 588–593, *589–591*
Glands of Brunner, 38
Glassman's gastrostomy, 337–341, *339–341*
Glossopharyngeal nerve, course and distribution of, *416*
Glover stitch, 563, *568–569*, 573
Gould inverted mattress suture, for enterorrhaphy, 573–574, *574*
Graham method, of total gastrectomy, 322–323, *323*
Grassi, nerve of, 371, *372*
Greater curvature, of stomach, 6, 7
Gunshot wounds. *See* Penetrating trauma.

H-2 receptor antagonists, as gastric secretion inhibitors, 26
Halsted, W. S., surgical contribution of, 580
Halsted interrupted quilt (mattress) suture, 563, *564*
Halsted stitch, Navy anastomosis versus, 577, *577*
Harris tube, 50, *54*
Hays–De Almeida reservoir, *329*
Head, of rib, 425
Healing, of intestinal wounds, 579–580
  mechanical sutures in, 580–581
Heineke-Mikulicz gastroplasty, for hourglass stomach, 192–193, *193*
Heineke-Mikulicz pyloroplasty, 288, 376–377, *376*, 383
  Gambee suture in, 576–577, *576*
  TA stapler in, 588
Hematemesis, after gastrointestinal anastomosis, 354–355
  methods of treatment for, 354–355
Hematoma, duodenal, intramural, 233–245
  clinical findings in, 235
  etiology of, 234
  incidence of, 234
  laboratory findings in, 234
  nonoperative treatment of, 236
  nonoperative versus operative treatment of, 237–241
  operative technics for, 242–243
  operative treatment of, 237
  pediatric, 243–245, *243*, 244t
  physical examination in, 235
  radiology studies for, 235–236
  stomach, intramural, 205
  wound, 532
Hemigastrectomy, for benign disease, 289

Hemorrhage. *See also* Bleeding.
  from duodenal ulcer, 261–263
  from gastric ulcer, 261–263
  in gastric volvulus, 177–178, *177–178*
  intraperitoneal, 354–355
  postoperative, 354–355
Hemostasis, in wound contamination, 530
Henroz, J. H. F., 579–580
Hernia(s), diaphragmatic, in gastric volvulus, 173–174
  repair of, 180
    upward extension of incision in, 491–493, *491–493*
  hiatal, esophageal, case report of, 126–128, *127–128*
    gastropexy for, 184–185, *185–187*
    repair of, incision for, *456*
      extension of, 495–497, *495*, *496*
      patient position in, *453*
  spigelian, 475
  thoracotomy for, 449
Hiatal hernia. *See* Hernia, hiatal.
Histamine, as gastric secretion stimulant, 25
  in gastric secretion, 20
Hoffman-Steinberg reservoir, *329*
Hofmeister modification, of Billroth II operation, *303*
Hofmeister-Finsterer operation, 288, 289
Hollander insulin gastric analysis, 29
Horsley modification, of Billroth I operation, 298, *300*, 300–301
  of Heineke-Mikulicz pyloroplasty, 377, *378–379*
Hourglass stomach, 188–195, *190*, *192–195*
  versus cascade stomach, 190
Hültl, Humer, 582
Hunger contractions, 34
Hunicutt-Lee reservoir, *329*
Hunt–Limo-Basto reservoir, *329*
Hydrochloric acid, in gastric juice, 17–18
  measurement of, 27–32
Hyoid bone, 403
Hypoglossal nerve, 415, *417*

IF (intrinsic factor), in gastric juice, 16
Ileum, terminal, as substitute gastric reservoir, 331, *331*
Iliac artery, 479–480, *479*
Iliac crest, *473*
Iliacus muscle, 480, *480*
Iliohypogastric nerve, 476–477, *477*
Ilioinguinal nerve, 477, *477*
Incision(s), 401–532. *See also* names of incisions.
  abdominal, 467–524
    anatomy of, 467–486
    choice of, 486–524
    comments on, 524
    oblique, lateral, *522*, *523*, *524*
    rupture of, 362
    transverse, 504–511
      closure of, 497
      extension by, 495–497, *496*
      modified, 506–508, *507*
      Singleton, 508–509, *509*
      upper, 504–506, *505*
    types of, 486–524
  abdominothoracic, 452–454, *453–454*
  axial, examination of stomach mucosa through, *463*
  Bevan, 523
  choice of, 486–488

Incision(s) (*Continued*)
  colectomy, right, 509–511, *510*
  Coller, 515
  complicated, *523*, 524
  complications of, 529–532, *531*
  disruption of, 532
  effect on pulmonary physiology of, 486
  epigastric, *488*
  gastrectomy, upward extension of, 491–494, *491–494*
  gastrotomy, transverse closure of, *465*
  Kammerer-Battle, 503–504, *504*
  Kocher, 515–519, *516–518*
    extension of, 519
    technic of, 515
  McBurney gridiron, 480, 484, 519–521, *520*
    extension of, 520
  midabdominal, transverse, 509–511, *510*
  midline, *455*, 455
    extension of, 455, *455, 456*
    lower, 497–499, *498, 499*
      closure in, 498, *499*
      comment on, 498
      methods of extension in, 498–499
      technic of, 497–498, *498*
    upper, 488–497, *488, 490–496*
      extensions of, 490–497, *491–497*
      technic of, 488–490
  midrectus, 502–503, *503*
    methods of extension of, 502–503
    technic of, 502, *503*
  oblique, 515–524
    Kocher, 515–519, *517, 518,* 522
    McBurney gridiron, 519–521, *520*
    Rockey-Davis, 521–524, *521*
    subcostal, 515–519, *517, 518*
  paramedian, 455, 499–502, *500, 501*
  pararectus, 503–504, *504*
  parascapular, right, *451*
  Pfannenstiel, 511–515, *512–514*
    methods of extension of, 513
    technic of, 512
  principles for, 402
  Rockey-Davis, 521–524, *521*
    technic of, 521
  rupture of, 362
  Singleton, 508
  special, 486
  subcostal (Kocher), 515–519, *516–518*
    extension of, 519
    technic of, 515
  thoracicoabdominal, 452–454, *453–454,* 455, *456*
  thoracotomy, 449–451, *450*
    closure of, 448–449, *448–449*
    enlargement of, 448, *448*
    extrapleural, 451–452, *451–452*
    major, 444–454, *445, 447–454*
    minor, 443–444, *443–444*
      for drainage, 443
    standard, *432,* 445–449, *445, 447–449*
  transrectus, 455, 502–503, *503*
    methods of extension of, 502–503
    technic of, 502, *503*
  transverse, 455, 486–487, *488,* 504
    advantages of, 486–487
    for excision of rectum, 515, *516*
    modified, 506
    vertical versus, 487
  types of, 486–524

Incision(s) (*Continued*)
  vertical, 486–487, *487*
    advantages of, 487
    transverse versus, 487
  Wangensteen's extension of, *309, 455*
Incisura, of stomach, 7
Incomplete membrane, versus hypertrophic pyloric stenosis, 119
Infantile hypertrophic pyloric stenosis, 117, *118,* 119
Infection, sutures in, 539–540
  wound, 532
Infraspinatus muscle, *436,* 437–438, *438*
Inhibitors, of gastric secretion, 26
Injuries, of duodenum, 219–245
    diagnosis of, 222–224
    treatment of, 224–245
    types of, 219–224
  of pancreas, 225–226, *226*
  of stomach, 197–218
    blunt trauma, 197
    corrosive, 217–218
    foreign bodies, 216
    penetrating trauma, 206
    stab wounds, 212
Instruments, mechanical. *See* Mechanical sutures; Stapling instruments.
Insulin, as gastric secretion stimulant, 25
Insulin infusion test, in gastric analysis, 30
Intercostal arteries, 427–428, *429,* 477–478
Intercostal fascia, external, 431, *432*
Intercostal method of thoracotomy, 446
Intercostal muscles, external, 431
  internal, 432, *432*
Intercostal nerves, 429–430, *429,* 476, 477, *477*
Intercostal spaces, 427, *428,* 428
Interrupted Lembert suture, 562–564, *563*
Interrupted quilt (mattress) suture, Halsted, *563,* 564
Interrupted sutures, 562
  single row of, 544
Intestinal phase of gastric secretion, 22, 23
Intramural duodenal hematoma, 233–245
Intramural gastric hematoma, 205
Intrinsic factor (IF), in gastric juice, 16
Intubation, gastric, peroral, 48–49
    indications for, 48
    lavage in, 49
    technic of, 48
    postoperative, omission of, 64–65
  gastroduodenal, 49–59
  gastrointestinal, 46–65
    indications for, 46
    lower, 49–59
  nasogastric, 49–59
    postoperative gastric decompression versus, 62–63
    routine, 63–65
Irrigation, wound, 530

Jaboulay gastroduodenostomy, 376
Jaboulay pyloroplasty, 344, 376
  GIA stapler in, 589
Janeway gastrostomy, 334–336, *336–337*
Jaundice, mechanical suturing and, 598
Jejunal interposition in gastric reconstruction, 328, *328*
Jejunoileal bypass, gastric bypass versus, 393–394, *393*

INDEX

Jejunojejunostomy, in gastric retention, 356–357
  in Graham method of total gastrectomy, 323
Jejunoplasty, 357–361
  advantages of, 361
  Finney pyloroplasty in, 357
  stoma closure in, 359–361, *359, 361*
  stoma enlargement in, 359, *360,* 361
  technic of, 357–361, *358–360*
Johnston tube, 50
Judd gastroduodenostomy, 383
Judd pyloroplasty, 381, 383
Jugular veins, 409–411, *409–411*

Kader gastrostomy, 342
Kammerer-Battle pararectus incision, 503–504, *504*
Kammerer-Finney gastroplasty, for hourglass stomach, 192, *193*
Kay augmented histamine test, of gastric acidity, 29
Kocher incision, 515, *522*
Kocher modification, of Billroth I operation, 289, *298,* 300–301
Kocher's maneuver, *40*
  in Billroth I operation, 296, *298*

Laceration, of gastric mucosa, 204
Lahey technic, of antecolic gastroenterostomy, *351*
  of total gastrectomy, 315, *315–320*
Langer's lines of cleavage, 468, *468*
Laparoscopy. *See* Peritoneoscopy.
Laryngeal nerves, 414, *414–416*
Latarjet, nerve(s) of, 371, 395
Latissimus dorsi muscle, 433, *470,* 471, *472, 473, 474,* 481
Lavage, of stomach contents, 49
Lawrence reservoir, 329
Layers, abdominal wall, 467–485, *467*
  sutures for, 489–490, *490*
  wound closure in, 489–490, *490*
LDS (ligating and dividing) stapler, 583, *584*
  complications with, 595
  surgical use of, *584,* 593
Leakage, from duodenal stump, 362
Lee operation for substitute gastric reservoir, 331, *331*
Leiomyomas, 246, 247
Leiomyosarcoma, gastric, 250
Lembert, surgical discoveries of, 579
Lembert stitch, purpose of, 556, 563
Lembert sutures, 303, 339, 465
  continuous, 563, 564
  interrupted, 562–564, *563*
Lesser curvature, of stomach, 6, 7
Levator scapulae muscle, *426,* 433–434
Levin tube, 49–50, *51*
  early use of, 60
  technic of, 50–51, *51*
Ligament, arcuate, external, 481, *483*
  falciform, 484
  lumbocostal, 481, *483*
  of Treitz, 40, *41,* 156–157, *157,* 325, *326*
    division in gastric bypass of, *384,* 385
    in duodenal exposure, 458, *460*
    in duodenojejunal obstruction, 152–155, *153*
    in SMA syndrome, 162–163, *163*
  Poupart's, 473

Ligamentum teres, closure of, 489
Ligating and dividing stapler (LDS), 583, *584*
Linea alba, *469, 472, 475, 476, 478,* 485–486, *485*
  closure of, 489
  incision in, 486
Linea semilunaris, 475
Lipomas, 247
Liver, biopsy of, in peritoneoscopy, 100–101, *100*
  peritoneoscopic visualization of, 102–103, *103*
Lock-stitch, 563, 568–569, 573
Longmire and Beal reservoir, 329
Longmire method, of total gastrectomy, 310–315, *310–314*
Lordosis, vascular compression of duodenum and, 171
Lumbar muscles, 480
Lumbocostal ligament, 481, *483*
Lumbodorsal fascia, *467,* 481–483, *482*
Lung abscess, minor thoracotomy incisions for, *443*
Lungs, thoracic relations of, 439
Lymph drainage, of stomach, 12
Lymph nodes, of stomach, 12, *12*
Lymphoma, gastric, 250

Maingot's method, for gastric volvulus, 182
Malformation, congenital, of stomach, 4–6
Mallory-Weiss syndrome, 204, 205
Mammary artery, 428–429, *429, 478, 479*
Mammary gland (breast), 432–433, *450*
  arterial supply of, 433, *434*
  of thorax, 430–438, *430–432, 434–438*
Mammary vein, 429
Mann-Williamson procedure, excluding gastric acid, 24
Marshall U-stitch, 465, 571, *571*
  through-and-through U-stitch versus, 566
Mason and Ito method of gastric bypass, 384 ff.
Materials, for gastrointestinal suturing, 559–562
Mattress suture, Halsted, 563, *564*
Mayo modification, of Billroth I operation, 297
McBurney gridiron incision, 519–521, *520*
McBurney's incision, 480, 484
Mechanical stapling instruments. *See* Stapling instruments.
Mechanical sutures, 579–600
  in Billroth II gastrectomy, *584–585*
  in healing of intestinal wounds, 580–581
  manual technics versus, 579, 581
Mediastinum, 439, 440–442
  anatomic structures of, *441*
  right surface, structures of, *373*
  superior, *411*
Megaduodenum, 147–152, *149*
  aganglionic, congenital, 147–150, *149*
  from absent musculature, 150
  hereditary, 150–152, *151*
Michel clip, 535
Microgastria, 5–6
Midline incision. *See* Incision, midline.
Midrectus (transrectus) incision, 502–503, *503*
Miller-Abbott tube, 46, 50, 53–54, *53*
Missile wounds, of stomach, 206–212, 206t, 207t, *212*
  diagnosis of, 207–208
  high-velocity, 209–210
  low-velocity, 209
  management of, 208–210
  operation for, 210–212, *212*

Monofilament sutures, 539
Morbid obesity, gastric partitioning for, 394–400, *395–399*
  gastric versus jejunoileal bypass in, 393–394, *393*
Moschel pyloroplasty, 381
Motor activity, gastric, 35
Moynihan closure of duodenum, 295
Moynihan's modification, in gastric plication, 185, 188, *188*
Mucosa-to-mucosa approximation, serosa-to-serosa closure versus, 579
Mucous neck cells, 13, *15*
Mucus, in gastric juice, 15
Multifilament sutures, 539
Murphy's button, 580
Muscle(s). *See also* names of muscles.
  back, *482*
    deep, *470*
  chest and arm, deep, *431*
  neck, *420*
  superficial, of back of neck and upper trunk, *438*
  thoracic, 430–438, *430–432, 434–438*
  trunk, *430, 472*
    right, *474*
Muscle layers, closure of, anatomic considerations in, 540–541
Muscle-bone layer, of abdominal wall, 469–483, *469, 470*
  abdominal muscles of, oblique, 471–480, *472–479*
    posterior, 480–483, *480, 482*
Musculature, extrinsic, of costal region of thoracic wall, 430

Nasogastric tube, in gastric blunt trauma injuries, 199
Navy anastomosis, 577–578, *577*
  Gambee versus, 577, *577*
Neck, anatomy of, 403–406, *404–408*
  arteries of, 412–413, *412*
  front, muscles of, *405*
  left side of, *422*
  muscles of, *420*
  nerves of, 413–418, *414–417*
  prevertebral region of, *411*
  veins of, 409–412, *409–411*
  visceral space of, 403, 408
Needles, in gastrointestinal suturing, 561–562
Neonatal gastric perforations, 274–276, *274*
Nerve(s). *See also* names of nerves.
  of abdominal wall, 476–477
  of Grassi, in vagotomy, 371, 372
  of Latarjet, in vagotomy, 371
    isolation of, in gastric partitioning, 395
  of neck, 413–418, *414–417*
  of stomach, 12, *12*
  of thorax, 427–430, *428–429*
Neurilemmomas, 247
Nonabsorbable material, for gastrointestinal suturing, 561
Nonabsorbable suture, 536–540, 537t, 538t
Nylon sutures, 536, 538t, 539

Obese patients, sutures for, 553–555, *553–555*
Obesity, morbid, gastric procedures for, 384–400
Oblique incisions, 515–524

Oblique muscles, 469–470, *469, 472*
  external, 471–473, *472, 473*
  internal, *472,* 473–475, *474*
  nerve supply of, 476, 478
Obstruction. *See also* Atresia.
  by duodenal ulcer, 260–261
  by gastric ulcer, 260–261
  combined gastric and duodenal, congenital, 120–122, *120–122*
  duodenal extrinsic, 130
    intrinsic, 129
  duodenojejunal junction, 152–155, *153*
  jejunoplasty for, 357–361, *358–360*
  postoperative, 355–361
Obstruction-like disorders, of stomach and duodenum, 184–196
Obstructive disorders, of stomach and duodenum, 111–183
Omentum, peritoneoscopic visualization of, *104,* 105, *105*
Operation(s). *See also* specific procedures.
  biliary tract, early history of, 59
  for antral mucosal diaphragm with hiatal hernia, 126
  for cascade stomach, 195
  for cast syndrome, 170, 171
  for combined congenital gastric and duodenal obstruction, 120–122
  for congenital antral membrane, 126
  for congenital duodenal stenosis, 142, 145
  for duodenal atresia, 132
    and biliary tract abnormalities, 136
  for duodenal hematoma, 242–243
  for duodenal injuries, 224–245
  for duodenal ulcer, 257–258
  for duodenojejunal junction obstruction, 154
  for freeing adhesions, 114
  for gastric hematomas, 205
  for gastric rupture, 285
  for gastric ulcer, 253–254
  for gastric volvulus, 179–183
  for gastritis, 286
  for gastrojejunocolic fistula, *271–272*
  for hourglass stomach, 192–195
  for laceration of gastric mucosa, 204
  for megaduodenum, 148
  for missile wounds of stomach, 210–212, *212*
  for morbid obesity, 384–393, 394–400
  for neonatal atresia of stomach, 119
  for neonatal gastric perforation, 275–276
  for obstruction from ulcer, 261
  for pyloric stenosis, 279–280, 281
  for SMA syndrome, 162, 163, 164, 165, 167, 170
  for stab wounds of stomach, 216
  for ulcer disease, 368–375
  for ulcer hemorrhage, 262–263
  for ulcer perforation, 260
  gastric, early history of, 59–60
  in stress ulcer, 267–268
  in Zollinger-Ellison syndrome, 265
  minor, during peritoneoscopy, 102
Opolzer's operation, for gastric volvulus, 183
Orr method, of total gastrectomy, 315–316, *321*

Pacemaker, gastric, 33
Pancreas, aberrant, 247

INDEX

Pancreas (*Continued*)
  blood supply of, *11, 459*
  injuries of, 225–226, *226*
Pancreaticoduodenectomy, 225–226
Papillotomy, endoscopic, 86–88, *86, 87*
Paracentesis, diagnostic, 202–204, *203*
Paramedian incision, 499
Pararectus incision, 503
Paré, Ambrose, 536
Parietal cell vagotomy, 258, 371
Parietal cells, in stomach, 13, *14*
Parker-Kerr stitch, 566, *567*
Pectoralis major, 430, *430,* 431
Pectoralis minor, 430–431, *430*
Pediatric. *See* Children.
Pelvic organs, peritoneoscopic visualization of, 106, *106*
Penetrating trauma, to duodenum, 220–221, *220*
  to stomach, 206–212, 206t, 207t, *212*
    missile wounds, 206
    stab wounds, 212
Pentagastrin, as gastric secretion stimulant, 25
Pepsinogens, in gastric juice, 15–16
Peptic ulcer disease. *See* Ulcer(s), peptic.
Perforation, following gastric bypass, 391–392, *391–392*
  gastric, neonatal, 274–276, *274*
  of duodenal ulcer, symptoms and diagnosis of, 259–260
    treatment of, 260
  of gastric ulcer, symptoms and diagnosis of, 259–260
    treatment of, 260
  transmural, 204–205
Perichondrium, 427
Periosteum, 427
Peristaltic waves, of stomach, 34
Peritoneal lavage, diagnostic, 200–202, *200–202,* 201t
Peritoneoscope, fiberoptic, description of, 94
Peritoneoscopy, 66–110
  advantages of, 91–92
  biopsy in, 100–101, *100*
  complications of, 88–89, 108–109
  contraindications of, 93–94
  indications for, 92–93
  limitations of, 91–92
  operative procedure with, 102
  postoperative care with, 108
  precautions with, 108
  regional examinations with, 102–107
  results with, 109–110
  special examinations with, 101–102
  technic of, 94–101, *96*
    abdominal inflation, 98
    anesthesia, 94–95
    instruments, 94
    needle insertion, 97–98, *97*
    preparation, 94
    site of puncture, 96
    trocar insertion, 98–99, *99*
    visualization, 99–100
  use in children of, 107–108
  wound closure in, 107
Peritoneum, 10, *10*
  closure of, 489, 490
    anatomic considerations in, 540
  parietal, 484–485
  peritoneoscopic visualization of, 107, *107*

Perthes' method, of gastropexy, 184, *186*
Petit's triangle, 472, *473,* 481
Pfannenstiel incision, 511
Pharmacologic stimulants, of gastric secretion, 25
Phrenic nerve, 414, *417, 418, 420*
Physiology, of duodenum, 38–45
  of stomach, 13–32
  pulmonary, effect of incisions on, 486
Platysma muscle, 406, *407*
Pleura(e), 439–440, *439*
  cervical, *439,* 440
  parietal, 439
  visceral, 439
Plication, gastric. *See* Gastric plication.
Polya modification, of Billroth II operation, *304–305*
Polya operation, 288, *289*
Polya-Balfour modification, of Billroth II operation, 306, *306*
Polya-type gastric reconstruction, 293
Polyester fiber, as suture material, 538t, 539
Polyglactin suture, 536, 537t, 549, 560
Polyglycolic acid sutures, 537t, 539, *548,* 549, 560
Polypropylene sutures, 536, 538t, 539
Polyps, gastric, 246
Portal vein, preduodenal, 42–45, *43*
Posterior extrapleural thoracotomy incision, 451–452, *451–452*
  technic of, 451
Posterolateral (standard) thoracotomy incision, *432,* 445–449
  closure of incisions in, 448–449, *448–449*
  technic of, 445–448, *445*
    incision enlargement in, 448
    intercostal method of, 446
    rib resection method of, 446–448, *447–448*
Pouch(es), gastric, reconstruction with, 328, *329*
  substitute, formation of, 331–332, *331*
  types of, *329*
Poupart's ligament, 473
Prepyloric membrane, *115. See also* Antral membrane.
  incomplete, 116
Prevertebral region, of neck, *411*
Procedure. *See also* Operation(s).
  Exalto, 24
  Mann-Williamson, 24
Prostaglandin analogues, as gastric secretion inhibitors, 26
Proximal gastric vagotomy. *See* Vagotomy, gastric, proximal.
Psoas major muscle, *470,* 471, *480, 480*
Pulmonary physiology, effect of incisions on, 486
Pursestring suture, *294, 295, 563,* 564–565, *565*
Pyeloduodenal fistula, traumatic, 228–230
Pyloric pump, 35–36
Pyloric stenosis, congenital, 277–281
  clinical signs and symptoms of, 278
  diagnosis of, 278
  in adults, 280–281
  incidence and etiology of, 277–278
  physical examination in, 278–279
  surgical procedure in, 279–280
  infantile, 117, *118, 119*
Pyloric vein, 7, *8*
Pyloroplasty, 375–383
  Balfour, 381, *381–382*
  comments on, 383
  Finney, 377–381, *380*

Pyloroplasty (*Continued*)
  Finney, Balfour modification of, 381, *381–382*
    GIA stapler in, 589, *592*
    in jejunoplasty, 357
    other types versus, 383
  Heineke-Mikulicz, 376–377, *376*
    Gambee suture in, 576–577, *576*
    Horsley modification of, 377, *378–379*
    TA stapler in, 588
    ulcer recurrence rate in, 383
    Weinberg modification of, 383
  indications for, 375–376
  Jaboulay, 344, 376
    GIA stapler in, 589
  Judd, 381, *383*
  Moschel, 381
  types of, 376–383, *376*, *378–383*
Pylorus, of stomach, 6, 7, *7*
Pyramidalis muscles, 469, 471, *478*
  left, *469*

Quadratus lumborum muscle, 470, 471, 480, *480*
Quilt sutures, Halsted, 563, *564*

Radiologic studies, diagnostic, in duodenal wounds, 222–223
  in stomach wounds, 199
  in gastric ulcer, 252
Receptive relaxation, 375
  definition of, 368
Reconstruction, Billroth I and II for, 289
  gastric. *See* Gastric resection.
Rectum, abdominoperineal excision of, incision for, 515, *516*
Rectus abdominis muscles, 469, 471, *472*, *478*
  in paramedian incision, 500, *501*
  nerve supply of, 476–477, *477*
  right, *469*
Rectus sheath, anterior, in paramedian incision, 500, *501*
  posterior, closure of, 489
Reflex, enterogastric, 23, 36
Resection, gastric. *See* Gastric resection.
  of nonviable duodenum, 243
  sleeve, 193–194, *194, 195*, 309
Reservoir(s), gastric, types of, 329
  gastric reconstruction with, 328, *329*
  State-Moroney, *329*
Retention bar, use in wound closure of, 552, *553*
Retention sutures, 549–555, *550–555*
Retroperitoneal rupture, 224–225
Rhazes of Baghdad, 535
Rhomboideus major muscle, 435, *473*
Rhomboideus minor muscle, 434–435
Rib(s), 424–427, *424–427*
  false, 424
  floating, 421
  head of, 425
  sternal, 424
  true, 424
  tubercle of, 426
Rib neck, 426
Rib resection method, of thoracotomy, 446–448, *447, 448*
  closure of, 448–449, *449*

Rienhoff modification, of gastroduodenostomy, 344
  of Roux-en-Y total gastrectomy, 325
Rockey-Davis incision, 521
Rosving's method, of gastropexy, 184–185, *187*
Roux operation, *288*
Roux-en-Y modification, of Billroth II operation, 308–309, *308*
Roux-en-Y reconstruction, 329
Roux-en-Y total gastrectomy, *324–327*, 325–328
  antiperistaltic segment of, 325
  indications for, 325
  isoperistaltic segment of, 327
Rupture, duodenal, 224–227
  with ampulla of Vater injury, 226–227
  gastric, celiotomy for, 285
    spontaneous, 281–285
  retroperitoneal, 224–225

Sacrospinalis (erector spinae) muscle, *470*, 471, 480–481
Sarcomas, gastric, 250
Scapula, 435, 436, *436*
Schoemaker modification, of Billroth I operation, 297, *298*
Schoemaker operation, 288, *289*
Scoliolordosis, vascular compression of dudodenum and, 171
Scoliosis, vascular compression of duodenum and, 171
Selective vagotomy. *See* Vagotomy, selective.
Semicircular line of Douglas, 469, 475, *475*, 479, 483
Serosa-to-serosa approximation, mucosa-to-mucosa closure versus, 579
Serratus anterior muscles, 431
Serratus posterior muscles, 435, *435*
Seventh layer, of abdominal wall, 484–485
SFM (skin and fascia) stapler, 587
Shaft (body), of rib, 426
Sheath, of rib, 427
Silk sutures, genesis of, 536
  in gastrointestinal suturing, 561
Silver wire, for sutures, 536
Singleton incision, 508
Sinography, in stab wounds of stomach, 214–215
Sixth (extraperitoneal fat) layer, of abdominal wall, 484
  incision in, 484
Skin, closure of, 541–544, *544*
  in abdominal incisions, 468, *468*
Skin and fascia (SFM) stapler, 587
Sleeve resection, for hourglass stomach, 193–194, *194–195*
  of stomach, 309
SMA syndrome. *See* Superior mesenteric artery syndrome.
Small intestine, peritoneoscopic visualization of, 106
Spinal accessory nerve, *416*, 418
Spleen, blood supply of, *11*, 459
  peritoneoscopic visualization of, 104
Splenectomy, lateral upper abdominal transverse incision for, 508
  upward extension of incision in, 491–492, *491, 492*
Splints, use in wound closure of, 552, *552*
Ssabanejew-Frank gastrostomy, 342–343
Stab wounds, of stomach, 212–216
  sinography in, 214–215
Stamm gastrostomy, 333–334, *333*, 342, 343

INDEX

Standard thoracotomy incision. *See* Incision, thoracotomy.
Staple partition, gastric, 394–400, *395–399*
    complications of, 396
Stapler. *See* name of stapler; Stapling instruments.
Stapling instruments. *See also* Mechanical sutures.
  advantages of, 594
  American, 583–587, *584–587*
  comments on, 600
  complications with, 598
  experiences with, 595–600
  history of, 581–583
  literature review of, 595–600
  precautions and safeguards with, 594–595
  Russian, 582–583
  surgical technics with, 587–600
  use in children of, 593
State-Moroney reservoir, *329*
Stay suture, *550*
Stenosis, duodenal, congenital, 141–147, *141–144*
    diagnosis of, 142
    pathology of, 141
    preoperative care of, 143
    surgical treatment of, 143
    symptoms of, 142
    treatment of, 143
  positions of, *142*
  postinfancy, 144–147
    surgical treatment of, 145
  types of, 141, *141*
  of stomach, 114–128, *115*
  pyloric. *See* Pyloric stenosis.
Sternal angle, 424
Sternal region, of thorax, 423–424
Sternocleidomastoid muscles, 403, *405, 406, 407*
Sternum, 424, *424*
  splitting of, in Wangensteen extension, 494–495, *495*
Stimulants, pharmacologic, of gastric secretion, 25
Stitch. *See also* Suture.
  Cushing, 566
  Czerny, 556
  Gambee, in Heineke-Mikulicz pyloroplasty, 377
  Glover, 563, 568–569, 573
  Lembert, purpose of, 556, 563
  Marshall U-, 465, 566, 571, *571*
  Parker-Kerr, 566, *567*
  U-, through-and-through, 566–571, *568–570*
Stoma, jejunoplasty, closure of, 359–361, *359, 361*
  enlargement of, *359, 360, 361*
Stomach. *See also* Gastric entries.
  adhesions of, freeing of, 113–114
  anatomy of, 3–13
    surgical, 6–12, *7–12*
  bilocular, 188–195, *190, 192–195*
  blood supply of, *459*
  cardia of, 7, *7*
  cardiac end of, 6
  cascade, 195–196, *196*
  circulation of, 8, 10–12, *11*
  coats of, 6
  cross sections of, in rotation, *5*
  "cup and spill," 195–196, *196*
  curvature of, greater, 6, 7
    lesser, 6, 7
  digestive function of, 32–37, *35*
  dilatation of, acute, 111–113, *113*
    clinical signs of, 112
    diagnosis of, 112
    etiology of, 111

Stomach (*Continued*)
  dilatation of, acute, treatment of, 112
  disorders of, obstruction-like, 184–196
    obstructive, 111–183
  divisions of, 6, 7
  embryology of, 3–4, *4, 5*
  emptying of, 34–37, *35*
  exposure of, 455–466
  features of, external, 7, *7*
  fixation points of, 9–10
  food mixing in, 34
  food propulsion through, 34
  functions of, 13
  fundus of, 7, *7*
  gastric secretion of, 13–32
  hematoma of, intramural, 205
  hourglass, 188–195, *190, 192–195*
    cascade stomach versus, 190
  identification of, 8, 12, 455, *456*
  incisura of, 7
  injuries of, 197–218
    blunt trauma, 197
    corrosive, 217–218
    foreign bodies, 216
    penetrating trauma, 206
    stab wounds, 212
  innervation of, 8, 10–12, *11*
    vagal, *12*
  laceration of, 204
  ligaments of, 9–10
  lymph drainage of, *12*
  lymph nodes of, 12, *12*
  lymphoma of, 250
  malformations of, congenital, 4–6
  malrotation of, 5–6, *5*
  missile wounds of, 206–212, 206t, 207t, *212*
  motor functions of, 33
  palpation of, bimanual, *464*
  perforation of, transmural, 204–205
  peristaltic waves of, 34
  peritoneal coverings of, 10, *10*
  peritoneoscopic visualization of, 104
  physiology of, 13–32
  position of, 7–9, *8*
  pylorus of, 6, 7, *7*
  relations to other organs of, 9, *9*
  rupture of, spontaneous, 281–285
    etiologic factors in, 282–284
  shape of, diagrams of, *5*
  skeletonization of, *292–293*
  stenosis of, 114–128, *115*
    diagnosis of, 117, *118, 119*
    history of, 116
    prognosis of, 120
    symptoms of, 117
    treatment of, 119
  storage function of, 33–34
  thoracic, 5
  transposition of, in abdomen, 5
  tubular, 5
  tumors of, benign, 246–247
    malignant, 247–250, *249*
  volvulus of. *See* Volvulus, gastric.
Stool, examination of, in duodenal ulcer, 256
Stress ulcer, 265–268, 266t, *267, 268*
  prevention of, 268
  treatment of, 267–268
Subcostal incision, 515

Subcutaneous tissues, closure of, anatomic
		considerations in, 541, *541-543*
	in abdominal incisions, 468
Subscapularis muscle, *431*, 436-437, *437*
Superior mesenteric artery (SMA) syndrome,
		155-162, *156-158*
	body casts and, 170-171
	burned children with, 168-169
	clinical characteristics of, 160-161
	diagnosis of, 161-162
	etiology of, 159-160
	in bedridden combat casualities, 169-170
	in pediatric patients, 167-168, *167-168*
	plus congenital duodenal diaphragm, 165-167,
		166
	treatment of, 162
	with peptic ulcer disease, 163-165
	without peptic ulcer disease, 162-163, *163*
Suprahyoid space, of neck, 408
Supraspinatus muscle, *436*, 437-438, *438*
Surgical cotton, 536, 538t, 539
Surgical gut, 536, 537t
Surgical silk, 536, 538t, 539
Surgical steel, 538t, 539
Surgical technics with stapling instruments, 587-600
Suspensory muscle of duodenum. *See* Ligament of
	Treitz.
Suture(s). *See also* names of sutures; Stapling
		instruments; Stitch; Suturing.
	absorbable, 536-540, 537t, 538t, *548*, *549*
		materials for, 536-540, 537t, 559-561
			synthetic, *548*, *549*, 560
		uses for, *548*, *549*
	Albert, 571-573, *572*
		for enterorrhaphy, 573-574, *574*
	Connell, *303*, *336*, 465, 563, *566*
	continuous, 546-547, *547*, 562
		overhand, simple, 571-573, *572*
		U-shaped, *566*
	cotton, in gastroinesinal suturing, 561
	Cushing, *303*, 563, 565-566
		in Finney pyloroplasty, *380*
	Czerny, 573, *573*
	for abdominal wall, 489-490, *490*
	for linea alba, 489, *490*
	for peritoneum, 490, *490*
	for skin, 490
	forms of, 562
	furrier, 571, *572*
	Gambee, in Heineke-Mikulicz pyloroplasty,
		576-577, *576*
	gastrointestinal, objectives of, 559
		purpose of, 559
		strength of, 559
		types of, 562-578
	in infected wounds, 539-540
	interrupted, 562
		Czerny, 573, *573*
		overhand, simple, 571-573, *572*
		single row of, 544-545, *545*
	Lembert, *303*, *339*, 465
		continuous, 563, *564*
		interrupted, 562-564, *563*
	mattress, *303*
		inverted, Gould, interrupted, 573-574, *574*
	mechanical. *See* Mechanical sutures; Stapling
		instruments.
	monofilament, 539
	multifilament, 539

Suture(s) (*Continued*)
	nonabsorbable, 536-540, 537t, 538t
	polyglactin, 536, 537t, 549, 560
	polyglycolic acid, 537t, 539, *548*, 549, 560
	polypropylene, 536, 538t, 539
	pursestring, *294*, *295*, 563, 564-565, *565*
		Doyen, *294*
	quilt, interrupted, Halsted, 563, *564*
	retention, 549-555, *550-555*
	selection of, principles of, 540
	silk, genesis of, 536
		in gastrointestinal suturing, 561
	silver wire, 536
	single row, in anastomosis, 558
		through all layers, 545-546, *546*
	stay, *550*
	through-and-through, continuous, 573-574, *574*
	Tom Jones far-and-near, 547-549, *547*
	types of, genesis of, 536
	wire, historical use of, 580
		through-and-through, use of, 545-546, *546*
Suture bridges, 555, *555*
Suture line, three-layer, 574
Suturing, gastrointestinal, 556-578, *557*
	materials for, 559-562
	standards for, 562
	types of, 562-578
	genesis of, 535-536
Sympathetic ganglion chain, cervical, *418*, *420*
Synthetic absorbable sutures, *548*, *549*
	in gastrointestinal suturing, 560

TA (thoracoabdominal) stapler, 465, 583
	complications with, 594
	surgical uses of, *584*, 587-588, *587*, *588*
"Tails" of wire, handling, 545, *545*
Televentroscope, 90
Thoracic alimentary tract, exposure of, 423-454
Thoracic duct, 413
Thoracic esophagus, approaches to, 442-443
Thoracic (mammary) artery, internal, 428-429, *429*,
	478, *479*
Thoracic (mammary) vein, internal, 429
Thoracic nerves, abdominal plexus of, *478*
Thoracic walls, 423-427, *424-427*
Thoracicoabdominal (abdominothoracic) incision,
	452-454, *453-454*
	technic of, 453
Thoracoabdominal (TA) stapler, 583
	in gastric bypass, 385, *386*, 387
	in gastric partitioning, 394-400, *395-398*
Thoracodorsal nerve, 481
Thoracotomy, intercostal method of, 446
	patient position in, 445
Thoracotomy incision(s), anterolateral, 449-451, *450*
	technic of, 449
	extrapleural, posterior, 451-452, *451-452*
	for cardiac operation, 449
	major, 444-454, *445*, *447-454*
	minor, 443-444, *443-444*
		comments on, 444
		selection of, 443
		technic of, 444, *444*
	standard, *432*, 445-449
Thorax, anatomy of, 423-442
	blood vessels and nerves of, 427-430, *428-429*
	contents of, 439-442, *439*, *440*

INDEX

Thorax (*Continued*)
  definition of, 423, *424, 425*
  diaphragm of, 440
  muscles and mammary gland of, 430–438, *430–438*
  walls of, 423–427, *424–427*
    fasciae of, 438–439
Three-layer suture line, 574
Through-and-through Albert suture, 573–574, *574*
Through-and-through monofilament closure, *552*
Through-and-through U-stitch, 566–571, *568–570*
Thyroid artery, inferior, 413, *420*
Thyroid cartilage, 403, *405*
Tissue trauma, avoidance of, in wound contamination, 529–530
TNM system, of tumor classification, 248
Tom Jones far-and-near sutures, 547–549, *547*
Torsion, volvulus versus, 171
Transrectus incision, 502
Transthoracic vagotomy, 372–374, *372–374*
Transversalis fascia, 483–484, *483*
  closure of, 489
Transversus abdominis muscles, *469,* 470, 475–476, *475, 476, 478*
  nerve supply of, 476, *477*
Trapezius muscle, *426, 433, 473*
Trauma. *See* Blunt trauma; Injuries; Penetrating trauma.
Travers, Benjamin, publication of, 579
Triangle, auscultatory, *473,* 481
  Petit's, *473,* 473, 481
Triangular areas, of neck, *406,* 408
Truncal vagotomy. *See* Vagotomy, truncal.
Trunk, muscles of, *430, 472*
  right, *474*
Tube(s), Cantor, description of, 46, *50,* 54
  Ewald, 47
    historical review of, 59–60
  feeding, 47
  gastroduodenal, bilumen, 52–53, *52*
  gastrointestinal, complications of, 54–59
  guidelines for, 58
  gastrojejunostomy, bilumen, 51–52, *52*
  gastrostomy, for pediatric patients, 341–342
  Harris, *50,* 54
  intestinal, for small bowel decompression, 46–47
  Johnston, *50*
  Levin, description of, 49–50, *51*
    early use of, 60
    technic of, 50–51, *51*
  Miller-Abbott, 53–54, *53*
    contraindications to, 53
    description of, 46, *50*
    indications for, 53
    technic of, 54
Tubercle, of rib, *426*
Tumors, duodenal, benign, 247
  malignant, 250
  gastric, benign, 246–247
    malignant, 247–250, *249*
    neurogenic, 247
    vascular, 247
  in Zollinger-Ellison syndrome, 263, 264

Ulcer(s), duodenal, 254–259
  clinical findings in, 255
  complications of, 259–263, 269

Ulcer(s) (*Continued*)
  duodenal, diagnostic studies in, 255–256
    etiology of, 254–255
    giant, 258–259
    hemorrhage of, 261–263
    medical treatment of, 256–257
    obstruction of, 260–261
    operative treatment of, 257–258, 269
    perforation of, 259–260
  experimental, procedures for, *24*
  gastric, 251–269
    clinical findings in, 252
    complications of, 259–263, 269
    diagnostic studies of, 252–253
    etiology of, 251
    hemorrhage of, 261–263
    obstruction of, 260–261
    operative treatment of, 269
    pathology of, 251–252
    perforation of, 259–260
    radiographic study in, 252
    treatment of, 253–254
    vagotomy versus gastric resection for, 374–375
  gastrojejunal, disconnection of gastrojejunostomy for, 364–366, *365–366*
  incidence of, after gastric bypass, 385–386
  jejunal, marginal, 362–363
    postoperative, 362–363
  marginal, as complication of gastric resection, 354, 361
    jejunoplasty for, 357–361, *358–360*
    postoperative, 354, 363–364
  peptic, absence in SMA syndrome of, 162–163, *163*
    experimental, Exalto procedure for, *24*
    SMA syndrome and, 163–165
      treatment of, 164
    vagotomy for, comments on, 374–375
    vagotomy versus gastrectomy for, 374
  recurrent, 354, 363–364
  stress, 265–268, 266t, *267, 268*
Ulcer-cancer relationship, of stomach, 253
Umbilicus, *472, 478, 486*
Urinalysis, diagnostic use in gastric blunt trauma, 199
U-shaped continuous suture, 566
U-stitch, Marshall, 465, 561, 571, *571*
  through-and-through, 561, 566–571, *568–570*

Vagal innervation of stomach, *12*
Vagal-antral phase inhibitors, of gastric secretion, 23
Vagotomy, 368–375
  abdominal, total. *See* Vagotomy, truncal.
  comments on, 374–375
  effects of, 368
  gastric, proximal, 258
    results of, 368, 372
    technic of, 371–372
  gastroenterostomy and, 344
  highly selective, 258, 371
  incision in, upward extension of, 491–493, *491–493*
  incomplete, 371
    evidence of, 368
      recurrent ulcer and, 363–364
      sequelae of, 375
  parietal cell, 258, 371
  postoperative complications of, 374
  results of, 368

Vagotomy (Continued)
  selective, results of, 368
    technic of, 371
  superselective, 258, 371
  supradiaphragmatic, technic of, 372–374, 372–374
  transthoracic, technic of, 372–374, 372–374
  truncal, results of, 368
    technic of, 370–371
  types of, 370–374, 372–374
Vagus nerve(s), 413–414, 415, 416
  anatomy of, 368–370, 369, 370
  distribution of, 369, 370
  gastric motility and, 368
  ligature and division of, 374
  physiology of, 370
  surgical isolation of, 373
Vascular compression of duodenum, 155, 158, 158
  scoliosis and, 171
Vein(s). See also names of veins.
  neck, 409–412, 409–411
  portal, preduodenal, 42–45, 43
  stomach, 8, 11, 11
Vertebral artery, 413
Vertebral vein, 411–412, 411
Visceral space, of neck, 403, 408
Vitamin B_{12}, in gastric juice, 16
Volvulus, definition of, 171
  gastric, 6, 171–183
    chronic, 176–177
    complex, acute, 175–176
    complications of, 177–178, 177–178
    diagnosis of, 176–177
    etiology of, 173–175
    gastropexy for, 184–185, 185–187
    idiopathic, 181–183
    in children, 183
    Maingot's method for, 182
    Opolzer's operation for, 183
    primary, 181–183
    surgical technics for, 178–180
    symptoms of, 175–176
    treatment of, 178–179
    types of, 171–172, 172
  idiopathic, 175
  mesenterioaxial, 171–172, 172
  organoaxial, 172, 172
  primary, 175
  secondary, 175, 180–181, 181
  types of, 173t
Von Haberer modification, 297–300, 298–300
Von Haberer operation, 287–289, 288

Von Haberer-Finney modification, of Billroth I operation, 298, 301, 302
Von Haberer-Finney operation, 288, 289
Von Petz instrument, for gastrointestinal tract stapling, 581–582

Wangensteen's extension, of incision, 309
  of midline incision, 455, 494–495, 495
Waves, constrictor, of stomach, 34
  mixing, of stomach, 34
Webs, antral, 116–117
Weir's modification, in gastric plication, 185, 187
Wilkie's syndrome, 155
Wire, "tails" of, handling, 545, 545
Wire sutures, historical use of, 580
  through-and-through, use of, 545–546, 546
Witzel gastrostomy, 333, 334, 335
Wölfler operation, 288, 350
Wound(s), abdominal, drainage of, 525–528, 525–527
  closure of. See Wound closure.
  contaminated, 529–530
    delayed closure in, 530–531, 531
    disruption in, 532
  hematomas in, 532
  high-velocity, 209–210
  infections in, 532
  intestinal, healing of, 579–580
    mechanical sutures in, 580–581
  low-velocity, 209, 216
Wound closure, 535–555
  anatomic considerations in, 540–544, 541–544
  buttons in, 554, 555
  delayed, 530–531, 531
  in peritoneoscopy, 107
  of upper midline incision, 489–490, 490
  splints in, 552, 552
  types of, 544–555

Xiphoid process, removal of, in incision extension, 491–492, 491–492

Zollinger-Ellison syndrome, 263–265
  gastrectomy for, 265
  recurrent ulcer and, 363–364